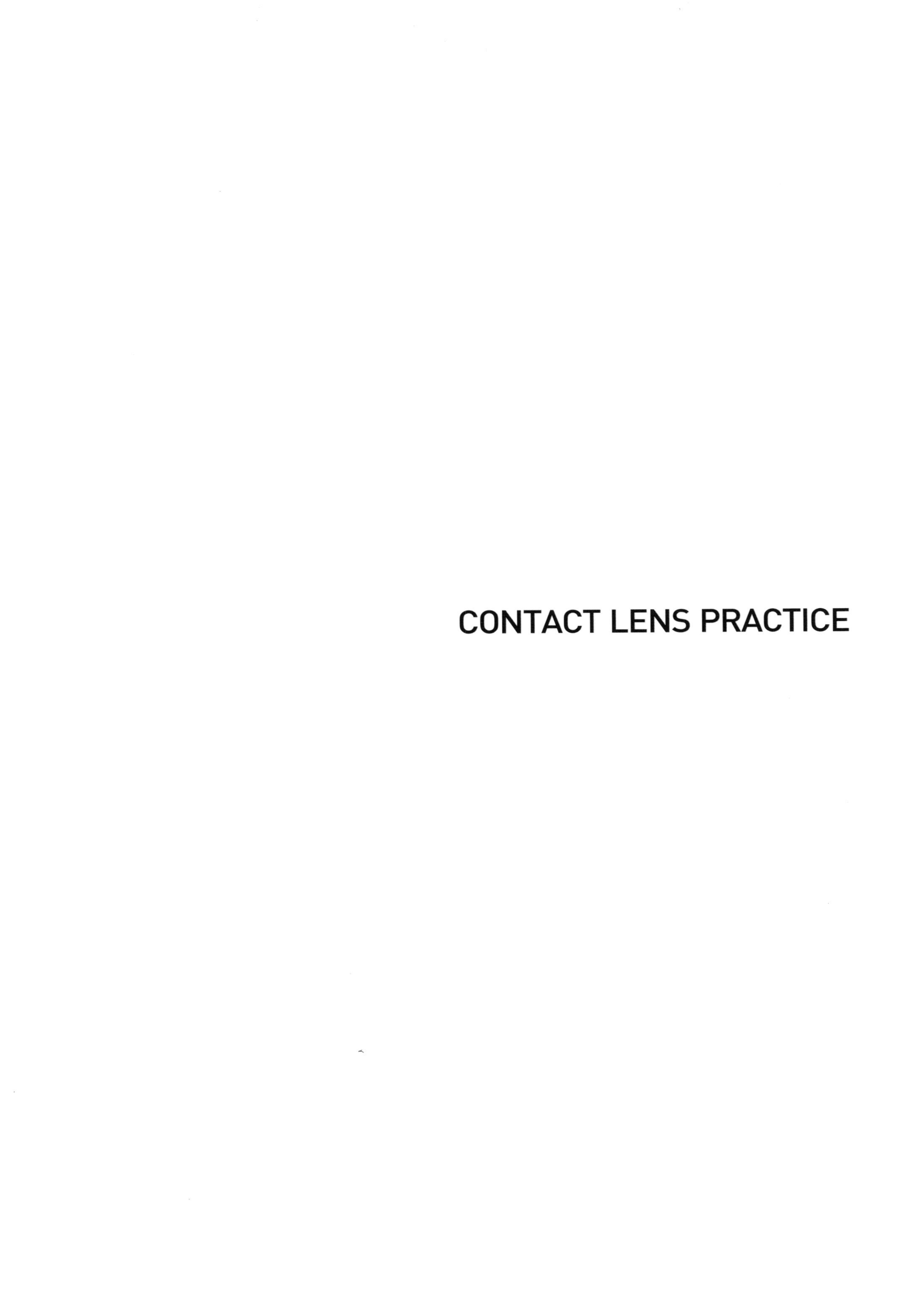

CONTACT LENS PRACTICE

To Suzanne, Zoe and Bruce

Commissioning Editor: *Russell Gabbedy*
Development Editor: *Alexandra Mortimer*
Project Manager: *Deepthi Unni*
Design: *Stewart Larking*
Illustration Manager: *Merlyn Harvey*
Grading scale artwork: *Terry R. Tarrant*
Schematic artwork: *Kathy Underwood and Lisa Dixon of J&L Composition Ltd*
New edition artwork: *Joanna Cameron and Oxford Illustrators*
Marketing Managers (UK/USA): *Richard Jones / Lynn Hoops*

CONTACT LENS PRACTICE

Second Edition

Edited by

Nathan Efron

BScOptom PhD (Melbourne) DSc (Manchester)
FAAO (Dip CCLRT) FIACLE FCCLSA FBCLA

Research Professor, School of Optometry,
Queensland University of Technology, Brisbane, Australia

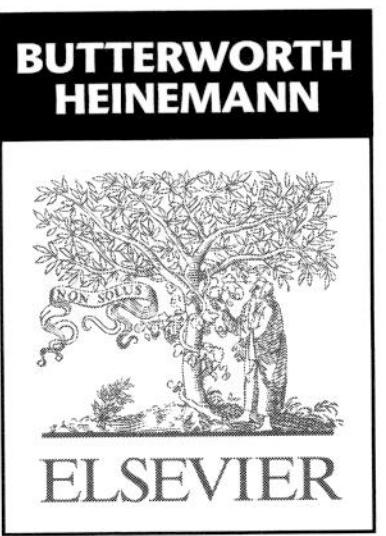

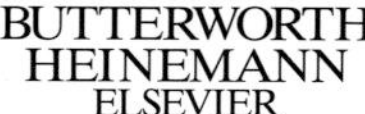

An imprint of Elsevier Limited

First published 2002
Reprinted 2005
Second edition 2010

ISBN 978-0-7506-8869-7

British Library Cataloguing in Publication Data
A catalogue record for this book is available from the British Library

Library of Congress Cataloging in Publication Data
A catalog record for this book is available from the Library of Congress

Notice
Medical knowledge is constantly changing. Standard safety precautions must be followed, but as new research and clinical experience broaden our knowledge, changes in treatment and drug therapy may become necessary or appropriate. Readers are advised to check the most current product information provided by the manufacturer of each drug to be administered to verify the recommended dose, the method and duration of administration, and contraindications. It is the responsibility of the practitioner, relying on experience and knowledge of the patient, to determine dosages and the best treatment for each individual patient. Neither the Publisher nor the author assume any liability for any injury and/or damage to persons or property arising from this publication.

The Publisher

The publisher's policy is to use **paper manufactured from sustainable forests**

Printed in China
Last digit is the print number: 9 8 7 6 5 4 3 2 1

Contents

Contributing authors

Joseph T. Barr OD, MS
Vice President, Clinical and Medical Affairs, Global Vision Care, Bausch & Lomb, Rochester, New York, USA
28 Keratoconus
29 High ametropia

Noel A. Brennan MScOptom, PhD, FAAO, FCCLSA
Chief Scientific Officer, Coles Brennan Pty Ltd, Melbourne, Victoria, Australia; Adjunct Professor, School of Optometry, Queensland University of Technology, Brisbane, Queensland, Australia
26 Continuous wear

Adrian S. Bruce BScOptom, PhD, FAAO, FACO
Senior Optometrist, Australian College of Optometry, Melbourne, Victoria, Australia; Senior Fellow, Department of Optometry and Vision Sciences, University of Melbourne, Melbourne, Victoria, Australia
37 Preliminary examination
41 Digital imaging

Roger J. Buckley MA, FRCS, FRCOphth, HonFCOptom, FBCLA
Professor of Ocular Medicine, Vision and Eye Research Unit and Department of Optometry & Ophthalmic Dispensing, Anglia Ruskin University, Cambridge, UK
31 Therapeutic applications

Leo G. Carney BAppSc, MSc, PhD, DSc, FAAO, FCCLSA
Professor Emeritus, School of Optometry, Queensland University of Technology, Brisbane, Queensland, Australia
34 Orthokeratology

Patrick J. Caroline COT, FCCLSA, FAAO (DipCCLRT)
Associate Professor of Optometry, Pacific University College of Optometry, Forest Grove, Oregon, USA
32 Post-refractive surgery

M-L. Chantal Coles BS, OD
Managing Director, Coles Brennan Pty Ltd, Melbourne, Victoria, Australia
26 Continuous wear

W. Neil Charman BSc, PhD, DSc, FOptSocAm, FCOptom (Hon)
Emeritus Professor of Visual Optics, Faculty of Life Sciences, University of Manchester, Manchester, UK
3 Visual optics
7 Soft lens optics
14 Rigid lens optics

Keith H. Edwards BSc, FCOptom, DipCLP, FAAO
Director, Clinical and Regulatory Affairs, LensAR Inc., Winter Park, Florida, USA
36 History taking

Nathan Efron BScOptom, PhD, DSc, FAAO (Dip CCLRT), FIACLE, FCCLSA, FBCLA
Research Professor, School of Optometry, Queensland University of Technology, Brisbane, Queensland, Australia
1 Historical perspective
6 Soft lens manufacture
13 Rigid lens manufacture
19 Unplanned lens replacement
20 Daily soft lens replacement
24 Tinted lenses
27 Sport
39 Aftercare
40 Complications
42 Compliance

Suzanne Efron BSc(Hons), MPhil, MCOptom
Private practice, Mermaid Beach, Queensland, Australia
24 Tinted lenses

Nizar K. Hirji JP PhD, MBA, BSc, FAAO, FCMI, FCOptom, FBCLA, Cert TP
Consultant Optometrist – Hirji Associates Birmingham, UK; Visiting Professor, University of Manchester, UK; Hon. Visiting Professor, City University, London, UK; Optometric Advisor, Dudley PCT, UK; Optometric Advisor, Wolverhampton City PCT, UK, London, UK
43 Practice management

Milton M. Hom OD, FAAO (DipCCLRT)
Private Practice, Azusa, California, USA
41 Digital imaging

Lyndon W. Jones BSc(Hons), PhD, FCOptom, DipCLP, DipOrth, FAAO (Dip CCLRT), FIACLE
Professor, School of Optometry, and Associate Director, Centre for Contact Lens Research, University of Waterloo, Waterloo, Ontario, Canada
4 Clinical instruments

John G. Lawrenson BSc, PhD, MCOptom
Professor of Clinical Visual Science, Department of Optometry and Visual Science, City University, London, UK
2 The anterior eye

Richard Lindsay BScOptom, MBA, FAAO(DipCCLRT), FCCLSA, FACO
Private Practice, East Melbourne, Victoria, Australia
10 Soft toric lens design and fitting
17 Rigid toric lens design and fitting

Carole Maldonado-Codina BSc(Hons), MSc, PhD, MCOptom, FAAO, FBCLA
Lecturer in Optometry, Faculty of Life Sciences, The University of Manchester, Manchester, UK
5 Soft materials

John Meyler BSc(Hons), FCOptom, DipCLP
Senior Director, Professional Affairs, Europe, Middle East & Africa, Johnson & Johnson Vision Care, Wokingham, Berkshire, UK
25 Presbyopia

Philip B. Morgan BSc(Hons), PhD, MCOptom, FAAO, FBCLA
Director, Eurolens Research; Senior Lecturer in Optometry, The University of Manchester, Manchester, UK
11 Soft lens care systems
18 Rigid lens care systems

Sarah L. Morgan BSc(Hons), MPhil, MCOptom, FAAO, FBCLA
Staff Development Consultant, Manchester, UK; Visiting Lecturer in Optometry, The University of Manchester, Manchester, UK
38 Patient education

Steve Newman
Vice President, Research and Development, Menicon, Co Ltd Singapore
6 Soft lens manufacture
13 Rigid lens manufacture

Clare O'Donnell BSc(Hons), MBA, PhD, MCOptom, FAAO
Lecturer in Optometry, Faculty of Life Sciences, University of Manchester, Manchester, UK
35 Diabetes

Sudi Patel PhD, M Phil, BSc(Hons), FCOptom, FAAO
Optometric Adviser, National Health Service, National Services, Scotland, UK; Visiting Professor, Vissum Institute of Ophthalmology, Alicante, Spain
8 Soft lens measurement
15 Rigid lens measurement

Kenneth W. Pullum BSc, FCOptom, DipCLP
Senior Optometrist, Moorfields Eye Hospital, London, UK; Senior Optometrist, Oxford Eye Hospital, Oxford, UK; Private Practice and Director, Innovative Sclerals Ltd, Hertford, Hertfordshire, UK
23 Scleral lenses

Sruthi Srinivasan PhD, BS Optom, FAAO
Post Doctoral Researcher, The Ohio State University, College of Optometry, Columbus, Ohio, USA
4 Clinical instruments

Loretta B. Szczotka-Flynn OD, PhD
Associate Professor of Ophthalmology, Department of Ophthalmology & Visual Science, Case Western Reserve University, Cleveland, Ohio, USA
39 Aftercare

Joe Tanner BOptom
Sales and Professional Services, CooperVision, Brisbane, Australia
21 Planned soft lens replacement

Brian J. Tighe BSc, PhD, CChem, FRSC
Professor of Polymer Science, Department of Chemical Engineering and Applied Chemistry, University of Aston, Birmingham, UK
12 Rigid lens materials

Cindy Tromans PhD, BSc(Hons), MCOptom, DipTp(AS), DipTp(SP)
Consultant Optometrist, Department of Optometry, Manchester Royal Eye Hospital, Manchester, UK
30 Paediatric fitting

Barry A. Weissman OD, PhD
Professor of Ophthalmology, Jules Stein Eye Institute, David Geffen School of Medicine at UCLA, Los Angeles; Adjunct Professor of Optometry, Southern California College of Optometry, California, USA
33 Post-keratoplasty

Craig A. Woods BSc (Hons), PhD PCerOcTher, MCOptom, DipCL, FAAO, FACO
Research Manager, Assoc Professor (Adjunct) School of Optometry, Centre for Contact Lens Research, University of Waterloo, Waterloo, Ontario, Canada
22 Planned rigid lens replacement

Graeme Young MPhil, PhD, FCOptom, DCLP, FAAO
Managing Director, Visioncare Research Ltd, Farnham, Surrey, UK
9 Soft lens design and fitting
16 Rigid lens design and fitting

Karla Zadnik OD, PhD, FAAO
Glenn A. Fry Professor in Optometry and Physiological Optics, and Associate Dean, The Ohio State University College of Optometry, Columbus, Ohio, USA
28 Keratoconus

Preface to the Second Edition

The aim of the second edition of this book has not changed from that of the first edition, which is to provide both students and clinicians with a substantial, evidence-based and balanced *overview* of the field of contact lenses. Many changes have occurred in the contact lens field since the first edition of this book was published – most notably, the remarkable advances in diagnostic technology in the consulting room being driven by digital technology, and the introduction of silicone hydrogel contact lenses for daily wear (the original silicone hydrogel lenses that entered the market were advocated for extended wear use only). This edition has been thoroughly revised and updated to reflect these changes and all other aspects of current contact lens practice.

As we enter the second decade of this millennium, there appears to be no dimunition of the demand for the various forms of vision correction to accommodate our work and leisure persuits. While spectacles will always be preferred by most, and advances in refractive surgery represents a viable option for some, many ametropes benefit from modern contact lens technology, which is widely recognised as a relatively safe, comfortable, convenient, non-permanent and cost-effective vision correction option. I trust that this book will serve to illustrate the many and varied approaches to contact lens fitting in such a way as to inform and inspire practitioners to continue to provide the best possible advice and service to the optically-challenged public. I hope you find this book as enjoyable as I found writing and editing it.

Nathan Efron

Acknowledgements

I am grateful to all of the contributors of this second edition of Contact Lens Practice. All have worked diligently to update their chapters and bring the latest clinically relevant information to the fore.

I have been privileged to enjoy the continued support of the long-standing publisher of all of my books - Elsevier. In particular, I am grateful to Russell Gabbedy (Comissioning Editor) and Alexandra Mortimer (Development Editor) for their encouragement and support during the planning and production of this book.

Editing a book of this size and scope is a monumental task, and I wish to pay special tribute to my lovely wife, Suzanne, who has served as a 'virtual co-editor' by way of spending many long hours assisting me in assembling, editing and organizing the contributed material. She has done a wonderful job. I really could not have completed this task without her assistance. I also thank Suzanne for co-authoring Chapter 24 with me. And thanks to my wonderful children, Zoe and Bruce, who did not complain (much) while mum and dad got on with the job of editing this book on weekends and evenings when we really should have been spending more time with them.

And finally, I would like to pay tribute to the photographers and illustrators, many of whom were not contributing authors of this book, for their extraordinary skills and insights in creating such fantastic imagery. I also thank them for giving me permission to use this material in the book. The clinical photographers and illustrators I refer to, and the images that they provided, are as follows:

A. L. Aan De Kerk (BLSC)*, Figure 25.9A; Anthony J. Aldave, Figures 33.3 and 33.4; Rosemary Austen (BLSC), Figure 40.30; Arthur Back (BLSC), Figures 19.2 and 26.18; Bausch & Lomb Slide Collection (unattributed authors), Figures 19.5, 19.10, 40.13, 40.19 and 40.20; Noel Brennan (BLSC), Figure 40.34; Bruce Bridgewater, Figure 25.13; Adrian Bruce, Figures 9.2, 9.4, 16.7 and 16.9; Ignacio Burgos (BLSC), Figure 31.1C; Hilmar Bussaker (BLSC), Figures 31.1A, 39.15 and 40.1; Patrick Caroline (BLSC), Figures 19.3, 19.4, 19.6, 26.16, 37.9B, 37.10B and 40.7; Mee Sing Chong (BLSC), Figure 40.25; Ruth Cornish (BLSC), Figures 28.10 and 40.31; V. K. Dada (BLSC), Figure 19.8; Leon Davids (BLSC), Figure 39.17; Kathy Dumbleton (BLSC), Figures 39.3 and 40.11; Suzanne Efron, Figure 39.12; Daniel Ehrlich, Figure 31.5; C. D. Euwijk (BLSC), Figures 40.17 and 40.18; Des Fonn (BLSC), Figures 33.5, 33.13 and 40.2; Charline Gauthier (BLSC), Figure 40.16; Tim Grant (BLSC), Figures 26.1 and 39.14; Michael Hare, Figures 24.6, 24.9, 24.14, 26.15, 40.8, 40.35, 40.43 and 40.47; Rolf Haberer (BLSC), Figures 39.1, 40.9 and 40.52; Arthur Ho, Figure 25.9; Brien Holden (BLSC), Figures 39.19 and 40.32; Debbie Jones, Figures 40.6, 40.21, 40.22 and 40.27; Lyndon Jones (BLSC), Figures 19.9, 26.21 and 40.4; Jan Kok (BLSC), Figure 31.6; Lourdes Llobet (BLSC), Figure 40.5; I. C. Lloyd, Figure 30.1; Russell Lowe, Figures 26.19 and 40.46; Florence Malet (BLSC), Figure 40.45; Pablo Gili Manzanaro (BLSC), Figure 37.7B; J. McCormick (BLSC), Figure 33.14; Charles McMonnies, Figure 40.48; J. Miller (BLSC), Figure 31.1B; I. Mojord, Figure 26.14; Philip Morgan, Figures 4.1, 4.2, 4.8, 4.12, 8.9, 8.12, 8.13, 8.15 and 15.6; Haliza Mutalib, Figures 40.37 and 40.39; Nghia Nguyen, Figure 41.2; Gary Orsborn (BLSC), Figures 40.26 and 40.33; Eric Papas, Figures 2.28 and 26.13; Richard Pearson, Figure 1.8; Frank Pettigrew, Figure 40.3; Nicola Pritchard (BLSC), Figure 19.11; Ken Pullum, Figures 31.3, 31.4 and 31.8; F. E. Ros (BLSC), Figure 40.38; David Ruston, Figures 25.12, 25.13B, 25.16 and 25.17; Marc Robboy (BLSC), Figure 40.14; Maki Shiobara (BLSC), Figure 26.20; Trefford Simpson, Figure 4.13; Luigina Sorbara, Figures 4.17, 4.20, 4.27 and 40.42; Sylvie Sulaiman (BLSC), Figures 37.11B and 39.22; Debbie Sweeney (CCLRU/CRCERT), Figure 1.9; Rob Terry (BLSC), Figures 33.6, 33.8 and 40.23; Brian Tompkins, Figures 40.10 and 40.12; C. van Mil (BLSC), Figure 31.10; C. Vervaet (BLSC), Figure 28.6; Jane Veys, Figure 42.1; Vistakon (division of Johnson & Johnson Vision Care), Figures 20.5 and 24.3; H. J. Völker-Dieben (BLSC), Figure 24.4; W. Vreugdenhil (BLSC), Figures 31.1D, 31.2, 31.7, 31.9 and 39.20; Jianhua Wang, Figures 4.21, 4.23 and 4.24; Barry Weissman, Figures 40.41 and 40.44; Craig Woods, Figure 40.28; and Steve Zantos, Figures 26.2, 26.17, 35.4, 40.29, 40.30, 40.49, 40.50 and 40.51.

(*BLSC = Bausch & Lomb Slide Collection)

PART: I

Introduction

CHAPTER 1

Historical perspective

Nathan Efron

Introduction

We cannot continue these brilliant successes in the future, unless we continue to learn from the past.

Calvin Coolidge, inaugural US presidential address, 1923

Coolidge was referring to the successes of a nation, but his sentiment could apply to any field of endeavour, including contact lens practice. As we continue to ride on the crest of a huge wave of exciting developments in the 21st century, we would not wish to lose sight of the past. Hence the inclusion in this book of this brief historical overview.

Outlined below in chronological order (allowing for some historical overlaps) is the development of contact lenses, from the earliest theories to present-day technology. Each heading, which represents a major achievement, is annotated with a year that is considered to be especially significant to that development. These dates are based on various sources of information, such as dates of patents, published papers and anecdotal reports. It is recognized, therefore, that some of the dates cited are open to debate, but they are nevertheless presented to give the reader a reasonable chronological perspective.

Early theories (1508–1887)

Although contact lenses were not fitted until the late 19th century, a number of scholars had given thought to the possibility of applying an optical device directly to the eyeball to correct vision. Virtually all of these suggestions were impractical.

Many contact lens historians point to Leonardo da Vinci's *Codex of the Eye, Manual D*, written in 1508, as having introduced the optical principle underlying the contact lens. Indeed, da Vinci described a method of directly altering corneal power – by immersing the eye in a bowl of water (Figure 1.1). Of course, a contact lens corrects vision by altering corneal power. However, da Vinci was primarily interested in learning of the mechanisms of accommodation of the eye (Heitz and Enoch, 1987) and did not refer to a mechanism or device for correcting vision.

In 1636, René Descartes described a glass fluid-filled tube which was to be placed in direct contact with the cornea (Figure 1.2). The end of the tube was made of clear glass, the shape of which would determine the optical correction. Of course, such a device is impractical since blinking is not possible; nevertheless, the principle of directly neutralizing corneal power used by Descartes is consistent with the principles underlying modern contact lens design (Enoch, 1956).

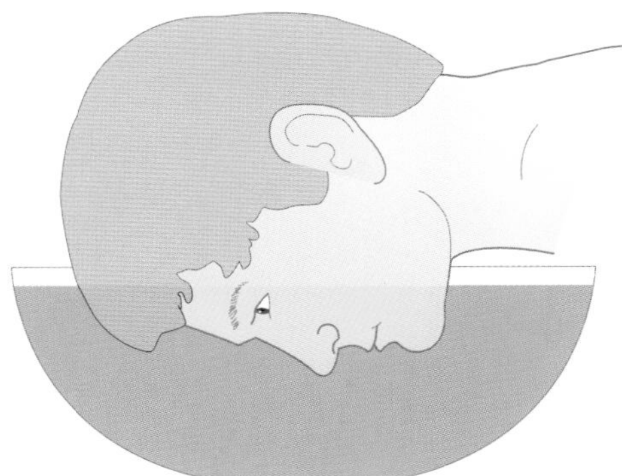

Figure 1.1 Idea of Leonardo da Vinci to alter corneal power.

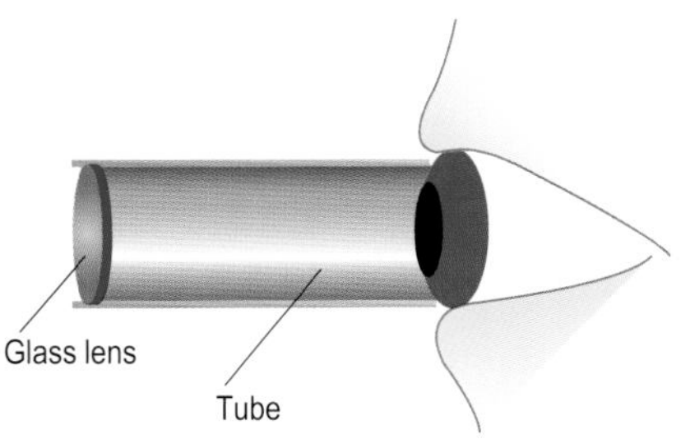

Figure 1.2 Fluid-filled tube described by René Descartes.

DOI: 10.1016/B978-0-7506-8869-7.00001-X

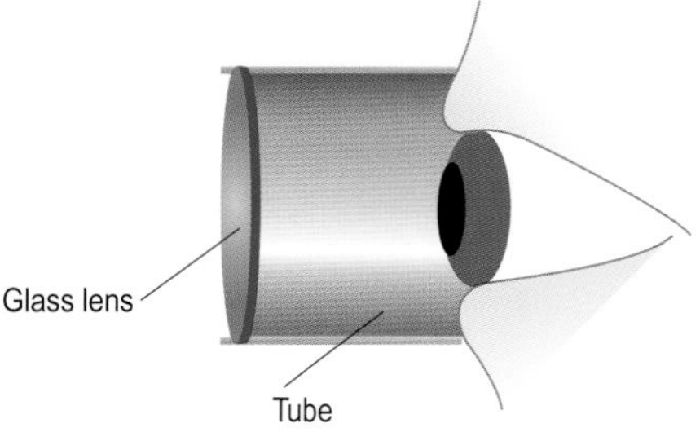

Figure 1.3 Eyecup design of Thomas Young.

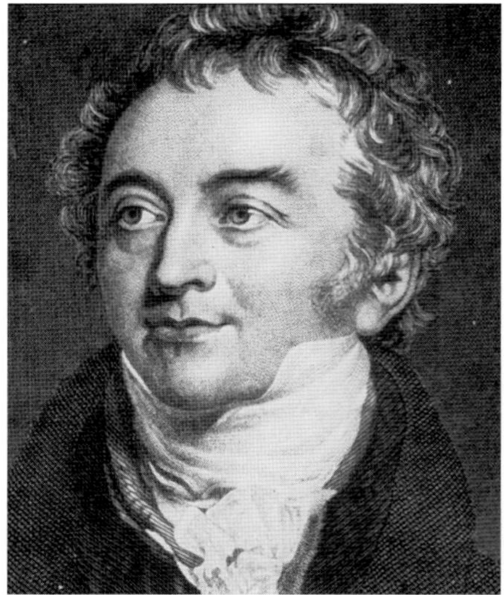

Figure 1.4 Thomas Young.

As part of a series of experiments concerning the mechanisms of accommodation, Thomas Young, in 1801, constructed a device that was essentially a fluid-filled eyecup that fitted snugly into the orbital rim (Young, 1801) (Figures 1.3 and 1.4).

A microscope eyepiece was fitted into the base of the eyecup, thus forming a similar system to that used by Descartes. Young's invention was somewhat more practical in that it could be held in place with a head band and blinking was possible; however, he did not intend this device to be used for the correction of refractive errors.

In a footnote in his treatise on light in the 1845 edition of the *Encyclopedia Metropolitana*, Sir John Herschel suggested two possible methods of correcting 'very bad cases of irregular cornea'. These were: (1) 'applying to the cornea a spherical capsule of glass filled with animal jelly' (Figure 1.5), or (2) 'taking a mould of the cornea and impressing it on some transparent medium' (Herschel, 1845). Although it seems that Herschel did not attempt to conduct such trials, his latter suggestion was ultimately adopted some 40 years later by a number of inventors, working independently and unbeknown to each other, who were all apparently unaware of the writings of Herschel.

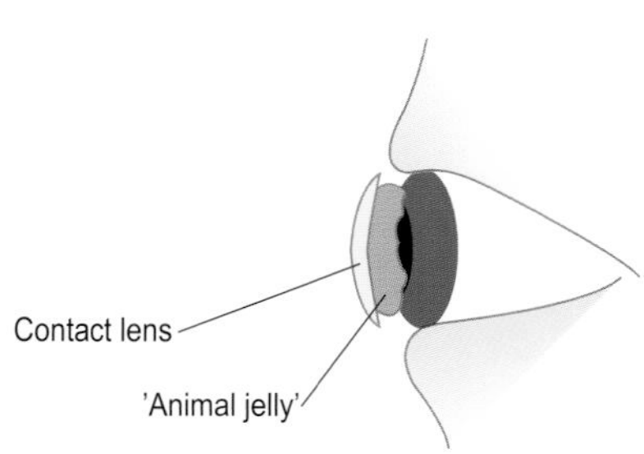

Figure 1.5 'Animal jelly' sandwiched between a 'spherical capsule of glass' (contact lens) and cornea, as proposed by Sir John Herschel.

Glass scleral lenses (1888)

There was a great deal of activity in contact lens research in the late 1880s, which has led to debate as to who should be given credit for being the first to fit a contact lens. Adolf Eugene Fick (Figure 1.6), a German ophthalmologist working in Zurich, appears to have been the first to describe the process of fabricating and fitting contact lenses; specifically, he described the fitting of afocal scleral contact shells first on rabbits, then on himself and finally on a small group of volunteer patients (Efron and Pearson, 1988). In their textbook dated 1910, Müller and Müller, who were manufacturers of ocular prostheses, described the fitting of a partially transparent protective glass shell to a patient referred to them by a Dr Sämisch (Müller and Müller, 1910). Fick's work was published in the journal *Archiv für Augenheilkunde* in March 1888, and must be accorded historical precedence over later anecdotal textbook accounts.

French ophthalmologist Eugène Kalt (Figure 1.7) fitted two keratoconic patients with afocal glass scleral shells and obtained a significant improvement in vision. A report of this work, presented to the Paris Academy of Medicine on March 20, 1888 by Kalt's senior medical colleague, Professor Photinos Panas, acknowledges and therefore effectively confirms that the work of Fick occurred earlier (Pearson, 1989).

Credit for fitting the first powered contact lens must be given to August Müller (no relation to Müller and Müller, mentioned above), who conducted his work whilst a medical student at Kiel University in Germany (Pearson and Efron, 1989). In his inaugural dissertation presented to the Faculty of Medicine in 1889, Müller described the correction of his own high myopia with a powered scleral contact lens. Paradoxically, Müller lost interest in ophthalmology and went on to practise as an orthopaedic specialist (Figure 1.8).

The lenses worn by Müller were made by an optical engineer, Karl Otto Himmler (1841–1903), whose firm enjoyed, until the outbreak of World War II, an international reputation for the manufacture of microscopes and their accessories. Himmler must therefore be acknowledged as the first manufacturer of optically ground contact lenses (Pearson, 2007).

Little development occurred in the 50 years subsequent to these early clinical trials. Improvements in methods of

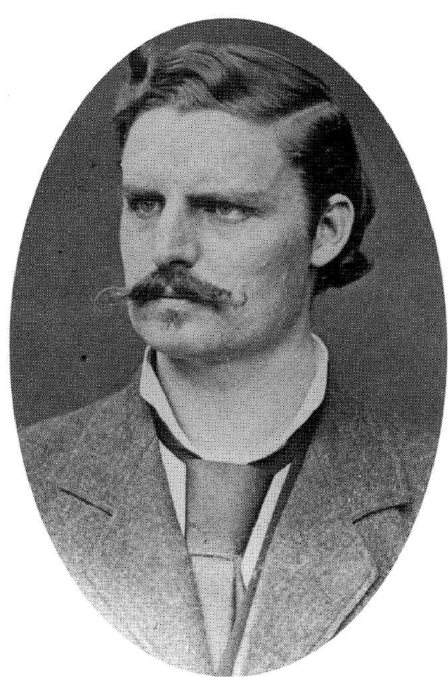

Figure 1.6 Adolf Eugene Fick.

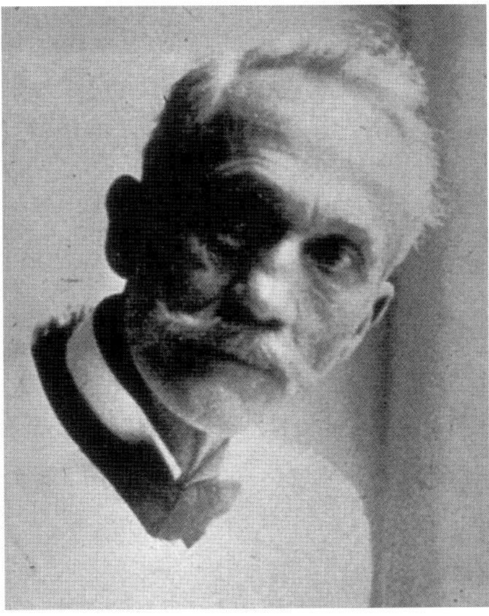

Figure 1.7 Eugène Kalt.

scleral lens fitting were described by clinicians such as Dallos, who emphasized the importance of designing the lens to facilitate tear flow beneath the lens (Dallos, 1936). Dallos also went on to develop techniques for taking impressions of the human eye and grinding the lenses from these impressions.

Plastic scleral lenses (1936)

The Rohm and Haas company introduced transparent plastic (polymethyl methacrylate: PMMA) into the USA in 1936, and in the same year Feinbloom (1936) described a scleral lens consisting of an opaque plastic haptic portion and a clear glass centre. Soon after, scleral lenses were fabricated entirely from PMMA using lathing techniques. A key rationale for using PMMA for the manufacture of contact lenses was that this material was considered to be biologically inert in the eye. This view was formed by military medical officers who examined the eyes of pilots who suffered eye injuries during the Second World War as a result of fragments from shattered cockpit windscreens (as would occur during aerial dogfights) becoming permanently embedded in the eye. These eyes remained unreactive years after such accidents. Other advantages of PMMA included light weight, break resistance and being easy to lathe and polish.

Plastic corneal lenses (1948)

The development of corneal lenses – or rigid lenses, as they are referred to today – began as the result of an error in the laboratory of optical technician Kevin Tuohy. During the lathing of a PMMA scleral lens, the haptic and corneal portions separated. Tuohy became curious as to whether the corneal portion could be worn, so he polished the edge, placed it in his own eye and found that the lens could be tolerated (Braff, 1983). Further trials were conducted, leading to the development of the rigid contact lens (rigid lenses were previously referred to as 'hard' lenses if they were manufactured from PMMA). Tuohy filed a patent for his invention in February 1948.

So began an era of popularization of the contact lens. The spherical Tuohy lens design suffered from two main drawbacks: considerable apical bearing, which caused central corneal abrasion and oedema, and excessive edge lift, which made the lens easy to dislodge. It was soon realized that these problems could be overcome by altering the peripheral curvature of the posterior lens surface, heralding the development of multicurve and aspheric designs, which remain in widespread use today, albeit with superior gas-permeable materials (PMMA is now virtually obsolete).

Silicone elastomer lenses (1965)

Silicone rubber forms a unique category amongst contact lens materials. It is a 'soft lens' in terms of its physical behaviour and lenses are fabricated from this material in the form of a soft lens. Unlike all other soft lens materials, silicone elastomer does not contain water and in this respect is analogous to a hard lens material. Silicone elastomer is highly permeable to oxygen and carbon dioxide and therefore provides minimal interference to corneal respiration; however, it is difficult to manufacture and its surface is hydrophobic and must be treated to allow comfortable wear. The considerable difficulties involved in enhancing surface wettability have limited the clinical application of this lens, and few advances have been made since it was originally fitted. The precise date of silicone elastomer lenses becoming commercially available is unclear. There

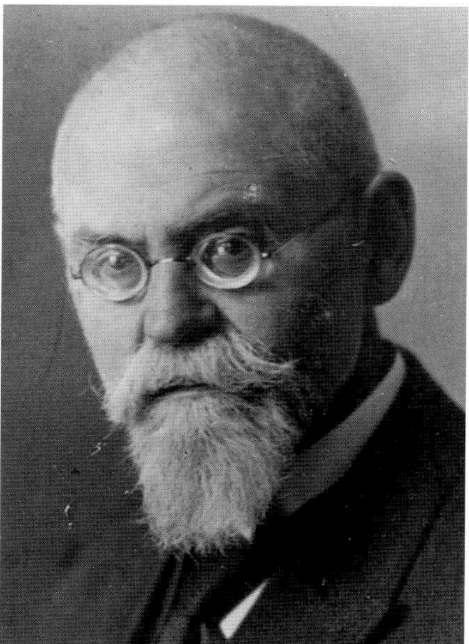

Figure 1.8 August Müller.

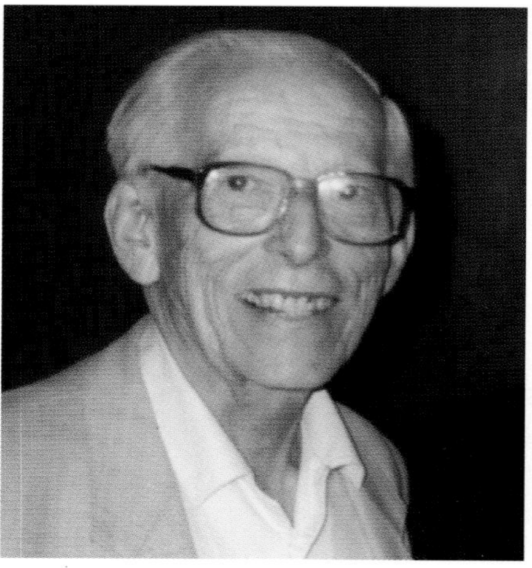

Figure 1.9 Otto Wichterle.

was some patent activity in the mid-1960s to early 1970s, and Mandell (1988) claims to have personally observed 10 patients who were wearing such lenses in 1965, noting very poor clinical results.

Soft lenses (1972)

Possibly the greatest understatement that can be found in the literature pertaining to contact lens development is the final sentence of a paper entitled 'Hydrophilic gels for biological use', published in *Nature* on January 9, 1960, by Wichterle and Lim (1960): 'Promising results have also been obtained in experiments in other cases, for example, in manufacturing contact lenses, arteries, etc.'

Initial attempts by Otto Wichterle (Figure 1.9) to produce soft lenses fabricated from hydroxyethyl methacrylate (HEMA), and manufactured using cast moulding, met with limited success.

Unable to attract support from the Institute of Macromolecular Research in Czechoslovakia (now the Czech Republic) where he worked, and indeed discouraged by his superiors, Wichterle was forced to conduct further secret experiments in his own home. Working with a childrens' mechanical construction kit, Wichterle developed the spin-casting technique (Figure 1.10) and eventually managed to persuade his peers to conduct further trials at the Institute. He claims to have produced 'the first suitable contact lenses' in late 1961 (Wichterle, 1978), which presumably approximates to the first occasion when a soft lens was actually worn on a human eye. The patent to develop soft contact lenses commercially was subsequently acquired by Bausch & Lomb in the USA, who introduced soft lenses into the world market in 1972.

Lenses manufactured from HEMA were an immediate market success, primarily by virtue of their superior comfort and enhanced biocompatibility. However, clinical experience and laboratory studies indicated that the poor physiological response of the anterior eye during wear of the early thick HEMA lenses could be enhanced by making soft lenses more permeable to oxygen – specifically, by making them thinner and of a higher water content. Much of the research and development in contact lenses up to the present time has been concerned with the development of materials and lens designs that optimize biocompatibility, primarily by enhancing corneal oxygenation and minimizing absorption of proteins, lipids and other tear constituents (McMahon and Zadnik, 2000).

Rigid gas-permeable lenses (1974)

In most respects, PMMA is considered to be an ideal contact lens material; however, its single drawback is its impermeability to gases that are exchanged at the corneal surface as part of aerobic metabolism. Specifically, oxygen is prevented from moving from the atmosphere into the cornea, and carbon dioxide efflux into the atmosphere is impeded. This drawback has been the major driving force in the development of rigid lens materials that are permeable to gases.

One of the first rigid gas-permeable materials to be tried was cellulose acetate butyrate, which afforded some oxygen permeability but was subject to warpage. In 1974, Norman Gaylord managed to incorporate silicone into the basic PMMA structure, heralding the introduction of a new family of contact lens polymers known as silicone acrylates (Gaylord, 1974). Subsequently, other ingredients such as styrene and fluorine have been incorporated into rigid materials in attempts to enhance material biocompatibility further.

Disposable lenses (1988)

In the early days of soft lens development, patients would typically use the same pair of lenses until the lenses became too uncomfortable to wear, caused severe eye reactions or

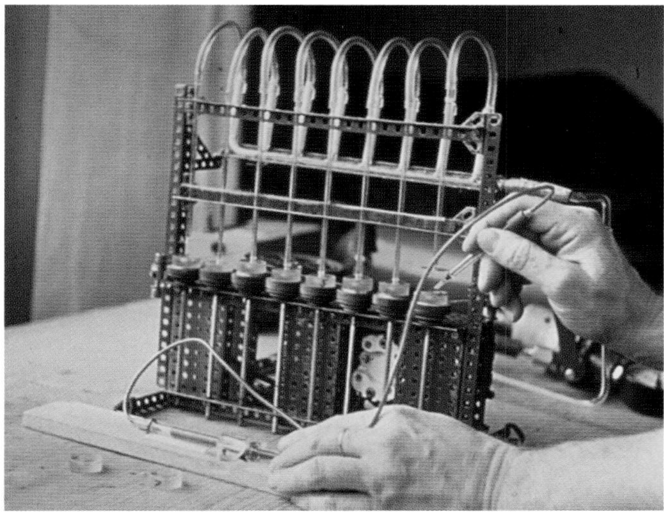

Figure 1.10 The prototype spin-casting machine built at home by Wichterle using his son's toy Meccano construction set.

were damaged or lost. It became apparent that lens deposition and spoilation over time were major impediments to successful long-term lens wear. Although regular lens replacement was an obvious solution to some of these problems, the high unit cost of lenses proved to be a significant disincentive. In the early 1980s, forward-thinking practitioners – notably Klas Nilsson of Gothenburg, Sweden – convinced patients of the benefits of replacing lenses on a regular basis (6-monthly in Nilsson's case) and began prescribing lenses in this way. A subsequent landmark scientific publication co-authored by Nilsson – known as the 'Gothenburg study' (Holden *et al.*, 1985) – unequivocally proved the benefits of regular lens replacement. So was born the concept of regular lens replacement, albeit relatively expensive for the patient at the time.

If regular lens replacement was to become the norm, something had to be done about lens cost. A group of Danish clinicians and engineers, led by ophthalmologist Michael Bay, developed a moulding process so that low-cost, multiple individual lens packs could be produced (Mertz, 1997). This product – known as 'Danalens' – was released into the Scandinavian market in 1984 and must be recognized as the first truly disposable lens. However, the initial manufacturing process was crude and numerous problems with the lenses and packaging were reported (Benjamin *et al.*, 1985; Bergmanson *et al.*, 1987).

The pharmaceutical giant Johnson & Johnson, which had not previously been involved in the contact lens business, purchased the Danalens technology in 1984 and completely overhauled the lens polymer formulation, packaging system and moulding technology (Mertz, 1997). The result was the Acuvue lens, an inexpensive weekly-replacement extended-wear lens, which was released in the USA in June 1988, and worldwide shortly thereafter. The success of this lens elevated Johnson & Johnson to a leadership position in the contact lens market. All other major contact lens companies followed suit, and today the vast majority of soft lenses prescribed (98% in the UK) are designed to be replaced monthly or more frequently (Morgan, 2009).

Daily disposable lenses (1994)

The ultimate frequency with which lenses can be replaced is daily. A Scottish company, Award (which was acquired by Bausch & Lomb in 1996), developed a manufacturing technique whereby the male half of the mould that formed the lens became the lens packaging. This technique further reduced the unit cost of a lens, making daily disposability a viable proposition. The 'Premier' daily disposable lens was launched in the UK in 1994. Johnson & Johnson released the '1-Day Acuvue' daily disposable lens into western regions of the USA around the same time, leading to an ongoing dispute as to which company (Award or Johnson & Johnson) was the first to release a daily disposable contact lens into the market (Meyler and Ruston, 2006). CIBA Vision entered the daily disposable lens market in 1997 with a product called 'Dailies'.

Silicone hydrogel lenses (1998)

The allure of a contact lens made from a material with a phenomenally high oxygen performance never escaped the contact lens industry. The development of such a lens would be critical to solving hypoxic lens-related problems, which severely limit the clinical utility of contact lenses, especially for extended wear. Silicone elastomers were the obvious answer, but for reasons outlined above, successful lenses could never be produced from this material. Polymer scientists in the contact lens industry had long recognized that many of the problems associated with silicone elastomers for contact lens fabrication could be theoretically overcome by creating a silicone–hydrogel hybrid.

After more than a decade of intensive research and development, two spherical-design silicone hydrogel lenses were introduced into the market in 1998: Focus Night & Day (CIBA Vision) and Purevision (Bausch & Lomb). The introduction of these lenses is considered by many to be the most significant advance in contact lens material technology since the development of HEMA by Wichterle in the 1960s. In the decade since these products entered the market, all major contact lens manufacturers have introduced silicone hydrogel lenses, which are now available in toric and multifocal designs and a range of replacement modalities, including daily disposable lenses.

Figure 1.11 presents a historical timeline of key developments in the contact lens field from the time contact (scleral) lenses were first fitted to human eyes in the late 1880s up to the present.

The future

Further refinements in material and manufacturing technology will be required to perfect silicone hydrogel lenses and optimize the performance of hydrogel lenses. Innovative approaches such as anti-infective and anti-inflammatory lenses (Weisbarth *et al.*, 2007; Zhu *et al.*, 2008) and lens surface modifications to include channels and patterns for improving postlens tear exchange (Weidemann and Lakkis, 2005; Lin *et al.*, 2006) are currently under development. Market competition may also lead to

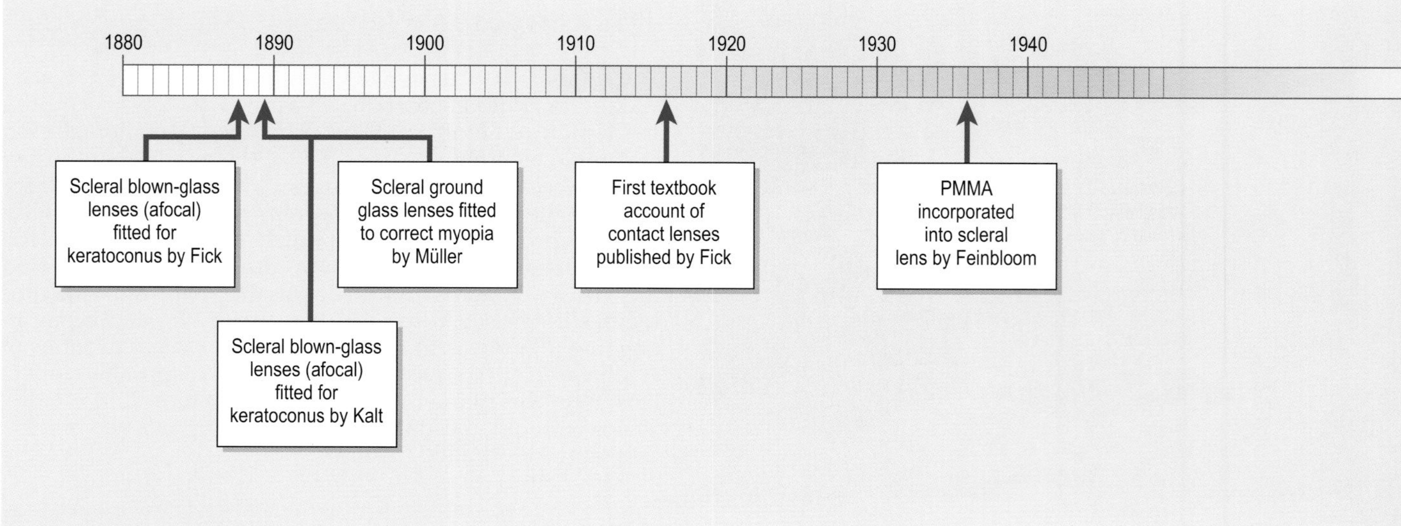

Figure 1.11 Historical timeline of contact lens development. PMMA = polymethyl methacrylate; HEMA = hydroxyethyl methacrylate.

improvements in manufacturing technology to drive the unit cost of lenses down even further. In the not-too-distant future, rigid lenses are likely to become virtually obsolete, especially in view of the recent development of custom-design aberration control soft lenses that are capable of correcting vision in patients with corneal distortions as in keratoconus (Marsack *et al.*, 2008). It is likely that all lenses prescribed in the future will be 'single-use' products, such as daily disposable or extended-wear lenses. In view of these developments, the need for contact lens solutions will continue to diminish.

References

Benjamin, W. J., Bergmanson, J. P. G. and Estrada, P. J. (1985) Disposable 'eight-packs'. *Int. Eyecare,* **1,** 494–499.

Bergmanson, J. P. G., Soderberg, P. G. and Estrada, P. (1987) A comparison between the measured and the desirable quality of hydrogel extended wear contact-lenses. *Acta Ophthalmol.,* **65,** 417–423.

Braff, S. M. (1983) The Max Schapero Lecture: Contact lens horizons. *Am. J. Optom. Physiol. Opt.,* **60,** 851–858.

Dallos, J. (1936) Contact lenses, the 'invisible spectacles'. *Arch. Ophthalmol.,* **15,** 617–623.

Efron, N. and Pearson, R. M. (1988) Centenary celebration of Fick's *Eine Contactbrille. Arch. Ophthalmol.,* **106,** 1370–1377.

Enoch, J. M. (1956) Descartes' contact lens. *Am. J. Optom. Arch. Am. Acad. Optom.,* **33,** 77–85.

Feinbloom, W. (1936) A plastic contact lens. *Trans. Am. Acad. Optom.,* **10,** 37–44.

Gaylord, N. G. (1974) Oxygen permeable contact lens composition methods and article of manufacture (to Polycon Lab Inc). *US Patent 3 808 178.*

Heitz, R. F. and Enoch, J. M. (1987) Leonardo da Vinci: An assessment on his discourses on image formation in the eye. In *Advances in Diagnostic Visual Optics.* (A. Fiorentini, D. L. Guyton and I. M. Siegel, eds) pp. 19–26, New York, Springer-Verlag.

Herschel, J. F. W. (1845) Of the structure of the eye, and of vision. Vol. 4, Section XII, Light. In: *Encyclopedia Metropolitana.* London.

Holden B. A., Sweeney, D. F., Vannas, A. *et al.* (1985) Effects of long-term extended contact lens wear on the human cornea. *Invest. Ophthalmol. Vis. Sci.,* **26,** 1489–1501.

Lin, M. C., Soliman, G. N., Lim, V. A. *et al.* (2006) Scalloped channels enhance tear mixing under hydrogel contact lenses. *Optom. Vis. Sci.,* **83,** 874–878.

Mandell, R. B. (1988) Historical development. Chapter 1, Section 1, Basic Principles. In: Mandell, R. B. (ed.) *Contact Lens Practice.* 4th edn. p. 19. Springfield, IL: Charles C. Thomas.

Marsack, J. D., Parker, K. E. and Applegate, R. A. (2008) Performance of wavefront-guided soft lenses in three keratoconus subjects. *Optom. Vis. Sci.* **85,** 1172–1178.

McMahon, T. T. and Zadnik, K. (2000) Twenty-five years of contact lenses – The impact on the cornea and ophthalmic practice. *Cornea,* **19,** 730–740.

Mertz, G. W. (1997) Development of contact lenses. Ch. 5, Section II., Contact Lenses. In *Corneal Physiology and Disposable Contact Lenses.* (H. Hamano and H. Kaufman, eds). pp. 65–99, Boston: Butterworth-Heinemann.

Meyler, J. and Ruston D. (2006) The world's first daily disposables. *Optician,* **231**(6053), 12.

Morgan, P. B. (2009) Trends in UK contact lens prescribing 2009. *Optician,* **237,** 20–21.

Müller, F. A. and Müller, A. C. (1910) *Das kunstliche Auge.* pp. 68–75. Wiesbaden: J. F. Bergmann.

Pearson, R. M. (1989) Kalt, keratoconus and the contact lens. *Optom. Vis. Sci.,* **66,** 643–646.

Pearson, R. M. (2007) Karl Otto Himmler, manufacturer of the first contact lens. *Cont. Lens Anterior Eye,* **30,** 11–16.

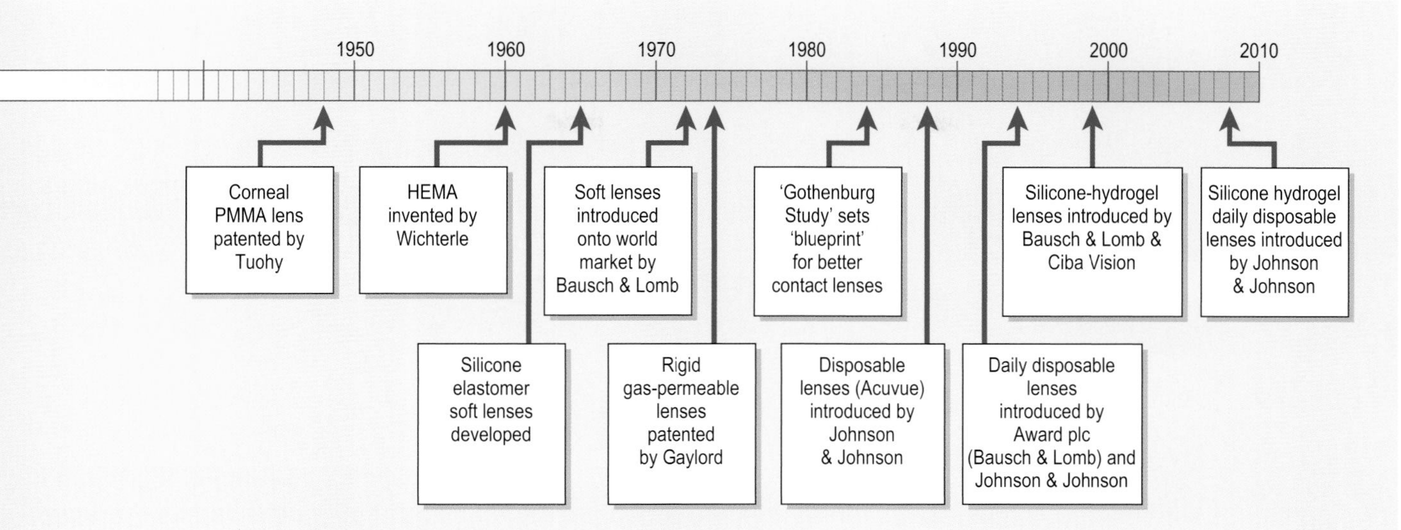

Pearson, R. M. and Efron, N. (1989) Hundredth anniversary of August Müller's inaugural dissertation on contact lenses. *Surv. Ophthalmol.,* **34,** 133–141.

Weidemann, K. E. and Lakkis, C. (2005) Clinical performance of microchannel contact lenses. *Optom. Vis. Sci.,* **82,** 498–504.

Weisbarth, R. E., Gabriel, M. M., George, M. *et al.* (2007) Creating antimicrobial surfaces and materials for contact lenses and lens cases. *Eye Contact Lens,* **33,** 426–429.

Wichterle, O. (1978) The beginning of the soft lens. Ch. 1, Section 1, Historical Development. In *Soft Contact Lenses. Clinical and Applied Technology.* (M. Ruben, ed.) pp. 3–5, Eastbourne: Baillière Tindall.

Wichterle, O. and Lim, D. (1960) Hydrophilic gels for biological use. *Nature,* **185**(4706), 117–118.

Young, T. (1801) On the mechanisms of the eye. *Phil. Trans. R. Soc. Lon. [Biol. Sci].,* **91,** 23–88.

Zhu, H., Kumar, A., Ozkan, J. *et al.* (2008) Fimbrolide-coated antimicrobial lenses: their in vitro and in vivo effects. *Optom. Vis. Sci.,* **85,** 292–300. Erratum in: Optom. Vis. Sci., **85**, 609.

The anterior eye

John G Lawrenson

Introduction

A critical aspect of contact lens practice is monitoring the ocular response to lens wear, which ranges from acceptable physiological changes to adverse pathology. In order to do this, practitioners must possess a thorough understanding of the normal structure and function of the anterior eye, which is the subject of this chapter. In the course of reading other chapters in this book, the reader might anticipate having to refer back constantly to descriptions of the functional anatomy of the anterior eye in order to develop a full understanding of the phenomena being described.

The cornea

The cornea fulfils two important functions: together with the sclera it forms a tough fibrous outer coat which encloses the ocular tissues and protects the internal components of the eye from injury. Significantly, the cornea also provides two-thirds of the refractive power of the eye. It is particularly well suited to its role: the cornea is curved and transparent, and the air–tear interface provides a refractive surface of good optical quality.

Corneal anatomy

Gross anatomy

The cornea is elliptical when viewed from in front, with its long axis in the horizontal meridian (Table 2.1). This asymmetry is produced by a greater degree of overlap of the peripheral cornea by opaque limbal tissue in the vertical meridian. The surface area of the cornea is 1.1 cm^2, which represents about 7% of the surface area of the globe (Maurice, 1984). Topographically, the cornea is conventionally divided into four zones (central, paracentral, peripheral and limbal). The central zone, which covers the entrance pupil of the eye, is spherical, approximately 4 mm wide, and principally determines high-resolution image formation on the fovea. The paracentral zone, which lies outside the central zone, is flatter and becomes optically important in dim illumination when the pupil dilates. The peripheral zone is where the cornea is flattest and most aspheric (Klyce *et al.*, 1998). Due to a difference in curvature between its posterior and anterior surfaces, the cornea shows a regional variation in thickness. Centrally the thickness is approximately 0.55 mm, increasing towards the periphery to 0.67 mm.

Microscopic anatomy

When the cornea is viewed in transverse section, five distinct layers can be resolved: epithelium, Bowman's layer, stroma, Descemet's membrane and endothelium (Figure 2.1).

Epithelium

The epithelium represents approximately 10% of the thickness of the cornea (55 μm) (Feng and Simpson, 2008). It is a stratified squamous non-keratinized epithelium, consisting of 5–6 layers of cells (Figure 2.2). Three distinct epithelial cell types are recognized: a single row of basal cells, 2–3 rows of wing cells and 2–3 layers of superficial (squamous) cells. In addition, several non-epithelial cells are present (e.g. lymphocytes, macrophages and Langerhans cells). The epithelium forms a permeability barrier to small molecules, water and ions as well as forming an effective barrier to the entry of pathogens. Further epithelial specialization enhances adhesion between cells, to withstand shearing and abrasive forces.

Superficial cells are structurally modified for their barrier function and interaction with the tear film. Scanning electron microscopy of surface cells shows extensive finger-like and ridge-like projections (microvilli and microplicae). Light, medium and dark cells can be distinguished depending on the number and pattern of surface projections (Pfister, 1973). It has been suggested that dark cells, which are relatively free of these surface features, are close to being desquamated into the tear film. By contrast, the newly arrived light cells possess a more extensive array of surface projections. In high-power transmission electron micrographs, microvilli and microplicae show an extensive filamentous covering known as the glycocalyx.

DOI: 10.1016/B978-0-7506-8869-7.00002-1

Table 2.1 Corneal dimensions and related measurements

Parameter	Value
Area	1.1 cm^2
Diameter	
Horizontal	11.8 mm
Vertical	10.6 mm
Radius of curvature	
Anterior central	7.8 mm
Posterior central	6.5 mm
Thickness	
Central	0.55 mm
Peripheral	0.67 mm
Refractive index	1.376
Power	42 D

(Data adapted from Bron *et al.*, 1997)

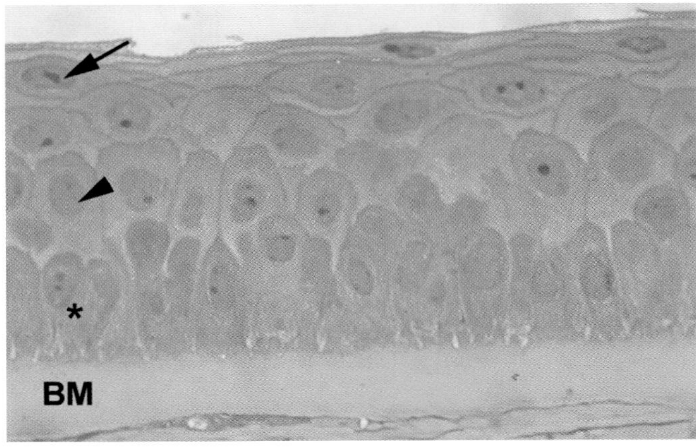

Figure 2.2 Corneal epithelium (detail). Three cell types are present: basal cells (asterisk), wing cells (arrow head) and squamous cells (arrow). BM= Bowman's membrane.

Figure 2.1 Transverse section through the cornea. The stroma, which represents 90% of the thickness of the cornea, is bounded by the epithelium (asterisk) and endothelium (arrow).

The glycocalyx is formed from membrane-bound glycoconjugates and is important for spreading and attachment of the precorneal tear film. In accordance with their barrier function, a complex network of tight junctions links superficial cells.

Wing cells are so named because of their characteristic shape, with lateral extensions and a concave inferior surface to accommodate the apices of the basal cells. Their nuclei tend to be spherical or elongated in the plane of the cornea. The cell borders of the polygonal wing cells show prominent infoldings which interdigitate with adjacent cells, and numerous desmosomes. This arrangement results in a strong intercellular adhesion. The cytoplasm contains prominent cytoskeletal elements (predominantly actin and cytokeratin intermediate filaments), and although the usual complement of organelles is present, they are few in number.

Basal cells consist of single-layer columnar cells with a vertically oriented oval nucleus. Ultrastructurally, they are similar in appearance to wing cells. The plasma membrane similarly shows pronounced infolding and the cytoplasm contains prominent intermediate filaments. A variety of cell junctions are present, including: desmosomes, which mediate adhesion between cells; hemidesmosomes, which are involved in the attachment of basal cells to the underlying stroma; and gap junctions, which allow for intercellular metabolic coupling. Basal cells form the germative layer of the cornea, and mitotic cells are often seen at this level.

Basal lamina and Bowman's layer

The basal lamina (basement membrane) is synthesized by basal cells. It varies in thickness between 0.5 and 1 μm, and under the electron microscope can be differentiated into an anterior clear zone (lamina lucida) and a posterior darker zone (lamina densa). The basal lamina is part of a complex adhesion system, which mediates the attachment of the epithelium to the underlying stroma (Figure 2.3). Hemidesmosomes link the cytoskeleton via a series of anchoring fibrils to anchoring plaques in the anterior stroma. The molecular components of this adhesion complex have been identified and include type VII collagen, integrins, laminin and bullous pemphigoid antigen (Gipson *et al.*, 1987).

Bowman's layer (anterior limiting membrane) varies in thickness between 8 and 14 μm. With the light microscope it appears as an acellular homogeneous zone. Ultrastructurally, it is composed of a randomly oriented array of fine collagen fibrils, which merge with the fibrils of the anterior

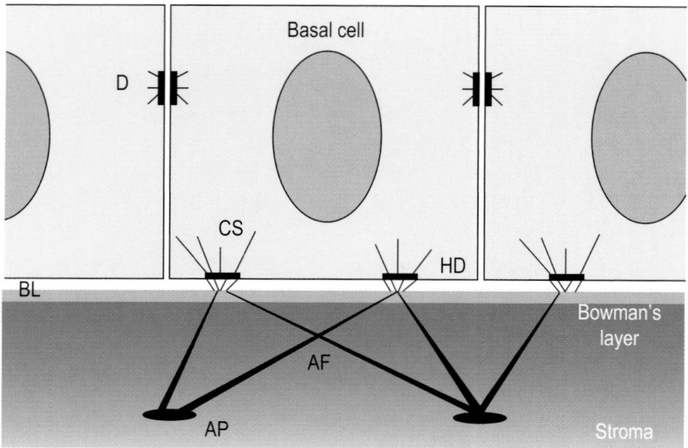

Figure 2.3 Schematic representation of the adhesion system of the corneal epithelium. Intermediate filaments in the cytoskeleton (CS) are linked through hemidesmosomes (HD) via anchoring fibrils (AF) to anchoring plaques (AP) in the anterior stroma. BL = basal lamina; D = desmosomes.

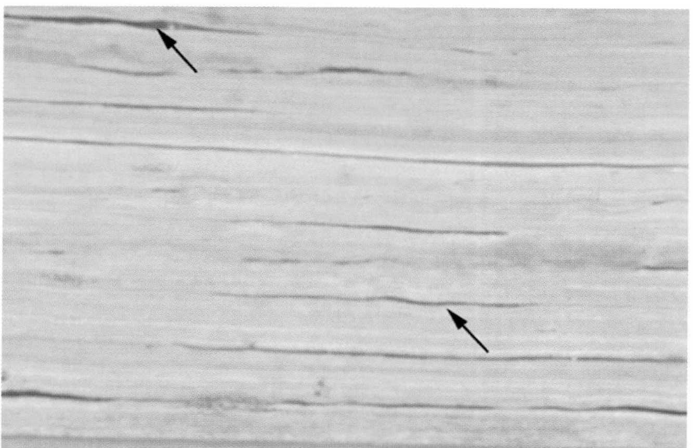

Figure 2.4 Section through the stroma. Keratocytes (arrowed) are located between lamellae.

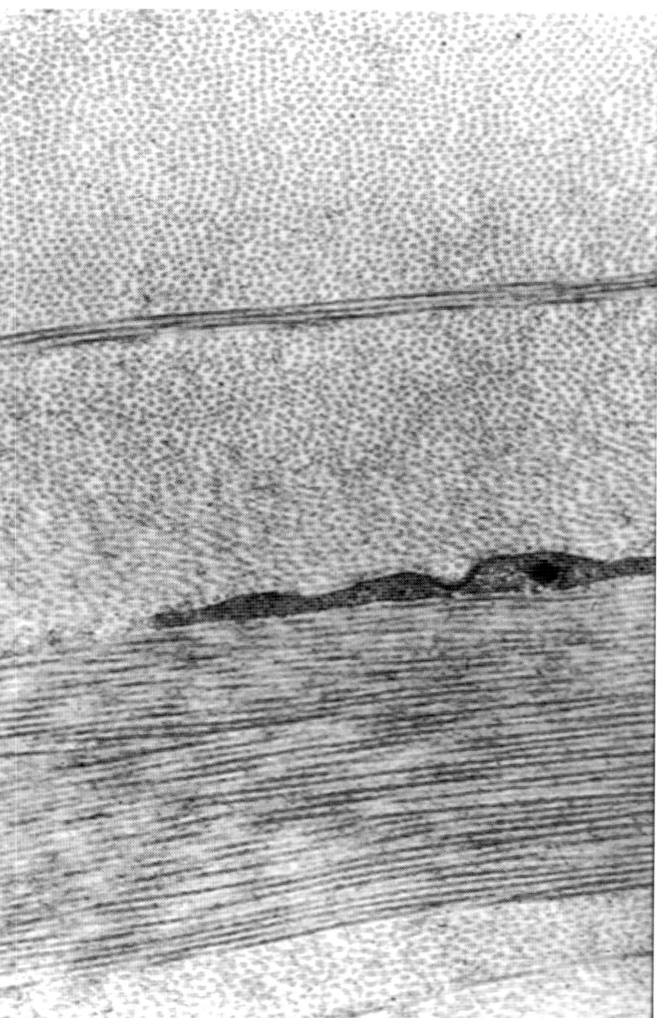

Figure 2.5 Electron micrograph of stromal lamellae which cross each other approximately at right angles. Note the regular arrangement of collagen fibrils within lamellae.

stroma (Hogan *et al.*, 1971). Fibrils are composed primarily of collagen types I, III and V. Collagen VII associated with anchoring fibrils is also present. There is evidence that Bowman's layer is formed and maintained primarily by the epithelium, although its function is unclear. The absence of Bowman's layer from the cornea of most mammals, and the fact that corneas devoid of this layer over the central cornea following PRK apparently function normally, suggest that it is not critical to corneal integrity (Wilson and Hong, 2000).

Stroma

The stroma is approximately 500 μm thick, and accounts for 90% of the thickness of the cornea. It is composed predominantly of collagen fibrils (68% dry weight) embedded in a highly hydrated matrix of proteoglycans. A variety of different collagen types have been identified. Type I is the major stromal collagen with lesser amounts of types III, V and VI (Meek and Leonard, 1993). A section taken perpendicular to the corneal surface reveals that the collagen fibrils are arranged in 200–250 layers (lamellae) running parallel to the surface (Figure 2.4). Lamellae are approximately 2 μm thick and 9–260 μm wide, and extend from limbus to limbus. Fibrils of adjacent lamellae make large angles with each other. In the superficial stroma angles are less than 90° but become orthogonal in this deeper stroma (Hogan *et al.*, 1971). This particular arrangement of collagen imparts a high tensile strength for corneal protection, which is important given its exposed position. Within lamellae, all collagen fibrils are parallel with uniform size and separation (Figure 2.5). Accurate physiological measurements of collagen fibre diameter and spacing can be obtained for the hydrated cornea with the aid of X-ray diffraction. Using this technique, the mean fibril diameter in the human cornea is 31 nm with an interfibrillar spacing of 55 nm (Meek and Leonard, 1993). This narrow fibril diameter and constant separation, which is a characteristic of corneal collagen, are necessary prerequisites for transparency.

The interfibrillar space contains a matrix of proteoglycans (approximately 10% of dry weight). Keratan sulphate and dermatan sulphate are the major corneal proteoglycans. These molecules are highly sulphated, and along with bound chloride ions create a polyanionic stromal interfibrillar matrix which induces osmotic swelling. As well as

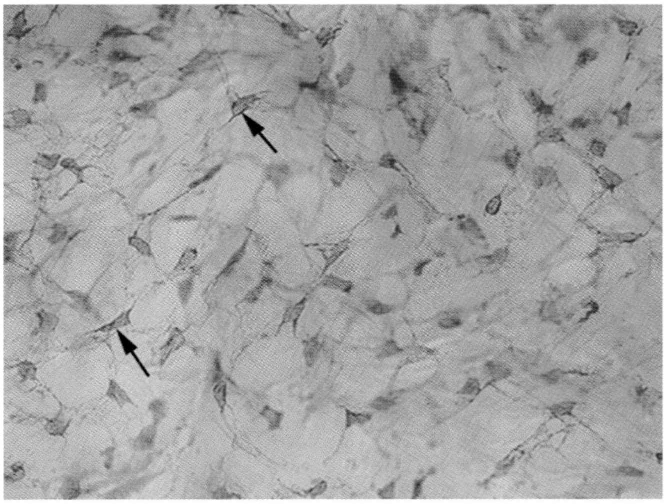

Figure 2.6 Flat section through the stroma stained with gold chloride. Keratocytes (arrowed) display a stellate appearance.

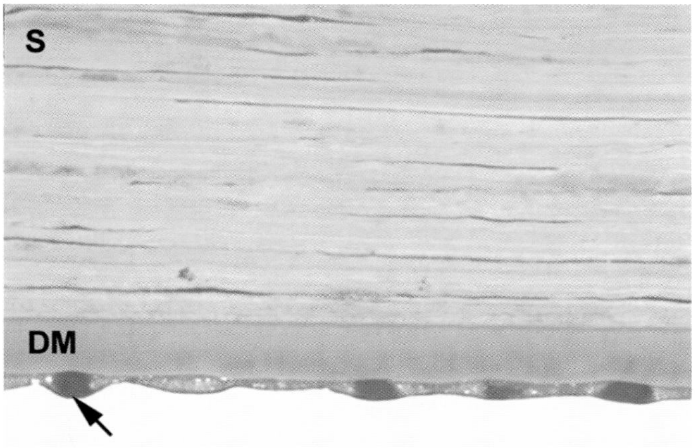

Figure 2.7 High-powered micrograph of the posterior stroma. Descemet's membrane (DM) is located between the stroma (S) and the endothelium (arrow).

playing a major role in the corneal hydration, collagen–proteoglycan interactions are important in determining the spatial arrangement of collagen fibrils (Scott, 1991).

Collagen and proteoglycans are maintained by keratocytes. These cells occupy 3–5% of stromal volume and lie between collagen lamellae, flattened in the plane of the cornea (Figure 2.6). Keratocyte density examined by confocal microscopy and biochemical methods (Møller-Pederson and Ehlers, 1995; Prydal *et al.*, 1998) is non-uniform. Density decreases from superficial to deep stroma (Hollingsworth *et al.*, 2001) and increases from centre to periphery. Keratocytes display a large central nucleus and long slender processes extend from the cell body. Processes from adjacent cells sometimes make tight junctions with each other. Cell organelles are not numerous but the usual complement of organelles, including endoplasmic reticulum, Golgi apparatus and mitochondria, can be observed (Hogan *et al.*, 1971).

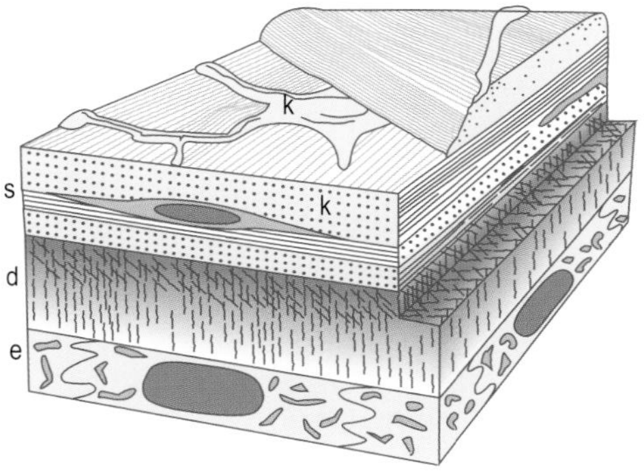

Figure 2.8 Three-dimensional representation of the posterior cornea showing the endothelium (e), Descemet's membrane (d) and stroma (s). A stromal lamella has been reflected to reveal an intralamellar keratocyte (k).

Descemet's membrane

Descemet's membrane is the basement membrane of the corneal endothelium. It lies between the endothelium and the overlying stroma (Figure 2.7). At birth it is 3–4 μm thick, and increases to a thickness of 10–12 μm in the adult. In the periphery of aged corneas, Descemet's membrane displays periodic sections of thickening, which are known as Hassall–Henle warts. The anterior one-third of Descemet's membrane represents that part produced in fetal life and, under the electron microscope, is characterized by a periodic banded pattern (Figure 2.8). The posterior two-thirds, which is formed postnatally, has a more homogeneous granular appearance. Descemet's membrane has a unique biochemical composition by contrast with other basement membranes (Lawrenson *et al.*, 1998). The major basement membrane collagen type is type IV, whereas in Descemet's membrane type VIII collagen predominates.

Endothelium

The endothelium is a monolayer of squamous cells that lines the posterior surface of the cornea (Figure 2.9). As it has a limited capacity for mitosis to replace damaged or

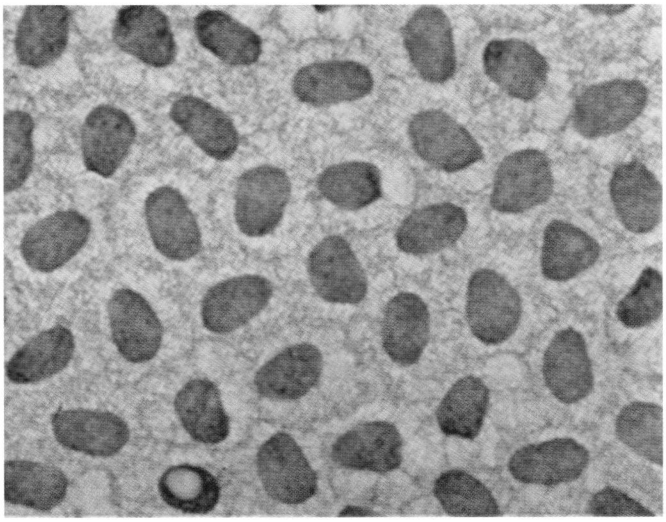

Figure 2.9 Tangential (flat) section through the corneal endothelium: a single layer of polygonal cells with irregular borders can be observed.

effete cells, there is a progressive reduction in endothelial cell number with age. At birth the cornea contains a total of approximately 500 000 cells, which represents a mean density of 4500 cells/mm^2. During infancy cell loss is particularly marked and a 26% reduction occurs in the first year (Sherrard *et al.*, 1987). Thereafter the rate of loss progressively declines into old age. Since grafted corneas appear to maintain transparency and functional normality with an endothelial cell density of less than 1000 cells/mm^2, it seems that normal cell density represents a considerable 'physiological reserve' (Klyce and Beuerman, 1998). When viewed *en face,* for example using a specular microscope, the endothelium appears as a mosaic of polygonal (typically hexagonal) cells (Efron *et al.*, 2001). In response to pathology, trauma, age and prolonged contact lens wear, the endothelial mosaic becomes less regular, and shows a greater variation in cell size (polymegethism) and shape (pleomorphism) as cells spread to fill gaps caused by cell loss. Under the electron microscope, the lateral borders of the cells are markedly convoluted and adjacent cells are linked by tight junctions (with less frequent gap junctions) (Hogan *et al.*, 1971). The complement of organelles seen in endothelial cells reflects their high metabolic activity, with numerous mitochondria and a prominent rough endoplasmic reticulum.

Corneal innervation

Source and distribution of corneal nerves

The cornea is the most richly innervated surface tissue in the body. It receives its predominantly sensory nerve supply from the nasociliary branch of the trigeminal nerve (Ruskell and Lawrenson, 1994). There is also evidence for the existence of a modest sympathetic innervation from the superior cervical ganglion (Marfurt and Ellis, 1993). Branches from the nasociliary nerve either pass directly to the eye as long ciliary nerves or traverse the ciliary ganglion, leaving as short ciliary nerves that enter the eye close to the optic nerve. Nerves destined for the cornea travel initially in the suprachoroidal space, before crossing the sclera to advance radially towards the cornea.

Most of the 50–80 precorneal nerve trunks, which contain a mixture of myelinated and unmyelinated fibre bundles, enter the cornea at mid stromal level. Myelin is soon lost and the unmyelinated nerve fibre bundles divide repeatedly and move anteriorly to form a rich plexiform network in the anterior one-third of the stroma. Axons are particularly dense immediately beneath Bowman's layer, forming an extensive subepithelial plexus (Oliveira-Soto and Efron, 2001). From this plexus, axons pass vertically through Bowman's layer, losing their Schwann cell sheath in the process. Upon entering the epithelium, axons turn through 90° and divide into a series of fine branches which course between basal cells (Figure 2.10). Some branches pass into the more superficial layers before terminating. Corneal nerves display a complex neurochemistry. A variety of neurotransmitters and neuromodulators have been identified, including acetylcholine, substance P, and calcitonin gene-related peptide. However, it is unclear how these particular neurochemicals correlate with function (Belmonte *et al.*, 1997).

Functional considerations

Corneal nerves serve important sensory, reflex and trophic functions. Interest in the sensitivity of the cornea dates back to the 19th century (Lawrenson, 1997), when the pioneering German physiologist von Frey concluded that pain was the only sensation perceived by the cornea. This was consistent with his theory of the specificity of sensory receptors, which maintained that each sensory modality was subserved by a separate anatomically distinct nerve terminal. In his experiments on the cornea von Frey could elicit only a sensation of pain, and since the cornea contained exclusively free (unspecialized) nerve endings, he concluded that free nerve endings were the exclusive receptors for pain. Although the specificity theory has subsequently been challenged, particularly with respect to its exclusivity, the question as to whether pain is the only sensory modality perceived by the cornea remains.

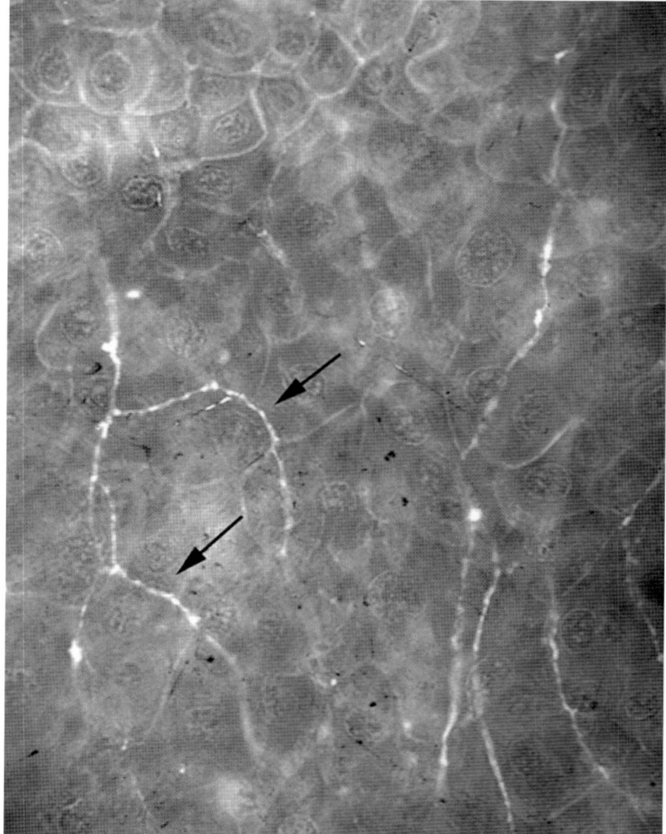

Figure 2.10 Whole-mount gold chloride-stained preparation of corneal nerves (arrowed) located at basal level.

Modern experiments using carefully controlled corneal stimulation, with a variety of mechanical, chemical and thermal stimuli, have evoked only sensations of irritation or pain. By contrast, electrophysiological studies of corneal afferent neurones have identified neurones which respond to mechanical, thermal and chemical stimulation. However, since the conscious perception of these sensations has not been demonstrated, it is likely that such specificity of modality is lost during central nervous system processing. Electrophysiological recording also allows for the mapping of receptive fields. These are often large and overlapping, which explains the inability of the cornea to localize a stimulus accurately (Belmonte *et al.*, 1997). The sensitivity of the cornea to mechanical stimulation is particularly acute, and acts as a trigger for the protective blink and lacrimal reflexes.

Cold receptors may be important in signalling evaporative cooling, which is a major determinant of spontaneous eye blink frequency (Tsubota, 1998).

Corneal afferent fibres also exert important trophic influences. Damage to corneal sensory nerves by surgery, trauma or infection produces neuroparalytic keratitis – a condition which is characterized by progressive epithelial cell loss and oedema. The mechanism of this trophic role is not fully understood, although the release of neuropeptides (e.g. substance P and calcitonin gene-related peptide) may be a factor. Sympathetic nerves also play a role in epithelial maintenance by regulating ion transport processes and cell proliferation and migration during wound healing.

Corneal metabolism

Source of oxygen and nutrients

In order to perform its vital functions the cornea requires a constant supply of oxygen and other essential metabolites (e.g. glucose, vitamins and amino acids). However, its avascularity dictates that alternative routes must exist for the provision of its metabolic needs. There are three possibilities: from the perilimbal vasculature, from the tear film or from the aqueous humour. In open-eye conditions the bulk of the oxygen required for the cornea is obtained from the atmosphere via diffusion across the precorneal tear film. Under steady-state conditions it can be assumed that the tears are saturated with oxygen, and therefore at an oxygen tension corresponding to the atmosphere (155 mm Hg at sea level). It has been estimated that the oxygen tension of the aqueous in the human eye lies between 30 and 40 mm Hg (Klyce and Beuerman, 1998).

Experiments using nitrogen-filled goggles or sealed scleral lenses have shown the corneal dependence on tear-side oxygen to avoid oedema and maintain normal function. The reason why the cornea swells during contact lens wear is explained in Figure 2.11. During eye closure the oxygen level in the tears is in equilibrium with the palpebral vasculature (55 mm Hg) (Efron and Carney, 1979).

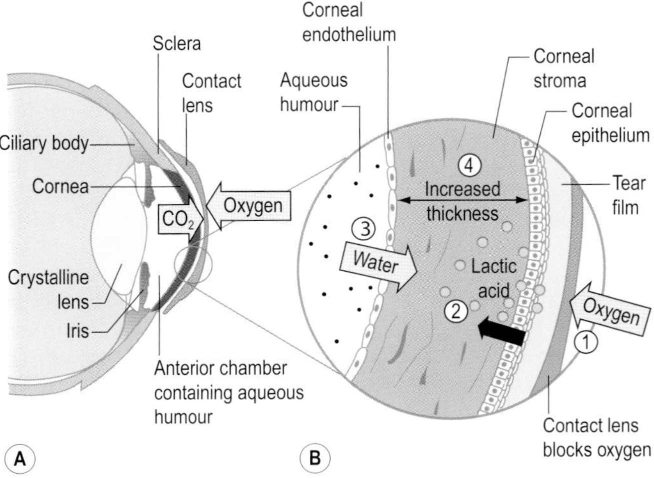

Figure 2.11 (A) Cross-section of an eye wearing a contact lens, which impedes ingress of oxygen into, and the egress of carbon dioxide from, the cornea. (B) The contact lens blocks oxygen supply to the cornea (1), causing lactic acid to accumulate in the stroma (2). This draws in water (3), leading to stromal oedema (4). (Adapted from Efron, N. (1997) Contact lenses and corneal physiology. Biol. Sci. Rev., **9**, 29–31.)

Significantly, corneal thickness increases by approximately 5% during sleep, and returns to baseline levels within 1 hour of eye opening. It has been suggested that overnight swelling is related to tear film tonicity rather than reduced oxygen availability (Klyce and Beuerman, 1998). Using polarographic oxygen sensors the oxygen flux into the cornea can be measured. For the cornea as a whole the oxygen flux is in the region of 6 $\mu l/cm^2/h$, although the consumption rate for its composite layers is not equal. Consumption rates have been estimated as 40 : 39 : 21 for the epithelium, stroma and endothelium respectively (Freeman, 1972).

Several lines of evidence indicate that the aqueous is the primary source of glucose and essential amino acids for the cornea (Maurice, 1984). The glucose concentration of tears is low compared to the aqueous, and the insertion of nutrient-impermeable implants into the stroma results in degeneration of the tissue lying anterior to the implant. Although exogenous glucose is primarily utilized, glycogen stores are present in all corneal cells to provide glucose in conditions of metabolic stress.

The role of the perilimbal vasculature in the provision of oxygen and nutrients appears limited and it is likely that it is only significant for the corneal periphery (Maurice, 1984).

Oxidative metabolism

The cornea derives its energy principally from the oxidative breakdown of carbohydrates (Riley, 1969). Glucose, which is the primary substrate for the generation of adenosine triphosphate (ATP), is catabolized by three metabolic pathways: glycolysis, tricarboxylic acid (Krebs) cycle and the hexose monophosphate shunt (Figure 2.12). Anaerobic glycolysis accounts for the majority of glucose metabolism. In this pathway, glucose is first oxidized to pyruvate and then subsequently reduced to lactate, with a net yield of two molecules of ATP. The TCA cycle results in a greater energy yield (36ATP). This pathway is most active in the corneal endothelium, which has the greatest energy requirement.

Metabolic waste products can be potentially damaging if allowed to accumulate. Although carbon dioxide can readily diffuse out of the cornea across its limiting layers,

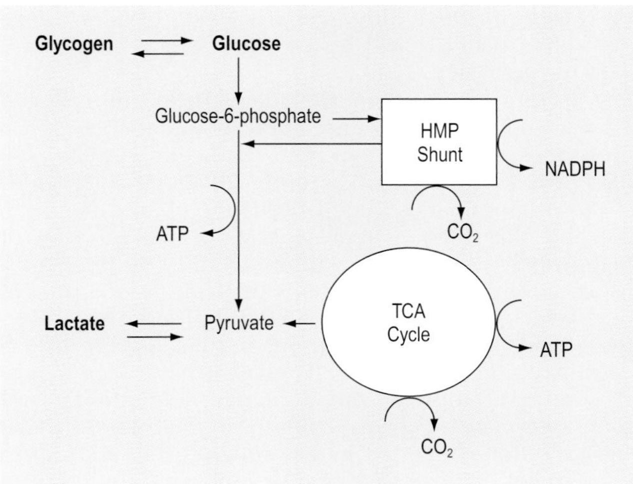

Figure 2.12 Metabolic pathways present in the cornea. HMP = hexose monophosphate shunt; TCA cycle = tricarboxylic acid (Krebs) cycle; ATP = adenosine triphosphate; NADPH = nicotinamide adenine dinucleotide phosphate (reduced form).

lactate is less easily eliminated. Under normoxic conditions lactate is able to diffuse slowly across the endothelium into the anterior chamber. However, during periods of hypoxia the proportion of glucose which is metabolized anaerobically increases. The resulting accumulation of lactate causes stromal oedema via an increased osmotic load (Klyce, 1981) and localized tissue acidosis (Klyce and Beuerman, 1998).

The hexose monophosphate shunt (also known as the pentose phosphate shunt) plays a significant role in the epithelium and endothelium, where it accounts for 35–65% of glucose utilization (Berman, 1981). It fulfils several important functions, including the generation of intermediates for biosynthetic reactions and the prevention of oxidative damage by free radicals.

Corneal transparency

Under normal conditions the cornea is highly transparent, transmitting more than 90% of incident light. Structurally, the cornea is a typical connective tissue consisting principally of a matrix of collagen and proteoglycans. Under normal circumstances such an arrangement would favour light scatter with consequent loss of transparency. This raises two fundamental questions. How is transparency achieved, and how is it maintained? To begin to answer these questions it is necessary to understand the spatial organization of the stromal matrix and the importance of corneal hydration control.

Stromal organization

Maurice (1957) explained the transparency of the cornea on the basis of the small diameter and regular separation of the stromal collagen. He suggested that the collagen fibrils of the stroma were disposed in a regular crystalline lattice, and light scattered by the fibrils is eliminated by destructive interference in all directions other than the forward direction. This situation will hold as long as the axes of the collagen fibrils are arranged in a regular lattice with a separation less than the wavelength of light. It has been suggested, however, that the fibrillar arrangement need not be in a perfect crystal lattice to maintain transparency (Maurice, 1984), although disruption of short-range order between fibrils will lead to increased scatter and a loss of transparency.

The factors involved in the maintenance of collagen fibril size and spatial order are not fully understood. It has been proposed that collagen fibril diameters may be controlled by the incorporation of minor collagens (e.g. type V) into the predominantly type I fibrils (Meek and Leonard, 1993) and that their spatial separation is a function of proteoglycan–collagen interactions (Scott, 1991). Proteoglycans are a family of glycoproteins that consist of a protein core to which are attached sugar chains of repeating disaccharide units termed glycosaminoglycans (GAG). In the corneal stroma two major proteoglycans have been identified – keratan sulphate and dermatan sulphate. Several keratan sulphate isoforms have been described in the cornea of different species. In the human cornea an isoform predominates that has been termed lumican (Funderburgh *et al.*, 1991; Funderburgh, 2000). In recent years a link between keratan sulphate content of the cornea and transparency has become apparent; for example, transgenic mice which lack the gene for lumican fail to develop a clear cornea (Funderburgh, 2000). Dermatan sulphate is the other main corneal proteoglycan which is present predominantly as decoran, a small proteoglycan with GAG side chains which are a mix of dermatan and chondroitin sulphates (Funderburgh *et al.*, 1991). In contrast to lumican, a clear role for decorin in corneal transparency has not been established, although it may be involved in determining fibre: fibre spacing. Cationic dyes such as cuprolinic blue can be used to stain proteoglycans for ultrastructural localisation. Using this technique corneal GAG filaments appear to be of an equal length and link adjacent collagen fibrils in a manner , suggesting that they regulate fibre spacing (Scott, 1991).

Hydration control

The state of corneal hydration is another important determinant of corneal transparency. The hydrophilic properties of the stroma are to a large part determined by proteoglycans, which contribute to the fixed negative charge of the stroma and produce a passive gel swelling pressure through electrostatic repulsion (Hodson, 1997). Physiologically, corneal hydration is maintained at approximately 78%. If the cornea is allowed to swell ± 5% of this value, it begins to scatter significant quantities of light (Hodson, 1997).

Maintenance of physiological corneal hydration is to a large part dependent on the corneal endothelium, which possesses both a barrier property and a metabolically driven pump. The endothelial barrier to the free passage of molecules from the aqueous is formed principally by focal tight junctions between adjacent endothelial cells. However, in contrast to other barrier epithelia, these junctions are of low electrical resistance and allow the passage of ions and small molecules. This leak is offset by the metabolically driven pumping of ions out of the stroma by the endothelium, which maintains a transcellular potential difference (aqueous side negative) to balance stromal swelling pressure (Maurice, 1984). Disruption of this osmotic gradient will result in stromal fluid imbibition.

The specific endothelial ion transport mechanisms responsible for the maintenance of physiological hydration are not fully understood. A simplified model representing our current level of knowledge is represented in Figure 2.13. There is compelling evidence that a flux of bicarbonate ions is the predominant component of the endothelial ion transport system (Hodson and Miller, 1976). The bicarbonate is generated either by a Na^+/HCO_3^- co-transporter located on the basolateral plasma membrane or via the intercellular conversion of carbon dioxide by the enzyme carbonic anhydrase. Bicarbonate leaves the cell via an apical bicarbonate ion channel. The driving force for the bicarbonate flux is generated by a sodium potassium ATPase which resides on the basolateral endothelial membrane. The energy associated with subsequent sodium re-entry (via Na^+/H^+ and Na^+/HCO_3^- transporters) is coupled to active HCO_3^- flux (Hodson *et al.*, 1991).

The epithelium also contributes to corneal hydration control (Klyce and Beuerman, 1998). The tight junctions between superficial epithelial cells form an effective permeability barrier to ions and polar solutes. For example, the anionic molecule sodium fluorescein does not penetrate an intact epithelium. Damage to the superficial cells allows fluorescein to enter the epithelium, with resulting corneal staining. In addition to its barrier properties the epithelium

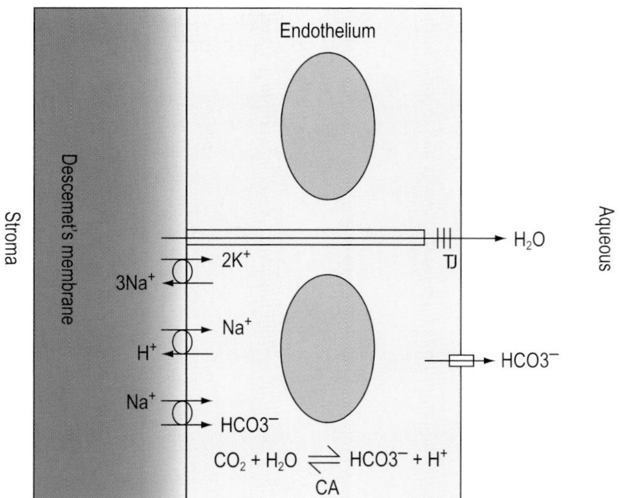

Figure 2.13 Schematic representation of the corneal endothelial pump. CA = carbonic anhydrase; TJ = tight junction.

also possesses active ion transport systems for Na^+ and Cl^-. Since these pumps contribute to the tonicity of the tear film, it is likely that they are involved in the maintenance of stromal hydration.

Response to oedema

When corneas swell, light scattering increases with an ensued transparency loss due to the disruption of the regular collagen matrix. The collagen fibrils themselves swell very little and most of the additional water goes into the interfibrillar spaces. Transmission electron micrographs of oedematous corneas show fibril aggregation, with the result that large areas are devoid of collagen fibrils (Stiemke *et al.*, 1995). There is evidence from several sources that collagen aggregation occurs as a result of loss of GAGs which previously had maintained fibre separation (Stiemke *et al.*, 1995).

Corneal epithelial wound healing

A smooth and intact corneal epithelium is necessary in order for the cornea to maintain clear vision. However, due to its exposed position the cornea is potentially vulnerable to a variety of external insults. The cornea possesses several protective mechanisms to avoid injury, but if tissue damage occurs it is capable of an effective wound-healing response (Gipson and Inatomi, 1995; Nishida and Tanaka, 1996). Corneal epithelial repair is a complex process involving an orchestrated interaction between cells and extracellular matrix, which is coordinated by a variety of growth factors. The process can be divided into three phases: (1) initial covering of the denuded area by cell migration; (2) cell proliferation to replace lost cells; and (3) epithelial differentiation to reform the normal stratified epithelial architecture.

Following a full-thickness epithelial defect, fibronectin, an adhesive glycoprotein, is synthesized and covers the surface of the bared stroma where it serves as a temporary matrix for cell migration. The adhesion between fibronectin and the epithelium is mediated by integrin–matrix interactions (integrins are a family of cell surface receptors which bind to certain extracellular matrix proteins). Several growth factors have been implicated in the control of the wound-healing response, including epidermal growth factor, transforming growth factor beta, platelet-derived growth factor and fibroblast growth factor (Gipson and Inatomi, 1995). Growth factors, which are produced by a variety of sources (e.g. ocular surface epithelia and the lacrimal gland), are able to regulate the process of epithelial migration, proliferation and differentiation. There is evidence that epithelial–stromal interactions play an important role in corneal wound healing (Wilson, 2000). Epithelial injury triggers keratocyte apoptosis (programmed cell death) in the anterior stroma, via the release of apoptosis-inducing cytokines from epithelial cells. Keratocyte apoptosis subsequently triggers a wound-healing cascade which influences epithelial repair.

Regeneration of the corneal epithelium is highly dependent on the integrity of the limbus. Cumulative evidence indicates that a proportion of limbal basal epithelial cells possess the properties of stem cells, which are ultimately responsible for corneal epithelial replacement (Dua and Azuara-Blanco, 2000). Stem cells have several unique characteristics – they are poorly differentiated, long-lived and have a high capacity for self-renewal. When these cells divide, one of the daughter cells replenishes the stem cell pool, whilst the other is destined to undergo further cell divisions before differentiating. Such a cell is referred to as a transient amplifying cell. Transient amplifying cells undergo several rounds of cell division before fully differentiating. These cells play an important role in epithelial wound healing, where their proliferative capacity is increased by shortening cycle times and increasing the number of times that the transient amplifying cells can divide before maturation.

The ocular adnexa

The ocular adnexa are those structures which support and protect the eye, and include the eyelids, conjunctiva and lacrimal system. They play an important role in the formation of the preocular tear film and collectively defend the eye against antigenic challenge.

Eyelids

The eyelids are two mobile folds of skin which perform several important functions: they act as occluders which shield the eyes from excessive light, and through their reflex closure they afford protection against injury. The lids also form a precorneal tear film of uniform thickness during the upturn phase of each blink. The action of blinking is important for tear drainage.

Gross anatomy

The eyelids are joined at their extremities, termed the canthi, and when the eye is open an elliptical space, the palpebral fissure, is formed between the lid margins. In the adult, the length of the fissure is approximately 30–31 mm, with a vertical height of 10–11 mm. In the primary position, the upper lid, which is the larger and more mobile of the two, typically covers approximately the upper third of the cornea, whilst the lower lid is level with the inferior corneal limbus (Figure 2.14). The eyelid margins are about

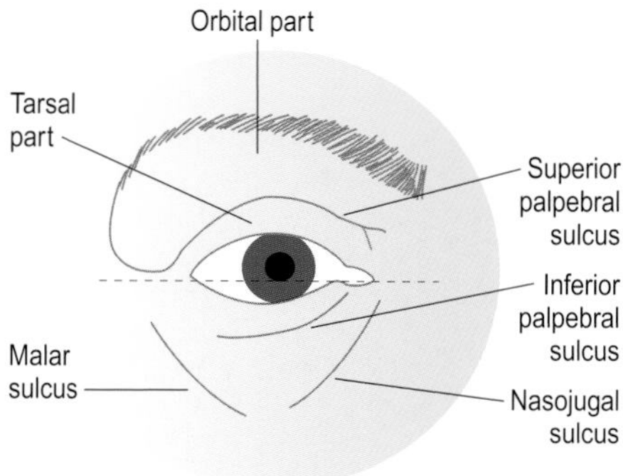

Figure 2.14 Surface anatomy of the eyelids. (Adapted from Bron , A. J., Tripathi, R. C. and Tripathi, B. (1997) Wolff's Anatomy of the Eye and Orbit. 8th Edition. Chapman and Hall.)

2 mm thick from front to back. The posterior quarter consists of conjunctival mucosa and the anterior three-quarters is skin. The junction between the two is referred to as the mucocutaneous junction. Two or three rows of eyelashes (cilia) arise from the anterior border of the lid margins. These are longer and more numerous in the upper lid. The lashes receive a rich sensory nerve supply, and their sensitivity provides an effective alerting mechanism.

The meibomian (tarsal) gland orifices emerge just anterior to the mucocutaneous junction (Figure 2.15). About 30–40 glands open onto the upper margin, and slightly fewer (20–40) onto the lower. On eversion of the lids the yellowish meibomian acini are visible as yellow clusters through the tarsal conjunctiva (Bron *et al.*, 1991). At the medial angle, the eyelid margins enclose a triangular space – the lacus lacrimalis – which contains the plica semilunaris and the caruncle. Lacrimal papillae are small elevations, located 5–6 mm from the medial canthal angle, which contains a small aperture (punctum) which is the opening to the lacrimal drainage system.

Muscles of the eyelids

Movements of the eyelids are governed by the coordinated action of several muscles.

Orbicularis oculi

The orbicularis oculi is the sphincter muscle of the eyelids, and anatomically can be divided into two main divisions – palpebral and orbital (Figure 2.16). Fibres of the palpebral division arise from the medial palpebral ligament and arc across the eyelids in a series of half-ellipses and meet at the lateral canthus to form a lateral raphe. The lateral palpebral ligament also acts as an anchor point. The palpebral division can be further subdivided into marginal, pretarsal and preseptal parts. The marginal part (pars ciliaris), which is also known as Riolans muscle, is responsible for maintaining the apposition of the lid to the cornea during lid closure. A third part of the muscle (pars lacrimalis) is closely associated with the lacrimal outflow pathway. The pars lacrimalis (also known as Horner's muscle) encloses the canaliculi and provides attachments to the lacrimal sac and its associated fascia.

The orbital part of the orbicularis oculi lies outside the palpebral division and extends for some distance beyond the orbital margins. Muscle fibres arise predominantly from bone at the medial orbital rim and appear to sweep around the lids without interruption as a series of complete ellipses. However, studies have shown that the muscle fibres of the

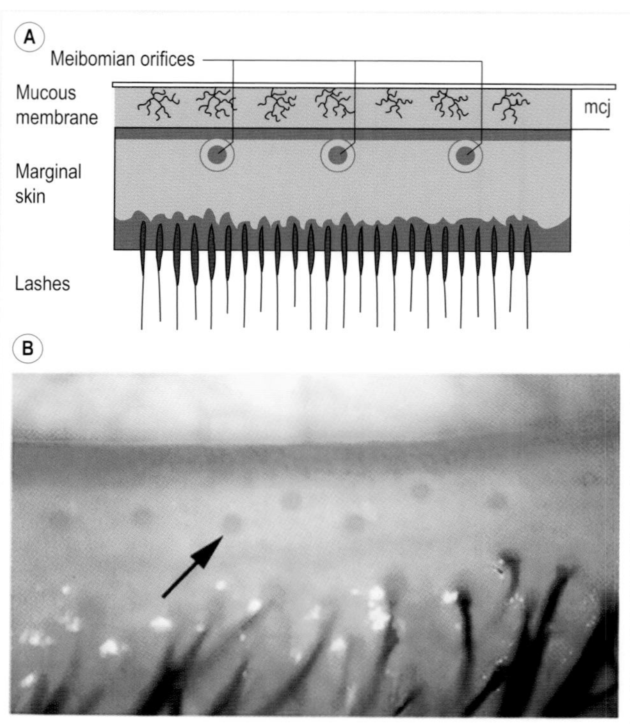

Figure 2.15 (A) Schematic representation of the eyelid margin. mcj = mucocutaneous junction. (B) Gross appearance of the eyelid margin. Openings of the meibomian glands are clearly visible (arrow). (Adapted from Bron , A. J., Tripathi, R. C. and Tripathi, B. (1997) Wolff's Anatomy of the Eye and Orbit. 8th Edition. Chapman and Hall.)

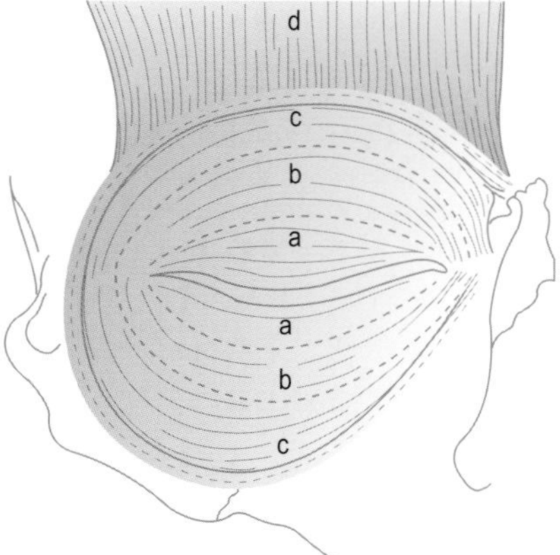

Figure 2.16 Schematic representation of the divisions of the orbicularis oculi and the frontalis. a = pretarsal; b = preseptal; c = orbital; d = frontalis. (Adapted from Bron , A. J., Tripathi, R. C. and Tripathi, B. (1997) Wolff's Anatomy of the Eye and Orbit. 8th Edition. Chapman and Hall.)

orbital and palpebral division of the orbicularis are relatively short (0.4–2.1 mm) and overlapping (Lander *et al.*, 1996). The regional divisions of the orbicularis also show a functional distinction. The action of the palpebral part of the muscle is to produce the reflex or voluntary closure of the lids during blinking. Contraction of the orbital division produces the forcible closure of the lids that occurs in sneezing or in response to a painful stimulus.

Levator palpebrae superioris

The levator palpebrae superioris is primarily responsible for elevating the upper lid during blinking and for

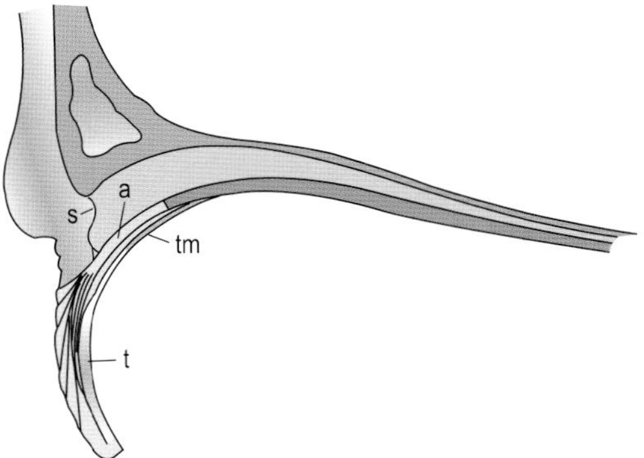

Figure 2.17 Diagram showing the relations of the levator palpebrae superioris. a = levator aponerosis; tm = superior tarsal muscle (of Müller); t = tarsal plate; s = orbital septum. (Adapted from Gray, H., Bannister, L. H., Berry, M. M. and Williams, P. L. (1995) Gray's Anatomy: The Anatomical Basis of Medicine and Surgery. 38th ed., Churchill Livingstone.)

maintaining an open palpebral aperture. The levator palpebrae arises from the lesser wing of the sphenoid, above and anterior to the optic canal, and runs forward along the roof of the orbit above the superior rectus before terminating anteriorly in a fan-shaped tendon (aponeurosis). Some fibres are attached to the anterior surface of the tarsal plate, whilst the remainder pass between fascicles of the orbicularis (Figure 2.17). The superior palpebral sulcus forms at the upper border of the attachment to the orbicularis.

Superior and inferior tarsal muscles (of Müller)

These smooth muscles arise from the lower border of the levator in the upper lid and the inferior rectus in the lower lid, and insert into the orbital margins of the tarsal plates. The role of the superior tarsal muscle is to assist the levator in maintaining the width of the palpebral aperture. A mild degree of ptosis results from damage to its sympathetic nerve supply (Horner's syndrome).

Control of eyelid movements

Movements of the eyelids occur through the coordinated action of several muscles – the levator palpebrae, tarsal muscles, the orbicularis oculi and the frontalis. The elevation of the upper lid and the control of its vertical position are mediated principally by the levator. In vertical gaze, lid position and eye movements are closely linked. During elevation the state of contraction of the levator is varied to maximize visibility. In extreme upgaze, lid retraction is augmented by the action of the frontalis which elevates the eyebrows. In downgaze, coordinated lid movements similarly occur through levator relaxation. In periodic and reflex blinks the levator is spontaneously inhibited prior to orbicularis contraction in lid closure. Similarly, in lid opening, the orbicularis relaxes, followed by contraction of the levator. Spontaneous eye blink activity is influenced by both central and peripheral factors (Tsubota, 1998).

Compared to the upper lid, the lower lid is relatively immobile and has no counterpart to the levator palpebrae. The depression of the lower lid which occurs in downgaze is due to the attachment of the sheaths of the inferior oblique and inferior rectus muscles to the tarsal plate via a fibrous extension.

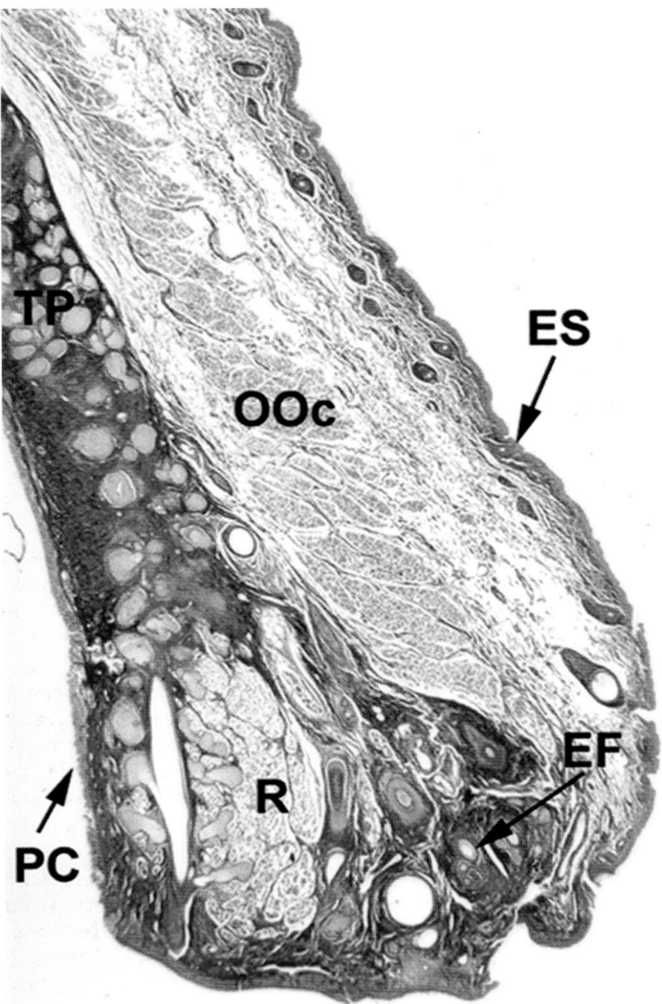

Figure 2.18 Sagittal section through the upper lid. TP = tarsal plate; Ooc = orbicularis oculi; R = Riolan's muscle; EF = eyelash follicles; PC = palpebral conjunctiva; ES = eyelid surface.

Microscopic anatomy

The histological appearance of the upper and lower lids is similar, and in sagittal section the following six tissue layers can be resolved: skin, subcutaneous connective tissue, muscle layer, submuscular connective tissue, tarsal plate and palpebral conjunctiva (Figure 2.18).

The eyelid skin is thin and very elastic. It is continuous with the palpebral conjunctiva at the lid margin, and keratinization is maintained up to this mucocutaneous junction. The subcutaneous connective tissue is composed of a loose areolar tissue and contains hair follicles and associated glands. The muscle layer consists of striated muscle fibres of the orbicularis oculi which are arranged in bundles (fascicles) separated by connective tissue. The orbicularis extends throughout the lid. The marginal part of the muscle (Riolan's muscle) is separated from the pretarsal portion by connective tissue which contains the eyelash follicles. The loose submuscular connective tissue layer lies between the orbicularis and the tarsal plate and contains the major nerves and vessels of the lid.

The tarsal plates (tarsi) are composed of dense fibrous connective tissue and provide support and determine lid

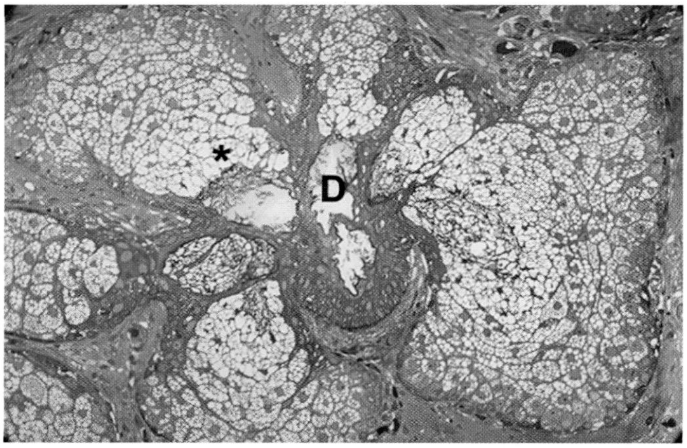

Figure 2.19 Histological section showing meibomian gland acini. Secretory cells degenerate (asterisk) as they approach the duct (D).

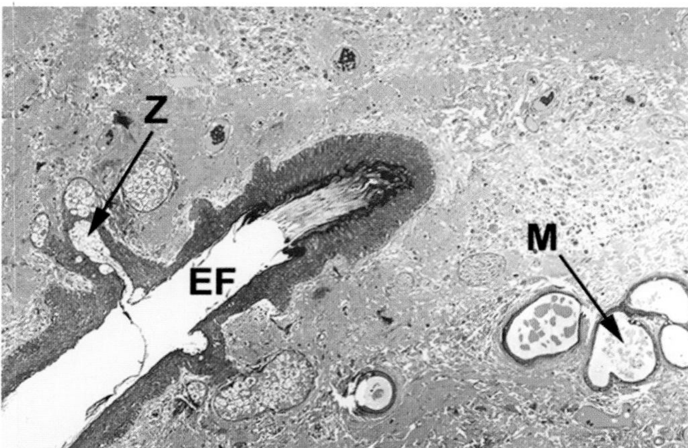

Figure 2.20 Histological section through the ciliary zone of the eyelid. Glands of Zeis (Z) discharge their contents into an eyelash follicle (EF) which contains the remnants of an eyelash. M = gland of Moll.

shape. They are anchored to the orbital margins by the medial and lateral palpebral ligaments. Each tarsus is approximately 25 mm long and 1–2 mm thick. The upper tarsus is semioval with a height of 11 mm at its midpoint, whereas the inferior tarsus is narrower (4 mm in height). The posterior surface of the eyelid is lined by the palpebral conjunctiva which is firmly adherent to the underlying tarsal plate.

Glands of the eyelids

Meibomian glands

The tarsal plates contain the acini and ducts of the meibomian (tarsal) glands. Ducts are vertically oriented with respect to the lid margins with multiple secretory acini which open laterally onto each duct. The glands occupy nearly the full length and width of each tarsus, and are fewer and shorter in the lower lid. Histologically, acini are lined by a layer of undifferentiated basal cells which divide, and cells are displaced from the basement membrane. As they progress towards the duct they gradually enlarge and develop lipid droplets in their cytoplasm (Figure 2.19). Ultimately, cell membranes rupture and cellular debris, together with the lipid product, is discharged into the duct.

The stimulus for meibomian gland secretion is unclear. Although a modest autonomic innervation of the meibomian glands has been demonstrated, there is still some doubt regarding a neuromodulation of glandular secretion, and it is likely that the principal control of the glands is hormonal. Androgens are known to regulate the development, differentiation and secretion of sebaceous glands throughout the body, and a study by Sullivan *et al.* (2000) has localized androgen receptor protein to meibomian acinar cells and was able to modulate the lipid profile of the gland by varying androgen levels.

Glands of Zeis and Moll

Ciliary glands of Zeis and Moll are found in association with eyelash follicles (Figure 2.20). Zeis glands are unilobular sebaceous glands which open directly into the follicle. The function of their oily secretion is to lubricate the lashes to prevent them from drying out and becoming brittle. Glands of Moll are modified sweat glands consisting of an unbranched spiral tubule. The exact function of these glands is unclear.

Blood and nerve supply

Nerves of the eyelids

The levator palpebrae and orbicularis oculi muscles are innervated by the oculomotor and facial nerves, respectively. The sensory supply of the upper lid derives from branches of the ophthalmic nerve (supraorbital, supratrochlear and lacrimal). The supply to the lower lid comes from branches of the maxillary nerve (zygomatic, infraorbital).

Blood and lymphatic supply to the eyelids

The arterial supply derives from branches of the ophthalmic, lacrimal and infraorbital arteries, which contribute to two palpebral arcades in the upper lid and one in the lower. Branches from these arcades supply the skin, orbicularis, tarsal glands and palpebral conjunctiva. Veins of the eyelids empty into veins of the forehead and temple and some into the ophthalmic vein. Lymphatics drain to the preauricular and submandibular lymph nodes.

The conjunctiva

Gross anatomy

The conjunctiva is a thin transparent mucous membrane which extends from the eyelid margins anteriorly, providing a lining to the lids, before turning sharply upon itself to form the fornices from where it is reflected onto the globe, covering the sclera up to its junction with the cornea. It thus forms a sac which opens anteriorly through the palpebral fissure. The conjunctiva is conventionally divided into the following regions: marginal, tarsal, orbital (these three collectively form the palpebral conjunctival), bulbar and limbal (Figure 2.21).

The static dimensions of the conjunctival sac in the primary position are illustrated in Figure 2.22 (Ehlers, 1965). The marginal zone extends from a line immediately posterior to the openings of the tarsal glands and passes around the eyelid margin from where it continues on the inner surface of the lid as far as the subtarsal fold (a shallow groove which marks the marginal edge of the tarsal plate).

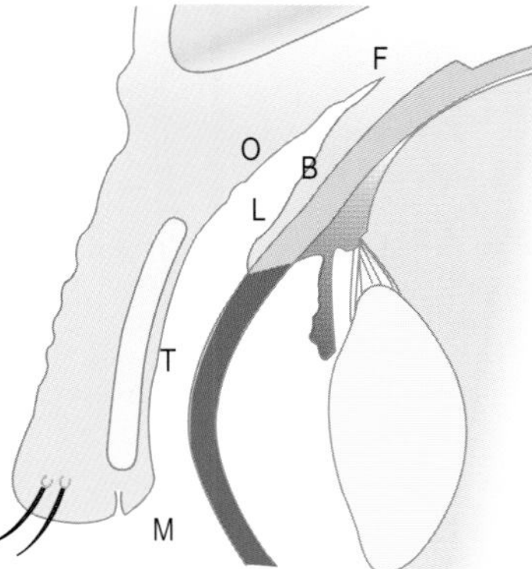

Figure 2.21 Schematic representation of a mid sagittal section through the eyelid and conjunctival sac showing the different conjunctival regions. M = marginal; T = tarsal; O = orbital; B = bulbar; L = limbal; F = fornical.

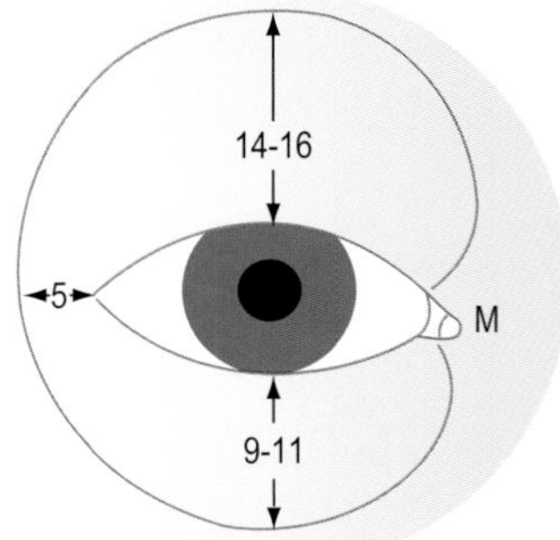

Figure 2.22 Static dimensions of the conjunctival sac in millimetres. M = medial canthus. (Adapted from Ehlers, N. (1965) On the size of the conjunctival sac. Acta Ophthalmol., 43, 205–210.)

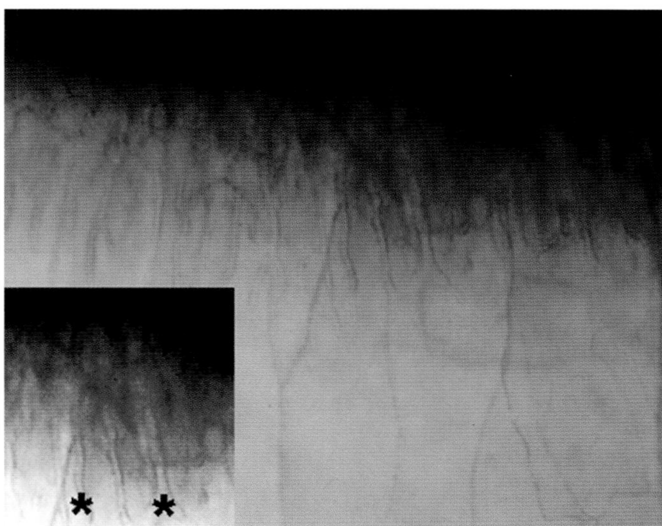

Figure 2.23 High-power slit-lamp view of the conjunctival palisades of Vogt (asterisks) at the lower limbus.

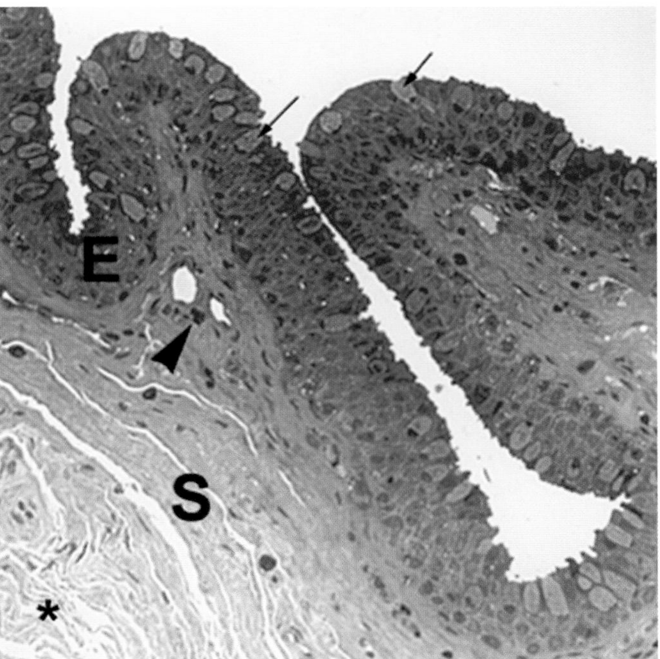

Figure 2.24 Histological section through the bulbar conjunctiva. E = epithelium; S = stroma. Goblet cells can be seen in the epithelium (arrows). The stroma can be resolved into an adenoid layer (arrow head) and a deep fibrous layer (asterisk).

The tarsal conjunctiva is highly vascular and is firmly attached to the underlying fibrous connective tissue. From the convex border of the tarsal plate the orbital zone extends as far as the fornices. Over this region the conjunctiva is more loosely attached to underlying tissues, and so readily folds. Elevations of the conjunctival surface in the form of papillae and lymphoid follicles are commonly observed in this region.

The transparency of the bulbar conjunctiva readily permits the visualization of conjunctival and episcleral blood vessels. Here, the conjunctiva is freely movable due to its loose attachment to Tenon's capsule (the fascial sheath of the globe). As the bulbar conjunctiva approaches the cornea its surface becomes smoother and its attachment to the sclera increases. The limbal conjunctiva extends approximately 1–1.5 mm around the cornea. Its junction with the cornea is ill defined, particularly in the vertical meridian, due to a variable degree of conjunctival/scleral overlap. The limbus has a rich blood supply, and in the majority of individuals a radial array of connective tissue elevations – the palisades of Vogt – can be seen adjacent to the corneal margin (Figure 2.23). The palisades are most prominent in the vertical meridian, and their visibility is enhanced in pigmented eyes.

Microscopic anatomy

In histological section two distinct layers can be resolved – an epithelium containing a variable number of goblet cells, and a vascular stroma which consists of a superficial lymphoid layer and a deep fibrous layer (Figure 2.24). The appearance of the conjunctiva shows a marked regional variability.

Epithelium

In the marginal zone the epithelium is stratified and squamous with few goblet cells. It has been suggested that a subpopulation of these cells, which lie close to the mucocutaneous junction, may be acting as stem cells for the

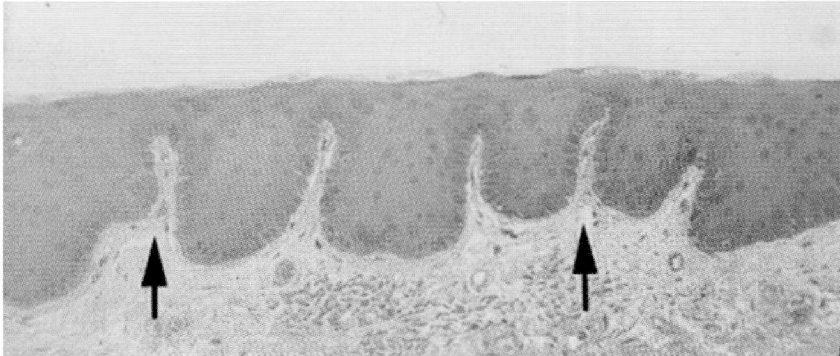

Figure 2.25 Histological section through the palisade region. Connective tissue ridges can be seen projecting into the overlying epithelium (arrows).

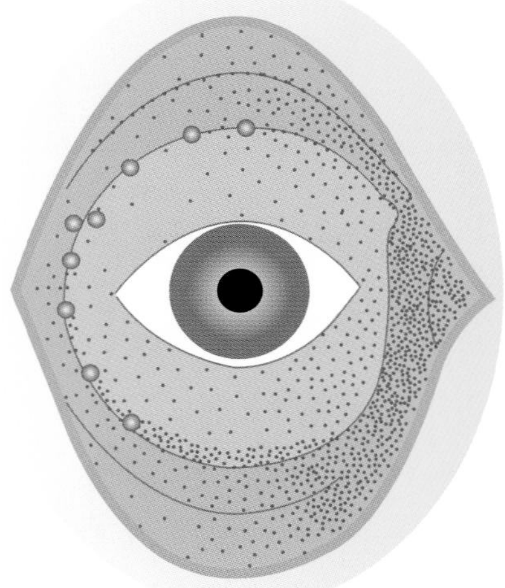

Figure 2.26 Diagram showing the regional variation in goblet cell density. Goblet cell density is greatest over the caruncle, plica semilunaris and inferior nasal palpebral conjunctiva. (Adapted from Bron , A. J., Tripathi, R. C. and Tripathi, B. (1997) Wolff's Anatomy of the Eye and Orbit. 8th Edition. Chapman and Hall. Reproduced from Bron, 1997.)

palpebral conjunctiva (Wirtschafter *et al.*, 1999). Approaching the tarsus, the epithelium thins to 2–3 layers of cuboidal cells with scattered goblet cells. The epithelium of the orbital zone is slightly thicker (2–4 cells) with more numerous goblet cells. The number of goblet cells declines over the bulbar conjunctiva and at the limbus the epithelium is again stratified squamous, and goblet cells are absent. The limbus contains a unique array of connective tissue ridges (the palisades of Vogt) which project into the overlying epithelium (Figure 2.25). Clinical and experimental evidence suggests that the palisades are the repositories of stem cells and therefore act as the regenerative organ of the corneal epithelium (Dua and Azuara-Blanco, 2000). The conjunctival epithelium additionally contains several non-native cells, including dendritic cells, melanocytes and lymphocytes.

Goblet and other secretory cells

Goblet cells provide the mucous component of the tear film. They arise in the basal cell layers and migrate to the surface, becoming fully differentiated. Mature goblet cells are larger than the surrounding epithelial cells and contain a peripherally placed nucleus. The cytoplasm is packed with membrane-bound secretory granules which discharge from the apical surface in an apocrine manner. The number

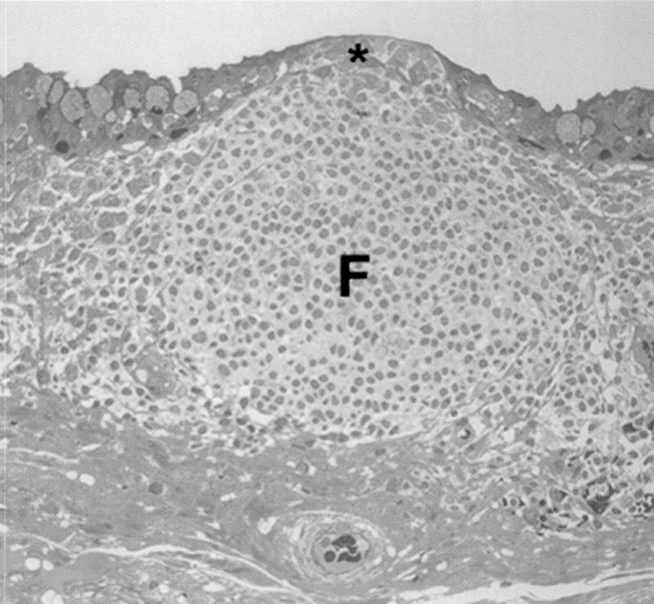

Figure 2.27 Histological section through a lymphoid follicle (F). Note the modification of the overlying epithelium (asterisk).

of goblet cells shows a marked regional variation in density (Kessing, 1968) (Figure 2.26) and they are occasionally seen lining intraepithelial crypts (of Henle).

The apices of many surface epithelial cells of the conjunctiva contain numerous carbohydrate-containing secretory vesicles, which are seen to migrate to the cell surface where they fuse with the plasma membrane (Dilly, 1985). It is likely that this represents a mechanism for recycling the cell surface glycocalyx rather than a secondary source of secretory mucin.

Conjunctival stroma

The conjunctival stroma (substantia propria) is variable in thickness. It can be resolved into two distinct layers: a superficial adenoid layer and a deeper fibrous layer (Figure 2.23). The adenoid layer contains numerous lymphocytes with local accumulations in the form of lymphoid follicles (Figure 2.27). Follicles represent aggregates of predominantly B cells which form part of the so-called conjunctiva-associated lymphoid tissue. The adenoid layer also contains a large number of mast cells which play a major role in ocular allergy (McGill *et al.*, 1998). The deep fibrous layer is generally thicker than the adenoid layer and contains the majority of conjunctival blood vessels and nerves.

Innervation and blood supply

Nerves

The conjunctiva receives nerves from sensory, sympathetic and parasympathetic sources. Sensory nerves, which are trigeminal in origin, reach the conjunctiva via branches of the ophthalmic nerve. The principal function of these fibres is to equip the conjunctiva with the ability to detect a variety of sensations – for example, touch, pain, warmth and cold. Sensory nerve terminals include both free (unspecialized) nerve endings and the more complex corpuscular endings (classically referred to as Krause end bulbs) (Lawrenson

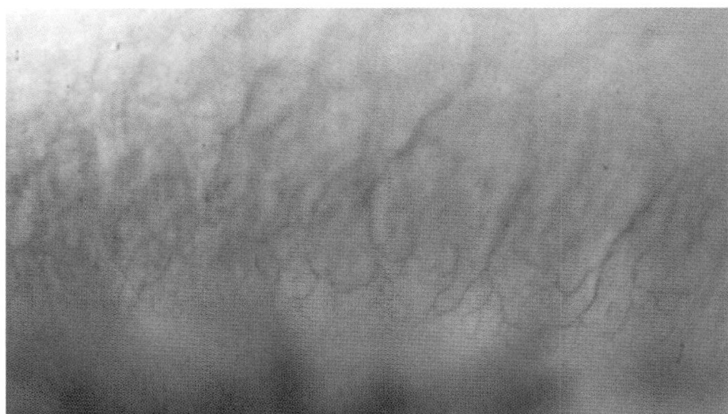

Figure 2.28 High-power slit-lamp photograph showing the limbal vascular arcades.

and Ruskell, 1991). Conjunctival blood vessels receive a dual autonomic innervation. Parasympathetic fibres, issuing from the pterygopalatine ganglion, and sympathetic fibres from the superior cervical ganglion are responsible for vasodilation and vasoconstriction, respectively.

Blood vessels and lymphatics

The arterial supply derives from two sources – palpebral branches of the nasal and lacrimal arteries, and anterior ciliary arteries.

Palpebral vessels serve two vascular arcades within the eyelid. The inferior (marginal) arcade sends branches through the tarsal plate to the eyelid margin and tarsal conjunctiva. The superior (palpebral) arcade supplies the tarsal, orbital, fornix and bulbar conjunctiva. The limbal zone, in contrast, is served by anterior ciliary arteries. The anterior ciliary arteries travel along the tendons of the rectus muscles and give off branches at episcleral level prior to dipping down into the sclera to link with the major iridic circle. Episcleral branches pass forward and loop back a few millimetres short of the cornea to become conjunctival vessels. Forward extensions of these vessels form the limbal arcades (limbal loops), which are a complex network of fine capillaries (Figure 2.28). Conjunctival veins are more numerous than arteries. They can be readily differentiated from arteries due to their larger calibre, darker colour and more tortuous path.

Functional considerations

The conjunctiva contributes the mucin component of the preocular tear film and plays an important role in the defence of the ocular surface against microbial infection. Mucins are a family of high-molecular-weight glycoproteins which include membrane-bound and secretory varieties (Corfield *et al.*, 1997; Gipson and Inatomi, 1997). Goblet cells are the primary source of secretory mucin whilst surface epithelial cells of both the conjunctiva and cornea possess mucin-like molecules within their glycocalyx. The conjunctiva also forms part of a common mucosal defence system which is an important component of the defence of the human body against microorganisms (McClellan, 1997). The conjunctiva possesses the immunological capacity for antigen processing, and cell-mediated and humoral immunity. Humoral immunity is provided by specific antibody (particularly immunoglobulin A (IgA)) produced by transformed B cells (plasma cells) in the stroma. T lymphocytes form the basis of cell-mediated immunity.

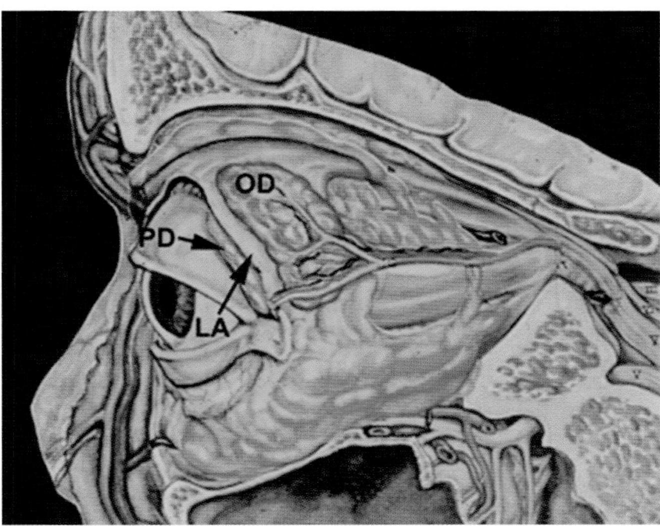

Figure 2.29 Lateral view of the orbit showing the position of the lacrimal gland. The levator aponeurosis (LA) partially divides the gland into an orbital (OD) and palpebral (PD) division. (Adapted from Kronfeld P., The Human Eye in Anatomical Transparencies. Bausch and Lomb Press, 1943.)

Lacrimal system

The lacrimal apparatus provides for the production and maintenance of the preocular tear film. The normal function of this system is essential for the integrity of the ocular surface and the provision of a smooth refractive surface. The lacrimal apparatus comprises a secretory system which includes the main and accessory lacrimal glands, and a drainage system which consists of the paired puncta and canaliculi, the lacrimal sac and the nasolacrimal duct.

Lacrimal gland

Gross anatomy

The main lacrimal gland is the key provider of the aqueous component of the tears. The gland is located in a shallow depression of the frontal bone behind the superolateral orbital rim (Figure 2.29). It is partially split by the aponeurosis of the levator palpebrae into an upper larger orbital lobe and a lower palpebral lobe, which can often be visualized through the conjunctiva upon lid eversion (Bron, 1986). The gland is pinkish in colour with a lobulated surface. Between 6 and 12 ducts leave the gland through the palpebral lobe and discharge into the conjunctival sac at the upper lateral fornix.

Microscopic anatomy

The lacrimal gland is tubuloacinar in form (Figure 2.30). Its secretory units (acini) contain secretory cells surrounded by myoepithelial cells (Ruskell, 1975). Acinar secretory cells show extensive folding of their plasma membrane and apical microvilli. Adjacent cells are linked by tight junctions which restrict diffusion between cells. The most prominent feature of these cells is the presence of abundant secretory

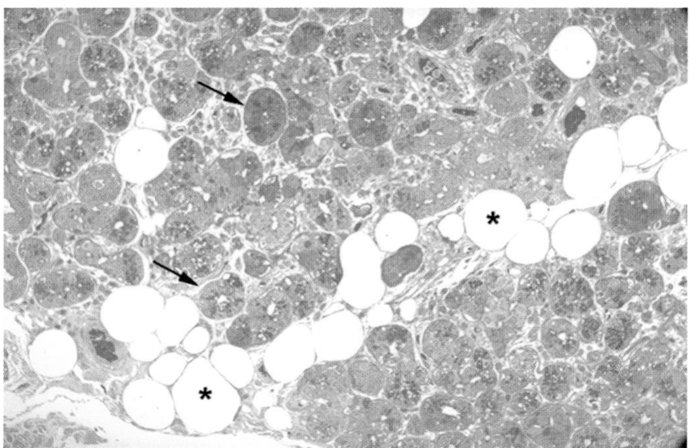

Figure 2.30 Low-power light micrograph of the lacrimal gland. Acini are arrowed. Adipose connective tissue (asterisks) extends across the gland.

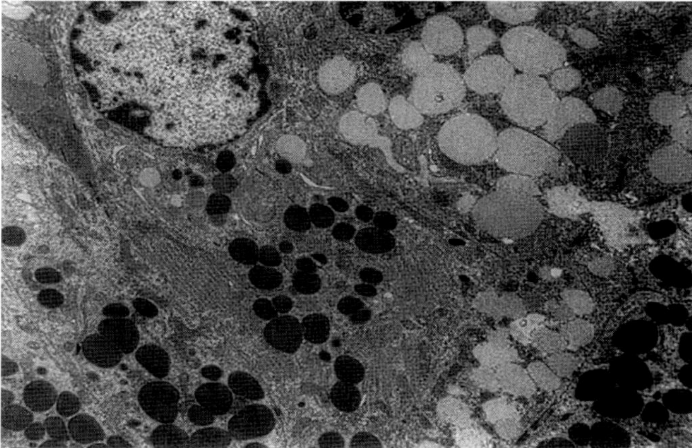

Figure 2.31 Electron micrograph of part of a lacrimal acinus showing light and dark secretory cells.

granules. Two principal secretory cell subtypes have been identified on the basis of their granule content (Figure 2.31). The majority of cells contain dark granules (dark cells), with a smaller number of cells containing light granules (light cells). The functional significance of this heterogeneity is uncertain at present. Ducts consist of a single layer of cuboidal cells which lack secretory granules. Myoepithelial cells are dendritic cells which are closely associated with the perimeter of acini and ducts. It is likely that these contractile cells play a role in the expulsion of tears from the gland. The interstices of the gland contain numerous blood vessels and nerves. A large population of immune cells (particularly IgA-secreting plasma cells) are also found between acini.

Blood and nerve supply

The arterial supply to the lacrimal gland is provided by the lacrimal artery which enters the posterior border of the gland. Venous drainage occurs via the lacrimal vein. A rich autonomic innervation includes secretomotor (parasympathetic) fibres which issue from the pterygopalatine ganglion and sympathetic (vasomotor) fibres from the carotid plexus. The lacrimal nerve traverses the gland to provide a sensory innervation to conjunctiva and lateral aspect of the eyelid.

Accessory lacrimal glands

Numerous small accessory lacrimal glands, which include the eponymous glands of Wolfring and Krause, are found within the conjunctival stroma. They have a particular predilection for the upper fornix and above the tarsal plate, and, on the basis of proportion of total lacrimal tissue, it has been estimated that they contribute 5–10% of aqueous tear volume. Structurally, they have a similar appearance to the lacrimal gland proper. However, true acini are absent and glands consist of elongated tubules which connect with ducts which open on to the conjunctival surface (Seifert *et al.*, 1993).

Functional considerations

In addition to its role as the principal provider of the aqueous phase of the tear film, the lacrimal gland is also a major component of the ocular sensory immune system, which acts as the first line of defence against microbial infection (Sullivan and Sato, 1994). The secretory immune system is mediated through secretory IgA. The lacrimal gland is the main source of tear IgA and the gland contains a large number of IgA-producing plasma cells. The mechanism by which an antigenic challenge of the ocular surface induces a lacrimal antibody response is not fully understood. However, since the administration of an antigen by a gastrointestinal route raises specific IgA levels in tears, one suggested mechanism is that ocular antigens - after drainage through the nasolacrimal duct - stimulate B cells in gut Peyer's patches. These sensitized B cells then populate the lacrimal gland where they transform into plasma cells (Figure 2.32).

Recent work has demonstrated that the lacrimal gland also secretes into the tears growth factors which are important for the maintenance of the ocular surface and epithelial wound healing (Pflugfelder, 1998). Prominent amongst these growth factors are epidermal growth factor and transforming growth factor-beta.

Lacrimal drainage system

Tears collect at the medial canthal angle where they drain into the puncta of the upper and lower lids. Each punctum is a small oval opening approximately 0.3 mm in diameter which is located at the summit of an elevated papilla. From each punctum the canaliculus passes first vertically for about 2 mm and then turns sharply to run medially for about 8 mm (Figure 2.33). At the angle, a slight dilation, the ampulla, can be seen. The canaliculi converge towards the lacrimal sac, usually forming a common canaliculus before entry. The lacrimal sac occupies a fossa formed by the maxillary and lacrimal bones. It measures 1.5–2.5 mm in diameter and approximately 12–15 mm in vertical length. From the lacrimal sac tears drain into the nasolacrimal duct, which extends for about 15 mm, passing through a bony canal in the maxillary bone, to an opening in the nose beneath the inferior nasal turbinate. A fold of mucosa is often observed at the termination of the duct: this has been termed the valve of Hasner, although there is no strong evidence that it functions as a valve.

The process of tear drainage is an active process mediated by the contraction of the orbicularis during blinking (Doane, 1981). Tears enter the canaliculi principally by capillary action. During the early part of the blink the puncta are

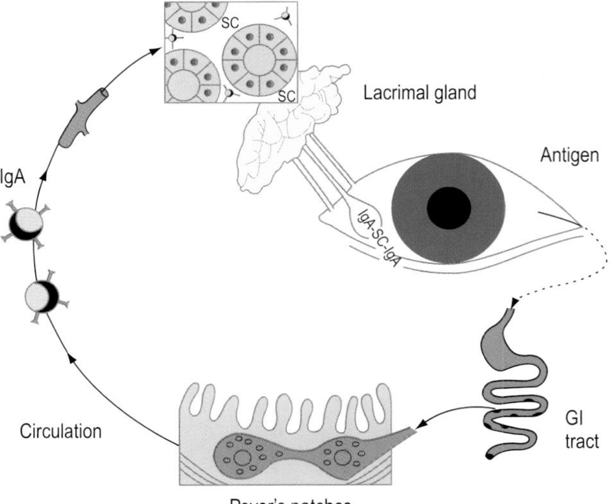

Figure 2.32 Diagram showing the role of the gastrointestinal tract generating specific immunoglobulin A (IgA) in the lacrimal gland. Antigens which challenge the ocular surface ultimately drain to the gastrointestinal (GI) tract where they stimulate B cells in Peyer's patches (gut-associated lymphoid tissue). Sensitized B cells then pass to the lacrimal gland via the circulation. SC= secretory component. (Adapted from Allansmith, M. R. (1992) The Eye and Immunology. Mosby. Copyright Elsevier 2002.)

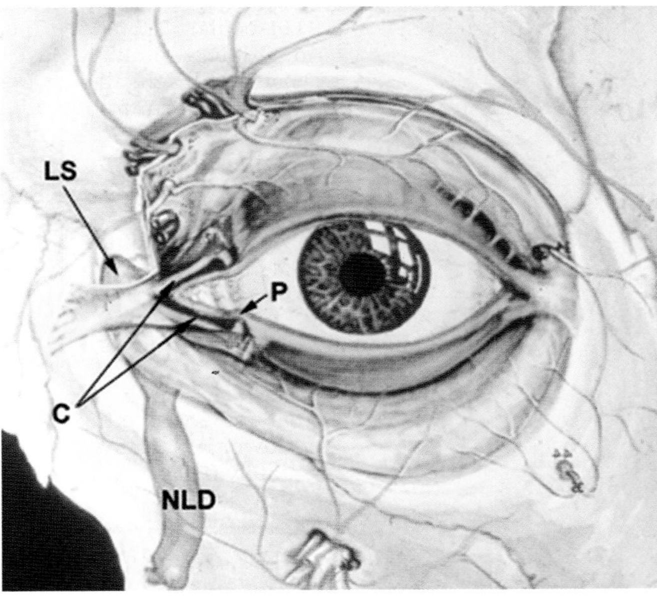

Figure 2.33 Illustration of the lacrimal drainage system. C = canaliculi; LS = lacrimal sac; P = punctum; NLD= nasolacrimal duct. (Adapted from Kronfeld P., (1943) The Human Eye in Anatomical Transparencies. Bausch and Lomb Press.)

occluded as the orbicularis further contracts. The canaliculi and lacrimal sac are also compressed, forcing fluid into the nose. An alternative hypothesis has been proposed, whereby orbicularis contraction dilates the sac, creating a negative pressure which draws in the tears from the canaliculi (Jones, 1961). An investigation by Paulsen *et al.* (2000) described a vascular plexus embedded in the wall of the lacrimal sac and duct which may influence tear outflow. It is postulated that opening and closing of the lumen of the lacrimal passages can be achieved by regulating blood flow within this plexus.

Table 2.2 Physical properties of the preocular tear film

Parameter	Value
Osmolarity	302 (±6.3) mmOsm/Kg smol/l
pH	7.45
Volume	7.0 (±0.2) μl
Rate of production	
Unstimulated	1–2 μl/min
Stimulated	>100 μl/min
Refractive index	1.336

The preocular tear film

Function and properties of the preocular tear film

The tear film is a complex fluid which covers the exposed parts of the ocular surface framed by the eyelid margins. The physical characteristics of this fluid are summarized in Table 2.2. Classically, the tear film has been regarded as a trilaminar structure, with a superficial lipid layer, secreted by the meibomian glands, which overlies an aqueous phase, derived from the main and accessory lacrimal glands, and an inner mucinous layer produced mainly by conjunctival goblet cells. The tear film performs several important functions, which can be broadly classified as optical, metabolic support, protective and lubrication.

By smoothing out irregularities of the corneal epithelium the tear film creates an even surface of good optical quality which is reformed with each blink. The air–tear interface forms the principal refractive surface of the optical system of the eye and provides two-thirds (43 D) of its total refractive power. Since the cornea is avascular it is dependent on the tear film for its oxygen provision. When the eye is open the tear film is in a state of equilibrium with the oxygen in the atmosphere, and gaseous exchange takes place across the tear interface. The constant turnover of the tear film also provides a mechanism for the removal of metabolic waste products.

Tears play a major role in the defence of the eye against microbial colonization. The washing action of the tear fluid reduces the likelihood of microbial adhesion to the ocular surface. Moreover, the tears contain a host of protective antimicrobial proteins. The tear film acts as a lubricant, smoothing the passage of the lids over the corneal surface and preventing the transmission of damaging shearing forces. To facilitate this, tear fluid displays non-Newtonian behaviour with respect to shear (Tiffany, 1991). Newtonian fluids maintain a constant viscosity with increasing shear rates. By contrast, tear fluid has a relatively high viscosity between blinks to aid stability, and with increasing shear rates, during the blink process, the viscosity falls dramatically, thereby easing the movement of the lids over the ocular surface.

Tear production

Jones (1966) first used the terms 'basic (basal)' and 'reflex' to describe tear flow. He proposed that the accessory lacrimal glands were the basic (minimal flow) secretors, and that reflex secretion (i.e. in response to strong physical or emotional stimulation) is mediated by the main lacrimal gland. However, Jordan and Baum (1980) questioned the concept of basic and reflex secretion, and suggested that it is more accurate to think of tear output as a continuum, whereby the rate of production is proportional to the degree of sensory or emotive stimulation. This concept would also mean that a functional distinction between main and accessory lacrimal glands, in terms of basal and reflex tear production, is unnecessary. Rather, it is more likely that tear flow is the combination of contributions from both glands, although the output from the accessory glands alone is sufficient to maintain a stable tear layer (Maitchouk *et al.*, 2000).

Sources and composition

Tears are a complex secretion which combine the products of several glands (Figure 2.34). Although the precise composition of tear fluid varies with collection method, flow rate and time of day, it can be considered as a watery secretion containing electrolytes and proteins, with lesser amounts of lipid and mucin.

Electrolytes

Human tears contain approximately the same range of electrolytes found in plasma (Tiffany, 1997). Table 2.3 gives typical values for the ionic composition of human tears. However, since the electrolyte content of tears varies with flow rate, there is significant variation in measured values. During the process of secretion by the lacrimal gland, there is a process of active electrolyte transport which is coupled to the passive movement of water by an osmotic process. Acinar-derived fluid is essentially an isotonic ultrafiltrate of plasma. Its composition is altered as it passes along the ductal system where further chloride and potassium ions are secreted. A variety of ion transport proteins have been identified in acinar cells, including sodium–potassium ATPase and potassium and chloride channels.

Proteins

Tear proteins are thought to originate from three main sources – the lacrimal gland, ocular surface epithelia and conjunctival blood vessels. The major lacrimal proteins include secretory IgA, lysozyme, lactoferrin and lipocalin (formerly known as tear-specific prealbumin) (Table 2.3). IgA, which is the major immunoglobulin in tears, is secreted as a dimer by plasma cells in the interstices between lacrimal acini. It then binds to a receptor on the basolateral aspect of acinar cells, and is transcytosed across the cell and secreted into tear fluid. IgA is a constitutively secreted lacrimal protein whose rate of secretion is independent of flow rate. During sleep, the levels of IgA increase as secretory IgA production continues and as acinar secretion declines (Sack *et al.*, 1992). IgA plays an important role in the defence of the ocular surface against microbial infection by preventing bacterial and viral adhesion, and inactivating bacterial toxins. Other immunoglobulins (e.g. IgG and IgM) are present in tears at much lower levels.

Lysozyme, lactoferrin and lipocalin, by contrast, originate from acinar cells and their rate of secretion roughly matches flow rate. Lysozyme is a well-known bacteriolytic protein which has the ability to lyse the cell wall of several Gram-positive bacteria. Lactoferrin serves an important bacteriostatic function by binding iron and making it unavailable for bacterial metabolism. It also acts as a free radical scavenger, thereby reducing free radical-mediated cell damage (Tiffany, 1997). Lipocalins are a family of lipid-binding proteins with an affinity for a broad array of lipids, including fatty acids, phospholipids and cholesterol. It has been suggested that tear lipocalins act as scavengers for a wide range of meibomian lipids, which could spill on to the corneal surface and perturb its wettability (Glasgow *et al.*, 2000). Furthermore, lipocalin may promote lipid solubility at the aqueous–lipid interface to facilitate the formation of a thin layer of lipid on the surface of the tear film.

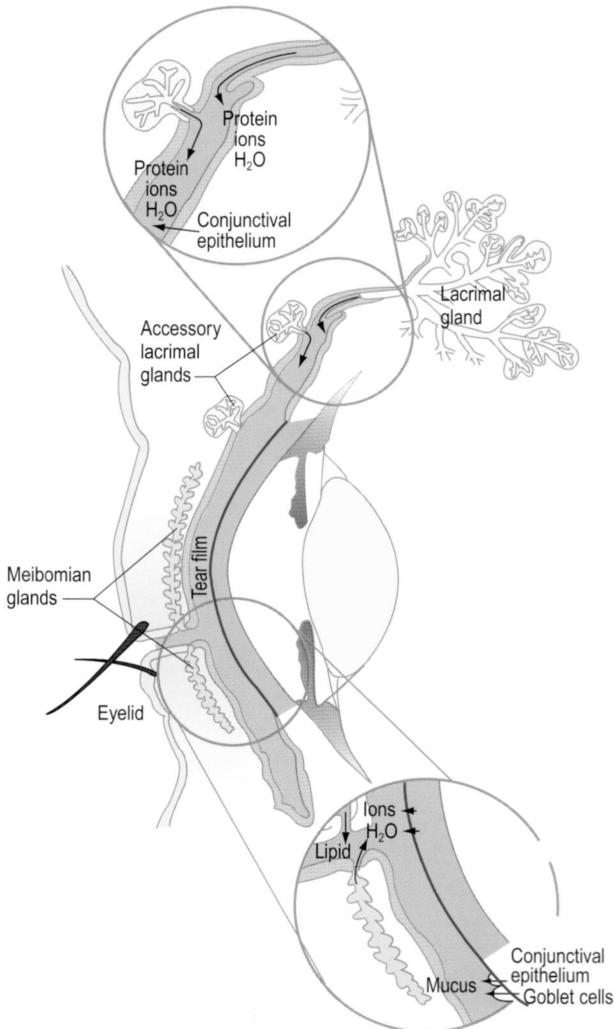

Figure 2.34 Schematic representation of the orbital glands which contribute the various components of the preocular tear film. (Adapted from Dart, D. A. (1992) Physiology of tear production In The Dry Eye: A Comprehensive Guide. (M. A. Lemp and R. Marquardt, eds.) Springer-Verlag.)

Mucins

Mucins are a family of high-molecular-weight glycoproteins, of which sugars contribute up to 85% of their dry weight. Structurally, they consist of a polypeptide backbone to which chains of sugar molecules attach via O-linkages to the amino acids serine and threonine. Mucins are a

Table 2.3 Biochemical composition of the preocular tear film

Component	Concentration
Electrolytes*	
Na^+	135 mEq/l
Cl^-	131 mEq/l
K^+	36 mEq/l
HCO_3^-	26 mEq/l
Ca^{2+}	0.46 mEq/l
Mg^{2+}	0.36 mEq/l
Major proteins*	
Lysozyme	2.07 g/l
Secretory IgA	3.69 g/l
Lactoferrin	1.65 g/l
Lipocalin	1.55 g/l
Albumin	0.04 g/l
IgG	0.004 g/l
Lipids†	
Wax esters	32.3% (dry weight)
Sterol esters	27.3%
Polar lipids	14.8%
Hydrocarbons	7.5%
Diesters	7.7%
Triacylglycerides	3.7%
Fatty acids	2.0%
Free sterols	1.6%
Mucin‡	
MUC1	nd
MUC5AC	nd
MUC4	nd
MUC16	nd

(Data from Tiffany, 1997)
Sources:
*Main and accessory lacrimal glands.
†Meibomian glands.
‡Epithelial cells/goblet cells.
nd = not determined.

heterogeneous group of molecules which can be subdivided into secretory and integrated-membrane varieties (Corfield *et al.*, 1997). So far, modern molecular biology techniques have identified eighteen mucin (MUC) genes, although only four of these (MUC1, MUC5AC, MUC4 and MUC16) are expressed on the human ocular surface (Gipson and Inatomi, 1997; McKenzie *et al.*, 2000; Pflugfelder *et al.*, 2000 , Mantelli and Argüesco 2008). The epithelia of the cornea and conjunctiva express the transmembrane mucins MUC1, and to a lesser extent MUC4 and MUC16, which attach to apical microvilli where they form a hydrophilic base to facilitate the spreading of the goblet cell-derived mucin MUC5AC. Mucins play a major role in stabilizing and spreading the tear film and provide protection against desiccation and microbial invasion (Gipson and Inatomi, 1997).

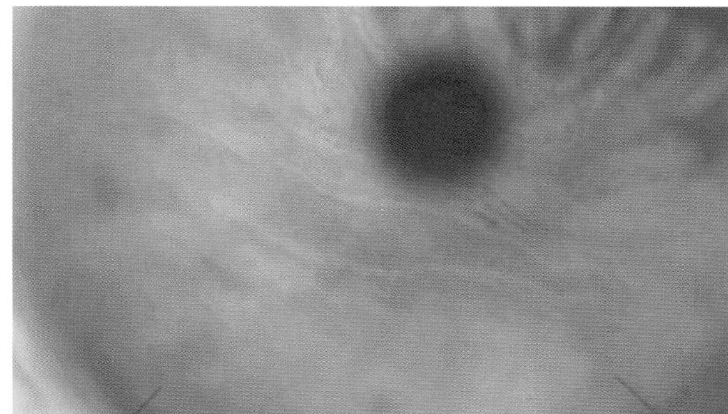

Figure 2.35 Lipid layer of the preocular tear film viewed in specular reflection. A 'wave' appearance can be seen which represents the most commonly observed lipid pattern in the population.

Lipids

The source of lipids in the tear film is the meibomian glands embedded within the tarsal plates of each lid. The blinking process is an important mechanism in the expulsion of the secretion from the glands (Tiffany, 1995). Lipid is delivered directly as a clear oil on to the lid margins and is spread over the tear film from the inner edge of the lid margins with each blink. The thickness of the lipid layer is variable (60–100 nm), and depending on thickness gives rise to characteristic interference patterns when viewed in specular reflection (Figure 2.35) (Guillon, 1998). Meibomian secretion consists of a complex mixture of lipids (Table 2.3), including wax esters, sterol esters, fatty acids and fatty alcohols (Tiffany, 1995). The primary functions of this secretion are to provide a hydrophobic barrier at the lid margin to prevent overspill of tears, and to cover the surface of the tear film to retard evaporation (Craig and Tomlinson, 1997).

Models of tear film structure

The classical trilaminar model of tear film structure in terms of a superficial lipid layer, a middle aqueous layer and deep mucin layer, first proposed by Wolff, and subsequently modified by Holly and Lemp (1977), has received broad acceptance. However, the results of recent studies have led to a re-evaluation of the nature of the aqueous and mucinous layers. Several pieces of evidence have suggested that the mucin contribution to the tear film is much greater than previously thought (Prydal *et al.*, 1992), and an alternative tear film model, which possesses a substantial mucinous phase, has been proposed (Figure 2.36). The nature of the mucinous phase has not been fully established but is thought to consist of a mixture of soluble and gel-forming mucins (Pflugfelder *et al.*, 2000). The greatest current uncertainty regards the thickness of the precorneal tear film. Published values, using several different techniques, lie in the range 3–40 μm. Invasive methods (e.g. using fine glass filaments) usually give rise to thickness estimates between 4 and 8 μm. However, the inherent disadvantage of such methods is that the invasive nature of the procedure may alter tear film thickness. By contrast, interferometry is a promising non-invasive method, that has estimated the thickness of the human tear film to be in the range 3–5 μm (King-Smith *et al.*, 2000).

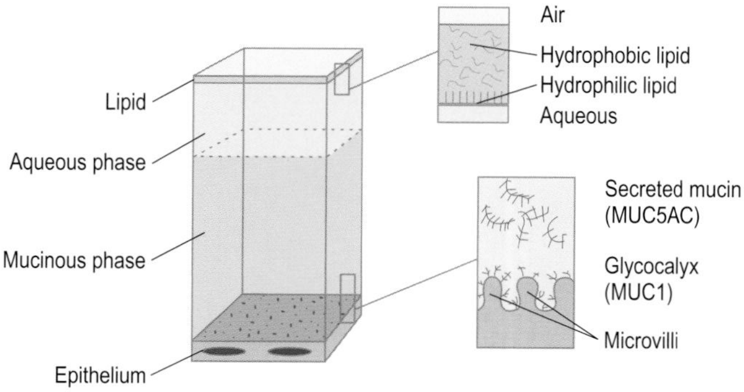

Figure 2.36 Diagram showing the composition of the preocular tear film. Insets show details of the glycocalyx and lipid–aqueous interface. (Adapted from Corfield, A. P., Carrington, S. D., Hicks, S. J. et al. (1997). Ocular mucins: purification, metabolism and functions. Prog. Ret. Eye Res., 16, 627–656.)

Conclusions

It is clear from the above account that our understanding of the structure and function of the anterior eye is far from complete. The consequence of uncertainties of such fundamental descriptors as the thickness of the precorneal tear film, and the factors that control tear film production, is that limits are placed on our understanding of clinical, contact lens-related phenomena. It is essential, therefore, that future research continues to focus on fundamental aspects of ocular anatomy and physiology, as well as the more applied clinical applications that are described in the remainder of this book.

References

Allansmith, M. R. (1992). *The Eye and Immunology*. St Louis, MO: Mosby.

Belmonte, C., Garcia-Hirschfeld, J. and Gallar, J. (1997). Neurobiology of ocular pain. *Prog. Ret. Eye Res.*, **16,** 117–156.

Berman, E. R. (1981). *Biochemistry of the Eye*. New York: Plenum Press.

Bron, A. J. (1986). Lacrimal streams: the demonstration of human lacrimal fluid secretion and the lacrimal ductules. *Br. J. Ophthalmol.*, **70,** 241–245.

Bron, A. J., Benjamin, L. and Snibson, G. R. (1991). Meibomian gland disease. Classification and grading of lid changes. *Eye*, **5,** 395–411.

Bron, A. J., Tripathi, R. C. and Tripathi, B. (1997). *Wolff's Anatomy of the Eye and Orbit*. 8th Edition. London: Chapman and Hall.

Corfield, A. P., Carrington, S. D., Hicks, S. J. *et al.* (1997). Ocular mucins: purification, metabolism and functions. *Prog. Ret. Eye Res.*, **16,** 627–656.

Craig, J. P. and Tomlinson, A. (1997). Importance of the lipid layer in human tear film stability and evaporation. *Optom. Vis. Sci.*, **74,** 8–13.

Dart, D. A. (1992). Physiology of tear production. In *The Dry Eye: A Comprehensive Guide*. (M. A. Lemp and R. Marquardt, eds), Berlin: Springer-Verlag.

Dilly, P. N. (1985). On the nature and the role of the sub-surface vesicles in the outer epithelial cells of the conjunctiva. *Br. J. Ophthalmol.*, **69,** 477–481.

Doane, M. G. (1981). Blinking and the mechanics of the lacrimal drainage system. *Ophthalmology*, **88,** 844–851.

Dua, H. S. and Azuara-Blanco, A. (2000). Limbal stem cells of the corneal epithelium. *Surv. Ophthalmol.*, **44,** 415–425.

Efron, N. (1997). Contact lenses and corneal physiology. *Biol. Sci. Rev.*, **9,** 29–31.

Efron, N. and Carney, L. G. (1979). Oxygen levels beneath the closed eyelid. *Invest. Ophthalmol. Vis. Sci.*, **18,** 93–95.

Efron, N., Perez-Gomez, I., Mutalib, H. A. *et al.* (2001). Confocal microscopy of the normal human cornea. *Cont. Lens Anterior Eye*, **24,** 16–24. Erratum in: *Cont. Lens Anterior Eye*, **24,** 83–85.

Ehlers, N. (1965). On the size of the conjunctival sac. *Acta Ophthalmol.*, **43,** 205–210.

Feng, Y. and Simpson, T. L. (2008). Corneal, limbal, and conjunctival epithelial thickness from optical coherence tomography. *Optom. Vis. Sci.*, **85,** 880–883.

Freeman, R. D. (1972). Oxygen consumption by the component layers of the cornea. *J. Physiol.*, **225,** 15–32.

Funderburgh, J. L. (2000). Keratan sulphate: structure, biosynthesis and function. *Glycobiology*, **10,** 951–958.

Funderburgh, J. L., Funderburgh, M. L., Mann, M. M. *et al.* (1991). Physical and biological properties of keratan sulphate proteoglycan. *Biochem. Soc. Trans.*, **19,** 871–876.

Gipson, I. K. and Inatomi, T. (1995). Extracellular matrix and growth factors in corneal wound healing. *Curr. Opin. Ophthalmol.*, **6,** 3–10.

Gipson, I. K. and Inatomi, T. (1997). Mucin genes expressed by the ocular surface epithelium. *Prog. Ret. Eye Res.*, **16,** 81–98.

Gipson, I. K., Spurr-Michaud, S. J. and Tisdale, A. S. (1987). Anchoring fibrils form a complex network in human and rabbit cornea. *Invest. Ophthalmol. Vis. Sci.*, **28,** 212–220.

Glasgow, B. J., Marshall, G., Gasymov, O. K. *et al.* (2000). Tear lipocalins: potential scavengers for the corneal surface. *Invest. Ophthalmol. Vis. Sci.*, **40,** 3100–3107.

Gray, H., Bannister, L. H., Berry, M. M. *et al.* (1995). *Gray's Anatomy: The Anatomical Basis of Medicine and Surgery*. 38th edn. New York: Churchill Livingstone.

Guillon, J. P. (1998). Non-invasive Tearscope Plus routine for contact lens fitting. *Contact Lens Ant. Eye*, **21,** S31–S40.

Hodson, S. A. (1997). Corneal stromal swelling. *Prog. Ret. Eye Res.*, **16,** 99–116.

Hodson, S. A. and Miller, F. (1976). The bicarbonate ion pump in the endothelium which regulates the hydration of the rabbit cornea. *J. Physiol.*, **263,** 563–577.

Hodson, S. A., Guggenheim, J., Kaila, D., *et al.* (1991). Anion pumps in ocular tissues. *Biochem. Soc. Trans.*, **19,** 849–852.

Hogan, M. J., Alvarado, J. A. and Weddell, J. E. (1971). *Histology of the Human Eye*. Philadelphia: Saunders.

Hollingsworth, J. Perez-Gomez, I., Mutalib, H. A. *et al.* (2001). A population study of the normal cornea using an in vivo, slit-scanning confocal microscope. *Optom. Vis. Sci.*, **78,** 706–711.

Holly, F. J. and Lemp, M. A. (1977). Tear physiology and dry eye. *Surv. Ophthalmol.*, **22,** 69–87.

Jones, L. T. (1961). An anatomical approach to problems of the eyelids and lacrimal apparatus. *Arch. Ophthalmol.*, **66,** 111–124.

Jones, L. T. (1966). The lacrimal tear system and its treatment. *Am. J. Ophthalmol.*, **62,** 47–60.

Jordan, A. and Baum, J. (1980). Basic tear flow: does it exist? *Ophthalmology*, **87,** 920–930.

Kessing, S. V. (1968). Mucus gland system of the conjunctiva: a quantitative normal anatomical study. *Acta Ophthalmol. (Suppl.)*, **95,** 1–333.

King-Smith, P. E., Fink, B. A., Fogt, N. *et al.* (2000). The thickness of the preocular tear film: evidence from reflection spectra. *Invest. Ophthalmol. Vis. Sci.,* **41,** 3348–3359.

Klyce, S. D. (1981). Stromal lactate accumulation can account for corneal oedema osmotically following epithelial hypoxia in the rabbit. *J. Physiol.,* **321,** 49–64.

Klyce, S. D. and Beuerman, R. W. (1998). Structure and function of the cornea. In *The Cornea.* (H. E. Kaufman, B. A. Barron and M. B. McDonald, eds.) 2nd ed., pp 3–50, Boston: Butterworth-Heinemann.

Klyce, S. D., Maeda, N. and Byrd, T. J. (1998). Corneal topography. In *The Cornea.* (H. E. Kaufman, B. A. Barron and M. B. McDonald, eds.) 2nd ed., pp 1055–1075. Boston: Butterworth-Heinemann.

Kronfeld, P. C., McHugh, S. L., Polyak, S. L. (1943) The Human Eye in Anatomical Transparencies. Rochester: Bausch and Lomb Press.

Lander, T., Wirtschafter, J. D. and McLoon, L. K. (1996). Orbicularis oculi muscle fibres are relatively short and heterogeneous in length. *Invest. Ophthalmol. Vis. Sci.,* **37,** 1732–1739.

Lawrenson, J. G. (1997). Corneal sensitivity in health and disease. *Ophthal. Physiol. Opt.,* **17,** S17–S22.

Lawrenson, J. G. and Ruskell, G. L. (1991). The structure of corpuscular nerve endings in the limbal conjunctiva of the human eye. *J. Anat.,* **177,** 75–84.

Lawrenson, J. G., Reid, A. R., and Allt, G. (1998). Corneal glycoconjugates: an ultrastructural lectin-gold study. *Histochem. J.,* **30,** 51–60.

Maitchouk, D. Y., Beuerman, R.W., Ohta, T. *et al.* (2000). Tear production after unilateral removal of the main lacrimal gland in squirrel monkeys. *Arch. Ophthalmol.,* **118,** 246–252.

Mantelli, F. and Argüesco, P. (2008). Functions of ocular surface mucins in health and disease. *Curr. Opin. Allergy Clin. Immunol.,* **8,** 477–483.

Marfurt, C. F. and Ellis, L. C. (1993). Immunohistochemical localisation of tyrosine hydroxylase in corneal nerves. *J. Comp. Neurol.,* **336,** 527–531.

Maurice, D. M. (1957). The structure and transparency of the cornea. *J. Physiol.,* **136,** 263–286.

Maurice, D. M. (1984). The cornea and sclera. In *The Eye. Vol. 1B.* (H. Davson ed.) 3rd ed., pp 1–158, Orlando: Academic Press.

McClellan, K. A. (1997). Mucosal defence of the outer eye. *Surv. Ophthalmol.,* **42,** 233–346.

McGill, J. I., Holgate, S. T., Church, M. K. *et al.* (1998). Allergic eye disease mechanisms. *Br. J. Ophthalmol.,* **82,** 1203–1214.

McKenzie, R. W., Jumblatt, J. E. and Jumblatt, M. M. (2000). Quantification of MUC2 and MUC5AC transcripts in the human conjunctiva. *Invest. Ophthalmol. Vis. Sci.,* **41,** 703–708.

Meek, K. M. and Leonard, D. W. (1993). Ultrastructure of the corneal stroma: a comparative study. *Biophys. J.,* **64,** 273–280.

Møller-Pederson, T. and Ehlers, N. (1995). A three-dimensional study of the human corneal keratocyte density. *Curr. Eye Res.,* **14,** 459–464.

Nishida, T. and Tanaka, T. (1996). Extracellular matrix and growth factors in corneal wound healing. *Curr. Opin. Ophthalmol.,* **7,** 2–11.

Oliveira-Soto, L. and Efron, N. (2001). Morphology of corneal nerves using confocal microscopy. *Cornea,* **20,** 374–384.

Paulsen, F. P., Thale, A. B., Hallmann, U. J. *et al.* (2000). The cavernous body of the human efferent tear ducts: function in tear outflow mechanism. *Invest. Ophthalmol. Vis. Sci.,* **41,** 965–970.

Pfister, R. R. (1973). The normal surface of the corneal epithelium: a scanning electron microscopic study. *Invest. Ophthalmol. Vis. Sci.,* **12,** 654–668.

Pflugfelder, S. C. (1998). Tear fluid influence on the ocular surface. *Adv. Exp. Med. Biol.,* **438,** 611–617.

Pflugfelder, S. C., Liu, Z., Monroy, D. *et al.* (2000). Detection of sialomucin complex (MUC4) in human ocular surface epithelium and tear fluid. *Invest. Ophthalmol. Vis. Sci.,* **41,** 1316–1326.

Prydal, J. J., Artal, P., Woon, H. and Campbell, F. W. (1992). Study of human preocular tear film thickness and structure using interferometry. *Invest. Ophthalmol. Vis. Sci.,* **33,** 2006–2011.

Prydal, J. J., Franc, F., Dilly, P. N. *et al.* (1998). Keratocyte density and size in conscious humans by digital image analysis of confocal images. *Eye,* **12,** 337–342.

Riley, M. V. (1969). Glucose and oxygen utilization by the rabbit cornea. *Exp. Eye Res.,* **8,** 193–200.

Ruskell, G. L. (1975). Nerve terminals and epithelial cell variety in the human lacrimal gland. *Cell Tiss. Res.,* **158,** 121–136.

Ruskell, G. L. and Lawrenson, J. G. (1994). Innervation of the anterior segment. In *Contact Lens Practice.* (M. Guillon and M. Ruben, eds), pp. 225–237, London: Chapman and Hall.

Sack, R. A., Tan, K. O. and Tan, A. (1992). Diurnal tear cycle: evidence for a nocturnal inflammatory constitutive tear fluid. *Invest. Ophthalmol. Vis. Sci.,* **33,** 626–640.

Scott, J. E. (1991). Proteoglycan: collagen interactions and corneal ultrastructure. *Biochem. Soc. Trans.,* **19,** 877–881.

Seifert, P., Spitznas, M., Koch, F. *et al.* (1993). The architecture of human accessory lacrimal glands. *Ger. J. Ophthalmol.,* **2,** 444–454.

Sherrard, E., Novakovic, P. and Speedwell, L. (1987). Age related changes of the corneal endothelium and stroma as seen in vivo with the specular microscope. *Eye,* **1,** 197–203.

Stiemke, M. M., Watsky, M. A., Kangas, T. A. *et al.* (1995). The establishment and maintenance of corneal transparency. *Prog. Ret. Eye Res.,* **14,** 109–140.

Sullivan, D. A. and Sato, E. H. (1994). Immunology of the lacrimal gland. In *Principles and Practice of Ophthalmology.* (D. M. Albert and F. A. Jakobiec, eds), pp. 479–486, Philadelphia: W.B. Saunders.

Sullivan, D. A., Sullivan, B. D., Ullman, M. D. *et al.* (2000). Androgen influence on the meibomian gland. *Invest. Ophthalmol. Vis. Sci.,* **41,** 3732–3742.

Tiffany, J. M. (1991). The viscosity of human tears. *Int. Ophthalmol. Clin.,* **15,** 371–376.

Tiffany, J. M. (1995). Physiological functions of the meibomian glands. *Prog. Ret. Eye Res.,* **14,** 47–74.

Tiffany, J. M. (1997). Tears and conjunctiva. In *Biochemistry of the Eye.* (J. J. Harding, ed), pp. 1–15, London: Chapman and Hall.

Tsubota, K. (1998). Tear dynamics and dry eye. *Prog. Ret. Eye. Res.,* **17,** 565–596.

Wilson S. E. (2000). Role of apoptosis in wound healing in the cornea. *Cornea,* **19,** S7–S12.

Wilson, S. E. and Hong, J. W. (2000). Bowman's layer structure and function. Critical or dispensable to corneal function? A hypothesis. *Cornea,* **19,** 417–420.

Wirtschafter, J. D., Ketcham, J. M., Weinstock, R. J. *et al.* (1999). Mucocutaneous junction as a major source of replacement palpebral conjunctival epithelial cells. *Invest. Ophthalmol. Vis. Sci.,* **40,** 3138–3146.

3 CHAPTER

Visual optics

W Neil Charman

Introduction

The human eye is a remarkable optical instrument. Its performance has been honed by millennia of evolution to meet admirably the needs of the neural system that it serves. At its best, few human-engineered photographic lens systems can match its semifield of more than 90°, its range of *f*-numbers from about *f*/11 to better than *f*/3, and its near diffraction-limited axial performance when stopped down under photopic light levels. Moreover, the focus of the eye of the young adult can be adjusted with reasonable accuracy for distances between about 0.1 m and infinity. Nevertheless, all eyes suffer from a variety of regular and irregular aberrations, while a substantial subset display clinically significant spherical and astigmatic refractive errors. In addition, the ability to change focus to view near objects is an asset that declines with age, to disappear entirely by the mid-50s, when presbyopia is reached.

The invention of spectacles in the 13th century, and their subsequent relatively slow refinement, followed by the more rapid development of contact lenses in the 20th century, has done much to provide solutions to the problems of both refractive error and presbyopia: improvements in the design of both types of lens continue to be made. Refractive surgical techniques, particularly laser-based methods, are beginning to compete with spectacle and contact lens corrections, although many unanswered questions still remain concerning the long-term efficacy and safety of the procedures used. In this chapter the basic optics of the eye and its components will first be reviewed. This will be followed by a discussion of the modifications that the correction of refractive error – particularly by contact lenses – produces in factors such as spectacle magnification, accommodation and convergence (Douthwaite, 2005).

The basic optics of the eye and ametropia

It is worthwhile briefly reviewing the basic optical configuration of emmetropic and ametropic eyes, and the characteristics of steady-state accommodation.

DOI: 10.1016/B978-0-7506-8869-7.00003-3

General optical characteristics

The familiar, and deceptively simple, optical layout of the eye is shown in Figure 3.1.

About three-quarters of the optical power comes from the anterior cornea, with the crystalline lens providing supplementary power that, in the pre-presbyope, can be varied to focus sharply objects at different distances. The actual optical design is, however, subtle, in that all the optical surfaces are aspheric, while the lens, and probably also the cornea, displays a complex gradient of refractive index. There is little doubt that such refinements play an important role in controlling aberration.

The distribution across the population of parameters such as surface radii, component spacing and refractive indices has been studied by a variety of authors (McBrien and Barnes, 1984; Charman, 1991a, 1995). Refractive indices of the media vary little between eyes, apart from the refractive index distribution across the lens, which changes with age as the lens grows throughout life (Pierscionek *et al.*, 1988; Pierscionek, 1995; Jones *et al.*, 2005). Each dimensional parameter appears to be approximately normally distributed amongst different individuals (Steiger, 1913; Stenstrom, 1946; Sorsby *et al.*, 1957). The values of the different parameters in the individual eye are, however, correlated so that the resultant distribution of refractive error is strongly peaked near emmetropia, rather than being normal (Figure 3.2).

This correlation is thought to be due to a combination of genetic and environmental factors, visual experience helping to 'emmetropize' the eyes actively (Troilo, 1992; Saunders, 1995; Wildsoet, 1997). Indeed, the apparently greater incidence of myopia in recent times has been attributed by some authors to the greater prevalence of near tasks biasing this active process towards myopia rather than emmetropia (Curtin, 1985; Rosenfield and Gilmartin, 1998).

Model eyes and ametropia

Many authors have produced paraxial models of the emmetropic eye, based on typical measured values of the ocular parameters (Rabbetts, 1998; Thibos and Bradley, 1999;

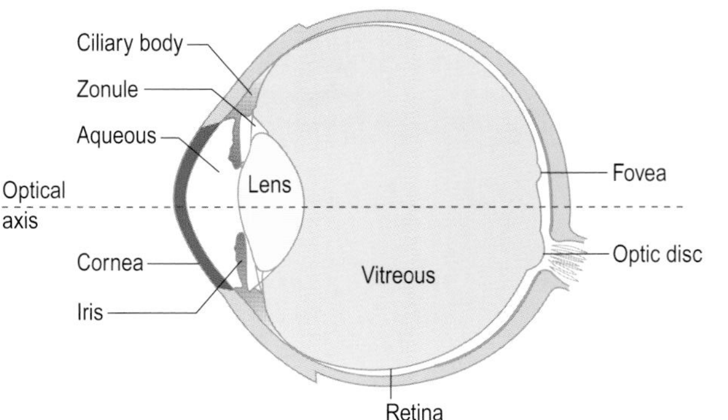

Figure 3.1 Schematic horizontal section of the human eye.

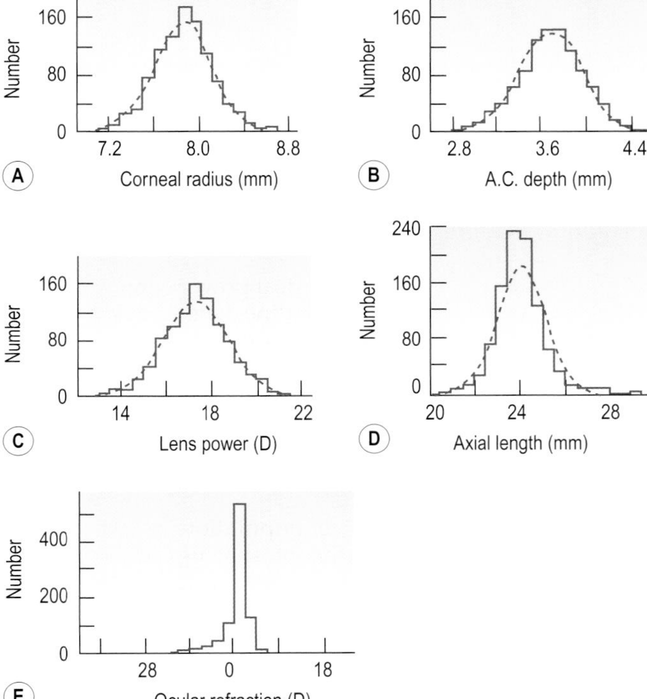

Figure 3.2 Distribution of some ocular parameters and of refractive error. (A) Radius of curvature of the anterior cornea. (B) Anterior chamber (A.C.) depth. (C) Lens power. (D) Axial length. (E) Spherical equivalent refractive error. In (A)–(D) the dashed curve represents the corresponding normal distribution. Note that, while individual parameters are distributed approximately normally, refractive errors are strongly peaked near emmetropia. (After Stenstrom, S. (1946) Untersuchungen uber der Variation und Kovaration der optische Elemente des menschlichen Auges. Acta Ophthalmol., 15(Suppl. 26), [Translated by Woolf, D.].)

Atchison and Smith, 2000). These simplify the optical complexities of the real eye while having approximately the same basic imaging characteristics. Some examples are given in Table 3.1; fuller details of these and other more elaborate eye models are given in the cited references.

Using the parameters of the model eyes it is straightforward to calculate the positions of the cardinal points, which, in thick lens theory, can be used to summarize paraxial imagery (Figure 3.3).

It is, however, important to stress that these eye models are only representative. In practice, an eye of shorter or longer axial length may still be emmetropic. This behaviour, and the various possible origins of refractive error, is easy to understand in terms of these basic models. Consider, for simplicity, the generic reduced eye shown in Figure 3.4, with a refractive surface of radius r, refractive index n' and axial length k'. The power of the eye, F_e, is given by:

$$F_e = (n' - 1)/r$$

For a distant object (zero object vergence) the image vergence n'/l' equals F_e. For emmetropia we require that the image of the distant object lies on the retina, i.e. $l' = k'$, implying that $F_e = n'/k' = K'$, where $K' = n'/k'$ is the dioptric length of the eye. There are, then, in principle an infinite number of matching pairs of values of F_e and K' that lead to emmetropia, so that eyes that are relatively larger or smaller than the 'standard' models may still be emmetropic.

In the case of ametropia F_e and K' are no longer equal. If the power of the eye is too high ($F_e > K'$) we get myopia; if too low ($F_e < K'$) we get hypermetropia. The ocular refraction K is given by:

$$K = K' - F_e$$

Thus, for example, myopia (K negative) can occur if K' is too low, corresponding to an axial length k' that is relatively too great (axial ametropia), or if F_e is relatively too large (refractive ametropia). A high F_e may arise as a result of either too small a corneal radius r or because n' is too large (note, however, that changes in n' affect both F_e and K'). Although more sophisticated eye models are characterized by more parameters, the possible origins of ametropia are essentially the same.

Astigmatism can arise either because one or more of the optical surfaces is toroidal or because of tilts of surfaces with respect to the axis, particularly of the lens.

How accurate do our models and associated calculations have to be? Although in the laboratory it may theoretically be possible to measure all the parameters of an individual eye, in general all that will be known in the consulting room is that the eye is ametropic. Thus, in clinical contact lens practice, precise calculation of the optical effects in the uncorrected or corrected eye is rarely possible: it is more important that the general magnitude of the effects be borne in mind and that the approximate changes brought about by correction be fully understood.

Accommodation and the precision of ocular focus

The decline in the subjective amplitude of accommodation (i.e. the reciprocal of the distance, measured in metres, of the nearest point at which vision remains subjectively clear to the distance-corrected patient) with age is illustrated in Figure 3.5A.

Few everyday tasks require accommodation in excess of about 4 D, so that it is normally only as individuals approach 40 years of age that marked problems with near vision start to appear. It is, however, important to recognize that, even for objects lying within the available range of accommodation, accommodation is rarely precise. 'Lags' of accommodation usually occur in near vision and 'leads' for distance vision (Figure 3.5B). Since the accommodation system is driven via the retinal cones, these lags increase if the environmental illumination is reduced to mesopic levels and

Table 3.1 Parameters of some paraxial models of the human eye. Dimensions are in millimetres (Adapted from Charman, W. N., 1991a Optics of the human eye. In Vision and Visual Dysfunction. Vol. 1: Visual Optics and Instrumentation (W. N. Charman, ed.), pp. 1–26, Macmillan.)

		Schematic eye	Simplified schematic eye	Reduced eye
Surface radii (mm)	Anterior cornea	7.80	7.80	5.55
	Posterior cornea	6.50	–	–
	Anterior lens	10.20	10.00	–
	Posterior lens	−6.00	−6.00	–
Distances from anterior cornea (mm)	Posterior cornea	0.55	–	–
	Anterior lens	3.60	3.60	–
	Posterior lens	7.60	7.20	–
	Retina	24.20	23.90	22.22
Refractive indices	Cornea	1.3771	–	–
	Aqueous humour	1.3374	1.333	1.333
	Lens	1.4200	1.416	–
	Vitreous humour	1.3360	1.333	–

(After Charman, 1991a)

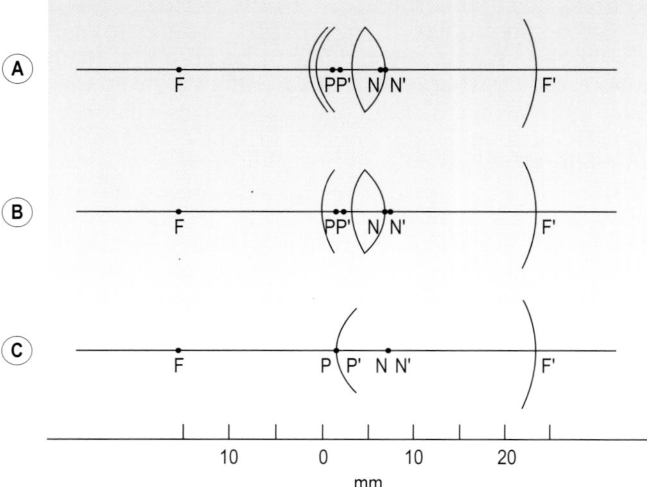

Figure 3.3 Examples of paraxial models of the human eye. In each case *F, F′* represent the first and second focal points, *P, P′* the first and second principal points and *N, N′* the first and second nodal points. (A) Unaccommodated schematic eye with four refracting surfaces. (B) Simplified, unaccommodated eye with three refracting surfaces. (C) Reduced eye with a single refracting surface. (Adapted from Charman, W. N. (1991a) Optics of the human eye. In Vision and Visual Dysfunction. Vol. 1: Visual Optics and Instrumentation (W. N. Charman, ed.), pp. 1–26, Macmillan.)

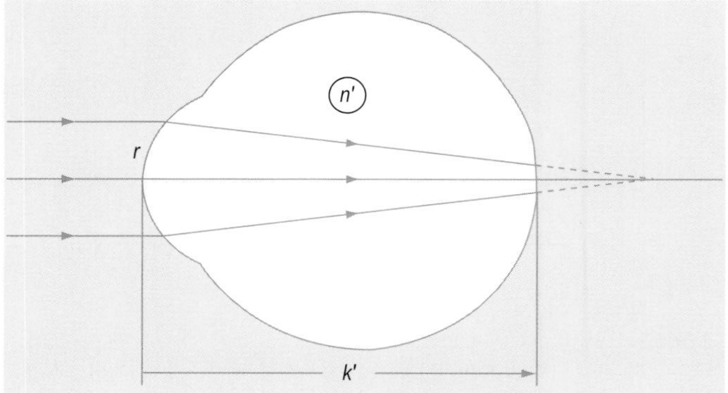

Figure 3.4 A generic reduced eye model, with parameters as indicated. *r* is the radius of curvature of the refracting surface, *k′* the axial length and *n′* the refractive index. The eye shown is hypermetropic.

the accommodation system is effectively inoperative at scotopic light levels, when the system reverts to its slightly myopic (around −1 D) tonic level (Ciuffreda, 1991, 1998).

Corneal topography

It has already been stated that the optical surfaces of the eye are not necessarily spherical. The topography of the anterior cornea is of particular interest since, as the dominant refractive surface, its form has a major influence on overall refractive error and ocular aberration. In contact lens work, it is of enormous importance to the fitting geometry.

We have already seen (Figure 3.2A) that the radius of curvature over the central region, as measured by conventional keratometers, shows considerable individual variation, and it has been recognized for more than a century that many corneas display marked astigmatism. Corneal astigmatism is not, of course, necessarily equal to the total ocular astigmatism, since additional astigmatism (residual astigmatism) may be contributed by the crystalline lens.

Earlier work on corneal topography using modifications of traditional keratometers concentrated on approximating the form of the corneal surface by a conicoid, in which each meridian is a conic section. In this approach the anterior corneal surface can be described by the following equation (Bennett, 1966, 1988):

$$x^2 + y^2 + pz^2 = 2r_0z$$

where the coordinate system has its origin at the corneal apex, z is the axial coordinate, r_0 is the radius of curvature at the cornea apex and the shape factor p is a constant

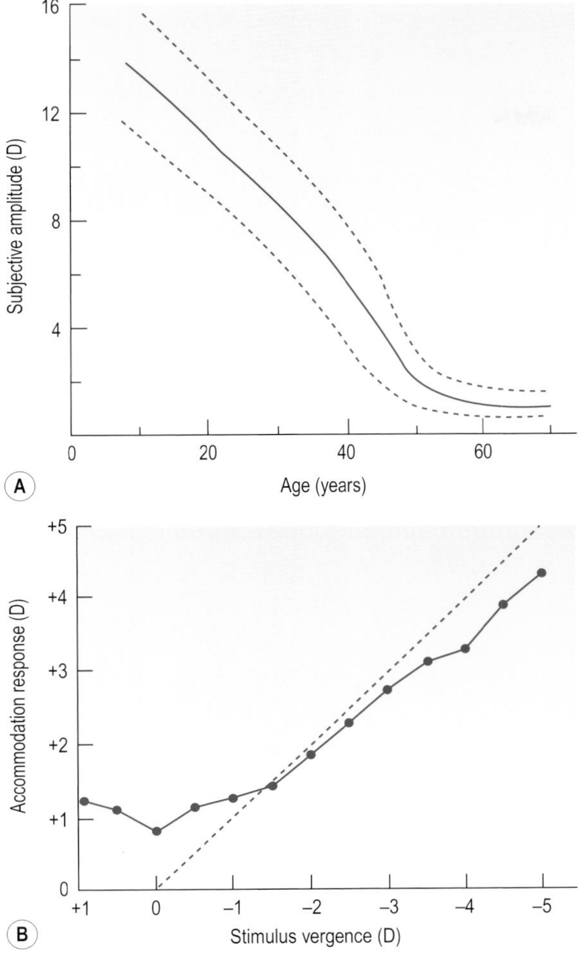

Figure 3.5 (A) The decline in monocular subjective amplitude of accommodation, referenced to the spectacle plane, with age. (After Duane, 1922.) (B) Typical steady-state accommodation response/stimulus curve, showing lags of accommodation for near stimuli.

parameter characterizing the form of the conic section for the individual eye. Values of $p < 0$ represent hyperboloids, $p = 0$ paraboloids, $0 < p < 1$ flattening (prolate) ellipsoids, $p = 1$ spheres and $p > 1$ steepening (oblate) ellipsoids. The same equation is sometimes written in terms of the Q-factor or the eccentricity e of the conic section, where:

$$p = 1 + Q = 1 - e^2$$

Kiely *et al.* (1982) found mean r_0 and p values of 7.72 ± 0.27 mm and 0.74 ± 0.18 respectively, these values being supported by the results of Guillon *et al.* (1986), that is, 7.85 ± 0.25 mm and 0.85 ± 0.15. Thus the typical general form of the cornea is that of a flattening ellipsoid, with the curvature reducing in the periphery. Evidently, however, not all corneas will have this form (Figure 3.6A).

Recent years have seen the introduction of a range of topographic instruments, marrying optical with electronic and computer technology, that can routinely give a much fuller picture of the corneal contour. These videokeratographic results show that the conicoidal model is only a first approximation to corneal shape and that individual eyes show a wide range of individual asymmetries. In particular, the rate of corneal flattening is often different in different meridians (Figure 3.6B), while the corneal cap of steepest curvature may be displaced with respect to the visual axis, on average lying about 0.8 mm below (Mandell *et al.*, 1995).

Currently the most popular form of output for the topographic data is probably a colour-coded map of the cornea, showing regions of different axial (sagittal) power (see Chapter 4). This may be slightly misleading, since each local area of the cornea is toroidal rather than spherical. For this reason both sagittal and tangential power maps are often used (Mountford *et al.*, 2004). It is possible that other forms of representation, such as those which plot local departures in height from a best-fitting sphere, will ultimately prove more useful, particularly in relation to the fitting of rigid contact lenses (Salmon and Horner, 1995; Horner *et al.*, 1998). The contribution of the cornea to the overall ocular wave aberration can be deduced from the videokeratogram (Hemenger *et al.*, 1995; Guirao and Artal, 2000).

Pupil diameter and retinal blur circles

As will be discussed below, although the retinal image is always blurred by both aberration and diffraction, in ametropia and presbyopia it is often defocus blur that is the major source of degradation. Defocus will occur whenever the object point lies outside the range of object distances embraced by the far and near points of the individual. As noted earlier, even within this range, small errors of focus will normally occur due to the steady-state errors that are characteristic of the accommodation system. Using a reduced eye model and simple geometric optical approximations (Smith, 1982, 1996; Rabbetts, 1998; Atchison and Smith, 2000) – which are normally valid for all errors of focus over about 1 D – such blur depends on the dioptric error of focus and the pupil diameter. From Figure 3.7 it can be seen that, for any object point and assuming that the eye pupil is circular, spherical defocus produces a 'blur circle' on the retina.

Using similar triangles, it is easy to show that the diameter (d, in mm) of this blur circle is:

$$d = \Delta F D / K'$$

where ΔF is the dioptric error of focus with respect to the object point, D is the pupil diameter in millimetres and K' is the dioptric length of the eye. If astigmatism is present, the blur patch is an ellipse, with major and minor axes corresponding to the focus errors in the two principal meridians.

We can express the blur circle diameter in angular terms as:

$$\alpha = \Delta F D\, 10^{-3} \text{ rads} = 3.44 \Delta F D \text{ min arc} \qquad \text{(Equation 3.1)}$$

Thus, for a 3 mm diameter pupil, the blur circle diameter increases by roughly 10 min arc per dioptre of defocus. Chan *et al.* (1985) measured blur circle diameters experimentally and found that results for pupil diameters between 2 and 6 mm and defocus between 1 and 12 D were quite accurately predicted by Equation 3.1.

The impact of blur on visual acuity depends somewhat on the acuity target chosen and the criteria and observation conditions used. We would expect the minimum angle of resolution (MAR) to be somewhat smaller than the blur circle diameter. Smith (1996) suggests that, for errors of focus above about 1 D, letter targets, a 50% recognition rate,

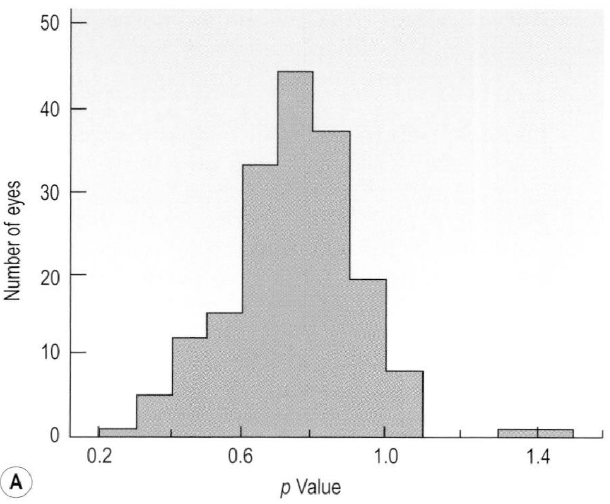

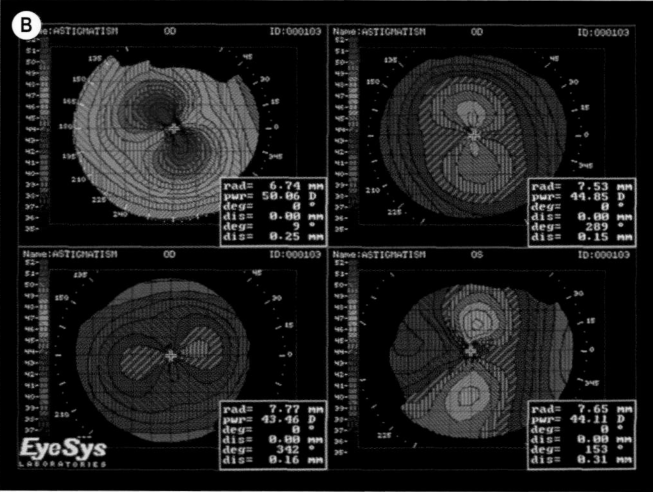

Figure 3.6 (A) Histogram showing the distribution of the shape factor, *p*, in 176 eyes. (B) Typical result from a topographic instrument, showing the local variation in nominal spherical power across four astigmatic corneas. (Adapted from Kiely, P. M., Smith, G. and Carney, L. G. (1982) The mean shape of the human cornea. Optica Acta, 29, 1027–1040.)

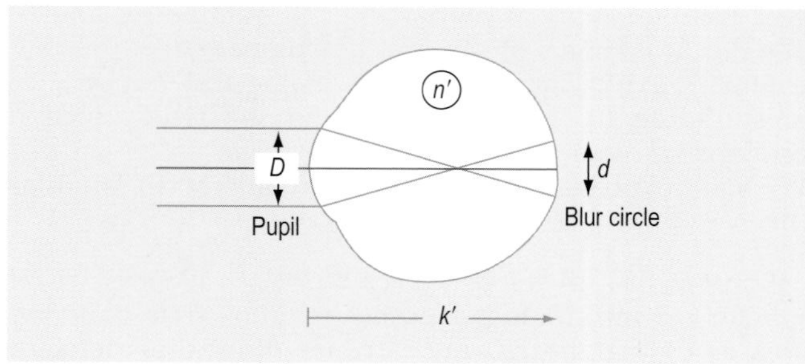

Figure 3.7 Formation of the retinal blur circle for a myopic eye.

and normal chart luminances of about 150 cd/m^2 (giving pupil diameters of about 4 mm):

$$\text{MAR} = 0.65\Delta FD \text{ min arc} \qquad \text{(Equation 3.2)}$$

With errors of focus smaller than about 1 D, diffraction, aberration and the neural capabilities of the visual system

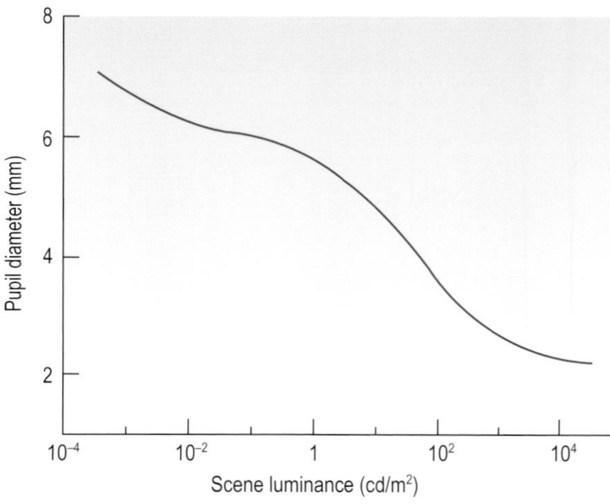

Figure 3.8 Dependence of pupil diameter on field luminance in young adults. (Adapted from Farrell, R. J. and Booth, J. M. (1984) Design Handbook for Imagery Interpretation Equipment, Sec. 3.2, p. 8, Boeing Aerospace Co.)

are more important than defocus blur and the MAR exceeds that predicted by Equation 3.2.

The natural pupil diameter is chiefly dependent on the ambient light level. Figure 3.8 shows typical results for this relationship in young adults.

Pupil diameters at any light level tend to decrease with age (senile miosis: Winn *et al.*, 1994) and with accommodation, as well as varying with a variety of emotional and other factors (Loewenfeld, 1998).

Clearly, reducing the pupil size results in smaller amounts of blur in the retinal image for any given level of defocus. Thus an uncorrected low myope may experience minimal levels of distance blur under good photopic levels of illumination but may notice considerable blur when driving at night, when the pupil is large.

Effects of diffraction and aberration

As noted above, these are chiefly important when the eye is close to its optimal focus. The point image for a spherical error of focus then no longer approximates to a blur circle (or a point in the absence of defocus) but has more complex form.

Diffraction

If the optical performance of the eye was limited only by diffraction, the in-focus retinal image of a point object would be an Airy diffraction pattern. The angular radius of the first dark ring in this pattern would be:

$$\theta_{min} = 1.22\,\lambda/D \text{ radians} = 4194\,\lambda/D \text{ min arc}$$

where the wavelength λ and the pupil diameter D are expressed in the same units. It is usually assumed that it will be possible to resolve the images of two identical point objects if their angular separation equals this value (the Rayleigh limit).

Monochromatic aberrations

Aberration obviously acts to introduce additional blur into both in- and out-of-focus images. Monochromatic aberration can arise from a variety of causes. The eye would be expected to display the classical Seidel aberrations (spherical aberration, coma, oblique astigmatism, field curvature and distortion) inherent in any system of spherical centred surfaces but, due to the various asphericities, tilts, decentrations and irregularities that may occur in its optical surfaces (Figure 3.6B), its aberrational behaviour is much more complex than that which would be expected on the basis of simple schematic eye models of the type illustrated in Figure 3.3 and Table 3.1.

Early authors attempted to analyse ocular aberration in terms of the individual Seidel aberrations. However, these attempts were of limited value because of the lack of rotational symmetry in the system. Monochromatic aberration is now most commonly expressed in terms of the wavefront aberration (Hopkins, 1950; Charman, 1991b). The behaviour of a 'perfect' optical system, according to geometrical optics, can either be visualized as involving rays radiating from an object point to be converged to a unique image point, or as spherical wavefronts diverging from the object point to converge at the image point, so that the object point is the centre of curvature of the object wavefronts and the image point that of the image wavefronts (Figure 3.9A).

The rays and wavefronts are everywhere perpendicular to one another. If we have aberration, the image rays fail to intersect at a single image point. Similarly, the wavefronts, which are still everywhere perpendicular to the rays, are no longer spherical (Figure 3.9B). It is usual to express the wavefront aberration at any point in the pupil as the distance between the ideal spherical wavefront, centred on the gaussian image point, and the actual wavefront, where both are selected to coincide at the centre of the exit pupil (Figure 3.9C).

Recent years have seen an explosion of interest in ocular aberrations, largely fuelled by the realization that the earlier excimer-laser refractive surgical techniques often resulted in poor vision because these procedures introduced high levels of aberration. As a result, a variety of commercial aberrometers have become available for measuring the wavefront aberration of the eye (Krueger *et al.*, 2004; Atchison, 2005). One of the more elegant designs involves the use of a Hartmann–Shack wavefront sensor (Liang *et al.*, 1994, 1997; Liang and Williams, 1997). A hexagonal array of identical microlenses allows the slope of the wavefront across a lattice of points in the pupil to be determined. The principle can be understood with reference to Figure 3.10.

Suppose we have a point source on the retina of a perfect emmetropic eye. The light leaving the eye can be envisaged either as a bundle of parallel rays or as a series of plane wavefronts (Figure 3.10A). We now place our array of microlenses in the path of the emerging light. Evidently each lens will converge the parallel rays to its second focal point, so that in the common focal plane we shall see an absolutely regular array of image points. If now the eye suffers from aberration, the emergent rays are no longer parallel and the associated wavefronts are no longer flat (Figure 3.10B). Thus the rays no longer come to a focus on the axes of the lenses: the lateral displacement from the focal point of each lens is directly proportional to the local inclination of the ray or the slope of the wavefront. It is, then, easy to calculate the form of the emergent wavefronts and the wavefront aberration from the distorted pattern of image points.

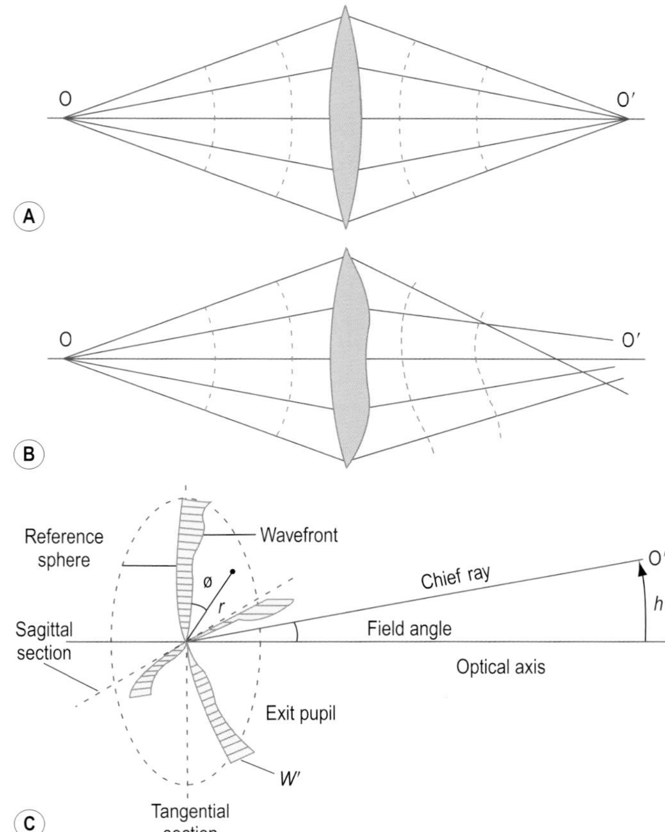

Figure 3.9 (A) With a perfect lens, rays from the object converge to a single image point. Alternatively we can visualize divergent spherical wavefronts (shown as dashed lines) from the object point converging as spherical wavefronts to the image point. (B) If the lens suffers from aberration, the imaging rays fail to converge to a single point and the corresponding wavefronts are not spherical. (C) The wavefront aberration, *W′*, is specified as the distance between the ideal wavefront, or reference sphere, centred on the gaussian image point, *O′*, and the actual wavefront in the exit pupil. It is usually adjusted to be zero at the centre of this pupil.

Examples of some typical results for normal eyes corrected for any spherocylindrical refractive error are shown in Figure 3.11. The wavefront error is usually expressed in microns.

Departures from the reference sphere (in this case of infinite radius) of more than a quarter of a wavelength (i.e. around 0.14 μm for the green region of the spectrum) would be expected to degrade image quality. What is striking is the wide variation between the aberrations shown by different eyes. The aberration in the central 2–3 mm of the pupil is usually modest but much larger amounts may be found in the periphery of dilated pupils. On the basis of wavefront aberration results, it is possible to calculate monochromatic point and line spread functions and also the ocular modulation and phase transfer functions for any pupil diameter (Hopkins, 1962).

Note that the wavefront maps shown in Figure 3.11 were obtained on axis with the eyes under cycloplegia. In each case ocular aberrations get worse nearer to the peripheral pupil, as with most optical systems. In practice, the

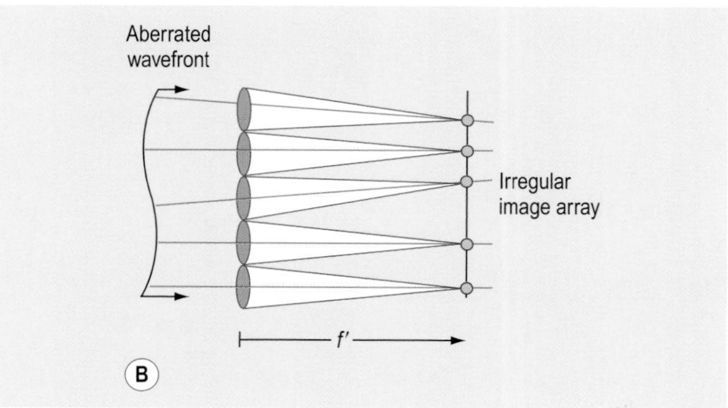

Figure 3.10 Principle of the Hartmann–Shack technique. (A) Effects with a perfect emmetropic eye, where the images are formed on the axis of each microlens and hence are regularly spaced. (B) Effects with an aberrated eye, where the image array is irregular since the images are no longer formed on the axes of the lenses (see text). f' is the focal length of the microlenses.

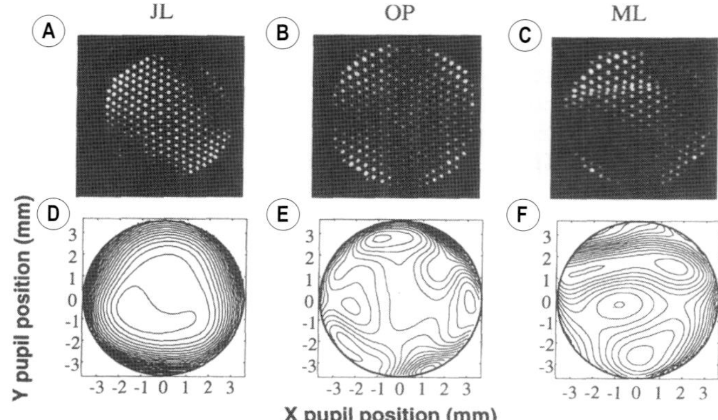

Figure 3.11 (A)–(C) Wavefront sensor images for three eyes with a pupil diameter of 7.3 mm. An aberration-free eye would give a regular hexagonal lattice of points. (D)–(F) Corresponding derived wavefront aberration. Contours are at 0.15 μm intervals for subject OP and at 0.3 μm intervals for subjects JL and ML. The peak-to-valley wavefront error for a 7.3 mm pupil is about 7, 4 and 5 μm for JL, OP and ML respectively. Note that for an aberration-free eye there would be a complete absence of contours. (Reproduced with permission from Liang, J. and Williams, D. R. (1997) Aberrations and retinal image quality of the human eye. J. Opt. Soc. Am. A., 14, 2873–2883.)

Table 3.2 Variation in the mean axial higher-order monochromatic root mean square (RMS) wavefront error and its standard deviation in the eyes of subjects aged 30–39 years. Also given is the typical ambient luminance level at which the natural pupil diameters occur (taken from Figure 3.8) and the equivalent defocus (see text)

Pupil diameter (mm)	Typical luminance level (cd/m²)	RMS wavefront error (μm)	Equivalent defocus (D)
3	400	0.052 ± 0.022	0.16
4	70	0.102 ± 0.041	0.18
5	7	0.174 ± 0.062	0.19
6	0.1	0.289 ± 0.091	0.22
7	0.0005	0.513 ± 0.138	0.29

(Based on Applegate *et al.*, 2007)

aberrations on the visual axis of each individual eye vary slightly with time due to factors such as accommodation fluctuations and tear layer changes after a blink (Hofer *et al.*, 2001; Cheng *et al.*, 2004; Montés-Micó *et al.*, 2004). There will also be variation in the measured wavefront errors due to the limited reliability of any aberrometer. It can be seen, for example, that in Figure 3.11 (A) to (C) the signal-to-noise of the Hartmann–Shack point images is poor in some cases: this may lead to errors in the estimates of the corresponding local slope and form of the wavefront.

Although the basic wavefront map gives a useful impression of the form and extent of the wavefront errors, it is helpful to be able to quantify this in some way. Various methods are available but those which are the most popular at the present time are the total root mean square (RMS) wavefront error and the values of the Zernike coefficients for the wavefront error.

The basic method for obtaining RMS wavefront error for any diameter of pupil is easily understood. We divide the pupil into equal small areas, and sum the squared values of the wavefront error for each small area. This sum is then divided by the number of areas and the square root of this result gives the RMS wavefront error. It can be shown that, if the RMS aberration is less than a 14th of a wavelength, i.e. about 0.04 μm, there is negligible loss in retinal image quality in comparison with an eye whose performance is limited only by diffraction. Obviously for any eye the RMS error will vary with pupil diameter: in general, since the wavefront aberration tends to increase in the outer zones of the dilated pupil, the RMS aberration increases with pupil diameter.

Applegate *et al.* (2007) have recently investigated axial RMS wavefront errors as a function of pupil diameter and age in a large sample of normal eyes which were corrected for spherical and cylindrical refractive error. Table 3.2 gives their mean data and their standard deviations for subjects aged 30–39 years.

It is interesting to note that the typical axial RMS wavefront error for a 3 mm pupil is close to the limit at which the image differs negligibly from that from an aberration-free system (about 0.04 μm). The luminance at which this pupil diameter is found, a few hundred cd/m^2, corresponds to that found on cloudy days in the UK. Thus in most eyes wavefront aberration can only play a minor role in vision under daylight conditions.

To give some clinical insight into the image degradation caused by these levels of RMS wavefront aberration, we can roughly evaluate the blurring effect of the RMS aberration by equating it with those of an 'equivalent defocus', that is, the spherical error in focus which produces the same magnitude of RMS aberration for the same pupil size. The equivalent defocus is given by:

$$\text{Equivalent defocus (D)} = 4.3^{1/2}[\text{RMS error}]/R^2$$

where the RMS aberration is measured in microns and the pupil diameter, R, in millimetres. Table 3.2 includes values for the equivalent defocus at each pupil diameter: except at the largest pupil diameter, the equivalent defocus is always less than 0.25 D. Although the assumption that equal RMS error produces equal degradation of vision is not completely justified (Applegate *et al.*, 2003), it is evident that, in normal eyes, the impact of optical blur due to monochromatic aberration is modest under most conditions. For comparison, the reliability of clinical refractive techniques is only around ±0.3 D (Bullimore *et al.*, 1998; O'Leary, 1988).

The second common way of specifying aberrations is in terms of Zernike coefficients (Atchison, 2004; Charman, 2005). The idea here is that, since very different forms of wavefront can have the same total RMS error yet still produce somewhat different effects on vision, it is better to break the complex wavefront patterns of the type shown in Figure 3.11 into a set of simpler 'building blocks'. Each 'block', mathematically described by a Zernike polynomial, corresponds to a specific type of wavefront deformation: some of these are closely related to the traditional Seidel aberrations. The set of polynomials, named after their originator Fritz Zernike (1888–1966), has the advantage that the individual polynomials are mathematically independent of one another. The overall complex wavefront can then be specified in terms of the size of the contributions made by each of these constituent wavefront deformations: the size of the contribution that each makes is given by the value of the coefficient of the corresponding polynomial. In the recommended formulation in current use, each coefficient gives the RMS wavefront error (in microns) contributed by the particular Zernike mode (Atchison, 2004; Charman, 2005): the overall RMS wavefront error is given by the square root of the sum of the squares of the individual coefficients. The relative sizes of the different Zernike coefficients thus give detailed information on the relative importance of the different aberrational defects of any particular eye.

The Zernike polynomials can be expressed in terms of polar coordinates (ρ, θ) in the pupil, where $\rho = R/R_{max}$ is the relative radial coordinate, R_{max} being the maximum pupil radius. θ is the azimuthal angle, defined in the same way as in the optometric notation, except that it can rise to 360°. Each polynomial, or wavefront building block, is defined by the highest power (n) to which ρ is raised (the radial order) and the multiple (m) for the angle θ (the angular frequency): $m = -2$, for example, means that θ appears as $\sin 2\theta$, while $m = +3$ means that it appears as $\cos 3\theta$. The polynomials and coefficients are, then, conveniently described as Z_n^m and C_n^m respectively. Figure 3.12 shows the first few levels of the 'Zernike tree' formed by the different polynomials, the levels corresponding to successively greater powers of n.

The top two rows of the tree ($n = 0$ and $n = 1$) are of no significance for image quality: piston ($n = 0$) just corresponds to a longitudinal shift of the wavefront and tilts ($n = 1$) to small prismatic shifts in the image point. The second-order terms ($n = 2$) all depend upon the square of the radius in the pupil. This is, of course, a familiar feature of the sag formula and in fact Z_2^0 represents spherical defocus and the other terms astigmatism in crossed-cylinder form, with the principal meridians either at 45/135 (Z_{-2}^{-2}) or 90/180 (Z_{-2}^{2}). Thus, collectively, the second-order terms correspond to our familiar spherocylindrical defocus and can be compensated for by an appropriate contact lens or other type of correction. The higher-order (third and greater) polynomials represent the residual aberrations which, in the past, it has not normally been possible to correct. Clinically these higher-order aberrations have often been described rather loosely by terms such as 'irregular astigmatism' and 'spherical aberration'. The third order includes vertical and horizontal primary coma and the fourth order primary spherical aberration.

What levels of Zernike aberrations are found on the visual axis in normal eyes? It must be remembered that, like the total RMS aberration, the values will tend to increase with pupil diameter but a variety of studies involving large numbers of subjects give very similar results (Salmon and van de Pol, 2006). The study by Applegate *et al.* (2007) generated mean values for the magnitudes of different types of third- and fourth-order Zernike aberration for different pupil sizes and age (coefficients for still higher-order Zernike modes are usually much smaller). Table 3.3 gives their values for 30–39-year-old eyes. Note that, where appropriate, the coefficients for similar, but differently oriented, Zernike polynomials have been combined.

It is evident that, at the smaller 3 mm pupil size, third-order coma and trefoil aberrations tend to dominate over fourth-order aberrations, including spherical aberration, although spherical aberration becomes comparable to coma for the larger 6 mm pupil.

A somewhat different picture emerges if we average the signed coefficients, rather than considering the RMS values. Figure 3.13 gives some typical data, in this case for a large sample (109) of normal eyes with a pupil diameter of 5.7 mm (Porter *et al.*, 2001). What is striking is that almost all the modes have a mean close to zero, although individual eyes may have substantial aberration, as shown by the relatively large standard deviations. A notable exception is the $j = 12$, Z_4^0 spherical aberration mode, where the mean is positive and differs significantly from zero. Thus, the picture that emerges is that most eyes have a central tendency to be free of all higher-order aberration, except for spherical aberration, which shows a significant bias towards slight positive (undercorrected) values. The Zernike coefficients of individual eyes vary randomly about these mean values in a way that presumably depends upon the idiosyncratic surface tilts, decentrations and other asymmetries of the individual eye.

Chromatic aberration

Since the refractive indices of all the ocular media vary with wavelength, the eye suffers from both longitudinal and transverse chromatic aberration. At the fovea, the former is more important – the amount of aberration approximating to that which would occur if the eye media were all water. Unlike the monochromatic aberrations, longitudinal chromatic aberration varies very little between individuals and equals about 2.5 D across the visible spectrum (Figure 3.14).

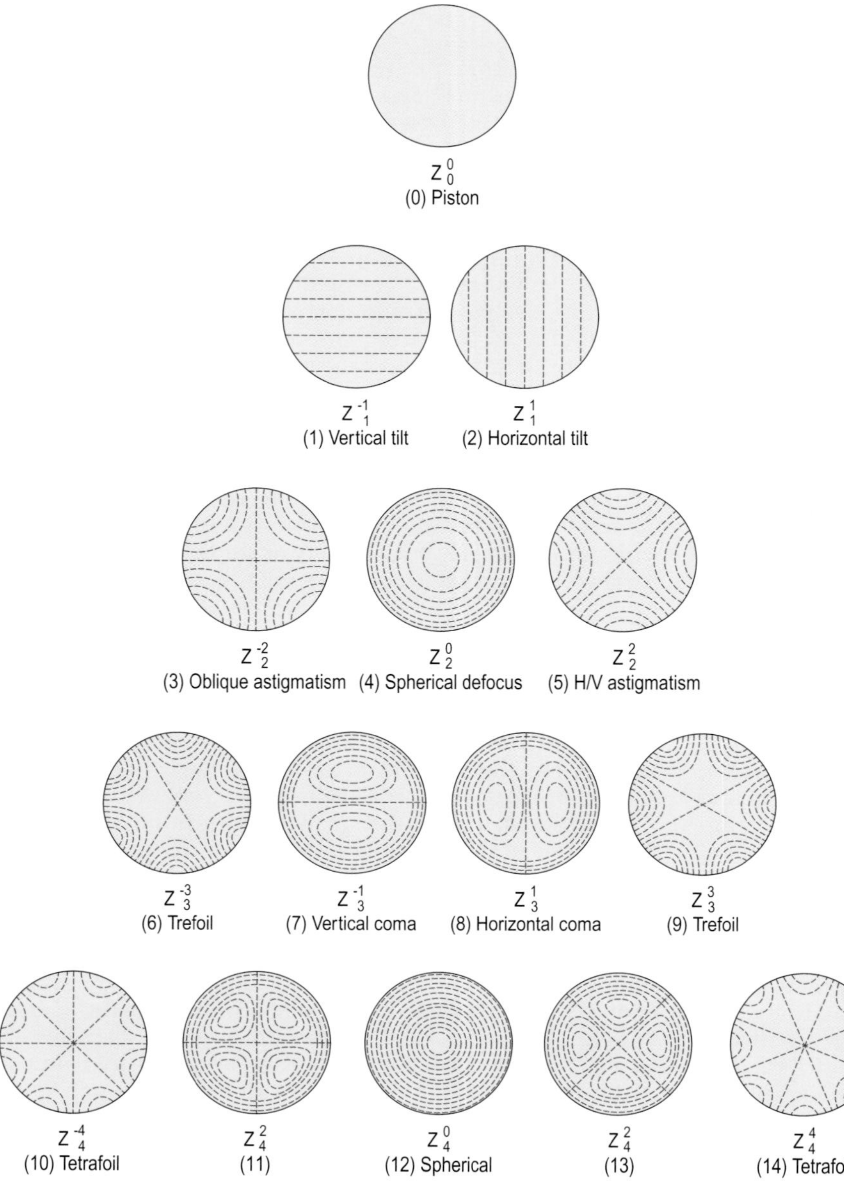

Figure 3.12 The first five levels of the Zernike 'pyramid' or 'tree' showing the contour maps corresponding to the first 15 Zernike polynomials (up to the fourth order). The contour scale is arbitrary and, in the individual eye, will vary with the coefficient of each polynomial. Rows represent successive orders, *n* (i.e. the maximal power to which the normalized pupil radius is raised) and columns different azimuthal frequencies, *m*. Also shown (in brackets) are the index numbers, *j*, of the polynomials and some of the names used to describe them: polynomials (11) and (13) are often called secondary astigmatism. H/V astigmatism = horizontal/vertical astigmatism.

Since the visual axis is usually displaced from the nominal optical axis of the eye by about 5°, some individually varying, transverse chromatic aberration is found at the fovea, typically amounting to about 0.8 min arc (Rynders *et al.*, 1995): this further degrades foveal image quality.

Overall optical performance of the eye in white light

Both monochromatic and chromatic aberration will degrade the in-focus retinal image in comparison with that which would be expected for an aberration-free eye with the same pupil size. Figure 3.15 illustrates this for the case of the image of a fine line, that is, the line spread function.

The experimental results are compared with the calculated profiles for the aberration-free case (Campbell and Gubisch, 1966). With small pupils, aberration has only minor effects but the performance deficit due to aberration steadily increases as the pupil diameter increases. It should, however, be borne in mind that under natural conditions large pupils are only found when field luminances are low and neural performance is poor. Thus diffraction-limited optical performance with large pupils would be of little value since the neural retina could not utilize the available information.

Ocular depth of focus

If the retinal image is gradually defocused, its quality will deteriorate due to defocus blur. Nevertheless, there is

Table 3.3 Mean absolute levels (root mean square (RMS) wavefront error (WFE)) of different types of higher-order Zernike aberration, and their standard deviations, for 30–39-year-old subjects and two pupil diameters

Aberration	Combination of coefficients	RMS WFE (μm) for 3 mm pupil diameter	RMS WFE (μm) for 6 mm pupil diameter
Trefoil (j = 6 and 9)	$\left[(C_3^{-3})^2+(C_3^{3})^2\right]^{1/2}$	0.027 ± 0.017	0.139 ± 0.089
Coma (j = 7 and 8)	$\left[(C_3^{-1})^2+(C_3^{1})^2\right]^{1/2}$	0.031 ± 0.022	0.136 ± 0.087
Tetrafoil (j = 10 and 14)	$\left[(C_4^{-4})^2+(C_4^{4})^2\right]^{1/2}$	0.010 ± 0.004	0.056 ± 0.030
Secondary astigmatism (j = 11 and 13)	$\left[(C_4^{-2})^2+(C_4^{2})^2\right]^{1/2}$	0.015 ± 0.008	0.055 ± 0.027
Spherical aberration	C_4^0	0.014 ± 0.010	0.130 ± 0.090
Total higher-order RMS (j = 12)	$\left[\Sigma(C_n^m)^2\right]^{1/2}$	0.052 ± 0.022	0.289 ± 0.091

(Based on Applegate *et al.*, 2007)

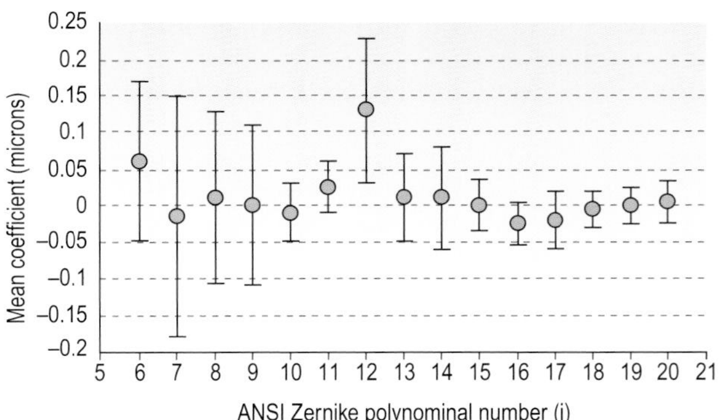

Figure 3.13 Typical data for the means of the signed values of the Zernike coefficients of eyes at a pupil diameter of 5.7 mm: among the higher-order coefficients only j = 12 (C_4^0), spherical aberration, has a value which differs significantly from zero. ANSI = American National Standards Institute. (Adapted from Porter J., Guirao, A., Cox, I. G. and Williams, D. R. (2001) The human eye's monochromatic aberrations in a large population. J. Opt. Soc. Am. A., 18, 1793–1803.)

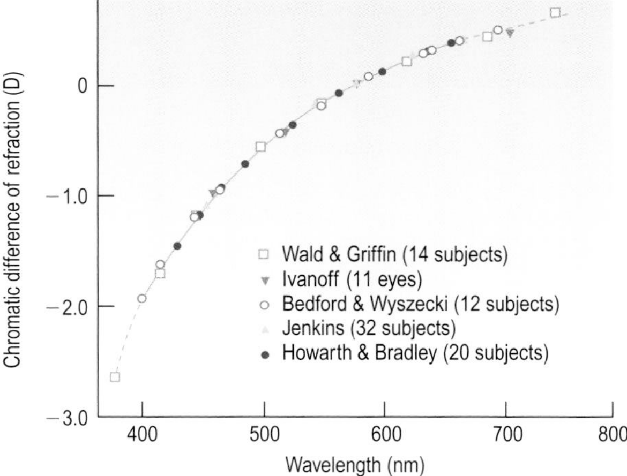

Figure 3.14 The longitudinal chromatic aberration of the eye as found by different investigators. (Adapted from Charman, W. N. (1991a) Optics of the human eye. In Vision and Visual Dysfunction. Vol. 1: Visual Optics and Instrumentation (W. N. Charman, ed.), pp. 1–26, Macmillan.)

a finite range of focus over which this blur causes no appreciable deterioration in visual performance. The precise value of the total depth of focus depends on how it is assessed but Figure 3.16 gives some representative photopic values from different studies. It can be seen that, for typical photopic pupils of about 4 mm diameter, visual performance will remain relatively unaffected provided that the spherical error of focus does not exceed about ±0.25 D.

Correction of higher-order ocular aberration

Conventional corrections are designed to compensate for the spherocylindrical errors of the eye. As noted earlier, in wavefront terms these corrrespond to second-order wavefront aberrations. Would it be possible to improve visual performance further by also correcting the higher-order aberrations of the eye, since we can now easily measure these under clinical conditions? Until recently, the irregular and individual nature of the monochromatic wavefront aberrations of the eye made it impossible to correct them fully, although some reduction could be achieved with appropriately aspheric contact lenses (see Chapters 7 and 14).

Longitudinal chromatic aberration can be corrected by a suitable achromatizing doublet lens, but the improvement in retinal image quality in white light is small and occurs mainly at intermediate spatial frequencies (Campbell and Gubisch, 1967): no improvement in conventional high-contrast, white-light visual acuity is normally detectable (Hartridge, 1947).

More recently, however, real progress has been made in correcting monochromatic aberration using either adaptive optics or liquid crystal phase plates (Liang *et al.*, 1997; Vargas-Martin *et al.*, 1998). While all these corrections are, at present, only feasible in the laboratory, they do show that marked improvements in spatial vision can be achieved over the uncorrected eye, particularly if both monochromatic and chromatic aberrations are corrected: if only monochromatic aberrations are corrected, perform-

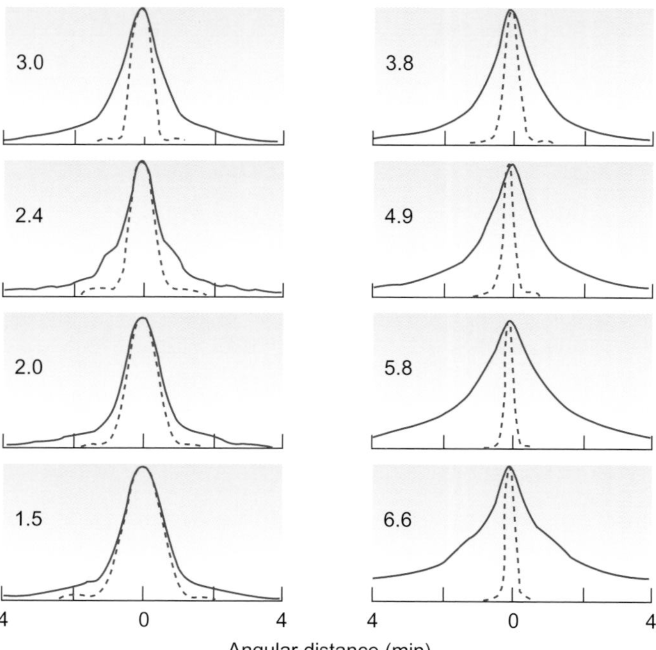

Figure 3.15 White-light optical line spread functions for eyes with different pupil diameters (mm) at optimal focus. The solid line curves give the experimental measurements, and the dashed curves the theoretical result for a diffraction-limited system. (Adapted from Campbell, F. W. and Gubisch, R. W. (1966) Optical quality of the eye. J. Physiol. (London), 186, 558–578.)

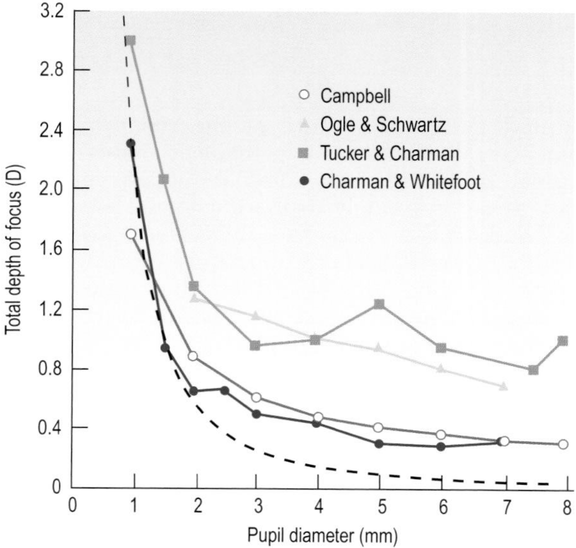

Figure 3.16 Examples of experimental measurements of photopic, total monocular depth of focus/field as a function of pupil diameter (optimal focus lies midway through the total depth of focus). (Adapted from Charman, W. N. (1991a) Optics of the human eye. In Vision and Visual Dysfunction. Vol. 1: Visual Optics and Instrumentation (W. N. Charman, ed.), pp. 1–26, Macmillan.)

ance in white light improves only modestly (Yoon and Williams, 2001).

Will it prove possible to correct ocular aberrations in everyday life? In theory, having measured the wave aberrations of the individual eye, the form of the cornea could be appropriately shaped, for example by a computer-controlled scanning spot excimer laser, to compensate for the aberrations. This has been the inspiration behind the development of many commercial aberrometers which, when coupled to suitably controlled excimer lasers, are used in wavefront-guided refractive surgery (Krueger *et al.*, 2004). In practice, rather than eliminating monochromatic aberrations, this approach has so far only been able to ensure that postsurgery aberrations are comparable to normal levels, partly because of our limited knowledge of regression effects associated with corneal healing.

Alternatively a tight-fitting, customized, contact lens with minimal transverse and rotational movement might be engineered to play the same role (Klein and Barsky, 1995; Klein, 1998; Schweigerling and Snyder, 1998). The lenses would lack rotational symmetry and would be customized so that their local optical thickness varied in such a way as to compensate for the wavefront aberration of the individual eye. To improve optical performance in eyes with normal levels of aberration, any lens decentration should be less than about 0.5 mm and any rotation less than 10° (Bara *et al.*, 2000; Guirao *et al.*, 2001). However, such approaches would only reduce the monochromatic aberrations, which, in any case, change with the level of accommodation (Ivanoff, 1956; Lopez-Gil *et al.*, 1998) and other factors (Charman and Chateau, 2003). The blur effects due to chromatic aberrations would remain uncorrected. Moreover, the worst monochromatic aberration occurs in the periphery of the dilated pupil, and pupil dilation only occurs when light levels are low and visual performance is largely limited by neural, rather than optical, factors. For these reasons correction of aberration only seems likely to be profitable in the case of individuals whose monochromatic aberration is particularly high. This problem is discussed further in Chapters 7 and 14.

Effectivity, spectacle magnification, accommodation and convergence effects with contact lens and spectacle corrections

Many patients may wish to change from a spectacle to a contact lens correction, and vice versa. Although the corrections may be equally effective in producing in-focus retinal images in both eyes, they do have a number of slightly different secondary effects, most of which are associated with the fact that, whereas contact lenses are placed directly on the cornea, spectacle lenses are placed at a significant distance, typically 10–20 mm, in front of this surface. Corrections achieved by corneal ablation using excimer lasers, such as photorefractive keratectomy (PRK), laser *in situ* keratomileusis (LASIK) or other corneal surgical procedures, such as radial keratotomy or intrastromal rings, produce broadly similar effects to contact lenses, although their effective optical zones are usually smaller.

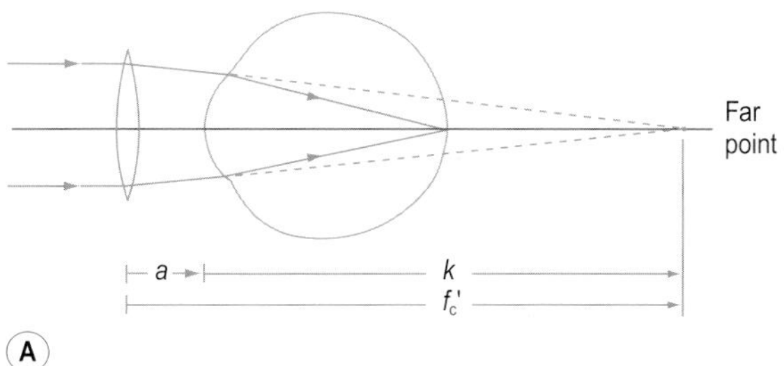

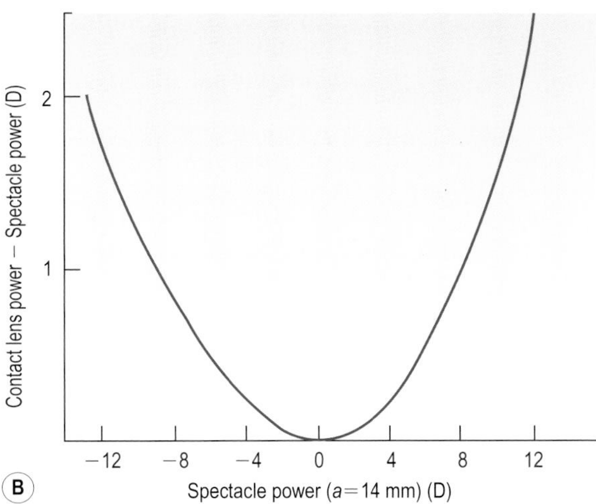

Figure 3.17 (A) Geometry relating the far point of an ametropic eye (hypermetropic in the case shown) and the correcting lens. (B) Difference between the required powers of contact lens and spectacle corrections, as a function of the spectacle correction, assuming that the vertex distance of the spectacle lens is 14 mm.

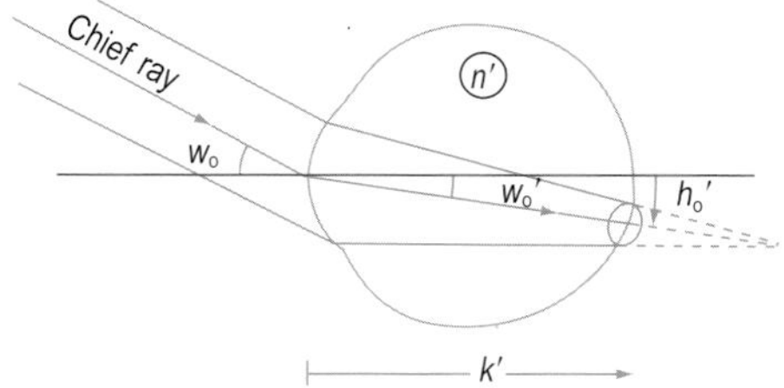

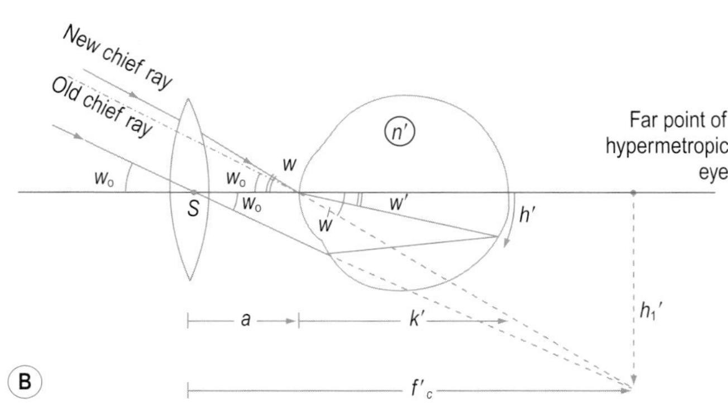

Figure 3.18 (A) Ray geometry in the case of an uncorrected hypermetrope. (B) Effect of a correcting spectacle lens. Note that the angle that the incident chief ray makes with the axis is increased from w_0 without correction to w with correction. Correspondingly, the angle of the chief ray with the axis after refraction is increased from w_0' to w' after correction.

Effectivity

The role of the distance correction is to produce an intermediate image at the far point of the particular eye. Due to the non-zero vertex distance of any spectacle correction, this far point will lie at slightly different distances from the two types of correcting lens. Thus the spectacle and contact lens powers required to correct a particular eye will differ.

From Figure 3.17A we can see that, using a reduced eye model, if the vertex distance is a (taken as positive) and the ocular refraction is K, giving a far point distance from the cornea $k = 1/K$, the second focal point of the correcting lens lies at a distance $a + k$.

Thus the power of the correcting lens (F_c) is:

$$F_c = 1/(a+k) = 1/(a+1/K) = K/(1+aK)$$

For a contact lens, a will be zero so that the required value of F_c equals the ocular refraction in this simple model. This does not apply with a spectacle lens. The result is that a hypermetrope will require a higher-powered contact lens than a spectacle lens, the reverse occurring for a myope. The difference between the two correcting powers is plotted as a function of the spectacle correction for a vertex distance of 14 mm in Figure 3.17B, from which it can be seen that the difference between the required powers of correction only becomes significant (i.e. greater than 0.25 D) when the magnitude of the ocular refraction exceeds about ±4 D. Appendix C provides a tabulation of ocular refraction values based on spectacle lens refractions for various vertex distances.

Spectacle magnification

Spectacle magnification, as its name implies, describes the ratio of the image size in the corrected ametropic eye to that in the uncorrected eye. It is particularly significant in cases of anisometropia, where after correction the differential magnification of the two retinal images may give rise to symptoms of aniseikonia, and with cylindrical errors, where the different magnifications in the two principal meridians caused by the correction may lead the patient to complain of distorted images.

The retinal images of any object in the eyes of an uncorrected ametrope have a scale that is governed by the chief rays passing from the extremities of the object through the centres of the entrance and exit pupils of the eye. Each image point will, of course, be blurred (Figure 3.18A).

Although placing a contact lens on the cornea does not affect the course of the chief ray, and hence does not alter the size of the retinal image, this is not the case with a spectacle lens. A positive correction increases the angle that the chief ray makes with respect to the axis, whereas a negative correction reduces it.

Figure 3.18B illustrates this effect for a positive, thin lens correction and a reduced eye with both entrance and exit pupils at the cornea. We define the spectacle magnification, SM, as the retinal image height in the corrected eye, h', divided by that in the uncorrected eye, h_0'. From the diagram it can be seen that, if all angles are assumed to be small:

$$SM = h'/h_0' = w'k'/w_0'k' = w'/w_0' = (w/n')/(w_0/n') = w/w_0$$

Since the role of the correcting lens is to form an image of height h_1' at the far point, we thus have (Figure 3.18B):

$$SM = \left[h_1'/(f_c' - a)\right]/\left[h_1'/f_c'\right] = 1/[1 - aF_c]$$

In this simple model, the spectacle magnification will be unity for contact lenses (vertex distance $a = 0$), less than unity for negative, myopic spectacle corrections and greater than one for positive corrections. Somewhat perversely, spectacle correction is often expressed as the percentage by which it differs from unity, so that a spectacle magnification of 1.05× would be described as '5% magnification'.

In practice we cannot strictly treat corrections as thin lenses and the entrance and exit pupils do not lie at the cornea. For practical purposes the pupils may be taken as being situated about 3 mm behind the cornea. Using a thick-lens extension of the arguments already used, it can then be shown that:

$$SM = [(1 - bF'_v)(1 - (t/n)F_1)]^{-1} \approx (1 + bF_v')(1 + (t/n)F_1)$$

where b is the vertex distance measured from the back surface lens to the entrance pupil, and t, n, F_1 and F'_v are the lens thickness, refractive index, anterior surface power and back vertex power, respectively. It can be seen that the magnification is a function of both lens design and vertex distance. Figure 3.19 shows typical values of spectacle magnification for both contact lens and spectacle corrections.

Note particularly that spectacle magnification is always close to unity for contact lenses, so that there are likely to be few magnification-related complaints from patients when moving directly from no correction to a contact lens correction or from one contact lens correction to another.

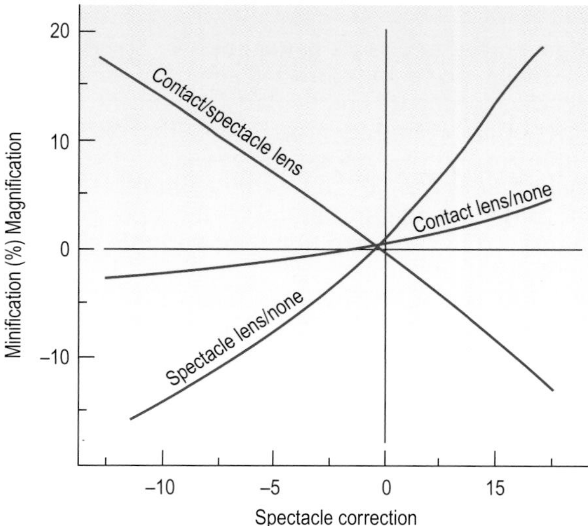

Figure 3.19 Typical values for spectacle magnification obtained with spectacle lens and contact lens corrections. The ratio of the two spectacle magnifications is also shown. Effectivity has been allowed for, so that points on any vertical line refer to the same ametropia. (Adapted from Westheimer, G. (1962) The visual world of the new contact lens wearer. J. Am. Optom. Assoc., 34, 135–138.)

Casual contact lens wearers who normally wear spectacle corrections may theoretically notice spatial distortion, although for myopes this is counterbalanced by the benefit of relatively larger retinal images, which may improve acuity. Spectacle magnification effects after corneal refractive surgery are similar to those with contact lenses (Applegate and Howland, 1993).

In addition to spectacle magnification as defined above, relative spectacle magnification (RSM) is sometimes discussed. This is the ratio of the retinal image size in the corrected ametropic eye to that in a specified emmetropic schematic eye. Theoretically it has the advantage of putting retinal image size on an absolute basis. However, in most clinical work it is the changes described by spectacle magnification that are of interest and RSM is of limited practical use.

When anisometropes are corrected by spectacle lenses, marked differences in spectacle magnification may occur between the two eyes, which may result in symptoms of aniseikonia. It is obvious that these are much reduced in the case of contact lenses, which therefore minimize the possibility of aniseikonic symptoms (Winn *et al.*, 1986). A closely related effect occurs when the anisometrope looks in different directions with the head in a fixed position. When ordinary spectacles are worn and the visual axes do not pass through the optical centres, prismatic effects are introduced, of magnitude given by Prentice's rule $P = cF_c$, where P is the induced prism power in prism dioptres, c the decentration in centimetres and F_c the lens power in dioptres. If the corrections are the same for both eyes, these prismatic effects cause no problems for the spectacle wearer. In anisometropia, however, the prismatic effects will be different for each eye. For example, in reading, the visual axes of a young anisometrope would normally intercept the lenses of the distance correction at some distance below the optical centres. Assuming this distance to be 8 mm and the corrections to be right eye (RE) −3.00 D, left eye (LE) −6.00 D, the prismatic effects would be RE −2.4 Δ and LE 4.8 Δ, both base-down. The difference in vertical prism power exceeds normal fusional abilities, so that, to avoid the problem, the spectacle-corrected anisometrope would have to execute head turns during reading rather than simply depress the visual axes. This problem is absent with well-centred contact lenses.

Accommodation demand

Just as the position of the correcting lens affects the correcting power required and the spectacle magnification, so it also influences the accommodation required to view a near object. The accommodation necessary with any particular correction can easily be calculated for any given object distance, lens position and correcting power by determining the difference between the vergence of the light striking the cornea when viewing a near object and that for a distant object. However, an adequate approximation for most purposes is that the accommodation demand (A, in dioptres) is given by:

$$A \approx -L(1 + 2aK)$$

where L is the object vergence (negative for real objects), a is the vertex distance and K is the ocular refraction. In this approximation, a is zero for a contact lens, so that we can see that for a myope (negative K) the accommodation

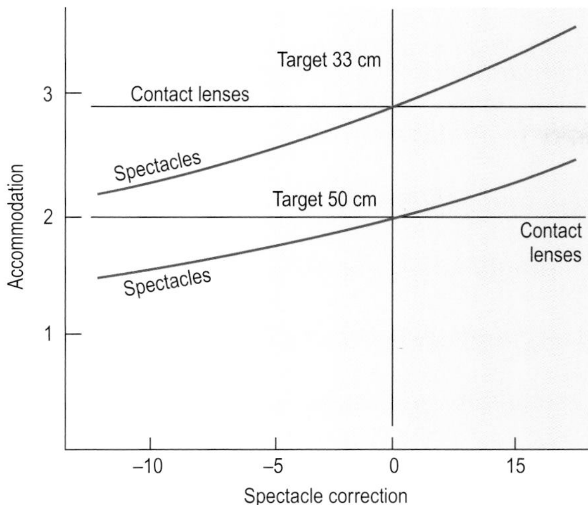

Figure 3.20 Ocular accommodation required when a patient with the spectacle ametropia given on the abscissa views targets at either 0.50 or 0.33 m (vergence, $L = -2$ or -3 D) when corrected with either spectacles ($a = 14$ mm) or contact lenses. (Adapted from Westheimer, G. (1962) The visual world of the new contact lens wearer. J. Am. Optom. Assoc., 34, 135–138.)

demand is higher with contact lenses than with spectacle lenses, whereas the reverse is true for hypermetropes. If we consider an object at 33 cm ($L = -3$ D) and a spectacle vertex distance $a = 14$ mm, we find that the difference in demand with the two types of correction becomes significant (>0.25 D) when the magnitude of the refractive error, K, is larger than about 3 D. Thus, higher myopes approaching presbyopia might slightly delay the need for a reading addition by wearing spectacles, whereas hypermetropes would find near vision easier with a contact lens correction.

Figure 3.20 shows results from a slightly more refined model for the accommodation demand at two object distances.

Convergence demand

Contact lenses move with the eyes, hence convergence demands when viewing near objects are identical to those applying in the uncorrected state. In contrast, myopes with a negative spectacle correction for distance observe near objects through base-in prisms, since they are no longer looking through the optical centres of their lenses (Figure 3.21).

The base-in prismatic effects reduce the convergence requirement, as compared to the naked eye or contact lens situation. Spectacle-corrected hypermetropes, however, experience a base-out effect at near, which increases the convergence demand. Allowing for a typical interpupillary distance of 65 mm and the centre of rotation of each eye being about 12 mm behind the cornea, application of Prentice's rule shows that, for an object distance of 33 cm, the convergence demand for each eye is reduced by about $0.25F_c$ prism dioptres for a negative spectacle correction and similarly increased for a positive correction. In most cases, then, the change in convergence demand is small as compared with the fusion reserves. Since both accommodation and convergence demands are higher for myopes with

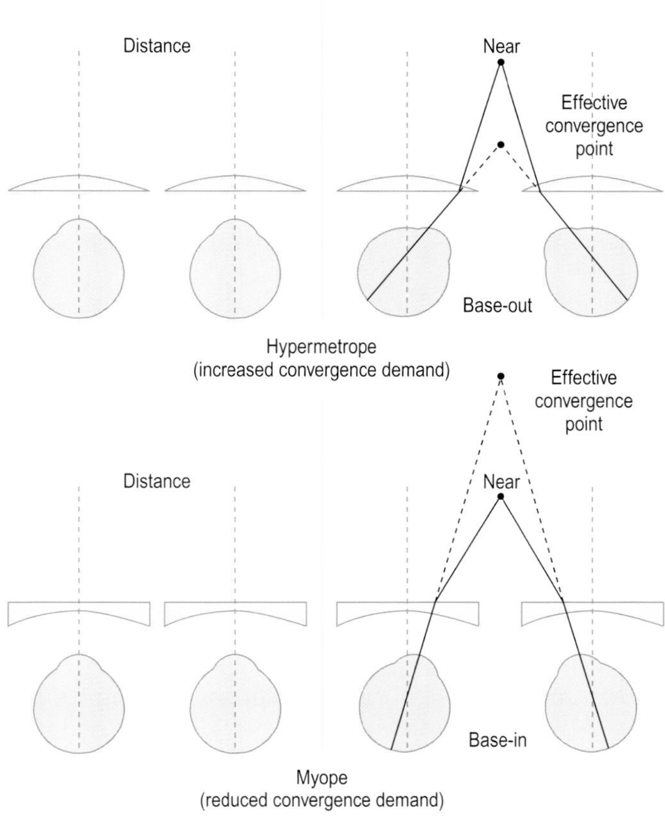

Figure 3.21 Prismatic effects of distance spectacle corrections during near vision.

contact lenses, and lower for hypermetropes, the accommodation–convergence links are minimally disturbed.

Other optical effects

There are certain additional phenomena related to prismatic effects of ophthalmic lenses that are not encountered by contact lens wearers. These phenomena, which are experienced by spectacle lens wearers, relate to the effective field of view in static gaze, the extent of eye movements required to maintain fixation and the appearance of the eyes as viewed by another person (or when looking in a mirror).

Fields of view and fixation

With spectacle lenses, the prismatic effects associated with the lens peripheries result, when the eyes are stationary, in an annular zone of the visual field being invisible (a ring scotoma) with a positive correction, and being seen diplopically with a negative correction. Analogously, when the eye is rotated to view objects away from the axis of the correction, a larger eye movement, in comparison with the uncorrected eye, is required with a negative spectacle lens and a smaller one with a positive correction. This can be seen in Figure 3.22.

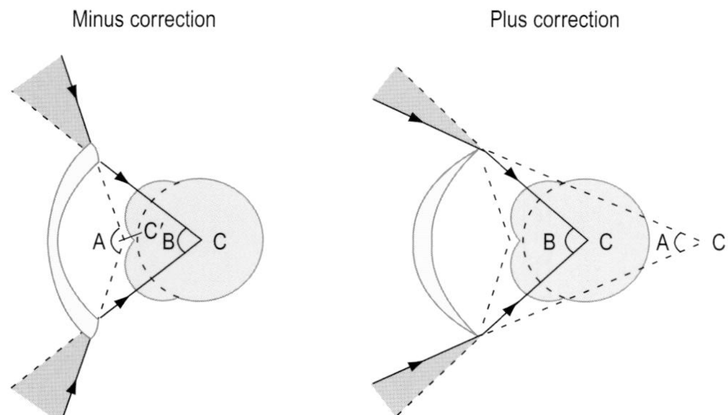

Figure 3.22 Fields of view as seen through spectacle lens corrections. The centre of rotation of the eye is at *C*, and its image as seen through the spectacle lens is at *C′*. *B* is the apparent macular field of view and *A* the actual field.

If *C* is the centre of rotation of the eye, the effective field of view as seen through the spectacle lens is governed by the position of its image, *C′*, as formed by the correcting lens.

These fixation effects are absent with contact lens corrections, since the lenses follow the movements of the eyes from fixation to fixation. The periphery of the static field of view may, however, be slightly affected if the contact lens or its optical zone is small, and in the case of rigid lenses flare or glare may occur due to discontinuities at the edge of the lens or optic zone affecting ray pencils from the periphery of the field. After laser refractive surgery, the optic zone diameter may be smaller than the dilated pupil, leading to complaints of haloes at night.

Apparent size of the eyes

A cosmetic disadvantage of spectacle lenses is that they alter the apparent size of the eyes of the wearer as seen by other people: the eyes appear larger with positive spectacle corrections and smaller with negative ones. Using a thin lens approximation, where the power of the correcting lens is F_c and the eye is at a distance l from the lens, it is easy to show that the paraxial magnification, M, of the anterior eye is given by:

$$M = 1/(1 + F_c l)$$

Since l is small (<0.02 m) this can be approximated by:

$$M = 1 - F_c l$$

Thus if l is −20 mm and F_c is −10 D, the eyes nominally appear to be only 80% of their true size. In fact for the viewer the apparent size will vary depending upon the viewing direction, since conditions will not necessarily be paraxial. These magnification effects can be reduced by minimizing the vertex distance with high-powered spectacle corrections.

Clearly, with contact lenses this cosmetic disadvantage is absent.

Summary

It has been shown that, although various types of correction all produce sharp retinal images in the ametropic eye, the sizes of the associated retinal images will differ, as will the demands on accommodation and convergence. A particular advantage of contact lenses is that they produce little change in the retinal image size in comparison with the uncorrected eye.

References

Applegate, R. A. and Howland, H. C. (1993) Magnification and visual acuity in refractive surgery. *Arch. Ophthalmol.* **111,** 1335–1342.

Applegate, R. A., Ballentine, C., Gross, H., *et al.* (2003) Visual acuity as a function of Zernike mode and level of root mean square error. *Optom. Vis. Sci.* **80,** 97–105.

Applegate, R. A., Donnelly, W. J., Marsack, J. D., *et al.* (2007) Three-dimensional relationship between higher-order root-mean-square wavefront error, pupil diameter, and aging. *J. Opt. Soc. Am. A* **24,** 578–587.

Atchison, D. A. (2004) Recent advances in representation of monochromatic aberrations of human eyes. *Clin. Exper. Optom.* **87,** 138–148.

Atchison, D. A. (2005) Recent advances in the measurement of monochromatic aberrations in human eyes. *Clin. Exper. Optom.* **88,** 5–26.

Atchison, D. A. and Smith, G. (2000) *Optics of the Human Eye,* Oxford: Butterworth-Heinemann.

Bara, S., Mancebo, T., Moreno-Barriuso, E. (2000) Positioning tolerances for phase plates compensating aberrations of the human eye. *Appl. Opt.* **39,** 3413–3420.

Bennett, A. G. (1966) Aspheric contact lens surfaces. Parts I, II and III. *Ophthal. Optician,* **8**(20), 1037–1040; **8**(23), 1297–1311; **9**(5), 222–230.

Bennett, A. G. (1988) Aspherical and continuous curve contact lenses. Parts I to IV. *Optometry Today,* **28,** 11–14; 140–142; 238–242; 433–444.

Bullimore, M. A., Fusaro, R. E. and Adams, C. W. (1998) The repeatability of automated and clinical refraction. *Optom. Vis. Sci.* **75,** 617–722.

Campbell, F. W. and Gubisch, R. W. (1966) Optical quality of the eye. *J. Physiol. (London),* **186,** 558–578.

Campbell, F. W. and Gubisch, R. W. (1967) The effect of chromatic aberration on visual acuity. *J. Physiol. (London),* **192,** 345–358.

Chan, C., Smith, G. and Jacobs, R. J. (1985) Simulating refractive errors: source and observer methods. *Am. J. Optom. Physiol. Opt.,* **62,** 207–216.

Charman, W. N. (1991a) Optics of the human eye. In *Vision and Visual Dysfunction. Vol. 1: Visual Optics and Instrumentation* (W. N. Charman, ed.) pp. 1–26, London: Macmillan.

Charman, W. N. (1991b) Wavefront aberration of the eye. *Optom. Vis. Sci.,* **68,** 574–583.

Charman, W. N. (1995) Optics of the eye. In *Handbook of Optics* (M. Bass, M. W. E. Van Stryland, D. R. Williams and W. L. Wolfe, eds) pp. 24.3–24.54, New York: McGraw Hill.

Charman, W. N. (2005) Wavefront technology: past, present and future. *Contact Lens & Ant. Eye* **28,** 75–92.

Charman, W. N., and Chateau, N. (2003) The prospects for super-acuity: limits to visual performance after correction of monochromatic aberrations. *Ophthal. Physiol. Opt.* **23,** 479–493.

Cheng, H., Barnett, J. K., Vilupuru, A. S., *et al.* (2004) A population study on changes in wave aberration with accommodation. *J. Vision* **4**(4), 3, 272-280.

Ciuffreda, K. J. (1991) Accommodation and its anomalies. In *Vision and Visual Dysfunction. Vol. 1: Visual Optics and Instrumentation* (W. N. Charman, ed.) pp. 231–279, London: Macmillan.

Ciuffreda, K. J. (1998) Accommodation, the pupil and presbyopia. In *Borish's Clinical Refraction* (W. J. Benjamin, ed.) pp. 77–120, Philadelphia: Saunders.

Curtin, B. J. (1985) *The Myopias: Basic Science and Clinical Management,* New York: Harper & Row.

Douthwaite, W. A. (2005) *Contact Lens Optics and Lens Design,* 3rd edn, Oxford: Butterworth-Heinemann.

Duane, A. (1922) Studies in monocular and binocular accommodation with their clinical implications. *Am. J. Ophthalmol.,* **5,** 865–877.

Farrell, R. J. and Booth, J. M. (1984) *Design Handbook for Imagery Interpretation Equipment,* Sec. 3.2, p. 8, Seattle, WA: Boeing Aerospace Co.

Guillon, M., Lydon, D. P. M. and Wilson, C. (1986) Corneal topography: a clinical model. *Ophthal. Physiol. Opt.,* **6,** 47–56.

Guirao, A. and Artal, P. (2000) Corneal wave aberration from videokeratography: accuracy and limitations of the procedure. *J. Opt. Soc. Am. A.,* **17,** 955–965.

Guirao, A., Williams, D. R., Cox, I. G. (2001) Effect of rotation and translation on the expected benefit of an ideal method to correct the eye's higher-order aberrations. *J. Opt. Soc. Am. A.,* **18,** 1003–1015.

Hartridge, H. (1947) The visual perception of fine detail. *Phil. Trans. Roy. Soc. B,* **232,** 519–671.

Hemenger, R. P., Tomlinson, A. and Oliver, K. (1995) Corneal optics from videokeratographs. *Ophthal. Physiol. Opt.,* **15,** 63–68.

Hofer, H., Artal, P., Singer, B., *et al.* (2001) Dynamics of the eye's wave aberration. *J. Opt. Soc. Am. A.,* **18,** 497–506.

Horner, D. G., Salmon, T. O. and Soni, P. S. (1998) Corneal topography. In *Borish's Clinical Refraction* (W. J. Benjamin, ed.) pp. 524–558, Philadelphia: Saunders.

Hopkins, H. H. (1950) *Wave Theory of Aberrations,* Oxford: Oxford University Press.

Hopkins, H. H. (1962) The application of frequency response techniques in optics. *Proc. Phys. Soc.,* **79,** 889–919.

Ivanoff, A. (1956) About the spherical aberration of the eye. *J. Opt. Soc. Am.,* **46,** 901–903.

Jones, C. E., Atchison, D. A., Meder, R. *et al.* (2005) Refractive index distribution and optical properties of the isolated human elens measured using magnetic resonance imaging. *Vision Res.* **45,** 2352–2366.

Kiely, P. M., Smith, G. and Carney, L. G. (1982) The mean shape of the human cornea. *Optica Acta,* **29,** 1027–1040.

Klein, S. A.(1998) Optimal corneal ablation for eyes with arbitrary Hartmann-Shack aberrations. *J. Opt. Soc. Am. A.,* **15,** 2580–2588.

Klein, S. A. and Barsky, B. A. (1995) Method for generating the anterior surface of an aberration-free contact lens for an arbitrary posterior surface. *Optom. Vis. Sci.,* **72,** 816–820.

Krueger R. R., Applegate R. A., MacRae S. M., editors. (2004) *Wavefront Customized Visual Correction: the Quest for Supervision II.* Thorofare, NJ: Slack.

Liang, J. and Williams, D. R. (1997) Aberrations and retinal image quality of the human eye. *J. Opt. Soc. Am. A,* **14,** 2873–2883.

Liang, J., Grimm, B., Goelz, S. *et al.* (1994) Objective measurement of wave aberrations of the human eye with the use of a Hartmann-Shack wavefront sensor. *J. Opt. Soc. Am. A,* **11,** 1949–1957.

Liang, J., Williams, D. R. and Miller, D. T. (1997) Supernormal vision and high-resolution retinal imaging through adaptive optics. *J. Opt. Soc. Am. A,* **14,** 2884–2892.

Loewenfeld, I. E. (1998) *The Pupil,* Boston, MA: Butterworth-Heinemann.

Lopez-Gil, N., Iglesias, I. and Artal, P. (1998) Retinal image quality in the human eye as a function of the accommodation. *Vis. Res.,* **38,** 2897–2907.

Mandell, R. B., Chiang, C. S. and Klein, S. A. (1995) Location of the major corneal reference points. *Optom. Vis. Sci.,* **72,** 776–784.

McBrien, N. A. and Barnes, D. A. (1984) A review and evaluation of refractive error development. *Ophthal. Physiol. Opt.,* **4,** 201–213.

Montés-Micó, R, Alio, J. L., Munoz, G., *et al.* (2004) Postblink changes in total and corneal aberration after a blink. *Ophthalmology* **111,** 758–767.

Mountford J., Ruston, D., Dave, T. (2004) Corneal topography and its measurement. In: Mountford J., Ruston, D., Dave, T. (eds) *Orthokeratology: Principles and Practice.* Butterworth Heinemann, Oxford, pp. 17–47.

O'Leary, D. J. (1988) Subjective refraction. In *Optometry,* edited by Edwards, K. and Llewellyn, R., Butterworths, London, pp. 111–139.

Pierscionek, B. K. (1995) Variations in refractive index and absorbance of 670 nm light with age and cataract formation in the human lens. *Exp. Eye Res.,* **60,** 407–414.

Pierscionek, B. K., Chang, D. Y. C., Ennis, J. P. *et al.* (1988) Non-destructive method of constructing three-dimensional gradient-index models for crystalline lenses: 1. Theory and experiment. *Am. J. Optom. Physiol. Opt.,* **65,** 481–491.

Porter J., Guirao, A., Cox, I. G. *et al.* (2001) The human eye's monochromatic aberrations in a large population. *J. Opt. Soc. Am. A.* **18,** 1793–1803.

Rabbetts, R. B. (1998) *Clinical Visual Optics,* 3rd edn, Oxford: Butterworth-Heinemann.

Rosenfield, M. and Gilmartin, B. (1998) *Myopia and Nearwork,* Oxford: Butterworth-Heinemann.

Rynders, M., Lidkea, B., Chisholm, W., *et al.* (1995) Statistical distribution of foveal transverse chromatic aberration, pupil centration, and angle psi in a population of young adult eyes. *J. Opt. Soc. Am. A.* **12,** 2348–2357.

Salmon, T. O. and Horner, S. D. G. (1995) Comparison of elevation, curvature and power descriptors for corneal topographic mapping. *Optom. Vis. Sci.,* **72,** 800–808.

Salmon, T. O. and van de Pol, C. (2006) Normal-eye Zernike coefficients and root-mean-square wavefront errors. *J. Cataract Refract. Surg.* **32,** 2064–2074.

Saunders, K. J. (1995) Early refractive development in humans. *Surv. Ophthalmol.,* **40,** 207–216.

Schweigerling, J. and Snyder, R. W. (1998) Custom photorefractive keratectomy ablations for the correction of spherical and cylindrical refractive error and higher-order aberration. *J. Opt. Soc. Am. A,* **15,** 2572–2579.

Smith, G. (1982) Ocular defocus, spurious resolution and contrast reversal. *Ophthal. Physiol. Opt.,* **2,** 5–23.

Smith, G. (1996) Visual acuity and refractive error. Is there a mathematical relationship? *Optometry Today* **36**(17), 22–27.

Sorsby, A., Benjamin, B., Davey, J. B. *et al.* (1957) *Emmetropia and its Aberrations.* Medical Research Council Special Reports Series, No. 293. London: HMSO.

Steiger, A. (1913) *Die Entstehung der sphaerischen Refraktionen des menschlichen Auges,* Berlin: Karger.

Stenstrom, S. (1946) Untersuchungen uber der Variation und Kovaration der optische Elemente des menschlichen Auges. *Acta Ophthalmol.,* **15**(Suppl. 26), [Translated by Woolf, D. (1948) as: Investigation of the variation and covariation of the optical elements of human eyes. *Am. J. Optom. Arch. Am. Acad. Optom.,* **25**, 218–232; 286–299; 340–350; 388–397; 438–449; 496–504.]

Thibos, L. N. and Bradley, A. (1999) Modelling the refractive and neurosensor systems of the eye. In *Visual Instrumentation* (P. Mouroulis, ed.) pp. 101–159, New York: McGraw Hill.

Troilo, D. (1992) Neonatal eye growth and emmetropisation – a literature review. *Eye,* **6,** 154–160.

Vargas-Martin, F., Prieto, P. M. and Artal, P. (1998) Correction of the aberrations in the human eye with a liquid-crystal spatial light modulator: limits to performance. *J. Opt. Soc. Am. A.,* **15,** 2552–2562.

Westheimer, G. (1962) The visual world of the new contact lens wearer. *J. Am. Optom. Assoc.,* **34,** 135–138.

Wildsoet, C. F. (1997) Active emmetropization – evidence for its existence and ramifications for clinical practice. *Ophthal. Physiol. Opt.,* **17,** 279–290.

Winn, B., Ackerley, R. G., Brown, C. A. *et al.* (1986) The superiority of contact lenses in the correction of all anisometropia. *Transactions of the British Contact Lens Association's Annual Clinical Conference,* **9,** 95–100.

Winn B., Whitaker D., Elliott D. B. and Phillips, N. J. (1994) Factors affecting light-adapted pupil size in normal human subjects. *Invest. Ophthamol. Vis. Sci.* **35,** 1132–1137.

Yoon, G-Y. and Williams, D. R. (2001) Visual performance after correcting the monochromatic and chromatic aberrations of the eye. *J. Opt. Soc. Am. A.* **19,** 266–275.

CHAPTER 4

Clinical instruments

Lyndon W Jones and Sruthi Srinivasan

Introduction

The purpose of this chapter is to review a number of the clinical instruments that are of considerable utility in the preliminary examination and ongoing care of contact lens patients. The emphasis will be on the design and principles of operation, with some comments on clinical use. Further details on the application of these instruments in contact lens practice can be found primarily in Chapter 37. The instruments discussed here form only a subset of the full range of instruments that should be available to primary eye care practitioners for examining all aspects of ocular health and visual function. General ophthalmic instruments that are used frequently (e.g. refracting equipment, retinoscopes, ophthalmoscopes) and periodically (e.g. tonometers, visual field analysers, colour vision and binocular vision assessment apparatus) in the course of a contact lens examination will not be considered here.

Observation of the eye

Perhaps the most fundamental procedure in a contact lens consultation is the examination of the anterior ocular structures. A general view of the eye can be obtained using low-optical-power hand-held devices, and the tear film can be assessed with a simple hand-held reflective instrument. The standard technique for examining the eye in detail is slit-lamp biomicroscopy, which has been available to practitioners since the invention of contact lenses over a century ago. More recently, high-powered observation tools have become available that allow examination of the living cornea at a cellular level.

Burton lamp

A number of manufacturers make a special hand-held magnifying device for contact lens work. This device is usually referred to as a 'Burton lamp', after the company that manufactured the original version (Burton Manufacturing Co., USA). The Burton lamp is essentially a large magnifying lens of about +5.00 D housed in a broad frame, within which are mounted a combination of 4 W white light and ultraviolet light fluorescent tubes, each 11 cm long. The operator can switch between the two light sources for white light and fluorescein stain examinations. A key advantage of this instrument is that both eyes of the patient can be viewed simultaneously, which facilitates interocular comparisons in the course of contact lens fitting. The Burton lamp is also useful for conducting an initial screening examination (Figure 4.1).

Non-invasive examination of the tear film

A full and healthy tear film is essential for successful contact lens wear, and a number of techniques are available for its assessment.

Tear morphology

The Tearscope-plus (Keeler, UK) can be used to observe certain characteristics of the tear film non-invasively (Guillon, 1997) (Figure 4.2A). This instrument takes the form of a small white dome with a central sight hole, surrounded by a cold cathode light source. It can be held directly in front of the eye, or used in conjunction with a slit-lamp biomicroscope to gain more magnification (Figure 4.2B). The thickness distribution, quality and freedom of movement of the tears can be assessed by observing the reflected light from the featureless white dome, and the integrity of the aqueous and lipid phases can be inferred from colour fringe interference patterns.

Tear break-up

Rapid tear break-up can lead to symptoms of dryness and discomfort in both lens wearers and non-lens wearers. Tear film break-up can be assessed by instilling fluorescein into the eye and timing how long it takes for breaks in the even fluorescent glow to appear. The problem with this approach is that it is 'invasive' in that the instillation of fluorescein in itself alters the quality and quantity of the tear film (Mengher *et al.*, 1985).

DOI: 10.1016/B978-0-7506-8869-7.00004-5

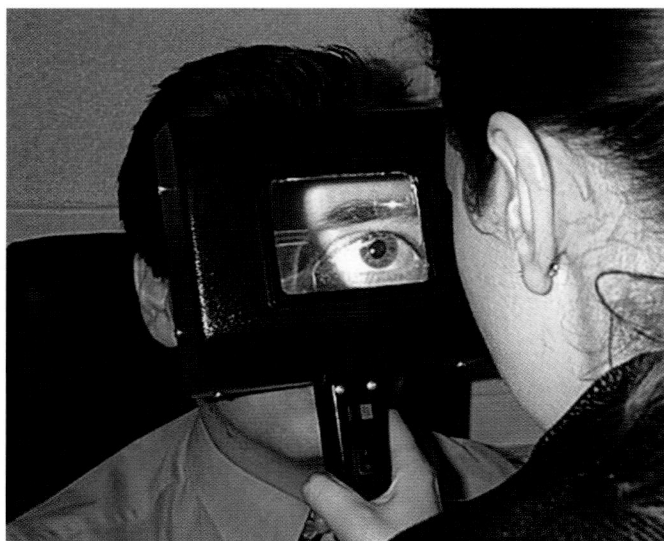

Figure 4.1 Examining the eyes using a Burton lamp.

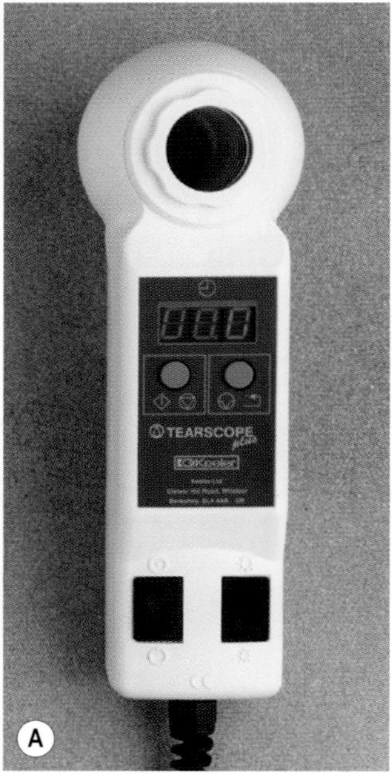

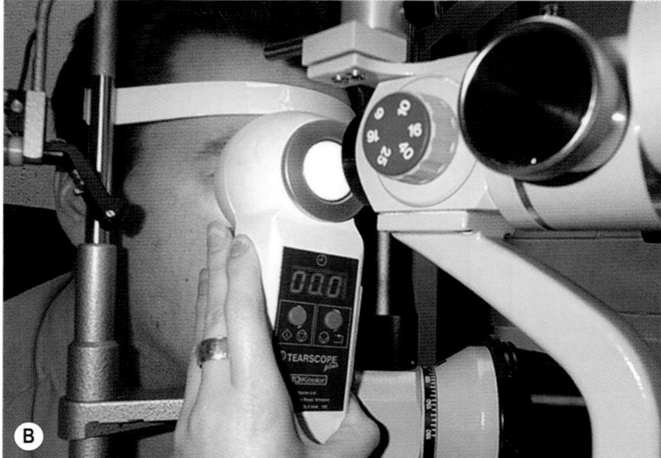

Figure 4.2 (A) The Tearscope-plus. (B) Examining the eye with the Tearscope-plus in conjunction with a slit-lamp biomicroscope to obtain higher magnification.

The preferred approach is to determine the non-invasive tear film break-up time (NIBUT). This can be achieved by optically projecting a grid pattern on to the cornea and timing how long it takes for the grid to become disrupted. Numerous devices employing this principle have been produced, including the instrument stand-mounted 'NIBUT dome' or 'Mengher grid' (Mengher *et al.*, 1985) and hand-held devices such as the keratometer-mounted Hir-Cal grid (Hirji *et al.*, 1989), the Loveridge grid (Loveridge, 1993) and the Tearscope-plus with NIBUT grid attachment (Guillon, 1997) (Figure 4.3).

Osmometry

A clinical test that has been suggested as being highly diagnostic involves measuring tear film osmolality (Tomlinson and Khanal, 2005; Khanal *et al.*, 2008). This is often considered a 'gold standard' in the evaluation of patients with dry eye (Farris *et al.*, 1986; Farris, 1994; Tomlinson and Khanal, 2005), due to the hypertonic tear film found in dry-eyed individuals (Gilbard *et al.*, 1978, 1987, 1989; Farris *et al.*, 1983; Lemp, 1995). A hypertonic tear film causes ocular surface damage and may lead to discomfort (Gilbard *et al.*, 1978, 1987; Lemp, 1995). Osmolality is a function of tear secretion, drainage, absorption and evaporation and can be regarded as a single parameter of tear film dynamics (Tomlinson and Khanal, 2005). Even though tear osmolality has been considered the 'gold standard' for diagnosing dry-eye syndrome, it is not widely used clinically due to the lack of available equipment and the fact that most osmometers require a large volume of tears, typically 5–10 μl (White *et al.*, 1993; Miller *et al.*, 2003), which limits its use in many dry-eye subjects, particularly those with severe disease (Nelson and Wright, 1986; White *et al.*, 1993).

Measuring tear film osmolality is often undertaken using a freezing-point depression method (Tomlinson and Khanal, 2005), typically using the Clifton instrument. However, this instrument requires considerable expertise, is time-consuming and the equipment is difficult to maintain (Farris *et al.*, 1986; Nelson and Wright, 1986; White *et al.*, 1993). New osmometers have recently become available that use microvolumes of fluid (<1 μl), which makes them ideally suited for use in clinical dry-eye research (Dalton and Jones, 2005; Sullivan, 2005). A novel freezing-point depression osmometer (model 3100 tear osmometer: Advanced Instruments, Norwood, MA, USA; Figure 4.4) requires only 0.5 μl of tears to evaluate tear osmolality (Dalton and Jones, 2005).

Tear meniscus height

An adequate volume of tears is a prerequisite for a healthy ocular surface (Holly and Lemp, 1977; Miller *et al.*, 2004) and a reduction in the volume of tears gives rise to a greater chance of symptoms of ocular dryness (Doughty *et al.*, 2001). Estimation of tear volume is often undertaken using Schirmer strips (Lamberts *et al.*, 1979; Yokoi *et al.*, 2000), phenol red threads (Tomlinson *et al.*, 2001) or estimating the volume of tears in the inferior tear meniscus (Lim and Lee, 1991; Golding *et al.*, 1997; Oguz *et al.*, 2000; Patel and Wallace, 2006; Santodomingo-Rubido *et al.*, 2006; Savini

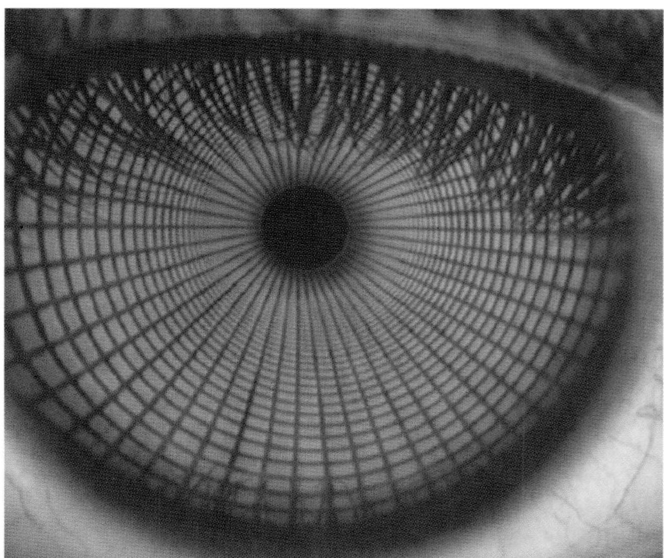

Figure 4.3 Reflection of the non-invasive tear film break-up time (NIBUT) grid attachment of the Tearscope-plus (shown in Figure 4.2) as seen in the precorneal tear film. The time taken from eye opening to distortion or break-up of the reflected grid pattern is recorded as the NIBUT.

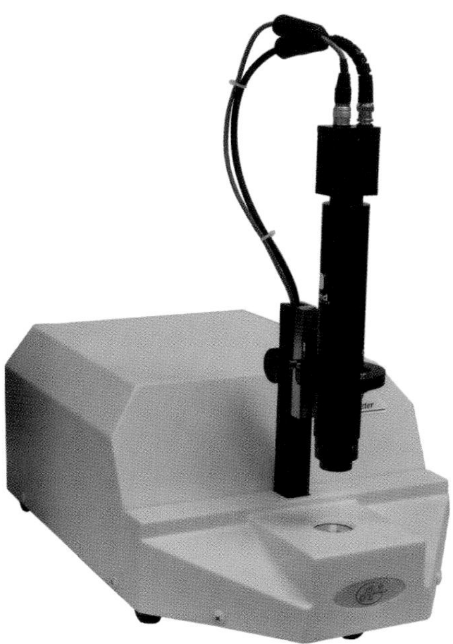

Figure 4.4 The model 3100 tear osmometer from Advanced Instruments.

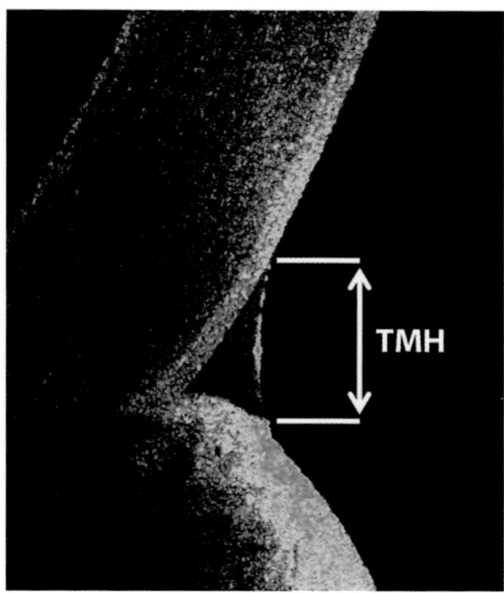

Figure 4.5 Optical coherence tomography (OCT) image of the lower-lid tear meniscus showing the tear meniscus height (TMH).

et al., 2006). The inferior tear meniscus contains about 90% of the tear volume (Holly, 1985) and tear meniscus volume is classically determined by estimating the tear meniscus height (TMH) (Patel and Blades, 2003; Patel and Wallace, 2006; Santodomingo-Rubido *et al.*, 2006; Savini *et al.*, 2006). Studies have shown that TMH estimation is a good clinical indicator in differentiating dry-eyed versus non-dry-eyed patients, as it is a direct measure of the quantity of the tear film (Lim and Lee, 1991; Mainstone *et al.*, 1996; Golding *et al.*, 1997).

The most common and simple method to determine TMH is visualizing the TMH using a slit-lamp biomicroscope with an eyepiece containing a graticule (Lamberts *et al.*, 1979; Lim and Lee, 1991; Papas and Vajdic, 2000; Miller *et al.*, 2004; Nichols *et al*, 2004; Patel and Wallace, 2006; Santodomingo-Rubido *et al.*, 2006). However, estimation of the upper border of the TMH is difficult and several studies have achieved this by adding a small volume of fluorescein to the tears (Lamberts *et al.*, 1979; Port and Asaria, 1990; Lim and Lee, 1991; Mainstone *et al.*, 1996; Golding *et al.*, 1997; Guillon *et al.*, 1997; Oguz *et al.*, 2000; Tomlinson *et al.*, 2001). Enhancing the visualization of the upper TMH border by the addition of fluorescein is clearly invasive and may interfere with the tear volume determined, resulting in a higher estimation of the TMH. To overcome such difficulties, a number of non-invasive approaches to measure TMH have evolved in the past decade. Studies have used videography of the meniscus (Oguz *et al.*, 2000), video assessments (Golding *et al.*, 1997; Doughty *et al.*, 2001, 2002), optical pachymetry (Port and Asaria, 1990; Patel and Port, 1991) and videoreflective dacryomeniscometry (Francis *et al.*, 2005) to measure the TMH non-invasively. Over the last few years, optical coherence tomography (OCT) has been used to determine TMH (Jones *et al.*, 2002; Johnson and Murphy, 2005; Savini *et al.*, 2006; Wang *et al.*, 2006a; Bitton *et al.*, 2007; Shen *et al.*, 2009). OCT offers an advantage in that it is the only available method to view the tear prism in cross-section in a non-invasive manner.

To measure TMH the scan beam, 2.00 mm high, is positioned on the lower lid margin. Once the tear prism is visualized, images can be scanned and stored as two-dimensional false-colour images. Analysis is performed using the caliper tool included in the integrated software, whereby the height within the OCT slice is calculated (Figure 4.5).

Slit-lamp biomicroscopy

The slit-lamp biomicroscope plays an essential role in the preliminary assessment and aftercare of the prospective and existing contact lens wearer. The opportunities for using the slit lamp within the routine eye examination are numerous and diverse. With the appropriate application of supplementary lenses and/or viewing techniques the

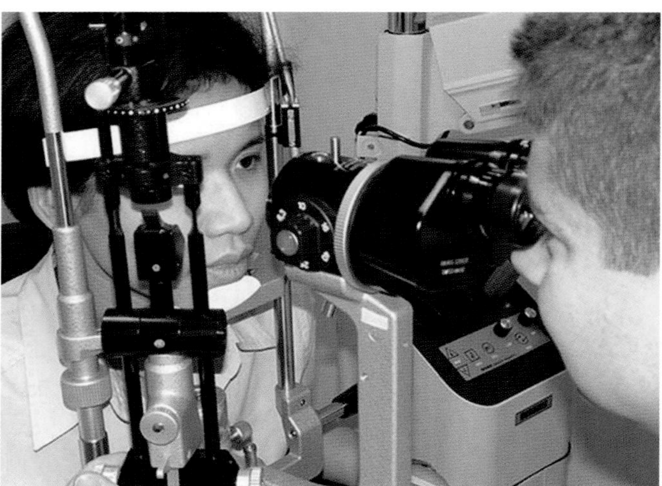

Figure 4.6 The slit-lamp biomicroscope. Note the separate controls for the illumination system and the magnification system.

instrument may be used to assess the condition of the vitreous, lens and retina from posterior pole to the ora serrata. Various ancillary instruments will permit examination of the anterior-chamber angle, measurement of intraocular pressure, corneal sensitivity and assessment of corneal thickness. This review will concentrate on the instrument itself: see Chapter 37 for an account of the use of the slit-lamp biomicroscope in contact lens practice.

The instrument consists of a separate illumination system (the slit lamp) and viewing system (the biomicroscope), which have a common focal point and centre of rotation (Figure 4.6).

A height control moves both systems simultaneously, whilst focusing and lateral movements are achieved via a joystick. This common control feature facilitates rapid and accurate positioning of the slit beam on the area of interest and ensures that the microscope and illumination system are simultaneously in focus.

Illumination system

Virtually all slit-lamp manufacturers have adopted the Koeller illumination system, which is optically almost identical to that of a 35 mm slide projector (Henson, 1996b). A bright illumination system (producing approximately 600 000 lux) is a fundamental requirement for a slit lamp if subtle conditions are to be seen clearly. Although halogen or xenon lamps are more expensive than tungsten lamps, they are the preferred illumination source as they provide a brighter light, last longer, have better colour rendering and generate less heat. Illumination brightness is controlled by a rheostat or multiposition switch such that brightness can be adjusted to obtain the correct balance between patient comfort and optimal visibility of the area of interest.

The slit within the illumination system must have sharply demarcated edges and desirable features include the following:

- The slit width and height must be easily adjustable such that any shaped patch from a slit to a circle may be projected, as this will increase the variety of illumination methods possible.
- A graduated slit width is particularly useful when measuring the size of a lesion.
- An ability to rotate the lamp housing such that the slit may be used in meridians away from the vertical is useful, particularly if a protractor scale is included. Such a system enables, for example, the angle of rotation of a soft toric lens away from the vertical to be accurately measured.
- The slit beam must have the facility to be displaced or offset sideways ('decoupled'). This ability to break the linkage between the illumination and observation systems facilitates indirect illumination techniques.

A number of filters can be incorporated into the illumination system; these serve to enhance the visibility of certain conditions:

- Green ('red-free') filter – enhances contrast when looking for corneal and iris vascularization, since red vessels appear black if viewed through such a filter. In addition, it may be used to increase the visibility of rose Bengal staining on both the cornea and conjunctiva.
- Neutral-density filter – reduces beam brightness and increases comfort for the patient.
- Polarizing filter – reduces unwanted specular reflections and can be useful to enhance the visibility of subtle defects.
- Diffusing filter – diffuses the illumination source over a wide area and is used to provide broad, unfocused illumination for low-magnification viewing of the general ocular surface.
- Cobalt blue filter – provides a suitable means of exciting sodium fluorescein for examination of ocular surface integrity. Illumination of fluorescein with cobalt blue light of 460–490 nm produces a greenish light of maximum emission 520 nm. Any abraded area will absorb fluorescein and display a fluorescent green area against a general blue background. The filter is occasionally used on its own to aid in the diagnosis of keratoconus. A frequent finding in this corneal ectasia is Fleischer's ring, which is formed by an annular iron deposition within the stroma at the base of the cone. The iron pigment is often difficult to see in white light but will usually appear in greater contrast when viewed through the cobalt blue filter.
- Kodak Wratten number 12 (yellow) filter – this filter is not contained within the illumination system but is used as a supplementary barrier filter that is placed in front of the viewing system. It significantly enhances the contrast of any fluorescent staining observed with the cobalt blue filter as it allows transmission of the green fluorescent light but blocks the blue light reflected from the corneal surface (Back, 1988). Some newer slit lamps incorporate it within the viewing system, but for most practitioners it is used as an 'add-on' system that is placed over the observation lens when required. Custom-made barrier filters for certain slit lamps are available from some manufacturers (Figure 4.7). Inexpensive hand-held versions may be constructed by using a cardboard mask and Lee filters number 101 yellow.

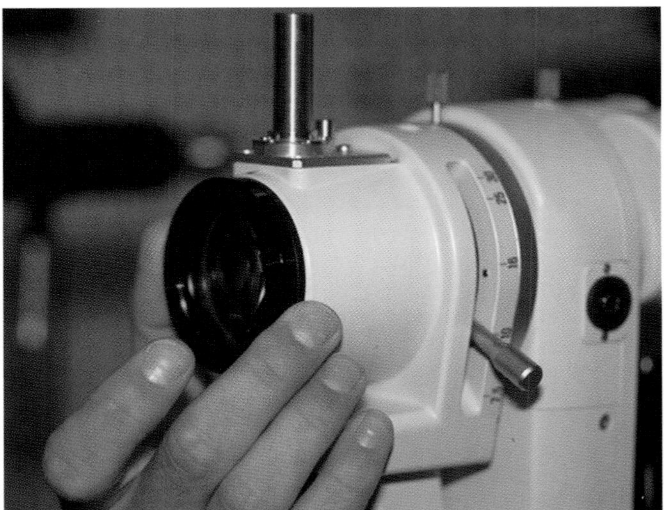

Figure 4.7 Custom-designed barrier filter in position on the Nikon FS3 slit-lamp microscope. The slider for the zoom magnification system is also clearly seen.

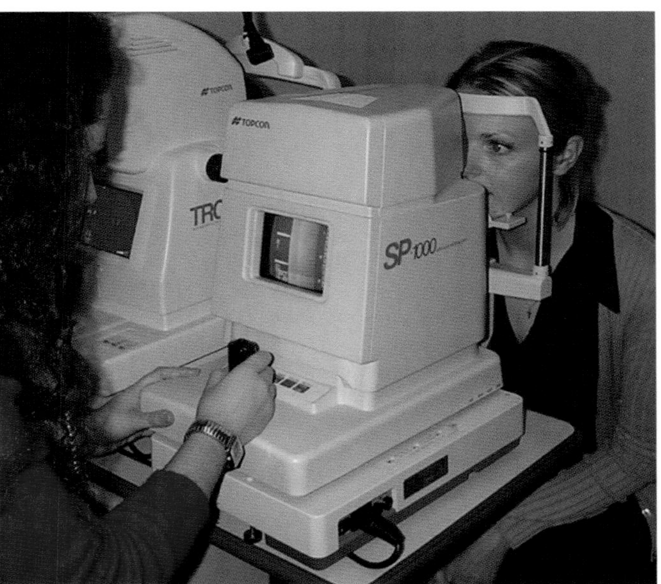

Figure 4.8 The Topcon SP1000 endothelial specular microscope.

The microscope

A key prerequisite for a slit-lamp biomicroscope is a viewing system that provides a clear image of the eye and has sufficient magnification for the practitioner to view all structures of interest. Magnification is an important consideration, and ideally magnifications of up to 40× should be possible; this may be achieved through interchangeable eyepieces and/or variable magnification of the slit-lamp objective (Henson, 1996b). Magnification greater than this level is usually unnecessary and is often counterproductive, as small involuntary eye movements will render the image too unstable to view. Ideally the practitioner should be able to change magnification swiftly and easily, which gives slit lamps with three or more objectives an advantage. Zoom systems have the added advantage of allowing the practitioner to focus on a particular structure without losing sight of it during changes in magnification.

Of course, the magnified image must also be clear, and the importance of choosing a slit lamp with a high-quality optical system cannot be overemphasized. Ideally the microscope should have excellent resolution and a good depth of field. However, these factors are inversely linked and so a compromise must be accepted.

Mastering all of the possible illumination techniques with the slit lamp is essential if the instrument is to be used to its full potential. Practice with the instrument is critical to becoming comfortable with its subtle but extensive variety of uses. Readers are advised to consult other texts for information concerning the use of the many and varied illumination techniques available with the slit lamp (Zantos and Cox, 1994; Jones and Jones, 2000).

High-powered microscopy

Conventional microscopy collects all the light reflected back through the object. As a result, information out of the focal plane, above and below areas of interest, creates noisy and blurred images in all but the thinnest specimens at high magnification (Cavanagh *et al.*, 2000). Over the past 25 years two techniques (specular and confocal microscopy) have emerged that have enabled researchers and clinicians to examine the structure of the cornea *in vivo* at very high magnification.

Specular microscopy

The specular microscope allows viewing of objects illuminated from above, and the objective lens also acts as the condenser lens. Light passes from inside the microscope out through the objective lens to arrive at a focus near the focal plane of the lens. If this position coincides with a reflecting surface then the focused light is reflected back through the objective lens and is viewed through the eyepiece of the microscope (Hodson and Sherrard, 1988). The first specular microscopes used for ophthalmic research were utilized by David Maurice in the 1960s in his work investigating corneal function. This technique enabled high-magnification images of both the epithelium and endothelium to be made, which had previously been difficult due to their transparency.

Early versions of the specular microscope used a contact dipping cone objective lens that was optically coupled to the cornea to provide higher magnification and resolution. However, most modern clinical specular microscopes can achieve equally high magnification without the need for ocular contact (Figure 4.8).

These instruments are primarily used to view and photograph the corneal endothelium and to monitor its morphology. By direct viewing with the specular microscope an overall impression of the condition of the endothelium can be established immediately. In addition, some of these instruments allow corneal thickness to be determined by measuring the distance between the epithelium and endothelium.

Typically the features looked for are the regularity of the endothelial mosaic, the size of the individual cells, the presence of intracellular vacuoles and abnormal features such as corneal guttae and keratic precipitates. From the images obtained factors such as the number of cells per unit area, cell shape and cell area can be calculated, enabling the clinician to assess the endothelial appearance compared with that expected of normal age-matched individuals. Results from these investigations (Hodson and Sherrard, 1988) have shown that the endothelial cell population density drops from approximately 4500 cells/m^2 at birth to 2000 cells/mm^2 in old age, and that their shape and size change dramatically over this time. At birth the endothelial mosaic is very regular and the cells are almost circular in shape. With time they become increasingly angular in shape and varied in size, a condition termed 'polymegethism' (see Chapter 40). In addition to age-related changes, the specular microscope has been used to investigate endothelial changes in a number of disease conditions, including posterior polymorphous dystrophy, Fuchs' dystrophy, corneal surgery, refractive surgery and contact lens wear (Hodson and Sherrard, 1988). In addition, deep stromal opacities such as glass foreign bodies, pigment deposits and corneal dystrophies can be imaged (Brooks *et al.*, 1992).

Confocal microscopy

Confocal microscopy is unlike conventional microscopy because defocus causes the image to disappear rather than appear as a blurred image. The properties of the confocal microscope stem from its ability to focus the illuminating light and the focal plane of the microscope objective on precisely the same point (Chan-Ling and Pye, 1994; Böhnke and Masters, 1999).

In most modern confocal microscopes (Figure 4.9) a point light source is focused on to a small volume within the specimen and a confocal point detector is used to collect the resulting signal. This results in a reduction of the amount of out-of-focus signal from above and below the focal plane, producing a marked increase in both lateral (x, y) and axial (z) resolution (Cavanagh *et al.*, 2000).

Only one tiny area of the specimen is observed by each point source, so a useful full field of view must be gained by mechanically scanning the area of interest. By varying the plane of focus of both the source and detector within the tissue, the specimen can be optically 'sectioned' non-invasively, and detailed information on corneal structure determined (Beuerman and Pedroza, 1996). Detailed descriptions of the optical principles involved in confocal microscopy have been published by Böhnke and Masters (1999), Cavanagh *et al.* (2000) and Efron *et al.* (2001).

The microscope objectives most commonly used are non-applanating water immersion objectives that are optically coupled to the cornea using a methylcellulose gel (Böhnke and Masters, 1999). To obtain the maximum axial resolution (and hence optical sectioning) it is necessary to use a microscope objective with a large numerical aperture (which describes the light-gathering ability of the objective). However, such devices have a reduced field of view and shorter free working distances, which reduces the distance that the microscope can focus into the specimen from the surface (Böhnke and Masters, 1999).

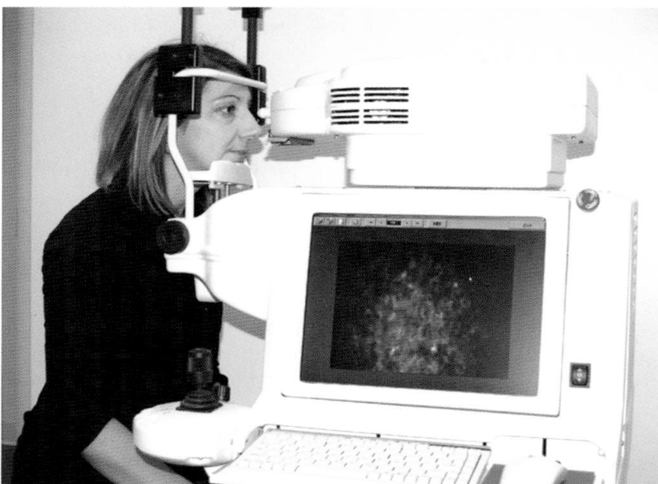

Figure 4.9 The NIDEK Confoscan 3 real-time confocal microscope.

Tandem scanning confocal microscopy

First-generation confocal microscopes used a modified Nipkow disc, which is a thin wafer with hundreds of pinholes that are arranged in a spiral pattern (Cavanagh *et al.*, 2000). When a portion of the disc is placed in the internal light path of the confocal microscope, the spinning disc produces a scanning pattern of the subject. As the subject is inspected, light is reflected back through the microscope objective. The light that was reflected from in front of or behind the focal plane of the objective approaches the disc at an angle rather than perpendicularly. The pinholes of the disc permit only perpendicularly oriented rays of light to penetrate. This enables the microscope to view a very thin optical section of tissue. Because the illumination and detection of light through conjugate pinholes occur in tandem, this microscope was named the tandem scanning confocal microscope.

The disadvantages of this system are a lack of a wide selection of objective lenses, an inability to control the signal-to-noise ratio directly at different tissue depths and the dramatic loss of light due to the fact that Nipkow discs transmit less than 1% of the available light (Cavanagh *et al.*, 2000). This latter problem necessitates the use of a low-light-level camera to acquire the images, which limits frame speed acquisition.

Slit scanning confocal microscopy

More recently, a variable-slit real-time scanning confocal microscope has been described (Masters *et al.*, 1994; Böhnke and Masters, 1999). In this design, two independently adjustable slits are located in conjugate planes. A rapidly oscillating two-sided mirror is used to scan the image of the slit over the plane of the cornea to produce optical sectioning in real time. This design has the advantages of optimal image contrast, enhanced clarity and decreased scan time, but it is more expensive than Nipkow-based systems, and z-axis quantification is not currently possible (Cavanagh *et al.*, 2000).

Confocal microscopy through focusing

Regardless of the technique used to obtain the images, the major problem associated with confocal microscopy relates to the interpretation and quantification of the data

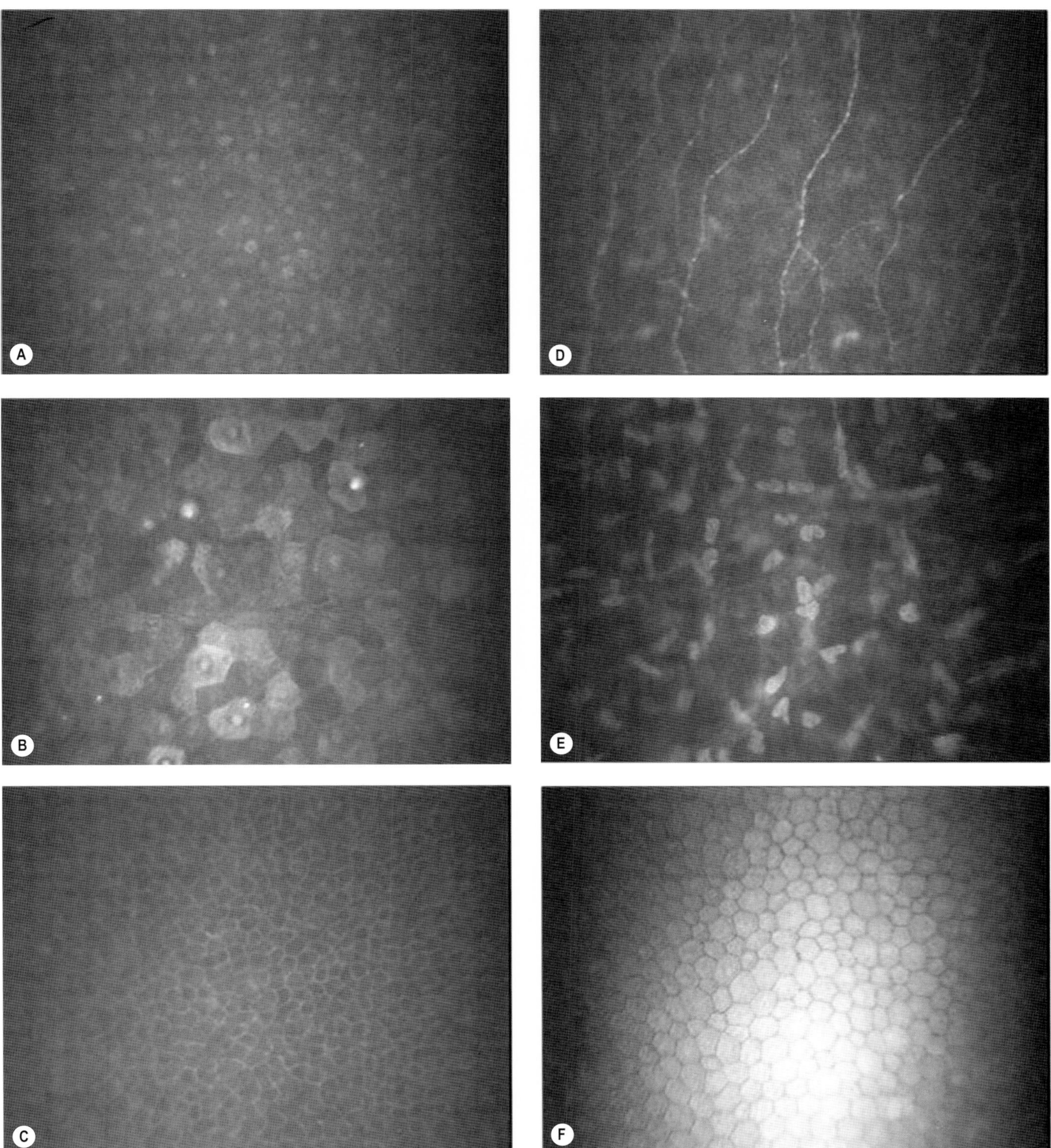

Figure 4.10 Confocal microscope images of the corneal layers of a normal eye of a human patient. (A) Superficial epithelium; (B) intermediate epithelium; (C) basal epithelium; (D) subbasal nerve fibre layer; (E) stroma; (F) endothelium.

obtained. A new technique called confocal microscopy through focusing attempts to overcome this by rapidly moving the focal plane of the objective lens through the entire cornea at a speed of approximately 80 µm/s while x–y images are acquired at the focal plane. This means that approximately 450 sequential images (which are separated by approximately 1 µm) are acquired over the time taken to traverse the cornea (approximately 15 s). The cornea is then reconstructed using image-processing techniques, and an image is produced that is similar to a histological section, albeit in three dimensions in a living cornea (Figure 4.10).

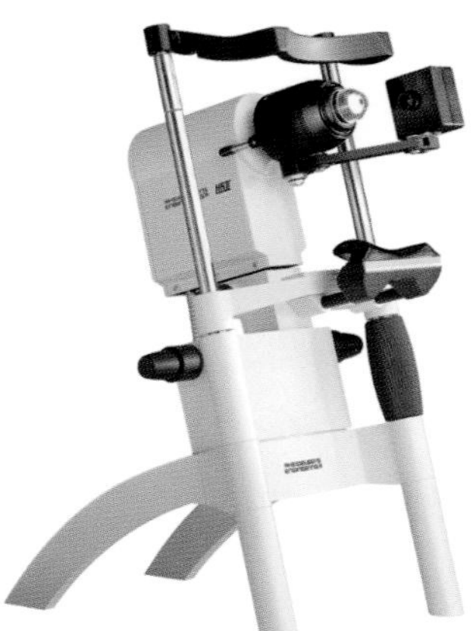

Figure 4.11 The HRT Rostock cornea module.

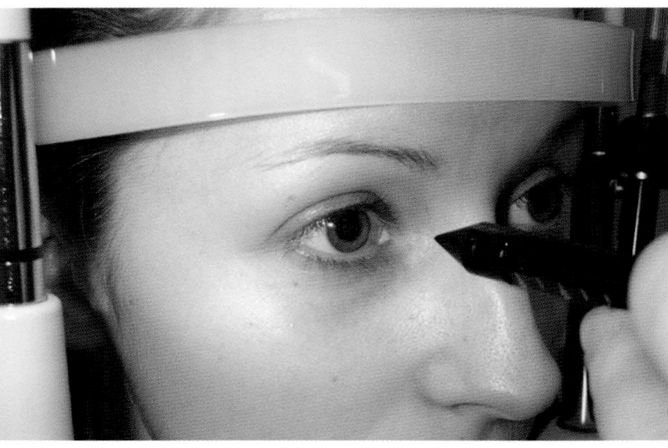

Figure 4.12 The Cochet–Bonnet aesthesiometer being used to measure corneal sensitivity. A fine nylon thread of a set length is advanced towards the eye and the patient is asked to report when he or she first feels the thread touching the corneal surface.

Rostock cornea module on HRT II

More recently, Heidelberg Engineering, in collaboration with Rostock University, Germany, has developed a novel digital confocal laser scanning microscope, a combination of Heidelberg retina tomograph II and the Rostock cornea module (RCM) (Stave *et al.*, 2002). The RCM uses the back-scattered light, similar to other confocal microscopes, with an interaction with the specimen producing a light signal that proceeds towards the detector. This device allows the operator to image sharply cellular structures and move through the different layers of the entire cornea, from epithelium to the endothelium. The RCM also enables the imaging of the peripheral areas of the cornea and conjunctiva. The instrument allows a scan depth of a maximum of 1500 μm, with an image size of 400 × 400 μm. The unit has an interchangeable 63× standard microscopic lens, offers a choice of manual depth position adjustment and has an automatic brightness adjustment system. The CCD camera allows a permanent monitoring of the corneal contact on the screen. The RCM technology provides better image quality and produces a precise depth measurement compared with confocal slit scanning microscopes (Eckard *et al.*, 2006) (Figure 4.11).

Using such techniques, confocal microscopy has provided valuable data on the structure and appearance of the cornea in many disease processes, including dystrophies, keratitis and endothelial disease. In addition, corneal changes following refractive surgery, keratoplasty (Moller-Pedersen *et al.*, 1997; Böhnke and Masters, 1999; Cavanagh *et al.*, 2000) and contact lens wear (Efron, 2007) have been documented.

Measurement of corneal sensitivity

The cornea is richly innervated and is one of the most sensitive tissues in the body. Corneal sensitivity is a useful indicator of corneal disease and can help to determine physiological stress from wearing contact lenses (Brennan and Bruce, 1991; Millodot, 1994). Interest in assessing corneal sensitivity has increased over recent years, particularly in light of new findings indicating that corneal sensitivity is significantly reduced in cases of dry eye (Xu *et al.*, 1996).

Contact aesthesiometry

Measurement of corneal sensitivity in the clinical setting has traditionally been achieved using a Cochet–Bonnet aesthesiometer (Figure 4.12).

This device can be hand-held or mounted on a slit lamp, and uses a single nylon thread to produce various forces, by varying its length in 0.5 cm steps (the longer the thread, the lighter is the force). The filament is lightly placed on to the cornea by the clinician using a support that allows manipulation in the x–y–z planes, whilst being viewed through the slit lamp. The subject reports when he or she can feel the thread touching the ocular surface, and the length of thread at which this occurs is recorded. The corneal touch threshold is defined as the length of the nylon filament at which the subject responds to 50% of the number of stimulations. This length is converted into pressure using a calibration curve and the reciprocal of this value gives the corneal sensitivity. Using this technique, it has been demonstrated that corneal sensitivity varies with surface location and is altered by age, iris colour, ambient temperature, time of day, contact lens wear and pregnancy (Millodot, 1994).

A number of factors complicate the use of such a device and can result in variations in the results obtained (Murphy *et al.*, 1998). These include physical aversion to the approach of the device, problems with mounting the device accurately in the slit lamp and the impact of ambient humidity on the stiffness of the thread (Brennan and Bruce, 1991).

Non-contact aesthesiometry

Over the last 10 years a number of devices have been tested and developed to overcome the problems described above with contact aesthesiometry. All of these devices use non-contact means of stimulating the cornea. Initially,

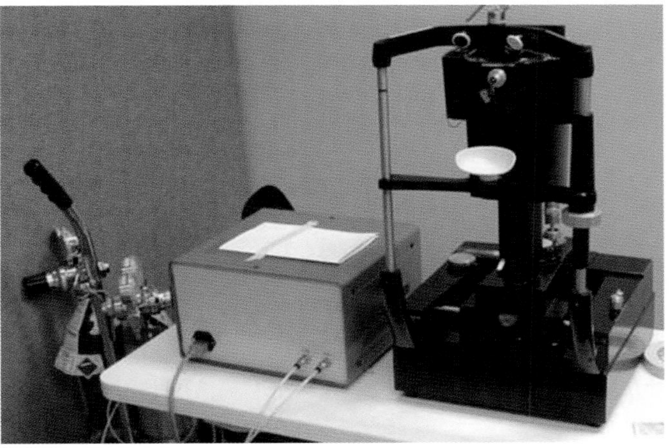

Figure 4.13 Custom-built non-contact aesthesiometer. This aesthesiometer is able to investigate a variety of mechanical, chemical and temperature responses of the conjunctiva and cornea.

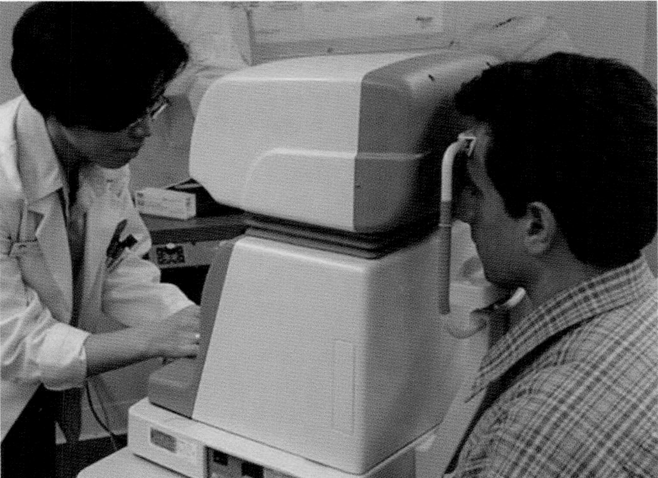

Figure 4.14 The Nikon autokeratometer/refractor in operation.

mechanical stimulation alone was investigated, but more recently aesthesiometers have been produced that stimulate the cornea using a variety of thermal, chemical or mechanical stimuli. These have included non-contact pneumatic devices, which deliver compressed air as the stimulus (Murphy *et al.*, 1998; Vega *et al.*, 1999); the application of a carbon dioxide laser to determine the threshold for the detection of an increase in corneal temperature (Ho and Brennan, 1993); and a device that measures chemical stimulation via the administration of varying concentrations of carbon dioxide (Belmonte *et al.*, 1999; Situ *et al.*, 2007) (Figure 4.13).

With time, it is likely that devices based on these approaches will become commercially available, and aesthesiometry will become an important technique in contact lens practice.

Assessment of corneal shape

Corneal shape assessment historically has been undertaken by determining the radius of curvature of the central cornea using a keratometer. However, over the last 10 years the development of sophisticated computer-driven corneal topographers has significantly improved the ability of both clinicians and researchers to measure subtle changes in corneal shape. The reduction in the cost of these latter devices has resulted in corneal topographers being used more commonly.

Keratometry

Knowledge of corneal curvature is primarily of interest as an aid in determining the initial contact lens to be placed on the eye in cases of rigid contact lens fitting. In addition, an indication of rapid changes in curvature can be indicative of a compromised cornea and also aid in the diagnosis of keratoconus. Measurement of the radius of curvature of the cornea is based on the fact that the front surface of the cornea acts as a convex mirror. The reflection of an object (or mire, from the French for 'target') of known size at a known distance is viewed using a short-focus telescope, and a relatively simple equation allows the corneal front surface radius of curvature to be determined directly from the instrument. The corneal power that results from a given radius is often also indicated on the keratometer; alternatively, this can be calculated (see Appendix D). The optical principles of keratometry, the various types of keratometer available and their specific mode of operation may be obtained from other sources (Stone and Rabbetts, 1994; Henson, 1996a). The actual region over which the standard keratometer measures corneal radius is that of two small areas approximately 1.5 mm on either side of the central fixation point (Stone and Rabbetts, 1994). Different types of keratometer use differently sized mires at differing separations. It is thus of no surprise that different keratometers may give differing radius values on the same eye.

The latest development in automated keratometry involves the use of infrared devices (Stone and Rabbetts, 1994) that rapidly and automatically determine central keratometry and refractive error simultaneously (Figure 4.14).

In addition to determining the central radius of curvature, it is useful to measure peripheral radius values, particularly in complicated conditions such as post penetrating keratoplasty and post refractive surgery. Conventional keratometers have traditionally been adapted by using peripheral fixation points (Stone and Rabbetts, 1994). However, in reality keratometers cannot be used to determine corneal curvature accurately if the surface being measured does not have a constant radius of curvature or is not radially symmetrical (Stone and Rabbetts, 1994). For this reason, dedicated instruments using other technologies have been developed to measure the overall corneal topography.

Corneal topographic analysis

The aim of corneal topography (or keratoscopy) is to describe accurately the shape of the corneal surface in all meridians (Mandell, 1992, 1996; Guillon and Ho, 1994).

In most cases, the technique uses a similar principle to keratometry, in that it determines the size of the image of a target reflected in the corneal surface, the primary difference relating to the fact that for keratoscopy a series of circular concentric targets are used (a Placido disc image). This arrangement allows both central and peripheral curvature to be determined. Historically, a photographic record of the corneal reflection images was made (photokeratoscopy) and measurements calculated subsequently (Veys and Davies, 1995). Modern-generation topographers capture the image electronically on a computer and use sophisticated image-processing software to provide immediate analysis of the reflected image (videokeratoscopy). Using this technique it has been clearly demonstrated that the cornea is aspheric and can best be described as a flattening ellipse, whose rate of flattening is asymmetrical about its centre (Guillon and Ho, 1994).

The history and detailed description of the development and operation of topographers and their clinical applications are described elsewhere (Guillon and Ho, 1994; Dave, 1998; Klyce *et al.*, 1998; Klyce, 2001).

Modern topographers can be categorized into two distinct forms – reflective devices and slit-scanning devices.

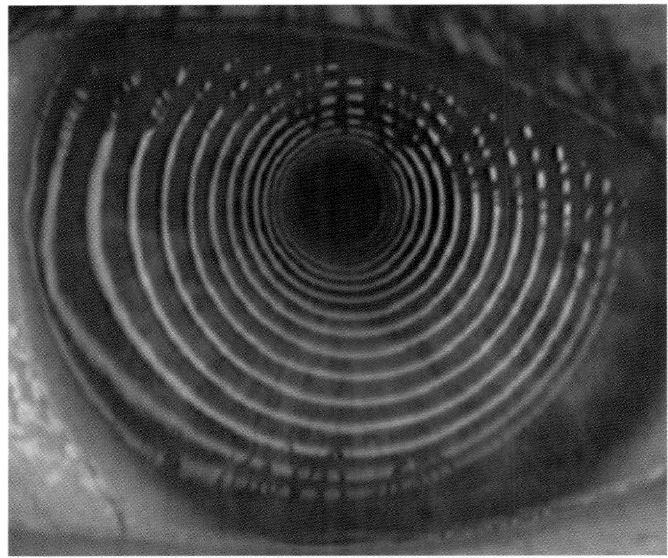

Figure 4.15 Reflection of the corneal topography grid attachment of the Tearscope-plus (shown in Figure 4.2) as seen in the precorneal tear film. Disturbances to the grid lines or overall deviations from a circular pattern may indicate gross alterations to corneal topography.

Reflective devices

Reflective devices measure topography based on the reflection of mires from the anterior surface tear film, which of course is essentially identical in shape to the corneal surface.

Qualitative assessment

The most basic reflective device for assessing corneal topography is the Placido disc, which is simply a series of concentric black and white rings on a flat circular disc with a central sight hole. The disc is positioned in front of the cornea and the reflections are observed. Using this method, only gross irregularities in the corneal surface and very high astigmatism can be detected. Improved versions of the Placido disc include the internally illuminated Klein keratoscope, Loveridge grid (Loveridge, 1993) and Tearscope-plus with corneal topography grid attachment (Guillon, 1997) (Figure 4.15).

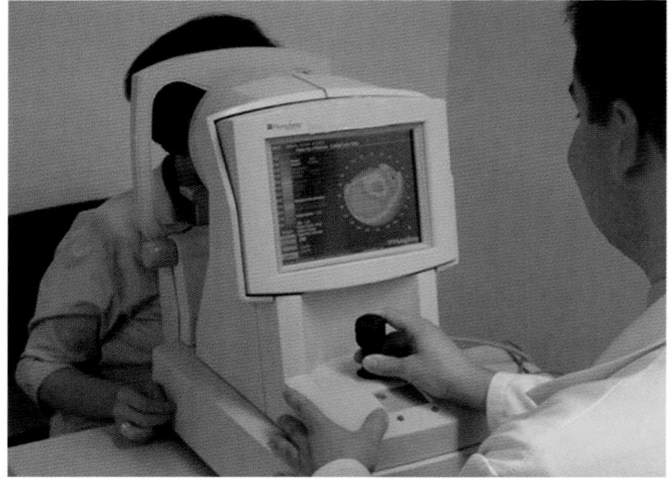

Figure 4.16 The Atlas corneal topographer from Humphrey-Zeiss. This is an example of a topographer that uses a reflective technique to obtain topographic data.

Quantitative assessment

Quantitative reflective devices (Figure 4.16) utilize the same basic principle of projecting a grid on to the cornea. The images are captured with a video camera and a computational approach is adopted to analyse the data and derive a description for the corneal shape.

The choice of computational method is important as this will largely dictate the accuracy and validity of the keratoscope. The most frequently utilized computational approach is the 'slope of surface' method, which is described in detail by Guillon and Ho (1994). Basically, devices that use this technology measure slope directly as a function of distance from a central reference axis and derive curvature from these results. It is important to note that these distance-based instruments are only estimating the average shape of the cornea, since the algorithms are based on a radially symmetrical surface, which does not accurately describe the cornea. These axial or sagittal measurements result in an underestimation of the radius of curvature in areas that may be steeper than the central cornea, and an overestimation in areas that are flatter. More recently, the algorithms have been modified and are now generally based on the radius of curvature, in an attempt to provide a better estimate of the local shape of the cornea.

The images (or 'maps') produced by reflective or Placido-based keratoscopes display the power distribution of the corneal surface using colour-coded displays, in which greens and yellows represent powers characteristic of those found in normal corneas, blues or cooler colours represent flatter areas (low powers) and reds or hotter colours represent steep areas (high powers) (Klyce *et al.*, 1998). These maps permit recognition of corneal shape through pattern recognition and swiftly reveal the presence of abnormal powers (Figure 4.17).

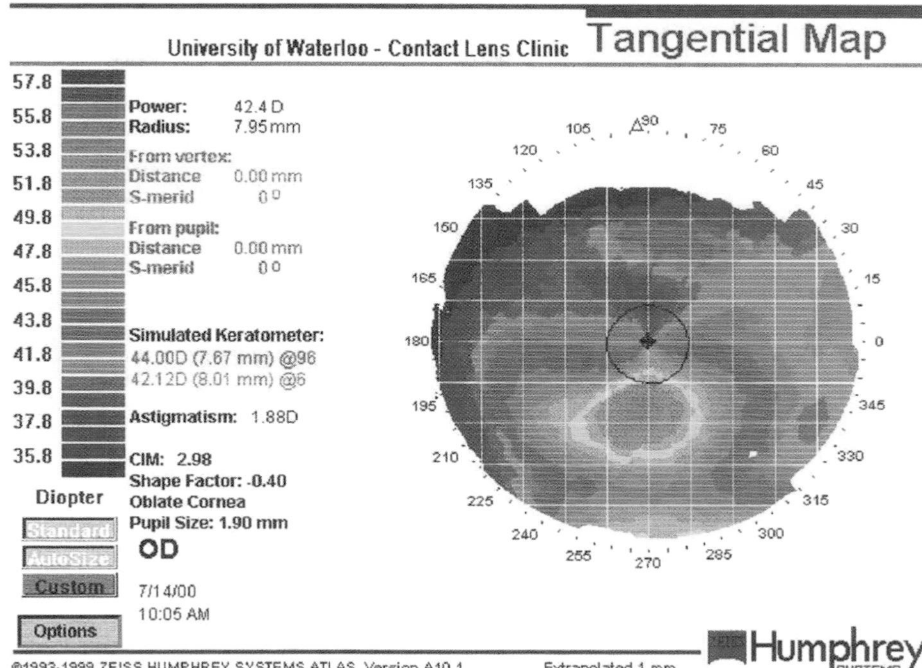

Figure 4.17 Corneal topography map of a patient with keratoconus obtained from the Atlas corneal topographer. The steep, inferiorly positioned conus is clearly seen on this tangential map.

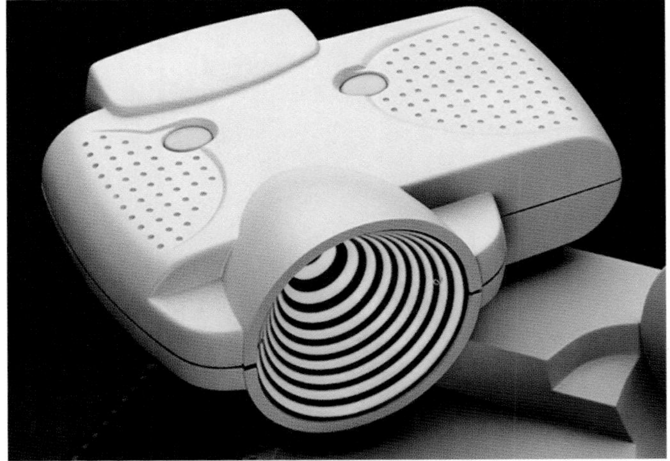

Figure 4.18 The Marco KM-500 hand-held corneal topographer.

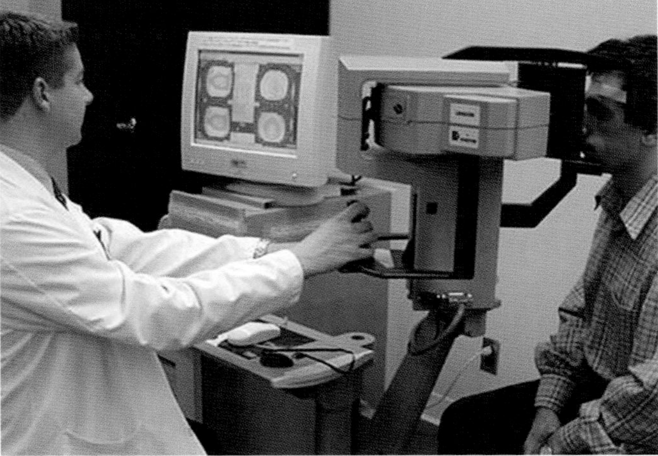

Figure 4.19 The Orbscan corneal topographer from Bausch & Lomb. This device uses a combination of reflective and slit-scanning techniques to obtain topographic and thickness data of the cornea.

All devices display simulated keratometry values, which are analogous to standard keratometry values, and simultaneously display the power and axis of the flattest meridian.

A number of manufacturers now produce hand-held topographers (Figure 4.18). These portable devices can prove very useful for examining children, the elderly and infirm, and for use in off-site consultations.

Slit-scanning devices

The latest development in corneal topography uses a slit-scanning device (the Orbscan II) to obtain topographic measurements of both anterior and posterior corneal surfaces, in addition to the anterior lens and iris (Figure 4.19).

The instrument scans across the anterior corneal surface, obtaining 40 sequential slit images, whilst simultaneously recording eye movements and reflection data from a Placido disc device. The data are then reassembled into a three-dimensional reconstruction of the anterior and posterior corneal surface. The overwhelming advantage of this system is that it allows for the measurement of multiple ocular surfaces (Liu *et al.*, 1999).

The instrument differs from traditional keratoscopes in that it uses a combination of slit-scan triangulation and surface reflection to determine corneal shape. Specifically, this instrument unifies triangulated and reflective data to obtain accurate measurements of elevation, slope and curvature. In addition to conventional axial and tangential

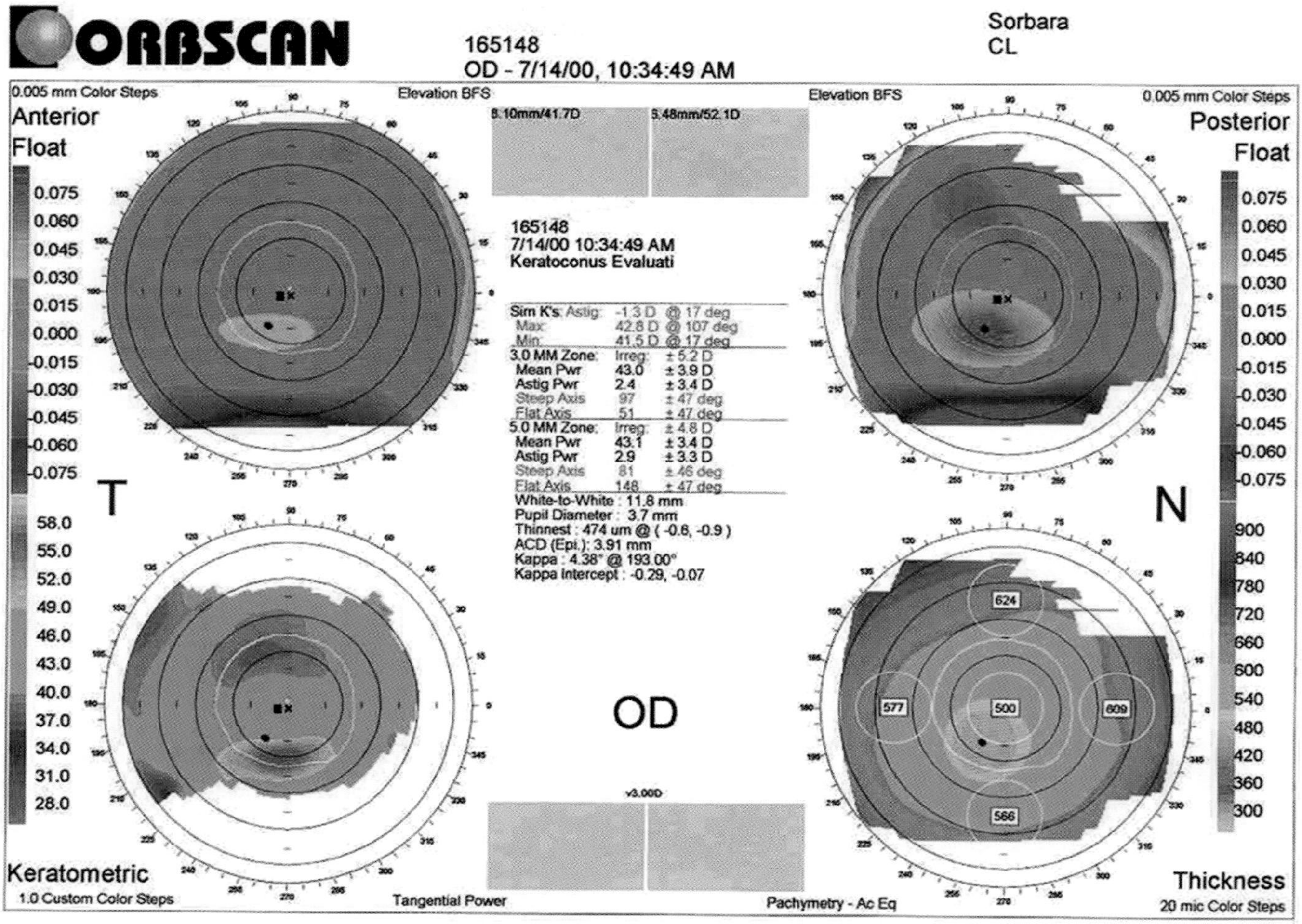

Figure 4.20 An Orbscan map of a keratoconic cornea. The top left plot describes the anterior surface shape using an elevation map and relates the shape to a reference sphere, as obtained by the Placido disc image. The bottom left plot describes the shape in terms of a tangential power plot and clearly shows the position of the conus. The top right plot describes the posterior corneal surface shape using an elevation model, derived from the slit-scanning image. The bottom right plot provides pachymetric data and indicates that the thinnest portion of the cornea is displaced inferiorly. The data in the centre provide simulated keratometry results and indicate the position and magnitude of the thinnest portion of the cornea.

maps, shape data can be displayed as an elevation map, in which the relative height of the cornea is compared to a spherical reference surface. Elevations above the reference sphere are red-coloured and depressions below the reference sphere are coloured blue (Figure 4.20).

Using such a device it has been suggested that changes in posterior corneal shape may be indicative of keratoconus prior to anterior changes being visible (Tomidokoro *et al.*, 2000). However, some authors have proposed that such findings should be interpreted with caution (Wilson, 2000).

Determination of corneal thickness

Measurement of corneal thickness is primarily used to assess corneal oedema following contact lens wear, corneal thickness prior to refractive surgery, and in keratoconic patients to monitor the progression of corneal thinning. In addition to obtaining central corneal thickness values, thickness measurements in the mid- and far-periphery of the cornea can be particularly useful in certain marginal thinning diseases. All of the techniques described below can be adapted to obtain such measurements, and these are explained in detail in the references provided.

Pachymetry

Historically, the principal instrument used to measure corneal thickness is the pachymeter, of which there are two major types, as described below.

Optical pachymetry

Optical pachymetry is based on the measurement of the apparent thickness of an optical section of the cornea, and its popularity is largely based on the commercial availability of a pachymeter attachment for the Haag–Streit slit lamp. Firstly, a split image device is inserted into one eyepiece of the slit lamp. The method depends upon the relative rotation of two glass plates, which are placed on top of each other. Rotation of the upper plate moves the upper half of the image of the cornea with respect to the fixed

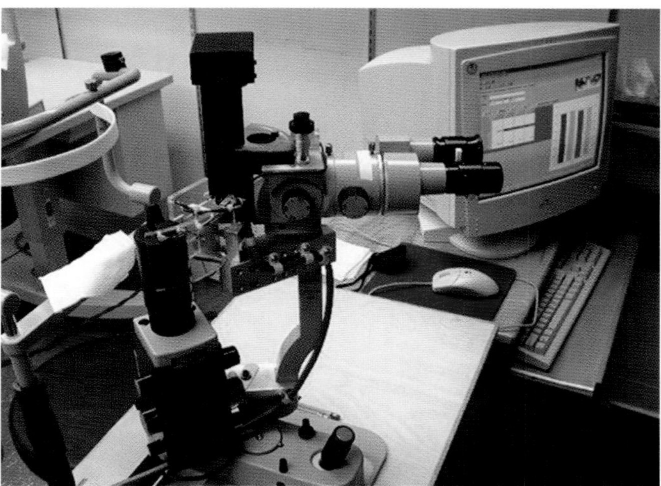

Figure 4.21 A computerized optical pachymeter. The pachymeter is connected to a potentiometer that is directly linked to a computer software program (Vistakon (division of Johnson & Johnson Vision Care)).

lower half. When the endothelium of the upper field is aligned with the epithelium of the lower field, the angle of rotation of the upper plate is read off an externally positioned scale. This measurement is proportional to the apparent thickness of the cornea, with true corneal thickness being determined by means of a conversion table.

Although perfectly acceptable for clinical purposes, the arrangement described above is too inaccurate for research purposes. A number of modifications to the technique (Chan-Ling and Pye, 1994) have resulted in an accuracy of approximately 5 μm being reported. Two such modifications include the use of two or four small light sources to ensure that the incident beam is normal to the corneal surface (Mishima and Hedbys, 1968), and an arrangement whereby the rotation of the glass plate is coupled to a potentiometer such that the angle of rotation is directly converted into an electrical signal, allowing it to be immediately input into a computer program (Figure 4.21).

This enables more rapid data collection, efficient file management and more accurate, repeatable data collection. More detailed information concerning these modifications and potential errors in optical pachymetry can be obtained from other sources (Chan-Ling and Pye, 1994; Henson, 1996a, b).

Ultrasonic pachymetry

With the rapid increase in interest in refractive surgery it has become necessary for refractive surgeons to obtain rapid, repeatable measurements of corneal thickness. In many cases this measurement is undertaken by support staff, who often have minimal slit-lamp skills. These factors have resulted in the development of simpler methods for the assessment of corneal thickness, and ultrasonic pachymetry has become the method of first choice in many practice settings.

The ultrasonic pachymeter is based on traditional A-scan ultrasonography, where the recording is in one dimension only, as compared with B-scan instruments, which provide a two-dimensional view of the eye. Ultrasound is transmitted to the eye from a transducer. Sound is reflected back to the transducer from tissue interfaces, which possess different acoustic impedances, enabling the distance from the ultrasound probe at the anterior epithelial interface to determine the distance between itself and the endothelium–aqueous interface. The transducer determines the time difference between the pulse signals obtained at the two interfaces and computes the corneal thickness based on this time delay and the velocity of sound in corneal tissue, which is approximately 1580 m/s at body temperature (Chan-Ling and Pye, 1994). A direct measurement of corneal thickness is then displayed on a digital readout.

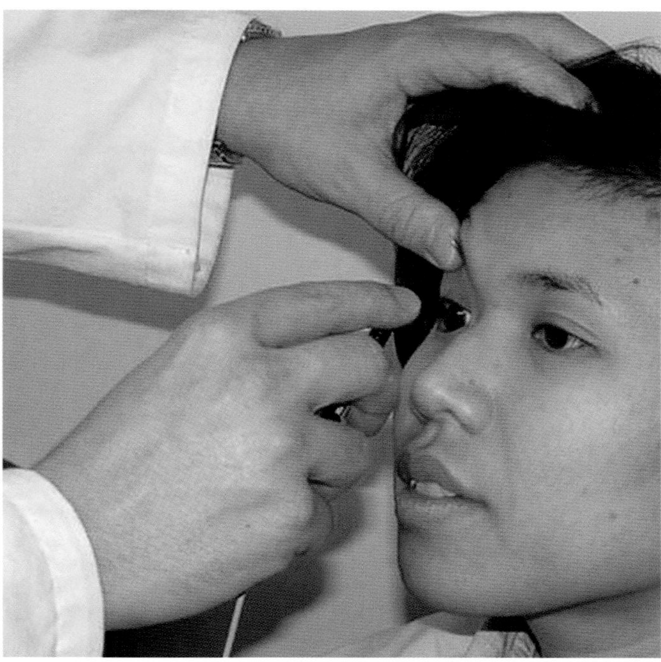

Figure 4.22 An ultrasonic pachymeter evaluation. The eye is anaesthetized and the probe touched to the cornea. Readings are digitally recorded once the angle of inclination of the probe is correct.

Prior to undertaking ultrasonic pachymetry, the cornea is anaesthetized and the patient slightly reclined (Figure 4.22).

Potential sources of error in measuring corneal thickness include holding the probe at an oblique angle to the cornea and measuring away from the central corneal apex, both of which would result in elevated readings of central corneal thickness (because corneal thickness increases from the centre to the periphery). The majority of modern instruments include a mechanism whereby a reading is not displayed if the probe is positioned such that there is excessive deviation from the perpendicular. The operator can use the pupil as a centring target, and using these adaptations the measurements obtained are valid for clinical use.

Optical coherence tomography

OCT is a relatively new non-contact optical imaging technique that is capable of high-resolution micrometer-scale cross-sectional imaging of biological tissue (Hrynchak and

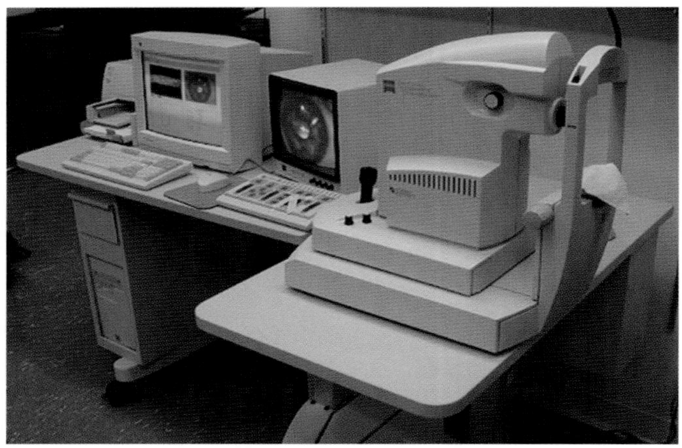

Figure 4.23 The Humphrey-Zeiss optical coherence tomographer (OCT).

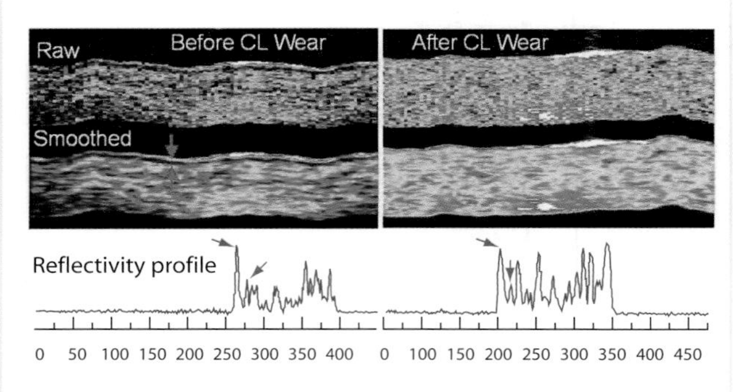

Figure 4.24 Optical coherence tomography (OCT) image, pre and post closed-eye wear of a thick poly(hydroxyethyl methacrylate) contact lens. The upper two-dimensional false-colour image indicates the plot obtained from the OCT, the smoothed image being that obtained once background noise is eliminated from the raw image. The lower plot indicates the reflectivity values obtained through the cornea. The data obtained indicate that the cornea has swollen substantially and that the water absorbed has resulted in increased thickness and reflectivity of the corneal tissue. By determining the distance between two peaks from the reflectivity profile, corneal and epithelial thickness can be obtained.

Simpson, 2000). The commercially available OCT (Figure 4.23) used for ophthalmic applications uses 843 nm wavelength near-infrared radiation, which provides a longitudinal resolution of 10–20 μm.

The technique uses Michelson interferometry to compare a partially coherent reference beam to one reflected from tissue. The two beams are combined and interference between the two light signals occurs only when their path lengths match to within the coherence length of light. The magnitude and distance within the tissue of the reflected or back-scattered light at a single point are determined using a mirror system (Izatt *et al.*, 1994; Fujimoto *et al.*, 1995, 1998). A tomographic image is generated by simultaneously displaying 100 adjacent scans, whose acquisition time is approximately 1 s. The technique of OCT is thus analogous to ultrasound B-mode imaging, except that it uses light rather than sound, and performs imaging by measuring the back-scattered intensity of light from structures within the tissue. Strong reflections occur at boundaries between materials of differing refractive indices. The OCT two-dimensional scans are subsequently processed by a computer, which corrects for any axial eye movement artefacts that have occurred during the acquisition time. The scans are displayed using a false colour representation scale in which warm colours (red to white) represent areas of high optical reflectivity, and cool colours (blue to black) represent areas of minimal optical reflectivity. The image obtained represents a cross-sectional view of the structure under investigation, similar in appearance to a histological section.

The OCT has traditionally been used to image retinal complications in which tissues have become separated or changed in structure. These include macular oedema, posterior vitreous detachment, macular holes, retinal detachment, retinoschisis and optic nerve head changes (Hrynchak and Simpson, 2000). More recently, OCT has been used to examine the cornea and has proven useful in determining epithelial and total corneal thickness changes following refractive surgery and in cases of corneal oedema (Figure 4.24), and in evaluating contact lens positioning on the ocular surface (Hrynchak and Simpson, 2000; Maldonado *et al.*, 2000; Wang *et al.*, 2002, 2006b; Haque *et al.*, 2004, 2008).

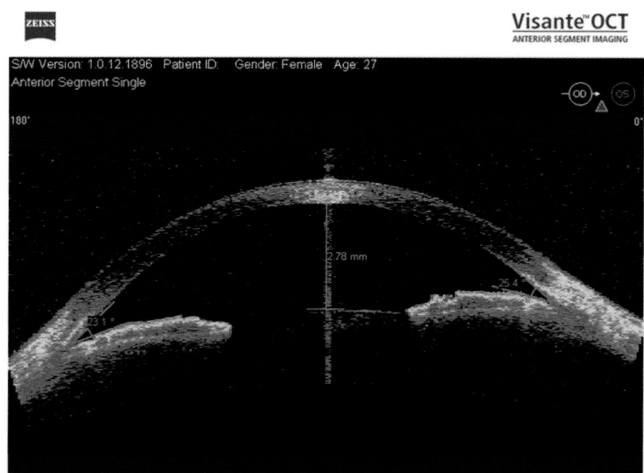

Figure 4.25 Imaging mode for the Visante optical coherence tomography (OCT), demonstrating various anterior-segment parameters.

All of the original papers using OCT to examine the anterior ocular surface relied upon the modification of OCT devices that were developed to image the retina. The recent release of the Visante anterior-segment OCT from Carl Zeiss Meditec has expanded the possibilities for examination of the anterior segment using this technology. Measurement tools incorporated into the device enable direct measurement of a variety of anterior-segment ocular structures, including corneal thickness, corneal flap thickness and residual stromal thickness following laser *in situ* keratomileusis (LASIK) surgery, anterior-chamber depth (ACD), anterior-chamber angles and anterior-chamber diameter (Figure 4.25).

Its potential value in detecting and imaging anterior-segment complications is significant (Figure 4.26).

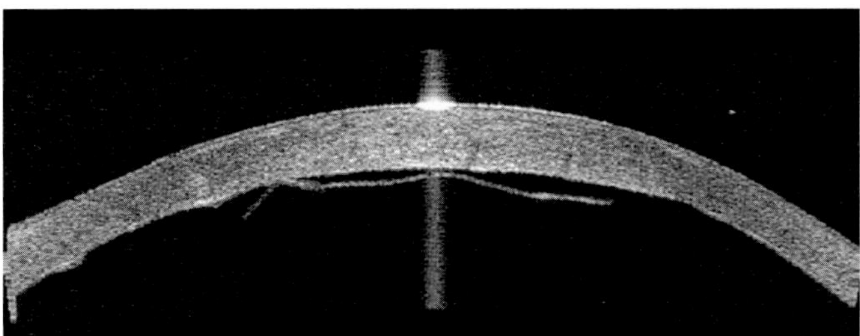

Figure 4.26 Use of the Visante optical coherence tomography (OCT) to record detachment of Descemet's membrane.

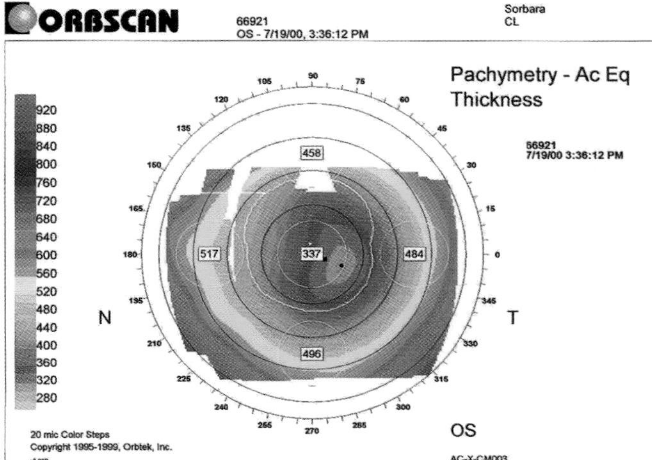

Figure 4.27 Orbscan pachymetry plot of a patient with keratoconus. The numbers represent the average thickness within the circles and clearly indicate that the corneal thinning in this patient is centralized.

In summary, OCT enables the non-excisional, *in situ*, real-time imaging of tissue microstructure, and is a powerful and promising technique for corneal imaging purposes.

Confocal microscopy

As previously described, the confocal microscope can obtain three-dimensional data by using the technique of confocal microscopy through focusing. Using a two-dimensional depth intensity profile, epithelial and corneal thickness can be estimated by measuring the distance between peaks corresponding to the epithelial and endothelial layers (Li *et al.*, 1997).

Orbscan

As previously described, in addition to assessing the shape of the anterior surface of the cornea, the Orbscan instrument determines posterior surface shape. A 'pachymetry map' (Figure 4.27) shows the differences in elevation between the anterior and posterior surfaces of the cornea.

The thickness at any point on the cornea can be determined (Liu *et al.*, 1999). The availability of full corneal pachymetry data offers significant advantages for refractive surgery, in that it allows surgeons to use regional blade settings, to measure the laser ablation depth from a fixed surface (the posterior cornea) and to assess the effect of the posterior surface on corneal power. In addition to the regular pachymetry values, the instrument calculates an 'acoustic equivalence' value, which gives theoretical ultrasound equivalence.

Conclusions

It is clear that the consulting room of the contact lens practitioner will become increasingly sophisticated as the emerging technologies described here gain increasing acceptance, leading to these instruments becoming more affordable. Notwithstanding these remarkable developments, it is likely that the slit-lamp biomicroscope will remain the cornerstone apparatus for the investigation of the contact lens-wearing eye.

Acknowledgements

We would like to thank our colleagues at the University of Waterloo – Trefford Simpson, Luigina Sorbara, Jianhua Wang, Simone Schneider and Stephanie Duench – for their assistance with the sections on non-contact aesthesiometry, OCT, confocal microscopy, HRT Rostock cornea module, topography and optical pachymetry.

References

Back, A. (1988) Corneal staining with contact lens wear. *J. Br. Contact Lens Assoc. Trans. Ann. Clin. Conf.*, **11**, 16–18.

Belmonte, C., Acosta, M. C., Schmelz, M. *et al.* (1999) Measurement of corneal sensitivity to mechanical and chemical stimulation with a CO2 esthesiometer. *Invest. Ophthalmol. Vis. Sci.*, **40**, 513–519.

Beuerman, R. W. and Pedroza, L. (1996) Ultrastructure of the human cornea. *Microsc. Res. Tech.*, **33**, 320–335.

Bitton, E., Keech, A., Simpson, T., *et al.* (2007) Variability of the analysis of the tear meniscus height by optical coherence tomography. *Optom. Vis. Sci.*, **84**, 903–908.

Böhnke, M. and Masters, B. R. (1999) Confocal microscopy of the cornea. *Prog. Retin. Eye Res.*, **18**, 553–628.

Brennan, N. and Bruce, A. (1991) Esthesiometry as an indicator of corneal health. *Optom. Vis. Sci.*, **68**, 699–702.

Brooks, A. M., Grant, G. and Gillies, W. E. (1992) Specular microscopy in the identification of deep corneal opacities. *Surv. Ophthalmol.*, **36**, 351–356.

Cavanagh, H. D., El-Agha, M. S., Petroll, W. M. *et al.* (2000) Specular microscopy, confocal microscopy, and ultrasound biomicroscopy: diagnostic tools of the past quarter century. *Cornea*, **19**, 712–722.

Chan-Ling, T. and Pye, D. (1994) Pachometry: Clinical and scientific applications. In *Contact Lens Practice*. (M. Ruben and M. Guillon, ed.) pp. 407–436, London: Chapman & Hall.

Dalton, K. and Jones, L. (2005) The performance of a novel nanolitre osmometer to investigate diurnal tear film osmolality. *Optom. Vis. Sci.*, **82**, E-abstract 055070.

Dave, T. (1998) Current developments in measurement of corneal topography. *Cont. Lens Anterior Eye,* **21,** Suppl 1, S13–30.

Doughty, M. J., Laiquzzaman, M. and Button, N. F. (2001) Video-assessment of tear meniscus height in elderly Caucasians and its relationship to the exposed ocular surface. *Curr. Eye Res.,* **22,** 420–426.

Doughty, M. J., Laiquzzaman, M., Oblak, E. *et al.* (2002) The tear (lacrimal) meniscus height in human eyes: a useful clinical measure or an unusable variable sign? *Cont. Lens Anterior Eye,* **25,** 57–65.

Eckard, A., Stave, J. and Guthoff, R. F. (2006) In vivo investigations of the corneal epithelium with the confocal Rostock Laser Scanning Microscope (RLSM). *Cornea,* **25,** 127–131.

Efron N. (2007) Contact lens-induced changes in the anterior eye as observed in vivo with the confocal microscope. *Prog. Retin. Eye Res.,* **26,** 398–436.

Efron, N., Hollingsworth, J. and Koh, H. H. (2001) Confocal microscopy. In *The Cornea: its Examination in Contact Lens Practice.* (N. Efron, ed.) pp. 86–135, Edinburgh: Butterworth-Heinemann.

Farris, R. L. (1994) Tear osmolarity–a new gold standard? *Adv. Exp. Med. Biol.,* **350,** 495–503.

Farris, R. L., Gilbard, J. P., Stuchell, R. N., *et al.* (1983) Diagnostic tests in keratoconjunctivitis sicca. *Contact Lens Assoc. Ophthalmol. J.,* **9,** 23–28.

Farris, R. L., Stuchell, R. N. and Mandel, I. D. (1986) Tear osmolarity variation in the dry eye. *Trans. Am. Ophthalmol. Soc.,* **84,** 250–268.

Francis, I. C., Chan, D. G., Papalkar, D. *et al.* (2005) Videoreflective dacryomeniscometry in normal adults and in patients with functional or primary acquired nasolacrimal duct obstruction. *Am. J. Ophthalmol.,* **139,** 493–497.

Fujimoto, J. G., Brezinski, M. E., Tearney, G. J. *et al.* (1995) Optical biopsy and imaging using optical coherence tomography. *Nat. Med.,* **1,** 970–972.

Fujimoto, J. G., Bouma, B., Tearney, G. J. *et al.* (1998) New technology for high-speed and high-resolution optical coherence tomography. *Ann. N. Y. Acad. Sci.,* **838,** 95–107.

Gilbard, J. P., Farris, R. L. and Santamaria, J., 2nd (1978) Osmolarity of tear microvolumes in keratoconjunctivitis sicca. *Arch. Ophthalmol.,* **96,** 677–681.

Gilbard, J. P., Rossi, S. R. and Gray, K. L. (1987) A new rabbit model for keratoconjunctivitis sicca. *Invest. Ophthalmol. Vis. Sci.,* **28,** 225–228.

Gilbard, J. P., Rossi, S. R. and Heyda, K. G. (1989) Tear film and ocular surface changes after closure of the meibomian gland orifices in the rabbit. *Ophthalmology,* **96,** 1180–1186.

Golding, T., Bruce, A. S. and Mainstone, J. (1997) Relationship between tear-meniscus parameters and tear-film breakup. *Cornea,* **16,** 649–661.

Guillon, J. P. (1997) The Keeler Tearscope-Plus. *Optician,* **213**(5594), 66–72.

Guillon, M. and Ho, A. (1994) Photokeratoscopy. In *Contact Lens Practice.* (M. Ruben and M. Guillon, ed.) pp. 313–357, London: Chapman & Hall Medical.

Guillon, M., Styles, E., Guillon, J., *et al.* (1997) Preocular tear film characteristics of nonwearers and soft contact lens wearers. *Optom. Vis. Sci.,* **74,** 273–279.

Haque, S., Fonn, D., Simpson, T., *et al.* (2004) Corneal and epithelial thickness changes after 4 weeks of overnight corneal refractive therapy lens wear, measured with optical coherence tomography. *Eye Contact Lens,* **30,** 189–193; discussion 205-186.

Haque, S., Jones, L. and Simpson, T. (2008) Thickness mapping of the cornea and epithelium using optical coherence tomography. *Optom. Vis. Sci.,* **85,** 963–976.

Henson, D. (1996a) Keratometry. In *Optometric Instrumentation.* (D. Henson, ed.) pp. 107–137, Oxford: Butterworth-Heinemann.

Henson, D. (1996b) Slit lamps. In *Optometric Instrumentation.* (D. Henson, ed.) pp. 138–161, Oxford: Butterworth-Heinemann.

Hirji, N., Patel, S. and Callander, M. (1989) Human tear film pre-rupture phase time (TP-RPT)–a non-invasive technique for evaluating the pre-corneal tear film using a novel keratometer mire. *Ophthalmic Physiol. Opt.,* **9,** 139–142.

Ho, S. M. and Brennan, N. A. (1993) Corneal sensitivity and contact lens wear. *Invest. Ophthalmol. Vis. Sci. (Suppl.),* **34,** 1007.

Hodson, S. A. and Sherrard, E. S. (1988) The specular microscope: its impact on laboratory and clinical studies of the cornea. *Eye,* **2,** Suppl., S81–97.

Holly, F. J. (1985) Physical chemistry of the normal and disordered tear film. *Trans. Ophthalmol. Soc. U. K.,* **104, (**Pt 4), 374–380.

Holly, F. J. and Lemp, M. A. (1977) Tear physiology and dry eyes. *Surv. Ophthalmol.,* **22,** 69–87.

Hrynchak, P. and Simpson, T. (2000) Optical coherence tomography: an introduction to the technique and its use. *Optom. Vis. Sci.,* **77,** 347–356.

Izatt, J. A., Hee, M. R., Swanson, E. A. *et al.* (1994) Micrometer-scale resolution imaging of the anterior eye in vivo with optical coherence tomography. *Arch. Ophthalmol.,* **112,** 1584–1589.

Johnson, M. E. and Murphy, P. J. (2005) The agreement and repeatability of tear meniscus height measurement methods. *Optom. Vis. Sci.,* **82,** 1030–1037.

Jones, L. and Jones, D. (2000) *Common Contact Lens Complications.* Oxford: Butterworth-Heinemann.

Jones, L., Leech, R., Rahman, S. *et al.* (2002) A novel method to determine tear prism height. *Optom. Vis. Sci.,* **79,** Suppl, 252.

Jones L, Rahman S, Leech R, *et al.* (2004) Determination of inferior tear meniscus height and inferior tear meniscus volume using optical coherence tomography. *ARVO* e-abstract 144.

Khanal, S., Tomlinson, A., McFadyen, A. *et al.* (2008) Dry eye diagnosis. *Invest. Ophthalmol. Vis. Sci.,* **49,** 1407–1414.

Klyce, S., Maeda, N. and Byrd, T. (1998) Corneal topography. In *The Cornea.* (H. Kaufman, B. Barron and M. McDonald, ed.) pp. 1055–1075, Oxford: Butterworth-Heinemann.

Klyce, S. D. (2001) Corneal topography. In *The Cornea: its Examination in Contact Lens Practice.* (N. Efron, ed.) pp. 178–199, Oxford: Butterworth-Heinemann.

Lamberts, D. W., Foster, C. S. and Perry, H. D. (1979) Schirmer test after topical anesthesia and the tear meniscus height in normal eyes. *Arch. Ophthalmol.,* **97,** 1082–1085.

Lemp, M. A. (1995) Report of the National Eye Institute/Industry workshop on Clinical Trials in Dry Eyes. *Contact Lens Assoc. Ophthalmol. J.,* **21,** 221–232.

Li, H. F., Petroll, W. M., Moller-Pedersen, T., *et al.* (1997) Epithelial and corneal thickness measurements by in vivo confocal microscopy through focusing (CMTF). *Curr. Eye Res.,* **16,** 214–221.

Lim, K. J. and Lee, J. H. (1991) Measurement of the tear meniscus height using 0.25% fluorescein sodium. *Korean J. Ophthalmol.,* **5,** 34–36.

Liu, Z., Huang, A. J. and Pflugfelder, S. C. (1999) Evaluation of corneal thickness and topography in normal eyes using the Orbscan corneal topography system. *Br. J. Ophthalmol.,* **83,** 774–778.

Loveridge, R. (1993) Breaking up is hard to do? *J. Br. Contact Lens Assoc.,* **16,** 51–55.

Mainstone, J. C., Bruce, A. S. and Golding, T. R. (1996) Tear meniscus measurement in the diagnosis of dry eye. *Curr. Eye Res.,* **15,** 653–661.

Maldonado, M. J., Ruiz-Oblitas, L., Munuera, J. M. *et al.* (2000) Optical coherence tomography evaluation of the corneal cap and stromal bed features after laser in situ keratomileusis for high myopia and astigmatism. *Ophthalmology,* **107,** 81–87; discussion 88.

Mandell, R. (1996) A guide to videokeratography. *Int. Contact Lens Clin.,* **23,** 205–228.

Mandell, R. B. (1992) Everett Kinsey Lecture. The enigma of the corneal contour. *Contact Lens Assoc. Ophthalmol. J.,* **18,** 267–273.

Masters, B., Thaer, A. and Geyer, O. (1994) Real time confocal microscopy of the *in vivo* human cornea. In *Contact Lens Practice.* (M. Ruben and M. Guillon, ed.) pp. 389–406, London: Chapman & Hall Medical.

Mengher, L. S., Bron, A. J., Tonge, S. R., *et al.* (1985) Effect of fluorescein instillation on the pre-corneal tear film stability. *Curr. Eye Res.,* **4,** 9–12.

Miller, W. L., Narayanan, S., Jackson, J. *et al.* (2003) The association of bulbar conjunctival folds with other clinical findings in normal and moderate dry eye subjects. *Optometry,* **74,** 576–582.

Miller, W. L., Doughty, M. J., Narayanan, S. *et al.* (2004) A comparison of tear volume (by tear meniscus height and phenol red thread test) and tear fluid osmolality measures in non-lens wearers and in contact lens wearers. *Eye Contact Lens,* **30,** 132–137.

Millodot, M. (1994) Aesthesiometry. In *Contact Lens Practice.* (M. Ruben and M. Guillon, ed.) pp. 437–452, London: Chapman & Hall.

Mishima, S. and Hedbys, B. O. (1968) Measurement of corneal thickness with the Haag-Streit pachometer. *Arch. Ophthalmol.,* **80,** 710–713.

Moller-Pedersen, T., Vogel, M., Li, H. F. *et al.* (1997) Quantification of stromal thinning, epithelial thickness, and corneal haze after photorefractive keratectomy using in vivo confocal microscopy. *Ophthalmology,* **104,** 360–368.

Murphy, P. J., Lawrenson, J. G., Patel, S. *et al.* (1998) Reliability of the non-contact corneal aesthesiometer and its comparison with the Cochet-Bonnet aesthesiometer. *Ophthalmic Physiol. Opt.,* **18,** 532–539.

Nelson, J. D. and Wright, J. C. (1986) Tear film osmolality determination: an evaluation of potential errors in measurement. *Curr. Eye Res.,* **5,** 677–681.

Nichols, K. K., Mitchell, G. L. and Zadnik, K. (2004) The repeatability of clinical measurements of dry eye. *Cornea,* **23,** 272–285.

Oguz, H., Yokoi, N. and Kinoshita, S. (2000) The height and radius of the tear meniscus and methods for examining these parameters. *Cornea,* **19,** 497–500.

Papas, E. B. and Vajdic, C. M. (2000) Inter-ocular characteristics of the pre-contact lens tear film. *Curr. Eye Res.,* **20,** 248–250.

Patel, S. and Blades, K. (2003) Assessment of Tear Volume. In *The Dry eye: A practical Approach,* (S. Patel and K. Blades, eds), pp. 37–41, Boston: Butterworth-Heinemann.

Patel, S. and Port, M. J. (1991) Tear characteristics of the VDU operator. *Optom. Vis. Sci.,* **68,** 798–800.

Patel, S. and Wallace, I. (2006) Tear meniscus height, lower punctum lacrimale, and the tear lipid layer in normal aging. *Optom. Vis. Sci.,* **83,** 731–739.

Port, M. J. and Asaria, T. S. (1990) Assessment of human tear volume. *J. Br. Contact Lens Assoc.,* **13,** 76–82.

Santodomingo-Rubido, J., Wolffsohn, J. and Gilmartin, B. (2006) Comparison between graticule and image capture assessment of lower tear film meniscus height. *Cont. Lens Anterior Eye,* **29,** 169–173.

Savini, G., Barboni, P. and Zanini, M. (2006) Tear meniscus evaluation by optical coherence tomography. *Ophthalmic Surg. Lasers Imaging,* **37,** 112–118.

Shen, M., Li, J., Wang, J., *et al.* (2009) Upper and lower tear menisci in the diagnosis of dry eye. *Invest. Ophthalmol. Vis. Sci.* **50,** 2722–2726.

Situ, P., Simpson, T. L. and Fonn, D. (2007) Eccentric variation of corneal sensitivity to pneumatic stimulation at different temperatures and with CO_2. *Exp. Eye Res.,* **85,** 400–405.

Stave, J., Zinser, G., Grummer, G. *et al.* (2002) [Modified Heidelberg Retinal Tomograph HRT. Initial results of in vivo presentation of corneal structures]. *Ophthalmologe,* **99,** 276–280.

Stone, J. and Rabbetts, R. (1994) Keratometry and specialist optical instrumentation. In *Contact Lens Practice.* (M. Ruben and M. Guillon, eds). pp. 283–311, London: Chapman & Hall.

Sullivan, B. (2005) Clinical resorts of a first generation lab-on-chip nanolitre tear film osmometer. *Ocul Surf,* **3,** s31.

Tomidokoro, A., Oshika, T., Amano, S., *et al.* (2000) Changes in anterior and posterior corneal curvatures in keratoconus. *Ophthalmology,* **107,** 1328–1332.

Tomlinson, A., Blades, K. J. and Pearce, E. I. (2001) What does the phenol red thread test actually measure? *Optom. Vis. Sci.,* **78,** 142–146.

Tomlinson, A. and Khanal, S. (2005) Assessment of tear film dynamics: quantification approach. *The Ocular Surface,* **3,** 81–95.

Vega, J. A., Simpson, T. L. and Fonn, D. (1999) A noncontact pneumatic esthesiometer for measurement of ocular sensitivity: a preliminary report. *Cornea,* **18,** 675–681.

Veys, J. and Davies, I. (1995) Assessment of corneal contour. *Optician,* **209**(5487), 22–27.

Wang, J., Fonn, D., Simpson, T. L. *et al.* (2002) Relation between optical coherence tomography and optical pachymetry measurements of corneal swelling induced by hypoxia. *Am. J. Ophthalmol.,* **134,** 93–98.

Wang, J., Aquavella, J., Palakuru, J. *et al.* (2006a) Repeated measurements of dynamic tear distribution on the ocular surface after instillation of artificial tears. *Invest. Ophthalmol. Vis. Sci.,* **47,** 3325–3329.

Wang, J., Thomas, J. and Cox, I. (2006b) Corneal light backscatter measured by optical coherence tomography after LASIK. *J. Refract. Surg.*, **22,** 604–610.

White, K. M., Benjamin, W. J. and Hill, R. M. (1993) Human basic tear fluid osmolality. I. Importance of sample collection strategy. *Acta Ophthalmol. (Copenh),* **71,** 524–529.

Wilson, S. E. (2000) Cautions regarding measurements of the posterior corneal curvature [editorial]. *Ophthalmology,* **107,** 1223.

Xu, K. P., Yagi, Y. and Tsubota, K. (1996) Decrease in corneal sensitivity and change in tear function in dry eye. *Cornea,* **15,** 235–239.

Yokoi, N., Kinoshita, S., Bron, A. J. *et al.* (2000) Tear meniscus changes during cotton thread and Schirmer testing. *Invest. Ophthalmol. Vis. Sci.,* **41,** 3748–3753.

Zantos, S. and Cox, I. (1994) Anterior ocular microscopy – part 1: Biomicroscopy. In *Contact Lens Practice.* (M. Ruben and M. Guillon, eds). pp. 359–388, London: Chapman & Hall.

PART: II

Soft contact lenses

CHAPTER 5

Soft lens materials

Carole Maldonado-Codina

Introduction

Soft contact lenses have had a massive impact on the global contact lens market since they became widely available in the early 1970s. Since their introduction, the number of soft contact lenses being prescribed around the world has steadily increased and it is mainly the sale of soft contact lenses which is responsible for an industry which is estimated to be worth around US$ 8 billion annually (this figure does not include the sale of contact lens solutions). A recent survey has indicated that soft lenses currently make up over 90% of all new contact lens fittings worldwide (Morgan *et al.*, 2009).

The saturation of the contact lens market with soft lenses has occurred primarily for two reasons. Firstly, soft lenses provide wearers with what they see as the two most important requirements for successful contact lens wear – good vision and good comfort. The major obstacle as far as rigid lenses are concerned is generally accepted as being their lack of comfort and, in particular, their initial discomfort (Polse *et al.*, 1999). Secondly, advances in manufacturing technology have directed the industry towards soft lenses, and still further, have directed it towards the concept of disposability.

Contact lens materials (both soft and rigid) are good examples of biomaterials. A biomaterial may be defined as a natural or synthetic material that is suitable for introduction into living tissue, especially as part of a medical device. The term encompasses a vast array of technologies, including tissue engineering, artificial organs, bioceramics, medical devices and implantable drug delivery systems. Contact lenses are classed as a medical device in most countries.

Very few of us are likely to get through life without having some kind of biomaterial introduced into our bodies. The most common examples in use today include dental fillings, contact lenses, intraocular lenses, heart valves, stents and the ubiquitous breast implant. This list in itself highlights just how diverse biomaterials must be in order to satisfy their very specific end application – for example, a contact lens material has very different properties to a material used for dental fillings.

If a biomaterial is to be successful in its application, it follows that it must also be biocompatible. Biocompatibility refers to the ability of a material to perform with an appropriate host response in a specific application. An 'appropriate host response' would include not having toxic or injurious effects on biological systems. Biomaterials manufactured for use as contact lenses must not only satisfy all these requirements for safe use within the eye but additionally they must also have very specific characteristics such as being transparent (and remain so on-eye), be comfortable and be relatively cheap to manufacture.

This chapter will review the building blocks, properties and characteristics of the materials which are used to manufacture soft contact lenses and provides some of the history of development of these materials. Most students and clinicians are familiar with the United States Adopted Name (USAN) of a particular lens material, e.g. etafilcon A or lotrafilcon A, but any further understanding about the material is generally lacking. This chapter aims to give meaning and background to these USAN names in order to help the reader understand and differentiate between different soft lens materials.

Polymers

All contact lens materials may be classified as polymers. The word 'polymer' is derived from ancient Greek, meaning 'many parts'. Polymers are solid materials (as opposed to gases or liquids) which are made up of high-molecular-weight chains (i.e. long chains) which in turn are made up from small repeating units. These repeating units are called monomers. Polymers are macromolecules (giant molecules) made from thousands of atoms. The term 'polymer' is therefore an umbrella term for materials which include plastics (e.g. polymethyl methacrylate (PMMA), used in the manufacture of 'hard' rigid lenses), fibres (e.g. nylon), elastomers (i.e. rubbers such as silicone rubber) and the materials being discussed in this chapter – hydrogels.

The term 'hydrogel' is often used interchangeably with the term 'soft' when referring to contact lenses. Soft lenses are so named because they are made from water-swollen, cross-linked, hydrophilic polymers which are flexible and

DOI: 10.1016/B978-0-7506-8869-7.00005-7

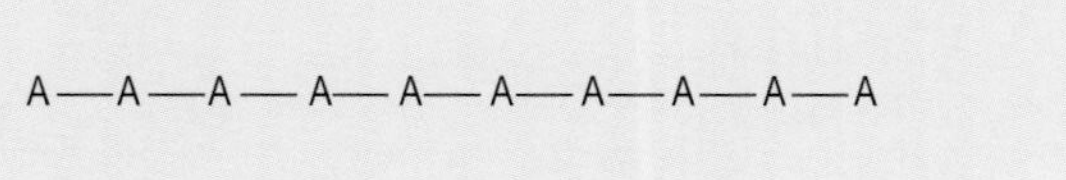

Figure 5.1 Linear homopolymer.

compliant. The term 'hydrophilic' is used to describe the fact that the networks from which these materials are made are 'water-loving'.

The widespread use of polymers in many areas of our everyday lives has become a common and accepted phenomenon – so much so that they have been referred to as the 'steel of the 21st century'. Polymers possess many properties which make them suitable for a wide range of applications, some of which are unique. These properties are in part due to the length of the molecules they are made from. Additionally, polymers also derive their unique characteristics from the ability of certain atoms to join together to form stable covalent bonds.

Many polymers are composed of hydrocarbons, i.e. carbon (C) and hydrogen (H) alone, such as polyethylene and polystyrene. However, even though the basic make-up of many polymers is carbon and hydrogen, other elements can also be involved. Oxygen (O), nitrogen (N), chlorine (Cl), fluorine (F) and silicon (Si) are other elements commonly found in the molecular make-up of polymers. Many polymers have carbon backbones (these are considered organic polymers) but some can also have silicon or phosphorous backbones (these are considered inorganic polymers).

The kinds of atoms making up a polymer as well as their geometric arrangement give each polymer its chemical distinctiveness, and thus, its particular use and function. Polymers themselves may be completely natural (e.g. cellulose), partly natural (e.g. cellulose acetate) or completely synthetic (e.g. PMMA). Most of the polymers used in the manufacture of soft contact lenses fall into this last category, i.e. they are man-made.

The structure of polymers

A polymer chain can be described by specifying the kind of repeating units present and their spatial arrangement. In this way, several broad categories of polymer can be described.

A homopolymer is one in which only one type of monomer is used, i.e. the units are chemically and stereochemically identical, with the exception of the end units. If the chain units are arranged in a linear sequence the polymer is referred to as a linear homopolymer. This is shown schematically in Figure 5.1. Departures from this simple array lead to structures of increasing geometric complexity. A non-linear or branched structure is shown in Figure 5.2.

The chemical differences between linear and branched polymers may be quite small, yet, because of the structural differences, the two molecules can have quite markedly different properties. A good example of these differences is found between low-density polyethylene (branched) and high-density polyethylene (linear). Low-density polyethylene is commonly used as a packaging film, e.g. cling film and for carrier bags, whereas high-density polyethylene is used for making pipes and durable plastic bottles because of its higher impact strength.

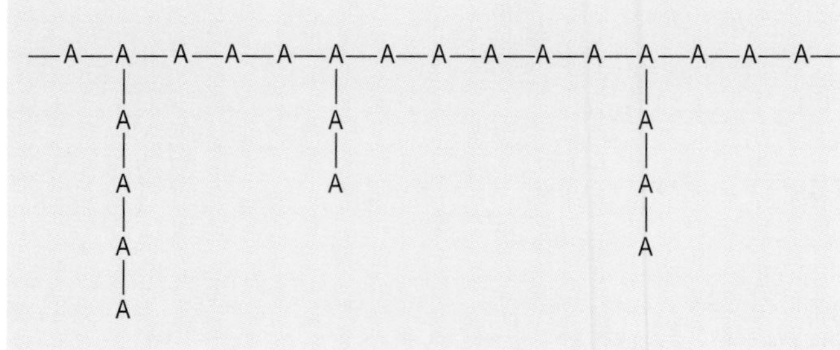

Figure 5.2 Branched homopolymer.

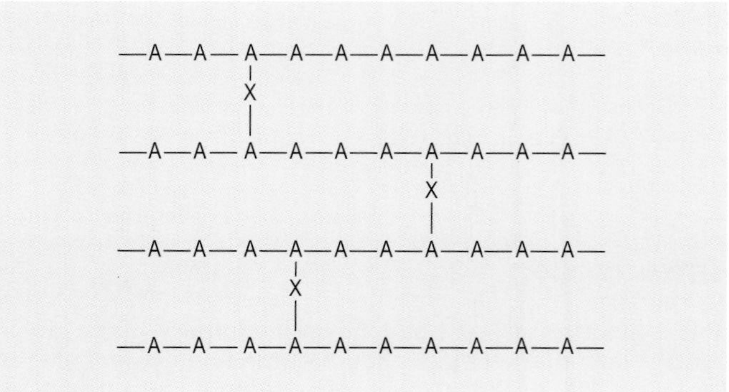

Figure 5.3 Cross-linked system.

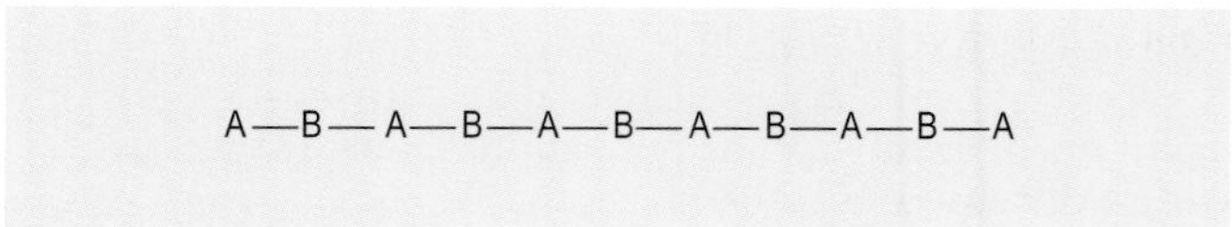

Figure 5.4 Alternating copolymer.

Non-linear and network structures can also be prepared from a collection of linear chains by covalently linking together chain units selected from different molecules. Such a system is said to be cross-linked. This is shown schematically in Figure 5.3. Here, X represents the chemical species (the cross-linker) that covalently links together the A units from different molecular chains. When a sufficient number of units are intermolecularly cross-linked, then an infinite network is formed. A cross-linker is an important ingredient in a soft contact lens monomer mix, which will be discussed later.

A copolymer is one in which more than one type of monomer is used. The properties of a copolymer depend not only on the chemical nature and amounts of the co-units, but also very markedly on how the units are distributed along the chain. For linear copolymers, three 'ideal' arrangements can be described. The first is an alternating copolymer of A and B, which is shown in Figure 5.4. In this scenario, each monomer prefers to react with the fellow monomer rather than itself.

At the opposite extreme is the ordered or block copolymer, where there is an overwhelming tendency for a unit to be succeeded by another of the same kind. Here, long

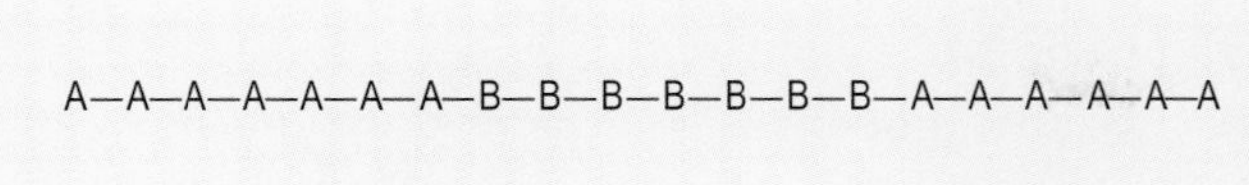

Figure 5.5 Block copolymer.

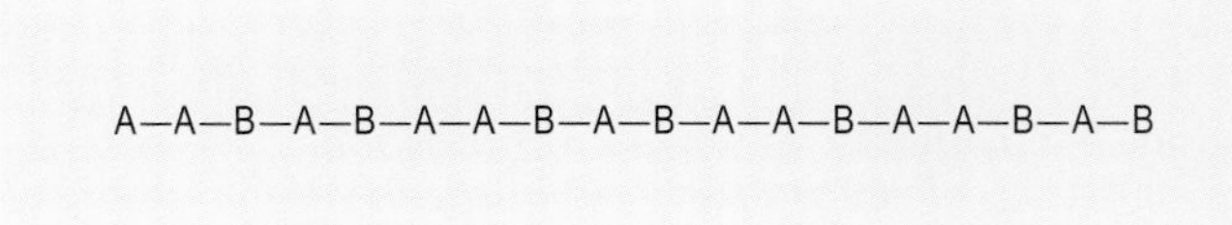

Figure 5.6 Random copolymer.

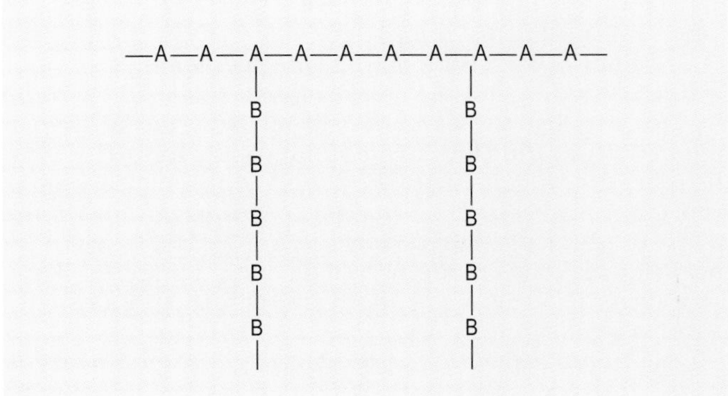

Figure 5.7 Graft copolymer.

sequences of one type of unit alternate with long sequences of the other kind (Figure 5.5).

The third major classification is the random copolymer. Here, different units are randomly distributed along the chain (Figure 5.6).

Departing from the restrictions of a linear array, branched copolymers, known as 'graft polymers', can also be prepared. The backbone of the molecule is composed of one type of unit, and the long side chains, or graft, are made up of another. More sophisticated types of graft polymers have backbones made up of different repeating units and several distinctly chemically different side groups. This type of polymer is represented schematically in Figure 5.7.

One final important classification is that of polymers into either amorphous or crystalline polymers (i.e. their macromolecular order) (Figure 5.8). Crystalline polymers have a geometrically regular structure and are generally stiff, resistant to chemicals and tough. They have limited use as materials for contact lenses due mainly to their poor optical qualities, i.e. they tend to be translucent and opaque. A good example of a semicrystalline polymer is polypropylene, which is often used to make the casts in the cast-moulded manufacturing process of contact lenses.

Amorphous polymers, on the other hand, do not have a regular structure. The polymer chains intermingle and are in random positions (imagine a pile of spaghetti on a plate), which gives these polymers better optical properties, i.e. they are usually transparent. Depending on their chain mobility, amorphous polymers can be classified as either 'plastic' or 'glassy' (Tighe, 1997).

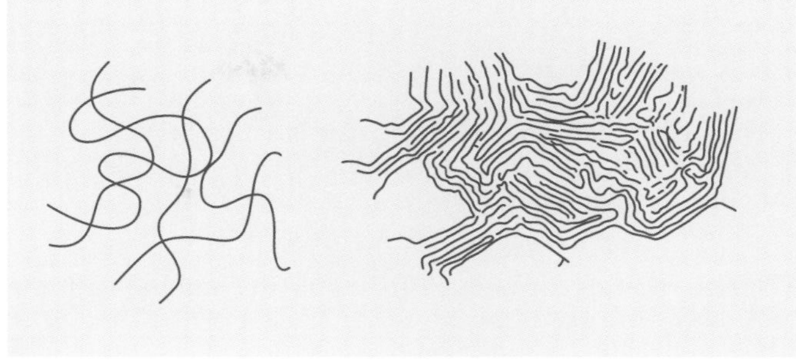

Figure 5.8 Schematic representation of macromolecular order showing an amorphous polymer (left) and a crystalline polymer (right). (Redrawn from Kastl, P. R., Refojo, M. F. and Dabezies, O. H. (1984) Review of polymerisation for the contact lens fitter. The CLAO Guide to Basic Science and Clinical Science. O. H. Dabezies. Grune & Stratton Inc., Orlando, USA.)

Polymerization

The chemical reaction which monomers undergo in order to form long-chained polymers is known as polymerization. Broadly speaking, monomers can be chemically joined together in two ways: by step growth (condensation) or chain growth (addition) processes. Condensation polymers are produced by the reaction of monomeric units with each other, resulting in the elimination of a small molecule, e.g. water. However, hydrogels are generally formed through chain growth (addition) polymerization.

Before entering into the intricacies of polymerization it is important to establish that in order to make a contact lens material, the following three basic 'ingredients' are required in the monomer 'mix': (1) the monomer(s); (2) a cross-linking agent; and (3) an initiator. In some cases a solvent is also added to the monomer mix. A solvent is used when lenses are manufactured by 'wet-casting', where the solvent is gradually replaced with saline. If a solvent is not used, the manufacturing process is often referred to as a 'dry casting', i.e. the contact lens is cast as a xerogel.

Chain polymerization

The monomers used in chain polymerization are unsaturated and are sometimes referred to as vinyl monomers. Essentially this means that the monomer has one or more carbon-to-carbon double bonds. During the polymerization process the monomer concentration decreases steadily with time, resulting in a reaction mixture that contains monomer, high-molar-mass polymer and a low concentration of growing chains. Chain polymerization is characterized by three distinct stages: initiation, propagation and termination.

Initiation

A hydrogel monomer mixture usually contains an initiator. This is a chemical whose role is to start off the polymerization process. Initiators readily fragment into free radicals (a highly chemically reactive atom, molecule or molecular fragment with a free or unpaired electron) when activated by heat or some other form of radiation, e.g. ultraviolet light.

The type of initiator used will depend on the manufacturing method. For example, a thermal initiator would usually be required in the manufacture of buttons or rods which will eventually form lathed lenses and a photo initiator would usually be required for spun-cast and cast-moulded lenses.

The fragmentation of the initiator is schematically represented by the following equation, where *I* represents the initiator molecule and $I^\bullet$ represents a free radical.

$$I - I \xrightarrow{\Delta} 2I^\bullet$$

The free radicals formed are then able to combine with the monomer (*M*), resulting in a free radical of the monomer (this is why the polymerization of hydrogels is sometimes referred to as free radical polymerization):

$$I^\bullet + M \rightarrow IM^\bullet$$

Propagation

The monomer radical, which is a transient compound, is now able to combine with another monomer unit, resulting in another new compound:

$$IM^\bullet + M \rightarrow IMM^\bullet$$

By the continuation of this process, the polymer chain is propagated. The resultant chain may consist of thousands of monomer units:

$$IM_n^\bullet + M \rightarrow IM^\bullet_{(n+1)}$$

Termination

Polymerization does not usually continue until all of the monomer has been used up because the free radicals involved are so reactive that they inevitably find a variety of ways of losing their reactivity. Polymerization can be terminated in two main ways. The first method is recombination. This occurs when two growing molecules containing free radicals meet, share their unpaired electrons and so form a stable covalent bond, thereby extinguishing their reactivity. The second method of termination is known as disproportionation. This occurs when two radicals interact via hydrogen abstraction, leading to the formation of two reaction products, one of which is saturated and one of which is unsaturated.

The conditions under which polymerization take place become important when one considers that soft contact lenses are currently made using three main methods of manufacture: lathing, spin-casting and cast-moulding. Lenses made by these different methods of manufacture will undergo very different polymerization conditions which are likely to have an effect on the resultant material. How a material is processed is likely to affect almost every aspect of a lens, from its clinical performance to its physical and chemical properties (Maldonado-Codina and Efron, 2004).

Properties of hydrogel materials

The ocular environment places significant demands on the performance of hydrogels as biomaterials. These materials must:

- Maintain a stable, continuous tear film.
- Be permeable to oxygen in order to maintain normal corneal metabolism.
- Be permeable to ions in order to maintain on-eye movement.
- Be comfortable.
- Provide clear, stable vision.

These essential properties are expanded upon below.

Optical transparency

A hydrogel to be used as a contact lens material needs to be transparent in order to achieve maximal visual performance. The light transmittance of polymers includes the description of materials as being transparent, translucent or opaque. Transparent polymers are those that you can see through, translucent polymers are those that you cannot see through but allow light to pass through and opaque polymers are those that you can neither see through nor allow light to pass through. Usually the optical clarity of contact lens materials is expressed as the percentage of transmission of the visible electromagnetic spectrum. Hydrogels which are useful as contact lens materials transmit over 90% of light in the visible part of the spectrum.

When a hydrogel loses its transparency it is likely to be due to microphase separation of water. This is due to regions of differing refractive index being formed within the gel. Hydrogels that show this type of behaviour (typically synthesized by making copolymers with large blocks or segments of hydrophobic and hydrophilic monomers rather than randomly dispersing them) do have advantages in terms of enhanced strength and permeability performance.

If the phase separation is limited (e.g. the phase size is shorter than the wavelength of light), transparent materials can still be obtained. Some hydrogels are known to lose their transparency when heated and this is an important consideration as there is an increase in temperature from lens packaging to eye and, additionally, some subjects still thermally disinfect their lenses, although this practice is seldom employed today.

Trying to combine hydrophilic conventional hydrogel monomers and hydrophobic silicone-based monomers into transparent hydrogels has been a major technical difficulty in the development of successful silicone hydrogel materials. Tighe (2004) likens this technical challenge to trying to mix oil with water.

Mechanical properties

The mechanical properties of hydrogel contact lenses are fundamentally important because they are directly related to factors such as the comfort, visual performance, fitting characteristics, physiological impact, durability and handleability of the lenses.

In the hydrated state most hydrogels are soft and flexible. When they are allowed to dehydrate they become hard and brittle. Lower-water-content polymers tend to become more hard and brittle than higher-water-content materials. Hydrogels take up water because they are hydrophilic, i.e. hydrogels swell in water (as well as many other liquids), which causes them to become soft with elastic properties (the water acts as a plasticizer).

Unlike perfectly elastic materials which deform under stress but return to their original size and shape when the stress is released, hydrogels are viscoelastic. This means that they deform time-dependently when a stress is applied to them and recover time-dependently when the stress is

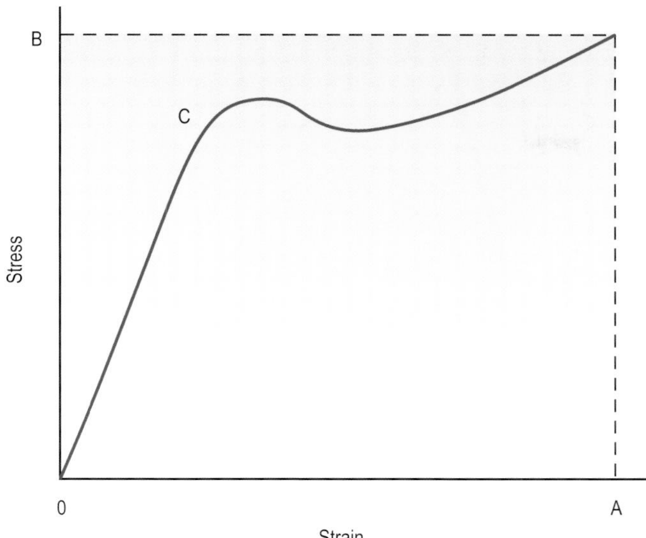

Figure 5.9 Typical tensile stress–strain curve for a theoretical material. Point *A* on the graph represents the elongation at break, point *B* represents the ultimate strength and point *C* represents the yield point of the material. A typical soft lens hydrogel does not demonstrate a yield; instead, it would break at point *C* on the graph.

removed. Theoretically, this can result in permanent deformation of the material.

One of the main difficulties in characterizing the mechanical properties of a contact lens is that there is no single property measurement which will accurately reflect its 'in-use' situation. Traditional material mechanical testing involves applying a deforming force (the 'stress') to a sample and observing the way that the sample responds (the 'strain').

Stress can be compression, tensile or shear. Compression is a stress that acts to shorten an object. Tension is a stress that acts to lengthen an object. Shear is a stress that acts parallel to a surface. Strain is defined as the amount of deformation an object undergoes compared to its original size and shape. When a tensile stress is applied to a material, the stress gradually builds up until the specimen breaks (fractures).

Some materials will go through a yield point (Figure 5.9), which is defined as the stress at which a material begins to deform plastically. Contact lens hydrogels typically do not demonstrate a yield point. A generalized stress–strain curve is shown in Figure 5.9 and provides several mechanical characteristics of the material under test. The strength of a material is defined as the force per cross-sectional unit area required to cause failure when the sample is subjected to a particular type of stress.

Young's modulus (E) or the elastic modulus is determined by the initial slope of the stress–strain curve and is, therefore, a constant (i.e. it is the stress divided by the strain). The Young's modulus and the thickness of the material (t) are related together in determining the stiffness of a lens. Just as Dk/t indicates the relative transmissibility of different lenses, so the stiffness factor multiplied by the thickness ($E \times t$) indicates the relative resistance to deformation of the lens.

It is important to note that several different moduli can be measured but Young's modulus is the one that is most commonly referred to in association with contact lenses. The elongation at break of the material, also referred to as the strain, is the fraction of its original length that a material stretches when placed under a load. It is a measure of how much the material can deform before breakage. Strain is dimensionless, i.e. it has no units attached to it.

A point of potential confusion in the literature is the lack of standardization of the units used for measuring stress. Stress is defined as force per unit area. The Système Internationale (SI) unit of stress is N/m^2 (newtons per square metre). One newton is the force required to give a mass of 1 kg an acceleration of 1 m/s/s. A newton spread out over a square metre is a pretty feeble force, so MN/m^2 (mega newtons per square metre or 10^6 N/m^2) is a more useful unit.

The pascal is also seen in the literature with reference to stress. The pascal is actually the SI unit of pressure. The units of pressure are defined in the same way as those for stress: force/unit area. One pascal is the pressure generated by a force of 1 N acting on an area of 1 m^2 (1 Pa = 1 N/m^2). Mega newtons/m^2 and mega pascals, therefore, have numerically equal values.

In US customary units, stress is expressed in pounds-force per square inch (psi). The conversion factor is as follows:

$$1\,\text{MPa} = 145.0377\,\text{psi}$$

The strength of a hydrogel gives some indication of the behaviour of the material during handling whilst the modulus indicates the extent to which the eyelid will deform it and has an impact on the fitting characteristics of the lens. Rigid lens materials have a relatively high modulus (in the region of 10^3 MPa) whereas soft lens materials have a much lower value when in the hydrated state. A lower value is associated with greater comfort, but can be offset by giving poor visual performance.

There has been renewed interest in the concept of 'modulus' as an important soft lens physical property since the introduction of silicone hydrogels in the late 1990s. These lenses (particularly the early 'stiffer' silicone hydrogel lenses) have a higher tensile modulus than conventional hydrogels (1.1–1.4 MPa compared with 0.2–0.6 MPa). The higher moduli of these materials have certain clinical implications, which are discussed in more detail in the silicone hydrogel materials section of this chapter, below.

The generally poor mechanical strength (including tear strength) of soft lenses is arguably the main reason why they have relatively short lifetimes. This problem has been somewhat overcome by the introduction of disposable lenses, which essentially means that the majority of soft lenses no longer need to last more than a day, 2 weeks or a month, depending on their intended replacement schedule.

Several factors can affect the mechanical properties of a hydrogel material and these can be broadly divided into: (1) material composition factors and (2) polymer processing factors. Examples of material composition factors include changing the co-monomers used in the hydrogel preparation. If the hydrogel is not a homopolymer, then increasing the relative amount of physically stronger component(s) will lead to an increase in the final mechanical strength of the material. This may have the effect of altering the mechanical strength by increasing the stiffness of the backbone polymer, for example by replacing acrylates with methacrylates, or it may alter the hydrophilicity of the polymer by replacing hydroxyethyl methacrylate (HEMA) with methacrylic acid (MAA). In general, as the equilibrium water content (EWC) of a hydrogel increases, its modulus decreases.

Another important material composition factor is that the mechanical properties of a hydrogel are dependent on the cross-link density in the system. Cross-links act as anchors or physical links and prevent the polymer chains from slipping past each other. In general, the strength of a hydrogel increases with increasing cross-link density, particularly when in the swollen state, where physical entanglements are low.

Cross-link density can be increased by the addition of larger amounts of cross-linking agent. Although increasing the cross-link density within a hydrogel network is beneficial in relation to its mechanical properties, it must also be considered that changes to other properties of the polymer will occur. The swelling capacity of the hydrogel is likely to be reduced with increasing cross-link density, and hence, its oxygen permeability will also be reduced, which is undesirable in a contact lens material. A balance of all the properties of a polymer is critical to its end application.

Polymer processing factors which can affect the mechanical properties of a hydrogel essentially refer to the fact that hydrogel materials are highly sensitive to the processing and fabrication conditions to which they are subjected. Lenses made by different methods of manufacture will undergo very different material processing, particularly polymerization. These different material processing steps may have an effect on the mechanical properties of the resultant lens. For example, lathed lenses are formed from solid buttons of dehydrated material. The buttons are usually bulk-polymerized over relatively long periods.

Thermal initiators are often used which have low activation energies, therefore allowing water baths or ovens to be set to relatively low temperatures. This type of polymerization is likely to lead to a polymer structure consisting of longer chains (higher molecular weights) and, therefore, more chains.

In the cast-moulding process a small amount of monomer is placed between two casts to form the lens directly. The polymerization process is typically very fast, which is one of the reasons why this is the method of choice for bulk (disposable) lens manufacture. Rapid polymerization times are likely to produce shorter chains, more chain ends and less efficient cross-links.

Surface properties

The surface characteristics of a hydrogel lens will directly affect its interactions with the tear film and consequently its biocompatibility in the ocular environment. 'Wettability' is used to describe the tendency for a liquid to spread on to a solid surface, and *in vivo* wettability in a contact lens context implies the ability of the tear film to spread and maintain itself over a contact lens surface. *In vivo* wettability is a key measure of clinical performance because the success of any contact lens is considered to be related to its ability to support a stable tear layer in the eye. General clinical consensus is that failure to meet this requirement is likely to result in a lens which is uncomfortable, has reduced visual performance and deposits rapidly. The quality of the pre-lens tear film will also have an effect on the friction between the eyelid and the lens surface. This in turn is thought to be important in the aetiology of physiologic responses such as contact lens-related papillary conjunctivitis (CLPC). The issue of wettability has received considerable attention since the introduction of silicone hydrogel materials at the turn of the century, in view of the potentially poor wettability of lenses manufactured from this material.

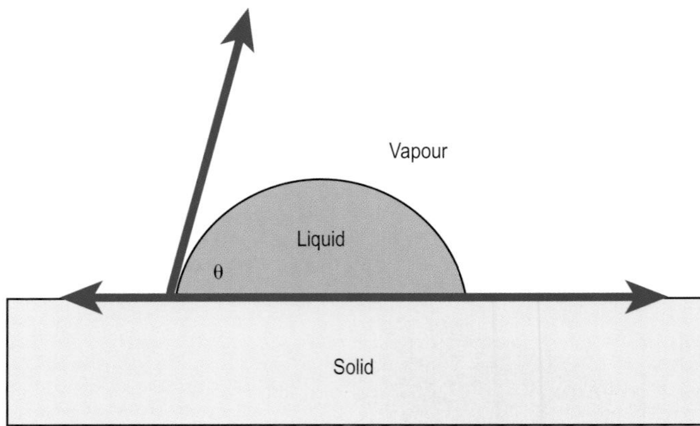

Figure 5.10 Schematic representation of the sessile drop technique showing the contact angle (θ) measured when a drop is placed on a solid surface.

In vivo wettability is generally assessed with a range of relatively crude tests which have been used for several decades. These include tear film break-up time (with or without the presence of fluorescein), interferometric techniques and various techniques based around specular reflection. Unfortunately, these methods frequently fail to differentiate adequately between lens surface types, even when relatively different lens surfaces are evaluated.

On the other hand, laboratory measures of wettability are well established and are better at differentiating lens surfaces. Wettability in relation to contact lenses has traditionally been assessed *in vitro* using contact angle analysis. When a drop of liquid is placed on a solid surface, an angle is formed at the solid–liquid–air interface (Figure 5.10). This angle is referred to as the contact angle.

Contact angles can be equilibrium, advancing or receding. The advancing contact angle is the angle formed when a liquid is advanced over an unwetted surface. The receding contact angle is the angle formed when a liquid is withdrawn over a previously wetted surface. There is usually a difference between the advancing and receding contact angles (the advancing angle is usually the larger one) for hydrogel materials and this difference is referred to as the hysteresis. Essentially, the smaller the contact angle, the better the liquid spreads over the solid surface and the more wettable the solid surface.

Figure 5.11 shows the contact angles of a conventional hydrogel and a silicone hydrogel. Note that the contact angle of the silicone hydrogel is considerably larger than that of the conventional contact lens. However, it is important to bear in mind that the wettability of a given surface depends on a number of factors, including the surface tension of the test liquid and, as such, it is a property of a liquid–solid combination rather than of the solid surface alone.

The most commonly used techniques applied to contact lenses include sessile drop and captive bubble techniques. In the sessile drop technique a drop of liquid (usually water) is applied to a dry or drying hydrogel lens surface

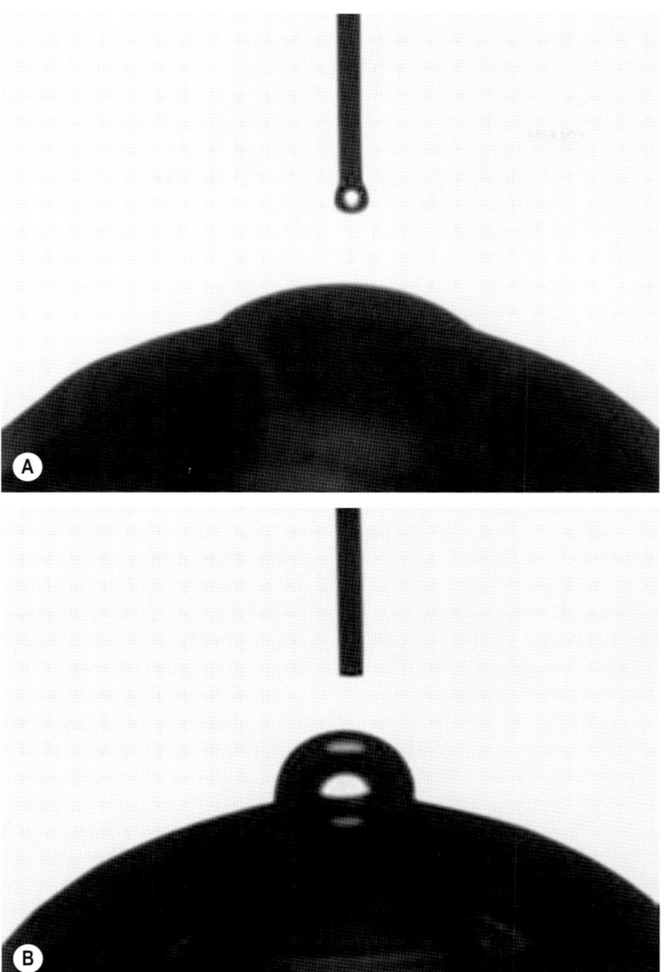

Figure 5.11 Sessile drop contact angle images of a conventional hydrogel lens (A) and a silicone hydrogel lens (B). Note the larger contact angle for the silicone hydrogel material.

in air (Figure 5.11). In the captive bubble technique, the hydrogel lens is submerged in liquid (usually water, saline or artificial tears) and a bubble of air is applied to the lens surface. The contact angles obtained for a lens–liquid combination are highly methodologically dependent (Maldonado-Codina and Morgan, 2007) and any reporting of contact angles should include the experimental details such as the method itself, the probe liquid and prior treatment of the material under test.

The sessile drop and the captive bubble techniques give discrepant results for a given sample because a different type of contact angle is measured in each technique: an advancing-type contact angle is measured in the sessile drop technique and a receding-type contact angle is measured in the captive bubble technique.

The receding contact angle obtained *in vitro* is especially relevant when considering the performance of a contact lens *in vivo*. The advancing angle corresponds more to the establishment of the tear film which is assisted mechanically by the eyelid. Conversely, the receding angle is thought to be important in the stability of the tear film between blinks.

Water content

The EWC of a hydrogel lens is defined as;

$$EWC = \frac{\text{weight of water in polymer}}{\text{total weight of hydrated polymer}} \times 100$$

The EWC of a hydrogel may vary depending on the environmental conditions. For example, pH, tonicity and temperature may alter the EWC of a hydrogel. Increased temperature is an important consideration because there is a significant increase in temperature when a contact lens is taken from its packaging solution (normally at room temperature) and placed on the eye. Most contact lens hydrogels will undergo a small change in EWC when placed in solutions of different pH and osmolality but these changes will be most pronounced in ionic lens materials.

The oxygen and ion permeability of a contact lens material are intimately associated with its EWC. This is discussed in more detail in the following sections.

The surface EWC of a contact lens can be measured using a soft contact lens refractometer (Efron and Brennan, 1987). This is a hand-held instrument which can be readily used in the clinical setting. It utilizes the inverse relationship between refractive index and EWC of hydrogel materials. The measured refractive index of a contact lens is converted to percentage water in sucrose using the Brix scale. This approach does, however, have limitations in that it assumes that dehydrated hydrogels all have the same refractive index (i.e. that of dry sucrose). However, this assumption is not strictly true and the difference in refractive index of a particular hydrogel material and sucrose will lead to the difference between Brix measures and manufacturer-reported water contents.

Difficulties are also encountered with this instrument when attempting to measure the EWC of silicone hydrogel lenses. These lenses have a lower refractive index compared to conventional hydrogels and their EWC is overestimated with the soft contact lens refractometer. Additionally, since it is surface EWC which is being measured with this instrument, it is unknown what effect the surface coatings on some of these lenses have on the final result. Despite these limitations it has become a popular instrument that is convenient and rapid to use for the determination of hydrogel EWC in the clinical setting.

British and International Organization for Standardization (ISO) standards specify both thermogravimetric and refractive index methods as valid techniques for measuring the EWC of a hydrogel lens (BSI, 2006b). The thermogravimetric method involves measuring the weight of a lens in the hydrated state and then re-measuring the lens in the completely dehydrated state. The disadvantages of this method are that it is time-consuming and essentially destroys the lens.

Oxygen permeability

Since the cornea receives most of its oxygen from the atmosphere, the oxygen transmissibility profile of a contact lens is one of its most important properties. Oxygen permeability is a property of the material itself and is described as the *Dk*, where *D* is the diffusivity of the material and *k* is the solubility of the material. The diffusivity is a measure of how quickly oxygen can move through a material whilst the solubility is a measure of how much oxygen the

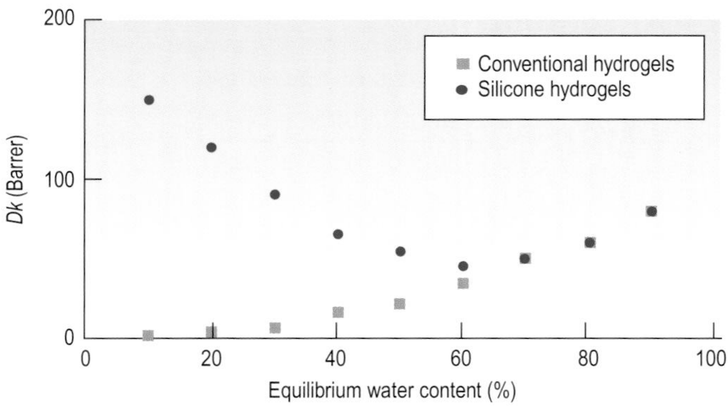

Figure 5.12 Relationship between *Dk* and equilibrium water content for conventional and silicone hydrogels.

material can hold. Oxygen permeability of a hydrogel will vary with temperature.

Oxygen permeability is essentially governed by EWC in conventional hydrogels. This relationship is based on the ability of oxygen to pass through the water rather than through the material itself. The relationship between EWC and oxygen permeability has been found to be (Morgan and Efron, 1998):

$$Dk = 1.67e^{0.0397\mathrm{EWC}}$$

where *e* is the natural logarithm (Figure 5.12).

In order to calculate the amount of oxygen which will move from the anterior to the posterior surface of a lens, the oxygen permeability (*Dk*) is divided by the thickness of the lens (*t*). The units of *Dk* have been traditionally known as Fatt units (after Professor Irving Fatt, who carried out much of the early work on oxygen permeability of contact lens materials) or Barrer, whereby:

$$Dk\ (\mathrm{Barrer}) = 10^{-11}(\mathrm{cm}^2 \times \mathrm{mlO_2})/(\mathrm{s} \times \mathrm{ml} \times \mathrm{mmHg})$$

$$Dk/t\ (\mathrm{Barrer/cm}) = 10^{-9}(\mathrm{cm} \times \mathrm{mlO_2})/(\mathrm{s} \times \mathrm{ml} \times \mathrm{mmHg})$$

However, the SI unit for pressure is the pascal (Pa). Because the unit mmHg is now becoming obsolete internationally, it is being advocated that the closest accepted metric unit of pressure – 100Pa, or hectopascal (hPa) – should replace mmHg (BSI, 2006a). The new units are referred to as '*Dk* units' in this latest British and international standard. When hPa is used, *Dk* and *Dk/t* values are quoted as below:

$$Dk \text{ in '}Dk\text{ units'} = 10^{-11}(\mathrm{cm}^2 \times \mathrm{mlO_2})/(\mathrm{s} \times \mathrm{ml} \times \mathrm{hPa})$$

$$(Dk/t) \text{ in '}Dk/t\text{ units'} = 10^{-9}(\mathrm{cm} \times \mathrm{mlO_2})/(\mathrm{s} \times \mathrm{ml} \times \mathrm{hPa})$$

The difficulty here is that converting from the traditional Barrer or Fatt units to ISO units involves multiplying *Dk* or *Dk/t* by the constant 0.75006. Thus, for example, a lens quoted with a traditional *Dk/t* of 40 units will have revised ISO *Dk/t* of 30 units. It is understandable that such a 'downsizing' will be resisted by contact lens manufacturers, because higher numeric *Dk/t* are perceived clinically as being 'superior'.

Fluid and ion permeability

The development of silicone hydrogel materials has highlighted the importance of the so-called hydraulic permeability or water transport of a contact lens material. Essentially, a minimum level of hydraulic (as well as ionic) permeability is necessary in order to maintain adequate lens movement. This is important in allowing the post-lens tear film to reform between blinks, thus reducing the likelihood of these quite elastic lenses from binding to the cornea. Water is able to move through a hydrogel in quite a different way to sodium ions, i.e. it is more difficult for sodium ions to travel through the gel since in order to do so they must be accompanied by a shell of water (Tighe, 2004). In the eye, the sodium ion permeability of contact lens materials is particularly important since it is a major constituent of the tear film. Sodium ion transport is impeded in gels with a water content below 20%.

Refractive index

Ideally hydrogels fabricated for contact lens materials should have refractive index similar to that of the cornea, i.e. near to 1.37. The variation of refractive index with EWC in conventional hydrogels is almost linear, with most hydrogel refractive indices falling within 1.46–1.48 at 20% water content and 1.37–1.38 at 75% water content, i.e. the refractive index decreases with increasing water content. Because of this relationship, it is possible to calculate the refractive index of a hydrogel if its EWC is known (and vice versa), which is the basis for the use of the soft contact lens refractometer, as discussed above. This relationship is well established for conventional hydrogel lenses but not so for silicone hydrogel lenses.

It is unlikely that a relationship between refractive index and water content will hold for all silicone hydrogel lenses on the market since many are based on completely different material chemistries. British and ISO standards recommend the use of an Abbé refractometer to measure the refractive index of a hydrogel contact lens (BSI, 2006b). However, other more automated instruments have been used for the assessment of hydrogel lens refractive index (Nichols and Berntsen, 2003; Lira *et al.*, 2008).

Swell factor and dimensional stability

The dimensional stability of a hydrogel lens refers to its ability to maintain its original dimensions under various conditions. It is dependent on any factor that will change the water content or swelling behaviour of the hydrogel. Factors that influence the swell factor include temperature, pH and tonicity. The swelling behaviour is particularly important during the manufacture of contact lenses in the dry state, e.g. when a soft contact lens is lathed. During the lathing process a smaller, steeper lens of greater power is made so that, when it is hydrated, it swells to the required dimensions and power required. It is vital, therefore, that the swell factors of the material are accurately known. The swell factor is described by the following relationship:

$$\text{Swell factor (SF)} = \text{wet dimension/dry dimension}$$

Initially it was thought that a hydrogel material swelled isotropically, that is, the same in all directions. With time it was found that the consistently anomalous swelling behaviour of hydrogels could only be explained by specifying two swell factors. These swell factors are those in the diameter and axial (thickness) directions. From these, the value of the radial swell factor of a contact lens can be calculated using the following equation:

$$SF_{rad} = (SF_{dia})^2/SF_{ax}$$

where SF_{rad} is the radial swell factor, SF_{dia} is the diametral swell factor and SF_{ax} is the axial swell factor.

Hydrogel materials

Hydrogel materials can be conveniently divided into two groups: (1) conventional hydrogel materials (now sometimes referred to as low-*Dk* materials) and (2) silicone hydrogels (high-*Dk* materials). In this chapter 'conventional' materials should not be taken to mean 'non-disposable' lens materials.

Conventional hydrogel materials

Hydrogel lenses were developed as a result of the extraordinary pioneering efforts of Professor Otto Wichterle and Dr Drahoslav Lim of the Institute of Macromolecular Chemistry of the Czechoslovak Academy of Sciences in Prague in the mid-1950s. Essentally, Wichterle and Lim were working on the synthesis of a new material that they hoped could be used for implantation into the human body. That material was poly(hydroxyethyl methacrylate) or pHEMA (Wichterle and Lim, 1960). They soon realized that the material had potential applications in the manufacture of contact lenses but were prevented from researching such a project by the directors of the Institute, who perceived this work as being a petty distraction from fundamental studies in chemistry. Wichterle was forced to carry out his experiments at home. Despite such difficult circumstances, he successfully managed to produce the first spun-cast lens (made from his son's toy construction set) in 1961 (Wichterle and Lim, 1961). The enormity of his breakthrough for the contact lens industry cannot be understated.

pHEMA is made by polymerizing 2-hydroxyethyl methacrylate monomer with a cross-linker such as ethylene glycol dimethacrylate (EGDMA) (Figure 5.13). Most of the hydrophilic behaviour of HEMA is due to the presence of the hydroxyl group (OH) at the end of the monomer. At this location in the resultant polymer hydrogen bonding with water molecules occurs, causing them to be drawn into the polymer matrix. The result is that contact lenses made from pHEMA contain approximately 40% water in the fully hydrated state.

Lenses fabricated from pHEMA were first distributed in western Europe in 1962 but sales were disappointing. In 1965 the National Patent Development Corporation bought the licence for the American rights to the technology from the Czechs. This was subsequently sold on to Bausch and Lomb who at that time manufactured ophthalmic equipment and spectacle lenses. Bausch and Lomb significantly refined Wichterle's spin-casting process and finally obtained approval from the US Food and Drug Administration (FDA) for their pHEMA lenses in 1971. This time, the lenses became very popular very quickly – both practitioners and patients enjoyed the benefits of increased comfort, reduced adaptation time and easier fitting procedures. With time, more companies developed their own pHEMA lenses; however, it soon became clear that these lenses were not problem-free. Most of these problems stemmed from the fact that the lenses caused hypoxia but other complications relating to solution toxicity and lens spoliation were also common.

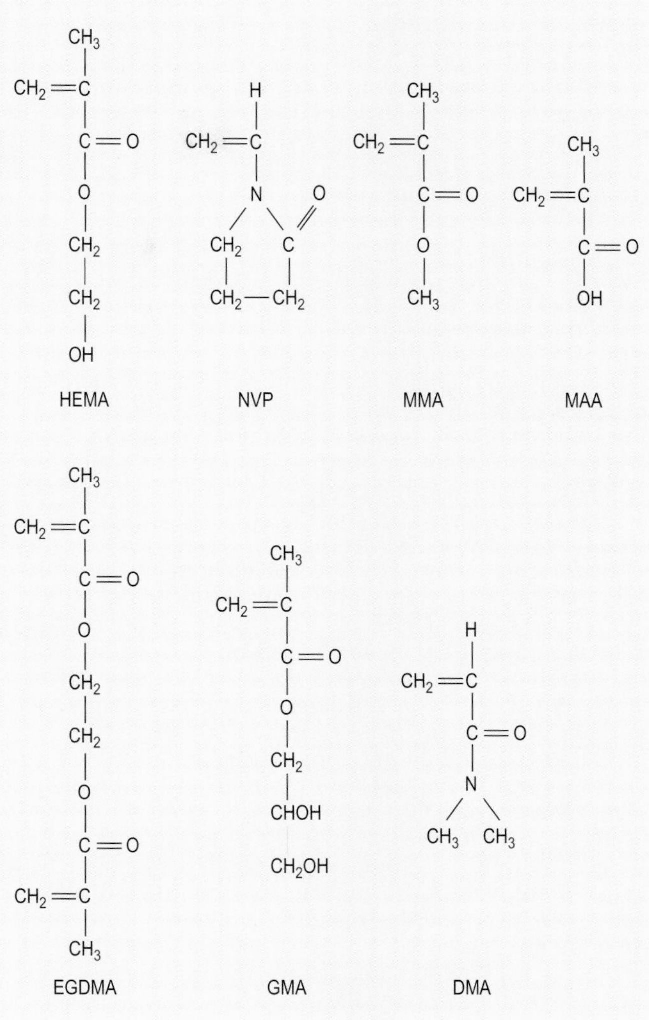

Figure 5.13 Some of the monomers used in conventional hydrogel lens materials. HEMA = hydroxyethyl methacrylate; NVP = *N*-vinyl pyrrolidone; MMA = methyl methacrylate; MAA = methacrylic acid; EGDMA = ethylene glycol dimethacrylate; GMA = glyceryl methacrylate; DMA = *N,N*-dimethyl acrylamide.

Contact lens manufacturers, therefore, had two possible avenues to follow to increase the oxygen transmissibility of lenses: develop 'hyperthin' lenses or develop materials with higher water contents. Producing lenses which were thinner was a relatively straightforward matter for lens designers and several such lenses were launched, e.g. the Hydrocurve thin lens (Soft Lenses) in 1977 and subsequently the O3 series (Bausch and Lomb). These lenses were in the region of 0.035–0.06 mm thick, which was less than half the thickness of the original Bausch and Lomb pHEMA lenses.

Developing materials with higher EWC led to the successful development of HEMA copolymers. One of the first successful copolymerizations was with *N*-vinyl pyrrolidone (NVP) (Figure 5.13). The amide (N–C=O) moiety is very polar and two molecules of water can become hydrogen-bonded to it. NVP-based copolymers lose the slippery feel of pHEMA and consequently can feel quite rubbery. These copolymers also tend to have relatively high evaporation rates of water, which may be seen as a problem for lens stability and comfort. This occurs because the amide group does not bind water as strongly as a hydroxyl group. In addition, these polymers are also significantly more temperature-sensitive than pHEMA-based materials, i.e. their parameters tend to change with increasing or decreasing temperature. This is important when fitting a lens as its parameters may change on-eye.

NVP-based lenses have also been associated with increased corneal staining and decreased comfort when used in conjunction with solutions containing higher levels of polyhexanide (Jones *et al.*, 1997, 2002). This does not mean that polyhexanide-based solutions cannot be used with NVP-containing lenses, rather the interaction should be borne in mind and, if any significant corneal staining or discomfort symptoms arise, these can usually be treated simply by changing the solution to one containing a lower level of polyhexanide or one free from polyhexanide.

Most contact lens practitioners are familiar with methyl methacrylate (MMA) as the material from which 'hard lenses' are made, i.e. PMMA (Figure 5.13). When MMA and NVP are copolymerized, a completely new material is obtained with very different characteristics to the HEMA/NVP (also known as HEMA/VP) copolymers. Depending on their composition, contact lenses made from MMA/VP copolymers can contain 60–85% water. MMA is very hydrophobic but is useful in soft lens hydrogels as it gives the resultant polymers increased mechanical strength.

Another hydrophilic monomer that has been very successfully used in contact lens hydrogels is MAA (Figure 5.13). When added to a soft lens polymer formulation, it results in a soft lens with ionized groups (negatively charged) within the polymer matrix, allowing the lens to absorb more water. The higher the amount of MAA, the higher the EWC of the resulting polymer. Amounts of MAA in the region of 1.5–2.5% will increase the water content of a HEMA material into the mid-water-content range of 50–60%, thereby allowing oxygen permeability to increase significantly.

Once HEMA/MAA lenses have been manufactured they need to be ionized (i.e. the hydrogen atom in the carboxyl group is removed). The conversion of the carboxyl group (CO_2H) to the more hydrophilic ionized form (the carboxylate anion, CO_2^-) produces an increase in water content. This is commonly achieved by washing the lenses in sodium bicarbonate solution or buffered saline and is referred to as 'expanding the matrix'. Unfortunately, using MAA to increase the water content of a polymer also has its disadvantages. These include:

- A lens which is extremely sensitive to changes in tonicity (McCarey and Wilson, 1982). The Na^+ ions present in saline solution have the effect of 'shielding' the carboxylate anions. In hypotonic solutions (e.g. pure water), since these shielding ions are present to a far lesser degree, more chain repulsion will occur, which increases the swelling of the network and consequently the EWC of the material. In hypertonic solutions, the reverse situation occurs and the material network shrinks, causing its EWC to decrease.
- A pH-sensitive lens (McKenney, 1990). If the pH of the solution in which the lens is immersed is decreased (i.e. the hydrogen ion concentration is increased), the carboxylate anions are more shielded and the network becomes less expanded. This will cause a decrease in the lens EWC.
- A very significant level of protein build-up both on the lens surface and within the lens matrix (Sack *et al.*, 1987; Maissa *et al.*, 1998). However, it is the biological activity of deposited proteins such as lysozyme which is thought to be most relevant in biocompatibility issues such as CLPC and comfort. Protein which remains active (as opposed to becoming denatured) is thought to be 'good' protein. The protein deposited on HEMA/MAA lenses has been found to denature to a significantly lower degree compared to other lens materials (Suwala *et al.*, 2007).
- Dimensional instability when the lens is heat-disinfected.

Glyceryl methacrylate (GMA) is more hydrophilic than HEMA due to the fact that the monomer contains two hydroxyl groups (Figure 5.13). This monomer has been used in contact lens materials in two main ways. The first method has used GMA in combination with MMA to produce materials which have water contents in the range of 30–42%. These materials are thought to be stiffer and stronger than pHEMA hydrogels but their oxygen permeabilities are not ideal for in-eye use.

The second method has been to use GMA in combination with HEMA to produce a high-water non-ionic contact lens material (up to approximately 70% has been possible). These contact lenses are said to be 'biomimetic', i.e. they are claimed to improve biocompatibility by imitating the hydrophilic properties of mucin. Manufacturers also suggest that these lenses show a low rate of dehydration and a rapid rate of rehydration, i.e. they have good 'water balance ratios'. In addition, the materials are thought to be relatively deposit-resistant and seem to be insensitive to pH changes in the range of pH 6–10. An example of such a lens is the hioxifilcon A material used in the Clear 1 Day lenses manufactured by Clearlab. Another example of a so-called biomimetic lens is the Proclear lens (Coopervision) which contains phosphoryl choline (PC) and HEMA. PC is said to mimic the natural chemistry of cell membranes.

In the early 1970s an English optometrist, John de Carle, proposed that if the EWC of hydrogel lenses could be sufficiently increased, then these lenses could be worn successfully on an overnight or continuous basis. He developed the first extended-wear lens to be distributed in the UK, known as Permalens (de Carle, 1975). The lens material had an EWC of 71% and was made from a HEMA/VP/MAA copolymer. In 1981 the lens was given FDA approval for 'extended wear' of up to 30 days along with another lens, the Hydrocurve II (Wesley Jessen).

Slowly, other lenses were given approval for extended wear during the 1980s but, along with the increase in demand for these lenses came an increase in complications. In 1989 studies were published which showed that the risk of microbial keratitis was 5–15 times greater for extended wear than daily wear (Poggio *et al.*, 1989; Schein *et al.*, 1989). As a result, the FDA recommended that extended wear be limited to 6 consecutive nights and with that, the enthusiasm for extended wear died down – that is, until the emergence of silicone hydrogel lenses in the late 1990s.

Table 5.1 lists some of the most common hydrogel lenses on the market and groups them into their appropriate FDA classification. See Appendix 5.1 for details on the classification of hydrogels.

Significant developments in conventional hydrogel materials have been relatively static for the past 20 years. Most of the work that has been carried out on 'improving' these lenses has been channelled towards developing them into disposable lenses and especially into daily disposable lenses. In order to achieve this, manufacturers have invested in more sophisticated automated manufacturing technologies to meet demand and make their production economically viable. This has been no easy task and it should be emphasized just how important these conventional hydrogel materials still are to the contact lens industry today.

Since convenience is such a big driving force, most of the lenses sold today are still made from conventional hydrogel materials, although daily disposable silicone hydrogel lenses have also recently entered the market. In recent years, so-called enhanced daily disposable lenses have been developed, such as 1 Day Acuvue Moist (Johnson and Johnson), Focus Dailes All Day Comfort (CIBA Vision) and SofLens daily disposable (Bausch and Lomb). These lenses utilize techniques of macromolecular entrapment and/or release of hydrophilic surface-active polymers at the lens surface in order to improve end-of-day comfort by stabilizing the pre-lens tear film.

The Focus Dailies All Day Comfort lens is manufactured from nelfilcon A which essentially consists of a cross-linked functionalized polyvinyl alcohol (PVA) macromer with the addition of non-functionalized PVA (Winterton *et al.*, 2007).

PVA and polyvinyl pyrrolidone (PVP) are common soluble polymeric components in comfort drops and artificial tears and have a viscous consistency at elevated concentrations and molecular weights, giving them good surface spreading characteristics. The 1 Day Acuvue Moist lens is manufactured from the etafilcon A polymer (HEMA/MAA) together with the incorporation of small concentrations of low-molecular-weight PVP into the ionic material network.

The Focus Dailies 'enhanced' lenses contain more unfunctionalized PVA than the original lenses. Unfunctionalized PVA is a non-cross-linked PVA macromer of a carefully selected molecular size which does not take part in the polymerization process and which is added to the monomer mix before polymerization. No imbibing step is required after the lens is polymerized. This unfunctionalized PVA macromer is thus free to elute from the lens into the tear film throughout the day with each blink. This PVA is thought to emerge from the lens matrix as 'strands' at the lens surface and it is this effect together with the effect of soluble PVA in the tear film which is referred to as the 'surface modification' of these lenses. The released PVA may improve lens comfort by decreasing the surface tension of the tears, or by mimicking mucin, found naturally in the tear film (Mahomed *et al.*, 2004).

In the 1 Day Acuvue Moist lens the PVP is 'locked' into the lens matrix and is not released from the lens during wear. The PVP is adsorbed on to the preformed lens surface after manufacture from solution. The lens packaging states that the lenses are supplied in 'buffered saline with povidone'. Povidone is another name for PVP. PVP is quite polar and it is likely to be relatively strongly attracted to the etafilcon material, potentially providing a mechanism for its retention on the lens surface. The persistence of the PVP at the lens surface during wear has been verified by Ross *et al.* (2007), who have also described the PVP as being in a predominantly 'looped structure' across the lens surface.

PVP decreases the coefficient of friction of the lens surface compared to its original counterpart. These changes are thought to improve comfort by reducing lens–lid interaction on blinking or, in much the same way as the Focus Dailies lens, by mimicking mucin found naturally in the tear film.

The new SofLens daily disposable lens is modified by the adsorption of Tetronic 1107 – a hydrophilic surface-active polymer composed of ethylene oxide/propylene oxide block copolymer – on to the lens surface. The Tetronic at the surface lowers the coefficient of friction of the lens but it has been shown to be progressively lost from the surface during wear (Ross *et al.*, 2007). It is likely, therefore, that the Tetronic is held by weak forces at the lens surface, which would explain the least in-eye persistence of the three 'enhanced' lenses (Ross *et al.*, 2007).

Silicone hydrogel materials

When Holden and Mertz (1984) defined the critical oxygen levels in order to avoid corneal oedema for daily and extended wear they concluded that 24.1 Barrer/cm was the oxygen transmissibility required for daily wear and 87 Barrer/cm was that required for overnight wear. These values were re-evaluated by Harvitt and Bonanno (1999), who found that the minimum oxygen transmissibility required to avoid anoxia throughout the entire cornea was 35 Barrer/cm for the open eye and 125 Barrer/cm for the closed eye.

Figure 5.12 shows the relationship between the EWC and the *Dk* of conventional hydrogels. From the graph, it is obvious that there is an upper limit to how much oxygen permeability can be attained simply by increasing the EWC of conventional hydrogel materials. A hydrogel with a theoretical EWC of 90% and a central thickness of 0.1 mm would have an oxygen transmissibility in the region of 60 Barrer/cm, which still falls far short of that required to avoid additional overnight corneal oedema. Such a lens would need to be in the region of 0.06 mm thick, which is unrealistic from both a manufacturing and a clinical point of view (Holden *et al.*, 1986).

If reducing the thickness of lenses made from conventional hydrogels was not an option for achieving success in extended wear, then polymer scientists had to come up with an altogether new kind of material. That material was silicone. The element silicon (Si) is the most abundant element on earth after oxygen (e.g. in the form of silicates or oxides such as sand and clay) and lies immediately below carbon in the periodic table. Silicones are organic compounds of silicon and oxygen.

Incorporating silicone into contact lens materials was not a new concept when scientists began trying to produce silicone hydrogels. Indeed, the first material to be used in contact lenses was silicone dioxide (glass). Additionally, silicone rubber (polydimethyl siloxane (PDMS)) (Figure 5.14) has been used with limited success as a contact lens material in the form of silicone elastomer lenses. These lenses have not become popular mainly due to lens tightening and surface wettability problems (PDMS is extremely hydrophobic) (Josephson and Caffery, 1987). PDMS has an oxygen permeability in the region of 600 Barrer but is unwettable by tears, deposits high degrees of lipid and needs to be surface-treated. Surface treatments of silicone elastomer lenses have not been particularly successful in

Table 5.1 Conventional soft (hydrogel) lenses

Name	Manufacturer/Supplier	Principal components	EWC (%)	USAN nomenclature
FDA group 1 (<50% EWC <0.2% ionic content)				
Biomedics 38	Coopervision	HEMA	38	Polymacon
CD	Ultra Vision	HEMA	38	Polymacon
Cibasoft	CIBA Vision	HEMA	38	Tefilcon-A
Classic	CIBA Vision	HEMA, VP, MMA	43	Tetrafilcon-A
CSI	CIBA Vision	GMA, MMA	38	Crofilcon-A
Durasoft	CIBA Vision	HEMA, EEMA, MA	30	Phemfilcon-A
Frequency 38	CooperVision	HEMA	38	Polymacon
Hydron Z4/Z6	Coopervision	HEMA	38	Polymacon
Ultra Vision 38	Ultra Vision	HEMA	38	Polymacon
Medalist 38	Bausch & Lomb	HEMA	38	Polymacon
Menicon Soft	Menicon	HEMA, VA, PMA	30	Mafilcon-A
Omega 38	Ultra Vision	HEMA	38	Polymacon
Optima 38	Bausch & Lomb	HEMA	38	Polymacon
Sauflon 38	Sauflon	HEMA	38	Polymacon
Seelite 38	Coopervision	HEMA	38	Polymacon
SeeQuence	Bausch & Lomb	HEMA	38	Polymacon
Soflens 38	Bausch & Lomb	HEMA	38	Polymacon
Softspin	Bausch & Lomb	HEMA	38	Polymacon
FDA group II (>50% EWC <0.2% ionic content)				
Actisoft 60	Coopervision	GlyMA	60	Hioxifilcon-A
Excelens	CIBA Vision	PVA, MMA	64	Atlafilcon
ES 70	Coopervision	AMA, VP	70	–
Focus Dailies	CIBA Vision	PVA	69	Nefilcon-A
Gentle Touch	CIBA Vision	MMA, DMA	65	Netrafilcon-A
Igel 67	Ultra Vision Optics	MMA, VP, CMA	67	Xylofilcon-A
Omniflex	Coopervision	MMA, VP	70	Lidofilcon-A
Medalist 66	Bausch & Lomb	HEMA, VP	66	Alphafilcon-A
Permaflex	CIBA Vision	MMA, VP	74	Surfilcon-A
Precision UV	CIBA Vision	MMA, VP	74	Vasurfilcon-A
Proclear	Coopervision	HEMA, PC-HEMA	62	Omafilcon-A
Rythmic	Coopervision	MMA, VP	73	Lidofilcon
Sauflon-55	Sauflon	HEMA, VP	55	–
Soflens One Day	Bausch & Lomb	HEMA, VP	65	Hilafilcon-A
Softlens 66	Bausch & Lomb	HEMA, VP	66	Alphafilcon-A
FDA group III (<50% EWC <0.2% ionic content)				
Accusoft	Ophthalmos	HEMA, PVP, MA	47	Droxifilcon-A
Comfort Flex	Capital Contact Lens	HEMA, BMA, MA	43	Deltafilcon-A
Durasoft 2	CIBA Vision	HEMA, EEMA, MA	38	Phemefilcon-A
Soft Mate II	CIBA Vision	HEMA, DAA, MA	45	Bufilcon-A
FDA group IV (>50% EWC >0.2% ionic content)				
Acuvue	Johnson & Johnson	HEMA, MA	58	Etafilcon-A
Durasoft 3	CIBA Vision	HEMA, EEMA, MA	55	Phemefilcon-A

Table 5.1 Conventional soft (hydrogel) lenses—cont'd

Name	Manufacturer/Supplier	Principal components	EWC (%)	USAN nomenclature
Focus 1-2 Week	CIBA Vision	HEMA, PVP, MA	55	Vifilcon-A
Focus Monthly	CIBA Vision	HEMA, PVP, MA	55	Vifilcon-A
Frequency 55	Coopervision	HEMA, MA	55	Methafilcon-A
Hydrasoft	Coopervision	HEMA, MA	55	Methafilcon-A
Hydrocurve II/3	CIBA Vision	HEMA, DAA, MA	55	Bufilcon-A
One Day Acuvue	Johnson & Johnson	HEMA, MA	58	Etafilcon-A
Permalens	CIBA Vision	HEMA, VP, MA	71	Perfilcon-A
Softcon	CIBA Vision	HEMA, PVP, MA	55	Vifilcon-A
Surevue	Johnson & Johnson	HEMA, MA	58	Etafilcon-A
Ultraflex 55	Coopervision	HEMA, MA	55	Ocufilcon-D

FDA, Food and Drug Administration; EWC = equilibrium water content; HEMA = 2-hydroxyethyl methacrylate; VP = *N*-vinyl pyrrolidone; MMA = methyl methacrylate; PC = phosphorylcholine; GMA = glyceryl methacrylate; EEMA = ethoxyethyl methacrylate; MA = methacrylic acid; VA = vinyl acetate; PMA = polymethyl acrylate; GlyMA = glyceryl, methacrylate; PVA = polyvinyl alcohol; AMA = alkyl methacrylate; DMA = *N,N*-dimethyl acrylamide; CMA = cyclohexyl methacrylate; PVP = polyvinyl pyrrolidone (i.e. graft copolymer); BMA = butyl (probably isobutyl) methacrylate; DAA = diacetone, acrylamide.
USAN = United States adopted name Council. Many USAN equivalents exist, e.g. Hefilcon (Unilens, Miracon); Deltafilcon (Amsoft, Aquasoft, Aquasight, Metrosoft, Soft Form, Softics, Softflow, Softact); Lidofilcon (CV 70, Genesis 4, Hydrosight 70, Q&E 70, Lubrisof. PDC 70, N&N 70); Tefilcon (Cibathin, Torisoft, Softint, Bisoft); Metafilcon (Kontur, Metro 55, Biomedics 55, Mediflex 55, Omniflex 55); Polymacon (CustomEyes 38, Vesoft, Versaflex, Synsoft, Cellusoft). Polymacon has become used as a generic term for polyHEMA and Lidofilcon for NVP-MMA copolymers. The SoftLens 2000 database (adp Consultancy, Bristol UK) provides clinically relevant information and brand equivalents on soft lenses in various modalities.

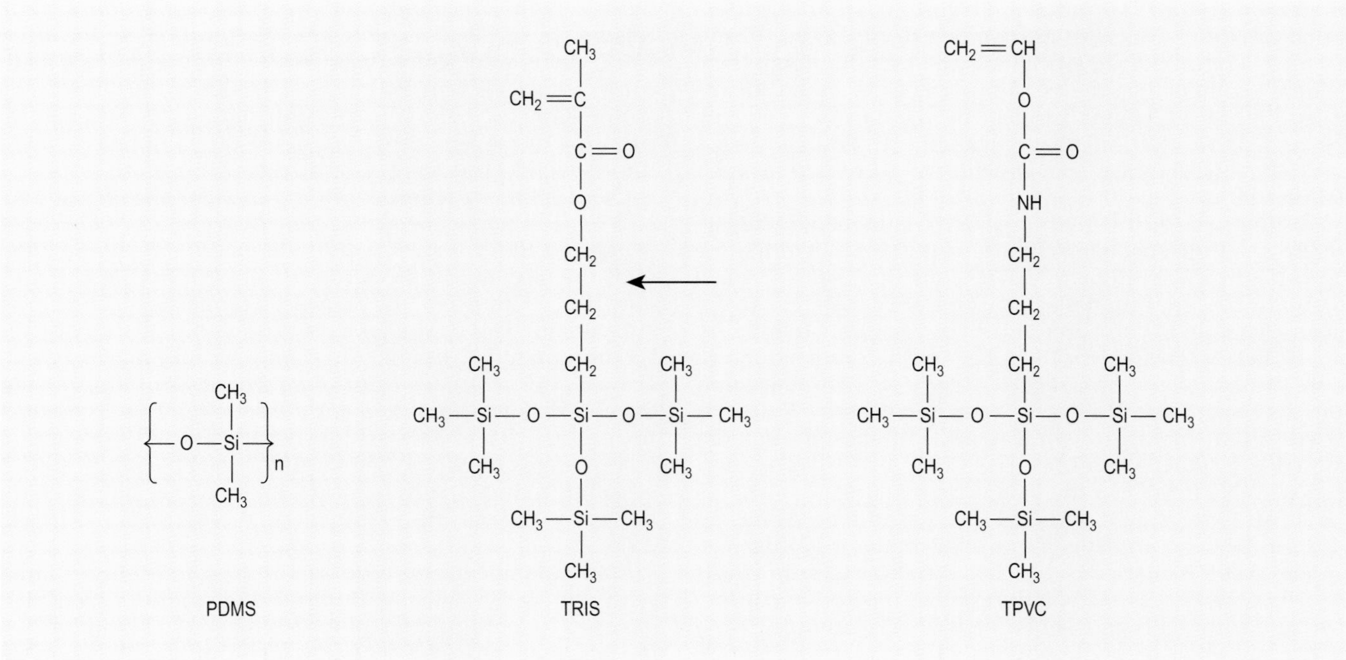

Figure 5.14 Silicone-based materials. PDMS = polydimethyl siloxane; TRIS = tris(trimethylsiloxy)-methacryloxy-propylsilane; TPVC = carbamate-substituted TRIS.

the past because Si–O chains have a tendency to rotate very easily and any hydrophilic parts of a newly treated surface tend to disappear inside the polymer.

Silicon, however, has been very successfully incorporated into rigid lens materials and it was this development which has proven to be a key milestone in the subsequent development of silicone hydrogel materials. The work of Norman Gaylord at Polycon Laboratories drove the development of the first siloxane-based rigid lens material which merged the properties of MMA with the increased oxygen

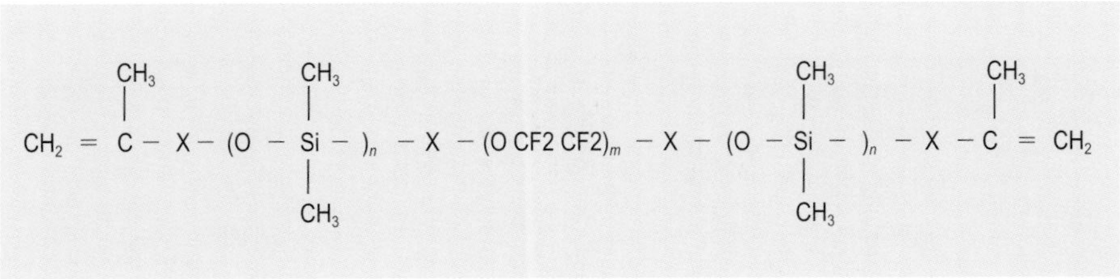

$$CH_2 = C(CH_3) - X - (O - Si(CH_3)_2 -)_n - X - (O\,CF2\,CF2)_m - X - (O - Si(CH_3)_2 -)_n - X - C(CH_3) = CH_2$$

Figure 5.15 Typical siloxy-containing macromer (macromonomer) structure.

performance of silicone rubber (Gaylord, 1974, 1978). The resultant siloxymethacrylate monomer was tris (trimethylsiloxy)-methacryloxy-propylsilane (Figure 5.14) and is more commonly referred to as TRIS.

The patent literature shows that combining silicone with conventional hydrogel monomers has been a goal for polymer scientists since the late 1970s. The biggest obstacle to this approach, however, is that silicone is hydrophobic and poorly miscible with hydrophilic monomers, resulting in opaque, phase-separated materials. In order to solve this problem, two main approaches have been utilized (Tighe, 2004). The first approach involves the insertion of polar groups into the section of the TRIS molecule, arrowed in Figure 5.14, in order to aid its miscibility with hydrophilic monomers (Tanaka *et al.*, 1979; Künzler and Ozark, 1994).

The second approach is that of utilizing macromers. Macromers are large monomers formed by preassembly of structural units that are designed to bestow particular properties on the final polymer (Tighe, 2004). This is illustrated in Figure 5.15 with an example from a CIBA Vision patent (Nicolson *et al.*, 1996) that contains poly(fluoroethylene oxide) segments and oxygen-permeable polysiloxane units. Figure 5.12 demonstrates the relationship between *Dk* and EWC for silicone-containing hydrogels based on TRIS, highlighting the benefits of increased oxygen performance.

The first two silicone hydrogels were launched in the late 1990s – the PureVision lens (Bausch and Lomb) and the Air Optix Night and Day lens (CIBA Vision). Both were licensed for 30 days of continuous wear. The PureVision lens (balafilcon A) has an EWC of 36% and an oxygen transmissibility of 110 Barrer/cm (at –3.00D). The exact compositions of these materials are proprietary but the USAN-registered components of the balafilcon A material show that it is based on a carbamate-substituted TRIS-based material known as TPVC (Figure 5.14). The TPVC is then copolymerized with NVP to form the balafilcon material.

The Air Optix Night and Day lens (lotrafilcon A) has an EWC of 24% and an oxygen transmissibility of 175 Barrer/cm (at –3.00D) and is described as 'biphasic'. Tighe (2004) describes the lens as being a fluoroether macromer copolymerized with TRIS and *N*,*N*-dimethyl acrylamide (DMA) in the presence of a diluent. Its biphasic (two-channel) structure means that oxygen and water permeability channels are not reliant on each other. The silicone-containing phase allows passage of oxygen whilst the water phase primarily allows the lens to move.

Without further treatment both of these lenses would be unsuitable for wear due to the fact that the resultant material surfaces are very hydrophobic. In order to overcome this problem, both lenses are surface-treated using gas plasma techniques. High-energy gases or gas mixtures (the plasma) are used to modify the lens surface properties without changing the bulk properties. The result for the balafilcon lens is that surface wettability is gained via plasma oxidation, which produces glassy silicate islands on the lens surface.

The lotrafilcon lens is coated with a dense 25-nm-thick coating. Both resultant surfaces have low molecular mobility, which minimizes the migration of hydrophobic silicone groups to the surface. However, despite these surface modifications, wettability problems with these lenses have been reported. It is generally accepted that these lenses have inferior wettability compared to conventional hydrogels, which occurs as a result of the hydrophobic interaction of silicone with the tear film.

Another important difference between these materials and conventional hydrogels is the fact that they have significantly greater elastic moduli, i.e. they are 'stiffer'. Such mechanical characteristics mean that the lenses are easy to handle but have also been implicated in the aetiology of a number of clinical complications (Dumbleton, 2003). These include higher incidences of superficial epithelial arcuate lesions, mucin balls and CLPC (in particular, localized CLPC compared with generalized CLPC), especially with continuous wear of these lenses (Skotnitsky *et al.*, 2002). The stiffness of the material may contribute to the mechanical irritation of the lens rubbing against the conjunctiva of the upper eyelid producing a localized response.

The design of the lens, and in particular the edges, may also have an impact on ocular compatibility. It has also been suggested that the design of the lens edge in conjunction with the mechanical properties of silicone hydrogel lenses may be responsible for increased conjunctival staining and conjunctival epithelial flaps observed with these lenses (Loftstrom and Kruse, 2005). A knife-point edge or chisel-shaped edge may cause more conjunctival staining and flap formation than a round edge by 'carving' into the conjunctival tissue (Back, 2006). It has been proposed that certain edge designs incorporating localized increases in posterior edge lift, reduced peripheral thickness or peripheral channels may reduce the pressure on the conjunctiva (Back, 2006).

In an attempt to improve on the problems encountered with the early silicone hydrogels, manufacturers have engaged in a programme of research aimed at manufacturing silicone hydrogel lenses with improved mechanical and surface characteristics. This has resulted in the gradual emergence of 'second-generation' silicone hydrogel lenses such as Acuvue Advance, Acuvue Oasys, TruEye, Avaira, Biofinity and Clariti. Table 5.2 compares the properties of all the silicone hydrogel lenses currently on the market.

The main advantage of these 'second-generation' silicone hydrogels compared to the early silicone hydrogels is that they have increased water contents, reduced moduli and they do not need to be surface-treated. The mechanical and surface properties can be thought of as being 'in between'

Table 5.2 Currently available silicone hydrogel lenses

Brand name	PureVision	Focus Night & Day	O_2 Optix	Avaira	Biofinity	Acuvue Advance	Acuvue Oasys	TruEye	PremiO	Clariti
Manufacturer	Bausch & Lomb	CIBA Vision	CIBA Vision	CooperVision	CooperVision	Johnson & Johnson	Johnson & Johnson	Johnson & Johnson	Menicon	Sauflon
USAN*	Balafilcon A	Lotrafilcon A	Lotrafilcon B	Enfilcon A	Comfilcon A	Galyfilcon A	Senofilcon A	Narafilcon A	Asmofilcon A	–
Water content (%)	36	24	33	46	48	47	38	46	40	58
Oxygen permeability (Barrers)†	91	140	110	100	128	60	103	100	129	60
Modulus (MPa)	1.50	1.52	1.00	0.50	0.75	0.43	0.72	0.66	0.91	0.50
Surface treatment	Plasma oxidation	Plasma coating	Plasma coating	None (internal wetting agent, undisclosed)	None (internal wetting agent, undisclosed)	None (internal wetting agent, PVP)	None (internal wetting agent, PVP)	None (internal wetting agent, PVP)	Plasma treatment	None (wetting process not disclosed)
Principal monomers‡	NVP, TPVC, NCVE, PBVC	DMA, TRIS, siloxane monomer	DMA, TRIS, siloxane monomer	NVP, VMA, IBM, TAIC, M3U, FM0411M, HOB	NVP, VMA, IBM, TAIC, M3U, FM0411M, HOB	MPDMS, DMA, HEMA, EGDMA, siloxane macromer, PVP	MPDMS, DMA, HEMA, siloxane macromer, TEGDMA, PVP	MPDMS, DMA, HEMA, siloxane macromer, TEGDMA, PVP	SIMA, SIA, DMA, pyrrolidone derivative	Not disclosed

* United States adopted name.
† Manufacturer-reported values.
‡ (Partly from Jones and Dumbleton, 2005)
PVP = polyvinyl pyrrolidone; NVP = *N*-vinyl pyrrolidone; TPVC = *tris*-(trimethyl siloxysilyl) propylvinyl carbamate; NCVE = *N*-carboxyvinyl ester; PBVC = poly(dimethysiloxy) di (silylbutanol) *bis* (vinyl carbamate); DMA = *N,M*-dimethylacrylamide; TRIS = trimethyl siloxysilyl; VMA = *N*-vinyl-*N*-methylacetamide; IBM = isobornyl methacrylate; TAIC = 1,3,5-triallyl-1,3,5-triazine-2,4,6(1*H*,3*H*,5*H*)-trione; M3U = *bis*(methacryloyloxyethyl iminocarboxy ethyloxypropyl)-poly(dimethylsiloxane)-poly(trifluoropropylmethylsiloxane)-poly(methoxy-poly[ethyleneglycol] propylmethylsiloxane); FM0411M = methacryloyloxyethyl iminocarboxyethyloxypropyl-poly(dimethylsiloxy)-butyldimethylsilane; HOB = 2-hydroxybutyl methacrylate; EGDMA = ethyleneglycol dimethacrylate; MPDMS = monofunctional polydimethylsiloxane; HEMA = hydroxyethyl methacrylate; TEGDMA = tetraethyleneglycol dimethacrylate; SIMA = siloxanyl methacrylate; SIA = siloxanyl acrylate.

those of conventional hydrogels and the early silicone hydrogels. Recent clinical work indicates that there may be a lower incidence of CLPC with these lenses (Maldonado-Codina *et al.*, 2004).

Some of the lenses in Table 5.2 are based on materials containing TRIS-like components. Acuvue Advance and Acuvue Oasys are based on Tanaka's original patent (following its expiration after 25 years) using a modified TRIS molecule, a silicone macromer and hydrophilic monomers such as HEMA and DMA. Alcohol is used as a solvent to aid the miscibility of these ingredients and is then extracted following polymerization. High-molecular-weight PVP is the internal wetting agent (the Hydraclear) used in these lenses which is entangled and therefore 'entrapped' within the lens matrix and which allows them to be manufactured without requiring a surface treatment (Maiden *et al.*, 2002; McCabe *et al.*, 2004). The PVP essentially works by shielding the silicone from the tear film at the lens interface.

The Biofinity lens (comfilcon A) is not based on TRIS chemistry. It is comprised solely of silicon-containing macromers and requires no surface treatment or wetting agent. The patents surrounding the material refer to a monofunctional macromer (which contains only one double bond which takes part in the polymerization process) being combined with another rubber-like siloxy macromer, resulting in a material with much longer chains (higher molecular weight) compared to the other silicone hydrogels (Iwata *et al.*, 2005, 2006). The patents also discuss other hydrophilic monomers which are presumably the key to why these materials do not need to be surface-treated. The material chemistry of this lens provides a higher than expected oxygen transmissibility for its water content. The introduction of these 'second-generation' lenses has also seen a significant rise in the number of silicone hydrogel lenses being prescribed on a daily-wear basis.

Classification of soft lens materials

There are three main classification systems for soft contact lens materials. Two are well established: the UK Association of Contact Lens Manufacturers (ACLM) classification system and the US FDA classification system. A third classification system has been put forward in a British and international standard (BSI, 2006a). These classification systems are expanded upon in Appendix 5.1.

Conclusion

A basic understanding of the materials from which contact lenses are made as well as their behaviour is vitally important to any contact lens practitioner since it is likely to form an important aspect of patient management. Soft contact lenses have come a long way since the pioneering efforts of Professor Otto Wichterle in the late 1950s in terms of material, design and in the way they are manufactured. Thick pHEMA lenses which were replaced every few years are now a thing of the past.

Hypoxia-related problems with conventional hydrogels have been solved by reducing the thickness of the lenses and/or utilizing more hydrophilic monomers to produce the highly successful (mainly disposable) lenses that dominate the market today. However, these materials still fall far short of the oxygen requirements needed for continuous wear.

Enter silicone. Although the various hypoxia-related problems associated with contact lens wear appear to have been resolved with the new breed of silicone hydrogel materials, a number of mechanical and surface material-related complications still remain, despite the introduction of 'second-generation' silicone hydrogel polymers. Future development of soft contact lens materials is likely to concentrate on trying to resolve the issues of inflammation and infection, improving lens comfort, enhancing post-lens tear exchange and improving surface wettability.

Acknowledgements

The author wishes to thank Andy Broad (Sauflon CL), Trevor Glasbey (Clearlab International), David Ruston (Johnson and Johnson Vision Care) and Guy Whittaker (CooperVision) for useful comments and discussions.

References

Back, A. (2007) Contact lenses and methods for reducing conjunctival pressure in contact lens wearers. CooperVision Inc. US patent 2007035693.

BSI (2006a) BS EN ISO 18369-1:2006. Ophthalmic optics – Contact lenses. Part 1. Vocabulary, classification system and recommendations for labelling specifications. London: British Standards Institution.

BSI (2006b) BS EN ISO 18369-4:2006. Ophthalmic optics – Contact lenses. Part 4. Physicochemical properties of contact lens materials. London: British Standards Institution.

de Carle, J.T. (1975) Hydrophilic polymers and contact lenses manufactured therefrom. GB patent 1385677.

Dumbleton, K. A. (2003) Noninflammatory silicone hydrogel contact lens complications. *Eye and Contact Lens,* **29,** S186–S189.

Efron, N. and Brennan, N. A. (1987) The soft contact lens refractometer. *Optician,* **194,** (5117), 29–41.

Gaylord, N. (1974) Oxygen permeable contact lens composition methods and article of manufacture. Polycon Lab. US patent 3 808 178.

Gaylord, N. G. (1978) Methods of correcting visual defects; compositions and articles of manufacture useful therein. Syntex USA. US patent 4 120 570.

Nicolson, P. C., Baron, R. C., Chabrecek, P. *et al.* (1996) Extended wear ophthalmic lens. Patent WO CIBA Vision 9631792.

Harvitt, D. M. and Bonanno, J. A. (1999) Re-evaluation of the oxygen diffusion model for predicting minimum contact lens *Dk/t* values needed to avoid corneal anoxia. *Optom. Vis. Sci.,* **76,** 712–719.

Holden, B. A. and Mertz, G. W. (1984) Critical oxygen levels to avoid corneal oedema for daily and extended wear contact lenses. *Invest. Ophthalmol. Vis. Sci.,* **25,** 1161–1167.

Holden, B. A., Sweeney, D. F. and Seger, R. G. (1986) Epithelial erosions caused by thin high water contact lenses. *Clin. Exp. Optom.,* **69,** 103–107.

Iwata, J., Hoki, T. and Ikawa, S. (2005) Long wearable soft contact lens. *Asahi Aime.* US patent 6867245.

Iwata, J., Hoki, T., Ikawa, S. *et al.* (2006) Silicone hydrogel contact lens. *Asakikasei Aime and CooperVision.* US patent 2006063852.

Jones, L. and Dumbleton, K. (2005) Contact lens fitting today. Silicone hydrogels Part 1: Technological developments. *Optometry Today,* November **18,** 23–29.

Jones, L., Jones, D. and Houlford, M. (1997) Clinical comparison of three polyhexanide-preserved multi-purpose contact lens solutions. *Contact Lens Ant. Eye,* **20,** 23–30.

Jones, L., MacDougall, N. and Sorbara, L. G. (2002) Asymptomatic corneal staining associated with the use of balafilcon silicone-hydrogel contact lenses disinfected with a polyaminopropyl biguanide-preserved care regimen. *Optom. Vis. Sci.,* **79,** 753–761.

Josephson, J. E. and Caffery, B. E. (1987) Progressive corneal vascularisation associated with extended wear of a silicone elastomer contact lens. *Am. J. Optom. Physiol. Opt.,* **64,** 958–959.

Kastl, P. R., Refojo, M. F. and Dabezies, O. H. (1984) Review of polymerization for the contact lens fitter. In: *The CLAO Guide to Basic Science and Clinical Science.* O. H. Dabezies (ed.). Grune and Stratton Inc., Orlando, FL, USA.

Künzler, J. and Ozark, R. (1994) Fluorosilicone hydrogels. US patent no. 5321108.

Lira, M., Santos, L., Azeredo, J. *et al.* (2008) The effect of lens wear on refractive index of conventional hydrogel and silicone-hydrogel contact lenses: a comparative study. *Contact Lens Ant. Eye,* **31,** 89–94.

Loftstrom, T. and Kruse, A. (2005) A conjunctival response to silicone hydrogel lens wear. *Contact Lens Spectrum,* **20**(9), 42–44.

Mahomed, A., Ross, G. and Tighe, B. (2004) Contact lenses and comfort enhancers: in vivo and in vitro release of soluble PVA. Poster presented at the BCLA International Conference and Exhibition, 21-23 May 2004, Birmingham, UK.

Maiden, A. C., Vanderlaan, D. G., Turner, D. C. *et al.* (2002) Hydrogel with internal wetting agent. *Johnson and Johnson Vision Care.* US patent 6367929.

Maissa, C., Franklin, V. J., Guillon, M. *et al.* (1998) Influence of contact lens material surface characteristics and replacement frequency on protein and lipid deposition. *Optom. Vis. Sci.,* **75,** 697–705.

Maldonado-Codina, C. and Efron, N. (2004) Impact of manufacturing technology and material composition on the clinical performance of hydrogel lenses. *Optom. Vis. Sci.,* **81,** 442–454.

Maldonado-Codina, C. and Morgan, P. B. (2007) In vitro water wettability of silicone hydrogel contact lenses determined using sessile drop and captive bubble techniques. *J. Biomed. Mater. Res. A.,* **83,** 496–502.

Maldonado-Codina, C., Morgan, P. B., Schnider, C. M. *et al.* (2004) Short-term physiological response in neophyte subjects fitted with hydrogel and silicone hydrogel contact lenses. *Optom. Vis. Sci.,* **81,** 911–921.

McCabe, K. P., Molock, F. F., Hill, G. A. *et al.* (2004) Biomedical devices containing internal wetting agents, Johnson and Johnson Vision Care US patent 6822016.

McCarey, B. E. and Wilson, L. A. (1982) pH, osmolarity and temperature effects on the water content of hydrogel contact lenses. *Contact Intraocul. Lens Med. J.,* **8,** 158–167.

McKenney, C. (1990) The effect of pH on hydrogel lens parameters and fitting characteristics after hydrogen peroxide disinfection. *J. Brit. Contact Lens Assoc.* (Trans BCLA Annual Clinical Conference), **13,** 46–51.

Morgan, P. B. and Efron, N. (1998) The oxygen performance of contemporary hydrogel contact lenses. *Contact Lens Ant. Eye,* **21,** 3–6.

Morgan, P. B., Woods, C. A., Jones, D. *et al.* (2009) International contact lens prescribing in 2008. *Contact Lens Spectrum,* **24**(2), 28–32.

Nichols, J. J. and Berntsen, D. A. (2003) The assessment of automated measures of hydrogel contact lens refractive index. *Ophthal. Physiol. Opt.,* **23,** 517–525.

Poggio, E. C., Glynn, R. J., Schein, O. D. *et al.* (1989) The incidence of ulcerative keratitis among users of daily-wear and extended-wear soft contact lenses. *N. Engl. J. Med.,* **321,** 779–783.

Polse, K., Graham, A., Fusaro, R. *et al.* (1999) Predicting RGP daily wear success. *Contact Lens Assoc. Ophthalmol. J.,* **25,** 152–158.

Ross, G., Mann, A. and Tighe, B. (2007) Disclosure: The true story of daily disposable lens surfaces. Poster presentation at the BCLA International Conference and Exhibition, May 31–June 3 2007, Manchester, UK.

Sack, R. A., Jones, B., Antignani, A. *et al.* (1987) Specificity and biological activity of the protein deposited on the hydrogel surface. Relationship of polymer structure to biofilm formation. *Invest. Ophthalmol. Vis. Sci.,* **28,** 842–849.

Schein, O. D., Glynn, R. J., Poggio, E. C. *et al.* (1989) The relative risk of ulcerative keratitis among users of daily-wear and extended-wear soft contact lenses. A case-control study. Microbial Keratitis Study Group. *N. Engl. J. Med.,* **321,** 773–778.

Skotnitsky, C., Sankaridurg, P. R., Sweeney, D. F. *et al.* (2002) General and local contact lens induced papillary conjunctivitis (CLPC). *Clinical and Experimental Optometry,* **85,** 193–197.

Suwala, M., Glasier, M. A., Subbaraman, L. N. *et al.* (2007) Quantity and conformation of lysozyme deposited on conventional and silicone hydrogel contact lens materials using an in vitro model. *Eye Contact Lens,* **33,** 138–143.

Tanaka, K., Takahashi, K., Kanada, M. *et al.* (1979) Copolymer for soft contact lens, its preparation and soft contact lens made therefrom. US patent 4139513.

Tighe, B. J. (1997) Contact lens materials. In *Contact Lenses,* 4th edn (A. J. Philips and L. Speedwell, eds), pp. 50-92, Oxford: Butterworth-Heinemann,.

Tighe, B. (2004) Silicone hydrogels: structure, properties and behaviour. In *Silicone hydrogels: continuous wear contact lenses.* D. F. Sweeney pp. 1-27, Oxford: Butterworth-Heinemann.

Wichterle, O. and Lim, D. (1960) Hydrophilic gels for biological use. *Nature,* **185,** 117–118.

Wichterle, O. and Lim, D. (1961) Method for producing shaped articles from three dimensional hydrophilic high polymers. Czeskoslovenska Akademie Ved. US patent 2 976 576.

Winterton, L. C., Lally, J. M., Sentell, K. B. *et al.* (2007) The elution of poly (vinyl alcohol) from a contact lens: the realization of a time release moisturizing agent/artificial tear. *J. Biomed. Mater. Res. B. Appl. Biomater.,* **80,** 424–432.

Appendix 5.1
Classification of soft lens materials

Food and Drug Administration (FDA) classification system

The FDA classification system for soft lens materials is shown in Table A.1. The classification system has four groups. The main drawback with this system is that different materials containing different monomers can be classified within the same material group.

Table A.1 FDA classification system for soft lens materials

Group	Material
I	Low-water-content (<50%), non-ionic polymers
II	High-water-content (>50%), non-ionic polymers
III	Low-water-content (<50%), ionic polymers
IV	High-water-content (>50%), ionic polymers

Association of Contact Lens Manufacturers (ACLM) classification system

The ACLM classification has two main groups: focon for rigid lens materials and filcon for soft lens materials. Each group is further subdivided depending on how much ionizable monomer is present in the material. The classification system is shown in Table A.2.

Table A.2 FDA classification system for soft lens materials

Group	Material
1a	Essentially poly 2-HEMA, but ≤0.2% by weight of any ionizable chemical (e.g. MA).
1b	Essentially poly 2-HEMA, but >0.2% by weight of any ionizable chemical.
2a	A copolymer of 2-HEMA and/or other hydroxyalkylmethacrylates, dihydroxyalkylmethacrylates and alkylmethacrylates, but ≤0.2% by weight of any ionizable chemical
2b	As in group 2a, but >0.2% by weight ionizable chemicals
3a	A copolymer of 2-HEMA with an *N*-vinyl lactam and/or an alkyl acrylamide but ≤0.2% by weight of any ionizable chemical
3b	As in group 3a, but >0.2% by weight of ionizable chemicals
4a	A copolymer of alkyl methacrylate and *N*-vinyl lactam and/or an alkyl acrylamide, but ≤0.2% by weight of any ionizable chemical
4b	As in group 4a but >0.2% by weight of ionizable chemical
5	Soft lens materials formed from polysiloxanes

BS EN ISO 18369-1: 2006

The specific classification of a contact lens or contact lens material is given as a six-part code as follows:

(prefix) (stem) (series suffix) (group suffix)
(*Dk* range) (modification code)

For soft lens materials, the classification denotes whether the material is ionic and the range in which the water content of the material lies. The presence or absence of surface modifications is also indicated.

The *prefix* is a term assigned to a material to designate a specific chemical formulation. Use of this prefix, which is administered by the United States Adopted Names (USAN) Council, is optional for all countries other than the USA.

Two types of *stem* are used. The filcon stem is affixed to the prefix and is applied for materials which contain ≥10% water by mass (hydrogel materials). Focon is applied to materials containing ≤ 10% water by mass (i.e. non-hydrogel materials).

The *series* suffix is also administered by the USAN council, and is used in cases in which the original ratio of the monomers of an existing contact lens polymeric material is changed to make a new material. In this case, the capital letter A is added after the stem designation. Subsequent changes in monomer ratio are designated by the next letter of the alphabet. These letters are used to differentiate copolymers of unchanged monomer units, but with different ratios.

The *group* suffix, represented by a Roman numeral, indicates the range of water content and ionic character of the material (Table A.3).

Table A.4 shows how the oxygen permeability of the materials is classified.

Table A.3 BS EN ISO hydrogel suffix groups

Group suffix	Material
I	Low-water-content, non-ionic: materials which contain less than 50% water and which contain 1% or less (expressed as mole fraction) of monomers that are ionic at pH 7.2
II	Medium- and high-water-content, non-ionic: materials which contain 50% water or more, and which contain 1% or less (expressed as mole fraction) of monomers that are ionic at pH 7.2
III	Low-water-content, ionic: materials which contain less than 50% water and which contain greater than 1% (expressed as mole fraction) of monomers that are ionic at pH 7.2
IV	Medium- and high-water-content, ionic: materials which contain 50% water or more, and which contain greater than 1% (expressed as mole fraction) of monomers that are ionic at pH 7.2

Table A.4 BS EN ISO hydrogel *Dk* groups

Group	*Dk* range (*Dk* unit)
0	<1
1	1–15
2	16–30
3	31–60
4	61–100
5	101–150
6	151–200
7 etc.	Increasing in increments of 50 *Dk*

The *modification* code, designated by a letter m, denotes whether the lens has a surface modification which renders the surface characteristics different to the bulk material. Such treatments include plasma treatment, acid/base hydrolysis and incorporation of a material which migrates to the surface. Certain types of tinted lens may also be considered surface-modified. In the case of an unmodified surface, this suffix is omitted.

Example

In order to demonstrate the BS EN ISO classification system, the Acuvue 2 lens would be classified as follows;

Prefix: eta
Stem: filcon
Series suffix: A
Group suffix: IV
Dk range: 1
Modification code: none

The lens can, therefore, be classified as (etafilcon A) (IV) (1).

6 CHAPTER

Soft lens manufacture

Nathan Efron and Steve Newman

Introduction

Three techniques can be employed to manufacture soft contact lenses – lathe cutting, spin casting and cast moulding. As medical devices that rest against the highly sensitive eyeball, contact lenses need to be of the highest quality in terms of their physical construction. As devices that correct optical defocus, the optical quality of contact lenses must also be of the highest order. At the same time, it must be recognized that companies will only manufacture contact lenses if they are profitable; the dominant forces in the market dictate that these high-quality products must be delivered at minimal cost, and one consequence of this is a simplification of lens parameters to streamline the high-volume process.

Methods of manufacture

A key requisite of any technology employed to manufacture a medical appliance is that the final product is safe, predictable and of high quality, so that it meets the intended need. The three technologies discussed below have been developed to meet these requirements.

Lathe cutting

This process essentially involves the use of a special contact lens lathe to cut an anhydrous cylindrical button of material (xerogel) into the required shape, and then hydrating this to form the finished soft lens. Lathe manufacture ranges from labour intensive, manual based cutting systems to sophisticated and fully automated manufacturing lines, depending on the capital budget or skill levels available (Figure 6.1). Even with the use of automation, however, the number and variability of manufacturing steps which are necessary for lathe cutting means that manufacturing soft lenses using this technology is necessarily more expensive than using spin casting or cast moulding.

Therefore, lathe cutting is generally reserved for the production of custom-ordered or extreme range lenses that contain design features not amenable to mass production, such as lenses of high spherical power and/or high toric power, and more recently, aberration-correcting soft lenses for keratoconus (Marsack *et al.*, 2008).

The raw xerogel is supplied to the lens manufacturer in the form of 'rods' or 'buttons'. A rod is a solid cylindrical piece of xerogel, about 16 mm in diameter and 400 mm long. The rod is then sliced, orthogonally to the long axis, into buttons about 10 mm thick. More commonly, the xerogels are fabricated and supplied in button form. When this occurs buttons have usually been pre-trimmed to an industry standard size so that they can be machined in most of the available lathes.

The button is first secured to a back surface lathe in a clamp or 'collet', and this assembly is set spinning at a high rate (typically 8000–12 000 rpm) about its central axis. A diamond-tipped tool cuts the posterior surface lens shape into the button. A second diamond tool advances from the side to reduce the diameter to the required size. The surface is rendered smooth by either fine machining or polishing. Modern sophisticated lathes are capable of cutting xerogel surfaces to a tolerance of 8–15 nm. Such smooth surface

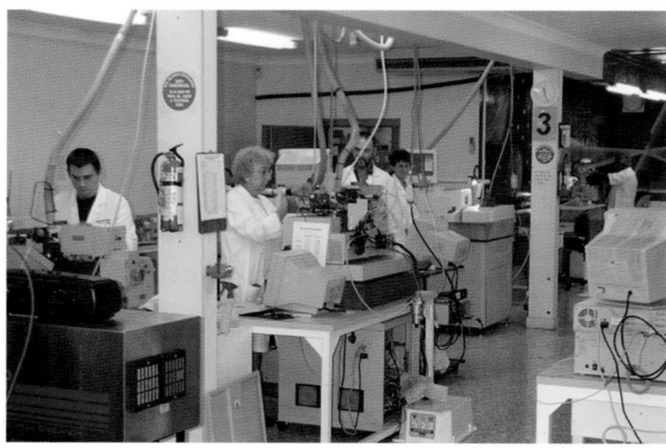

Figure 6.1 A laboratory using the labour-intensive method of lathe cutting to manufacture soft contact lenses.

DOI: 10.1016/B978-0-7506-8869-7.00006-9

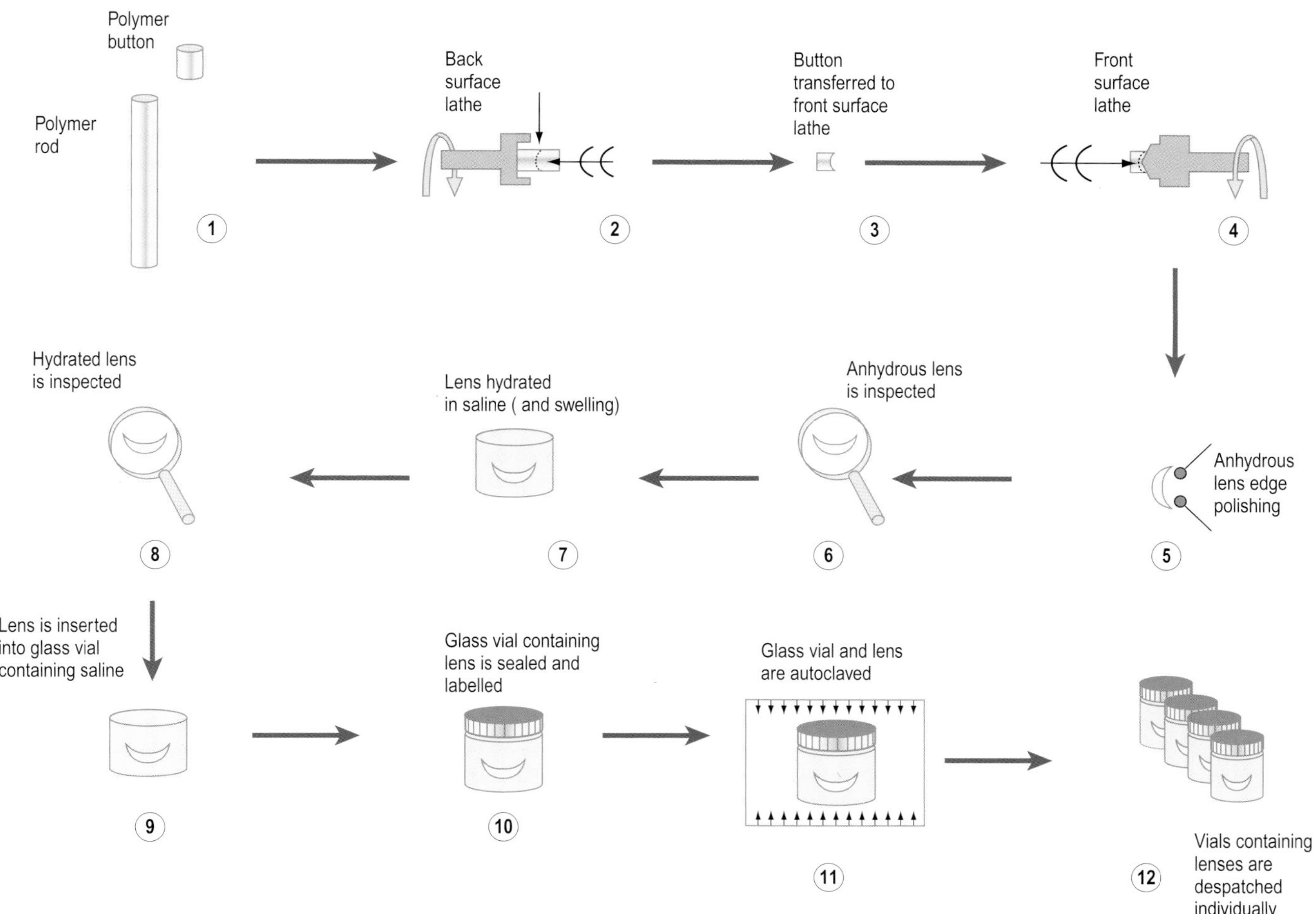

Figure 6.2 The process of manufacturing a soft contact lens by lathe cutting. (1) The dry polymer is supplied as a rod or button. (2) A polymer button is placed on a lathe; the button spins and a diamond tool is advanced towards the button to generate the lens back surface. (3) The button is released from the back surface lathe. (4) The button is mounted on a front surface lathe with adhesive wax; the button spins and a diamond tool is advanced towards the button to generate the lens front surface. (5) The dry lens is removed from the lathe and the edges are polished. (6) The lens is inspected at 17× magnification. (7) The dry lens is placed in saline to hydrate the lens, which swells to its final soft lens form. (8) The hydrated soft lens is inspected at 10× magnification. (9) The soft lens is inserted into a glass vial containing saline. (10) The glass vial is sealed and labelled. (11) The sealed glass vial containing the lens is sterilized in an autoclave. (12) The individual glass vials are despatched.

finishing precludes the need for polishing and is preferred when non-spherical surface geometries are being generated. This approach also serves to preserve the consistency of one surface to the next. The dimensions of the lathed surface are calculated to allow for eventual expansion when the xerogel is later hydrated.

The button is removed from the collet and the cut posterior surface of the button is mounted onto a support tool of a front surface lathe, using low melting point wax. It is essential during this process that the button is mounted and fixed in an absolutely concentric and level aspect to the support tool in order to minimize unwanted prsim being introduced by the front surface cutting. A diamond-tipped tool cuts the anterior surface down to the required thickness, and the surface is smoothed. The most advanced lathes now offer 'W' axis cutting options that can generate rotationally non-symmetric surfaces whilst the primary front surface is being cut. Polishing tools may be used to smooth the lens edge, although some advanced lathes obviate this step.

After inspecting and measuring all relevant dry lens parameters, the lens is hydrated in normal, unpreserved saline until it is fully equilibrated and impurities have been extracted. The hydrated lens is re-inspected for final wet parameter conformity, sealed in small glass vials and autoclaved at 120°C for at least 15–20 minutes to effect sterilization. Advances in lathing technology and computer-controlled processing have led to the development of semi-automatic systems whereby stacks of buttons are automatically fed into lathes; however, even this technology cannot match the mass-production capabilities of cast moulding.

Figure 6.2 is a schematic flow diagram illustrating the process of manufacturing a soft contact lens using lathe cutting technology.

The process of manufacturing rigid contact lenses by lathe cutting is very similar to the process described above – the key difference being that, with soft lens manufacture, the xerogel must eventually be hydrated and sterilized, whereas rigid lenses only need to be cut to their final shape and polished. Other notable manufacturing differences concerning materials of high gas permeability are tighter manufacturing tolerances and the requisite for more critical control of cutting and mounting temperatures in order to preserve their in vivo wetting properties. A pictorial account of this process of rigid contact lens manufacture, and an explanation of how toric lenses are made using lathe cutting, is given in Chapter 13.

Spin casting

In this process, a convex 'male-shaped' stainless steel tool, or 'insert', is produced on a high-precision engineering lathe and lapped to provide an accurate surface that matches the dry dimensions of the proposed anterior surface of the contact lens. Modern non-ferrous materials are also suitable for producing the mould tool and these materials can be generated on 'nano-accurate' single point turning lathes. These lathes can cut mould tools to a surface finish which renders polishing unnecessary. The final surface shape of the master mould tool is verified using interferometry or other similar non-contact measuring methods. Any given tool is used to make hundreds of thousands of moulds.

The metal tool is impressed against heated liquid polypropylene or polyvinyl chloride (PVC), which then cools and sets to form a solid plastic concave female mould. A multiple number of metal tools (typically 8×–12×) of about eight tools is used to produce the same number of plastic moulds simultaneously. The moulding methods and tooling used must be very accurate in order to preserve the concentricity of the resultant plastic part. Any moulding runout will create unwanted prism in the lens during the spinning process. This type of injection cast moulding is generally conducted in a controlled environment (usually to a class 100K level). It is imperative for a spin cast manufacturing process to control the level of potential contaminants to a minimum as it is an open moulding system.

The xerogel lens form is created by pouring liquid monomers into the concave moulds, which spin at a controlled rate about the central mould axis.

This spinning takes place in a controlled atmosphere of nitrogen or similar oxgen deprived atmosphere (Figure 6.3). This is necessary as the spin mould is an open system and thus exposes one surface of the lens (posterior) to air as it is being cured. Oxygen in air is a natural scavenger of the initiatior and will ultimately inhibit the polymerization process.

The speed of rotation, combined with both the mould tool shape and monomer dose ultimately determines the final lens parameters. The shape of the back surface is primarily governed by centrifugal force generated by the rate of spin of the mould, surface tension forces between the mould and polymer, and the effects of gravity. A greater speed of rotation of the mould will result in more polymer mass being shifted towards the lens periphery, and more negative lens power. Due to this system of manufacture, certain process controls such as monomer dosing, must be more accurate than those found in full cast moulding of contact lenses.

As the mould spin rate stabilizes, ultraviolet radiation and/or heat is introduced to initiate polymerization. The lens is removed from the mould, and the mould is discarded. Certain spinning processes hydrate the lens in the original plastic mould and it is never removed. This process has been proven advantageous and cost-effective for the mass production of daily disposable lenses.

Other spinning systems still require that the edges of the lens are polished and that the lens be inspected, hydrated, re-inspected, packaged and autoclaved. Spin casting can produce a much higher output volume than lathe cutting, and in the latest systems can match the high volume of lenses that can be produced by cast moulding. The primary restriction of spincast manufacture lies in its inability to generate a fully formed edge from the posterior to anterior surface; however, sophisticated design modelling, combined with accurate tooling has largely mitigated this limitation. The process of spin casting is illustrated in Figure 6.4.

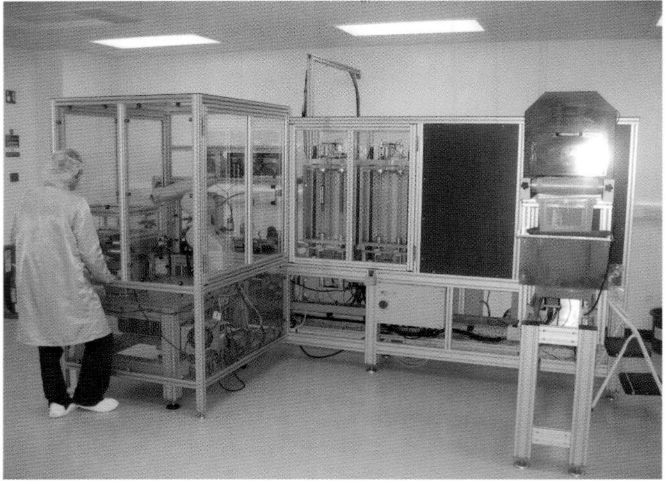

Figure 6.3 A manufacturing line for spin casting soft contact lenses.

Cast moulding

Cast moulding has become the dominant technology in high-volume lens manufacture. As with spin casting, a series of highly polished steel tools is used to fabricate polypropylene moulds; however, matching male and female moulds are required for cast moulding. Again, modern non-ferrous materials are suitable for producing the mould tool and can be generated to extremely fine levels of accuracy and surface finish. These master tools are used to make hundreds of thousands of male and female moulds (Figure 6.5).

The variations found in different manufacturing facilities around the world, however, attest to significant development in challenging this norm. Modern moulding machines can create reproducible results (a critical requirement for the high volume production of contact lenses, particularly daily disposable lenses) with higher numbers of tools. Some machines can successfully carry as many as 36 cavities (18 males and 18 females) in one mould base. Moulding parameters, tool accuracy, cooling and balancing are critical if this is to be successful. The manufacturer will seek a balance between output and accuracy with the moulding process.

Cast moulding generally takes place in a continuous, automated production line (Figure 6.6). Monomer in liquid form is introduced into a concave female mould, which defines the shape of the lens front surface. An ultraviolet-transparent male mould is mated to the female mould and the two are clamped together in a carefully controlled environment.

The contact lens edge is formed when the two sides of the mould come together. There is considerable science and art in the control of the polymerization process and the

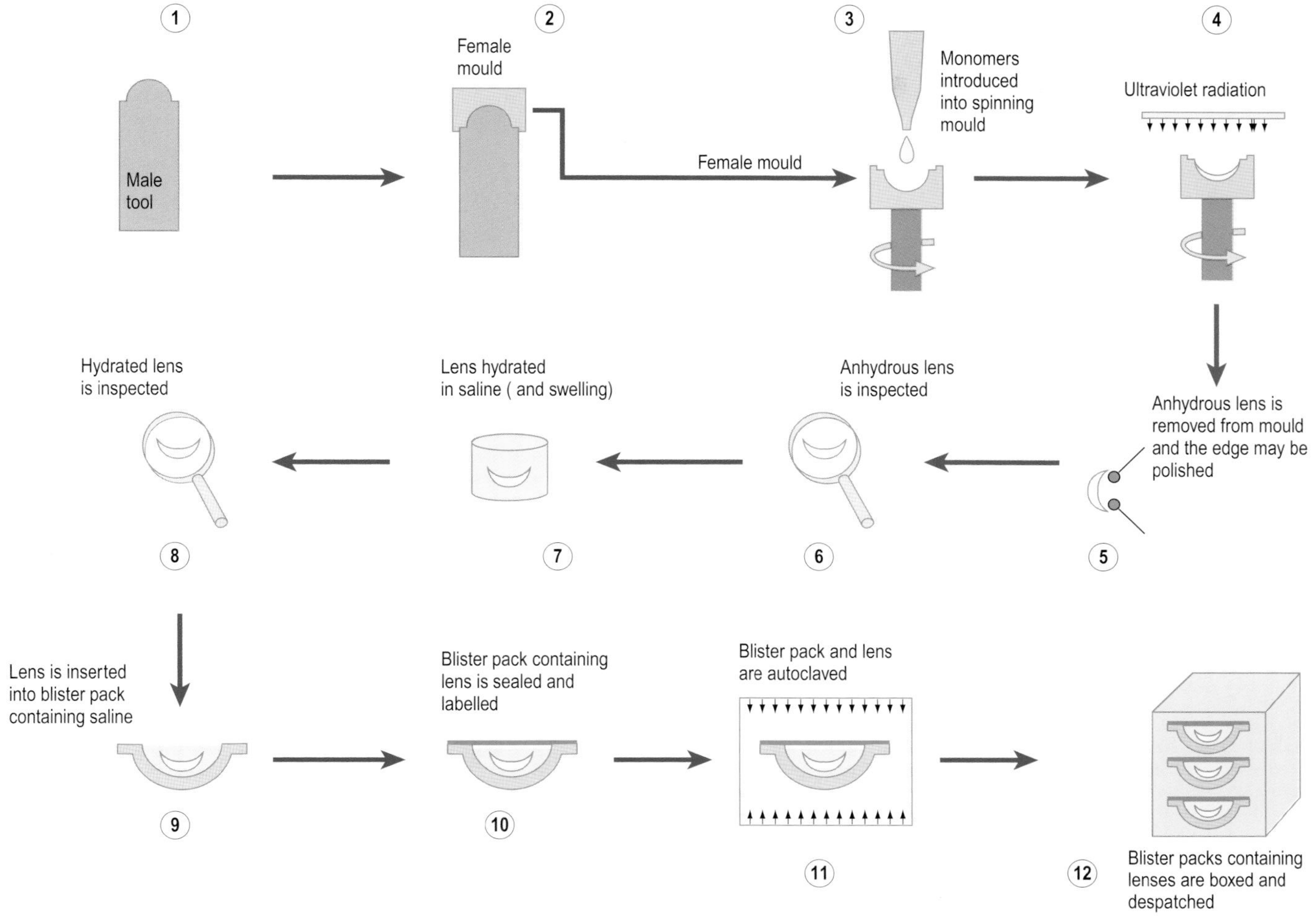

1 Male tool

2 Female mould

Female mould

3 Monomers introduced into spinning mould

4 Ultraviolet radiation

5 Anhydrous lens is removed from mould and the edge may be polished

6 Anhydrous lens is inspected

7 Lens hydrated in saline (and swelling)

8 Hydrated lens is inspected

9 Lens is inserted into blister pack containing saline

10 Blister pack containing lens is sealed and labelled

11 Blister pack and lens are autoclaved

12 Blister packs containing lenses are boxed and despatched

Figure 6.4 The process of manufacturing a soft contact lens by spin casting. (1) A male tool is machined from stainless steel; the contour of the tool head will define the shape of the anterior lens surface. The same tool is used to make hundreds of thousands of moulds. (2) A female mould is made by pressing the male tool into molten polypropylene, which cools and sets. (3) The female mould is mounted, with the concavity facing upwards, in a spindle that spins about the lens axis, and liquid monomers are introduced into the spinning mould. (4) The monomers in the spinning mould are irradiated with ultraviolet light to initiate lens polymerization. (5) The dry lens is removed from the mould, the lens edge may be polished and the mould is discarded. (6) The edge of the dry lens is inspected at 10× magnification. (7) The dry lens is placed in saline, which hydrates the lens, causing it to swell to its final soft lens form. (8) The hydrated soft lens is inspected at 10× magnification. (9) The soft lens is inserted into a blister pack containing saline. (10) The blister pack is sealed with a special foil, and a label is stuck on to this. (11) The sealed blister pack containing the lens is sterilized in an autoclave. (12) The individual blister packs are inserted into packages, typically in multiples of either three or six lenses.

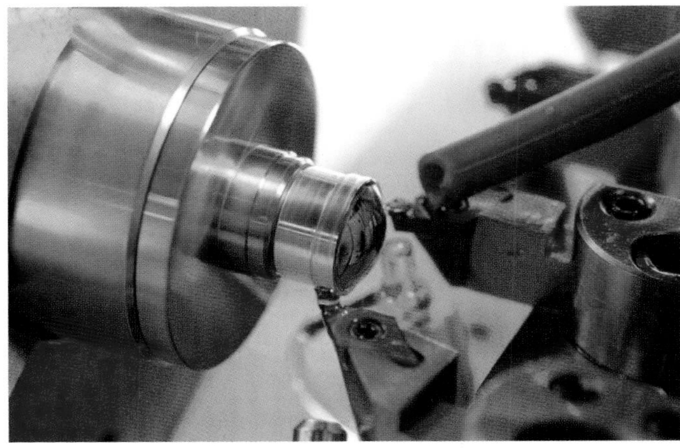

Figure 6.5 Generating a metal master tool.

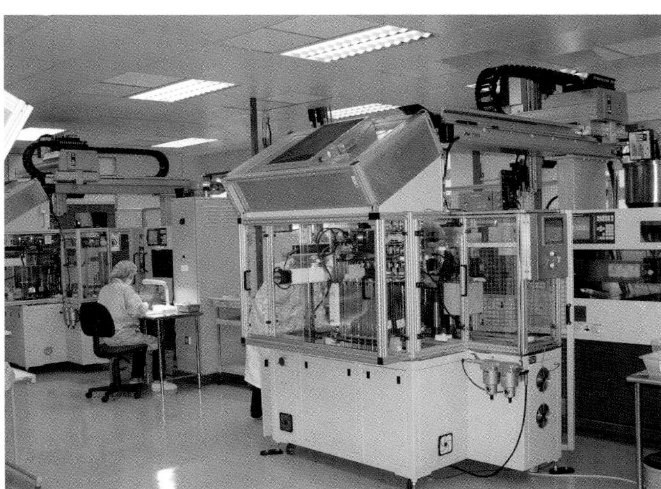

Figure 6.6 A manufacturing laboratory for cast moulding soft contact lenses.

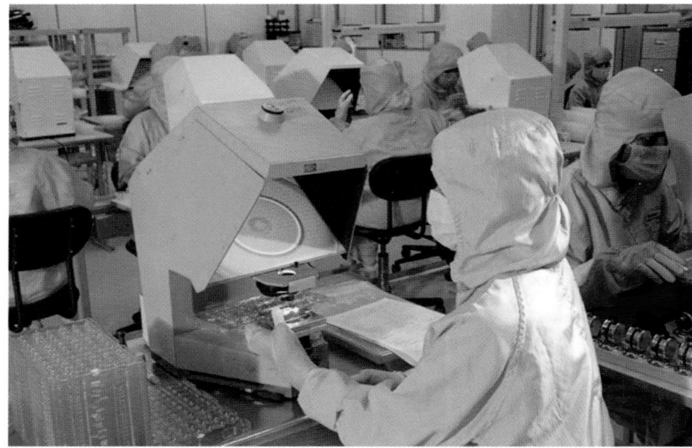

Figure 6.7 An inspection laboratory for quality checking soft cast moulded contact lenses.

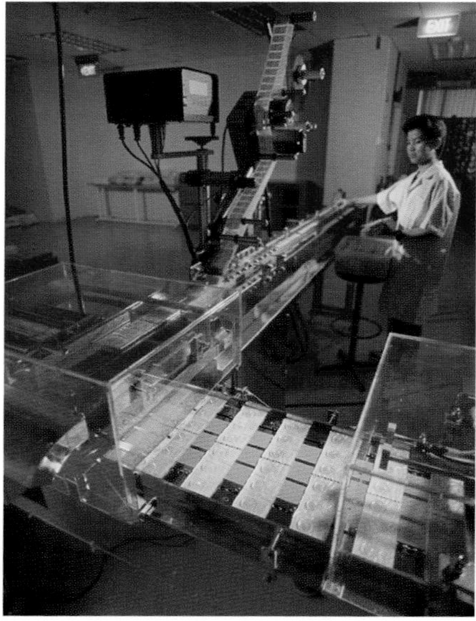

Figure 6.8 A blister packing line for packing and labelling soft cast moulded contact lenses.

pressure that is applied to the mould to form the lens. A crucial aspect of this process is to arrange for the excess polymer (so-called 'flash') to be squeezed out while leaving the edge intact.

Once the polymer is encapsulated in the mould, it is 'cured' – a process in which the assembled moulds are exposed to either UV light or thermal radiation, or a combination of both, to effect polymerization so as to form the dry contact lens. Most cast moulding processes are designed so that when the dry lens is removed from the mould there is no need to polish the edge. The moulds are disassembled and discarded, and the lens that is released from the moulds – still in rigid form – is hydrated in saline.

Inspection is undertaken either manually (Figure 6.7) or using automated video-based computer-controlled image analysis. Finally, the lens blister packs are sealed, labelled (Figure 6.8), autoclaved, and packaged in boxes. Figure 6.9 is a flow diagram of the cast mouding **process.**

It should be recognized that the above descriptions are highly simplified accounts of sophisticated engineering processes. Various manufacturers have introduced a number of unique variations, such as wet-state polymerization, the employment of reusable glass moulds (Hough, 1998), and use of the male half of the mould for final lens packaging. Also, toric and bifocal lenses can be manufactured using either spincasting or cast moulding technology by engineering the master tools to contain the desired lens forms; these design elements will then be faithfully transposed to the moulds and then to the final lens.

Reproducibility and quality of mass-produced lenses

Practitioners who prescribe lenses, and patients who wear lenses, need to be assured of the reproducibility of lenses that have been manufactured using mass-production techniques. Young *et al.* (1999) determined the reproducibility of 24 lenses in three lens powers (–1.00 D, –3.00 D and –6.00 D) of eight common frequent replacement spherical soft contact lens types. They found that the mean power of all the lenses was higher than their labelled powers, although all were within the tolerance ranges. Reproducibility was observed to be worse for all lenses at higher powers. All but two lens types had mean diameters within tolerance. A slight reduction of optical quality at high powers was noted. Measures of back optic zone radius, centre thickness and overall diameter showed reasonably good repeatability.

In a similar study conducted on three brands of daily disposable contact lenses, Efron *et al.* (1999) found that 450 lenses of –3.00 D in power displayed an overall high degree of accuracy and reproducibility. They concluded that, with a single inconsequential exception, all measured parameters were found to fall well within clinically acceptable limits for providing wearers of these lenses with consistent vision and fit.

Efron and Veys (1992) examined the quality of three types of early-generation disposable lenses at 17× magnification using an Optimec JFC Contact Lens Analyzer. An overview of the observed defects revealed that they could be divided into two broad categories – edge defects and non-edge (body) defects (Figure 6.10).

Each of these categories could be further divided into four subcategories, as follows:

Edge defects

- Nick – small piece of lens material missing from lens edge.
- Tear – partial or full separation of lens material continuous with lens edge (Figure 6.11).
- Roughness – uneven edge profile.
- Excess material or flash – lens mass or surplus material extending beyond lens circumference.

Non-edge (body) defects

- Split – partial or full separation of lens material that is not continuous with lens edge.
- Blemish – hazy, low-transparency region of lens, on lens surface or within lens.
- Eccentric optic zone – optic zone not concentric with lens perimeter.
- Multiple pieces – lens separated into sections.

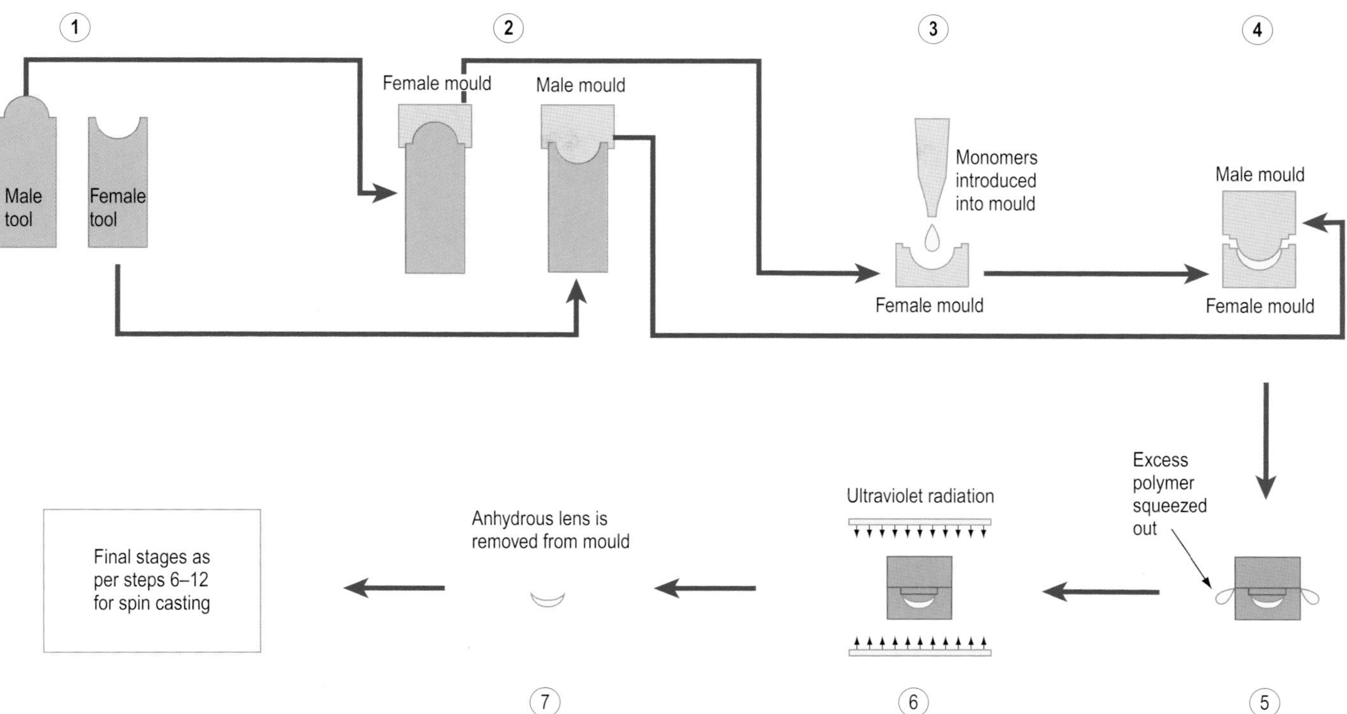

Figure 6.9 The process of manufacturing a soft contact lens by cast moulding. (1) Male and female tools are machined from stainless steel; the contour of the male tool head will define the shape of the anterior lens surface, and the contour of the female tool head will define the shape of the posterior lens surface. The same tools are used to make hundreds of thousands of moulds. (2) Male and female moulds are made by pressing the tools into molten polypropylene, which cools and sets. (3) The female mould is mounted in an accurate aligning fixture, with the concavity facing upwards, and liquid monomers are introduced into the concavity. (4) The male mould is registered over the female mould and the two moulds are clipped together. (5) Excess polymer is squeezed out from the sides of the mould. (6) The monomers inside the mould assembly are irradiated with ultraviolet light or thermal energy to initiate lens polymerization. (7) The dry lens is removed from the mould and the moulds are discarded. The final stages of lens production are essentially the same as for spin casting, which is illustrated in steps 6–12 in Figure 6.4.

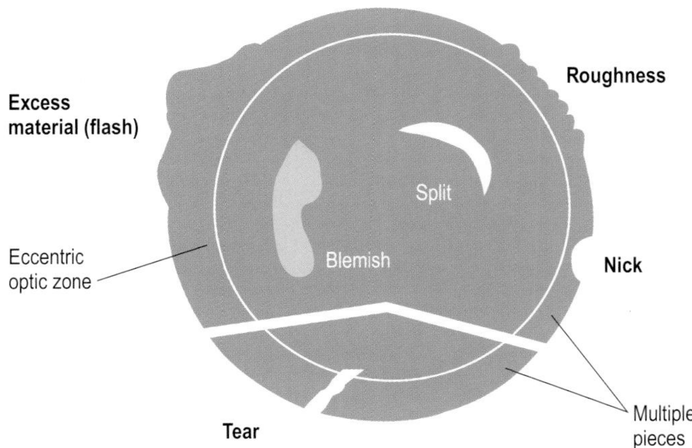

Figure 6.10 System for classifying the types of defects that can be observed on contact lenses. Edge defects are indicated in bold font, and body defects in plain font.

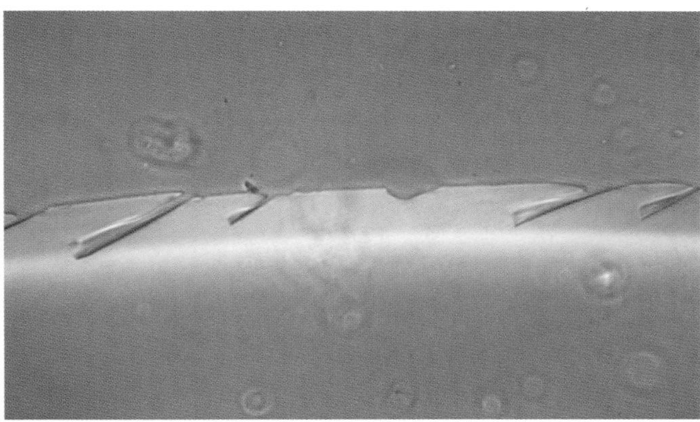

Figure 6.11 Tears in the edge of a disposable soft lens observed at 100× magnification. Such edge defects are uncommon with modern cast-moulding technology.

Some lenses contained more than one defect, and a high prevalence of nicks, tears, roughness and blemishes was observed. At the time, other authors reported similar findings (Wodis *et al.*, 1990; Holden *et al.*, 1991; Lowther, 1991). These studies accorded a valuable service to the contact lens industry in the early 1990s as they focused attention on the importance of the quality of mass-produced lenses, especially edge quality. Advances in cast moulding manufacturing technology over the past two decades, fuelled by the attention drawn to the above issues, has led to a substantial overall improvement in lens quality.

At a microscopic, subclinical level, it can be observed that different manufacturing techniques can have a significant effect on the finished lens surface. Fine concentric rings can often be seen on the surface of soft lenses that have been manufactured by lathe cutting; these 'lathe marks' are often visible under high magnification using the slit-lamp biomicroscope. Using atomic force microscopy, Bhatia *et al.*

(1997) observed that the surface of unused cast-moulded lenses varied from smooth to rough with surface features unique to the polymers and manufacturing process.

Maldonado-Codina and Efron (2005) investigated the impact of manufacturing method and material composition on the surface characteristics of five types of hydrogel contact lenses: three polyhydroxyethyl methacrylate (pHEMA) lenses, each manufactured by a different technique, namely, lathing, spin-casting and cast-moulding, a HEMA/methacrylic acid cast-moulded lens and a HEMA/glycerol methacrylate cast-moulded lens. Front and back lens surfaces were examined using scanning electron microscopy (SEM) and atomic force microscope (AFM). The surfaces of the lathed lenses were covered in lathing/polishing marks. In general, at a microscopic level, the anterior surface appeared more rough. All three cast-moulded lenses had more processing debris than the lathed and spun-cast pHEMA lenses. Overall, the surfaces of the lathed lens were 'rougher' than those of the cast-moulded lens. Maldonado-Codina and Efron (2005) concluded that surface topographies of hydrogel contact lenses are dependent on method of manufacture. They also noted that cast-moulded lenses are associated with apparently 'stickier' surfaces, which may be indicative of surface degradation or cure related issues during the manufacturing process.

Maldonado-Codina and Efron (2004) measured high- and low-contrast visual acuity, and the level of protein deposition, in patients wearing HEMA lenses made by three manufacturing methods. They found that spun-cast HEMA lenses deposited less protein than cast-moulded or lathed HEMA lenses; however, the differences in the amount of protein deposited did not affect visual function.

The impact of manufacturing method on pre-lens tear film of soft HEMA contact lenses was also investigated by Maldonado-Codina and Efron (2004). Manufacturing method was found to have only a minor effect on the quality and stability of the pre-lens tear film (PLTF) in HEMA lenses. The authors concluded that PLTF structure is likely to be more related to material and patient characteristics than manufacturing method.

Conclusion

The three primary methods of manufacturing soft contact lenses are lathe cutting, spin casting and cast moulding. The technique of cast moulding has become the dominant form of soft contact lens manufacture, because it is capable of producing sufficient quantities of high-quality lenses so as to meet the intense clinical demand for affordable planned replacement and disposable lens wearing modalities. Practitioners can be reassured that modern soft lens manufacturing techniques produce lenses of high quality and good reproducability.

References

Bhatia, S., Goldberg, E. P. and Enns, J. B. (1997) Examination of contact lens surfaces by atomic force microscope (AFM). *Contact Lens Assoc. Ophthalmol. J.,* **23,** 264–269.

Efron, N. and Veys, J. (1992) Defects in disposable contact lenses can compromise ocular integrity. *Int. Contact Lens Clin.,* **19,** 8–18.

Efron, N., Morgan, P. B. and Morgan, S. L. (1999) Accuracy and reproducibility of one day disposable contact lenses. *Int. Contact Lens Clin.,* **26,** 168–173.

Holden, B. A., Sulaiman, S. and Cornish, R. (1991) Acuvue 'imperfections' study. Discussion paper presented at the 25th/30th Jubilee Conference of the Netherlands Association of Contact Lens Specialists (ANVC) and the Netherlands Optometric Association (OVN), Maastricht, Holland, November 16–18.

Hough, T. (1998) Shedding light on a new high-volume contact lens manufacturing process. *Contact Lens Spectrum,* **13,** 42–44.

Lowther, G. E. (1991) Evaluation of disposable lens edges. *Contact Lens Spectrum,* **5,** 41–43.

Maldonado-Codina, C. and Efron, N. (2004) Impact of manufacturing technology and material composition on the clinical performance of hydrogel lenses. *Optom. Vis. Sci.,* **81,** 442–454.

Maldonado-Codina, C. and Efron, N. (2005) Impact of manufacturing technology and material composition on the surface characteristics of hydrogel contact lenses. *Clin. Exp. Optom.,* **88,** 396–404.

Marsack, J.D., Parker, K.E. and Applegate, R.A. (2008) Performance of wavefront-guided soft lenses in three keratoconus subjects. *Optom. Vis. Sci.,* **85,** 1172–1178.

Wodis, M., Hodur, N. and Jurkus, J. (1990) Disposable lens safety: The reproducibility factor. *Int. Contact Lens Clin.,* **17,** 96–102.

Young, G., Lewis, Y., Coleman, S. *et al.* (1999) Process capability measurement of frequent replacement spherical soft contact lenses. *Contact Lens Ant. Eye,* **22,** 127–135.

CHAPTER 7

Soft lens optics

W Neil Charman

Introduction

Single-vision soft contact lenses have a number of optically attractive features. They centre well on the cornea with only small amounts of lateral movement and hence introduce little additional asymmetric aberration into the lens–eye system. The diameter of their optic zone normally exceeds that of the entrance pupil of the eye under all lighting conditions; thus, the 'haloes' around light sources that are observed at night following excimer refractive surgery or during wear of some rigid lenses are avoided. Their large overall diameter, greater than that of the cornea, ensures the absence of the discontinuities, flare and stray light effects that can arise with smaller-diameter rigid lenses in the peripheral visual field, due to refractive and scattering effects at the lens edges. Their refractive index (about 1.37–1.48) is quite close to that of the cornea, so that Fresnel reflection losses are comparable to those in the natural eye. They shape themselves so that their back surface conforms closely to the anterior surface of the cornea, thus minimizing fitting problems.

On the other hand, the tendency to drape to conform to the corneal surface and the consequent near-elimination of tear lens effects mean that, unlike rigid lenses, soft lenses cannot compensate for modest amounts of corneal astigmatism. Only by using a well-stabilized toric lens can the latter be corrected (see Chapter 10). Other possible disadvantages from the optical point of view include lens flexure and hydration variations, which may result in on-eye power changes. This chapter will primarily be concerned with such on-eye power changes and aberration effects, insofar as they apply to the optic zone of spherical corrections.

On-eye power changes

Before being placed on the eye, the back vertex power of a soft lens is normally checked when the lens is at room temperature in a fully hydrated state (see Chapter 8). As has already been noted, when the soft lens is worn its inherent flexibility allows it to 'drape', so that the shape of the posterior surface approximates closely to that of the anterior cornea. While this greatly simplifies fitting, any associated changes in the curvatures of the lens surfaces and lens thickness may result in the on-eye power of the lens differing slightly from that measured off-eye.

Although draping implies that the tear lens between the contact lens and the cornea ought to have zero power, this may not always be the case. Wechsler *et al.* (1979) found no evidence for a significant tear lens, and several subsequent authors agreed with this result (Chaston and Fatt, 1980; Holden and Zantos, 1981; Plainis and Charman, 1998). However, Weissman and Zisman (1979) and Michaels and Weissman (1982) suggested that a tear lens about 10 μl in volume may sometimes exist and contribute about −0.15 D of power to the combined lens–eye system. Weissman and Gardner (1984) went on to propose that, although low-minus lenses may entrap only a small volume of tears (about 5.5 μl), thicker, low-plus lenses may entrap a greater volume (about 9.5 μl), giving a correspondingly greater tear lens effect (up to −2.00 D).

Changes in hydration, which are a function of the lens design and material (Andrasko and Schoessler, 1980; Andrasko, 1983; Brennan and Efron, 1987), the wearer, the visual task and the environmental conditions (Efron *et al.*, 1987; Brennan *et al.*, 1988) will affect the refractive index and geometry of any soft lens, and hence its power. Typically, hydration may fall by around 5–10% after the first hour of lens wear (Wechsler *et al.*, 1982; Andrasko, 1983; Efron and Morgan, 1999). Thinner lenses reach equilibrium after about 5 min, whereas thicker, high-power positive lenses may continue to dehydrate for 30 min or more after insertion. Effects appear to be material-dependent (Brennan and Efron, 1987); in particular, high-water-content lenses dehydrate more and reach equilibrium sooner than lower-water-content lenses of comparable thickness. There is a strong suggestion that greater dehydration may occur during near work, due to reduced blinking, and when atmospheric humidity is low. Water loss can occur by several pathways, including evaporation into the atmosphere, drainage into the nasolacrimal system and, possibly, absorption into the conjunctival capillaries.

As the corneal temperature is around 32–35°C (Efron *et al.*, 1989), while the room temperature is normally about

DOI: 10.1016/B978-0-7506-8869-7.00007-0

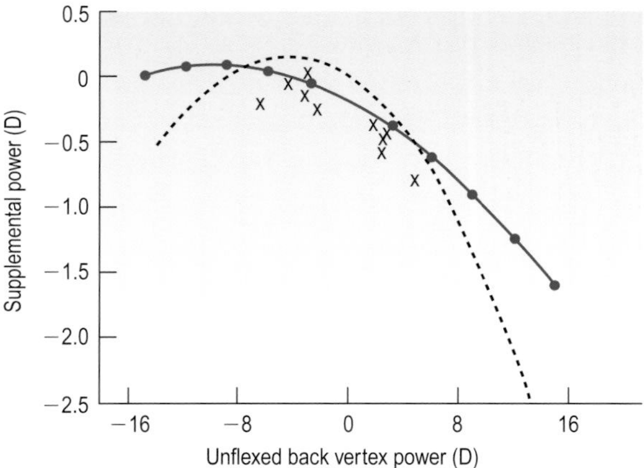

Figure 7.1 Supplemental lens power (i.e. difference between on-eye power and *in vitro* power) as a function of *in vitro* power. The smooth curves are from Holden *et al.* (1976; continuous line) and Weissman (1984; dashed line); the crosses are experimental data obtained by Plainis and Charman (1998).

20°C, there is a change in temperature when the lens is put on the eye: this affects all the lens parameters (Fatt and Chaston, 1980a, b; Purslow *et al.*, 2005), including hydration and refractive index. The measurements made on a variety of soft lens materials by Fatt and Chaston (1980b), however, suggest that the maximum increase in ($n_L - 1$), where n_L is the refractive index, for a temperature rise of 14°C is only about 1 part in 40, so that the associated power change in a lens of this material would only be about 0.25 D for a ±10 D lens.

Many authors have attempted to develop either theoretical or empirical models to allow overall on-eye power changes to be predicted (Ford and Stone, 1997; Patel *et al.*, 1998; Plainis and Charman, 1998). Among the more mathematically sophisticated models of flexure alone are those based on the concept that the flexed lens always retains constant volume (Bennett, 1976) or that the arc length of the back optic zone of the lens remains constant (Holden *et al.*, 1976). Experimental studies, whose results include the effects of all the factors mentioned, not just those of flexure, agree in indicating that any power changes are small for negative lenses but that larger, clinically significant changes, which increase with the lens power, occur for positive lenses.

This can be seen in Figure 7.1, which compares a smooth continuous curve derived from best fits to a substantial body of experimental data by Holden *et al.* (1976), with more recent experimental data obtained by Plainis and Charman (1998).

Also shown (dashed) is a curve based on the empirical equation proposed by Weissman (1984), that is:

$$\Delta r_1/\Delta r_2 = 1 - 0.05F$$

Here Δr_1 and Δr_2 are the on-eye changes in the front and back surface radii of the contact lens and F is the unflexed back vertex power. For the purpose of Figure 7.1 it has been assumed that the initial value of r_2 is 0.8 mm flatter than the corneal radius of 7.8 mm, and that the lens index is 1.43. It can be seen that, while there is reasonable agreement, to within about 0.25 D, between the formula's predictions for corrections up to about ±6 D, those for high-powered corrections are less consistent.

More recent work by Dietze and Cox (2003) suggests that the paraxial power of contemporary thin, disposable, soft lenses does not change when the lens is placed on the eye, and that any small apparent discrepancies in the expected subjective correcting effect might be associated with the spherical aberration of the lens and eye. This would be expected to shift the optimal focus away from the paraxial value towards the marginal focus in a way that depended upon the pupil diameter and the sign and magnitude of the aberration.

It should be mentioned that unusually thick (up to 0.6 mm) soft lenses have occasionally been suggested for the correction of keratoconus (Kaufman et al., 1970; Koliopoulos and Tragakis, 1981; Campbell and Caroline, 1995). These show less draping during wear and might be expected to be accompanied by substantial tear lens effects and effective on-eye power changes.

Thus at the present time neither modelling nor experimental data provide fully convincing predictions for on-eye power changes. All the earlier models involve inadequately justified assumptions and it is probable that additional factors such as material, lens design, fitting philosophy, patient tear flow and lens–lid interactions also influence the results occurring in practice. It may be that the greater thickness of the first generation of soft lenses unduly influenced the early results. Although predictions based on Figure 7.1 should give a general guide to the magnitude of the on-eye power changes to be expected, for practical work it still seems more sensible to follow the conventional approach of trial lens fitting, since after suitable equilibration the trial lens will display similar on-eye effects as the ordered lens of the same design and power (Efron, 1991).

Aberration

Westheimer (1961) pointed out that, for foveal vision and well-centred, rotationally symmetric contact lenses having steeply curved surfaces, the classical lens aberration of greatest potential importance would be spherical aberration, in which the power of the contact lens varies with distance from its axis. This is in contrast to spectacle lenses where, since the eye moves with respect to the lens, oblique astigmatism, distortion and field curvature are all introduced whenever the visual axis moves away from the optical centre of the lens. Indeed, spherical aberration is of little importance in spectacle lenses whereas control of the off-axis aberrations is a major design aim. Since for primary spherical aberration, the wavefront aberration varies with the fourth power of the radius in the pupil and the change in zonal power with the square of the radius, the greatest optical impact of spherical aberration is likely to occur when the pupil diameter is large, that is, under mesopic and scotopic conditions.

With the exception of diffractive lenses for presbyopes (see Chapter 25), longitudinal chromatic aberration is normally of negligible importance in either spectacle or contact lens design, since any contribution from the correcting lens is much smaller than that of the eye itself (see Chapter 3). While transverse chromatic aberration associated with prismatic effects during oblique viewing is of great significance in relation to spectacle lens materials and their dispersion, it plays little role in relation to well-centred contact lenses.

Early work in this area concentrated on exploration of the benefits of aspheric lens surfaces in reducing the

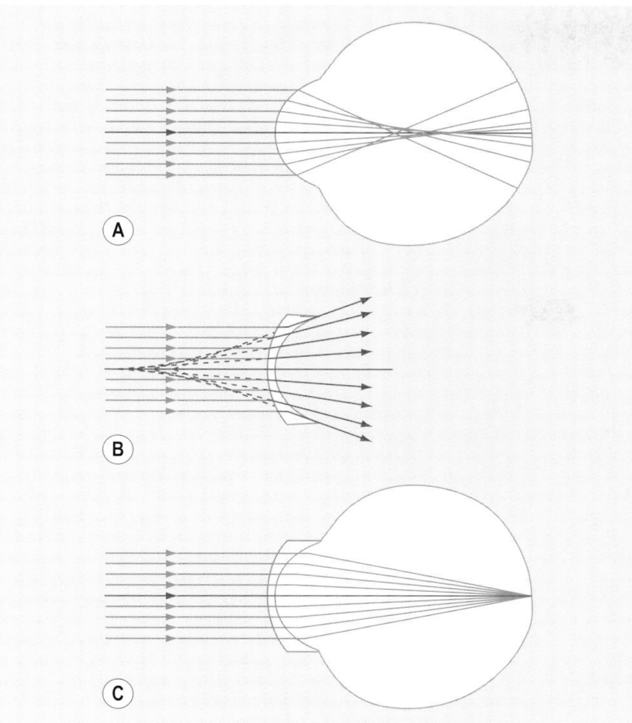

Figure 7.2 Concept of balancing the positive spherical aberration of a myopic eye with a negative lens having negative spherical aberration. (A) Eye alone; (B) lens alone; (C) combined corrected lens–eye system.

spherical aberration of the contact lens in isolation (Bauer and Lechner, 1979; Bauer, 1980). More recently, it has been realized that what matters is the combined aberration of the lens–eye system and that a contact lens with minimal spherical aberration does not necessarily lead to the best visual performance (Campbell, 1981). In principle, ideally the aberration of the lens should balance that of the eye, so that the combined system has minimal aberration (Figure 7.2).

It is clear that, if any series of aspheric lenses designed to have a fixed level of spherical aberration for all lens powers is to offer useful improvements in the vision of patients by compensating for the eye's own spherical aberration, several conditions must be fulfilled:

- The spherical aberration of the eye should be consistent from patient to patient.
- Spherical aberration should be the major ocular aberration, so that its neutralization produces a substantial reduction in root mean square (RMS) wavefront error.
- The on-eye spherical aberration introduced by the lenses should not differ from the off-eye aberration due to flexure or other factors, or, if it does, it should vary in a systematic, predictable way.
- Lens wear should not induce any change in the ocular aberrations, for example through corneal warpage.
- Any decentration of the aspheric contact lens with respect to the axis of the eye should not itself introduce significant aberration.
- The neural components of the visual system should be capable of appreciating any benefits in optical image quality that correction might provide.

Although various early attempts were made to assess the impact on visual performance of soft lenses designed to have different levels of spherical aberration (Cox, 1990; Cox and Holden, 1990; Chateau *et al.*, 1998; De Brabander *et al.*, 1998), they produced somewhat mixed results, with some patients showing improvements, some no change and others a loss in visual performance. Under photopic conditions, with relatively small pupils, mean high- and low-contrast visual acuities produced with spherical and aspherical versions of the same lens showed no significant differences (Vaz and Gundel, 2003). Chateau *et al.* (1998) were, however, able to demonstrate that if the aberration of the lens was systematically varied, mesopic contrast sensitivity at 12 c/° passed through a peak for each patient: the optimal spherical aberration of the correcting lens tended to become more negative with age. Two groups of subjects aged between 20 and 45 years were used: one consisted of emmetropes and the other of myopes with corrections between −5.00 and −10.00 D. The range of lenses used was designed to display varying amounts of primary spherical aberration of the form:

$$P(r) = P_0 + Ar^2$$

where P_0 is the paraxial power, $P(r)$ is the power at a distance r mm from the lens axis and A is a constant (D/mm^2). The values of A used ranged from −0.27 to +0.19 D/mm^2. For comparison the values of A can be converted to the Zernike coefficient C_4^0 used to describe primary spherical aberration in Chapter 3, for any pupil radius, R, by substitution in the equation:

$$C_4^0 = (AR^4)/(24\sqrt{5})$$

Use of the parameter A to describe the spherical aberration has the advantage that it is independent of pupil diameter. Under the conditions of the visual measurements of Chateau *et al.* (1998), pupil diameters were typically around 6 mm.

Figure 7.3A gives examples of the way in which the contrast sensitivity for individual subjects varied with the value of A, whereas Figure 3.7B plots the variation in the value of A for optimal contrast sensitivity, A_{opt}, against the age of the subjects in the emmetropic and myopic groups.

It appears that A_{opt} becomes more negative with age, with, at any age, the value always being more negative for myopes. In subjects of all ages the average value of A_{opt} was −0.16 D/mm^2 in myopes and −0.054 D/mm^2 in emmetropes. It is of interest that these values are similar in magnitude but of opposite sign to the mean values of ocular spherical aberration of about +0.05 D/mm^2 found by Charman and Walsh (1985) or +0.07 D/mm^2 found by Radhakrishnan and Charman (2007) as a result of averaging available ocular wavefront aberration data across all meridians from various studies. This suggests that best visual performance may indeed involve a balance between lens and ocular aberration.

Unfortunately, interpretation of these earlier studies was hampered by the lack of information on the ocular aberrations of the individual subjects. Such information would have allowed each subject's visual results to be interpreted in terms of the combination of their ocular aberration with that of the lens. In recent years, the growing availability of effective aberrometers capable of rapidly estimating a patient's ocular aberration under clinical conditions has transformed this situation. As a result, a much clearer picture of the possible benefits of lenses designed to have

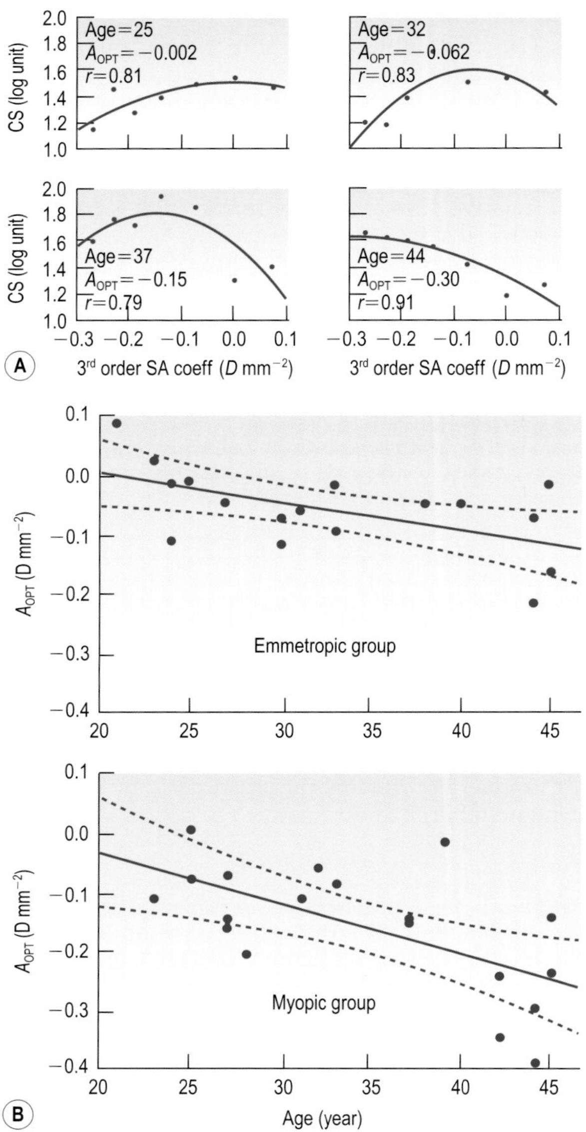

Figure 7.3 (A) Contrast sensitivity (CS) at 12 c/° for four myopes corrected by soft lenses having different amounts of spherical aberration (SA), as specified by the third-order coefficient *A*. (B) Variation in the value of the optimal SA coefficient A_{OPT} for the correcting soft lens, as a function of age for emmetropic and myopic subjects. (Adapted from Chateau, N., Blanchard, A. and Baude, D. (1998) Influence of myopia and aging on the optimal spherical aberration of soft contact lenses. J. Opt. Soc. Am. A., 15, 2589–2596.)

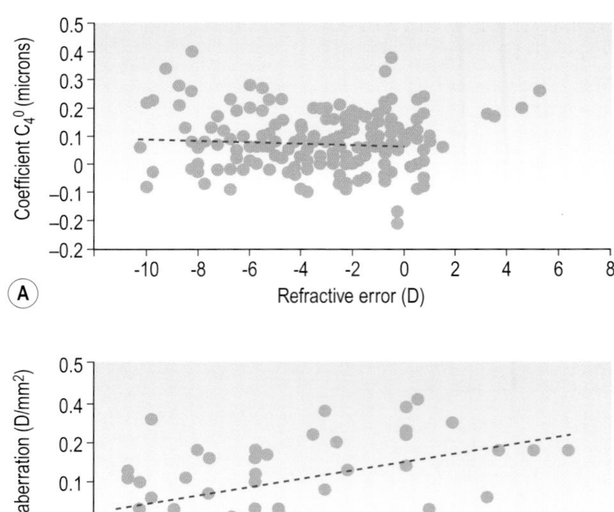

Figure 7.4 (A) Root mean square primary spherical aberration, C_4^0, for a 6 mm pupil as a function of refractive error. (Adapted from Cheng, X., Bradley, A., Hong, X. and Thibos, L. N. (2003) Relationship between refractive error and monochromatic aberrations of the eye. Optom. Vis. Sci., 80, 43–49.) (B) Primary spherical aberration, expressed in D/mm², for a 4.5 mm pupil as a function of age. (Adapted from Radhakrishnan, H. and Charman, W. N. (2007) Age-related changes in ocular aberrations with accommodation. J. Vision, 7, 1–21.) In both plots right-eye data are shown.

a specific level of spherical aberration can now be obtained (Efron *et al.*, 2008).

Summarizing this recent work in relation to the conditions discussed earlier:

- As outlined in Chapter 3, individual eyes show substantial variation in their levels of spherical aberration and in their overall higher-order aberrations. Although Chateau *et al.* (1998) appeared to find differences between myopes and emmetropes, the consensus view is now that mean spherical aberration does not seem to change systematically with refractive error (Figure 7.4A). However, it does change with age, the mean value becoming progressively more positive (Figure 7.4B; Salmon and van de Pol, 2006). This evidently explains the finding of Chateau *et al.* (1998) that the optimal aberration of the correcting contact lens became more negative with age. At any particular age there is a wide spread in the individual levels of spherical aberration (Figure 7.4B; see Chapter 3). No aspheric lens series with a fixed level of spherical aberration can, then, correct the spherical aberration of all patients. While negative spherical aberration in the contact lens may benefit the majority of patents, after 'correction' the minority of younger eyes with negative aberration will have that level increased.
- Even if spherical aberration is corrected, substantial levels of other higher-order wavefront aberrations remain, as well as additional blur due to chromatic aberration and residual spherocylindrical refractive errors. If, for example, we take RMS wavefront aberration values for a 6 mm pupil diameter from the meta-analysis by Salmon and van de Pol (2006), the mean RMS in the fourth-order Zernike spherical aberration mode, Z_4^0, is 0.128 μm, in comparison with a total RMS aberration (third- to sixth-order) of 0.327 μm. Thus eliminating the spherical aberration would only reduce the total RMS to 0.301 μm, a relatively small improvement. For comparison, for this pupil diameter, an RMS wavefront error of 0.327 μm corresponds to an equivalent spherical defocus of about 0.25 D, which is about the level of reliability for clinical refraction techniques. In fact, as a generalization in soft lens work, it is often assumed

that astigmatism only needs to be corrected when it exceeds 0.75 D, so that RMS wavefront errors due to uncorrected residual spherocylindrical errors often exceed those due to higher-order aberrations.

- It appears that the on-eye spherical aberration of thin soft contact lenses is similar to that found off-eye. Any changes due to lens flexure or change in hydration are small (Lopez-Gil *et al.*, 2002; Dietze and Cox, 2003). Comparative studies in which the same subjects wore either standard soft or rigid gas-permeable contact lenses suggest that levels of total lens–eye wavefront aberration are generally lower with rigid lenses (Hong *et al.*, 2001; Lu *et al.*, 2003).
- Hydrogel lenses can undoubtedly, over time, cause marked corneal warpage and consequently changes in aberration (Schornack, 2003) in a minority of patients. As yet, the question of whether more subtle levels of change occur in the majority of patients or with different lens materials remains to be explored.
- If an aspheric lens with significant levels of spherical aberration decentres, it will introduce coma (Dietze and Cox, 2004). It may, however, be possible to modify aspheric design to minimize the aberrations associated with decentration (Suzaki *et al.*, 2007).
- The greatest optical improvements associated with correction of any form of monochromatic wavefront aberration are likely to be obtained when the pupil is large, that is, under natural mesopic and scotopic conditions. However, under such conditions, much of the observed degradation of spatial vision is caused by neural rather than optical factors. Thus even an ideal correction can only improve visual performance to a limited extent: such improvement is likely to be primarily in contrast sensitivity rather than high-contrast acuity (Charman and Chateau, 2003).

Overall, then, any claim that all normal patients would benefit markedly from an aspheric lens series with some fixed level of spherical aberration, as compared to standard spherical lenses, is unlikely to be valid. This does not mean of course that the vision of specific individual patients, particularly those with unusually high levels of aberration, might not be usefully improved by some form of customized correction. The improvements in individual mesopic contrast sensitivity given by selecting the optimal lenticular spherical aberration in Figure 7.3 illustrate this, although the improvement in contrast sensitivity over that for a lens with zero spherical aberration rarely exceeds about 0.2 log units (1.6×).

It seems likely that, in future, aberrometry will be a standard procedure in many clinical practices, since relatively low-cost, multi-role instruments capable of aberrometry, topography and autorefaction are becoming increasingly available. As discussed below, true customization of lenses to correct individual aberrations raises a number of problems. It may be that aberrometry followed by the selection of a suitable lens from a commercial series with several levels of spherical aberration for each paraxial power might allow practitioners to offer useful improvements in vision to at least some patients, particularly at mesopic levels where the pupil is large.

As discussed briefly in Chapter 3, there is, in fact, continuing scientific and commercial interest in the possibility of fully customized soft contact lens corrections, particularly for those patients having high levels of ocular aberration. The optical thickness of the lens would be varied across its area in such a way as to compensate for all the higher-order aberrations of the eye, not just the spherical aberration. Although the required lenses lack rotational symmetry, their production by suitable excimer laser or asymmetric lathe-cutting techniques has already been successfully demonstrated (Lopez-Gil *et al.*, 2002; Chernyak and Campbell, 2003; Jeong *et al.*, 2005). The major problem is, however, that to be effective, any wavefront-correcting lens must undergo minimal rotation or translation on the eye (Bara *et al.*, 2000; Guirao *et al.*, 2001). The tolerances get smaller as the pupil diameter increases. Bara *et al.* (2000) suggest that, for a 6.5 mm pupil, permissible limits to rotation and translation are about 10° and 0.5 mm respectively. The tolerances are larger for abnormal eyes, such as those of keratoconics (De Brabander *et al.*, 2003).

Preliminary trials with customized soft contact lenses suggest that first-generation customized lenses can match the acuity achieved with their habitual rigid lens correction (Marsack *et al.*, 2008). No useful gains have been found for normal or postpenetrating keratoplasty patients, perhaps because of the difficulties in maintaining lens registration with the eye (Lopez-Gil *et al.*, 2003; Sabesan *et al.*, 2007). Nevertheless, this is an area where rapid developments may be expected to occur within the next few years.

Conclusion

The advent of clinical aberrometers is leading to rapid progress in our understanding of the way in which the optical design of soft contact lenses interacts with the second-order spherocylindrical refractive error and higher-order aberrations of the eye. At present it appears that, for photopic vision, making proper allowance for the possibility of on-eye power change is more important than concern about correcting aberration. Aspheric lens series offering a fixed level of spherical aberration appear to offer little general optical advantage over conventional designs with spherical surfaces. However, the availability of aberrometry, combined with aspheric lenses with different levels of spherical aberration, could allow a near-optimal lens to be offered to each patient and hence yield useful visual benefits under mesopic conditions if the lens remains well centred. Fully customized lenses based on aberrometric measurements may be particularly useful for keratoconic and other eyes with unusually high levels of aberration.

References

Andrasko, G. (1983) Hydrogel dehydration in various environments. *Int. Contact Lens Clin.*, **10,** 22–28.

Andrasko, G. and Schoessler, J. (1980) The effect of humidity on the dehydration of soft contact lenses on the eye. *Int. Contact Lens Clin.*, **7,** 210–212.

Bara, S., Mancebo, T. and Moreno-Barriuso, E. (2000) Positioning tolerances for phase plates compensating aberrations of the human eye. *Appl. Opt.* **39,** 3413–3420.

Bauer, G. T. (1980) Longitudinal spherical aberration of modern ophthalmic lenses and its effect on visual acuity. *Appl. Opt.*, **19,** 2226–2234.

Bauer, G. T. and Lechner, H. B. (1979) Measurement of the longitudinal spherical aberration of soft contact lenses. *Optics Letters*, **4,** 224–226.

Bennett, A. G. (1976) Power changes in soft contact lenses due to bending. *Ophthal. Optician,* **16,** 939–945.

Brennan, N. A. and Efron, N. (1987) Hydrogel lens dehydration: a material-dependent phenomenon? *Contact Lens Forum,* **12,** 28–29.

Brennan, N. A., Efron, N., Bruce, A. S. *et al.* (1988) Dehydration of hydrogel lenses: Environmental influences during normal wear. *Am. J. Optom. Physiol. Opt.*, **65,** 277–281.

Campbell, C. E. (1981) The effect of spherical aberration of contact lens to the wearer. *Am. J. Optom. Physiol. Opt.,* **58,** 212–217.

Campbell, R. and Caroline, P. (1995) A soft lens alternative for keratoconus correction. *Spectrum,* **8,** 56.

Charman, W. N. and Chateau, N. (2003) The prospects for super-acuity: limits to visual performance after correction of monochromatic aberration. *Ophthal. Physiol. Opt.*, **23,** 479–493.

Charman, W. N. and Walsh, G. (1985) The optical phase transfer function of the eye and the perception of spatial phase. *Vis. Res.,* **25,** 619–623.

Chaston, J. and Fatt, I (1980) The change in power of soft lenses. *Optician,* **180**(4663), 14–21.

Chateau, N., Blanchard, A. and Baude, D. (1998) Influence of myopia and aging on the optimal spherical aberration of soft contact lenses. *J. Opt. Soc. Am. A.,* **15,** 2589–2596.

Cheng, X., Bradley, A., Hong, X. *et al.* (2003) Relationship between refractive error and monochromatic aberrations of the eye. *Optom. Vis. Sci.*, **80,** 43–49.

Chernyak, D. A. and Campbell, C. E. (2003) System for the design, manufacture, and testing of custom lenses with known amounts of high-order aberrations. *J. Opt. Soc. Am. A.,* **20,** 2016–2021

Cox, I. (1990) Theoretical calculation of the longitudinal spherical aberration of rigid and soft contact lenses. *Optom. Vis. Sci.,* **67,** 277–282.

Cox, I. and Holden, B. A. (1990) Soft contact lens-induced longitudinal spherical aberration and its effect on contrast sensitivity. *Optom. Vis. Sci.,* **67,** 679–683.

De Brabander, J., Chateau, N., Bouchard, F. *et al.* (1998) Contrast sensitivity with soft contact lenses compensated for spherical aberration in high ametropia. *Optom. Vis. Sci.,* **75,** 37–43.

De Brabander, J., Chateau, N., Marin, G., *et al.* (2003) Simulated optical performance of custom wavefront soft contact lenses for keratoconus. *Optom. Vis. Sci.* **80,** 637–643.

Dietze, H. H. and Cox, M. J. (2003) On- and off-eye spherical aberration of soft contact lenses and consequent changes of effective lens power. *Optom. Vis. Sci.* **80,** 126–134.

Dietze, H. H. and Cox, M. J. (2004) Correcting ocular spherical aberration with soft contact lenses. *J. Opt. Soc. Am. A.,* **21,** 473–485.

Efron, N. (1991) Contact lens correction. In *Vision and Visual Dysfunction. Vol. 1: Visual Optics and Instrumentation* (W. N. Charman, ed), p. 99, London: Macmillan.

Efron, N. and Morgan, P. B. (1999) Hydrogel contact lens dehydration and oxygen transmissibility. *Contact Lens Assoc. Ophthalmol. J.,* **25,** 148–151.

Efron, N., Brennan, N. A., Bruce, A. S. *et al.* (1987) Dehydration of hydrogel lenses under normal wearing conditions. *Contact Lens Assoc. Ophthalmol. J.,* **13,** 152–156.

Efron, N., Young, G. and Brennan, N. A. (1989) Ocular surface temperature. *Curr. Eye Res.,* **8,** 901–906.

Efron, S., Efron, N. and Morgan, P.B. (2008) Optical and visual performance of aspheric soft contact lenses. *Optom. Vis. Sci.,* **85,** 201–210.

Fatt, I. and Chaston, J. (1980a) Temperature of a contact lens on the eye. *Int. Contact Lens Clin.,* **7,** 195–198.

Fatt, I. and Chaston, J. (1980b) The effect of temperature on refractive index, water content and central thickness of hydrogel contact lenses. *Int. Contact Lens Clinic.,* **7,** 37–42.

Ford, M. W. and Stone, J. (1997) Practical optics and computer design of contact lenses. In *Contact Lenses,* 4th edn (A. J. Phillips and L. Speedwell, eds), pp. 154–231, London: Butterworth-Heinemann.

Guirao, A., Williams, D. R., Cox, I. G. (2001) Effect of rotation and translation on the expected benefit of an ideal method to correct the eye's higher-order aberrations. *J. Opt. Soc. Am. A.,* **18,** 1003–1015.

Holden, B. A. and Zantos, S. G. (1981) On the conformity of soft lenses to the shape of the cornea. *Am. J. Optom. Physiol. Opt.,* **58,** 139–143.

Holden, B. A., Siddle, J. A., Robson, G. *et al.* (1976) Soft lens performance models: the clinical significance of the lens flexure effect. *Aust. J. Optom.,* **59,** 117–129.

Hong, X., Himebaugh, N. and Thibos, L. N. (2001) On-eye evaluation of optical performance of rigid and soft contact lenses. *Optom. Vis. Sci.,* **78,** 872–880.

Jeong, T. M., Menon, M. and Yoon, G. (2005) Measurement of wavefront aberration in soft contact lenses by a Shack-Hartmann wave-front sensor. *Applied Optics,* **44,** 4523–4527.

Kaufman, H. E., Uotila, M. H., Gasset, A. R. *et al.* (1970) The medical uses of soft contact lenses. *Trans. Am. Acad. Ophthalmol.,* **75,** 361-373.

Koliopoulos, J. and Tragakis, M. (1981) Visual correction of keratoconus with soft contact lenses. *Am. J. Ophthalmol.,* **13,** 835–837.

Lopez-Gil, N., Castejon-Mochon, J. F., Benito, A., *et al.* (2002) Aberration generation by contact lenses with aspheric and asymmetric surfaces. *J. Refract. Surg.,* **18,** S603–S609.

Lopez-Gil, N., Chateau, N., Castejon-Monchon, J. *et al.* (2003) Correcting ocular aberrations by soft contact lenses. *S. Afr. Optom.,* **62,** 173–177.

Lu, F., Mao, X., Qu, J., *et al.* (2003) Monochromatic wavefront aberrations in the human eye with contact lenses. *Optom. Vis. Sci.,* **80,** 135–141.

Marsack, J. D., Parker, K. E. and Applegate, R. A. (2008) Performance of wavefront-guided soft lenses in three keratoconus subjects. *Optom. Vis. Sci.,* **85,** E1172–E1178.

Michaels, D. and Weissman, B. A. (1982) Calculating tear volumes under thin hydrogel contact lenses. In *Advances in Diagnostic Visual Optics* (G. M. Breinin and J. M. Siegel, eds), pp. 131–136, Berlin: Springer-Verlag.

Patel, S., Plainis, S. and Charman, W. N. (1998) Correspondence: on-eye power characteristics of soft contact lenses. *Optom. Vis. Sci.,* **75,** 558–559.

Plainis, S. and Charman, W. N. (1998) On-eye power characteristics of soft contact lenses. *Optom. Vis. Sci.,* **75,** 44–54.

Purslow, C., Wolffsohn, J. S., Santodomingo-Rubido, J. (2005) The effect of contact lens wear on dynamic ocular surface temperature. *Contact Lens Ant. Eye,* **28,** 29–36.

Radhakrishnan, H. and Charman, W. N. (2007) Age-related changes in ocular aberrations with accommodation. *J. Vision,* **7,** 1–21.

Sabesan, R., Jeong, T. M., Carvalho, L., *et al.* (2007) Vision improvement by correcting higher-order aberrations with customized soft contact lenses in keratoconic eyes. *Optics Letters,* **32,** 1000–1002.

Salmon, T. O. and van de Pol, C. (2006) Normal-eye Zernike coefficients and root-mean-square wavefront errors. *J. Cataract Refract. Surg.,* **32,** 2064–2074.

Schornack, M. (2003) Hydrogel contact lens-induced corneal warpage. *Contact Lens Ant. Eye,* **26,** 153–159.

Suzaki, A., Kobayashi, A., Maeda, N. *et al.* (2007) A new design of contact lens to reduce higher-order aberrations in decentred position. *Invest. Ophthalmol. Vis. Sci.,* **48,** E5374

Vaz, T. C. and Gundel, R. E. (2003) High- and low-contrast visual acuity measurements in spherical and aspheric contact lens wearers. *Contact Lens Ant. Eye,* **26,** 147–151.

Wechsler, S., Perrigin, J. and Farris, D. (1979) Further investigations of lens power change due to flexure. *Am. J. Optom. Physiol. Opt.,* **56,** 512–520.

Wechsler, S., Prather, D. and Sosnowski, J. (1982) *In vivo* hydration of gel lenses. *Int. Contact Lens Clin.,* **9,** 154–158.

Weissman, B. A. (1984) A general relation between changing surface radii in flexing soft contact lenses. *Am. J. Optom. Physiol. Opt.,* **61,** 651–653.

Weissman, B. A. and Gardner, K. M. (1984) Power and radius changes induced in soft contact lens systems by flexure. *Am. J. Optom. Physiol. Opt.,* **61,** 239–245.

Weissman, B. A. and Zisman, F. (1979) Approximate tear volumes under flexible contact lenses. *Am. J. Optom. Physiol. Opt.,* **56,** 727–733.

Westheimer, G. (1961) Aberrations of contact lenses. *Am. J. Optom. Arch. Am. Acad. Optom.,* **38,** 445–458.

Soft lens measurement

Sudi Patel

Introduction

With the advent of mass-produced planned replacement and disposable soft lenses there is little practical need for the clinician to check the parameters of a prescription lens – just as a physician prescribing a mass-produced drug has no need to analyse the prescribed drug chemically. Nevertheless, in a fully integrated automatic soft lens manufacturing facility it is essential to monitor continuously the quality and progress of the emerging lens at key stages of manufacture, and automated checking facilities are often built into manufacturing assembly lines. Most of these checking devices evolved from the techniques developed during the infancy of soft lens technology. Some of the early techniques are now obsolete.

Notwithstanding the above, it is still necessary to maintain a capability for checking the parameters of soft contact lenses. Examples of reasons why a practitioner may wish to make such measurements include the following:

- To 'sample' features of a prescribed mass-produced lens.
- To check individual custom-made prescription and cosmetic lenses.
- To establish if certain parameters have changed with handling or maintenance.
- To reconcile observed ocular pathology with any lens defects.
- To uncover features of an otherwise unidentifiable lens being worn by a patient who is new to the practice.

The parameters of soft lenses are physically unstable once they are removed from the storage solution. This is most noticeable with thin, high-water-content lenses. An aqueous environment is required to give the lens physical support when not placed on the eye; thus, small saline-containing receptacles ('wet cells') have been developed for purposes of evaluation. Soft lens parameters are greatly influenced by temperature, pH and tonicity of the bathing solution. British and international standards (ISO 10344) for testing soft lenses advise that, when using a wet cell for checking a soft lens, the lens be immersed in 0.9% saline at $20 \pm 0.5°C$.

DOI: 10.1016/B978-0-7506-8869-7.00008-2

The chief parameters of a finished soft lens which can be assessed are:

- back optic zone radius (BOZR)
- overall diameter
- edge profile
- surface quality
- back vertex power (BVP)
- water content
- surface wettability.

Material-specific properties (e.g. specific gravity, optical transmission, elasticity and oxygen permeability) are typically measured in research or manufacturing laboratories. It is neither practical nor essential for these properties to be checked in the clinic.

Back optic zone radius

The back surface of a soft lens can be measured directly using a keratometer or radiuscope, and indirectly using the techniques of profile matching, apical height/sag measurement or interferometry.

Keratometry

Keratometers are designed and calibrated for estimating the curvature of the convex corneal surface. With slight modification, they can be adapted for measuring any reflective concave surface, as shown in Figure 8.1. In conjunction with a wet cell, this is a precise though cumbersome method for measuring the BOZR of a soft lens. Keratometer scales are calibrated for corneal radius and/or corneal surface power; thus, the keratometer scale needs to be recalibrated when used for estimating the BOZR of a soft lens. Recalibration can be achieved using rigid contact lenses of known BOZR.

Soft lenses are temperature-sensitive; raising the temperature of the fluid supporting system causes the lens to steepen. High-water-content lenses are more susceptible to temperature effects compared with low-water-content lenses. Several other factors can affect measurement, such

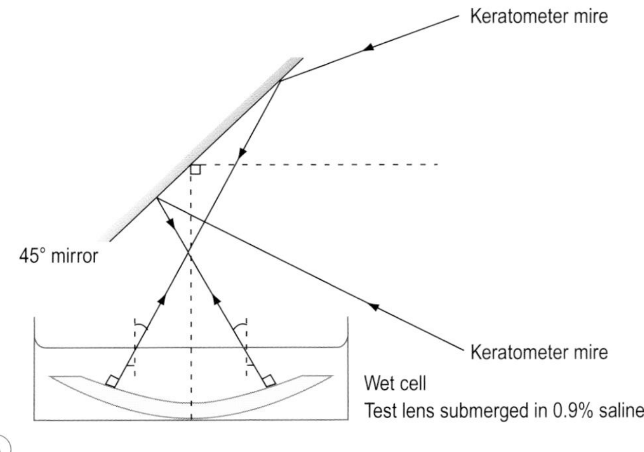

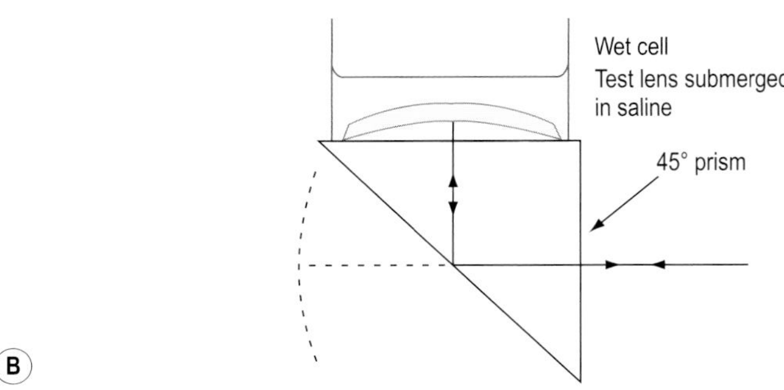

Figure 8.1 Keratometer attachments for checking the back optic zone radius (BOZR) of soft contact lenses. (A) Mirror system. (B) Prismatic system.

as the formation of air bubbles, vibrations and lens decentration. These potentially confounding influences must be overcome before finalizing the measurement (Holden, 1975; Chaston, 1977). Several soft lens wet cell attachments have been marketed (e.g. for the Zeiss keratometer), but most are no longer produced.

Radiuscopy

Although the radiuscope was originally developed for measuring the surface curvature of rigid lenses (see Chapter 15), it can also be used for soft lenses. Essentially, the radiuscope is a travelling microscope relying on the concave reflective properties of the lens back surface. The lens front surface is placed on a concave support with saline between this surface and the support surface. This helps to reduce the effects of unwanted reflections generated by the front surface. Droplets of saline are gently removed from the back surface and care must be taken to ensure the lens is not distorted in any way. The back surface of the test lens is focused with the instrument; then the aerial image of a target formed by reflection from this surface is focused. This time-consuming technique is rarely used for soft lens measurement.

Profile matching

The lens is placed with its circular edge in contact with an optical flat. The lens is illuminated from the side using a cold light projector. A magnified profile of the lens back surface is projected on to a series of curves of varying radii.

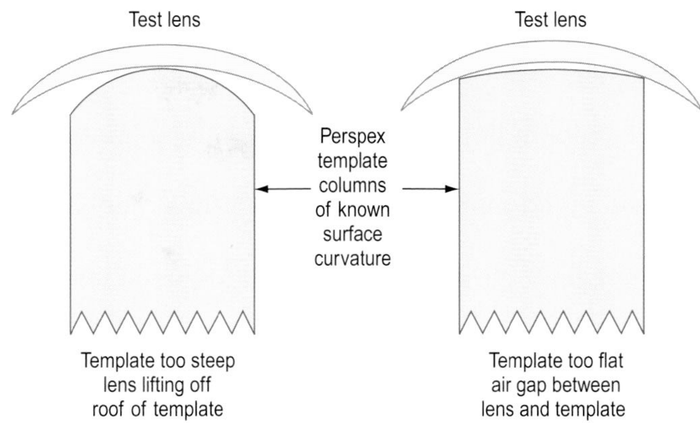

Figure 8.2 Template method for determining back optic zone radius.

After correcting for magnification, the radius of the curve best fitting the profile is an indication of lens BOZR (Loran, 1974). Another similar technique – but one requiring contact with the lens – involves placing the lens on a series of perspex domes of known and varying curvature. This has been termed the 'template method' (Harris *et al.*, 1973). If the lens is steeper than the dome, an air bubble will appear between the lens and dome and/or central lens warpage will be observed. The lens is placed on progressively steeper domes until the air bubble is no longer observed and the lens surface is smooth. If the lens is flatter than the dome, a section of the lens edge will be seen to lift off the periphery of the dome. This is a very crude though rapid method of radius assessment (Figure 8.2).

The 'sag' method

The radius of curvature of a circle can be calculated by measuring the height, or sag, of the curve over a fixed chord diameter. In Figure 8.3,

$$R = (y^2 + s^2)/2s \qquad \text{(Equation 8.1)}$$

where R is the radius, s is the sag height and y is half the chord diameter. By differentiating this formula, the minimum change or difference in s required to detect a change or difference in R of +0.05 mm can be calculated as:

$$dR/ds = 0.5 - (y^2/2s^2) \qquad \text{(Equation 8.2)}$$

For y = 5 mm and s = 2 mm, ds = –0.019 mm. Hence, sag methods should be capable of measuring apical height to within a tolerance of 0.019 mm. Clearly, if y is reduced, then ds will also reduce in order to maintain the tolerance in R.

Instrument manufacturers have used this approach to develop several devices for determining lens back surface radius. Using an appropriate calibration curve, the BOZR can be estimated. The apical height can be measured using mechanical or ultrasonic probes (Koetting, 1981; Patella *et al.*, 1982), either in air or saline. In ultrasonic devices, the sound beam is reflected from the back surface. Referring to Figure 8.3, the time taken for the sound beam to pass point A, reach point B, and back again, is directly proportional to the apical height of the lens. Using one such ultrasonic system (Panametrics model 25DL, USA), Young *et al.* (1999) were able to measure the BOZR of mass-produced disposable lenses to within ±0.1 mm of the stated value.

Mechanical probe devices are operated by 'zeroing' the probe at point A and then raising the probe until it touches

Diagram of 'sag' theory

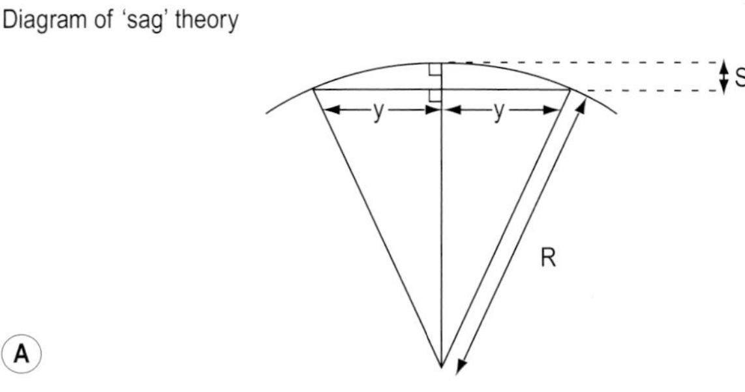

Mechanical sag-based system (in air; wet cell systems are available)

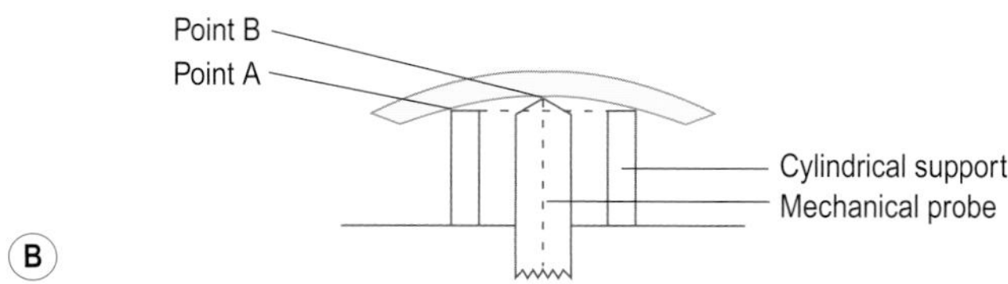

Figure 8.3 Sag method for determining back optic zone radius. (A) Sag theory; (B) mechanical sag-based system.

point B (Figure 8.3). The Optimec contact lens analyser (Chiltern, UK) incorporates such a mechanical probe. The lens is immersed in saline, the temperature of which can be internally controlled in some models. A magnified side-view profile of the lens is projected on to a viewing screen. The mechanical probe is manually raised until the observer witnesses slight lens movement, indicating that the probe has come into contact with the posterior pole of the lens. This device tends to measure BOZR slightly less than stated when used on most lenses (Port, 1982; Patel *et al.*, 1988).

The BC Tronic (Medicornea, France) also features a mechanical probe, but in this instrument, the sag height is measured in air and relies on completing a weak electrical circuit through the lens. The lens is placed on a cylindrical column and a central probe is gently raised until it touches the back surface of the lens. On contact, an electrical circuit is completed. The height of the probe is electronically monitored and displayed; once the probe touches the lens back surface, the displayed figure is 'frozen'. This figure is the sag height of the lens, and using a calibration chart the BOZR corresponding to the recorded sag height can be determined. The lens is measured in air, using one of two columns (10- or 12-mm diameter). For low-water-content soft lenses the BC Tronic has a tendency to indicate a flatter BOZR than stated (Patel *et al.*, 1988).

The sag method assumes the lens back surface is spherical over the chord diameter of measurement. If the surface is aspheric, the estimated BOZR can be noted as the 'equivalent sphere'. If it is suspected that a particular lens design has an aspheric back surface, it is possible to estimate the asphericity of the surface by measuring the apical height over more than one chord diameter. Consider a curve that is rotationally symmetrical about the x-axis passing through the Cartesian coordinates 0,0. This curve can be described using Baker's equation as follows:

$$y^2 = 2rx - px^2 \qquad \text{(Equation 8.3)}$$

where r is the radius of the curve at the origin 0,0 and p is the shape factor, a numerical indicator of asphericity. When p is less than 1, the curve is a flattening (prolate) ellipse. When $p = 0$, the curve is a parabola. When p is greater than 1, the curve is a steepening (oblate) ellipse. When p is negative the curve is hyperbolic.

Let the sag height x_1 be measured over a hemichord diameter y_1 and repeated (x_2) for a second hemichord diameter of y_2. Then it follows:

$$p = [y_2^2 x_1 - y_1^2 x_2]/[x_1^2 x_2 - x_2^2 x_1] \qquad \text{(Equation 8.4)}$$

In a study using the BC Tronic to measure BOZR for two lens designs, the estimated radius using a 10 mm diameter column was greater than the estimate using a 12 mm diameter column (Patel *et al.*, 1988). Extrapolating the published data, and using Equation 8.4, it can be shown that soft lens back surfaces used in that study were aspheric with a back surface akin to a steepening ellipse with a p value of approximately 1.3.

Interferometry

There are two types of interferometry, optical and geometric. Both have been applied to assess soft contact lenses.

Optical interferometry

Optical interferometry is one of the most precise methods for estimating the shape of a reflecting surface relative to a test surface of known parameters. Using Newton's rings, or a similar optical arrangement, the resolution of the technique is of the order $\lambda/2$, where λ is the wavelength of light. A Newton's rings arrangement is cumbersome, time-consuming and difficult to use with unstable devices such as soft lenses. This has limited its popularity. The technique is eminently suitable for checking non-spherical surfaces (El Nashar *et al.*, 1979) and for any minute imperfections on either the front or back surface of a contact lens.

In keeping with current technology for quantifying corneal topography, the interference pattern could be computer-grabbed, digitized and analysed to create a topographic map of contact lens surface architecture; however, the economic viability and practical value of such a system designed for soft lens measurement are questionable. An interference pattern can be generated from a pair of reflecting optical interfaces. When a soft lens with its front surface pointing upwards is placed in a wet cell with saline just covering the front surface, there are four optical interfaces that can potentially generate up to six separate interference patterns (Figure 8.4). These patterns can overlap and can be troublesome with regard to analysis. The interference pattern directly related to the surface of interest – the lens back surface – could be improved using a variety of optical modifications and computer-assisted image enhancement techniques. Another limitation of this technique is that slight movements or vibrations can upset the relevant interference pattern, resulting in significant problems in both image detection and measurement.

Geometric interferometry

'Moiré fringes' are geometric interference patterns produced when two gratings overlap (Oster and Nishijima, 1963). An example of this enigmatic pattern is shown in Figure 8.5, where two gratings consisting of parallel dark and clear lines are inclined by an angle θ relative to each other.

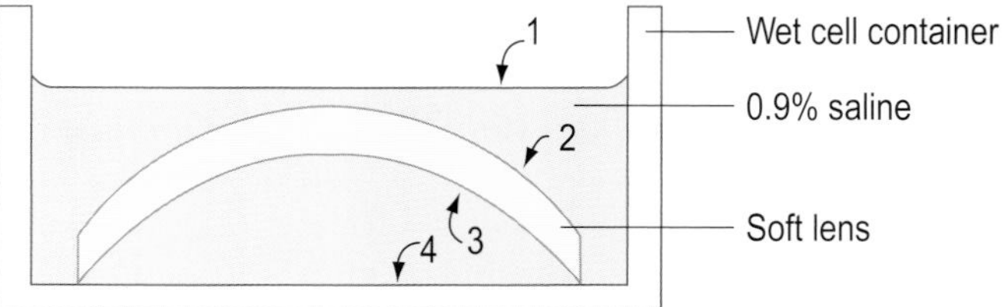

Figure 8.4 Optical interferometry used to determine the surface shape of soft lenses in saline. The surfaces labelled 1–4 are capable of generating troublesome interference patterns.

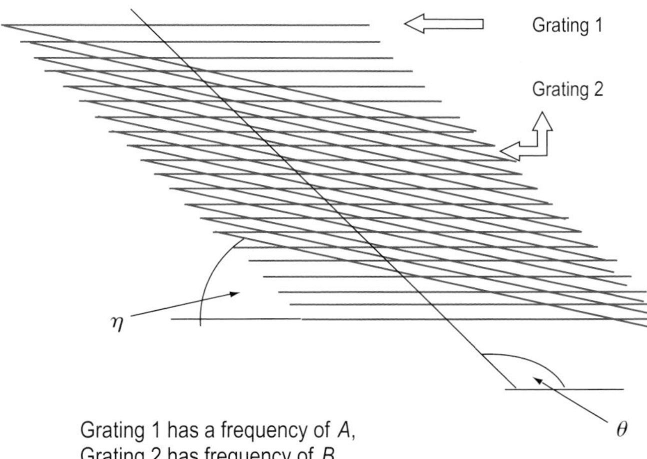

Figure 8.5 Moiré pattern resulting from an overlap of two gratings.

The angular direction of the resultant pattern (φ) depends on the ratio of the frequency of one grating relative to the other and the angular separation of the two gratings (θ). The ratio of frequencies is the same as the ratio of the apparent sizes of the gratings. If the apparent size of one grating is known for a particular Moiré pattern, as well as the values of θ and φ, then the apparent size of the other grating can be calculated as follows:

$$B/A = [\sin\theta/\tan\varphi] + \cos\theta \quad \text{(Equation 8.5)}$$

where A is the apparent size of the lines in grating 1, and B is the apparent size of the lines in grating 2 at the viewing plane. In Figure 8.5, $A = B$. However, keeping θ constant and separating the gratings along the viewing axis (i.e. out of the plane of the paper), the direction of the Moiré pattern (φ) would change because A would no longer equal B at the plane of observation. A curved reflecting surface has magnifying properties depending on radius. If the image of a grating of known frequency is formed by reflection from the back surface of a soft lens, and this image is analysed in a Moiré pattern arrangement, it is possible to create an optical system whereby the radius of the unknown surface is a relatively simple function of φ. The Visionix system (Rotlex, Israel) is a commercially available soft lens-measuring device with a built-in program that analyses the resulting Moiré pattern; it offers a unique tool for assessing aspheric lens surfaces and power over a central 5 mm aperture. Moiré pattern systems are valuable for checking non-spherical surfaces in multifocal lenses.

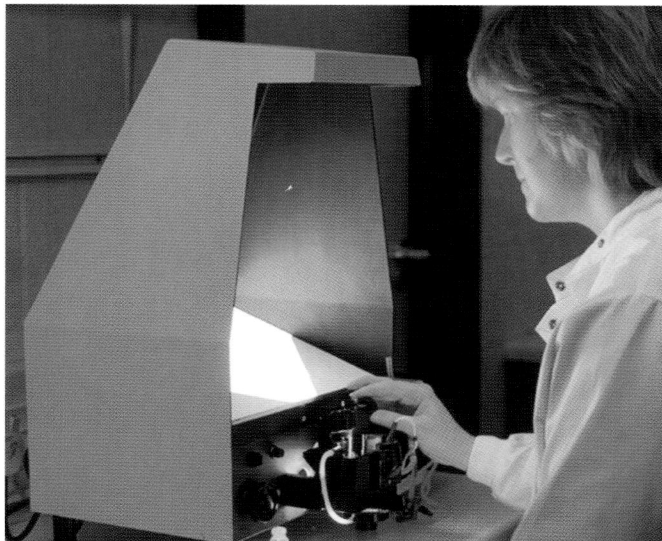

Figure 8.6 The Optimec soft contact lens analyser, which allows an optical projection of the lens to be viewed at 17× magnification.

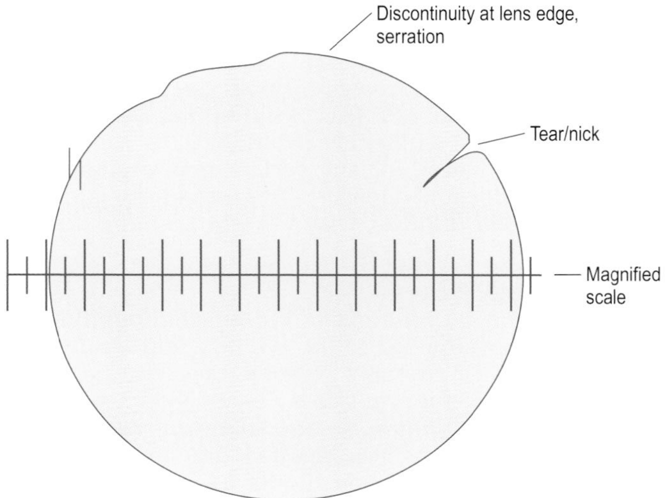

Figure 8.7 Projection technique for checking lens diameter and quality.

Overall diameter, optic zones, edge profile and surface quality

The overall diameter of soft lenses is best measured using a projection magnifier and a graduated scale. The Optimec soft contact lens analyser (Chiltern, UK) is one such device; it has a magnification of 17× (Figure 8.6). The lens is placed in saline, illuminated with a cold light source, and the projected image is focused on to a fixed scale (Figure 8.7). The projected image can be checked for any optical defects and regularity of the circumference. Using this system, it was shown by Young *et al.* (1999) that certain frequent-replacement lens designs tended to be larger than quoted by the manufacturer.

The same device can be used to check the optic zones (Figure 8.8), and the body of the lens and the lens periphery for physical defects.

During the early days of frequent-replacement lenses up to 75% of brand new lenses were found to have edge

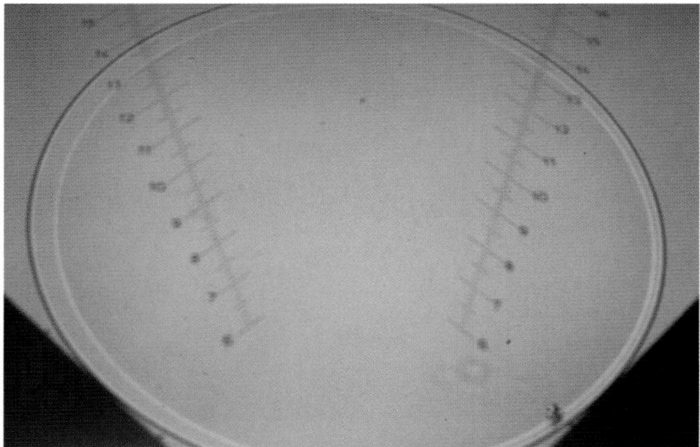

Figure 8.8 A lens with an eccentric optic zone (decentred to the right), viewed using the Optimec soft contact lens analyser.

defects using this device (Efron and Veys, 1992). For toric, truncated lenses, the smoothness of edge transition can also be checked. It is essential that the lens is assessed at fixed temperature. The measuring device should be calibrated regularly and the overall diameter of the lens should be measured to a precision of ±0.05 mm.

The overall diameter can also be measured *in vivo* using a video slit-lamp biomicroscope. This is useful for quantifying the effects of *in vivo* lens bending and dehydration. Projection systems with either a dark or light background can be used to check for any surface imperfections (e.g. scratches, residue and deposits). This assessment is vital in the case of either printed or hand-finished cosmetic lenses.

Back vertex power

The true power supplied to the eye by a soft lens can be easily checked by subjective or objective refraction after placing the lens on the eye. This is a relatively simple practical procedure that bypasses some of the factors that can affect the power of the lens, e.g. dehydration and flexure. Furthermore, the distribution of optical power supplied by the lens to the eye over the pupil can now be checked *in vivo* using corneal topographic systems. Subtracting the corneal surface topographic map from the map of the lens surface after placing on the eye results in a point-by-point picture of the actual power supplied to the eye over the pupil. This clinical procedure is particularly useful for checking the optical performance of toric, aspheric, bi- or multifocal soft lenses. For more advanced and customized lens designs, optical wavefront analysis can be used to assess the quality of the optics the lens is delivering to the eye *in vivo*. Optical wavefront systems are gradually entering mainstream practice as the emerging designs become more practical and affordable. These techniques are ideal for *in vivo* lens power checking, but what about *in vitro* checking? The remainder of this section is devoted to bench tests for lens power.

A standard optical focimeter can be used to measure soft lens BVP (Figure 8.9). An automatic focimeter can also be used. Any surface droplets, distortions or lens surface deposition (even fingerprints) will decrease the quality of the viewed image and this increases the likelihood of an error in assessing BVP. The recommended technique, therefore, is to surfactant-clean the lens, dab the lens dry with a

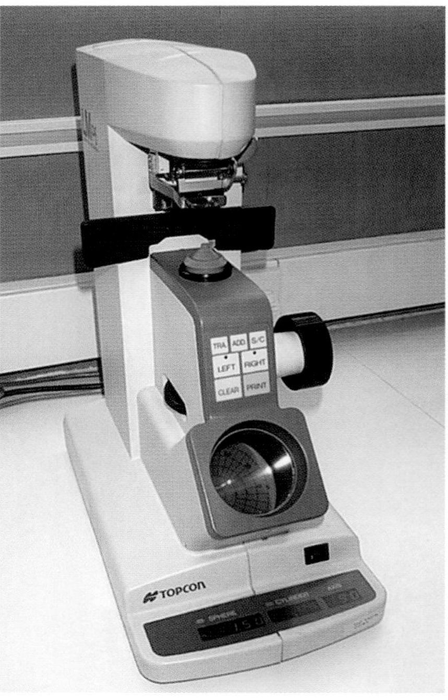

Figure 8.9 A vertically oriented optical focimeter with reduced aperture to support a soft lens.

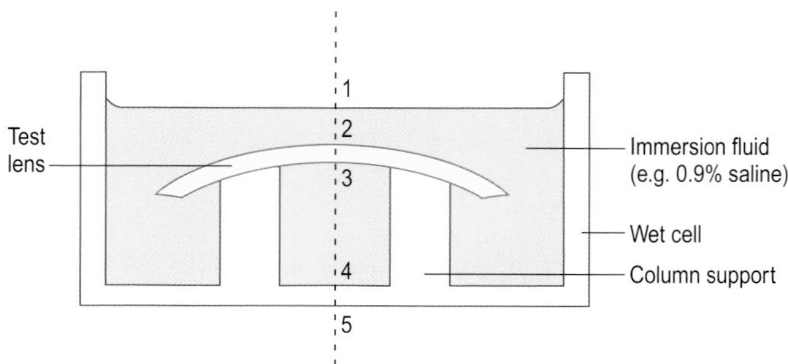

Figure 8.10 Wet cell for measuring back vertex power. Refraction takes place at the five interfaces (labelled 1–5) where there is a change in refractive index.

lint-free tissue and place the lens on the focimeter support using rubber-tipped tweezers.

A potential problem when measuring BVP in air is that lens dehydration can influence the result. Placing the lens in a wet cell filled with saline would obviate these difficulties (Figure 8.10). The BVP of the lens–saline complex is measured and the BVP of the lens in air can be calculated. The BVP of a lens is a function of the front and back surface radii, central thickness and refractive index of the lens material in relation to ambient temperature. In saline, the effective BVP of the lens is reduced. Using 'thin' lens optical approximations, it can be shown that, for a hydroxyethyl methacrylate lens of refractive index 1.43, a ±0.25 D uncertainty in saline wet cell focimetry yields a ±1.00 D error in deriving lens BVP in air (Harris *et al.*, 1973). This error increases to ±2.50 D for a lens of refractive index 1.37. Placing the lens in an optically clear liquid medium of relatively high refractive index can improve the accuracy of wet-cell focimetry. Ideally, the refractive index of the medium should be 0.2 units greater or lower than the

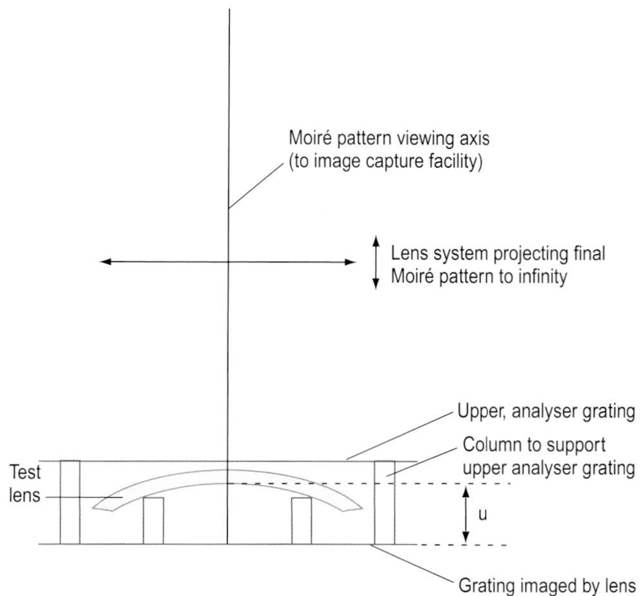

Figure 8.11 Technique for checking back vertex power using Moiré patterns projected to infinity.

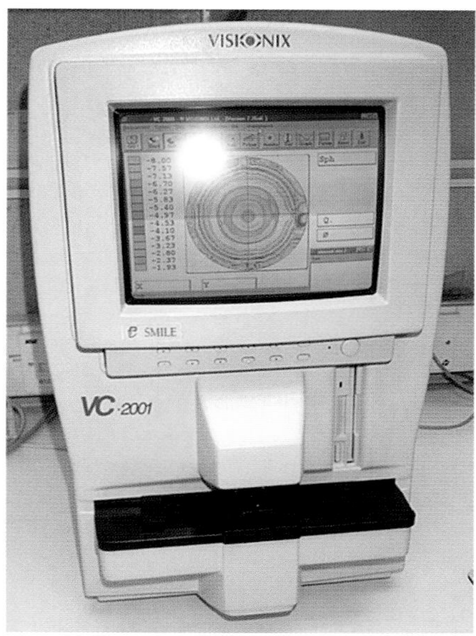

Figure 8.12 The Visionix system (model VC2001), which is used to obtain a plot of the power distribution across a soft lens.

refractive index of the lens (Patel *et al.*, 1985). Unfortunately, most non-toxic media with acceptable optical properties can damage soft lenses. Cinnamaldehyde, with a refractive index of 1.62, has been used as a destructive test for checking soft lens power and as such, can be used as a quality control procedure (Patel *et al.*, 1985).

The BVP can be calculated after measuring each individual dependent parameter featured in the BVP formula, but the cumulative effect of errors in the measurement of each of the dependent parameters limits the value of this approach (Pearson, 2008). Nevertheless, the results from a saline-filled wet cell can be improved; using a double aperture (Scheiner disc), Plakitsi and Charman (1992) demonstrated that the reliability of the wet cell could be improved when checking the power distribution of low-water-content multifocal lenses.

Moiré pattern technology can be adapted to check lens BVP. In Figure 8.5, when a lens is placed between the gratings the angle of the resulting pattern would change because the image of the grating would be affected by the magnifying power of the lens. Such an arrangement is shown in Figure 8.11. It can be shown (Patel, 1985), assuming the lens is 'thin', that the power can be calculated as follows:

$$F = (1/u) \times (\{(\tan\varphi_1/\tan\varphi_0) \times [(\sin\theta + \cos\theta\tan\varphi_0)/(\sin\theta + \cos\theta\tan\varphi_1)]\} - 1) \quad \text{(Equation 8.6)}$$

where F is the lens power in air, u is the distance between the lens and the imaged grating, φ_1 is the angular direction of the pattern in the aperture of the lens, φ_0 is the direction outside the limits of the lens and θ is the angular separation of the gratings.

When the final Moiré pattern is viewed at infinity, Equation 8.6 reduces to:

$$F = (1/u) \times ([\tan\varphi_1/(\sin\theta + \cos\theta\tan\varphi_1)] - 1) \quad \text{(Equation 8.7)}$$

These expressions are based on thin-lens theory and further considerations are required for relatively thick lenses. Oster and Nishijima (1963) advocated using Moiré patterns for determining lens focal length, describing an optical arrangement for viewing the Moiré pattern at infinity. Indeed, any optical system that changes the apparent size of one grating in a Moiré pattern arrangement can be analysed to quantify its optical properties. The Visionix system (Rotlex, Israel) (Figure 8.12) has the facility for checking soft lens power in saline. The built-in pattern analysis software program can display lens power over a 5 mm central zone (Figure 8.13). This is a relatively fast, user-friendly tool, which is very useful for checking aspheric and multifocal lenses.

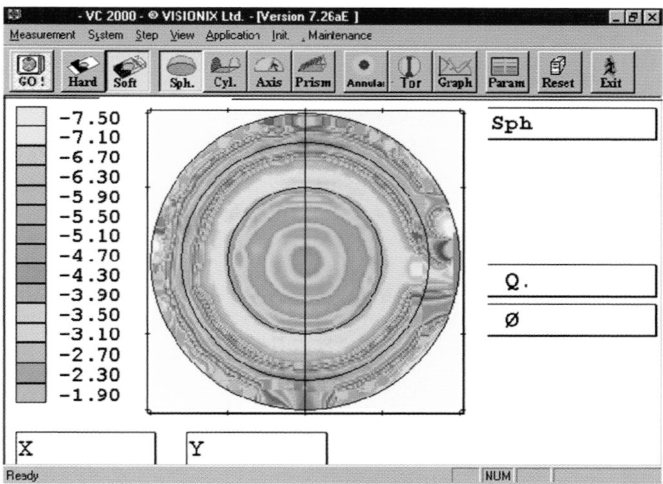

Figure 8.13 Power distribution plot from the Visionix system (model VC2001). Featured here is the power distribution across an Acuvue bifocal contact lens, clearly showing the concentric bifocal power zones.

Water content

Checking the water content of soft lenses is necessary because, for the bulk of hydrogel lens materials, the oxygen permeability is exponentially equated with water content (Fatt and Chaston, 1982; Morgan and Efron, 1998). To understand how a particular contact lens hydrogel responds to factors that in turn will affect oxygen permeability, a suitable clinical technique is required to quantify water content.

The water content of the lens can be estimated by the gravimetric method: weighing the sample in air at 20°C (W_1), completely dehydrating the lens in a suitable oven and then reweighing the dried sample (W_2). The water content is defined by $(W_1 - W_2)/W_1 \times 100\%$. Alternatively, dehydration can be achieved by placing the lens above an active desiccant such as anhydrous calcium sulphate ($CaSO_4$). This technique may also be used for silicone hydrogel lenses. Efron *et al.* (2007) found good agreement between their measured values and those stated by the manufacturers for five different silicone hydrogels lens types. Although the above technique is a useful approach in a research environment, it is destructive and therefore of no value to the clinician. Nuclear magnetic resonance techniques are non-destructive, and can be applied to determine the proportion of water in the lens, but this is not viable economically.

The refractive index of a hydrogel is directly related to its water content. In theory, this is based on the simple Gladstone–Dale law (Gladstone and Dale, 1863). The Gladstone–Dale law, originally proposed for liquid mixtures, is a simple way of predicting the final refractive index of a solution (N) based on the refractive indices of the solvent (N_1), the solid (N_2) and their relative proportions, as follows:

$$N = N_1X_1 + N_2X_2 \qquad \text{(Equation 8.8)}$$

where X_2 is the relative proportion of solid present in the mixture as a percentage (a), and X_1 is the relative proportion of solvent in the mixture ($100 - a$).

Measurement of soft lens refractive index to infer water content is an accepted simple, rapid, non-destructive technique with universal appeal. Of the several ways one can measure refractive index, a hand-held optical refractometer is probably the simplest and most viable (Atago Soft Lens Refractometer, Atago, Japan) (Figure 8.14). This refractometer features a scale where refractive index values are replaced with percentage water content. It is a subjective device whereby the observer has to make a conscious decision when observing the instrument's scale concerning the water content of the lens being checked. In keeping with all subjective tests the measurements using this refractometer are prone to operator bias. An automated electronic refractometer suitable for soft lenses is also available offering objective measurements by circumventing such sources of bias (Index Instruments, Huntingdon, UK).

The resolution of refractometry to infer lens water content indirectly can be very high. A unit increase in refractive index of +0.001 is equivalent to a 0.7% drop in water content (Mousa *et al.*, 1983; Efron and Brennan, 1987; Patel, 1989). Because this is a surface-measuring technique, it is assumed that the refractive index at the surface is the same as the refractive index throughout the lens matrix. Deposits (e.g. protein or lipid) on a worn soft lens could increase the refractive index at the lens surface, which in turn could be misinterpreted as a fall in water content (Mousa *et al.*, 1983; Patel, 1989). Furthermore, it is not possible to measure the water content of certain types of cast-moulded lenses, which, as a result of the curing process, end up with a slight refractive index variation throughout the lens matrix.

The water content of silicone hydrogel lenses cannot be inferred directly from measurement of its refractive index. Hand refractometry overestimates the equilibrium water content of silicone hydrogel materials and this bias is related to the proportion of siloxane moieties in the material (González-Méijome *et al.*, 2006). Correction factors may be applied. The water content of silicone hydrogel lenses is of less relevance to the practitioner than that of hydrogel lenses as the oxygen transmissibility is not so closely tied to water content.

Thickness

Standard mechanical contact thickness-measuring systems are too robust for the delicate soft lens. In the Rehder electromechanical gauge (Rehder, USA), the force of contact is reduced to 0.015 N and thickness can be measured to a resolution of 0.01 mm (Figure 8.15).

The device still tends to compress the lens; thus, the result is typically lower than expected (Young *et al.*, 1999). The

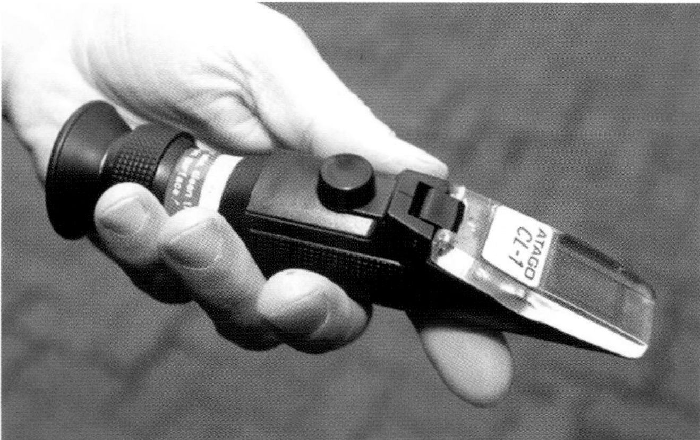

Figure 8.14 The Atago CL-1 soft lens refractometer, which is used to determine the water content of soft contact lenses.

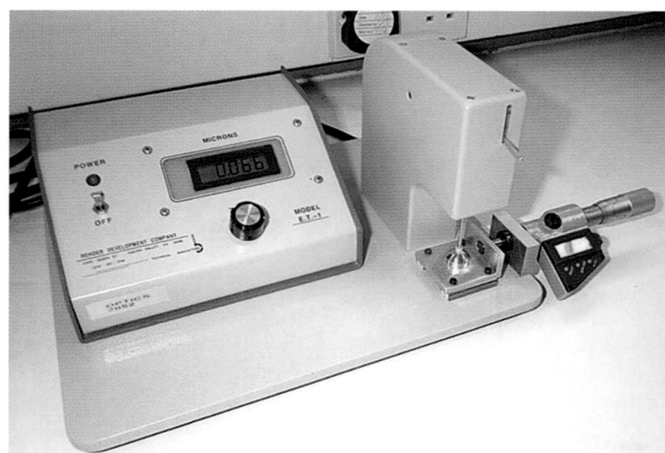

Figure 8.15 Rehder electromechanical gauge for measuring soft lens thickness. The lever is lowered until the vertical probe rests lightly in the surface of the lens, which rests on the support dome underneath. The instrument shown here has been modified for determining the thickness profile of a soft lens.

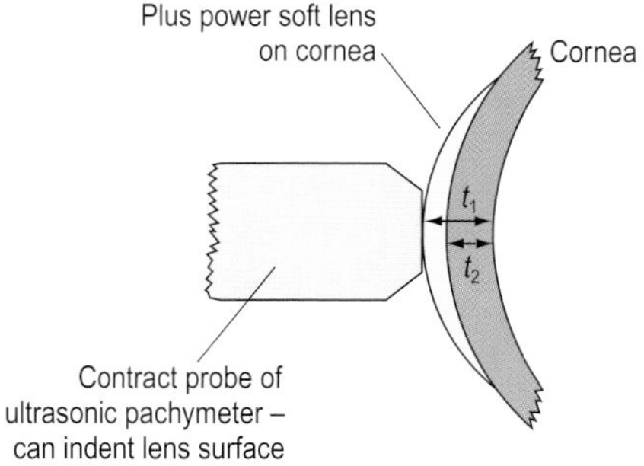

Figure 8.16 Ultrasonic pachymeter used to measure lens thickness *in vivo*.

thickness of a soft lens can be measured using a travelling microscope. In air or in saline, the microscope is focused on one surface and then the other at specific locations over the surface.

Electronic contact systems relying on the electrical conductivity of soft lenses have been developed. Using appropriate magnifying systems, the lens is centred on an electrical contact. Another contact is gradually lowered on to the lens; its position relative to the first contact is monitored using a Vernier scale. On contact with the lens, a flow of electrical current is detected, and the Vernier scale is read.

Using a slit-lamp biomicroscope, the lens can be carefully supported in air or in saline, and a side-view profile of the lens can be visualized. This allows for a qualitative assessment of the thickness distribution over a single 'slice' of the lens. It is possible to monitor lens thickness *in vivo*. With sufficient magnification on a video slit lamp, an optical section through the lens can be produced, video-captured, digitized and analysed.

Optical and ultrasonic pachymeters, although designed for measuring corneal thickness, can also be used for measuring soft lens thickness (Ruben, 1974). For example, as shown in Figure 8.16, a solid probe ultrasonic pachymeter can be used to measure the thickness of a lens–cornea complex at the centre of cornea (t_1). The lens is then removed and central corneal thickness (t_2) is measured after anaesthetizing the cornea. The difference ($t_1 - t_2$) is the relative thickness of the lens. The exact thickness depends on the velocity setting for the particular model of ultrasonic pachymeter, and any indentation of the lens surface. With practice, this can be a very effective way of checking lens thickness *in vivo*.

The average thickness of a lens can be easily calculated by measuring lens weight (w) and overall diameter ($2r$) in air. From the material density (ρ), lens volume $v = w/\rho$. Assuming the lens is a circular disc, with volume $= t\pi r^2$, then the average thickness $t = w/\rho\pi r^2$. This simple approach is useful in attempts to quantify the typical oxygen transmissibility of a lens. Appendix F allows calculation of soft lens average thickness.

Surface wettability

The wettability, or surface affinity for water, of a biological polymer can be measured using several techniques, such as the sessile drop method (Fatt, 1984; Knick and Huff, 1991). This laboratory test is difficult to perform in a clinical environment and it does not predict how well a material will perform on a specific eye. Evaluating the stability of the pre-lens surface *in vivo* is a particularly valuable indirect measure of lens wettability in association with the tear properties of the individual patient. This feature can be assessed during a routine aftercare examination to indicate any variations in lens performance. The wettability can be quantified indirectly by measuring the stability of the pre-lens tear film using a specular reflection from the illumination source of a slit-lamp biomicroscope, keratometer or Tearscope (Patel, 1987; Guillon and Guillon, 1989; Golding *et al.*, 1990). In a well-fitted clean lens, after a blink, the keratometer mire reflex should be crisp and clear. With the eye remaining open after a few seconds, the quality of the mire will develop a localized blur, split or general discontinuity, as shown in Figure 8.17. These changes result from a breakdown in the pre-lens tear film. The time between the blink and depreciation in quality of the reflected mire is an indication of surface wetting. This technique is very suited for tracking changes in wettability with the duration of lens wear and resulting from lens care systems (Patel, 1987; Patel *et al.*, 1996).

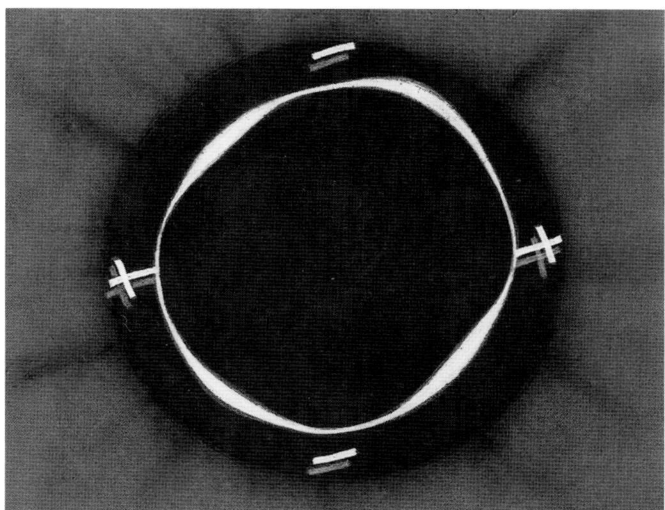

Figure 8.17 Distorted keratometer mire on a normal cornea can indicate poor surface wettability.

With either the Keeler Tearscope or Bausch & Lomb keratometer, significant intersubject and interlens variations in lens wettability are observed. *In vivo*, assessment of wettability is a useful indicator of the physiological behaviour of the lens. Poor wetting can adversely affect visual performance and facilitate lens deposition. Shearing optical interferometry using a low-power He-Ne laser has also been applied to observe the dynamics of the tear film over the soft lens *in vivo* and, as such, quantify the surface wettability of individual finished lenses on individual eyes (Licznerski *et al.*, 1998). This is an excellent and promising laboratory technique. However, this procedure has met with limited success with industry and leading clinicians.

Conclusion

Several advanced systems have been developed for checking the parameters and physical integrity of soft lenses. Many of these techniques can be easily included in a busy contact lens practice. Finer details, tolerances and physical limits of precision of the essential measurements are listed in a range of British and international standards. The key standards applicable to soft lens technology are summarized in Appendix B.

References

Chaston, J. (1977) In office measurement of soft contact lenses. *Am. J. Optom. Physiol. Opt.*, **54,** 286–291.

Efron, N. and Brennan, N. A. (1987) The soft contact lens refractometer. *Optician,* **194,** 29–41.

Efron, N. and Veys, J. (1992) Defects in disposable contact lenses can compromise ocular integrity. *Int. Contact Lens Clin.,* **19,** 8–18.

Efron, N., Morgan, P. B., Cameron, I. D. *et al.* (2007) Oxygen permeability and water content of silicone hydrogel contact lens materials. *Optom. Vis. Sci.,* **84,** 328–337.

El Nashar, N., Brookes, C. and Larke, J. (1979) The measurement of the Bausch and Lomb Soflens contact lens by interferometry. *Am. J. Optom. Physiol. Opt.,* **56,** 10–15.

Fatt, I. (1984) Contact lens wettability. Myths, mysteries and realities. *Am. J. Optom. Physiol. Opt.,* **61,** 419–430.

Fatt, I. and Chaston, J. (1982) Measurement of O_2 transmissibility and permeability of hydrogel lenses and materials. *Int. Contact Lens Clin.,* **9,** 76–88.

Gladstone, J. M. and Dale, T. P. (1863) Research in the refraction, dispersion and sensitiviness of liquids. *Phil. Trans. Roy. Soc. (Lond.),* **153,** 317–337.

Golding, T. R., Efron, N. and Brennan, N. A. (1990) Soft lens lubricants and prelens tear film stability. *Am. J. Optom. Physiol. Opt.,* **67,** 461–465.

González-Méijome, J. M., Lira, M., López-Alemany, A. *et al.* (2006) Refractive index and equilibrium water content of conventional and silicone hydrogel contact lenses. *Ophthalmic Physiol. Opt.,* **26,** 57–64.

Guillon, M. and Guillon, J-P. (1989) Hydrogel lens wettability during overnight wear. *Ophthal. Physiol. Opt.,* **9,** 355–359.

Harris, M. G., Hall, K. and Oye, R. (1973) Measurement and stability of hydrophilic lens dimensions. *Am. J. Optom. Arch. Am. Acad. Optom.,* **50,** 546–552.

Holden, B. A. (1975) An accurate and reliable method of measuring soft contact lens curvatures. *Aust. J. Optom.,* **58,** 443–449.

Knick, P. D. and Huff, J. W. (1991) Effects of temperature and conditioning on contact lens wetting angles. *Contact Lens Assoc. Ophthalmol. J.,* **17,** 177–180.

Koetting, R. A. (1981) Use of the Medicornea B.C. Tronic unit. *Am. J. Optom. Physiol. Opt.,* **58,** 631–632.

Licznerski, T. J., Lechna, M. I., Kasprzak, H. T. (1998) Application of interferometry for in-vivo testing of the stability of the tera film on the contact lens. *Proc SPIE.,* **3579,** 152–157.

Loran, D. F. C. (1974) Determination of hydrogel contact lens radii by projection. *Ophthalmic Optician.,* **14,** 980–985.

Morgan, P. B. and Efron, N. (1998) Oxygen performance of contemporary hydrogel contact lenses. *Contact. Lens Ant. Eye.,* **21,** 3–6.

Mousa, G. Y., Callender, M. G., Sivak, J. G. *et al.* (1983) The effects of the hydration characteristics of hydrogel lenses on the refractive index. *Int. Contact Lens. Clin.,* **10,** 31–37.

Oster, G. and Nishijima, Y. (1963) Moiré patterns. *Sci. Am.,* **208,** 54–64.

Patel, S. (1985) *Refractive index and power of the cornea in relation to hydration and thickness.* M. Phil thesis, Glasgow Caledonian University.

Patel, S. (1987) The constancy of the front surface desiccation times for Igel 67 lenses in vivo. *Am. J. Optom. Physiol. Opt.,* **64,** 167–171.

Patel, S. (1989) Apparent changes in the refractive index of hydrogel lenses. *Ophthal. Physiol. Opt.,* **9,** 222–225.

Patel, S., Kayani, N., Birbeck, F. *et al.* (1985) An improved immersion method of soft lens power assessment. Parts I, II, III. *J. Brit. Cont. Lens. Assoc.,* **8,** 53–70.

Patel, S., MacKay, C. and McCallum, G. (1988) The clinical evaluation of hydrogel lens back optic zone radius according to 3 commercially available procedures. *J. Brit. Cont. Lens. Assoc.,* **11,** 17–24.

Patel, S., Thomson, A. and Raj, S. (1996) Tear Stability With Planned Replacement Soft Lenses. *Optician – Contact Lens Monthly* **212**(No. 5558) July 5, pp 28–30.

Patella, M. J., Harris, M. G., Wong, V. A. *et al.* (1982) Ultrasonic measurement of soft contact lens base curves. *Int. Contact Lens. Clin.,* **9,** 41–53.

Pearson, R. M. (2008) Aspects of wet cell measurement of back vertex power of contact lenses. *Clin. Exp. Optom.* **91,** 461–468.

Plakitsi, A. and Charman, W. N. (1992) On the reliability of focimeter measurements of simultaneous vision varifocal contact lenses. *J. Brit. Cont. Lens. Assoc.,* **15,** 115–124.

Port, M. J. A. (1982) Comparison of two soft lens radiuscopes. *J. Brit. Cont. Lens. Assoc.,* **5,** 107–116.

Ruben, M. (1974) Soft lenses: the physico-chemical characteristics. *Contacto,* **18,** 11–23.

Young, G., Lewis, Y., Coleman, S. *et al.* (1999) Process capability of frequent replacement spherical soft contact lenses. *Contact. Lens. Ant. Eye.,* **22,** 127–135.

CHAPTER 9

Soft lens design and fitting

Graeme Young

Introduction

Assessment of soft contact lens fit is probably the most commonly undertaken task in contact lens practice but is also one of the least discussed, possibly because it is regarded as a relatively straightforward exercise. However, soft lens fitting is not just a process of finding a soft lens that fits but of determining the soft lens and wearing regimen that will provide the patient with the most comfortable, convenient and safe contact lens wear.

There is a traditional view that fitting soft lenses is a poor second choice to the much safer and technically challenging option of rigid lenses; however, this view is no longer sustainable. Studies of frequent-replacement soft lenses have shown little difference in the complication rates between soft and rigid lenses (Hamano *et al.*, 1994; Nilsson, 1997; Dart *et al.*, 2008). Furthermore, the increased choices of materials, wearing regimens, care systems and lenses themselves make the decision-making process as complex for soft lenses as rigid lenses. Since these decisions rely on clinical judgement rather than measurement, soft lens fitting, when done well, is a skilled activity.

Ocular measurement

Contrary to popular belief, keratometry is of little help in the fitting of soft lenses because the curvature of the central cornea is only one of a number of relevant ocular parameters governing soft lens fit. If soft lens fitting is a process of identifying the optimum lens sagittal depth for a given eye, then the sagittal height of the eye is the key biometric parameter. Normal variations in corneal asphericity and diameter have a greater effect on corneal sagittal height than the normal variation in corneal curvature (Young, 1992). Thus, keratometry alone is a poor predictor of the optimum soft contact lens back optic zone radius (BOZR). Since there is a positive correlation between corneal diameter and corneal curvature (i.e. a tendency for flatter corneas to be larger in diameter), any change in sagittal height due to varying corneal radius is nullified by corresponding variation in corneal diameter (Garner, 1982). This would suggest that corneal asphericity is the most important determinant of soft lens fit.

One caveat applies, however, with atypical combinations of corneal diameter and curvature which may indicate extremes of sagittal height. For instance, a large cornea showing a relatively steep keratometry measurement is likely to have a relatively large sagittal height and will probably require a soft contact lens with a correspondingly large sagittal depth (i.e. steep). Conversely, a small flat cornea is likely to have a small corneal sagittal height and require a relatively flat BOZR. When viewed from the side, these corneas often seem abnormally deep or shallow, even to the naked eye.

Measurement of the horizontal visible iris diameter (HVID) provides a useful guide to whether a large or small lens is required. However, this is only a rough indicator because the true corneal diameter is significantly larger than the iris diameter. The horizontal corneal diameter has been shown to be, on average, 1.25 mm larger than the HVID (Martin and Holden, 1982). This can be measured to the nearest half-millimetre with a PD rule or, more accurately, using a slit-lamp graticule.

Palpebral aperture does not have the same relevance as in the fitting of rigid lenses but extreme cases are worth noting. A narrow palpebral aperture may increase difficulties of insertion and so, given the choice, a smaller lens may be appropriate. Larger palpebral apertures are often associated with incomplete blinking. This might influence the choice of lens material, particularly when noted in combination with signs of corneal desiccation staining.

Basic principles

Forces acting on a soft lens

A range of forces act on a soft lens, keeping the lens in place on the eye but allowing it to move a small amount between blinks (Figure 9.1).

Soft lenses are usually required to flex in two directions in order to align to the shape of the cornea and sclera. Since soft lenses are usually flatter than the central corneal

DOI: 10.1016/B978-0-7506-8869-7.00009-4

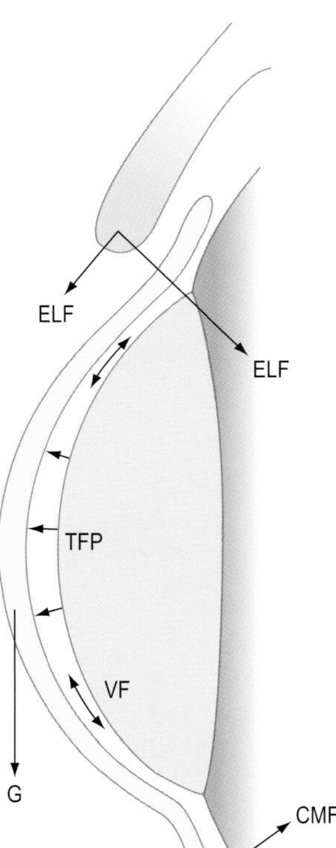

Figure 9.1 Forces acting on a soft lens. CMF = circumferential membrane force; ELF = eyelid force; G = gravity; MMF = meridional membrane force; TFP = tear fluid pressures; VF = viscous forces. (Adapted from Martin, D. K., Boulos, J., Gan, J. et al. (1989) A unifying parameter to describe the clinical mechanics of hydrogel contact lenses. Optom. Vis. Sci., 66, 87–91.)

curvature, they steepen in order to align with the cornea but, at the periphery, they are required to flatten so as to align with the sclera. The stresses formed in the lens are proportional to the mechanical properties of the material as well as the dimensions of the lens. Due to the viscous nature of the tear fluid, this deformation of the lens to match the shape of the eye results in pressures being developed in the post-lens tear film that Martin and Holden (1986) have termed 'squeeze pressure'. This squeeze pressure is related to the amount of force required to move the lens across the eye and therefore lens fit (Martin and Holden, 1986; Martin *et al.*, 1989). The amount of force required to move the lens is also related to the viscosity of the post-lens tear film (Martin, 1989). This helps to explain why the movement of a soft lens can vary markedly during a given wearing period.

Soft lens retaining forces are relatively large compared with those of rigid lenses and therefore gravitational force has less of an effect.

Ideal soft lens fit

The appropriate soft lens, as far as possible, should be indiscernible to the patient during wear. In other words, there should be no discomfort or disturbance of vision throughout the wearing period. Any effect on ocular physiology should be minimal and within acceptable limits. A well-fitting soft contact lens should fulfil the criteria listed in Table 9.1.

Table 9.1 Requirements of a well-fitting soft lens

Requirement	Significance
Good comfort	Patient satisfaction
Constant corneal coverage	Avoidance of peripheral corneal staining Comfort
Good centration	Corneal coverage Stable peripheral vision
Movement on blink or version	Adequate post-lens lubrication Exchange of metabolic waste Avoidance of conjunctival staining
Optimum tightness on push-up	Avoidance of discomfort through excessive movement or excessive mechanical squeeze force Avoidance of adherence with dehydration Avoidance of conjunctival indentation
Good peripheral fit (i.e. alignment)	Avoidance of conjunctival indentation Avoidance of edge stand-off; comfort
Good and stable vision	Patient satisfaction

Soft lens design

Contact lens practitioners have little direct control over lens design. Custom-made soft lenses can be ordered from specialist laboratories; however, these are relatively expensive. The practitioner is therefore dependent on the judgement of the manufacturer.

Most lenses are offered in a limited range of specifications, e.g. two BOZRs in a single diameter. Despite the relatively wide range of corneal diameters in the population, most spherical soft lenses are specified within a relatively narrow range of diameters: 14.0–14.5 mm.

The design of proprietary soft lenses is governed by a number of factors in addition to geometry, including material, method of manufacture and lens power.

Lens material and water content

The selection of contact lens material is relevant to several aspects of lens performance:

- oxygen transmission
- deposit resistance
- surface wetting
- rigidity (and therefore fitting characteristics).

Nowadays, there is little justification for using low-*Dk* lenses such as poly(hydroxyethyl methacrylate) (poly-HEMA) lenses. The effects of hypoxia with conventional low-water-content (i.e. <50%) lenses are well documented (Bruce and Brennan, 1990). Based on estimates of corneal swelling, complications such as corneal striae can be expected to affect a high proportion of wearers (Holden and Mertz, 1984; Efron, 1996). An exception to this rule is in those rare cases where it proves impossible to fit patients with higher-*Dk* products.

The prime decision, therefore, is whether to use a silicone hydrogel or conventional hydrogel material in mid- (50–60%) or high-water-content (>60%) lenses. All silicone hydrogel lenses will provide superior oxygen transmission compared with conventional lenses; however, they may incorporate disadvantages in relation to mechanical properties and surface wetting (see Chapter 5).

Comparing conventional hydrogels, a higher-water-content material does not necessarily guarantee that the lens will produce better oxygen transmissibility (Morgan and Efron, 1998). Different material categories (e.g. ionic and non-ionic) have differing strengths and weaknesses which can be taken into account when selecting a lens type for a given patient.

Higher-water-content lenses tend to be thicker for two reasons. Firstly, higher-water materials have a lower modulus and therefore tend to be less easy to handle in equivalent thicknesses. Secondly, there is a minimum thickness threshold for any material below which lenses tend to induce corneal desiccation staining. There is some variation between patients and precise material types; however, for a 70% water content material, the critical thickness is approximately 0.12 mm whereas with 38% polyHEMA it would be approximately 0.03 mm.

Method of manufacture

The method of lens manufacture can influence the edge design. Lathing allows a greater range of parameters and may be the best choice for patients who are otherwise hard to fit. Lathe-cut lenses, however, tend to incorporate a thicker edge design than moulded lenses as the lathing and polishing involved in lathe-cut lens manufacture do not allow the manufacture of thin lenses without high levels of breakage. Most moulding processes, on the other hand, allow extremely thin knife edges to be formed.

Back optic zone radius

Soft lenses are specified by BOZR or base curve, total diameter, centre thickness, back vertex power and material. If the lens is only available in a single specification (i.e. a one-fit lens), the lens brand name and power may be enough to specify the lens prescription. However, this apparent simplicity belies the complexity and importance of soft lens design. Lenses with apparently similar specifications can show widely differing fitting characteristics (Young *et al.*, 1997), for instance, due to variations in back surface design (Young *et al.*, 1993).

Traditionally, BOZR is the main parameter to be modified when attempting to optimize lens fit; a steepening of BOZR is required to tighten lens fit and vice versa. However, even with relatively thick polyHEMA lenses, large changes in BOZR are required in order to have a significant effect on lens movement (Lowther and Tomlinson, 1981). With thinner high-water lenses, changes in BOZR have even less effect. The labelled BOZR is therefore of little help in soft lens fitting.

BOZR is also not helpful when comparing different brands of lens. Lenses of similar BOZR can show widely differing sagittal depths because of differences in back surface design (Burki, 1997). This and differences in materials' mechanical properties means that widely differing lens fits may be observed from seemingly similar lenses. With silicone hydrogel lenses the high modulus of elasticity of many lenses means that even small (0.2 mm) changes in base curve can have a significant impact on lens fit and comfort (Dumbleton *et al.*, 2002).

Total diameter

Unfortunately, the labelled total diameter is often as unhelpful as the labelled BOZR. The fact that the water content, and therefore the dimensions, of some lens materials varies with temperature makes it difficult to compare the labelled diameter of one lens with another. Most non-ionic lenses, particularly those containing *N*-vinyl pyrrolidone, shrink by approximately 0.5 mm when raised from room to eye temperature. Ionic lenses are also temperature-sensitive although they shrink much less than non-ionic lenses (Young and Grewel, 1999). Some lenses are made larger in diameter to compensate for this.

A further complicating factor is that the on-eye diameter is affected by the sagittal depth of the lens. Lenses of similar nominal diameter can vary in sagittal depth by as much as 1 mm (Burki, 1997) and, since the periphery of a soft lens flattens to align with the scleral conjunctiva, the sagittal depth can have a significant effect on effective diameter.

Back vertex power

Some modifications are often made to the lens design at the extremes of the power range. At the lower end of the minus power range (<–1.50 D) the centre thickness is usually increased to improve lens handling. At the higher end of the power range, the centre thickness is often reduced and the optic zone diameter kept to a minimum in order to maximize oxygen transmission.

The thickness of high-minus lenses can be further reduced and the optical performance improved by incorporating aspheric optics in order to overcome lens spherical aberration (Cox, 1990). Aspheric optics can also be incorporated to reduce the spherical aberration of the eye (Kollbaum & Bradley, 2005). A number of designs are available which claim to use aspheric optics in order to improve visual performance (e.g. Bausch & Lomb PureVision, CooperVision Biomedics Premier); however, the published data suggest there is little benefit to be gained from these designs (Morgan *et al.*, 2005; Efron *et al.*, 2008).

With plus-power lenses, the optic zone diameter is again minimized in order to minimize centre thickness. Some manufacturers have utilized a larger diameter in order to accommodate the anticipated greater movement; however, hyperopic eyes tend to be smaller in diameter and therefore this is of doubtful benefit.

There tends to be little difference in lens fit between low-minus and higher-minus lenses of similar design. However, plus-power lenses tend to show significantly more post-blink movement than minus lenses, probably due to greater interaction with the upper lid (Young *et al.*, 1993).

Centre and edge thickness

Lens centre thickness is relevant to ease of lens handling and susceptibility to dehydration. Mid-water-content lenses (50–59%) are generally manufactured with centre thicknesses in the range 0.06–0.10 mm whereas high-water-content lenses (60%) generally have centre thicknesses in the range 0.10–0.18 mm.

Due to poor measurement repeatability, soft lens peripheral thickness is not the subject of an ISO standard and is not always routinely verified during lens manufacture. Nevertheless, variations in peripheral thickness can have a significant effect on lens fit; contrary to expectations, thicker-edged lenses often show a looser fit than thinner lenses of similar basic design (Young *et al.*, 1993).

Soft lens fitting options

Many soft lenses show an acceptable fit on a wide range of eyes but an acceptable fit is not necessarily the optimal or most comfortable fit. As well as finding the most appropriate lens design, selecting the optimal lens involves finding the lens material, lens replacement schedule and wearing regimen which best suit the individual patient. In order to achieve this, it is necessary to use a wide range of soft lens types and brands.

Trial lens fitting

Initial lens selection

As discussed earlier, without understanding the material and design characteristics of a particular lens, it is not possible to predict its clinical fitting performance. Even with this information, it is difficult to predict from keratometry and HVID measurements which lens is likely to be the most suitable.

The selection of first trial lens can take into account HVID, particularly if the cornea appears to be unusually large or small. The selection of BOZR is a process of trial and error unless there is useful information from the patient's previous lenses. If, for instance, the patient previously required a steeper-fitting lens in order to achieve a successful fit, this will suggest the need for a lens with relatively tight fitting characteristics.

Lens material and wearing regimen are also key factors in the selection of the initial trial lens. While compromises occasionally have to be made, these should be selected based on an assessment of the patient's requirements rather than prescribing habits or practice policy.

Soft lens insertion

1. Before inserting a soft lens, place it between the index and middle fingers and rinse with saline to remove any debris.
2. Allow the excess saline to drain before placing the lens on a dry index finger.
3. With the thumb of the other hand, hold open the patient's top lid while holding open the bottom lid with the middle finger of the other hand (Figure 9.2).
4. With the patient looking to the opposite side, place the lens on the bulbar conjunctiva, allowing it to stick by capillary force rather than pressure from the finger.
5. Slide the lens laterally on to the cornea. Continue to hold the lids open for a few seconds to allow the lens to settle.

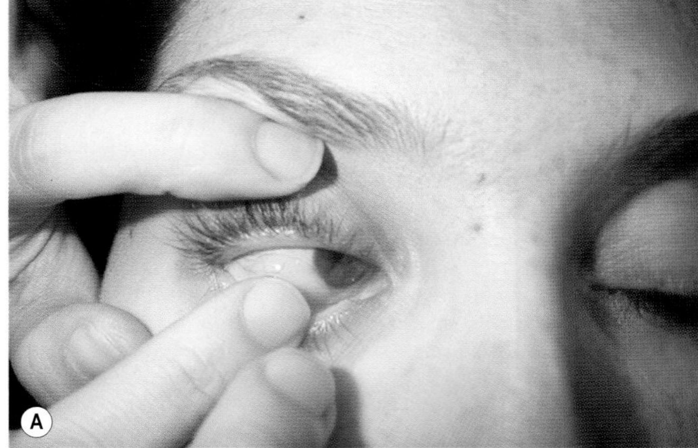

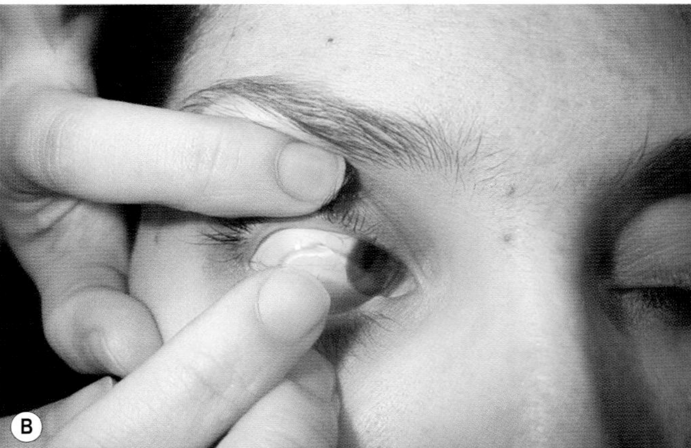

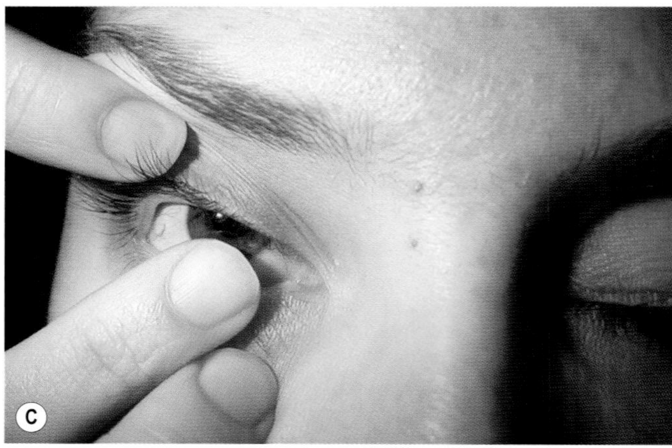

Figure 9.2 Inserting a soft lens. (A) Direct the gaze of the patient nasally to expose the bulbar conjunctiva. Retract the upper eyelid with your left forefinger, and the inferior eyelid with the middle finger of the right hand. (B) With your right forefinger, apply the lens to the bulbar conjunctiva of the patient. (C) Slide the lens laterally on to the cornea. Once the lens is centred on the cornea, and without air bubbles beneath it, your finger can be removed.

6. Ask the patient to look down then let go of the lids. With thin soft lenses the lens can be easily folded or dislodged if it has not properly settled.
7. If the patient finds the lens uncomfortable, this may be due to post-lens debris, in which case temporarily dislodging the lens on to the sclera may remove this (Figure 9.3).

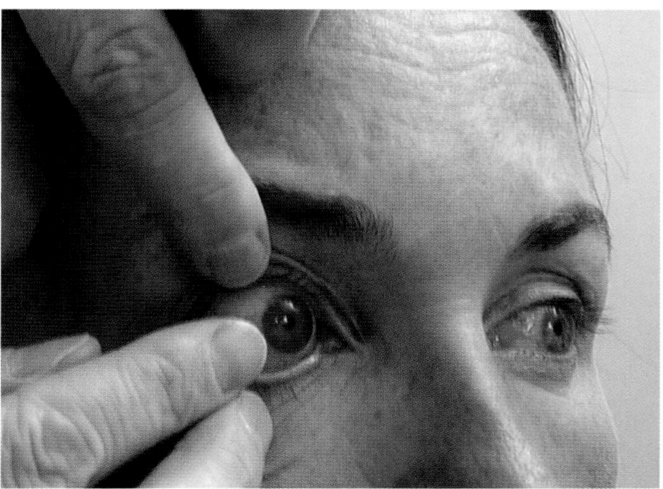

Figure 9.3 Displacing a soft lens to dislodge a foreign body.

Soft lens removal

1. Ask the patient to look up.
2. Hold down the patient's bottom lid with the middle finger of the left hand.
3. Slide the lens on to the lower sclera.
4. Pinch and remove the lens with the thumb and forefinger (Figure 9.4).

Settling time

Lenses alter their fitting characteristics during a period of equilibration due to differences in temperature, pH and osmolarity between the lens vial and eye. Lenses tend to show less movement after this period of settling. In some cases, lenses exhibit gross tightness immediately after insertion and are unlikely to show sufficient improvement on settling. The post-lens tear film appears to settle within minutes while the pre-lens tear film can take 30 minutes to thin to its equilibrium state (Nichols and King-Smith, 2004). A fast blink rate appears to quicken lens settling (Golding *et al.*, 1995), possibly because the thickness of the post-lens tear film is an important factor in lens movement (Little and Bruce, 1994).

Many fitting guides recommend a long settling period before assessing lens fit, particularly in the case of high-water-content lenses (e.g. 30 minutes); however, this is frequently impractical and unnecessary. Martin and Holden (1983), however, showed that high-water ionic lenses stabilize within a 10–15-min period. Brennan *et al.* (1994) noted that the most effective time to predict the final fitting characteristics was approximately 5 min after lens insertion; however, they also noted that a proportion of patients show a relatively long settling time (>25 min) and hence the importance of reassessing lens fit at the first aftercare check.

Lens fit characteristics

Soft lenses rarely show the idealized fit described in textbooks and fitting guides (Young, 1996). Table 9.2 summarizes the factors affecting soft lens fit.

A summary of the characteristics of tight, loose and optimally fitting soft lenses can be seen in Table 9.3. It should be noted, however, that soft lenses rarely show all of the classic characteristics of a given type of lens fitting. Loose lenses, for instance, often show good centration despite excessive movement (Young, 1996).

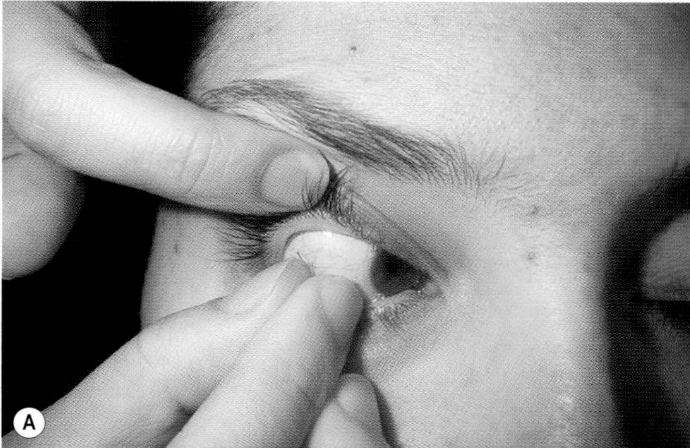

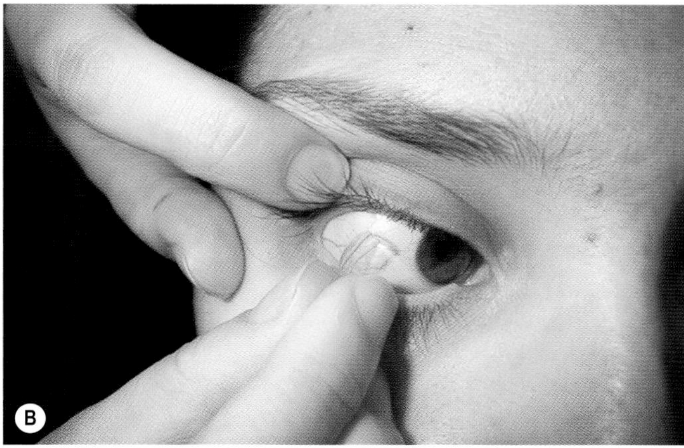

Figure 9.4 Removing a soft lens. (A) The lens is slid off the cornea on to the inferior or temporal bulbar conjunctiva and light pressure is applied on to the lens surface using the thumb and forefinger. (B) The fingers are pinched together to lift the lens off the eye.

Table 9.2 Factors affecting soft lens fit

- Corneal geometry: corneal asphericity, curvature and diameter
- Contact lens geometry: back optic zone radius, peripheral thickness, central thickness
- Contact lens material: mechanical properties
- Post-lens tear film: non-invasive break-up time (NIBUT)
- Extraneous factors: pingueculae, lid tension

Optimum soft lens fit

The ideal soft lens will:

- Be comfortable.
- Be perfectly centred, overlapping the limbus by at least 1 mm.
- Show approximately 0.3 mm of movement with a blink and a similar amount of lag on version gaze.
- Show easy movement on push-up followed by smooth recentring.
- Have edges that align with the sclera without indenting the conjunctiva.

Table 9.3 Typical soft lens fitting characteristics

Criterion	Tight	Optimum	Loose
Comfort	Initially good, although eyes may feel tired later in wearing period	Good	Poor
Centration	Can be good or poor	Good	Possibly decentred
Post-blink movement	Little or none	0.2–0.4 mm	>0.4 mm
Lag on version or upgaze	Little or none	0.2–0.4 mm	>0.4 mm
Tightness on push-up	Difficult to dislodge and slow to recover	Easy to dislodge and smooth recovery	Very easy to dislodge and fast recovery
Peripheral fit	Conjunctival indentation	Aligned	Edge stand-off
Vision	Stable or possibly clearer after a blink	Stable	Variable

The minimum requirements of an acceptable-fitting soft lens are as follows:

- Full corneal coverage at all times.
- Some movement on blink and/or version.
- Absence of excessive movement.
- No conjunctival indentation or edge stand-off.

Tight soft lens fit

A typical tight soft lens fitting will:

- Be initially comfortable but may ache or feel tired later in the wearing period.
- Display minimal or no movement with a blink.
- Be difficult to dislodge by the push-up test and will be slow to recover.

In extreme cases, there will be indentation of the scleral conjunctiva. The centration of the lens is not a helpful indicator of whether a lens is tight.

Loose soft lens fit

A typical loose-fitting soft lens will:

- be uncomfortable due to excessive lens movement or decentration
- sometimes show decentration and excessive movement on blinking (≥0.5 mm)
- be easily dislodged on push-up and fall quickly when the lower lid is retracted
- have an edge that may show some stand-off, especially at the inferior temporal edge.

Assessment of fit

The visual assessment of soft lens fit should be undertaken with the aid of a slit lamp rather than a Burton lamp. Only a slit lamp can give the magnification required to view the finer details of soft lens fit, for instance, the fit of the lens periphery.

Comfort

The patient's reaction to the lens in terms of comfort is the first clue to the lens fit. A well-fitting soft lens is a comfortable lens. Tight-fitting lenses are also usually comfortable but some discomfort or lens awareness may indicate a loose-fitting lens. One study found that 63% of loose-fitting lenses were graded relatively uncomfortable (Young, 1996). Due to the overlapping distribution of corneal nerves, it is difficult for patients to locate precisely the source of any discomfort; however, it is worth asking the patient to describe the discomfort, with questions such as:

- Can you feel the edge of the lens?
- Is the discomfort at the top or bottom edge of the lens?
- Is it more noticeable when you blink?
- Does the lens feel as if it is moving about in your eye?

Also, gauge the severity of any discomfort by observing the patient. Clearly, excessive lacrimation or blepharospam would tend to suggest a more severe reaction.

It is wrong to think that new wearers require a prolonged adaptation period to the comfort of soft lenses in similar fashion to rigid lenses. Well-fitting soft lenses, once settled, should be virtually indiscernible to the patient.

Centration

Some decentration is acceptable provided the lens shows corneal coverage at all times and does not appear to compromise comfort. Remember that the cornea extends beyond the HVID and that some overlap of the visible iris is necessary, ideally by about 1 mm.

As expected, loose-fitting lenses tend to show greater decentration. In one study, three-quarters of loose-fitting lenses showed decentration greater than 0.3 mm (Young, 1996). Tight lenses show similar centration characteristics to those of well-fitting lenses. In other words, tight lenses do not necessarily show perfect centration but can vary from perfect to noticeably decentred.

With most higher-power lens designs, the optic zone diameter will be reduced in order to minimize lens thickness. In these cases, it is important to ensure that any decentration does not compromise peripheral vision.

Movement

Some lens movement is necessary to maintain post-lens lubrication and, in turn, ensure a complete post-lens tear film. Excessive movement can cause unnecessary discomfort and disrupt vision. Post-blink movement is a more important indicator of tight rather than loose-fitting lenses as virtually all tight-fitting lenses show little or no movement (Young, 1996). Loose-fitting lenses do not necessarily

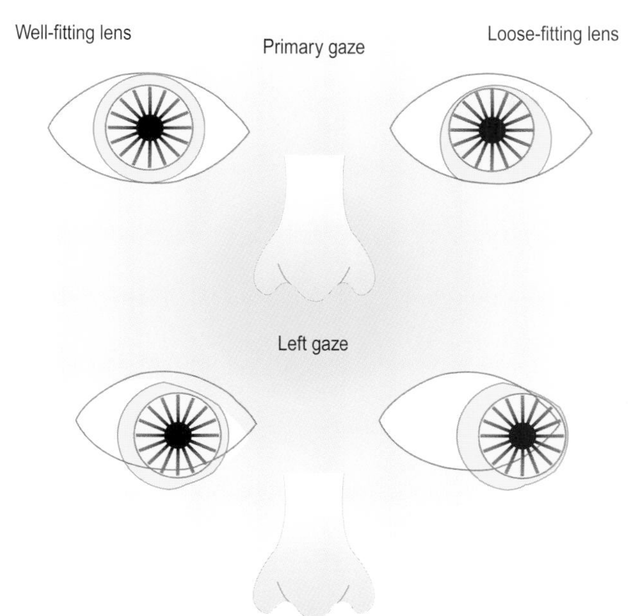

Figure 9.5 Loose and well-fitting lenses in primary gaze and on version.

show excessive movement and therefore the assessment of lens movement on its own is an inadequate measure of lens fit.

In a normal fit, the lens usually remains stationary when the lid moves downward during the first part of the blink but then moves upwards by a small amount during the second part of the blink, returning to its original position immediately after the blink and hence the description 'post-blink movement'. Some loose fittings show a type of movement reminiscent of lid attachment with rigid lenses. The lens shows some downwards movement as soon as the lid starts to blink before showing the normal up and downwards movement. In some cases, the lens can be seen to move with the lid even during small changes in lid position.

Soft lens movement correlates surprisingly poorly with the pressure that the lens exerts on the eye, except where the lens exerts pressure above a certain threshold. In these cases, the lens tends to show no movement (Martin *et al.*, 1989). In addition, Little and Bruce (1994) have shown that lens movement is affected by the state of the post-lens tear film. Depletion of the post-lens tear film due to lens dehydration may even result in lens adherence. In cases where patients present with lenses showing no movement, it is therefore wrong to assume that this is due to the lens itself and other factors such as the patient's tear film and working environment should be considered.

Movement on sideways gaze (version lag) can be as sensitive an indicator of fit as post-blink movement. The assessment of upgaze lag is less useful and, in fact, a large proportion of well-fitting lenses show no movement on upgaze lag (Figure 9.5).

Tightness on push-up

The assessment of lens fit using the push-up test is the most useful single test of lens fit (Figure 9.6). This is undertaken

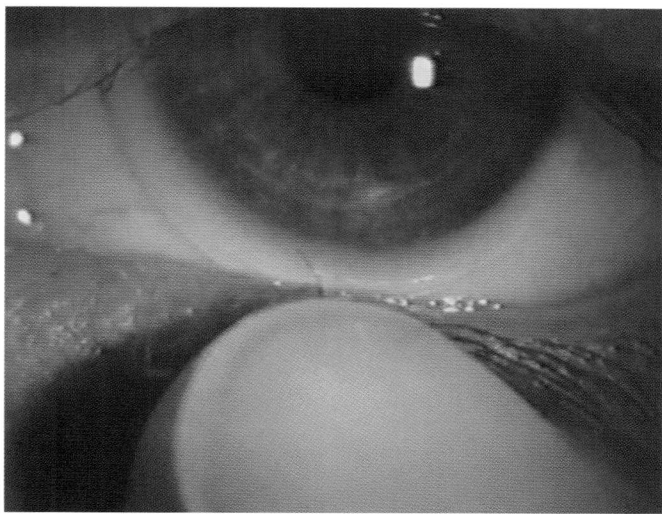

Figure 9.6 Assessment of fit by the push-up test.

by digitally moving the lens upwards by pushing the lower lid against the lens edge. The test consists of an assessment of the amount of force necessary to dislodge the lens upwards coupled with the speed of recentration of the lens from its dislodged position. Crude as it sounds, the push-up test has been shown to correlate closely with 'squeeze pressure', which is a measure of the mechanical properties of the lens and an index of the force exerted by lenses on a given eye (Martin *et al.*, 1989). The test shows high predictive value and is equally sensitive for both tight and loose fits (Young, 1996).

If the lens is already decentred upwards it may be difficult to dislodge, thus giving the false impression of tightness. In this situation, lens fit can be checked by using the top lid to recentre the lens before performing the push-up test in the normal way. Lenses can also give the false impression of tightness because of post-lens dryness causing the lens to adhere to the eye. This is rarely seen during trial lens fitting but is occasionally seen in patients attending aftercare visits, particularly if the patient is prone to dry eye or has been in a dry atmosphere. In these cases, once the lens has been forcibly dislodged by push-up and the post-lens tear film is able to reform, the lens resumes its normal fitting appearance.

A variant of the test, the spring-back test, involves digitally displacing the lens sideways and observing the speed of recentration. However, this test is unnecessarily disruptive and is not recommended.

Peripheral fit

The peripheral fit is an important, but often overlooked, aspect of soft lens fit. A lens can show good centration and tightness on push-up but still show poor edge alignment. Even slight, barely visible edge stand-off can cause discomfort due to interaction with the lids (Figure 9.7). Edge stand-off is often more easily disclosed by moving the lens closer to the limbus by push-up (Josephson, 1977).

The opposite case of excessive peripheral tightness is rarely seen with conventional hydrogel lenses due to their relatively thin edges but is common with higher-modulus silicone hydrogel lenses. The type of constriction described

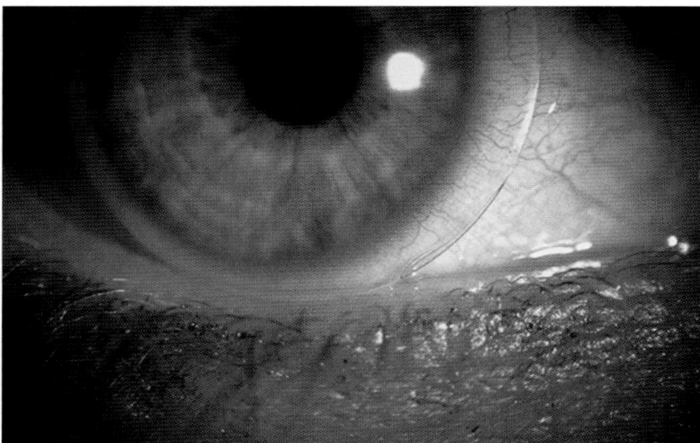

Figure 9.7 Gross edge stand-off; even slight edge stand-off can cause discomfort.

in textbooks as vessel blanching is extremely rare and would only occur with a thick lens that was tightly fitting in every respect. Particularly with silicone hydrogel lenses, it is useful to examine the periphery under magnification for signs of indentation of the bulbar conjunctiva. When present, this may also be visible on lens removal through pooling of fluorescein in the indentation.

Vision

An over-refraction is usually unnecessary as part of the fitting procedure. Spherical soft lenses, because of their thinness and flexibility, rarely support a tear lens between the lens and cornea. In the case of with-the-rule astigmatism, the required contact lens power corresponds to the vertex distance-corrected spectacle sphere (assuming minus cylinder); thus, no adjustment is necessary for cylinder power. On the other hand, with against-the-rule astigmatism, the required power will incorporate approximately half of the cylinder power. Where an over-refraction yields an unexpected result, this can usually be explained by checking the lens power with a focimeter (see Chapter 8).

Unstable vision may indicate a loose, relatively mobile fit. In rare cases, unstable vision that clears with a blink indicates a steep central fit. However, this was more common with relatively thick or high-modulus lens designs, but even then is rarely seen.

Other methods of fit assessment

Other techniques for assessing lens fit have been suggested; however, the basic methods described above are usually sufficient. These other methods include:

- Assessing keratometry mires – the keratometry mires tend to distort when the lens is not aligned with the lens surface. Mire distortion tends to clear immediately after a blink with tight-fitting lenses and between blinks with loose-fitting lenses.
- Videokeratoscopy – this gives a more detailed picture than keratometry. The final contour map, however, unlike keratometry is a static assessment.
- Retinoscopy – this can be useful in confirming that the optic zone gives proper coverage of the pupil, which may be particularly useful with some bifocal designs.

Soft lens fitting problems

Discomfort

Two aspects of the lens design can affect comfort: diameter and edge design. However, other possibilities should be ruled out first, such as:

- foreign body
- lens inside out
- lens damage
- lens spoilation.

Since there is a relatively wide transition zone between cornea and sclera, a soft lens may appear just to cover the cornea when in reality the lens edge is irritating the peripheral cornea. If the lens decentres so that the edge is close to the limbus, the patient is usually able to localize the discomfort to that part of the limbus.

Many larger corneas show marginal corneal coverage with standard-diameter soft lenses. Since most soft lens brands are offered in one diameter only, the obvious remedy is not available and it is necessary to try a different lens type. However, since lenses with a steeper BOZR have a slightly larger surface area than their equivalent flatter versions, changing BOZR can sometimes overcome the problem.

Relatively large changes in peripheral thickness can be made to a lens design without affecting comfort (Young *et al.*, 1993). Nevertheless, some thinner-edged designs do appear to give better comfort than others. As with rigid lenses, there does appear to be an adaptation effect. However, since comfort appears to be the characteristic that patients most value, the best approach is to find a design that is immediately comfortable for a particular patient. As noted earlier, some cases of edge sensation may be related to the peripheral fit.

In case of dryness-related discomfort, an alternative approach is to change to a more wettable material and/or dehydration-resistant material such as omafilcon A or senofilcon A (Lemp *et al.*, 1999; Riley *et al.*, 2006).

Inappropriate diameter

Too large

Greater than usual coverage of the sclera is not in itself a clinical problem. However, the fact that the lens is required to flex close to the optic zone junction in order to align with limbus and sclera can result in areas of increased mechanical pressure. When concentrated at the edge, this can result in conjunctival indentation. When too large a diameter results in poor flexure in the midperiphery, this can lead to superior arcuate staining (Young and Mirejovsky, 1993).

Another problem with large lenses is that the lens may be visible on the eye, particularly if the lens has a thick periphery or incorporates a deep handling tint.

Unfortunately, there are few soft lenses available in diameters smaller than 14.0 mm. Also, as noted earlier, comparing the labelled diameters of soft lenses is not necessarily a reliable guide to their on-eye performance. It is therefore necessary for practitioners to gain an appreciation of which lenses are relatively small on-eye; current examples are Ciba Vision Night & Day and CooperVision Actifresh 400.

Too small

Lenses that are too small can cause peripheral corneal staining as well as discomfort. Again, it is necessary to have an appreciation of which lenses are relatively large once equilibrated on the eye; current examples of relatively large lenses are CooperVision Proclear and CooperVision Frequency 55 AB.

Conventional as opposed to frequent-replacement soft lenses are often available in a wide range of diameters (e.g. Lunelle ES70) and can be useful alternatives.

Inappropriate fit

Too loose

Loose-fitting lenses can also cause peripheral corneal staining and symptoms of discomfort and variable vision. Patients may also complain of lenses being displaced from the cornea during wear.

The first possibility to consider is whether the lens is inside out. Switching to a similar lens of steeper BOZR may not always overcome the problem, particularly with thin lens designs. It may be necessary therefore to change to a lens with a tendency towards tight fitting, e.g. Vistakon 8.30 Acuvue Advance.

Too tight

Tight lenses induce greater levels of staining than well-fitting lenses and the prevalence of staining increases with increasing degree of tightness. Tight-fitting lenses tend to be comfortable but patients occasionally complain of aching eyes later in the wearing period. Relatively loose-fitting lenses include CooperVision 8.90 Frequency 55.

Poor vision

Occasionally, soft lenses fail to give acceptable vision even when the optimum power appears to have been selected.

Possible reasons for poor vision include the following:

- uncorrected astigmatism
- lens deposits
- poor surface wetting
- lens imperfections.

Slit-lamp inspection of the lens on the eye will indicate whether poor surface wetting as a result of spoilation or merely poor tear quality is to blame. Generally, if these are severe enough to affect vision, they will be easily visible on slit-lamp examination.

As with spectacle lenses, contact lenses very occasionally show optical imperfections that, in turn, affect vision. These include waves, distorted optics and multiple zones of power. The focimeter image may give an indication but the lens optics can also be inspected by dabbing the lens dry with a tissue wipe and viewing through the lens with the naked eye while holding it towards a light source.

In the event of no obvious cause, the best remedy is to replace the lens to see whether this overcomes the problem.

Variable vision

When the visual acuity is normal but the patient complains of variable vision, the following causes may be suspected:

- Incorrect back vertex power, e.g. over-minus, under-plus.
- Poor binocular balance.
- Excessive lens movement, i.e. loose fit.
- Poor pre-lens tear film.

Conclusions

As will be seen from reading this chapter, the fitting of soft contact lenses is not a simple formulaic task. Careful thought needs to be given to selecting a lens of appropriate material, dimensions and wearing modality to match the ocular characteristics and lifestyle preferences of the individual patient. Using a range of lens brands gives greater flexibility and increases the chance of arriving at the best solution expeditiously.

References

Brennan, N. A., Lindsay, R. G., McGraw, K. *et al.* (1994) Soft lens movement: Temporal characteristics. *Optom. Vis. Sci.*, **71,** 359–363.

Bruce, A. S. and Brennan, N. A. (1990) Corneal pathophysiology with contact lens wear. *Surv. Ophthalmol.*, **35,** 25–58.

Burki, E. (1997) Erweiterte anpassmoglichkeiten van austauschlinsen (Expanding the fitting possibilities of disposable lenses). *Contactologia,* **19,** 108–112.

Cox, I. (1990) Theoretical calculation of the spherical aberration of rigid and soft contact lenses. *Optom. Vis. Sci.*, **67,** 277–282.

Dart, J. K., Radford, C. F., Minassian, D. *et al.* (2008) Risk factors for microbial keratitis with contemporary contact lenses: a case-control study. *Ophthalmology,* **115,** 1647–1654, 1654.

Dumbleton, K. A., Chalmers, R. L., McNally, J. *et al.* (2002) Effect of lens base curve on subjective comfort and assessment of fit with silicone hydrogel continuous wear contact lenses. *Optom. Vis. Sci.*, **79,** 633–637.

Efron, N. (1996) Contact lens-induced corneal oedema. *Optician,* **211**(5540), 18–26.

Efron, S., Efron, N. and Morgan, P. B. (2008) Optical and visual performance of aspheric soft contact lenses. *Optom. Vis. Sci.*, **85,** 201–210.

Garner, L.F. (1982) Sagittal height of the anterior eye and contact lens fitting. *Am. J. Optom. Physiol. Opt.*, **59,** 301–305.

Golding, T. R., Bruce, A.S., Gaterell, L. L. *et al.*, (1995). Soft lens movement: effect of blink rate on lens settling. *Acta Ophthalmol. Scand.*, **73,** 506–511.

Hamano, H., Watanabe, K., Hamano, T. *et al.* (1994) A study of the complications induced by conventional and disposable contact lenses. *Contact Lens Assoc. Ophthalmol. J.*, **20,** 103–108.

Holden, B.A. and Mertz, G.W. (1984) Critical oxygen levels to avoid corneal edema for daily and extended wear contact lenses. *Invest. Ophthal. Vis. Sci.*, **25,** 1161–1167.

Josephson, J.E. (1977) Techniques for determining lens fit acceptability prior to dispensing hydrophilic semi-scleral lathed lenses. *Int. Contact Lens Clin.*, **4,** 52–54.

Kollbaum, P. and Bradley, A. (2005) Aspheric contact lenses: fact and fiction. *Contact Lens Spectrum* **20**(3), 34–38.

Lemp, M., Caffery, B., Lebow, K. *et al.* (1999) Omafilcon A (Proclear) Soft Contact Lenses in a Dry Eye Population. *Contact Lens Assoc. Ophthalmol. J.*, **25,** 40–47.

Little, S. A. and Bruce, A. S. (1994) Hydrogel (Acuvue) lens movement is influenced by the postlens tear film. *Optom. Vis. Sci.,* **71,** 364–370.

Lowther, G. E. and Tomlinson, A. (1981) Critical base curve and diameter interval in the fitting of spherical soft contact lenses. *Am. J. Optom. Physiol. Opt.* **58,** 355–360.

Martin, D. K. and Holden, B. A. (1982) A new method for measuring the diameter of the in vivo human cornea. *Am. J. Optom. Physiol. Opt.*, **59,** 436–441.

Martin, D. K. and Holden, B. A. (1983) Variations in tear fluid osmolarity, chord diameter and movement during wear of high water content hydrogel contact lenses. *Int. Cont. Lens Clin.*, **10,** 332–341.

Martin, D. K., Holden, B. A. (1986) Forces developed beneath hydrogel contact lenses due to squeeze pressure. *Phys. Med. Biol.*, **31,** 635–649.

Martin, D. K., Boulos, J., Gan, J. *et al.* (1989) A unifying parameter to describe the clinical mechanics of hydrogel contact lenses. *Optom. Vis. Sci.,* **66,** 87–91.

Morgan, P. B. and Efron, N. (1998) The oxygen performance of contemporary hydrogel contact lenses. *Contact Lens and Anterior Eye,* **21,** 3–6.

Morgan, P. B., Efron, S. E., Efron, N. *et al.* (2005) Inefficacy of aspheric soft contact lenses for the correction of low levels of astigmatism. *Optom. Vis. Sci.,* **82,** 823–828.

Nichols, J. J., King-Smith, P. E. (2004) The impact of hydrogel lens settling on the thickness of the tears and contact lens. *Invest. Ophthalmol. Vis. Sci.*, **45,** 2549–3554.

Nilsson, S.E.G. (1997) Ten years of disposable contact lenses – a review of benefits and risks. *Contact Lens and Anterior Eye,* **20,** 119–128.

Riley, C., Young, G. and Chalmers, R. (2006) Prevalence of ocular surface symptoms, signs, and uncomfortable hours of wear in contact lens wearers: the effect of refitting with daily wear silicone hydrogel lenses (senofilcon A). *Eye and Contact Lens,* **32,** 281–286.

Young, G. (1992) Ocular sagittal height and soft contact lens fit. *J. Br. Contact Lens Assoc.,* **15,** 45–49.

Young, G. (1996) Evaluation of soft contact lens fitting characteristics. *Optom. Vis. Sci.,* **73,** 247–254.

Young, G. and Grewel, I. (1999) How relevant are the labelled diameters of soft lenses? *Optom. Vis. Sci.,* **76,** 171.

Young, G. and Mirejovsky, D. (1993) A hypothesis for the aetiology of soft contact lens induced superior arcuate keratopathy. *Int. Contact Lens Clin.,* **20,** 177–180.

Young, G., Holden, B. and Cooke, G. (1993) The influence of soft contact lens design on clinical performance. *Optom. Vis. Sci.,* **70,** 394–403.

Young, G., Allsopp, G., Inglis, A. and Watson, S. (1997) Comparative performance of disposable soft contact lenses. *Contact Lens and Anterior Eye,* **20,** 13–21.

CHAPTER 10

Soft toric lens design and fitting

Richard Lindsay

Introduction

The use of soft toric lenses (in preference to spherical soft lenses) is indicated when there is ocular astigmatism present, be it corneal or non-corneal, that warrants correction. Unlike rigid lenses, soft lenses do not mask corneal astigmatism but rather conform to the shape of the cornea. Consequently, correcting ocular astigmatism with soft lenses requires that cylinder be incorporated into the back vertex power (BVP) of the lens.

Numerous manufacturers of soft contact lenses have made extremely optimistic claims of their spherical lenses being able to correct satisfactorily astigmatism of between 1.00 and 2.00 D. Only rarely is this achieved. Bernstein *et al.* (1991) showed that there was no statistically significant masking of corneal cylinder with standard-thickness soft spherical lenses. Indeed, the most helpful indication of the likely residual astigmatism found while wearing a spherical soft contact lens is the ocular astigmatism determined from an accurate subjective spectacle refraction.

For many years it was held that prospective contact lens wearers with clinically significant astigmatism could not be successfully fitted with soft lenses. Since the early 1980s, however, notable advances in soft toric lens technology have been made such that the correction of astigmatism with soft lenses is now a viable option for the majority of these patients.

Criteria for use of soft toric lenses

When deciding whether or not to prescribe a soft toric lens, practitioners should avoid using criteria such as 'all patients with cylinders greater than a certain amount should be fitted with soft toric lenses'. Instead, each patient should be assessed separately, taking into account the following factors.

Degree of astigmatism

As a generalization, 1.00 D or more of astigmatism should be corrected, although there will be significant variability between patients. Holden (1975), in discussing the criteria for the prescribing of toric lenses, showed that 45% of the population required a cylindrical correction of up to 0.75 D and 25% of the population required a correction of 1.00 D or more.

Cylinder axis

The axis of the ocular cylinder is also an important factor. For example, an uncorrected cylinder with an oblique axis will cause greater degradation of visual image compared with an equivalent amount of uncorrected with-the-rule or against-the-rule astigmatism (Lindsay, 1998).

Ocular dominance

Uncorrected astigmatism is far more likely to be accepted by the patient if it is in the non-dominant eye. For example, patients may tolerate uncorrected cylinder of up to 2.00 D in their non-dominant eye, while at the same time requiring that cylinder as small as 0.50 D be corrected in their dominant eye. Related to this is the situation where a patient has unequal visual acuities. In this case, higher degrees of uncorrected astigmatism will usually be tolerated in the eye with the poorer acuity.

Viability of other alternatives

The practitioner also needs to consider whether soft toric lenses are the best option or if the patient would be better off with spectacles or rigid lenses. For example, a patient with high degrees (>5.00 D) of both corneal and spectacle astigmatism would most likely achieve better acuities with a rigid toric lens.

Visual needs of the patient

Usually, the less critical the visual task, the greater the amount of astigmatism that can be left uncorrected (and vice versa). For example, a musician may require that a

DOI: 10.1016/B978-0-7506-8869-7.00010-0

cylinder as small as 0.50 D be corrected to enable music to be read. On the other hand, a person with no specific critical visual tasks may be happy with a cylinder as high as 2.00 D left uncorrected so long as the spherical component of the refractive error is corrected.

Design of soft toric lenses

Satisfactory visual performance with soft toric lenses is dependent upon two key design components – surface optics and lens stabilization.

Surface optics

The two principal categories of surface optics are as follows:

1. Toroidal back surface with a spherical front surface
2. Spherical back surface with toroidal front surface.

With soft toric lenses, regardless of which of the above optical configurations is prescribed, the end result on the eye will be a bitoric lens form due to the wrapping of the front and back surface of the lens on to the cornea.

The optical considerations for soft toric lenses are different from those encountered when using rigid lenses. This is primarily because a soft toric lens will tend to wrap on to the cornea such that a negligible tear lens forms between the back surface of the lens and the front surface of the cornea. Consequently, the optical principles of rigid toric lenses do not apply. There are no tear lens calculations to perform and all the ocular astigmatism will usually be corrected by incorporation of cylinder into the BVP of the soft toric lens.

The choice of design (i.e. toric back surface versus toric front surface) is generally based more on considerations relating to manufacture, lens stability and physiological performance. Currently, the majority of soft toric lenses prescribed globally are of a planned-replacement form and virtually all of these lenses are mass-produced by a process of cast moulding. All other soft toric lenses are custom-made for the patient by a process of either crimping or generating, the latter being a specific form of lathe cutting devoted to the production of toric surfaces. As a general rule, generated toric lenses will be thinner and show better reproducibility than those made from crimping techniques.

Stabilization techniques

All forms of soft toric lenses need to be stabilized so that the toric optics of the lens can be maintained in the desired orientation so as to correct the ocular astigmatism. The aim is to minimize rotation from the ideal in-eye orientation. The orientation of a soft toric lens on the eye must be predictable and consistent, otherwise suboptimal vision will result. The development of the technique of dynamic stabilization in the 1980s has resulted in an overall improvement in the performance of soft toric lenses.

Toroidal back surface

Some practitioners and laboratories believe that a soft toric lens with a toric back surface will generally locate better than a front surface toric lens, because it is believed that the back toric surface is more likely to align, or 'lock on', to the matching toroidal corneal surface. However, experience has shown that a toroidal back surface alone is insufficient to achieve lens stabilization.

Prism ballast

The theory of prism ballast is that base-down prism is incorporated into the lens so that the lens will be heavier at the prism base (due to excess lens mass). Gravity then acts to cause the prism base to locate inferiorly.

Prism ballast has long been used as a technique for stabilizing toric forms of lenses, but it does have certain disadvantages when applied to soft lens designs. The additional thickness brought about by the use of a prism can be a problem in that it reduces oxygen transmissibility in the thick prism zone and can also cause physical discomfort in patients with sensitive lids. In addition, soft toric lenses incorporating prism ballast often show excessive downward mislocation on the eye. The thicker edge in the region of the prism base can be thinned during the manufacturing stage to form a 'comfort' chamfer (Edwards, 1999), although this will slightly negate the intended thickness differential along the vertical axis of the lens. The problem here is finding an acceptable compromise between comfort and lens stability.

One of the difficulties that arises with the use of prism ballast is that if it is going to be prescribed monocularly it may cause vertical prismatic effects that can make the patient uncomfortable. This then requires the use of a similar prism for the other eye, which can prove difficult if the other eye requires a spherical lens or is emmetropic. Fortunately, however, prism ballast does not often give rise to binocular problems (Gasson, 1977).

This design feature is perhaps considered inferior to dynamic stabilization (see below) for maintaining the orientation of a soft toric lens on the eye; nevertheless, prism ballast is the method of stabilization that is used predominantly in disposable toric lens designs, which have proved to be reasonably successful in clinical practice.

Peri-ballast

This method of lens stabilization features a lens with a minus carrier (peripheral zone), with the carrier being thicker inferiorly. In other words, the prismatic thickness profile changes are confined to the lens carrier, where the carrier is thicker inferiorly (prism base-down). This design is fabricated simply by removing the high-minus lenticular carrier from the superior portion of the lens. In effect, it is similar to prism ballast except that with peri-ballast all the prism is outside the region of the optic zone.

Truncation

Truncation refers to the technique of slicing off the bottom of the lens, so as to form a 'shelf' that will rest upon – and therefore align with – the lower lid. This is a reasonably successful method of stabilizing lenses with thick edges, especially when combined with prism ballast (Figure 10.1). Either a single lower truncation, or a double truncation (where both the top and bottom of the lens are sliced off), can be used (Strachan, 1975). With the former, the truncated section of the lens that is removed can be anywhere between a sag of 0.5 and 1.5 mm.

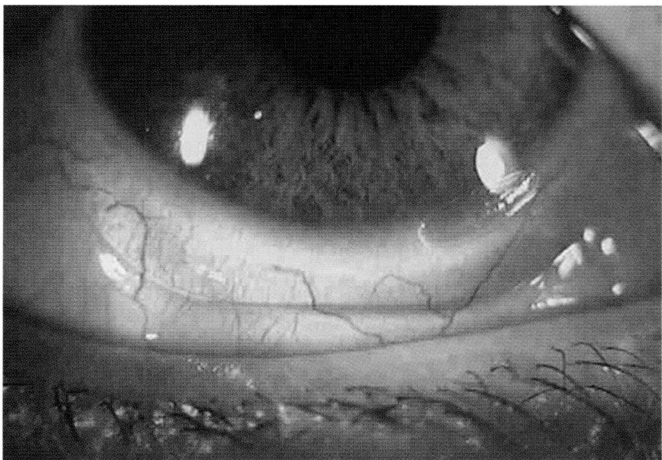

Figure 10.1 A prism-ballasted soft toric lens with a single (inferior) truncation. The truncation has been cut at the angle of the middle third of the lower lid, but in this photograph the patient had to look up in order to bring the truncation near the lower lid. The lid margin may thus only have a limited effect on the truncation in this patient. Note the prominent bubble under the lens near the truncation – a common problem with these lenses. (Adapted from Tan, J., Papas, E., Carnt, N. et al. (2007) Performance standards for toric soft contact lenses. Optom. Vis. Sci., 84, 422–428.)

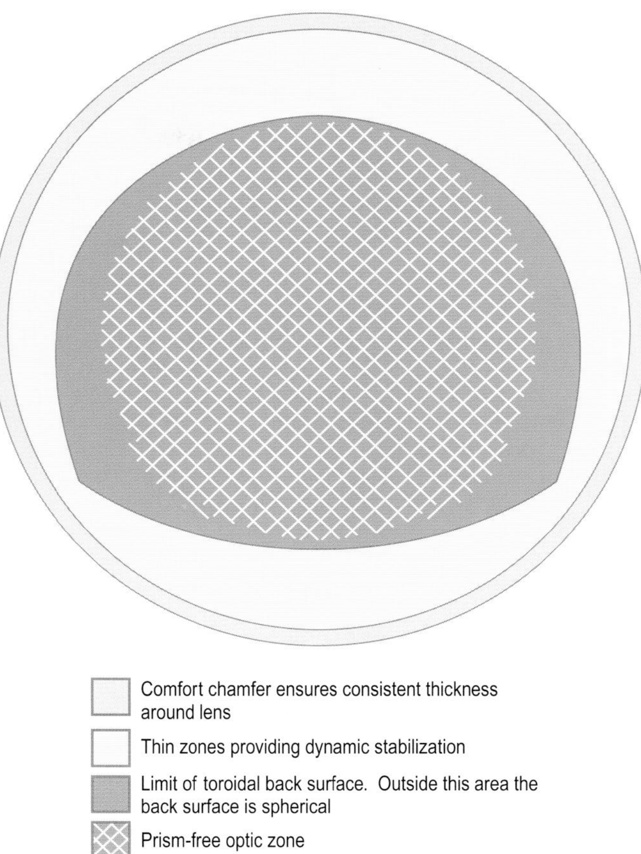

Figure 10.2 Design features of a soft toric lens which help to minimize lens rotation. Note the prism-free optic zone in the toroidal region of the lens.

There are problems with the use of truncation in soft toric lens fitting. The truncated edge can make the soft lens uncomfortable to wear. The measurement of the lid angle can be difficult and imprecise. Quite often the truncation does not work, with the lid angle appearing to have no effect on the positioning or location of the truncated lens. Another difficulty with truncations (and prism ballasting) is the instability that can occur with oblique cylinders. The uneven thickness produced by oblique cylinders can make lens stabilization very difficult. For these reasons, soft toric lens truncation is rarely used today.

Dynamic stabilization

The technique of dynamic stabilization was initially developed by Fanti (1975) and this is currently the most commonly used method of stabilization for soft toric lenses. With this technique, the dominant lens orientation effect is achieved by pressure from the upper lid (primarily) and the lower lid. Hanks (1983) used the analogy of the 'watermelon seed' to illustrate how dynamic stabilization works. Simply put, pressure applied to the thin end of a watermelon seed by the fingers (i.e. the pressure exerted on a thin zone of a lens between the upper lid and globe) causes the watermelon seed to move away from the fingers (i.e. causes the lens to orient away from the squeezing force of the eyelid and globe). Hanks (1983) demonstrated that the effect of gravity is insignificant, and that the effect of the thickness profile interaction with the upper lid as described above is the dominant stabilizing component.

With dynamic stabilization, the contact lens toricity is confined to the central portion of the lens. The superior and inferior ('dynamic stabilization') zones of the lens incorporate a thickness differential. The action of the lids on these superior and inferior lens chamfers serves to stabilize the lens in the correct orientation. Such a design is shown in Figure 10.2. Many similar approaches, referred to as 'double slab-off', 'thin-zone' or 'reverse prism' designs, are manufactured throughout the world.

Dynamic stabilization avoids the complications of truncation and prism ballast. Oxygen transmissibility is not reduced as additional thickness is generally not incorporated into the lens. Indeed, the excessive thickness of prism ballast lenses can be avoided and, by producing toroidal back surfaces, the average lens thickness is only slightly greater than that of equivalent spherical designs. The main disadvantage of this design is that the thickness differential which can be achieved at the edge of the lens is dependent on the spherical power of the lens. Lower-powered lenses will have a reduced thickness differential and, for this reason, a design incorporating prism ballast is often more effective in stabilizing a soft toric lens that has a low spherical power component (Snyder, 1998).

The orientation in which a lens incorporating dynamic stabilization is inserted into the eye is generally not important since the action of the lids during blinking will quickly stabilize the lens in the correct orientation. With some designs a larger, thinned zone is provided superiorly to utilize the fact that most of the blink action is performed by the upper eyelid. With these designs it is more important that the lens is inserted the correct way up. To facilitate this – and to assist the practitioner in determining the degree of in-eye lens rotation – such lenses will generally have some form of marking at the 6 or 12 o'clock position.

Principles of correction

It is clear that to produce a stable ocular correction for the astigmatic eye, the lens must align closely over the central cornea in front of the pupil. It must provide the correct power while it is *in situ* and must stabilize effectively to prevent the rotation of the meridional powers away from their intended orientation.

Fitting

The fitting principles for soft toric lenses are very similar to those for soft spherical lenses, as outlined in Chapter 9. A well-fitting lens is comfortable in all directions of gaze, gives complete corneal coverage and appears properly centred. On blinking there should be about 0.25–0.5 mm of vertical movement when the eye is in the primary position. On upwards gaze or lateral movements of the eye, the lens should lag by no more than 0.5 mm.

The total diameter of the lens is very important because this parameter will influence both lens centration and lens stability. Generally, when specifying the lens diameter, the practitioner should err on the large side, as a larger diameter means that more area is available for the stabilization zones to take effect in the periphery of the lens.

Some practitioners advocate fitting soft toric lenses very steep (tight) with minimal lens movement, on the assumption that this will aid stability and reduce lens rotation. With the designs available today, however, this is not necessary. If a lens is too tightly adherent to the eye, it will not be affected by the locating forces designed to stabilize lens orientation (Holden, 1976). Consequently, a steeply fitting lens may decrease stability and lead to undesirable factors such as limbal indentation and fluctuating vision – the latter being caused by the soft lens vaulting the corneal apex.

A well-fitting lens will reveal stable lens orientation with a quick return to axis if mislocated. A tight-fitting lens will show stable lens orientation but a slow return to axis if mislocated. A loose-fitting lens will demonstrate an unstable and inconsistent lens orientation (Hanks and Weisbarth, 1983).

Back vertex power determination

The determination of BVP for a soft toric lens is much easier than that for a rigid toric lens. Due to the absence of a tear lens, the BVP for a soft toric lens should be similar to the spectacle refraction (or ocular refraction if the vertex distance effect is significant).

The BVP of the lens can either be determined empirically or by performing a spherocylindrical over-refraction (SCO) over a diagnostic lens. With empirical prescribing, the BVP ordered for the soft toric lens will be equal to the ocular refraction of the patient, based on the assumption of an afocal tear layer under the soft toric lens. For the latter method, an SCO may be performed over either a spherical or toric trial lens. Use of a spherical trial lens is generally preferred, as an SCO with a toric trial lens may require complex calculations involving oblique cylinders in order to determine the required lens power. When using a spherical trial lens, the resultant toric lens power is simply calculated by adding the SCO to the BVP of the trial lens. With both methods, some arbitrary allowance for lens rotation may have to be incorporated into the final lens prescription.

Table 10.1 Recommended performance standards

	Excellent	Acceptable	Poor
Comfort (1–100)	≥90	80–89	<80
Mean lens mislocation	≤±6°	±7° to ±10°	>10°
SD of lens location	<±6°	±6° to ±10°	>±10°
Rotational recovery/10 blinks	>10°	6–10°	<6°
% Lenses within ±10°	≥90	70–89	<70

(Reproduced from Tan *et al.*, 2007)

Effect of lens rotation

A considerable degree of cylindrical error can be induced when a lens does not stabilize satisfactorily and rotates away from the intended orientation (Lindsay *et al.*, 1997); this phenomenon is demonstrated in Appendix I. For example, if the contact lens correction incorporates a power of plano/−2.00 DC × 180, Appendix I reveals that a mislocation of the axis by 10° results in a spherocylindrical error of +0.35/−0.69 DC × 40. A useful rule of thumb here is that a lens made to specification but mislocating on the eye will produce an over-refraction with a spherical equivalent equal to zero. Where the sphere or cylinder power is incorrect, the spherical equivalent of the over-refraction will not equal zero (Long, 1991).

Predicting lens rotation

Hanks and Weisbarth (1983) showed that, on average, soft toric lenses will tend to rotate nasally by about 5–10°, where nasal rotation is designated as rotation of the inferior aspect of the lens towards the nose. They also showed, however, that there was significant variability between soft toric lens wearers in the actual amount and direction of lens rotation; variations also occur between different lens designs.

The nature of both contact lens materials and their associated designs is continually changing; performance characteristics that were typical for toric soft contact lenses of a decade ago may be of questionable relevance today. Tan *et al.* (2007) have examined the performance of several lenses with differing methods of stabilization and have developed recommended performance standards for toric soft contact lenses (Table 10.1).

The variability in performance of soft toric lenses can be due to the following factors.

Lid anatomy

Variation in lid tension (tightness), lid location, lid angle and lid symmetry can all have a significant effect on the location and stability of a toric lens on the eye. Tight lids are more likely to affect lens movement and location than loose lids. Measurements made by Young (2003), from high-speed video recordings of toric soft lenses during reorientation, indicate that lid-induced rotation takes place during rather than between blinks.

Lens–eye relationship

The optimal fitting relationship between the lens and the eye may vary from one patient to the next. The type of fit

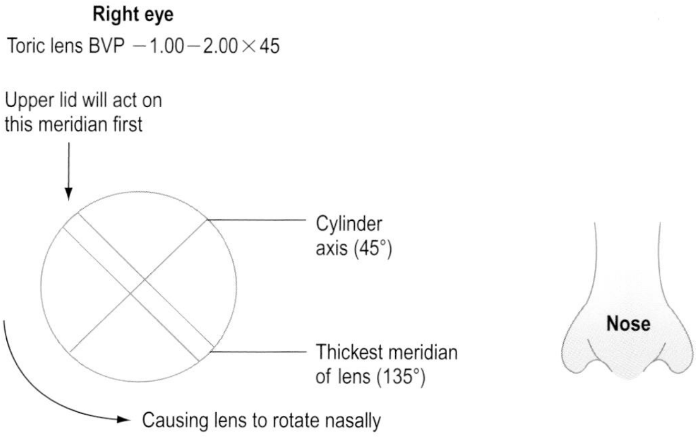

Figure 10.3 The effect of lid action on lens rotation for a soft toric lens with the prescription of −1.00/−2.00 × 45 being worn in the right eye. As the upper lid comes down, it will first act on the lens (and the 135° meridian) at around the 10 o'clock position on the cornea. The downward motion on the lens at this point will cause it to rotate nasally. BVP = back vertex power.

(steep, alignment or flat) will, in turn, have a significant bearing on lens position. For example, the degree of adherence between lens and eye is a very important factor (Holden, 1976). If a lens is too tightly adherent to the eye, it will not be affected by the locating forces designed to stabilize lens orientation.

Lens thickness profile

It has been noted previously that with dynamic stabilization the thickness profile interaction with the upper lid is the dominant stabilizing component. While most soft toric lenses manufactured today have the contact lens toricity confined to the central portion of the lens, a thickness differential due to the astigmatic correction can still have a significant effect on lens location.

The lens thickness profile is determined by the power of the lens, in particular the axis and magnitude of the astigmatic correction. For soft toric lenses incorporating dynamic stabilization, Gundel (1989) showed that rotational influence is greatest for lenses with cylinders at oblique axes (either between 30 and 60° or 120 and 150°), followed by lenses incorporating correction for with-the-rule astigmatism (150 to 30°), and is least for lenses with against-the-rule axes (60 to 120°).

Gundel (1989) postulated that the principal factor affecting lens rotation is the initial point of contact between the upper lid and the thicker meridian of the lens. For toric lenses with oblique axes, the implication is that there will be notable rotational effects as contact from the upper lid will always affect one edge of the thicker meridian before the other. As the upper lid comes down, it will force the lens down at this first point of contact, causing it to rotate in a certain direction. This principle is illustrated by the example shown in Figure 10.3. A mislocating effect also occurs with lenses correcting for with-the-rule astigmatism as the lid contraction angle will usually be at a slight angle to the thickest axis of the lens (Holden, 1975). For toric lenses incorporating a correction for against-the-rule astigmatism, upper-lid contact with the thicker (horizontal) meridian will be fairly symmetrical and so the rotational effect is minimal. However, the influence of the lower lid can override that of the upper lid depending on its position, tightness and amount of lateral movement (Young, 2003).

Allowing for lens rotation

If it is expected that the soft toric lens to be ordered will rotate when placed on the eye of the patient, then an allowance must be made for this rotation, otherwise the cylinder axis of the lens *in situ* will not adopt the correct orientation for the ocular correction. When allowing for nasal rotation in the right eye, the amount of rotation should be subtracted from the required cylinder axis and vice versa for the left eye. When allowing for temporal rotation in the right eye, the amount of rotation should be added to the required cylinder axis and vice versa for the left eye. Hence:

- If left eye and nasal rotation: add.
- If left eye and temporal rotation: subtract.
- If right eye and nasal rotation: subtract.
- If right eye and temporal rotation: add.

The acronym LARS (left add, right subtract) - relating to nasal rotation of the inferior aspect of the lens - can be quite useful.

Many practitioners work on the principle that clockwise rotation necessitates adding the allowance for rotation to the required cylinder axis, and anticlockwise rotation requires subtracting the allowance for rotation to determine the final cylinder axis. Hence:

- If clockwise rotation: add.
- If anticlockwise rotation: subtract.

If, at the dispensing or aftercare visit, the lens rotation is not what was expected (but the lens location is stable), simply reorder the lens with the revised allowance for lens rotation. Generally, rotational stability is a more important factor than the degree of rotation. Lenses that give sub-optimal but stable acuity are more likely to be acceptable than those that give moments of clear vision followed by moments of poor vision as the lens rotates.

Measurement of lens rotation

Soft toric lenses will usually have markings on the lens at a specific reference point so the degree of rotation can be assessed when the lens is on the eye. The markings may be in the form of laser trace, scribe lines (Figure 10.4), engraved dots or ink dots (Figure 10.5).

The lens markings do not represent the cylinder axis; they are simply a point of reference with regard to which the rotation of the lens can be assessed. They may either be at the 6 o'clock position of the lens or in the horizontal lens meridian at the 3 and 9 o'clock positions. The latter situation is preferable as the markings can then be observed without having to retract the lower eyelid (which would interfere with the dynamic stabilizing forces that normally act to orient the lens). In addition, having two widely spaced markings about 14 mm apart at the 3 and 9 o'clock positions, as opposed to one mark or a set of marks at the 6 o'clock position, makes it easier to quantify the angle of rotation. Many laboratories that opt for the 6 o'clock indication provide three lines on their lenses, each separated by the same known angle, thus also facilitating a determination of lens rotation. Generally, lenses with markings at the 6 o'clock position are those with asymmetrical dynamic

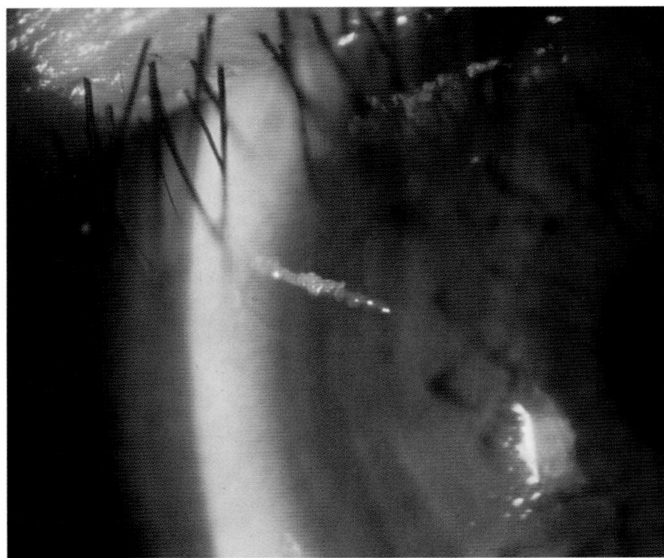

Figure 10.4 Scribe line on soft toric lens. This lens has two scribe lines as markers with the reference points being at the 3 and 9 o'clock locations (only the 9 o'clock mark is visible here). Debris has accumulated in the scribe line – a common site for deposit formation.

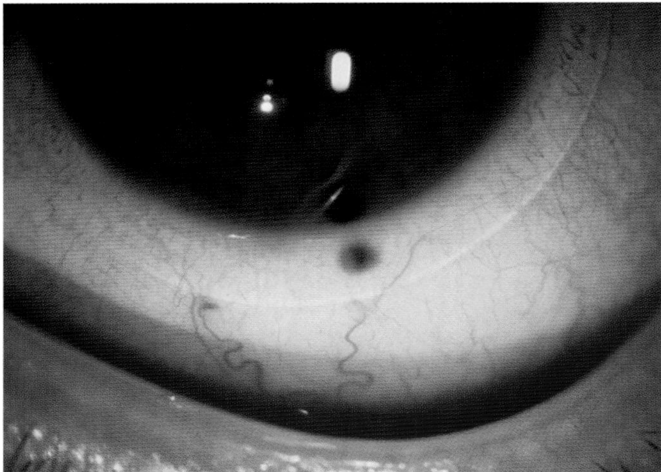

Figure 10.5 Soft toric lens with two ink dots, one above the other, as markers for the 6 o'clock reference point. The upper ink dot is only just visible against the dark iris. Two dots are used to help with lens identification; the lens in the other eye has just one ink dot. This lens is exhibiting about 10° nasal rotation.

stabilization where it is important for the larger, thinner peripheral zone to be oriented superiorly for optimal lid interaction.

Estimation is a straightforward and reasonable technique for assessing the degree of lens rotation, made simpler if the practitioner remembers that there is 30° between each hour on a clock face. Clinical experience has shown that this is a satisfactory method of assessing lens rotation, with errors more likely to occur when evaluating higher amounts of lens rotation (Snyder and Daum, 1989).

When assessing lens rotation, it is important to realize that it is the angular orientation of the marker on the lens that is significant and not the position of the marker on the cornea. Figure 10.6 shows a soft toric lens on a left eye with

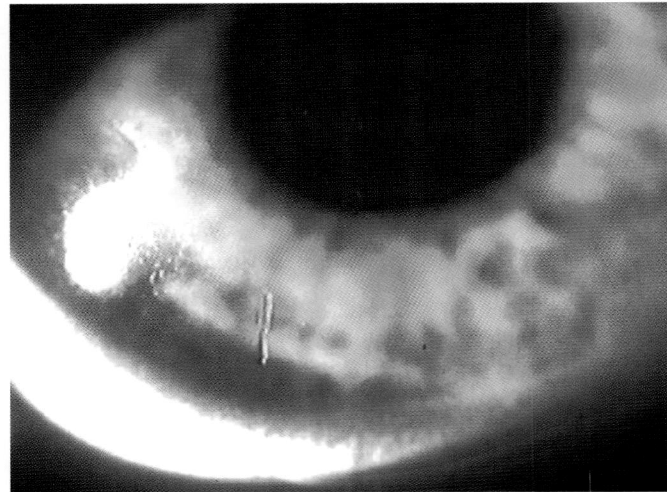

Figure 10.6 Misleading lens rotation resulting from a decentred contact lens.

the marker indicating that the lens is rotating nasally by about 20° (given that the reference point for the marker is the 6 o'clock position). However, a closer look at the marker reveals that it is vertically oriented, the expected orientation if the lens was not rotating. In this case, the apparent nasal rotation is due to a nasal decentration of the contact lens.

Determining lens misalignment

The usual method of determining lens misalignment is simply to estimate the degree of lens rotation by observing the location of the soft toric lens on the eye. This value is then compared with the expected lens rotation that has been incorporated into the BVP of the contact lens. The difference between the actual and expected values represents the degree of lens misalignment.

An SCO can also be used to determine the degree of lens misalignment. The lens misalignment is deduced by calculating the effective BVP of the lens on the eye ($BVP_{in\ situ}$). The *SCO* obtained over the mislocating soft toric lens is subtracted from the ocular refraction (*Oc Rx*) of the patient (Lindsay *et al.*, 1997). That is:

$$BVP_{in\ situ} = Oc\ Rx - SCO$$

Calculating the $BVP_{in\ situ}$ will require the resolving of obliquely crossed cylinders and this is best done by matrix optics (Long, 1976; Keating, 1980) using the following method:

1. Express both the spherocylindrical ocular refraction and the *SCO* in dioptric power matrix form (*F*), whereby:

$$F = \begin{vmatrix} S + C\sin^2\theta & -C\sin\theta\cos\theta \\ -C\sin\theta\cos\theta & S + C\cos^2\theta \end{vmatrix}$$

where *S* is the sphere power, *C* is the cylinder power and θ is the axis (in radians) of the cylinder.

2. Subtract the dioptric power matrix for the over-refraction from the dioptric power matrix for the ocular refraction, to obtain the dioptric power matrix, F_r, for the $BVP_{in\ situ}$:

$$F_r = \begin{vmatrix} S_r + C_r\sin^2\theta_r & -C_r\sin\theta_r\cos\theta_r \\ -C_r\sin\theta_r\cos\theta_r & S_r + C_r\cos^2\theta_r \end{vmatrix}$$

	A	B	C	D	E
1		SPHERE	CYLINDER	AXIS	
2					
3	Oc Rx	−3	−2	10	=D3/57.2958
4	MATRIX	=B3+C3*(SIN(E3)^2)	=−C3*SIN(E3)*COS(E3)		
5		=−C3*SIN(E3)*COS(E3)	=B3+C3*(COS(E3)^2)		
6	OR	0.5	−1	47.5	=D6/57.2958
7	MATRIX	=B6+C6*(SIN(E6)^2)	=−C6*SIN(E6)*COS(E6)		
8		=−C6*SIN(E6)*COS(E6)	=B6+C6*(COS(E6)^2)		
9	SUM	=B4-B7	=C4-C7		
10		=B5-B8	=C5-C8		
11	TRACE	=B9+C10			
12	DET	=(B9*C10)−(B10*C9)			
13	BVPin situ	=(B11-C13)/2	=−SQRT((B11^2)−4*B12)	=IF(57.2958*ATAN((B13-B9)/C9)>0, 57.2958*ATAN((B13-B9)/C9), 180+57.2958*ATAN((B13-B9)/C9))	
14					

Figure 10.7 Spreadsheet for determining soft toric lens misalignment.

3. Convert the matrix form of the $BVP_{in\ situ}$ back to spherocylindrical notation using the following formulae:

If the lens power matrix is $\begin{vmatrix} a_{11} & a_{12} \\ a_{21} & a_{22} \end{vmatrix}$

trace $(t) = a_{11} + a_{22}$ and

determinant $(d) = (a_{11}a_{22}) - (a_{12}a_{21})$

To convert the matrix form of the $BVP_{in\ situ}$ back to spherocylindrical notation, the sphere power, cylinder power and cylinder axis of the $BVP_{in\ situ}$, S_r, C_r and θ_r, can be determined as follows:

$$S_r = \frac{(t - C_r)}{2}$$

$$\theta_r = a\tan\frac{(S_r - a_{11})}{a_{12}} \times \frac{180}{\pi} \text{(where } \theta_r \text{ is in degrees)}$$

$$C_r = -\sqrt{t^2 - 4d}$$

The minus sign before the radical symbol simply means that the final solution will be in minus cylinder form.

These formulae can easily be incorporated into a spreadsheet (Figure 10.7) which can then be quickly utilized in clinical practice.

Once the $BVP_{in\ situ}$ has been determined, any degree of lens misalignment can then be identified along with any errors in the power of the manufactured lens by comparing the $BVP_{in\ situ}$ with the BVP specified for the contact lens.

For example, consider a soft toric lens being fitted to the left eye of a patient. The ocular refraction is –3.00/–2.00 × 10. The specified BVP of the contact lens is –3.00/–2.00 × 20, so this prescription incorporates an allowance for 10° nasal rotation. An SCO with this lens yields +0.50/–1.00 × 47.5. Solving for $BVP_{in\ situ}$ gives –3.00/–2.00 × 175. The specified cylinder axis was 20°; however the effective cylinder axis on the eye is 175°. Therefore the lens is exhibiting 25° nasal rotation on the eye (instead of the expected 10° nasal rotation). To allow for this 25° nasal rotation, the contact lens would now have to be reordered with a cylinder axis of 35° to achieve the target cylinder axis on the eye of 10°.

If visual acuity is not improved by the SCO, the cause of the suboptimal acuity may be a poorly fitting lens, a lens of poor quality (possibly due to significant deposition on the lens surface) or some form of ocular pathology (Myers *et al.*, 1990).

Planned replacement of soft toric lenses

Many clinicians initially treated planned-replacement (i.e. disposable) soft toric lenses with scepticism because of concerns about on-eye performance and reproducibility (Lindsay, 2006). However presently most soft toric contact lenses are prescribed on a disposable basis, with a recent survey revealing that less than 1% of new soft toric lens fits did not involve any planned lens replacement (Morgan *et al.*, 2009). The majority of disposable lenses are replaced at monthly, 2-weekly or daily intervals and disposable soft toric lenses are available in these three modalities, as well as in both conventional hydrogel and silicone hydrogel materials. The rationale for the planned replacement of soft contact lenses is based on the tenet that cleaner lenses should produce fewer adverse ocular effects.

Virtually all disposable soft toric lenses are produced as a stock range of lenses encompassing a certain number of cylindrical powers (such as –0.75, –1.25 and –1.75 D), a set choice of spherical powers (for example, from +6.00 to –9.00) and cylinder axes in 5 or 10° steps – usually the latter – most often covering the complete spectrum from 0° to 180°. The choice of back optic zone radius and total lens diameter for these lenses is also usually limited, hence, given that the contact lens practitioner has chosen to use a particular type of disposable soft toric lens, the main decision in fitting and prescribing these lenses generally relates to the specification of BVP.

One of the advantages associated with the use of disposable soft toric lenses is that it is usually possible to undertake a lens-wearing trial on a prospective patient using a disposable soft toric lens with the appropriate BVP. This allows the practitioner to ascertain more accurately if the cylinder axis of the soft toric lens *in situ* will adopt the correct orientation for the ocular correction. At the same time, the practitioner is also able to determine if the patient can wear the lens comfortably without any adverse effect on the eye.

Limitations of toric soft lenses

There will be a certain number of cases encountered in clinical practice where soft toric lenses are either less likely to be successful or do not represent the best option for the prospective contact lens patient. In these situations, the practitioner should take extra care when prescribing soft toric lenses.

Low spherical components

Patients who are fitted with soft toric lenses that contain a low spherical component, for example +0.25/−2.50 × 180, are often very critical of axis alignment because the astigmatism is the most significant component of their refractive error. In addition, with some of the older soft toric lens designs, the thickness differentials (to aid lens location) that can usually be achieved are reduced with small spherical components (Hanks and Weisbarth, 1983).

Oblique cylinders

As previously discussed (Holden, 1975; Gundel, 1989), soft toric lenses incorporating oblique cylinders, for example −2.00/−2.00 × 45, may show poorer stability due to complex lid lens interactions.

Large cylindrical components

Lens rotation becomes more significant as the degree of cylinder is increased. For example, a patient with a toric lens incorporating a 1.25 D cylinder may be able to tolerate a 5° rotation from the expected lens location, whereas a toric lens patient with a 3.50 D cylinder will probably notice a significant drop in vision for the same degree of rotation off-axis.

Irregular astigmatism

No form of soft toric lens is able to correct irregular astigmatism. Patients with astigmatic errors of this nature are usually corrected with some form of rigid contact lens.

Physiological considerations

Improvements in toric lens design have led to an overall reduction in the thickness of most soft toric lenses. This decrease in lens thickness has led to a reduction in the number of physiological problems encountered with soft toric lenses. Despite this, the overall thickness of a soft toric lens can be significantly greater than that of a soft spherical lens because of the addition of cylinder and the creation of thickness differentials throughout the toric lens form. Consequently, oxygen transmissibility will be reduced and mechanical irritation increased in the thicker regions of the lens, with the result that compromises to ocular health are more likely to occur.

Conditions seen quite often with soft toric lens wear include the following:

- Corneal oedema – especially in patients with hyperopic astigmatism.
- Corneal neovascularization – usually inferior and superior and more likely in myopic patients.
- Superior limbic keratoconjunctivitis – especially with large lenses.
- Conjunctival indentation – especially with tight-fitting lenses.

If corneal hypoxia is a suspected cause of any ocular changes seen with soft toric lens wear, then a sensible strategy would be to refit the patient with a soft toric lens incorporating a silicone hydrogel material so as to improve the oxygen transmissibility of the lens.

Conclusions

A large variety of soft toric lens designs are available today, incorporating a number of different stabilization techniques. As a result, the visual requirements of most astigmatic patients are readily satisfied. The fact that these products are often supplied in frequent replacement and disposable modalities means that it is also possible to make soft toric lens wear convenient and tailored to the lifestyle requirements of the patient.

References

Bernstein, P. R., Gundel, R. E. and Rosen, J. S. (1991) Masking corneal toricity with hydrogels: Does it work? *Int. Contact Lens Clin.*, **18,** 67–70.

Edwards, K. (1999) Problem-solving with toric soft contact lenses. *Optician,* **217**(5695), 18–19, 22, 24–25, 27.

Fanti, P. (1975) The fitting of a soft toroidal contact lens. *Optician,* **169**(4376), 8–9, 13, 15–16.

Gasson, A. P. (1977) Back surface toric soft lenses. *Optician,* **174**(4491), 6–7, 9, 11.

Gundel, R. E. (1989) Effect of cylinder axis on rotation for a double thin zone design toric hydrogel. *Int. Contact Lens Clin.*, **16,** 141–145.

Hanks, A. J. (1983) The watermelon seed principle. *Contact Lens Forum,* **9,** 31–35.

Hanks, A. J. and Weisbarth, R. E. (1983) Troubleshooting soft toric contact lenses. *Int. Contact Lens Clin.*, **10,** 305–317.

Holden, B. A. (1975) The principles and practice of correcting astigmatism with soft contact lenses. *Aust. J. Optom.*, **58,** 279–299.

Holden, B. A. (1976) Correcting astigmatism with toric soft lenses – an overview. *Int. Contact Lens Clin.*, **3,** 59–61.

Keating, M. P. (1980) An easier method to obtain the sphere, cylinder, and axis from an off-axis dioptric power matrix. *Am. J. Optom. Physiol. Opt.*, **57,** 734–737.

Lindsay, R. G. (1998) Toric soft contact lens fitting. *Optician,* **216**(5671), 18–20, 22, 24.

Lindsay, R. G. (2006) Determining power for disposable soft torics. *Contact Lens Spectrum,* **21**(7), 36–40.

Lindsay, R. G., Bruce, A. S., Brennan, N. A. *et al.* (1997) Determining axis misalignment and power errors of toric soft lenses. *Int. Contact Lens Clin.,* **24,** 101–107.

Long, W. F. (1976) A matrix formalism for decentration problems. *Am. J. Optom. Physiol. Opt.,* **53,** 27–33.

Long, W. F. (1991) Lens power matrices and the sum of equivalent spheres. *Optom. Vis. Sci.,* **68,** 821–822.

Morgan, P. B., Woods, C. A., Tranoudis, I. G. *et al.* (2009) International contact lens prescribing in 2008. *Contact Lens Spectrum,* **24**(2), 28–32.

Myers, R. I., Jones, D. H. and Meinell, P. (1990) Using over-refraction for problem solving in soft toric fitting. *Int. Contact Lens Clin.,* **17,** 232–234.

Snyder, C. (1998) Overcoming toric soft lens challenges. *Contact Lens Spectrum,* (suppl), 2–4.

Snyder, C. and Daum, K.D. (1989) Rotational position of toric soft contact lenses on the eye – clinical judgements. *Int. Contact Lens Clin.,* **16,** 146–151.

Strachan, J. P. F. (1975) Correction of astigmatism with hydrophilic lenses. *Optician,* **170** (4402), 8–11.

Tan, J., Papas, E., Carnt, N. *et al.* (2007) Performance standards for toric soft contact lenses. *Optom. Vis. Sci.,* **84,** 422–428.

Young, G. (2003) Toric contact lens designs in hyper-oxygen materials. *Eye and Contact Lens,* **29,** S171–S173; discussion S190–S191, S192–S194.

11 CHAPTER

Soft lens care systems

Philip B Morgan

Introduction

With the notable exception of daily disposable lenses and extended-wear lenses that are discarded after each period of continuous wear, all contact lenses must be subjected to some form of maintenance procedure after each use. The key elements of lens maintenance are cleaning and disinfection. Contact lenses must also be safely stored in solution until they are next worn. This chapter will explore the rationale for undertaking these tasks, and will review current lens care maintenance options.

A rationale for disinfecting contact lenses

Contact lens practitioners are acutely aware that an eye wearing a contact lens is more likely to become infected than an eye not wearing a contact lens. Brennan and Coles (1997) estimated the risk of contact lens-associated infection as being 60 times greater in a contact lens wearer than in a non-lens wearer. The reasons for this increase in risk are multifactorial, and it is worth considering these factors in the first instance as they essentially form the rationale for contact lens disinfection.

The eye has a number of inherent protective mechanisms to resist infection. These are generally successful, as can be seen in the light of work by Fleiszig and Efron (1992), who estimated that potential pathogens are present in the tear film of 5% of a population at any time, yet the prevalence of ocular-surface infection falls far short of this value. The tear film and the blinking process play an important role in the resistance of infection. Basal tear production is of the order of 1–2 μl/min and the overall tear volume is about 7 μl, which confirms the rapid turnover of tears at the ocular surface with the consequent removal of microorganisms.

Bacteria in the tear film must also breach the defence provided by proteins in the tear film such as lysozyme, lactoferrin and transferrin. Furthermore, immunoglobulins such as secretory IgA, IgG, IgE and IgM can act to resist infection.

A microorganism which is able to defeat all the above systems is still hampered in its quest to invade and infect the cornea because of the various defences of the corneal epithelium. These include: tight junctions which prevent the migration of microorganisms between epithelial cells; sloughing of cells from the epithelial surface to remove infected cells before any further harm is caused to the rest of the cornea; the active release of antibacterial factors from the corneal epithelium; and the 'filter-like' barrier provided by the basal lamina which prevents bacteria reaching the underlying stroma (Fleiszig, 2006).

Contact lens wear adversely affects a number of these defence mechanisms. Perhaps the most significant effect is the prevention of clearance of debris and microorganisms from the ocular surface by the blinking mechanism due to the protection offered by the contact lens. It has also been postulated that the level of fibronectin is reduced during contact lens wear, thereby increasing the likelihood of bacterial attachment to the epithelium (Fleiszig *et al.*, 1992).

A key reason for the increase in ocular infections amongst contact lens wearers is the bioburden of microorganisms introduced to the ocular surface when lenses are inserted. Indirect evidence for this is provided by the work of Radford *et al.* (1998), who analysed the risk factors associated with contact lens-related infections. They found that the risk of infection was significantly increased in those wearers only undertaking irregular disinfection with their contact lenses. The association of inappropriate use of the contact lens storage case (Seal *et al.*, 1999) and a lack of handwashing (Stapleton *et al.*, 2007) with an increased risk of contact lens-related infections also supports the notion that contact lens wear presents an increased microbial challenge to the ocular-surface defence systems. As such, it seems clear that whilst contact lens wear renders the eye at greater risk of infection, there is good evidence that the appropriate use of suitable contact lens disinfection systems will reduce the magnitude of this increased risk.

A rationale for cleaning contact lenses

There are two key reasons why a contact lens should be cleaned prior to disinfection. First, a wide variety of intrinsic and extrinsic debris can adhere to the surface of a

DOI: 10.1016/B978-0-7506-8869-7.00011-2

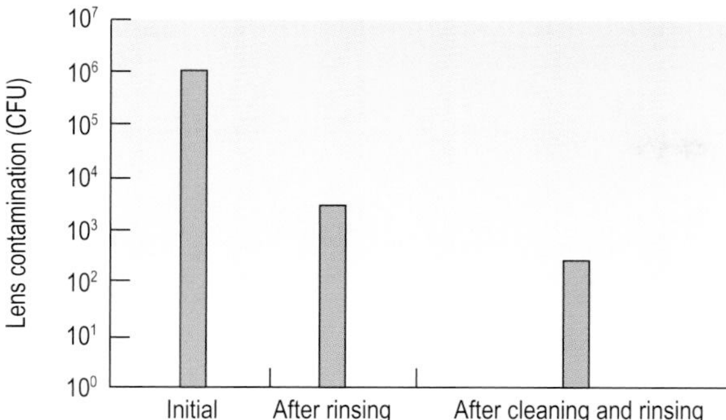

Figure 11.1 Effect of lens rinsing and cleaning on bacterial bioburden. (Adapted from Shih, K. L., Hu, J. and Sibley, M. (1985) The microbiological benefit of cleaning and rinsing contact lenses. Int. Contact Lens Clin., 12, 235–242.)

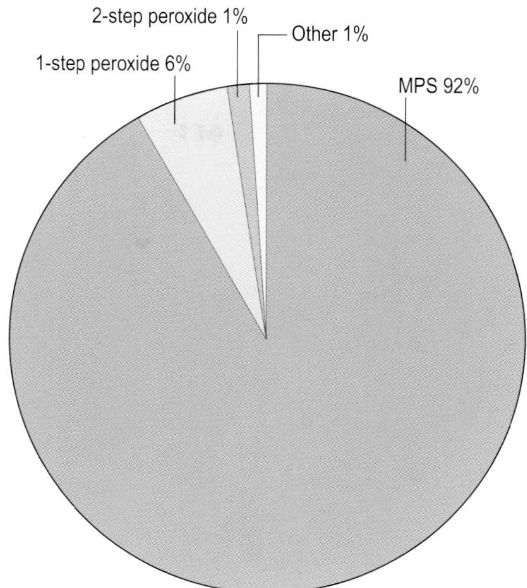

Figure 11.2 Soft lens solutions prescribed in 19 countries. MPS = multipurpose solutions.

contact lens. This can lead to lens distortion, discomfort, an unsightly cosmetic appearance (as soiled lenses can show marked discolouration clearly visible to an onlooker), ocular-surface and eyelid pathology and vision loss (Gellatly *et al.*, 1988). Lens cleaning can mitigate against these problems. Cho *et al.* (2009) found rinsing to be ineffective in removing loosely bound deposits on lenses compared to rubbing. Lens deposits are discussed in depth in Chapter 19. Second, cleaning acts to enhance the disinfection process by reducing the levels of microorganisms on the contact lens. Shih *et al.* (1985) demonstrated this by contaminating contact lenses with an organic load plus live cells of *Pseudomonas aeruginosa* or *Staphylococcus epidermidis*. When lenses were rinsed for 10 seconds, contamination was reduced from 1 million colony-forming units (cfu) per lens to less than 3000 cfu per lens. When the lenses were rubbed with the index finger in the palm of the hand for 10 seconds with three drops of cleaner on each side before the rinsing process, there was a reduction to less than 300 cfu per lens (Figure 11.1). The importance of contact lens cleaning is supported by the epidemiological work of Radford *et al.* (1995) who demonstrated that the risk of infection was about three times greater in patients who cleaned their lenses less than twice per week compared with those who achieved at least this frequency of cleaning. Kilvington and Lonnen (2009) have demonstrated that the use of a manual rubbing step is more effective than rinsing or soaking alone in removing pathogenic microbes from silicone hydrogel lenses. Accordingly, it would seem prudent to recommend that all contact lens care systems include a rub step as part of the hygiene regimen.

The evolution of soft lens care systems

Historically, the care of a soft contact lens was a complex and time-consuming activity for the wearer. The various steps of the lens care process were divided into separate activities with a different bottle or tablet for each. This has changed over time for two reasons: first, the introduction of multipurpose products has meant that more than one component of the lens care process could be undertaken with a single solution. Second, the commercial success of disposable and planned-replacement soft lenses in the 1990s – with the associated emphasis on patient convenience – acted as a powerful incentive for the lens care industry to reduce the complexity of the lens care process as much as possible. In some respects, such as a reduced requirement for regular enzymatic cleaning of soft lenses, this was justified. In others, such as the omission of any form of lens surface cleaning, there appeared to be a related increase in the incidence of microbial keratitis (Sarwar *et al.*, 1993).

The great majority of soft contact lens wearers are prescribed multipurpose products. Figure 11.2 shows the results of a survey, conducted in 2006, of over 22 000 contact lens fits in 19 countries. It was found that 92% of soft lens wearers were prescribed a multipurpose product, 6% a one-step hydrogen peroxide system, 1% a two-step hydrogen peroxide system and 1% some other care system (Morgan *et al.*, 2007).

Lens care systems

Physical methods

The various physical methods of soft lens disinfection rely on energy being imparted to microorganisms to cause lethal cell changes. Heating was the first soft lens disinfection method approved by the US Food and Drug Administration (FDA) in 1972. Disinfection using this approach requires a temperature of 80°C to be maintained for at least 10 min. A representative example of one of the heating units available at this time was the Bausch & Lomb system (Figure 11.3), which reached 96°C for a period of about 20 min (Mote *et al.*, 1972). In terms of lens disinfection, the heating systems were recognized as being highly effective (Busschaert *et al.*, 1978), even against the protozoan *Acanthamoeba* (Ludwig *et al.*, 1986). Furthermore, after the initial purchase of the heat unit, the ongoing costs of operation were minimal.

There were a number of disadvantages associated with heat disinfection. In normal circumstances, the protein which spoils the surface of a soft contact lens does not

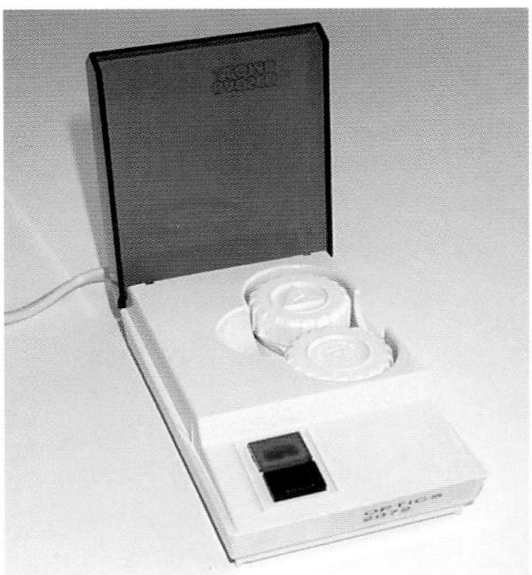

Figure 11.3 The Bausch & Lomb lens heat unit.

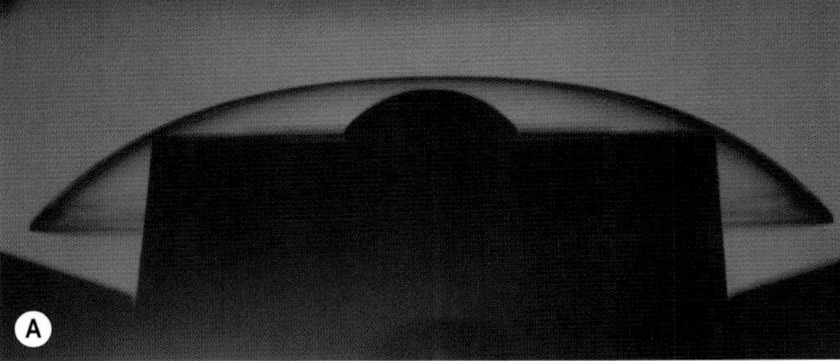

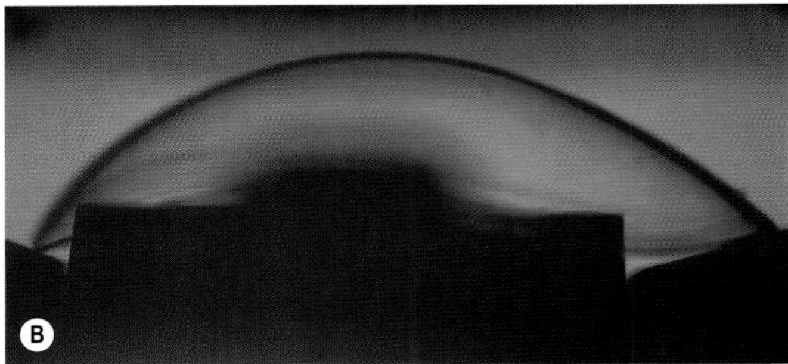

Figure 11.4 Profile view of an ionic, high-water-content contact lens. (A) Following 1 week of extended wear. (B) Same lens as shown in (A) after one cycle of heat disinfection, which has resulted in discolouration and distortion.

denature; however, heating the lens tends to denature protein with adverse clinical consequences such as reduced acuity, the potential for ocular surface reactions such as giant papillary conjunctivitis and altered physical lens parameters. With the popularity of low-water-content, non-ionic lenses in the early and mid-1970s, this was not as significant a problem as with the use of these systems with more modern, high-water-content and ionic materials which absorb much greater quantities of proteins (Maissa *et al.*, 1998). Figure 11.4 demonstrates how a standard single heat disinfection cycle – performed on an ionic, high-water-content lens that had been worn for 8 h – causes the lens to turn yellow and become deformed.

The heating process was also inconvenient for many wearers. Not only did this method require a nearby source of electricity, but the system used unpreserved saline which did not offer any antimicrobial activity. The opportunity for microbial contamination arose if the lenses remained in the cooled saline for a prolonged period, so this disinfection system required the process to be repeated each day with fresh solution if the lenses were not used.

With the advent of planned-replacement lenses, which were generally of high water content and often manufactured from ionic materials more prone to parameter changes, the popularity of heat disinfection waned, and this technique is rarely used today.

Microwave irradiation has been proposed as a potentially cheap and effective method of soft lens disinfection. Harris *et al.* (1993c) demonstrated that, although there are some parameter changes when lenses are repeatedly irradiated with a standard 650-W microwave oven, none of these changes are clinically significant. However, as patients often need to care for their lenses in locations remote from a microwave oven, this approach is often impractical or inconvenient.

Studies on the efficacy of ultraviolet radiation for contact lens disinfection have provided equivocal results. Using radiation at 253.7 nm at an energy of 44.3 $\mu W/cm^2$, Kilvington and Scanlon (1991) found that pathogenic *Acanthamoeba* cysts and trophozoites survived irradiation of 22 min duration. Similarly, Palmer *et al.* (1991), using an identical system, concluded that although the numbers of microorganisms were reduced by ultraviolet irradiation, the level of survivors was unacceptably high. On the other hand, Harris *et al.* (1993b) demonstrated that disinfection could be achieved at the same wavelength for a panel of bacteria using an ultraviolet lamp with a higher energy output, 950 $\mu W/cm^2$. Harris *et al.* (1993a) concluded that any parameter changes with this method were not clinically important.

The use of ultrasound systems for lens disinfection has also been proposed. Although such devices can be shown to have a limited disinfection effect (Efron *et al.*, 1991b), the efficacy of ultrasound energy is limited by the physical similarity between lens material and solution, meaning that the relatively large amount of energy required to clean the lens successfully would probably damage its surface (Fatt, 1991).

Chlorhexidine and thiomersal preserved systems

After the problems associated with heat systems became known, alternative disinfection systems were required which allowed for the simple storage of contact lenses without affecting the lens or causing irritation to the eye. Suitable early candidates were products which contained chlorhexidine gluconate or thiomersal.

Chlorhexidine is probably the most widely used biocide in antiseptics, especially for handwashing and oral products. Its action has been closely studied, and it is believed that its uptake by both bacteria and yeast is extremely rapid. Chlorhexidine damages cell walls and subsequently attacks the bacterial cytoplasmic or inner membrane, or the yeast plasma membrane (McDonnell and Russell, 1999).

Thiomersal is considered to be a less effective antimicrobial agent overall, although its action against fungi is better than that of chlorhexidine. Due to this, a combination of chlorhexidine gluconate and thiomersal became common in disinfectants for soft contact lenses. However, due to the absorption of these agents on to soft lenses, toxic and hypersensitivity reactions were reported when they were used clinically (Wilson *et al.*, 1981). The build-up of these preservatives, and the subsequent leeching on to the ocular surface over time, had the potential to cause discomfort and discontinuation of lens wear (Hind, 1975). These products were ultimately superseded by others which offered a similar level of convenience and antimicrobial efficacy, and a lower adverse reaction rate.

Anthony *et al.* (1991) described a novel approach for a chlorhexidine system, known as OptimEyes (Bausch & Lomb). They developed a tablet which, when dissolved in tap water, provided a solution with a chlorhexidine concentration of 0.004%. The solution was shown to be effective against a panel of challenge microorganisms and also against most of the microorganisms found in tap water. This was a controversial development because this product was specifically designed for use with tap water and practitioners were concerned that contact lens wearers would consider standard tap water as an acceptable component of lens care generally. The product was simple and cheap to use, and it provided action against *Acanthamoeba*. Its disadvantages included the reliance on a supply of rising mains tap water and, importantly, it was contraindicated for use with FDA group IV lenses because the action of chlorhexidine is reduced with ionic lenses. With the increasing popularity of group IV lenses throughout the 1990s, the OptimEyes product did not become a mainstream soft lens care product.

Chlorine

Chlorine-releasing agents are long established as disinfection systems for swimming pools, baby feeding equipment and medical instrumentation. In the 1980s, chlorine-releasing systems were developed for the disinfection of contact lenses. These were seen as being highly convenient due to their ease of use, portability and low adverse reaction rate. In markets which did not have access to multipurpose solutions (MPS) when planned-replacement lenses were introduced at the end of the 1980s, these systems became very popular. Pearson (1992) reported that 26% of soft lens wearers in the UK used chlorine systems in 1991. No chlorine-releasing products are available today in the UK.

Two chlorine-releasing systems achieved market success. Alcon introduced the Softab product in the early 1980s (Figure 11.5). This was a tablet of sodium dichloroisocyanurate which was dissolved in saline to form 3 parts per million (ppm) chlorine. Sauflon developed the Aerotab product in the mid-1980s which released 8 ppm chlorine. Laboratory studies suggested that these solutions were effective at destroying a range of microorganisms, including bacteria and fungi (Rosenthal *et al.*, 1992). The killing action was thought to be due to the direct effect of the chlorine on some vital constituent of the cell of the microorganism, such as its protoplasm or enzyme system (Copley, 1989). However, these products became associated with an increase in contact lens-related microbial keratitis (Radford *et al.*, 1995, 1998). For example, the optimal use of a chlorine system was associated with about a 15-fold increase in the likelihood of *Acanthamoeba* keratitis compared with hydrogen peroxide or other solutions.

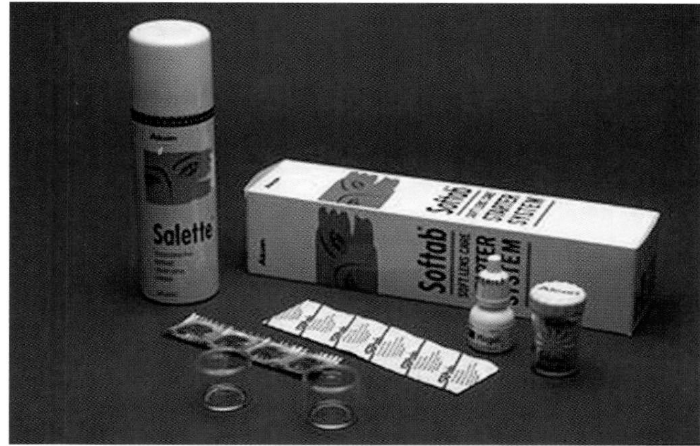

Figure 11.5 The Softab chlorine system.

The association of ocular infections with chlorine solutions, despite satisfactory laboratory performance, suggests that there were problems with the efficacy of these systems with normal day-to-day usage. One issue was that the overnight dissipation of chlorine resulted in a loss of disinfecting power, so prolonged storage was not appropriate with these products. There was also evidence that the antimicrobial performance was severely reduced when lenses were soiled (Copley, 1989); this factor would not have been addressed when antimicrobial efficacy was determined by the licensing authorities. Overall, there was little margin for error when using these products; for example, Efron *et al.* (1991c) and Sarwar *et al.* (1993) reported a number of cases of corneal infection in patients who had failed to use surfactant cleaning solutions prior to chlorine disinfection. The negative publicity generated by such cases of microbial keratitis, and the widespread availability of MPS which were also very easy to use, led to a great reduction in the use of chlorine-releasing systems throughout the 1990s.

Hydrogen peroxide

Hydrogen peroxide has been used as an antimicrobial agent for about 200 years. It is widely used medically for disinfection and sterilization and is generally available in concentrations from 3% to 90%, depending on its purpose. Hydrogen peroxide has a broad-spectrum efficacy against bacteria, viruses and yeast by producing hydroxyl free radicals which attach essential cell components such as lipid and proteins (McDonnell and Russell, 1999), and is often considered to be the 'gold standard' in terms of soft contact lens disinfection. For example, 3% hydrogen peroxide will kill trophozoites and cysts of *Acanthamoeba castellanii* in 3 min and 9 h of soaking, respectively (Zanetti *et al.*, 1995). It can be chemically broken down into oxygen and water, and is therefore considered to be environmentally friendly. Hydrogen peroxide tends to decompose on standing, and it therefore needs to be stabilized, typically with phosphates or phosphorates. The use of stannate as a stabilizer has been associated with hazing of ionic lenses due to an interaction between the stannate ions, methacrylic acid groups in the lens material and tear-derived lysozyme (Sack *et al.*, 1989).

Although hydrogen peroxide has a high efficacy in terms of its antimicrobial action, it is toxic to the eye, and requires neutralization before a lens which has been placed in hydrogen peroxide can be worn comfortably. Paugh *et al.* (1988) demonstrated that conjunctival hyperaemia was induced by levels of hydrogen peroxide greater than 200 ppm and that concentrations in excess of 100 ppm were associated with subjective stinging. Interestingly, these authors could not demonstrate any corneal or conjunctival staining with the highest concentration of hydrogen peroxide studied in their study (800 ppm). Changes in epithelial cell activity have been noted in the presence of concentrations as low as 30 ppm (Tripathi and Tripathi, 1989).

Storage in hydrogen peroxide has been reported to alter lens parameters. Bruce (1989) noted a temporary reduction in lens hydration after prolonged lens storage in hydrogen peroxide. High-water ionic lenses (FDA group IV) appear to be most susceptible to changes in diameter and base curve (McKenney, 1990), although the clinical consequences of these changes are generally not significant because of their temporary nature; for example, a soaking period of 20 min in neutralizer returns lens parameters to their original specification within 1 h of lens wear (Jones *et al.*, 1993).

The approaches to neutralization have varied since the introduction of hydrogen peroxide as a contact lens disinfectant. The initial approach was to allow for the storage of the lenses in hydrogen peroxide with neutralization undertaken as a secondary process before lens insertion.

These two-step systems are still considered to provide the best antimicrobial action, especially when the lens is exposed to 3% hydrogen peroxide overnight; however, the complexity of using these systems has led to a cessation of their use in many markets.

The two most popular approaches for neutralization in a two-step hydrogen peroxide system are the catalytic and reactive methods. For example, in the Oxysept system (Advanced Medical Optics), a solution containing the enzyme catalase is added to the lens storage case after the hydrogen peroxide has been discarded. This quickly breaks down the remaining hydrogen peroxide into water and oxygen, with the production of the latter requiring a vented storage case (Figure 11.6). With this system, no hydrogen peroxide is detectable 1 min after the introduction of the neutralizer (Gyulai *et al.*, 1987). In products adopting the reactive method, the lens case is filled with a solution containing sodium pyruvate after the hydrogen peroxide has been discarded. This completely neutralizes the peroxide in about 6 min (Christie and Meyler, 1997).

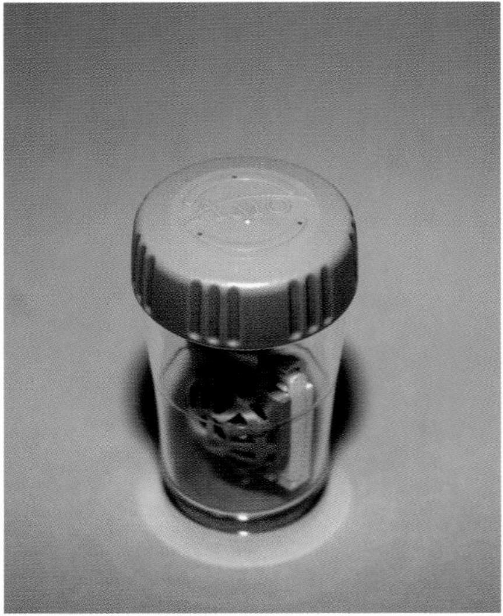

Figure 11.6 The release of oxygen in some systems requires the use of a vented contact lens storage case, or a case with gas release holes.

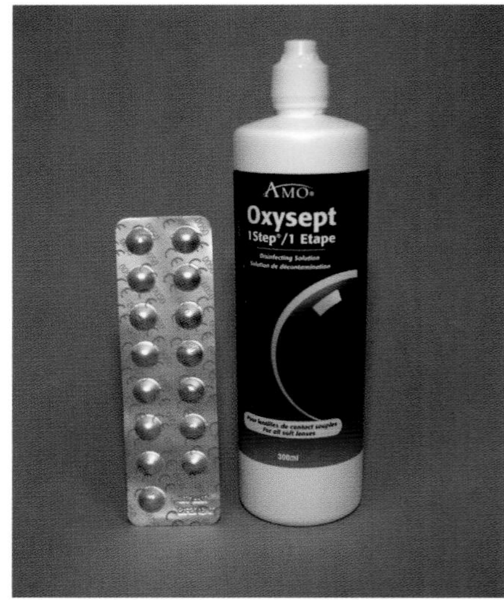

Figure 11.7 One-step hydrogen peroxide systems which use a tablet for neutralization.

Essentially, the one-step hydrogen peroxide systems negate the requirement for a separate neutralization process by the contact lens user. After the lens storage case is closed, the disinfection and neutralization steps take place without further intervention. Two approaches are common. In the first, such as in the Oxysept 1-step system (Advanced Medical Optics), the lens case is filled with hydrogen peroxide, and a coated tablet containing catalase is added (Figure 11.7). As the coating of the tablet dissolves, catalase is released into the solution, leading to neutralization of the hydrogen peroxide within about 2 h (Christie and Meyler, 1997). A number of products use a second method of neutralization: a platinum disc (Figures 11.8 and 11.9). In this approach, the disc is either attached as an integral part of the lens holder or is permanently lodged in the base of the storage case. There is a rapid neutralization over the first 2 min – from the original 30 000 ppm, or 3% concentration, to about 9000 ppm – followed by a slower phase to 50 ppm after 3 h (Gyulai *et al.*, 1987) and 15 ppm after 6 h (Christie and Meyler, 1997) (Figure 11.10).

The trade-off for the increased convenience of a one-step system is twofold. First, as the lenses are held only in neutralized solution within a few hours of entering the case, long-term storage is not advisable as the residual solution has no antimicrobial properties. Second, the reduced time in relatively high-concentration hydrogen

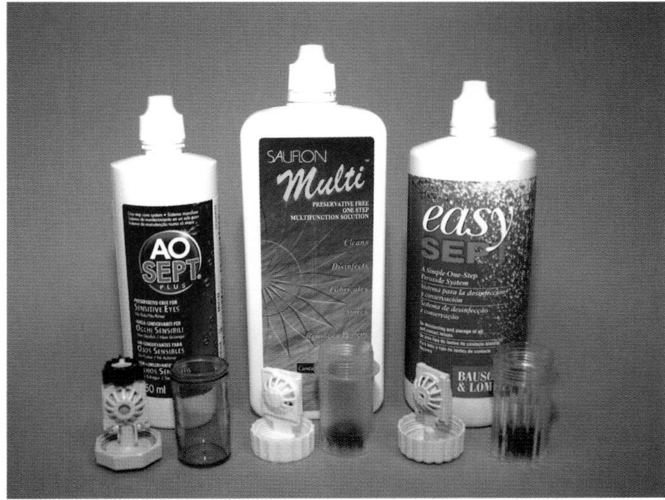

Figure 11.8 One-step hydrogen peroxide systems which use a platinum disc for neutralization.

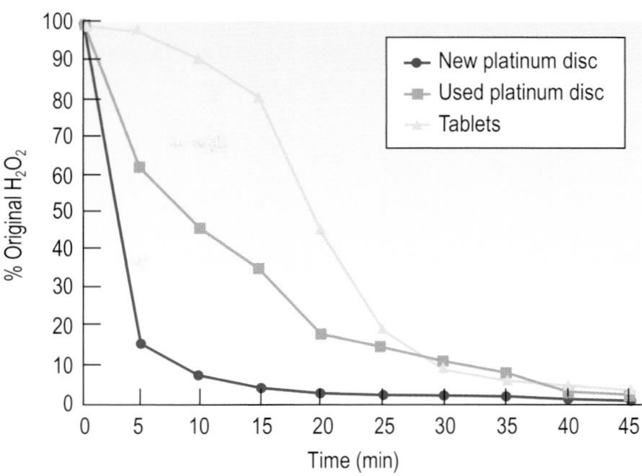

Figure 11.10 Hydrogen peroxide is neutralized more rapidly with platinum disc systems than with tablet systems. (Adapted from Christie, C. L. and Meyler, J. G. (1997) Contemporary contact lens care products. Contact Lens Ant. Eye, 20, S11–17.)

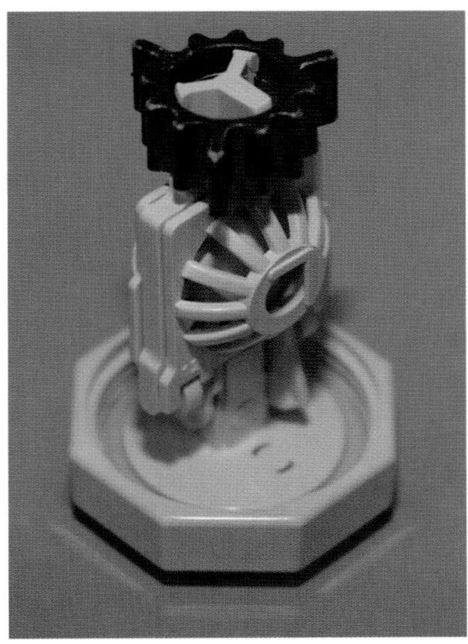

Figure 11.9 The platinum disc in this one-step hydrogen peroxide system is attached to the lens holder. In other systems it is fixed in the base of the case.

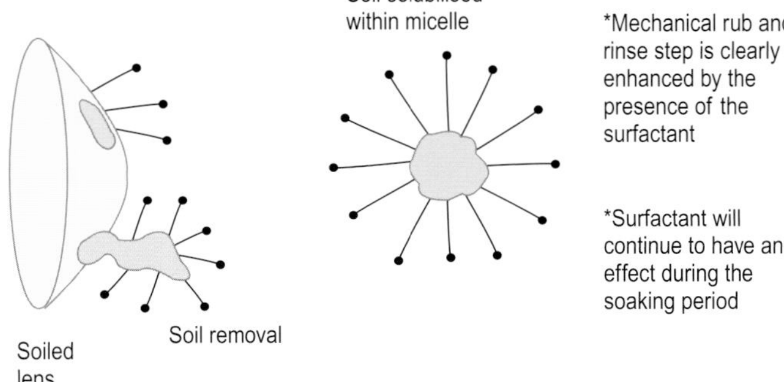

Figure 11.11 Schematic representation of the action of a surfactant cleaner on a soft lens.

peroxide compared with the two-step systems affords a reduced antimicrobial power to the system. Furthermore, the speed of hydrogen peroxide neutralization differs between the tablet systems and the platinum disc systems (Figure 11.10). Although activity against bacteria is likely to be adequate with these systems (Stokes and Morton, 1987), the storage period is unlikely to be sufficient for efficacy against *Acanthamoeba* cysts (Zanetti *et al.*, 1995). However, antimicrobial efficacy can be enhanced by appropriate lens cleaning and rinsing (Cancrini *et al.*, 1998). It is noteworthy that the use of one-step hydrogen peroxide systems has not been associated with an increased risk of *Acanthamoeba* keratitis in case-control studies (Radford *et al.*, 1995).

Lens cleaning

Some one-step hydrogen peroxide systems are used with a separate cleaner which rids the lens surface of mucus, proteins and lipids from the tear film and of other debris, such as pollutants and cosmetics, from the environment. Lens cleaning of this type has numerous clinical benefits, and wearers should be advised to clean their lenses after each use.

Typically, this cleaner is a stand-alone surfactant (surface-active agent) which solubilizes debris from the lens surface. Furthermore, because the surfactant molecules have a hydrophilic end and a hydrophobic end, a monolayer is formed around lipid droplets created after physical dispersion of any lipid spoilation, creating a micelle. With the hydrophobic end of the surfactant molecule 'buried' in the lipid droplet, and the hydrophobic end exposed, recoalescence of the lipid due to repulsion of the electrical charges is prevented. As the hydrophilic region is water-soluble, the lipid spoilation can be emulsified (Figure 11.11).

Surfactants also act to wet hydrophobic surfaces. This is an important consideration for silicone hydrogel lenses as they are typically less wettable than conventional hydrogels. For contact lens care, non-ionic surfactants from either the poloxamer or poloxamine family are employed. Few stand-alone surfactants are currently available due to the popularity of multipurpose contact lens solutions. One example is Miraflow (CIBA Vision), which also contains 20% isopropyl alcohol as a lipid solvent. Some one-step peroxide systems (Sauflon Multi and CIBA Vision AOSept Plus) incorporate a surfactant in the peroxide solution to eliminate the requirement for a separate product.

Historically, lenses were often subjected to enzymatic cleaning, which required the use of tablets or solutions which attempted to remove protein from soft lenses. With the domination of daily disposable and frequent-replacement lenses worldwide, the use of such products is very limited.

Multipurpose solutions

MPS account for over 90% of prescribed care regimens in Europe, Canada and Australia (Morgan *et al.*, 2007). By definition, these products (Table 11.1) do not require the use of other auxiliary components in the lens care process. The first such products were made available for use with contact lenses in the 1980s and their popularity has increased steadily since that time.

Polyhexanide-based MPS

Most MPS contain polyhexanide (polyhexamethylene biguanide) which was originally developed as a presurgery antimicrobial scrub and then marketed for the sanitization of swimming pools and spas. Polyhexanide is part of the same pharmaceutical family as chlorhexidine, and is active against a wide range of bacteria. The action of polyhexanide is thought to be due its rapid attraction towards the negatively charged phospholipids at the bacterial cell surface, followed by impairment of membrane activity with the loss of potassium ions and the precipitation of intracellular constituents. Polyhexanide has a larger molecular weight than chlorhexidine, which means that it is not able to enter the matrix of soft lens materials. In turn, this reduces the likelihood of the preservative reaching the ocular surface, with the potential for toxic or hypersensitivity reactions (Figure 11.12). MPS contain polyhexanide at a range of concentrations from 0.6 to 1.0 ppm (Figure 11.13).

A number of enhanced versions of polyhexanide-based MPS are available. In ReNu MultiPlus (Bausch & Lomb), hydranate has been incorporated as a sequestering agent to reduce protein deposition. This chemical forms complexes with calcium, which can act as a bridge between the lens surface and proteins. Complete Comfort Plus (Advanced Medical Optics) contains the viscosity agent hydroxypropyl methylcellulose, which is claimed to improve ocular comfort. Cyclean (Sauflon Pharmaceuticals) also contains a viscosity agent and uses a novel design of lens case which allows the lens baskets to be rotated within the case to provide a cleaning action.

Polyquaternium-1-based MPS

Some MPS have polyquaternium-1 or polyquad as the preservative. This compound is derived from the same pharmaceutical family as polyhexanide – the polyquats. It is a

Table 11.1 Constituents of soft lens multipurpose solutions

Company	Product	Preservative (ppm)	Surfactant cleaner	EDTA (%)	Buffer	Other components
Abatron	Quattro	Polyhexanide (1)	Lubricare	0.1	Phosphate	
Advanced Eyecare Research	Regard	Sodium chlorite Hydrogen peroxide (100)	Pluronic			Hydroxypropyl methylcelluylose (wetting agent)
Advanced Medical Optics	Complete Comfort Plus	Polyhexanide (1)	Poloxamer	0.02	Phosphate	Hydroxypropyl methylcelluylose (wetting agent)
Alcon	Opti-Free Express	Polyquad (10) and myristamidopropyl dimethylamine (5)	Poloxamine	0.5	Borate	Sorbitol Amino alcohol
Alcon	OptiFree Replenish	Polyquad (11) and myristamidopropyl dimethylamine (5)	Poloxamine + nonanoyl EDTA		Borate	
Bausch & Lomb	ReNu	Polyhexanide (0.6)	Poloxamine	0.1	Borate	
Bausch & Lomb	ReNu MultiPlus	Polyhexanide (1)	Poloxamine	0.1	Borate	Hydranate (sequestering agent)
CIBA Vision	Solocare soft	Polyhexanide (1)	Poloxamer and Triklens	0.025	Phosphate	
Sauflon	All-in-One	Polyhexanide (5)	Poloxamine	0.3	Borate	
Sauflon	Synergi	Oxipol	Poloxamer		Phosphate	Hydroxypropyl methylcellulose (wetting agent)

EDTA, ethylenediamine tetraacetic acid.

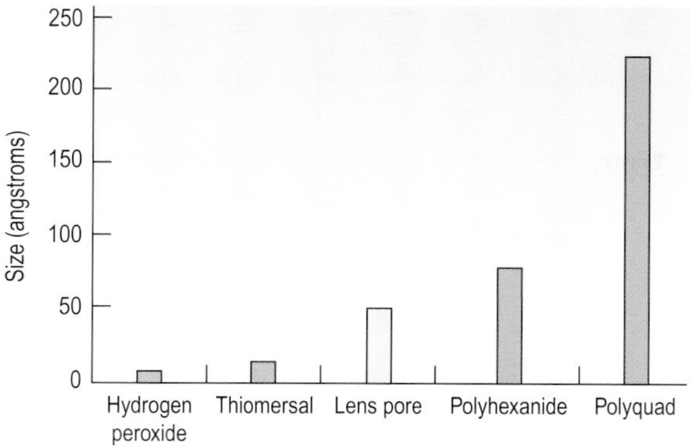

Figure 11.12 Some active agents are smaller than a typical soft lens pore size whereas others are larger.

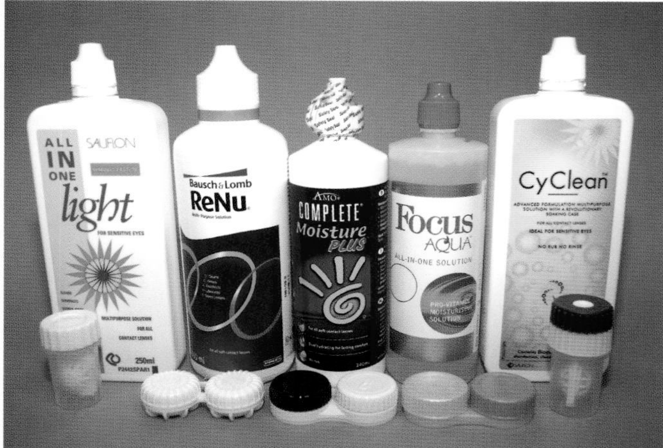

Figure 11.13 Polyhexanide-based soft lens solutions.

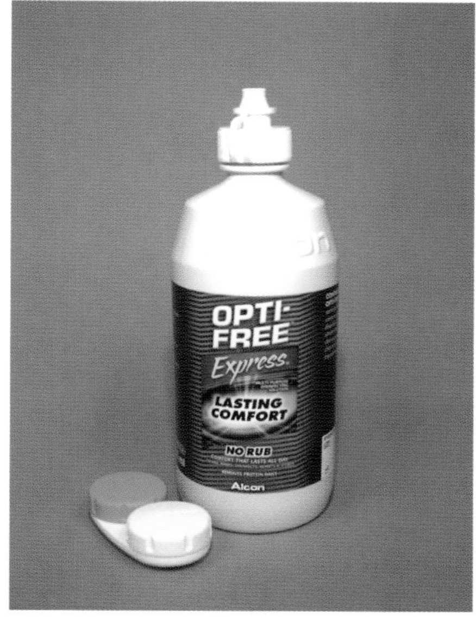

Figure 11.14 OptiFree Express.

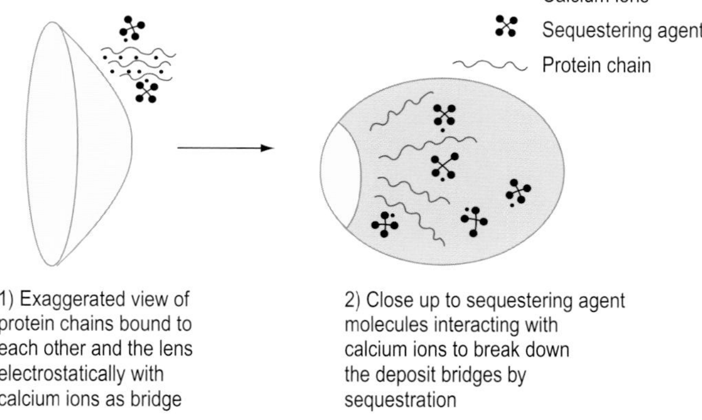

Figure 11.15 Schematic action of a chelating agent.

large molecule, and has a long history of use in the cosmetics industry.

The most widely used polyquad product is OptiFree Express, which contains polyquad and another antimicrobial agent, myristamidopropyl dimethylamine (MAPD) (Figure 11.14). This contains a citrate buffer instead of phosphate or borate buffers which are generally found in polyhexanide-based MPS. This negatively charged buffer is included in the polyquad products to reduce the adherence of polyquad to the surface of some ionic lens materials; this same property can reduce the protein deposition on soft lenses because positively charged proteins, such as lysozyme, can bind with the citrate rather than with the lens surface (Hong *et al.*, 1994). However, citrate is not effective against lipid spoilation (Franklin *et al.*, 1995). The antimicrobial performance of this product is claimed to be similar to disinfection with a one-step hydrogen peroxide system (Rosenthal *et al.*, 1999).

A surfactant is typically included in MPS (both polyhexanide and polyquad-based) so that they can offer a cleaning action in addition to their disinfection properties. These solutions also contain ethylenediamine tetraacetic acid (EDTA), or one of its salts, as a chelating agent. A chelating agent is a substance comprised of molecules which can form several coordinate bonds to a single metal ion (Figure 11.15). In the case of contact lens care, EDTA removes ions such as calcium, resulting in a lens-cleaning effect (protein can bind to calcium on the lens surface, and therefore increase deposition) and an antimicrobial effect (calcium ions are required for cell wall metabolism by microorganisms).

Multipurpose solutions and silicone hydrogel lenses

The MPS products discussed above were all developed and launched when conventional hydrogels dominated the daily-wear contact lens market. Since the launch of the first silicone hydrogels specifically marketed for daily wear in 2004, there has a been a dramatic increase in their use for this modality – from 6% of soft contact lenses prescribed as non-daily disposable spherical daily-wear lenses in the UK in 2004 to about 70% in 2007. Over a similar time period, there has been a strong move towards recommending to contact lens wearers that lens rubbing or rinsing is no longer required, such that a majority of wearers do neither step (Morgan, 2007).

A silicone hydrogel material presents different challenges compared to conventional hydrogels for lens cleaning. The non-ionic nature of silicone hydrogels means that the lenses attract increased amounts of lipid and reduced quantities of protein compared with conventional hydrogels (the majority of which are ionic in nature) (Jones *et al.*, 2003). Additionally, there have been reports of asymptomatic corneal staining when some MPS have been used with daily-wear silicone hydrogels (Jones *et al.*, 2002), although the clinical significance of such staining is not clear.

Given the different material composition of silicone hydrogel lenses, a number of manufacturers have developed MPS for this family of lens materials. One such development was ReNu MoistureLoc (Bausch & Lomb) which incorporated alexidine as the preservative. This agent has been used in mouthwashes for many years, but this was its first application in a contact lens solution. Another feature of the product was the unique combination of polymers, designed for lens cleaning and wettability. Despite being licensed worldwide by meeting the disinfecting criteria set by the various regulatory agencies, the product was associated with an outbreak of *Fusarium* keratitis in Singapore and the USA. Further analysis found that, in circumstances when wearers had not replaced all their solution, but who had simply 'topped up' with new solution, and/or when some of the solution had evaporated, the mix of polymers tended to provide protection for some strains of *Fusarium* which presumably contributed to the infections (Levy *et al.*, 2006).

A factor that has perhaps led to the withdrawal of Complete Moisture Plus is the increased viscosity of the solution, introduced in an attempt to enhance lens comfort. Dalton *et al.* (2008) measured the average viscosity of several solutions at room temperature and all were between 0.95 and 1.26 cP, except for Complete Moisture Plus (3.02 cP). These withdrawals from the market, and controversies concerning corneal staining with some lens–solution combinations (Andrasko and Ryen, 2008), have led to an undermining of patient and practitioner confidence in MPS (Efron and Morgan, 2008).

Another product which has been advocated for use with silicone hydrogels is Regard (Advanced Vision Research) which offers a very different chemistry to other MPS products. Regard contains sodium chlorite and low-concentration hydrogen peroxide (100 ppm) for disinfection, a wetting agent and a surfactant cleaner. When exposed to light, sodium chlorite breaks down to sodium chloride and oxygen, thereby making this product autoneutralizing. Another product which shares some similar characteristics is Synergi (Sauflon Pharmaceuticals) which has also been developed for silicone hydrogels. This product is based around the oxochlorite complex which is used in other industries for disinfection. This complex has appropriate disinfection properties and breaks down in light into sodium chloride and oxygen. Synergi also contains a surfactant cleaner and hydroxypropyl methylcellulose as a wetting agent (Figure 11.16). Alcon has launched OptiFree Replenish for use with silicone hydrogel lenses. This new product contains the same disinfectant ingredients as OptiFree Express (polyquad and MAPD) but has a different range of surfactants (termed Tearglyde) (Figure 11.17).

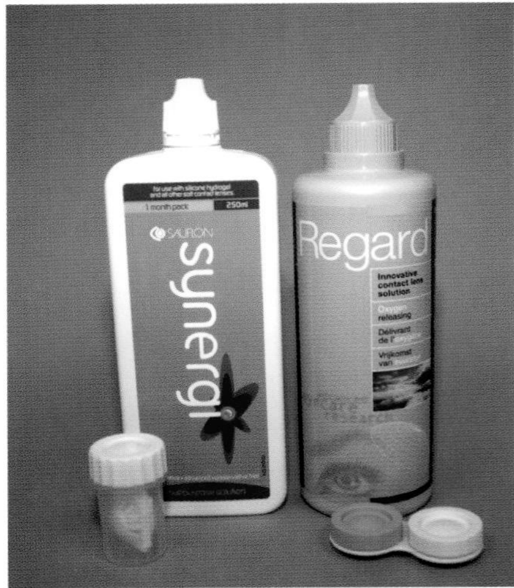

Figure 11.16 Multipurpose products available after the launch of silicone hydrogel lenses.

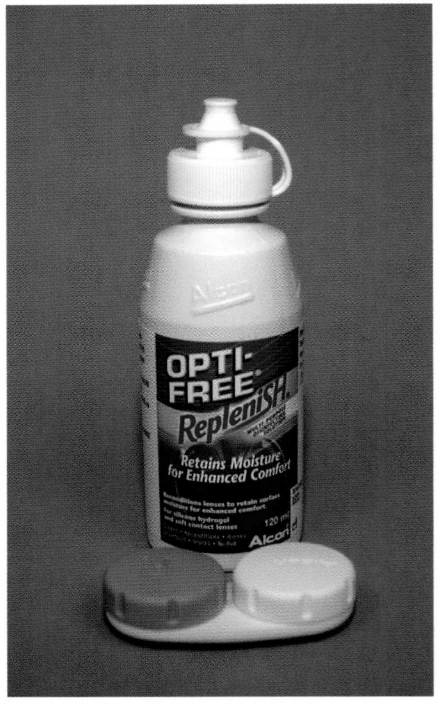

Figure 11.17 OptiFree Replenish.

Rewetting solutions

Contact lens wearers may complain of numerous symptoms, including dryness and general discomfort; such symptoms are the primary reasons for the discontinuation of contact lens wear (Vajdic *et al.*, 1999). A common method

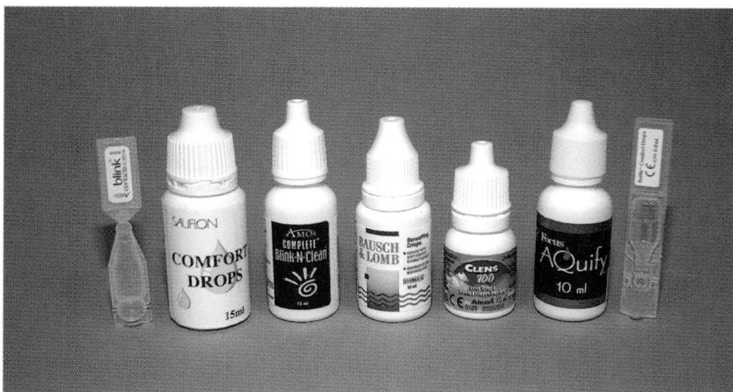

Figure 11.18 Contact lens rewetting solutions.

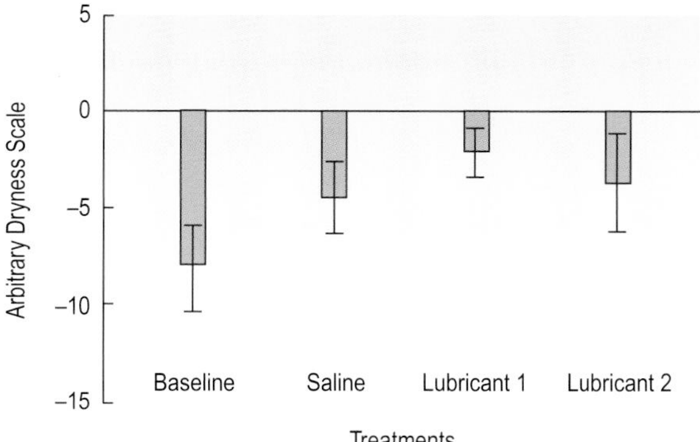

Figure 11.19 Dryness symptoms improve with both saline and prescribed rewetting solutions. (Adapted from Efron, N., Golding, T. R. and Brennan, N. A. (1991a) The effect of soft lens lubricants on symptoms and lens dehydration. Contact Lens Assoc. Ophthalmol. J., 17, 114–119.)

of clinical management of ocular discomfort is the prescription of soft lens rewetting solutions, which are also known by the synonyms of 'lubricants' and 'comfort drops' (Figure 11.18). Efron *et al.* (1991a) found that, although these products were often well received by wearers, and comfort was improved for at least 6 h after their instillation, there was little evidence that their effect was greater than that of saline (Figure 11.19). Furthermore, the mechanism of symptomatic relief is not clear; Golding *et al.* (1990) demonstrated that this was not due to an enhancement of the pre-lens tear film.

A number of products contain viscosity-increasing agents such as methylcellulose which increase the adherence of the solution to the lens and enhance the contact time of the solution at the ocular surface. Other components which are commonly found in rewetting solutions include sodium chloride and buffering agents.

Saline solutions

Many contact lens wearers are prescribed a saline rinsing solution when they first commence contact lens wear. These products are particularly helpful to new wearers as they tend to handle lenses more frequently, and require more attempts at lens insertion, leading to increased contamination from the fingers. Some hydrogen peroxide users remove any residual hydrogen peroxide with a rinsing product to reduce any stinging on insertion. The rinsing process can also play a significant role in the removal of microorganisms from the lens surface (Cancrini *et al.*, 1998).

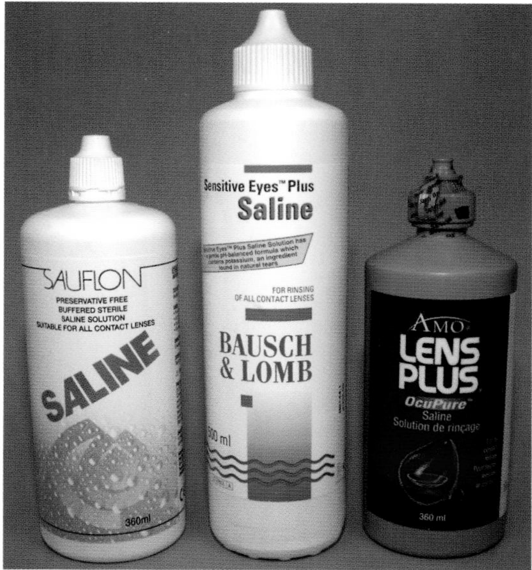

Figure 11.20 Preserved 'squeezy' bottle salines.

Home-made and unpreserved saline have been associated with serious ocular-surface infections and are not recommended (Sweeney *et al.*, 1992). Previously, contact lens solution manufacturers provided saline primarily in aerosol canisters with the pressure within the canisters preventing contamination, although it was recommended that the user ejects a small amount of saline before use as contamination of the spray tip has been associated with corneal infections (Donzis, 1997). However, this was an expensive approach to supplying saline and preserved saline solutions have gained popularity in their 'squeezy' bottle format (Figure 11.20). With these products, the active ingredient serves only to prevent contamination of the solution, rather than play any active role in contact lens disinfection. Examples of these products include Lens Plus saline (Advanced Medical Optics), which contains a stabilized oxychloro complex, Bausch & Lomb saline, preserved with a low concentration of polyhexanide (0.3 ppm) and Sauflon saline, which contains low-concentration hydrogen peroxide (50 ppm).

Relative performance measures

An important consideration for the contact lens practitioner when dispensing a care product is its performance in terms of cleaning and, perhaps more importantly in terms of wearer safety, disinfection efficacy.

The first safeguard for the practitioner is that, in many parts of the world, contact lens disinfectants are required to meet a number of criteria before they can be labelled and

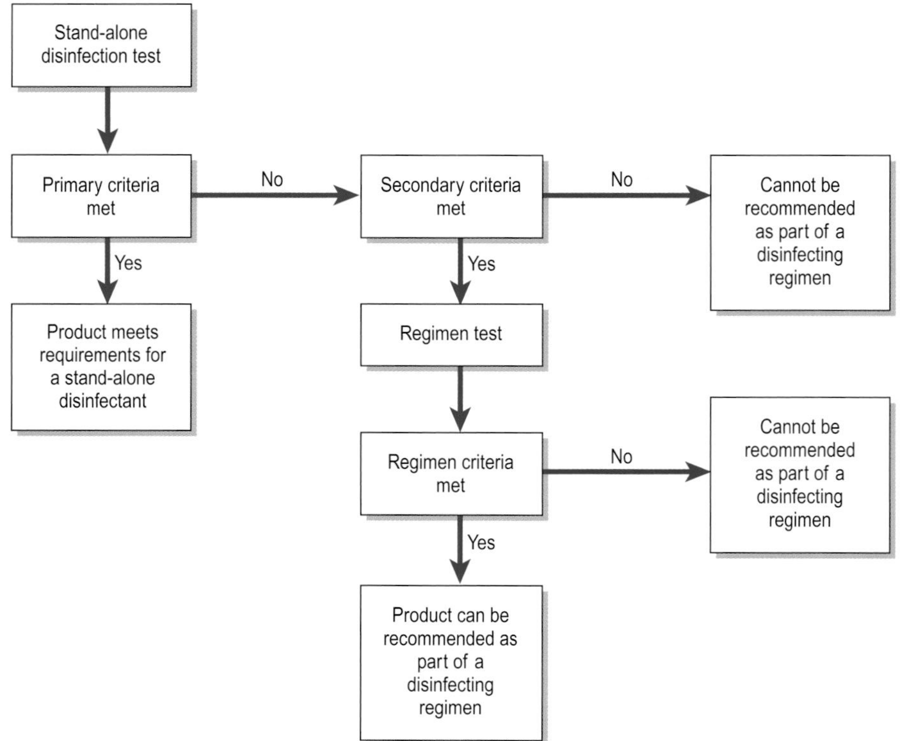

Figure 11.21 Flow chart indicating the path by which disinfectant products are tested for ISO 14729:3.

sold as such. For example, in the European Union, all such products are required to display the CE mark, which indicates that the product has displayed a minimum level of disinfecting performance and that a number of other criteria (such as satisfactory manufacturing conditions) have been met. The CE mark requires a contact lens disinfectant to meet the performance requirements of the international standard ISO 14729:3 (Microbiological requirements for products and regimens for hygienic management of contact lenses). To achieve this, the product must show activity against three bacteria (*Pseudomonas aeruginosa*, *Staphylococcus aureus* and *Serratia marcescens*) and two forms of yeast (*Candida albicans* and *Fusarium solani*) (Figure 11.21).

Products are first tested on a stand-alone basis. Here, the disinfectant must be able to reduce the population of each of the bacteria by 99.9% (or a three log reduction) and the yeast by 90% (a one log reduction). This testing is performed in laboratory conditions without the use of contact lenses; that is, there is a mixing of the test organisms with a fixed quantity of the solution under test.

If the product fails to meet the stand-alone criteria, the regimen procedure can be invoked whereby the performance of the product in a more 'real-world' situation is analysed. However, to proceed to this stage, solutions must at least have demonstrated that they are able to achieve stasis for yeast in the stand-alone test, and an overall combined five log reduction for the three bacteria, with at least one log reduction for each of the bacteria.

In the regimen procedure, contact lenses are inoculated with the panel of test organisms, and then treated according to the instructions provided by the manufacturer for cleaning, rinsing and soaking. To satisfy the criteria, there must be at least a four log reduction for all the test organisms.

In order to reach the marketplace, therefore, contact lens solutions are required to achieve a set standard of performance. However, of further interest is the relative performance of the various products which are available. Although this might seem to require simply generating comparative data for a range of care products, this area is fraught with problems. For example, an approach which has been used in the past to demonstrate the disinfection capabilities of disinfectant systems is the D-value. This parameter denotes the time taken for a disinfectant product to reduce the population of an organism to 10% of its original level (a one log reduction).

Although this appears to be a useful indication of solution performance, there are a number of problems with its use. The D-value assumes a linear relationship between the logarithm of the number of survivors and time. However, the action of contact lens disinfectants tends to be non-linear, which suggests that the use of D-values is inappropriate and can lead to misleading representations of product performance (Sutton *et al.*, 1991).

Another drawback to the D-value approach is that no account is made of the minimum recommended disinfection time (MRDT) recommended by the manufacturer. For example, a product may offer a one log reduction in 20 min, and a three log reduction in 1 h; the clinical success of this product, however, must depend to some extent on the MRDT, which could be 10 min or 6 h. Lowe *et al.* (1992) proposed a new measure of solution potency – solution power – to overcome this problem. This parameter was defined as the MRDT divided by the D-value.

A difficulty with this sort of approach is that no account is made of any cleaning or rinsing (as distinct from disinfecting) which may be employed as part of the overall care system. Some wearers may tend to omit these steps with some systems and not with others; this must have an impact on the overall disinfecting capabilities of the regimen.

Another significant problem when assessing differences between products is that different laboratory conditions and techniques can be employed. A relevant example here is the effectivity of disinfectants against *Acanthamoeba*. A number of variables exist when analysing the performance of products against *Acanthamoeba*, including the strain of *Acanthamoeba* used, growth conditions and contact time of the disinfectant. Indeed the results in this area are highly dependent on methodology, which has led, in part, to the efficacy of contact lens disinfectants against *Acanthamoeba* being omitted from ISO 14729:3.

Despite this, the effectiveness of contact lens disinfectants against *Acanthamoeba* is of considerable interest to contact lens practitioners. On a stand-alone basis, hydrogen peroxide is effective at destroying both *Acanthamoeba* trophozoites and cysts, with overnight storage in 3% hydrogen peroxide providing better performance in this regard than the shorter contact time with a one-step system (Zanetti *et al.*, 1995). MPS have poor antiacanthamoebal efficacy (Davies *et al.*, 1990), although the combination of MAPD and polyquad may improve this (Rosenthal *et al.*, 2000). In a clinical setting, cleaning and rinsing are likely to remove some *Acanthamoeba* (Cancrini *et al.*, 1998). Furthermore, *Acanthamoeba* is thought to require the presence of bacteria to survive and grow, so antibacterial efficacy of a contact lens disinfectant will have an effect on acanthamoebal contamination.

The lens storage case

An important component of the complete lens care system is the case in which the lenses and disinfecting solutions are stored. Surveys have reported that up to 77% of lens cases are contaminated with bacteria and 8% with *Acanthamoeba* (Gray *et al.*, 1995). Contamination appears to be unrelated to solution type, and it is now clear that the development of microbial biofilms in contact lens cases can reduce the effect of a disinfecting solution (Figure 11.22). Indeed, it has been speculated that long-term use of a solution might select a naturally resistant population of microbes which adapt to survive exposure to a disinfectant (Gray *et al.*, 1995). Interestingly, some bacteria release catalase when their cell membranes are disrupted; this release could potentially act to neutralize local hydrogen peroxide and protect other bacteria within the biofilm.

The careful cleaning of lens cases has been advocated by some practitioners. This can include measures such as cleaning the case – with a cotton wool bud or new toothbrush – with cooled boiled water, or submersing the case in boiling water on a regular basis. However, with compliance acknowledged to be poor in a high proportion of lens wearers, this approach might be unrealistic. Certainly, after lens insertion, rinsing the contact lens case with fresh disinfecting solution, and leaving the case open to air-dry fully, is likely to be helpful. It is clear, however, that the regular replacement of contact lens cases is an effective method of reducing this potential problem. Many manufacturers assist practitioners in this regard by supplying a new contact lens case with each bottle of disinfecting solution.

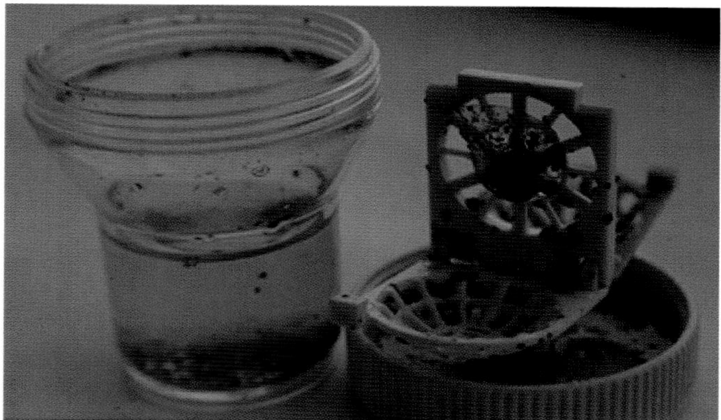

Figure 11.22 The correct use of prescribed care systems is very important for efficient cleaning and disinfecting.

Conclusions

With the growing popularity of daily disposable and extended-wear lenses, there has been a commensurate reduction in the use of contact lens solutions. Nevertheless, the vast majority of lenses prescribed still require lens care systems, and various options are available to satisfy the needs of patients. In the current climate of strict regulatory control in most markets, practitioners and patients can use these products with confidence. An important caveat is that patients use these lens care systems – as simple as they may appear – in precise accordance with the instructions supplied by the manufacturer. As discussed in Chapter 42, the prevalence of non-compliance with contact lens care systems is uncomfortably high, and practitioners are obliged to encourage patients constantly to use these systems as directed, in order to maximize their efficacy.

References

Andrasko, G. and Ryen, K. (2008) Corneal staining and comfort observed with traditional and silicone hydrogel lenses and multipurpose solution combinations. *Optometry*, **79,** 444–454.

Anthony, Y., Davies, D. J. G., Meakin, B. *et al.* (1991) A chlorhexidine contact lens disinfection tablet: design criteria and antimicrobial efficacy in potable tap water. *J. Br. Contact Lens Assoc.*, **14,** 99–108.

Brennan, N. A. and Coles, M-L. C. (1997) Extended wear in perspective. *Optom. Vis. Sci.*, **74,** 609–623.

Bruce, A. S. (1989) Hydration of hydrogel contact lenses during hydrogen peroxide disinfection. *J. Am. Optom. Assoc.*, **60,** 581–582.

Busschaert, S. C., Good, R. C. and Szabocsik, J. (1978) Evaluation of thermal disinfection procedures for hydrophilic contact lenses. *Appl. Environ. Microbiol.*, **35,** 618–621.

Cancrini, G., Iori, A. and Mancino, R. (1998) *Acanthamoeba* adherence to contact lenses, removal by rinsing procedures, and survival to some ophthalmic products. *Parassitologia*, **40,** 275–278.

Cho, P., Cheng, S. Y., Chan, W. Y. *et al.* (2009) Soft contact lens cleaning: rub or no-rub? *Ophthalmic Physiol. Opt.*, **29,** 49–57.

Christie, C. L. and Meyler, J. G. (1997) Contemporary contact lens care products. *Contact Lens Ant. Eye,* **20,** S11–S17.

Copley, C. A. (1989) Chlorine disinfection of soft contact lenses. *Clin. Exp. Optom.*, **72,** 3–7.

Dalton, K., Subbaraman, L. N., Rogers, R. *et al.* (2008) Physical properties of soft contact lens solutions. *Optom. Vis. Sci.*, **85,** 122–128.

Davies, D. J. D., Anthony, Y., Meakin, B. J. *et al.* (1990) Evaluation of the anti-acanthamoebal activity of five contact lens disinfectants. *Int. Contact Lens Clin.*, **17,** 14–20.

Donzis, P. B. (1997) Corneal ulcer association with contamination of aerosol spray tip. *Am. J. Ophthalmol.*, **124,** 394–395.

Efron, N. and Morgan, P. B. (2008) Soft contact lens care regimens in the UK. *Cont Lens Anterior Eye,* **31,** 283–284.

Efron, N., Golding, T. R. and Brennan, N. A. (1991a) The effect of soft lens lubricants on symptoms and lens dehydration. *Contact Lens Assoc. Ophthalmol. J.,* **17,** 114–119.

Efron, N., Lowe, R., Vallas, V. *et al.* (1991b) Clinical efficacy of standing wave and ultrasound for cleaning and disinfecting contact lenses. *Int. Contact Lens Clin.*, **18,** 24–29.

Efron, N., Wohl, A., Toma, N. *et al.* (1991c) *Pseudomonas* corneal ulcers associated with daily wear of disposable hydrogel contact lenses. *Int. Contact Lens Clin.*, **18,** 46–52.

Fatt, I. (1991) Physical limitation to cleaning soft contact lenses by ultrasonic methods. *J Br. Contact Lens Assoc.*, **14,** 135–136.

Fleiszig, S. M. J. (2006) The pathogenesis of contact lens-related keratitis. *Optom. Vis. Sci.*, **83,** 866–873.

Fleiszig, S. M. and Efron, N. (1992) Microbial flora in eyes of current and former contact lens wearers. *J Clin. Microbiol.*, **30,** 1156–1161.

Fleiszig, S. M., Efron, N. and Pier, G. B. (1992) Extended contact lens wear enhances *Pseudomonas aeruginosa* adherence to human corneal epithelium. *Invest. Ophthalmol. Vis. Sci.*, **33,** 2908–2916.

Franklin, V., Tighe, B. and Tonge, S. (1995) Disclosure - the true story of multipurpose solutions. *Optician,* **209**(5500), 25–28.

Gellatly, K. W., Brennan, N. A. and Efron, N. (1988) Visual decrement with deposit accumulation on HEMA contact lenses. *Am. J. Optom. Physiol. Opt.*, **65,** 937–941.

Golding, T. R., Efron, N. and Brennan, N. A. (1990) Soft lens lubricants and prelens tear film stability. *Optom. Vis. Sci.*, **67,** 461–465.

Gray, T. B., Cursons, R. T. M., Sherwan, J. F. *et al.* (1995) *Acanthamoeba*, bacterial, and fungal contamination of lens storage cases. *Br. J. Ophthalmol.*, **79,** 601–605.

Gyulai, P., Dziabo, A., Kelly, W., *et al.* (1987) Relative neutralization ability of six hydrogen peroxide disinfection systems. *Contact Lens Spectrum,* **2,** 61–68.

Harris, M. G., Buttino, L. M., Chan, J. C. *et al.* (1993a) Effects of ultraviolet radiation on contact lens parameters. *Optom. Vis. Sci.*, **70,** 739–742.

Harris, M. G., Fluss, L., Lem, A. *et al.* (1993b) Ultraviolet disinfection of contact lenses. *Optom. Vis. Sci.*, **70,** 839–842.

Harris, M. G., Gan, C. M., Grant, T. *et al.* (1993c) Microwave irradiation and soft contact lens parameters. *Optom. Vis. Sci.*, **70,** 843–848.

Hind, H. W. (1975) Various aspects of contact lens solutions for hard and soft lenses. *Optician,* **149**(4380), 13–29.

Hong, B. S., Bilbault, T. J., Chowhan, M. A. *et al.* (1994) Cleaning capability of citrate-containing vs. non-citrate contact lens cleaning solutions: an in vitro comparative study. *Int. Contact Lens Clin.*, **21,** 237–241.

Jones, L., Davies, I. and Jones, D. (1993) Effect of hydrogen peroxide neutralization on the fitting characteristics of group IV disposable contact lenses. *J. Br. Contact Lens Assoc.*, **16,** 135–140.

Jones, L., MacDougall, N. and Sorbara, L. G. (2002) Asymptomatic corneal staining associated with the use of balafilcon silicone-hydrogel contact lenses disinfected with a polyaminopropyl biguanide-preserved care regimen. *Optom. Vis. Sci.,* **79,** 753–761.

Jones, L., Senchyna, M., Glasier, M. A. *et al.* (2003) Lysozyme and lipid deposition on silicone hydrogel contact lens materials. *Eye Contact Lens,* **29,** S75–S79.

Kilvington, S. and Lonnen, J. (2009) A comparison of regimen methods for the removal and inactivation of bacteria, fungi and *Acanthamoeba* from two types of silicone hydrogel lenses. *Cont. Lens Anterior Eye,* **32,** 73–77.

Kilvington, S. and Scanlon, P. (1991) Efficacy of an ultraviolet light contact lens disinfection unit against *Acanthamoeba* keratitis isolates. *J Br. Contact Lens Assoc.*, **14,** 9–11.

Levy, B., Heiler, D., and Norton, S. (2006) Report on testing from an investigation of *Fusarium* keratitis in contact lens wearers. *Eye Contact Lens,* **32,** 256–261.

Lowe, R., Vallas, V., and Brennan, N. A. (1992) Comparative efficacy of contact lens disinfection solutions. *Contact Lens Assoc. Ophthalmol. J.,* **18,** 34–40.

Ludwig, I., Meisler, D., and Rutherford, I. (1986) Susceptibility of *Acanthamoeba* to soft contact lens disinfection systems. *Invest. Ophthalmol. Vis. Sci.*, **27,** 626–630.

Maissa, C., Franklin, V., Guillon, M. *et al.* (1998) Influence of contact lens material surface characteristics and replacement frequency on protein and lipid deposition. *Optom. Vis. Sci.*, **75,** 697–705.

McDonnell, G. and Russell, A. D. (1999) Antiseptics and disinfectants: activity, action and resistance. *Clin. Microbiol. Rev.*, **12,** 147–179.

McKenney, C. (1990) The effect of pH on hydrogel lens parameters and fitting characteristics after hydrogen peroxide disinfection. *Trans. Br. Contact Lens Assoc. Ann. Clin. Conf.*, 46–51.

Morgan, P. B. (2007) Contact lens compliance and reducing the risk of keratitis. *Optician,* **234**(6109), 20–25.

Morgan, P. B., Woods, C. A., Jones, D., *et al.* (2007) International contact lens prescribing in 2006. *Contact Lens Spectrum,* **22**(1), 34–38.

Mote, E. M., Filppi, J. A. and Hill, R. M. (1972) Does heating arrest organisms in hydrophilic cases? *J. Am. Optom. Assoc.*, **43,** 302–304.

Palmer, W., Scanlon, P. and McNulty, C. (1991) Efficacy of an ultraviolet light contact lens disinfection unit against microbial pathogenic organisms. *J. Br. Contact Lens Assoc.*, **14,** 13–16.

Paugh, J. R., Brennan, N. A. and Efron, N. (1988) Ocular response to hydrogen peroxide. *Am. J. Optom. Phys. Opt.*, **65,** 91–98.

Pearson, R. M. (1992) Contact lens trends in the United Kingdom in 1991. *J. Br. Contact Lens Assoc.*, **15,** 17–23.

Radford, C. F., Bacon, A. S., Dart, J. K. G. *et al.* (1995) Risk factors for *Acanthamoeba* keratitis in contact lens users: a case control study. *Br. Med. J.*, **310,** 1567–1570.

Radford, C. F., Minassian, D. C. and Dart, J. K. (1998) Disposable contact lens use as a risk factor for microbial keratitis. *Br. J. Ophthalmol.*, **82,** 1272–1275.

Rosenthal, R. A., Schlitzer, R. L., McNamee, L. S. *et al.* (1992) Antimicrobial activity of organic chlorine releasing compounds. *J. Br. Contact Lens Assoc.*, **15,** 81–84.

Rosenthal, R. A., Buck, S., McAnally, C. *et al.* (1999). Antimicrobial comparison of a new multipurpose disinfecting solution to a 3% hydrogen peroxide system. *Contact Lens Assoc. Ophthalmol. J.*, **25,** 213–217.

Rosenthal, R. A., McAnally, B. S., McNamee, L. S. *et al.*, (2000) Broad spectrum antimicrobial activity of a new multipurpose disinfecting solution. *Contact Lens Assoc. Ophthalmol. J.*, **26,** 120–126.

Sack, R. A., Harvey, H. and Nunnes, I. (1989) Disinfection associated spoilage of high water content ionic matrix hydrogels. *Contact Lens Assoc. Ophthalmol. J.*, **15,** 138–145.

Sarwar, N., Griffith, G. A. P., Loudon, K. *et al.* (1993) *Acanthamoeba* keratitis associated with disposable hydrogel contact lenses disinfected daily with a chlorine-based care system. *J. Br. Contact Lens Assoc.*, **16,** 15–18.

Seal, D. V., Kirkness, C. M., Bennett, H. G. B., *et al.* (1999) *Acanthamoeba* keratitis in Scotland: risk factors for contact lens wearers. *Contact Lens Ant. Eye,* **22,** 5868.

Shih, K. L., Hu, J. and Sibley, M. (1985) The microbiological benefit of cleaning and rinsing contact lenses. *Int. Contact Lens Clin.*, **12,** 235–242.

Stapleton, F., Keay, L., Jalbert, I., *et al.* (2007) The epidemiology of contact lens related infiltrates. *Optom Vis Sci.* **84,** 257–272.

Stokes, D. J. and Morton, D. J. (1987) Antimicrobial activity of hydrogen peroxide. *Int. Contact Lens Clin.*, **14,** 146–149.

Sutton, S. V., Franco, R. J., Porter, D. A. *et al.* (1991) D-value determinations are an inappropriate measure of disinfecting activity of common contact lens disinfecting solutions. *Appl. Environ. Microbiol.*, **57,** 2021–2026.

Sweeney, D. F., Taylor, P., Holden, B. A. *et al.* (1992) Contamination of 500 ml bottles of unpreserved saline. *Clin. Exp. Optom.*, **75,** 67–75.

Tripathi, B. J. and Tripathi, R. C. (1989) Hydrogen peroxide damage to human corneal epithelial cells in vitro. Implications for contact lens disinfection systems. *Arch. Ophthalmol.*, **107,** 1516–1519.

Vajdic, C., Holden, B. A., Sweeney, D. F. *et al.* (1999) The frequency of ocular symptoms during spectacle and daily soft and rigid contact lens wear. *Optom. Vis. Sci.*, **76,** 705–711.

Wilson, L. A., McNatt, J. and Reitshcel, R. (1981) Delayed hypersensitivity to thimerosal in soft contact lens wearers. *Ophthalmology,* **88,** 804–809.

Zanetti, S., Fiori, P. L., Pinna, A. *et al.* (1995) Susceptibility of *Acanthamoeba castellanii* to contact lens disinfecting solutions. *Antimicrobiol. Agents Chemo.*, **39,** 1596–1598.

CHAPTER 12

Rigid lens materials

Brian J Tighe

Introduction

It is interesting to speculate whether the present rigid lens materials would be invented and brought to market now if they did not already exist. Given the competitive situation that exists in relation to production costs and pricing policy, against the high background costs of product development in the biomedical field, the answer is probably, no. They have, however, played an important role in the development of contact lens materials and occupy a small but significant place in the range of currently available products. Much of the relevant information is contained in the patent literature, which is analysed in some detail elsewhere (Kishi and Tighe, 1988; Künzler and McGee, 1995; Tighe, 1997).

Poly(methyl methacrylate)

To appreciate the way in which rigid, as distinct from soft, materials have developed it is necessary to go back to the period following the Second World War. The new availability of plastics materials, specifically poly(methyl methacrylate), commonly known as PMMA, led to the design and development of the first corneal lens as a replacement for glass corneoscleral lenses. The PMMA lenses were prepared by polymerization of methyl methacrylate with a free radical initiation system (Figure 12.1) to form rods or buttons from which a lens was obtained by lathing and polishing. Figure 12.1 represents the assembly of n methyl methacrylate units to form a PMMA chain n units long. PMMA was an ideal candidate for use as a hard contact lens material because it had similar appearance and ease of fabrication to glass, acceptable surface wettability and excellent durability. The lenses compared favourably with scleral lenses in that they were thin and light-weight, could be worn more comfortably and gave excellent visual correction.

The need for oxygen

By the 1960s a greater appreciation of the effects of contact lens wear on the anterior eye was developing and the fact that PMMA is essentially a barrier to oxygen transport became widely recognized. Corneal physiologists at that time were not only able to carry out theoretical calculations on the effect of contact lenses on corneal respiration, but were also able to carry out well-differentiated experiments using PMMA and a very different material, silicone rubber (Figure 12.2).

Some aspects of the structure and behaviour of polymers, including these two materials, have been outlined in Chapter 5. The most important property to consider in the context of the present discussion is the difference in their oxygen permeabilities. PMMA is a glassy thermoplastic material, which has advantageous optical clarity, processability and ease of sterilization, but the disadvantage, as a contact lens material, of virtual impermeability to oxygen. Silicone rubber, on the other hand, belongs to a group of materials known as synthetic elastomers, which are not only flexible but show rubber-like behaviour, i.e. they are capable of being compressed or stretched and when the deforming force is removed they instantaneously return to their original shape. They consist of polymer chains that possess high mobility and which are cross-linked at intervals along the polymer backbones. Because of this chain mobility, oxygen is able to diffuse rapidly through the structure. These polymers have oxygen permeabilities more than 100 times greater than that of PMMA. Silicone rubber is the most significant member of the group, with an oxygen permeability around 1000 times greater than PMMA. This extremely high oxygen permeability arises from the backbone of alternate silicone and oxygen atoms which confers not only great freedom of rotation but a much higher solubility for oxygen than rubbery polymers with simple carbon backbones.

Silicone rubber lenses, surface-treated to give acceptable wettability, were developed in the mid-1960s (McVannel *et al.*, 1967) and found clinically to have little deleterious effect on corneal respiration (Hill and Schoessler, 1967). The problems of maintaining adequate surface properties, which were initially encountered in its routine clinical use, have never been fully overcome, however, and silicone rubber lenses are used only rarely. The uniquely high oxygen permeability of the silicon–oxygen backbone has, however, been harnessed in two distinct types of contact lens material: silicone hydrogels (Chapter 5) and the so-called rigid gas-permeable (RGP) materials described here. Because PMMA is now essentially redundant as a contact lens material, the term 'rigid gas-permeable' is equally redundant. All rigid lenses manufactured today

DOI: 10.1016/B978-0-7506-8869-7.00012-4

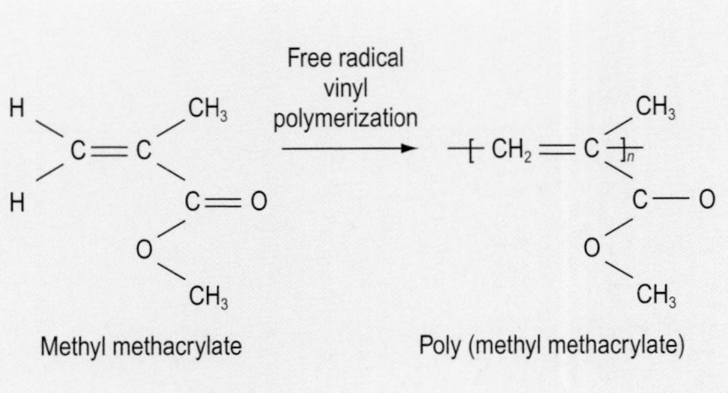

Figure 12.1 Schematic representation of free radical polymerization of methyl methacrylate.

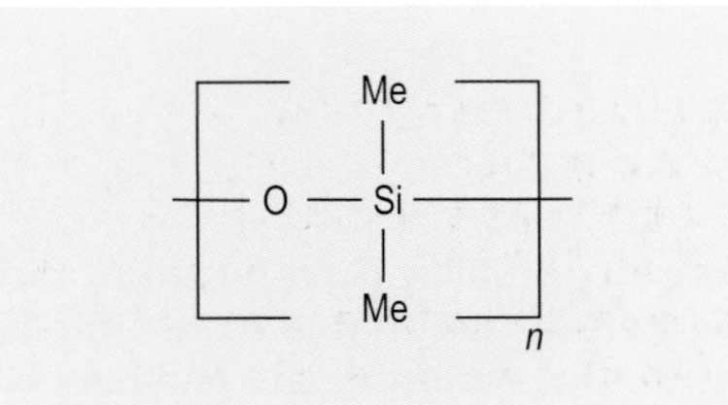

Figure 12.2 Structure of silicone rubber. Me = CH_3.

(aside from PMMA) are gas-permeable. For this reason, the term 'rigid lens' is used throughout this book, and is intended to refer to all rigid lenses apart from PMMA, unless the latter is specifically designated.

The problem of hydrophobic surfaces

Elastomers, such as silicone rubber, are in many ways intermediate between thermoplastics such as PMMA and hydrogels such as poly(hydroxyethyl methacrylate) (polyHEMA). Thus, they possess to a degree the toughness associated with the former group of materials and the softness of the latter, and in this sense they are ideal candidates for contact lens usage. Unfortunately, however, they all possess the same inherent disadvantage. The molecular features required for true elastic behaviour invariably produce polymers with hydrophobic surfaces. All polymers in this group – not only the silicone-based materials – require some form of surface treatment to render them sufficiently hydrophilic for use as contact lenses, but because of the ease of chain rotation, the surfaces slowly revert to their untreated state. This problem is made worse by the virtually instantaneous elastic recovery of the materials, which causes them to 'grab' the cornea after being deformed by the blink. This in turn displaces the posterior tear film and leads to lens binding. Despite the attempts to harness almost every available elastomeric material, as witnessed by the patent literature, no true elastomer has been successfully used as a commercial contact lens material.

The search for better materials

Once the need for a contact lens material with higher oxygen permeability than PMMA was established, a wide-ranging search began. There was, additionally, some belief that a more flexible material than PMMA would confer enhanced comfort. At first sight the task of finding an improved material would not seem too difficult since almost all thermoplastics are less rigid and more oxygen-permeable than PMMA. Several flexible thermoplastics materials have been suggested as being suitable for contact lens manufacture in the patent literature, but none of these has achieved clinical significance. The most promising results were obtained with poly (4-methyl pent-l-ene), a form of which is known commercially as TPX, and with cellulose esters such as cellulose acetate butyrate (CAB). TPX and CAB resemble each other in many ways. Both polymers are less rigid and less brittle than PMMA – they can conveniently be described as 'tougher'. The oxygen permeability of both materials is appreciably (of the order of 20 times) greater than that of PMMA (Kamath, 1969; Refojo *et al.*, 1977) and both were capable of being fabricated by moulding techniques, which are inherently cheaper than lathe cutting, this still being the most widely used method of contact lens fabrication in the 1970s. Even the fact that TPX required a surface treatment step and that both materials (especially CAB) lacked the dimensional stability of PMMA did not seem to be inhibitors to their commercial future. The fact that they became, fairly quickly, curiosity materials was largely due to the appearance, and almost instant success, of the silicone acrylates.

Hybrid rigid gas-permeable materials

The logic of silicone acrylate materials is inescapable. They combine, to a degree, the ease of preparation of PMMA and the oxygen permeability of silicone rubber. When the need to modify PMMA to improve its oxygen permeability arose, there was, therefore, no difficulty in recognizing that fact. The problem lay in combining such polymers to achieve a balance of properties. The origin of the problem is the fact that different types of reaction are used in the formation of the two materials. This can be illustrated by using the picture of polymers such as PMMA and hydrogels as 'washing line' polymers. The principle is that polymers of this type have a long backbone (i.e. the string or 'washing line') from which a variety of chemical groups may be suspended (the 'washing').

Other types of polymer, of which silicone rubber is one example, can be regarded as 'poppet bead' polymers. The individual units are joined just like the individual beads on a 'poppet bead' necklace. There is no 'washing' hanging from the chain and the properties of the polymer are controlled by the structure of the poppet beads themselves. The fundamental problem that prevented simple PMMA–silicone rubber combinations from being prepared is that the 'washing line' and 'poppet bead' chemistries are incompatible and beads cannot be inserted into the washing line. The requirement is that, in order to insert an individual monomer unit into an acrylate or methacrylate polymer such as PMMA, it is necessary that the monomer should have a carbon-to-carbon double bond (as shown in Figure 12.1). Without the double bond the washing cannot be pegged on to the washing line. The siloxymethacrylates that form the basis of current gas-permeable technology get round this problem in a well-recognized, but nevertheless quite ingenious, way. Short segments of the poppet bead chain are turned into 'washing' by attaching them to a chemical intermediate that contains the necessary double bond. This can be seen in the structure of the siloxymethacrylate monomer (Figure 12.3) which in essence consists of the individual units of silicone rubber structure

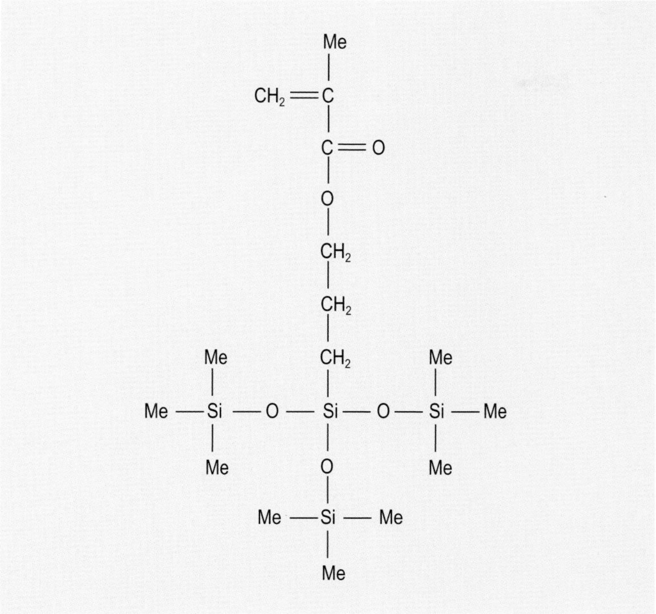

$$\begin{array}{c} CH_2{=}C(Me){-}C({=}O){-}O{-}CH_2{-}CH_2{-}CH_2{-}Si[O{-}Si(Me)_3]_3 \end{array}$$

Figure 12.3 Tris(trimethyl-siloxy)–methacryloxy-propylsilane (TRIS) monomer. Me = CH_3.

pasted on to a modified methyl methacrylate molecule. On the basis of this simple picture, the story of gas-permeable lenses can be unfolded.

The Gaylord patents – harnessing silicon

The major advance that enabled the development of rigid contact lens materials is found in the work of Norman Gaylord at Polycon Laboratories, described in a series of patents (Gaylord, 1974, 1978). There are two distinct aspects of this work that are worth noting. The first is the development of what has become the industry standard siloxy methacrylatemonomer, tris(trimethyl-siloxy)–methacryloxy-propylsilane (Figure 12.3), commonly referred to as TRIS. The second is the recognition of the value of incorporating fluoroalkyl methacrylates (e.g. 1,1,9-trihydroperfluoro-nonyl methacrylate; Figure 12.4) principally to enhance oxygen permeability. It is important to recognize that the bonds between individual carbon atoms are not disposed at right angles to each other and that molecules are not flat but have three-dimensional shapes. Although this point, which has been discussed in Chapter 5, is reflected in Figure 12.1, it is impractical to do so in the representation of more complicated molecules such as the siloxy and fluoro methacrylates shown in Figures 12.3 and 12.4. Both these aspects of the work of Gaylord have been subsequently developed, and together form the basis of most existing commercial rigid contact lens materials. Although TRIS is still the most widely used siloxymethacrylate monomer in rigid lens manufacture, the fluoromethacrylate monomers employed in current commercial materials are much simpler than that initially used by Gaylord.

It is important to note that the concept of a fluorine-containing contact lens was not new. Fluorocarbons dissolve more oxygen than do hydrocarbons and give rise to polymers with somewhat higher oxygen permeabilities than their hydrocarbon equivalents. It was over 10 years after the first description of the advantages of contact lenses

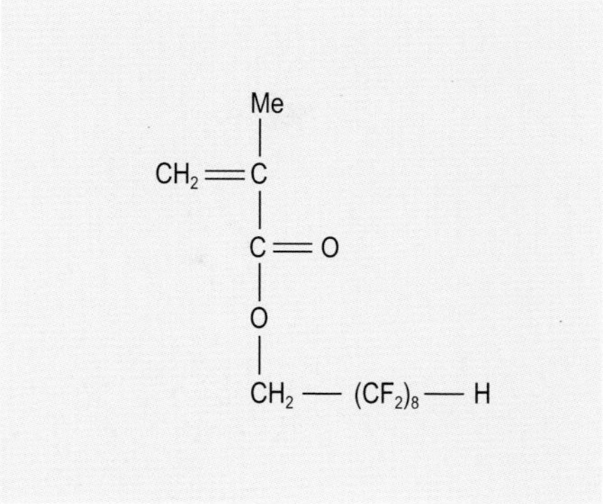

$$CH_2{=}C(Me){-}C({=}O){-}O{-}CH_2{-}(CF_2)_8{-}H$$

Figure 12.4 1,1,9-trihydroperfluoro-nonyl methacrylate monomer. Me = CH_3.

prepared from polymers derived from perfluoroalkylethyl methacrylates, in a series of DuPont patents, that significant commercial use was made of fluorocarbon-based contact lenses (Tighe, 1997). The reason is straightforward. There is a huge advantage in oxygen permeability of the siloxy-methacrylates over fluorocarbon methacrylates, which on their own do not produce a clinically significant balance of advantages over PMMA. The great advantage of the fluorinated methacrylates comes when they are used partially to replace methyl methacrylate in copolymers with TRIS. The balance of the three components (fluoro methacrylate, methyl methacrylate and TRIS) is adjusted to optimize oxygen permeability, hardness (which influences processability) and wettability. Although the Gaylord patents marked the beginning of the inventive thread, several other workers made significant contributions to the development of lenses with advantages in clinical practice by identifying ways of optimizing the balance of oxygen permeability, wettability and mechanical behaviour.

Within a 12-month period in 1978 and early 1979, at about the time of appearance of the third patent of Gaylord's, three workers began to file their separate series of patents related to siloxymethacrylate-based contact lens materials. These were, in advancing order of the priority date for the first written filing, Kyoichi Tanaka (Toyo Contact Lens), Edward Ellis (Polymer Technology) and Nick Novicky, whose later patents (and presumably rights to the earlier patent) were assigned to Syntex (USA). The Ellis and Novicky patents form a clear line of continuation from the early work of Gaylord and, because of this, are best considered together (Ellis and Salamone, 1979; Novicky, 1980). The work of Tanaka – for which parallel filings exist in Japan and the USA – has some slight and significant differences mainly concerned with the inclusion of a hydroxyl group into the siloxy monomer to improve wettability (Tanaka *et al.*, 1979). This was a significant early step in overcoming the technical obstacles to the development of silicone hydrogels, as separately discussed in Chapter 5.

The Ellis and Salamone patents used the basic concept of Gaylord with slight but significant modifications. The more important of these uses the basic composition – described by Gaylord – based on TRIS, but claiming novelty in the additional use of methacrylic acid (Figure 12.5 – a hydrophilic monomer referred to but not exemplified by Gaylord) to improve surface wettability, and by the incorporation of an itaconate ester (e.g. dimethyl itaconate: Figure 12.6). This composition formed the basis of the influential early range of Boston rigid lens materials.

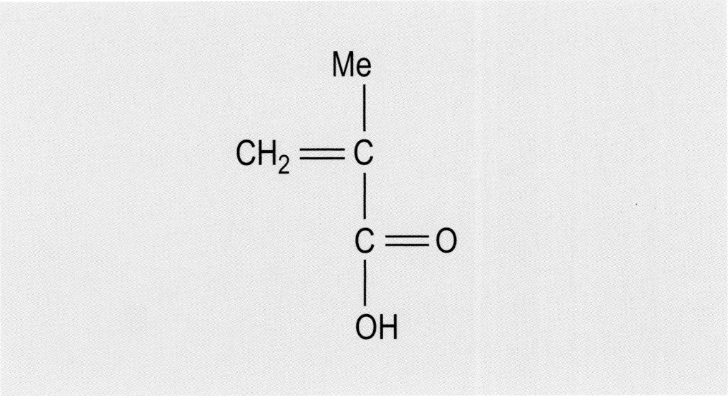

Figure 12.5 Methacrylic acid monomer. Me = CH_3.

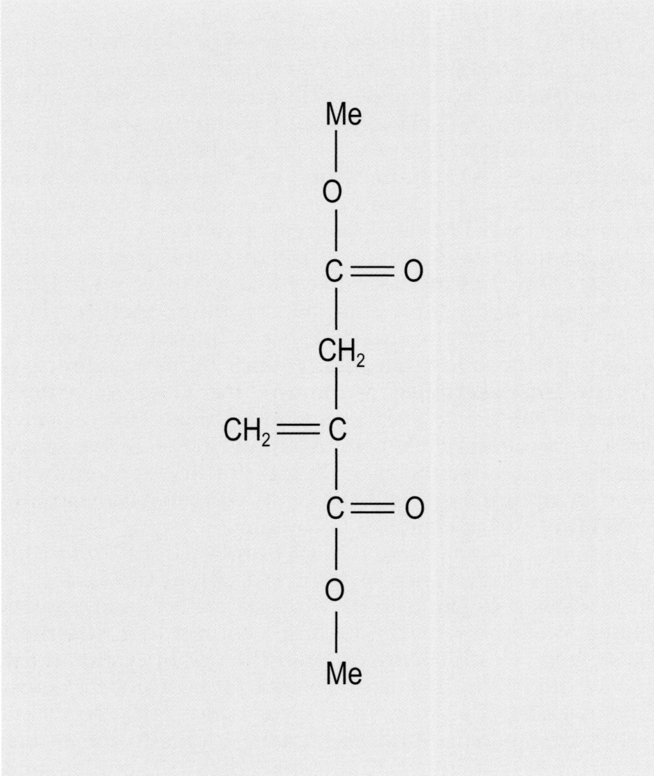

Figure 12.6 Dimethyl itaconate monomer. Me = CH_3.

The early Japanese patent of Tanaka marked the beginning of a rapid growth in Japanese patent activity, principally as a result of work assigned to Hoya Lens and Toyo Contact Lens. The subsequent clinical interest in the use of rigid lenses for extended wear in Japan stimulated particular interest in means of enhancing *Dk*. This interest was paralleled by a series of patents, which provide valuable information on the use of fluoroalkyl methacrylates in conjunction with siloxymethacrylates, and the properties of fluoroalkyl methacrylates themselves. The properties, specifically the permeabilities of the individual homopolymers, are carefully described. It is in the Japanese patent literature, for example, that the relative permeability along the series of homopolymers of methyl methacrylate, trifluoroethyl methacrylate (Figure 12.7) and hexafluoroisopropyl methacrylate (Figure 12.8), is disclosed: (1:60:100). This indicates the relative advantage, in terms of permeability, of replacing methyl methacrylate by either of these two fluoro monomers. The ground is clearly seen in this patent for the development of fluorine-containing siloxy-methacrylate gas-permeable materials (e.g. Equalens, Fluoroperm, Menicon SP) which penetrated the UK and US markets towards the mid-1980s. It is in the Japanese patents, however, that the relationship between composition and permeability of these materials is described (Tarumi and Komiya, 1982).

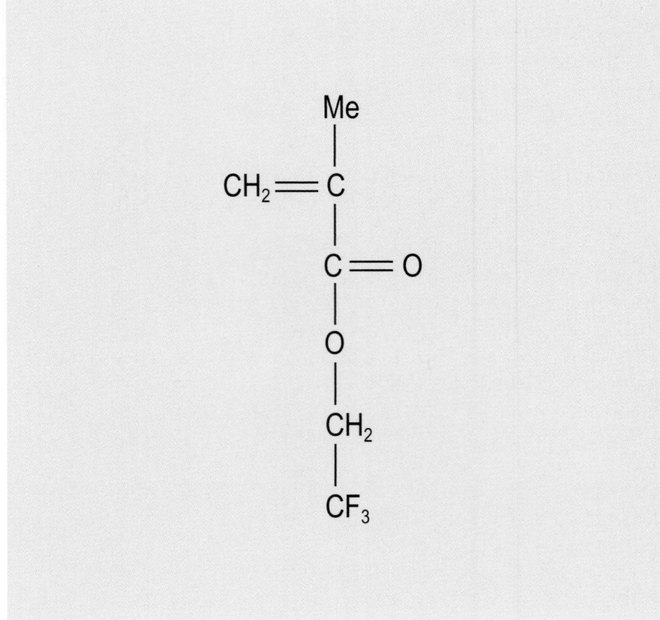

Figure 12.7 Trifluoroethyl methacrylate monomer. Me = CH_3.

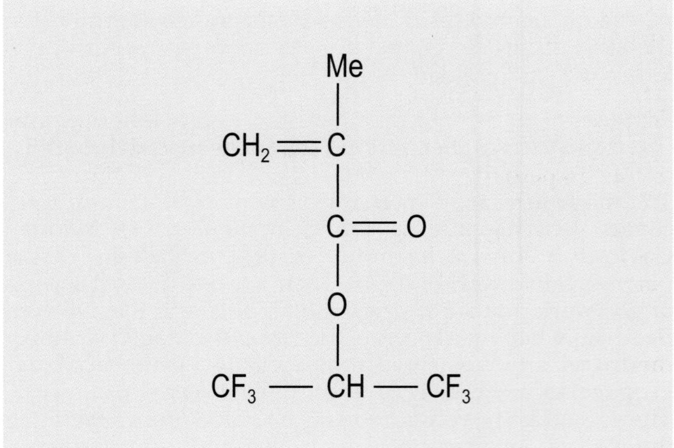

Figure 12.8 Hexafluoroisopropyl methacrylate monomer. Me = CH_3.

The readily discernible trend in the development of rigid contact lens materials described in the patent literature and discussed here is one of increasing oxygen permeability balanced against the retention of acceptable dimensional stability and ocular compatibility (characterized by wettability and deposit resistance). The essential structural developments have centred around four areas:

1. The TRIS component, characterized by attempts to incorporate higher proportions of more highly branched siloxy derivatives.

2. The use of fluorocarbon co-monomers in the place of hydrocarbon-based components such as methyl methacrylate.
3. The improvement of wettability by incorporation of hydrophilic co-monomers, or subsequent surface modification of the formed lens.
4. The development of cross-linking technology: rigid lens materials necessarily contain much higher levels of cross-linking agents than do soft lenses.

Much attention has been paid in the patent literature to the comprehensive coverage of all possible structural variants disclosed in the original patents won by Gaylord, published in 1974. Despite this, little that is truly new has appeared since then, and certainly nothing to match the leap forward brought by the identification of TRIS as a means of producing rigid contact lens materials with *Dk* values many times greater than PMMA. The process since that time has been one of refinement and improvement, based on the underlying principles that are contained in the patents described above.

One recent refinement to increase both oxygen permeability and material strength has been the introduction by Menicon of novel siloxanylstyrene monomers into the polymer backbone. Unlike its previous lenses (SFP and EX), which relied on silicone-containing methacrylate compounds for enhanced oxygen permeability, the Menicon Z material features tris (trimethylsiloxy) silyl styene as the key monomer to fluoromethacrylate. This chemical structure results in excellent mechanical properties, allowing the lens to be significantly thinner than a typical rigid lens (Szczotka, 2004). It is the first rigid lens material classified in the 'hyperoxygen transmissibility' category with a *Dk* of 175, and is the only rigid lens that is approved by the US Food and Drug Administration for 30 days of continuous wear. This is a variation of the styrene-HEMA polymer used in the Softperm hybrid lens. The use of styrene adds a greater resistance to flexure and a lower specific gravity.

Plasma coating has been used to good effect in silicone hydrogel materials to overcome inherent hydrophobicity. The lenses are enclosed in an ionized gas with an equal number of positively and negatively charged species. The highly charged species within the gas plasma bombard the surface of the material, and the resulting energy causes a number of changes on the surface of the material. It is used in a wide variety of applications, including highly efficient surface cleaning, or increasing hydrophilicity and even hydrophobicity. A plasma oxidation surface treatment process has been developed for the treatment of rigid contact lenses produced from the Optimum range of materials (Contamac). The manufacturers claim the processes have been optimized to produce significant improvements in the wetting characteristics, without requiring a lengthy treatment procedure.

Silicone hydrogel polymers have been very successful in the form of soft lenses but can be made with a range of water contents from 0 to 60%. At low water contents (<10%), the polymers are rigid. There are two types of rigid silicone hydrogel materials. In one type, the water content and expansion are constrained by decreasing the ratio of hydrophilic monomers and increasing the cross-link density. Thus the polymer cannot absorb water into the interior of the matrix, but the surface can hydrate like a hydrogel lens. In the second type, a reactive hydrolysable monomer is included in the formulation. This means that, when the lens is placed in water, the reactive monomer hydrolyses, producing a hydrophilic surface like a hydrogel lens. The reaction cannot proceed into the interior since expansion is constrained by cross-linking. This type also has the novel property of regenerating the hydrophilic surface if the lens surface is damaged or the lens is repolished. The Comfort O2 material contains a unique blend of both hydrophilic and reactive monomers.

Commercial rigid materials and their properties

The influence of the disclosures contained in the patent literature and outlined here is reflected in the nature and the properties of commercially available contact lens materials. Some commercially available rigid lens materials, together with information on chemical type, oxygen permeability, wettability, mechanical properties and refractive index are shown in Table 12.1. This information has been compiled from various sources, including literature from manufacturers, reviews, results of other workers and measurements made in the laboratories of the author. In addition, values for PMMA, cellulose acetate butyrate and a silicone rubber lens are included for comparison.

There has been some movement in recent years towards the standardization of experimental procedures for measurement techniques. It is by no means certain, however, that all quoted measurements have been made to such standards. This is particularly true of the wide range of rigid lenses supplied, as they are, from such a variety of sources. This fact, coupled with the debatable relevance of existing measurements to the clinical performance of materials, presents a major problem to the clinician in selecting materials on the basis of listed information. Some cautionary comments are included here.

Oxygen permeability

Several different experimental procedures for determining oxygen permeability may be distinguished. In each case, oxygen at a known effective concentration passes from the donor side of the cell through the membrane (of known thickness and cross-sectional area) to a receiver side, also of known volume, where it is sensed. In the case of rigid polymers it is possible to use both gas-to-gas and liquid-to-liquid systems. This has the advantage that reference values for standard materials can be obtained in the gas-to-gas system which does not suffer from some of the shortcomings of the liquid-to-liquid cell, in which the liquid is ideally stirred on both sides of the membrane.

The polarographic electrode technique, which is usually used for lens measurement, has several shortcomings. First, the cell is unstirred (thereby giving rise to boundary layer problems); secondly, the thickness of the contact lens normally shows a centre-to-edge variation (which produces uncertainties in the calculation); and thirdly, because the lenses vary in curvature, the volume of the receiver side is not accurately fixed. In principle, this last point should be less important, because the technique is not usually operated in the manner that measures rate of increase in oxygen concentration of the receiver side of the cell, but rather the resultant equilibrium oxygen consumption by the electrode. The ability to do this relies on the assumption that oxygen transported to the receiver side is

Table 12.1 Properties of typical commercial rigid lens materials

Name (manufacturer/ supplier)	Material type	*Dk* (Barrer, 34°C)	Contact angle (dry)	Contact angle (soaked)	Hardness	Refractive index
Alberta S (Progressive Optical)	Polysulphone Copolymer	28(a), 45(c)	65°(a)	28°(a), 9°(c)	85SD	1.475
Aquila (CIBA Vision)	Siloxy – fluoromethac Copolymer (Aquifocon)	143(c)		39°(c)	78SD	1.431
Boston II (B&L/ Polymer Tech)	Siloxy – methac – itaconate Copolymer (Itafocon-A)	12–14(a,b,c)	65°(a)	25°(b), 20°(c)	85SD, 119R (c)	1.471
Boston IV (B&L/ Polymer Tech)	Siloxy – methac – itaconate Copolymer (Itafocon-B)	21(a), 28(b), 22(c)	79°(a) 90°(b)	25°(b), 17°(c)	80SD, 117R (c)	1.469
Boston RXD (B&L/ Polymer Tech)	Siloxy – fluoromethac Copolymer (Itabisflufocon-A)	27,45(b), 24(c)		39°(b), 39°(c)	85SD, 121R (c)	1.435
Boston ES (B&L/ Polymer Tech)	Siloxy – fluoromethac Copolymer (Enflufocon-A)	31(b), 18(c)		52°(b), 52°(c)	118R (c)	1.443
Boston EO (B&L/ Polymer Tech) Fluoromethac – Fluoromethac –	Siloxy – fluoromethac Copolymer (Enflufocon-B)	82(b), 58(c)		49°(c)	83SD, 114R (c)	1.429
Boston XO (B&L/ Polymer Tech)	Siloxy – fluoromethac Copolymer (Hexafocon-A)	100(b),(c)		49°(c)	81SD, 112R (c)	1.415
Boston XO_2 (B&L/ Polymer Tech)	Siloxy – fluoromethac Copolymer (Hexafocon B)	141(c)		38°(c)	78SD	1.424
Comfort O2	Rigid silicone hydrogel (Onsifocon A)	56(c)		7°(c)	85SD	1.452
Equalens (B&L/ Polymer Tech)	Siloxy – fluoromethac Copolymer (Itafluorofocon-A)	47,72(b) 47(c)	65°(a)	30°(c)	81SD, 115R (c)	1.439
Equalens II (B&L/ Polymer Tech)	Siloxy – fluoromethac Copolymer (Oprifocon-A)	125(b), 85(c)	65°(a)	40°(b), 30°(c)	114R (c)	1.423
Fluorocon 30,60,92,151 (CIBA Vision)	Siloxy – fluoromethac Copolymer (Paflufocon)	30,60,92,151(c)		As Fluoroperm range	As Fluoroperm range	As Fluoroperm range
Fluoroperm 30 (Paragon Vision Sci)	Siloxy – fluoromethac Copolymer (Paflufocon-A)	24(b), 30(c)		13°(c)	84SD	1.466
Fluoroperm 60 (Paragon Vision Sci)	Siloxy – fluoromethac Copolymer (Paflufocon-B)	47(b), 60(c)		15°(c)	83SD	1.453
Fluoroperm 92 (Paragon Vision Sci)	Siloxy – fluoromethac Copolymer (Paflufocon-C)	50(b), 92(c)		16°(c)	81SD	1.453
Fluoroperm 151 (Paragon Vision Sci)	Siloxy – fluoromethac Copolymer (Paflufocon-D)	151(c)		42°(c)	79SD	1.442
Hybrid FS, FS Plus (Contamac)	Siloxy – fluoromethac Copolymer with fluid surface (Hybufocon A)	31(c),60(c)			79SD, 79SD	1.446, 1.446
Menicon SFP (Menicon)	Siloxy – fluoromethac Copolymer	102(c)		18°(c)	80SD(b), 7.6V(c)	N/A
Menicon Z (Menicon)	Siloxy – fluoromethac Copolymer (Tisilfocon A)	163,175(a)		23°(c)	83SD	1.440
Optacryl 60 (Paragon Vision Sci)	Siloxy – methac Copolymer	12, 14(b), 18(c)	70°(a)	25°(c)	83SD(b), 88SD	1.467
Optacryl K (Paragon Vision Sci)	Siloxy – methac Copolymer	21(b), 32(c)	82°(a)	25°(c)	81SD(b), 84SD	1.467

Table 12.1 Properties of typical commercial rigid lens materials—cont'd

Name (manufacturer/ supplier)	Material type	*Dk* (Barrer, 34°C)	Contact angle (dry)	Contact angle (soaked)	Hardness	Refractive index
Optimum Classic (Contamac)	Siloxy – fluoromethac Copolymer (Roflufocon A)	26(c)		12°(c)	83SD	1.450
Optimum Comfort (Contamac)	Siloxy – fluoromethac Copolymer (Roflufocon B)	65(c)		6°(c)	79SD	1.437
Optimum Extra (Contamac)	Siloxy – fluoromethac Copolymer (Roflufocon C)	100(c)		3°(c)	75SD	1.431
Optimum Extreme (Contamac)	Siloxy – fluoromethac Copolymer (Roflufocon D)	125(c)		6°(c)	77SD	1.432
Optimum HR 1.51, 1.53 (Contamac)	(Hirafocon A, Hirafocon B)	50(c), 20(c)		33°(c), 42°(c)	79SD, 82SD	1.51, 1.53
Paragon HDS (Paragon Vis Sci)	Siloxy – methac Copolymer (Paflufocon B)	58(c)		13°(c)	84SD	1.449
Paragon HDS 100 (Paragon Vis Sci)	Siloxy – fluoromethac Copolymer (Paflufocon D)	100(c)		42(c)		
Paragon HDS HI 1.54 (Paragon Vis Sci)	Siloxy – fluoromethac Copolymer (Pahrifocon A)	22(c)	77°(c)		84SD	1.54
Paraperm 02 (Paragon Vis Sci)	Siloxy – methac Copolymer	12(b), 15(c)	80°(a)	30°(b), 25°(c)	86SD	1.473
Paraperm EW (Paragon Vis Sci)	Siloxy – methac Copolymer (Pasifocon)	40(b), 56(c)	68° 82° (a)	26°(c)	10.6V(b), 82SD	1.467
Persecon 92E (CIBA Vision)	Siloxy – fluoromethac Copolymer (Paflufocon-C)	50(b), 92(c)		16°(c)	81SD	1.453
Polycon II (CIBA Vision)	Siloxy – methac Copolymer (Silafocon-A)	10(a), 12(c)	77°(a)	12°(c)	84.5SD	1.467
Polycon HDK (CIBA Vision)	Siloxy – methac Copolymer	30(b), 40(c)		40°(c)	85SD	1.469
Silicone Rubber (e.g. Silsoft, B&L)	Silicone rubber	340–450(a,c)	80–105° (a)			1.43
PMMA (Various)	Poly methyl methacrylate	0.1(a)	63–67°(a)	15–35°(a,b)	>90SD(b)	1.49
CAB [e.g. Persecon E, (CIBA Vision)]	Cellulose acetate-butyrate	7–9(a,c)	60–65°(a)	15–30°(a,c)	77.5SD	1.476

(a) Independent laboratories; (b) competitor laboratories; (c) manufacturers' information.
Hardness: V = Vickers, SD = Shore, R = Rockwell (R).
Contact angles: dry = sessile water droplet on cleaned and dried surface, soaked = captive air bubble in soaking solution (not identified).
Material type: siloxy – methac = copolymer includes siloxy compound (usually tris (trimethyl-siloxy) – methacryloxy-propylsilane (TRIS)) and conventional methacrylate; siloxy – fluoromethac = copolymer includes siloxy compound (usually TRIS) and fluorinated methacrylate; other components include, wetting agents (e.g. *N*-vinyl pyrrolidone, methacrylic acid), cross-linking agents, itaconate esters (Boston materials).
Extensive rebranding occurs for various reasons. For example, lens manufacturers may use original name (e.g. Boston), own name (e.g. AL 01,02 … , Eureka, Novagas etc.) or rebranded materials name (e.g. Optacryl range also made as Vistacryl; Fluoroperm becomes Fluorocon, Oxyflow, Persecon).

efficiently consumed by the electrode sensor, and that, as a result, the partial pressure of oxygen on the receiver side is always effectively zero. With very permeable samples, however, these assumptions are not justified. In all cell configurations, it is important to have an oxygen-tight seal of the membrane separating donor and receiver chambers, but this again is difficult to achieve with the format and samples involved in contact lens measurement and edge effect corrections must be made. A great deal of effort has gone into standardization of procedures and cross-correlation of results but only when results have come from specialist laboratories can they be relied upon (Holden *et al.*, 1990; Weissman and Fatt, 1991; Tranoudis and Efron, 1995; Benjamin and Cappelli, 2002).

Because in hydrogels, water is the oxygen transport medium through the lens, boundary layer effects are more readily analysed and eliminated. In rigid lenses however, although measurements are easily made, the deviations from ideal behaviour increase with increasing permeability and are dependent upon the surface properties of the individual lens. It has been recognized for many years that, even in stirred cells, boundary layer effects produce greater problems with non-hydrophilic materials (Hwang *et al.*, 1971). As a result of the various factors identified here, wide variations exist between reported *Dk* values for the same lens material. This is particularly problematical for the clinician, as there is no readily measured property (such as the water content of a hydrogel) that gives an independent guide to the permeability value. These issues have been discussed at length by Brennan *et al.* (1987).

Mechanical properties

The problems associated with the use of increasing quantities of siloxymethacrylates to achieve high oxygen permeabilities are twofold. First, incompatibility, phase separation and deterioration in mechanical properties – particularly dimensional stability – limit the proportion of such monomers that can be incorporated. Secondly, their use requires the incorporation of hydrophilic monomers containing hydroxyl, carboxyl, amide or lactam groups to improve wettability. These monomers tend to reduce oxygen permeability and produce low levels of water uptake that in turn reduce dimensional stability. It is well recognized that developments that have produced higher oxygen permeabilities have led to problems with mechanical properties, and that such problems are quite common. Despite this, the currently used mechanical property measurements, such as hardness, do not indicate any clear distinction between materials, which is evident from Table 12.1. Although materials are recognized to fail because of inadequate mechanical behaviour, there is certainly no accepted basis upon which the performance of lenses in a clinical setting can be correlated with presently used test measurements (Kerr and Dilly 1988; Jones *et al.*, 1996).

Flexure

Lens flexure causes induced residual astigmatism on toric corneas. Polycon lenses have been shown to undergo significantly more flexure, and alter residual astigmatism more, than PMMA lenses at all centre thicknesses (Harris *et al.*, 1982). For both lens types, lenses thinner than 0.15 mm flexed significantly more than thicker lenses. This critical centre thickness should be considered when fitting these lens types on toric corneas (Harris *et al.*, 1987). However, it is not correct to assume that all gas-permeable lenses flex more than PMMA. Lin and Snyder (1999) compared flexure in low- (15), medium- (60) and high- (150) *Dk* materials, as measured by keratometry over the lenses. No significant differences were found within or between lens materials when comparing magnitude of flexure. The flexure of both PMMA and Boston XO materials were investigated by Collins *et al.* (2001) in three centre thicknesses (0.05, 0.10 and 0.15 mm) using a videokeratoscope; they also found no significant differences in flexure. Methods of flexure measurement are discussed in Chapter 15.

Hardness

Little work is carried out on the measurement of clinically relevant mechanical properties at present, and the values quoted are almost invariably related to the hardness of the material. Although hardness tests have some place in contact lens characterization, they do not reflect the type of mechanical failure or problems that normally arise, which are usually associated with fracture, chipping or splitting, or distortion. In the absence of agreed standards for suitable methods, manufacturers' quoted data are usually obtained with one or other of the standard hardness test methods.

Hardness can be defined as resistance to penetration. In a hardness test, an indenter is pressed on the surface of the material under test, and the extent to which it sinks into the material for a given pressure and time is an inverse measure of the hardness. There are many hardness testers available commercially which are suitable for plastics and rubbers, including the Vickers indenter, the Rockwell hardness tester and the Shore durometers. These may be divided into three categories:

1. Hardness tests that measure the resistance of a material to indentation by an indenting probe (e.g. Brinell, Vickers and Shore durometers). Some tests measure the indentation with the load applied and some measure the residual indentation after the load is removed.
2. Hardness tests that measure the resistance of a material to scratching by another material (e.g. the Bierbaum scratch test, the Moh hardness test). Similar techniques are commonly used in paint testing and involve pulling the sample beneath a loaded indenter.
3. Hardness tests that measure recovery efficiency or resilience (e.g. the various Rockwell testers).

There is no common method of measurement in these tests. For example, the Rockwell A-scale hardness test measures the depth of penetration with the load applied, whereas the Rockwell R, L, M and E scale tests measure depth caused by a spherical indenter after most of the load has been removed. In these methods the amount of rebound or recoverable deformation is important. The Vickers Microhardness test differs again, in that a microscope is used to measure the diagonals of the pits left by a diamond-shaped indenter on a square base. There is a linear relationship between the depth of impression and the hardness number. Each of the hardness methods uses an arbitrary scale and, although the scales can be approximately compared, precise correlation is not possible.

Surface properties

Similar problems arise with the measurement of wettability by contact angle techniques. In this case, the effect of soaking on water uptake and thus the wettability of materials, coupled with the use of the inverted or captive air bubble technique in solutions other than water, combine to produce wide variations, because of the different methodologies, in the reported values for a given material. The field of contact lens surface properties has also become more complex with the passage of time. The water wettability of materials provides a good primary indication of the ability of tears to form a coherent and stable layer on the surface of the material. It tells nothing of the compatibility of the material with tears.

Unfortunately, the inverted (captive) air bubble technique has been identified as a standard in contact lens work. The measurement is made after an air bubble is allowed to impinge, from underneath, on to the surface of the sample, which is suspended in an aqueous liquid. This is the most difficult type of contact angle to measure correctly since it involves judging where the base of a distorted sphere just impinges on a surface. More importantly, the air bubble has to displace water from the surface of the sample, which is frequently pre-soaked. Since all the siloxymethacrylate materials contain appreciable amounts of hydrophilic monomer to improve surface wettability, they all retain a strongly adsorbed water layer at the surface under these conditions. Not surprisingly, therefore, with this method very similar and very low so-called wetting angles are obtained with current rigid lens materials. What is measured in each case is the value for a diffuse layer of water on a polymer surface. The values are similar to those obtained by this technique with hydrogels. The biological and biochemical surface events, on the other hand, occur at a molecular level and do not recognize the diffuse water layer barrier that is sensed by macroscopic droplet techniques. This is the underlying reason for the lack of relevance to clinical practice of the wetting angle, as presently measured.

Well-established techniques exist which enable the wetting hysteresis and the detailed surface energy components, rather than a single wetting angle, to be determined. Biomaterials science makes widespread use of such methods; the contact lens community could profitably do the same.

Refractive index

Fluorosilicone acrylate lenses are likely to have a refractive index between 1.420 and 1.460, whereas an index of 1.460 or greater usually indicates a silicone acrylate material. The refractive index of PMMA is 1.49. Unlike in spectacle lens dispensing, refractive index has rarely been a factor in the choice of rigid lens material. However, manufacturers are starting to introduce lenses with higher refractive indices. Contamac's Optimum HR material and Paragon Vision Sciences' Paragon HDS HI material have refractive index values ranging from 1.51 to 1.54. A benefit of these higher-index materials is the enhanced refractive effect the materials might have when used in aspheric multifocal designs. With the same amount of asphericity, a higher-index material will produce an increased add effect (Pence, 2009).

Conclusions

This chapter provided an outline of the basic chemistry of rigid plastics used in the contact lens industry, and has traced the successive developments in rigid lens materials primarily with reference to the patent literature. All stages of development have been driven by a parallel growth of information relating to the biocompatibility (the need for oxygen permeability and surface wettability) and the clinical performance of the lenses.

Predicting compatibility *in vivo* from tests *in vitro* is never entirely successful. Increasingly, however, it enables differences between the performance of materials to be successfully predicted. In addition the use of biological probes, such as animal cells, and interaction with biological sera, provide useful information in the development of new biomaterials. The area is complex, but offers several approaches that will improve considerably on current techniques, and will have some relevance to the clinical performance of rigid contact lenses.

References

Benjamin, W. J. and Cappelli, Q. A. (2002) Oxygen permeability (*Dk*) of thirty-seven rigid contact lens materials. *Optom. Vis. Sci.*, **79,** 103–111.

Brennan, N. A., Efron, N., Holden, B. A. *et al.* (1987) A review of the theoretical concepts, measurement systems and application of contact lens oxygen permeability. *Ophthal. Physiol. Opt.*, **7,** 485–490.

Collins, M. J., Franklin, R., Carney, L. G. *et al.* (2001) Flexure of thin rigid contact lenses. *Cont. Lens Anterior Eye,* **24,** 59–64.

Ellis, E. J. and Salamone, J. C. (1979) (to Polymer Technology Corp). Silicone-containing hard contact lens material. US patent 4 152 508.

Gaylord, N. G. (1974) (to Polycon Lab Inc). Oxygen-permeable contact lens composition methods and article of manufacture. US patent 3 808 178.

Gaylord, N. G. (1978) (to Syntex USA Inc). Methods of correcting visual defects: compositions and articles of manufacture useful therein. US patent 4 120 570.

Harris, M. G., Kadoya, J., Nomura, J. *et al.* (1982) Flexure and residual astigmatism with Polycon and polymethyl methacrylate lenses on toric corneas. *Am. J. Optom. Physiol. Opt.*, **59,** 263–266.

Harris, M. G., Gale, B., Gansel, K. *et al.* (1987) Flexure and residual astigmatism with Paraperm O_2 and Boston II lenses on toric corneas. *Am. J. Optom. Physiol. Opt.*, **64,** 269–273.

Hill, R. M. and Schloessler, J. (1967) Optical membranes of silicone rubber. *J. Am. Optom. Assoc.*, **38,** 480–483.

Holden, B. A., Newton-Howes, J., Winterton, L. *et al.* (1990) The DK project – an interlaboratory comparison of DK/L measurements. *Optom. Vis. Sci.*, **67,** 476–481.

Hwang, S. T., Kammermeyer, K. and Tang, T. E. (1971) Transport of dissolved oxygen through silicone rubber membrane. *J. Macromol. Sci. Phys. (B),* **5,** 1–10.

Jones, L., Woods, C. A., and Efron, N. (1996) Life expectancy of rigid gas permeable and high water content contact lenses. *Contact Lens Assoc. Ophthalmol. J.*, **22,** 258–260.

Kamath, P. M. (1969) Physical and chemical attributes of an ideal contact lens. *Contacto,* **13,** 29–34.

Kerr, C. and Dilly, P. N. (1988) Problems of dimensional stability in RGPs. *Optician,* **195**(5134), 21–23.

Kishi, M. and Tighe, B. J. (1988) RGP materials: a review of the patent literature. *Optician,* **195**(5134), 21–23.

Künzler, J. F. and McGee, J. A. (1995) Contact lens materials. *Chem. Ind.*, **21,** 651–653.

Lin, M. C. and Snyder, C. (1999) Flexure and residual astigmatism with RGP lenses of low, medium, and high oxygen permeability. *Int. Contact Lens Clin.*, **26,** 5–9.

McVannel, D. E., Mishler, J. L. and Polmanteer, K. E. (1967) (to Dow Corning Corp) Hydrophilic contact lens and method of making same. US patent 3, 350, 216.

Novicky, N. N. (1980) Oxygen permeable hard and semi-hard contact lens compositions, methods and articles of manufacture. US patent 4 242 483.

Pence, N. (2009) GP materials offer new options and convenience to patients. *Contact lens Spectrum,* **24**(3), 26.

Refojo, M. F., Holly, F. J., and Leong, F. L. (1977) Permeability of dissolved oxygen through contact lenses I. Cellulose acetate butyrate. *Contact Intraoc. Lens Med. J.*, **3,** 27–33.

Szczotka, L. B. (2004) The future of GP continuous wear. *Contact lens Spectrum,* **19**(2), 21.

Tanaka, K., Takahashi, K., Kanada, M. et al. (1979) (to Toyo contact Lens Co Ltd, Japan) Methyl di(trimethylsiloxy) silylpropyl glycerol methacrylate. US patent 4 139 548.

Tarumi, N. and Komiya, S. (1982) (to Hoya Lens KK) Contact lens with high oxygen permeability. Jap Kokai 57-182718.

Tighe, B. J. (1997) Contact lens materials. Ch. 3 in *Contact Lenses* 4th edn. (A. J. Phillips and L. Speedwell, eds.) pp. 50–92, Oxford: Butterworth-Heinemann.

Tranoudis, I. and Efron, N. (1995) Oxygen permeability of rigid contact lens materials. *J. Br. Contact Lens Assoc.*, **18,** 49–53.

Weissman, B. A. and Fatt, I., (1991) Contact-lens wear and oxygen permeability measurements. *Curr. Opin. Ophthalmol.*, **2,** 88–94.

13 CHAPTER

Rigid lens manufacture

Nathan Efron and Steve Newman

Introduction

Although lathing technology has been used to fabricate contact lenses since their invention over a century ago, developments over the past two decades in precision engineering, materials technology and computer control systems have resulted in a capability to manufacture lenses of almost any imaginable shape – from basic spherical lens forms to highly complex aspheric designs. These developments have resulted in renewed interest in rigid lenses, which despite representing a small minority of lenses sold, are still a very important alternative form of vision correction – and indeed the only form of contact lens that will provide adequate vision in cases of corneal distortion (as occurs in keratoconus). The type of use or design of rigid lenses prescribed has shifted substantially over time (Morgan and Efron, 2008). In 1996, 80% of rigid lenses were of spherical design; this had dropped to 47% in 2007. The proportion of lenses requiring more specialized manufacturing techniques has risen accordingly (Figure 13.1).

This chapter will explain the process of rigid lens manufacture and will present an analysis of the impact of regulatory constraints on the rigid lens sector.

Rigid lens manufacture

The process of lathe cutting soft lenses has already been outlined in Chapter 6. Here, a more comprehensive illustrative account of the process of lathe cutting will be presented in the context of rigid lens manufacture.

Raw materials

The raw material is supplied to the lens manufacturer in the form of flat cylindrical buttons of 12.7 mm diameter and circa 4.3 mm thickness. Some types are sold with a concave depression in one surface as preparation for base curve cutting. These are supplied in various colours and the tradename of the product is typically imprinted on one surface of the button (Figure 13.2). The choice of material is largely dictated by clinical needs, with oxygen permeability being a key consideration. The latest range of rigid materials are designed as 'super' gas-permeable with *Dk* values of over 150 Barrers. These materials typically require some postproduction surface treatment in order to ensure a wettable surface. There has been renewed interest in achieving extended-wear approvals for lenses made from these polymers, for use in overnight orthokeratology. From the standpoint of the manufacturing laboratory, however, consideration needs to be given to the 'machinability' of the material, as some materials are more susceptible to surface deterioration and degradation of optical quality compared to other materials when subjected to the same manufacturing processes (Meyers, 1997). Manufacturing laboratories that wish to make lenses from the latest rigid materials need to use only the best types of lathes available. Typically these lathes will use hydrostatic X,Y slides and air-bearing spindles, all under sophisticated computer control.

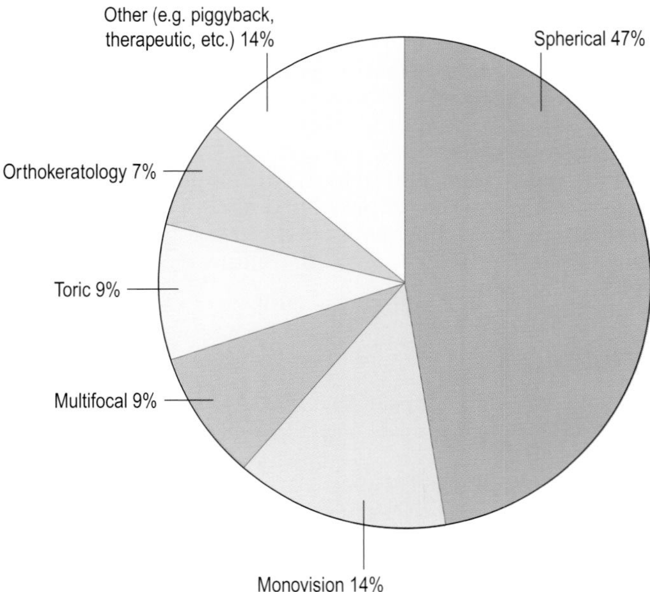

Figure 13.1 Rigid lens prescribing. (After Morgan and Efron, 2008.)

DOI: 10.1016/B978-0-7506-8869-7.00013-6

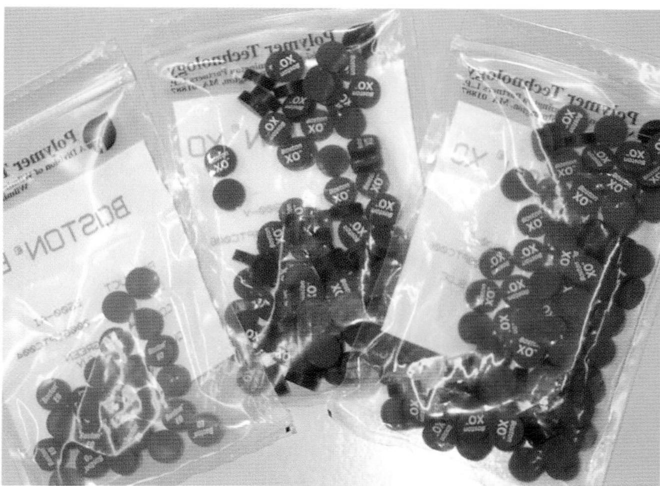

Figure 13.2 Rigid lens buttons.

Generating the lens back surface

Some lathes are configured so that they can be used to generate both the front and back surface of the lens; however, in practice, separate lathes are used in order to optimize the lens production process. Figure 13.3A shows a lathe configured for generating the lens back surface.

The button is first secured in a carrier, or dolly, which is a small hollow cylinder lined with plastic (Figure 13.3B). This assembly is secured to a back surface lathe in a clamp, or collet (Figure 13.3C) and this assembly is set spinning at a high rate about its central axis. Orssengo *et al.* (1997a) have demonstrated that the accuracy in achieving the desired back optic zone radius can be increased by minimizing the pressure applied to the button when fixing it into the collet of the lathe.

A 'rough' or preparation diamond-tipped tool is automatically advanced towards the spinning button and the posterior surface lens shape is cut by advancing the diamond cutter from the edge to the centre of the button (because the button is spinning around its central axis, a cut on only one side of the button will result in the full width of the button being cut) (Figure 13.3D). The waste plastic that is lathed away (swarf) is extracted via an air vacuum tube mounted above the lathe assembly. Some laboratories will strive to improve swarf and surface management by the use of suitable cutting fluids. These cutting fluids or sprays maintain a cooler surface and assist the swarf to peel away cleanly from the button surface. Any clogging of swarf around the diamond tool will very quickly result in a pitted and overheated surface. A fine diamond tool is used to make the final surface cut so as to render a smooth, high-quality finish. With some lathes, the fine cut can be so precise as to obviate the need for polishing. This can be achieved with the use of gem-quality diamond tools, air-bearing spindles and slides and nanometer surface control. The best of these lathes can achieve a surface roughness (Ra) close to 3–8 nm.

A diamond tool advances from the side to reduce the button diameter to the required size of the finished lens. The button is released from the lathe and the cut surface is given a brief polish – typically for about 5–30 seconds, depending on the lathe/material combination (Figure 13.3E). The thickness of the button is measured at its thinnest point (centrally) and this information is programmed into the front surface lathe so that the final lens will be cut to the desired thickness.

In the process of lathing and polishing, care must be taken to avoid overheating the lens material, because the generation of excess heat can result in warpage, surface crazing (Sanford, 1987) (Figure 13.4) and errors in generating the desired surface curvature (Orssengo *et al.*, 1997c).

Strategies employed to avoid this problem include programming the lathe to make incremental cuts rather than one continuous cutting action, and passing a constant flow of air/cutting fluid over the lathing assembly to keep it cool.

Generating the lens front surface

In order to generate the lens front surface, the button needs to be fixed on to a mount, or arbour (which will later be secured to a front surface lathe). This process of mounting the button on to the arbour is known as blocking. The arbour can be a metal or plastic cylindrical tool, one end of which is dome-shaped so that the curve of the dome approximately matches the form of the posterior lens surface that has previously been generated. The operator heats the arbour to approximately 80°C and applies low-melting-point wax to the dome end or, in the case of a plastic tool, applies a UV sensitive glue which can be cure to a hard form after centering. The newly cut back surface of the button is mounted on to the wax-surfaced dome of the arbour and carefully centred (Figure 13.5A) via either a centrifugal means or by some form of precision alignment jig.

The arbour–button assembly is clamped into a front surface lathe (Figure 13.5B) and the button is inspected under magnification while spinning at low speed to confirm that it is properly centred; if this were not the case, the front and back surfaces would not be co-concentric, and both prism power and uneven edge thicknesses would inadvertently be introduced into the lens. Once centration is confirmed, the thickness of the button is determined by a computer-controlled thickness gauge. A series of incremental cuts is made from the edge to the centre with a rough preparation diamond-tipped cutter, then with a fine diamond-tipped cutter, in precisely the same manner as for the back surface (Figure 13.5C). As front surface cutting requires that the spindle spins in the opposite direction of back surface face cutting, however, the diamond holders are mounted on the front surface lathe in different configurations to the back. This specific configuration allows for optimal swarf and surface management. The front surface is cut to a depth that will result in a finished lens of desired thickness. The arbour–button assembly is released from the lathe and mounted in a support in a polishing machine. The front surface is polished for about 30 s to 2 min with a soft pad impregnated with a water-based polishing compound (Figure 13.5D).

Engraving, marking and fenestration

At this juncture in the manufacturing process – with the near-finished lens still mounted on the arbour (Figure 13.6A) – the lens can be engraved or marked. Engraving can be undertaken using a pantographic device, whereby the operator traces the desired letters to be engraved on the lens against a stainless-steel master template into which the

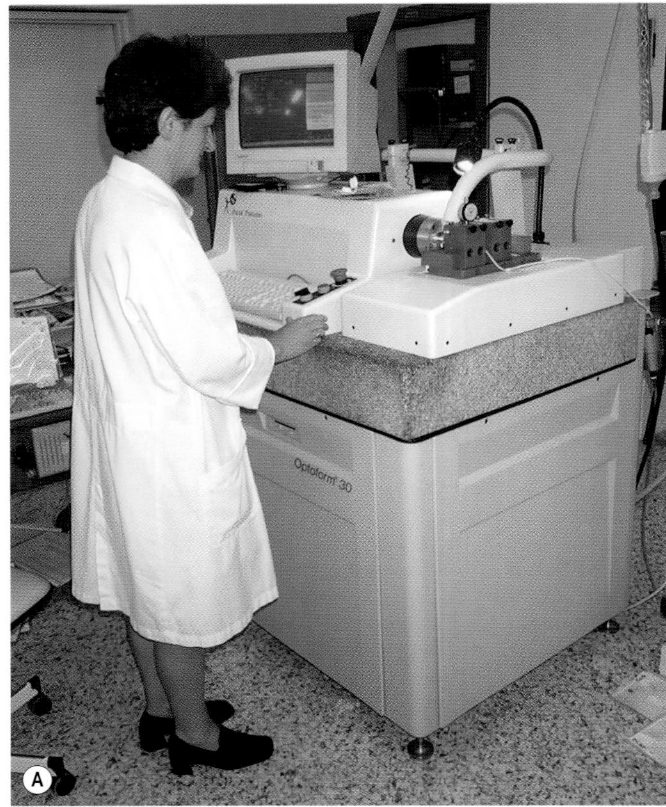

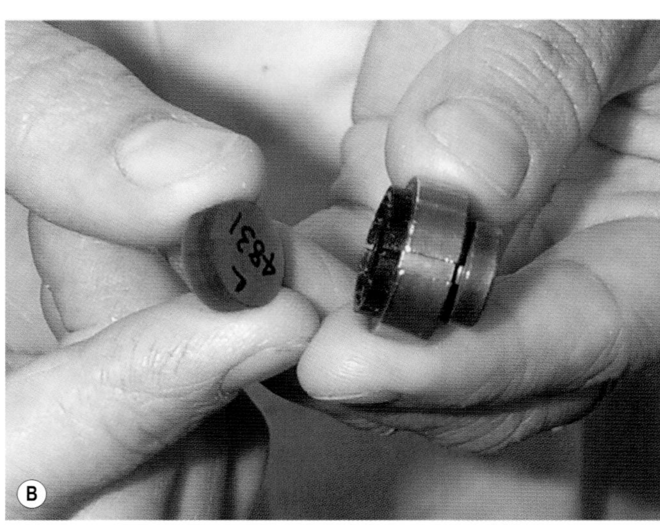

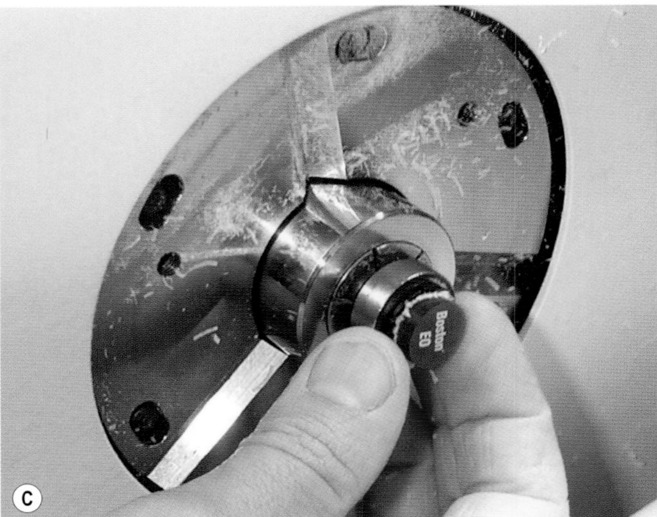

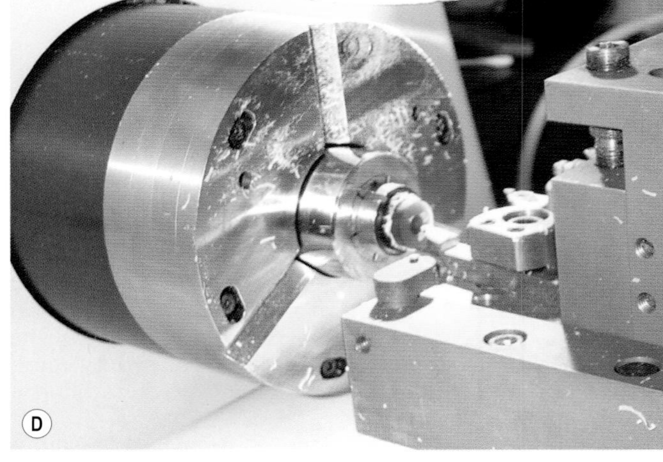

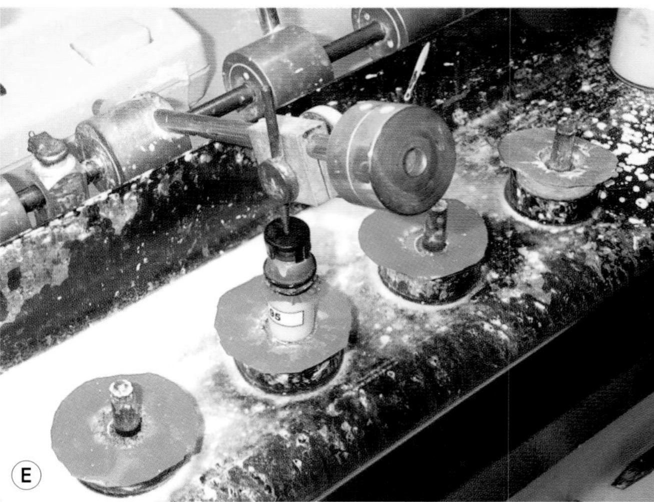

Figure 13.3 Generating the rigid lens back surface. (A) Back surface lathe. (B) Button about to be mounted in dolly. (C) Button–dolly assembly is colleted in lathe. (D) Back surface curve being cut into the button with a diamond-tipped tool. (E) Back surface polishing.

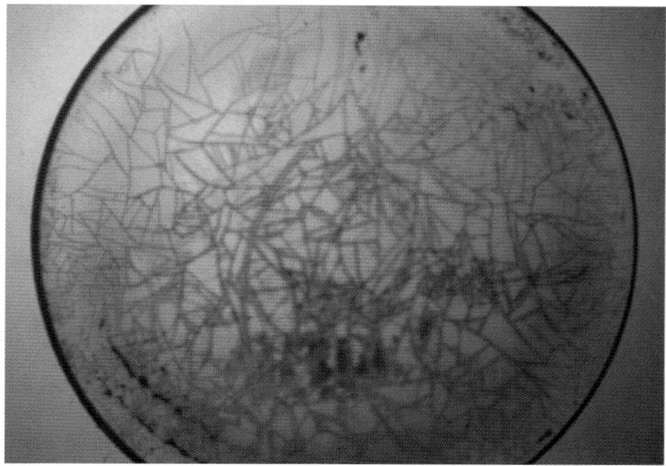

Figure 13.4 Crazing and cracking appearing in a rigid lens that has been improperly manufactured; this could be due to overheating during lathing or use of an inappropriate solvent.

letter forms are impressed; such a device is illustrated in Figure 13.6B. Typical engravings might include 'R' and 'L' to indicate the right and left eyes, the back optic zone radius, total lens diameter or a lens identification code.

If requested by a practitioner, fenestrations (small holes) can be introduced into the lens using a laser (Figure 13.6C). This procedure is usually done to the finished lens. Both lens surfaces are given a light manual polish following these procedures.

Edge polishing and final inspection

The lens is released by either ultrasonic or manual means from the arbour and washed in detergent to remove any excess wax remaining on the lens surface. Edge polishing can be carried out using a polishing machine such as that illustrated in Figure 13.7A. (With certain lens designs and lathes, the lens edge can be finished with a smooth, fine cut so that polishing is not required.) The lenses are fixed to a support arm by placing the lens front surface on to a concave

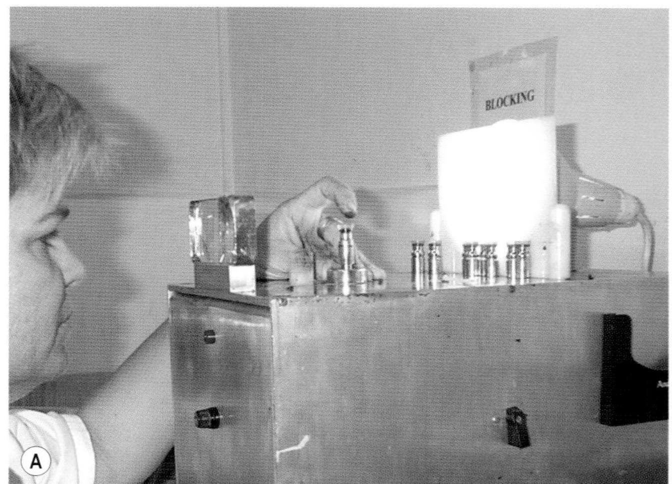

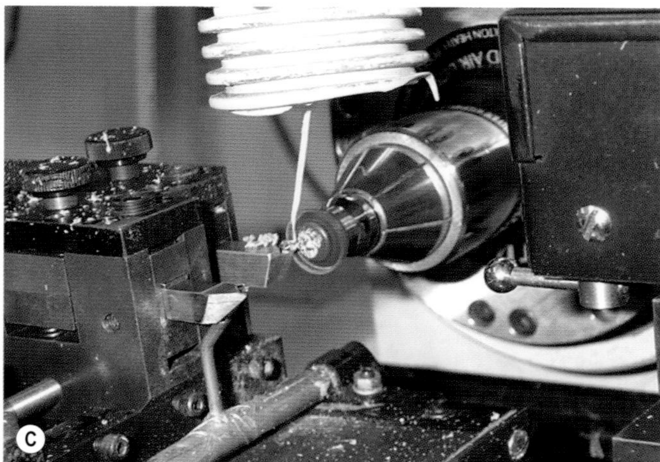

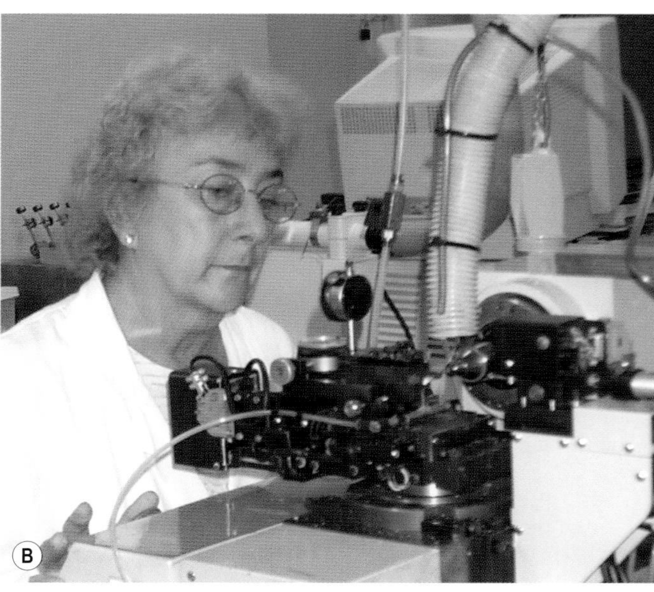

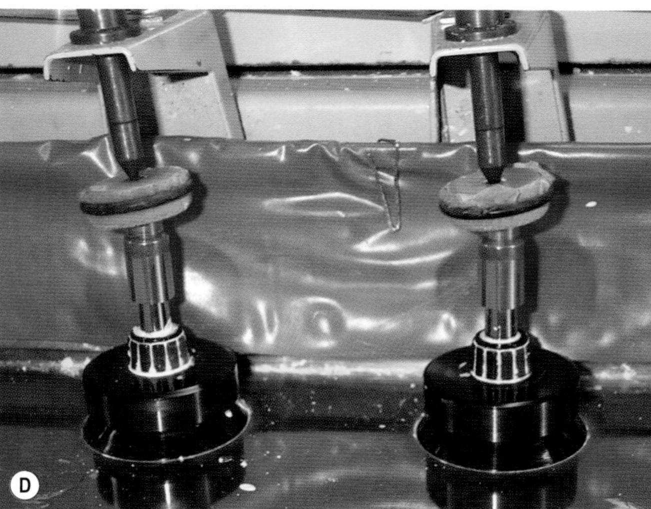

Figure 13.5 Generating the rigid lens front surface. (A) Blocking the button on to a brass arbour. (B) Front surface lathe. (C) Front surface curve being cut into the button with a diamond-tipped knife. (D) Front surface polishing.

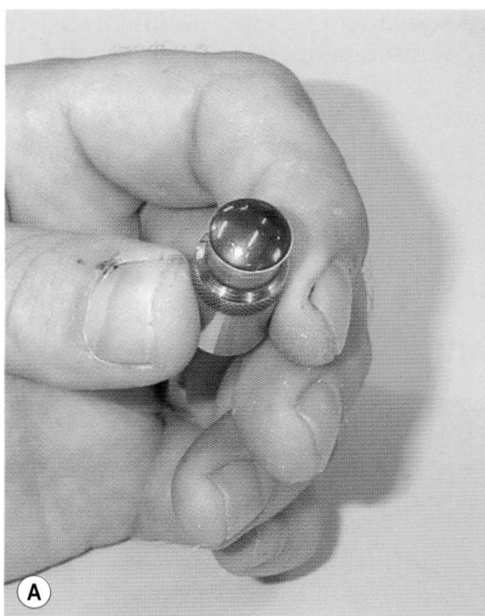

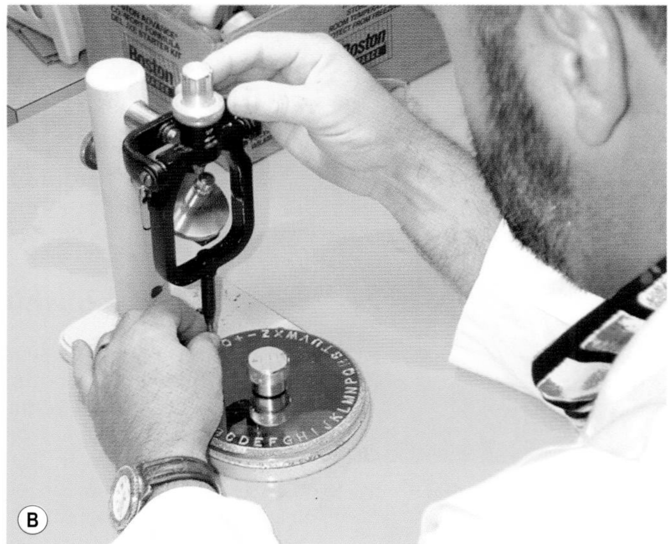

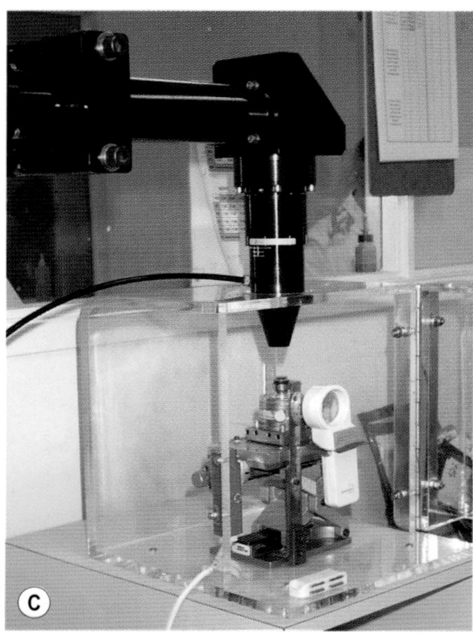

Figure 13.6 Custom modification. (A) Near-finished lens form wax-mounted on the brass arbour. (B) Pantographic system for lens engraving. (C) Laser system for toric lens scribe marking and introducing fenestrations.

rubber cup support, through which air is drawn to 'suck' the lens firmly in place. The spindle rotates around its long axis, and the spinning lens is lowered on to a flat rotating polishing pad and moved slowly from side to side. By doing this, the polishing pad alternately brushes towards the anterior and posterior edges, creating a smooth, rounded edge.

After polishing, the lens is supported in a small suction holder and the edges are inspected using a 10× hand magnifier (Figure 13.7B). Any irregularities can be rectified manually by polishing the lens – again supported in a suction holder – against a small rotating polishing pad (Figure 13.7C). Ehrmann *et al.* (1999) have described an optical profilometer that can accurately portray the edge profile of rigid lenses; such a system may pave the way to a more exact approach to the edge finishing of rigid lenses in the future. Modern digital optical inspection devices can also provide a highly accurate and detailed image of the lens edge and surface.

The key parameters of the lens – power, back optic zone radius, total diameter, optic zone diameter and thickness – are checked (see Chapter 15), to ensure that these fall within expected tolerances (see Appendix B). If all is well, the lens is cleaned and dispatched to the customer. Proctor (1997) advises that rigid lenses should be soaked for 24 h prior to checking the lens parameters because certain lens forms may display a small amount of flattening upon hydration (Proctor and Efron, 1997).

Lenses may be dispatched in solution or dry. If supplied dry, the practitioner should soak the lenses for at least 4 h before dispensing them to the patient, to ensure optimal lens surface wettability.

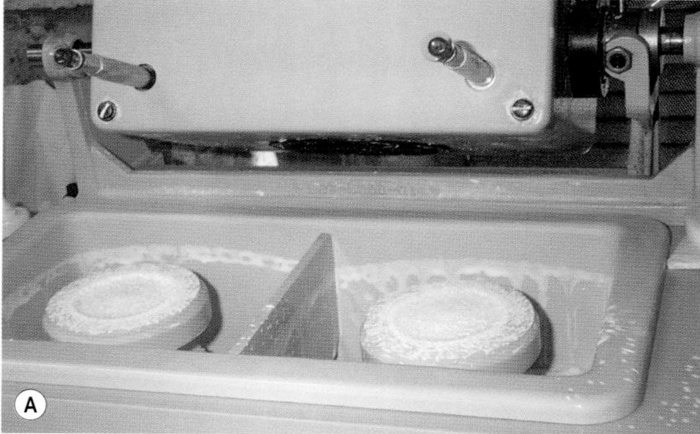

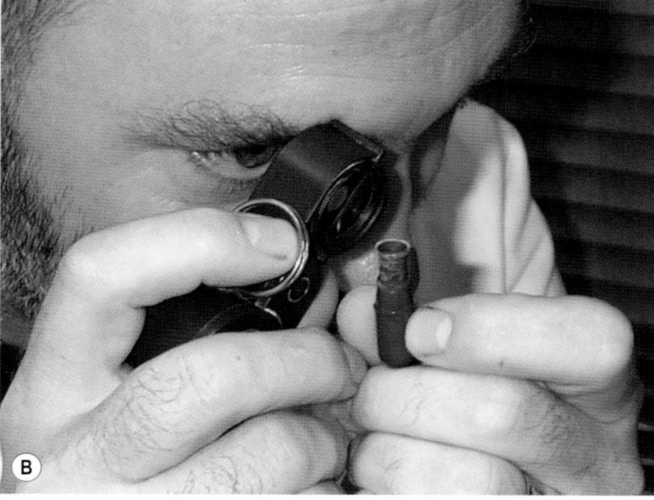

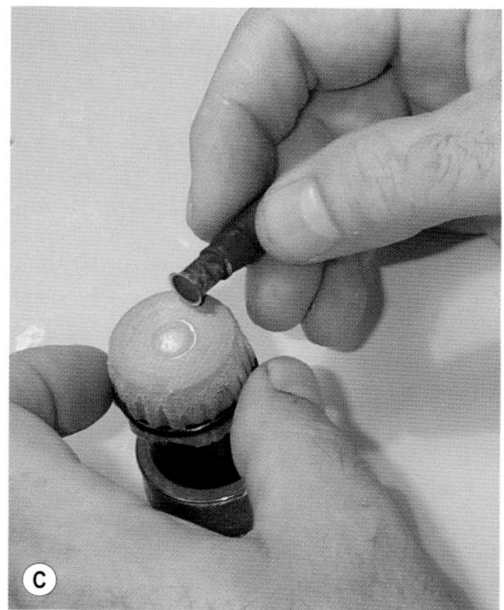

Figure 13.7 Edge polishing and inspection. (A) Two lenses suction-mounted to the spindles of an edge-polishing machine, ready to be lowered on to rotating pads. (B) Inspecting the lens edges using a 10× hand magnifier. (C) Manual polishing of the lens edge.

Merindano *et al.* (1998) used the techniques of interferential shifting-phase microscopy and scanning electron microscopy to examine the surfaces of unworn rigid lenses manufactured using lathe cutting. They found a higher degree of surface irregularities in lenses made from materials of higher oxygen permeability. These results may give insights into factors such as surface wettability and propensity for deposit formation, but are unrelated to lens comfort as the irregularities were measured on a nanometre scale and therefore could not be detected by the human cornea.

Specialty rigid lens manufacture

Computer numerically controlled lathes have ushered in a new era in which virtually any curve a practitioner wants can be cut. The lathes are controlled from a centre point to achieve the desired rate of change from centre to edge. They have also reduced the need for excessive polishing. This helps to ensure that the lenses produced are consistent and easily duplicated. From the desired base curve, the computer mathematically calculates the spline curve, which starts at the optical zone and ends at the tip of the lens.

Toric rigid lens manufacture

Either surface of a rigid lens will sometimes require a toric form for the correction of astigmatism and/or to achieve rotational stabilization. This can be achieved by directly lathing a toric surface on to the button, or by a technique known as crimping. The process of directly lathing a toric back surface on to the lens button is achieved by using a fly-cutter, which is a diamond tool that has its cutting tip set at right angles to the axis of its support shank. The positions of the fly-cutter and lens blank are reversed, so that the lathe manoeuvres the lens button in an arc around the fly-cutter, which spins in a fixed position. A similar principle is applied for generating a front toric surface. An alternative direct cutting technique involves the principle of pulsing either the diamond tool or the spindle containing the lens itself in an orthogonal axis to the lens surface that is to be cut. By adjusting the stroke length of the pulses in conjunction with the spindle revolution and feed rate, rotationally non-symmetrical shapes can be generated.

To generate a toric back surface using the technique of crimping, a spherical back curve is cut into the button in the usual way, except that a stepped rim is also engraved into the base of the blank. The curvature of this surface is the average of the required toric radii of the finished lens. The button is machined down to about 0.20 mm thick so that it can be flexed to the desired amount. The button is placed in a crimping tool with the concave surface facing upwards; this tool is a form of clamp that allows pressure to be incrementally applied to the rim of the button until it bends by a measured amount. The extent of bending is monitored optically using a conventional radiuscope.

The crimping assembly containing the flexed button is fixed to the spindle of a lathe and set spinning. A spherical surface is cut into the rotating flexed button. When the button is eventually released from the crimping tool, it reverts to its natural shape and the lathed surface assumes a toric form. The lens is blocked and a spherical curve can be generated on the front surface. Crimping is used again to generate a toric front surface if required. Orssengo *et al.* (1997b) have described how variations in crimping pressure and the preliminary radius of curvature of the back lens surface prior to crimping can influence the average back surface curvature and degree of toricity achieved.

Aspheric rigid lens manufacture

Aspheric surfaces can be generated for two main purposes:

1. To provide an enhanced lens fit, by more closely matching the aspheric surface of the cornea.
2. To provide a progressively changing power profile across the lens to correct longitudinal spherical aberration or presbyopia.

Modern lathing techniques enable these complex curves to be generated accurately and in a consistant manner.

Reverse-geometry lens manufacture

Reverse-geometry designs, in which the peripheral curves are steeper, rather than flatter than the base curve, were not possible with older lathe technology. The ability to generate such profiles is required to produce lenses suitable for orthokeratology, where the flatter central curve is used to flatten the cornea, but the steeper periphery aids centration (see Chapter 34). It is now possible to generate steeper or flatter curves just in the periphery of the inferior quadrant to minimize or eliminate edge stand-off. Previously this might have been done manually, but the lenses were inherently almost impossible to reproduce.

Industry regulation

In Europe, the control of contact lenses and contact lens care products is regulated by the European Medical Devices Directive. This directive sets out requirements to which each device must conform – there are thousands of medical devices covered by the directive – and the associated trade then devises appropriate management mechanisms to ensure the conformity of its products. Devices conforming to the directive should carry the European standard CE mark. Since June 1998, it has been illegal either to sell or buy a contact lens that does not have the CE mark affixed to it.

The CE marks are dispensed through what are called notified bodies. Companies wishing to affix the CE mark to their products must be registered as an approved manufacturer with a notified body, which will provide them with authority to use the mark. In order to get on the approved list of a notified body, manufacturers of contact lenses are generally required to have: (1) implemented a quality system, typically ISO 9002; and then (2) applied the medical device-specific CE requirements in the form of a further layer of bureaucratic controls set out in EN 46002. This procedure has become the *de facto* approach used by UK contact lens manufacturers who have obtained the CE mark for their products, and looks set to be the normal pathway for complying with the regulations. A principal activity of the notified bodies is to audit the device manufacturer to make sure that the procedures in use are such that devices made in the system comply with the directive.

An unfortunate outcome of working within a regulated industry is that new product development will in future be a slower and more expensive process. Such regulations do not provide for the 'fast-track' approach of the 1980s, when new materials and designs moved rapidly from research and development to the clinic. Certainly, there has been a noticeable decline in the pattern of frequent releases of new highly permeable materials and innovative back surface designs into the marketplace since the new European regulatory framework came into being (Hough, 1997).

Conclusions

There is ever-increasing commercial pressure in the average optical practice to prescribe soft contact lenses, and a certain amount of peer pressure to do the same (Efron, 2000). Mass media consumer advertising by major soft lens manufacturers reinforces this trend by continuously highlighting the clear benefits of the comfort and convenience of disposable soft lenses. Modern contact lens lathes based on the latest developments in computer control systems and precision engineering have resulted in sophisticated designs that can address the most complex of ocular disorders.

The huge numbers of soft lenses produced to meet the requirements of disposable and frequent-replacement wearing modalities could easily give the impression that rigid lenses form a very minor part of contact lens practice: indeed, between 1996 and 2005, rigid lens new fits decreased from 22% to 4% in the U.K. (Morgan and Efron, 2006). However, even though rigid lens manufacture is labour-intensive and expensive, the survival of this sector attests to the fact that there is an ongoing clinical requirement for rigid lenses. Other forces serving to preserve rigid lens sales include inertia in the prescribing habits of more traditional practitioners, demand from existing wearers who are satisfied with the product, trends towards frequent rigid lens replacement (see Chapter 22), but perhaps most importantly, the willingness of some practitioners to embrace the challenges of specialty rigid lens fitting to achieve the best possible outcomes for their patients. Fortunately there appears to be a sufficient market for rigid lenses to enable the small specialized manufacturers to survive.

Acknowledgements

The authors would like to thank Joe Tanner and Bruce Workman for their assistance in writing and illustrating this chapter.

References

Efron, N. (2000) Guest editorial. Contact lens practice and a very soft option. *Clin. Exp. Optom.*, **83,** 243–245.

Ehrmann, K., Ho, A. and Schindhelm, K. (1999) A novel method to quantify the edge contour of RGP contact lenses. *Contact Lens Ant. Eye,* **22,** 19–25.

Hough, T. (1997) Rigid lens manufacture in the 1990s. *Optician,* **214**(5612), 24–28.

Merindano, M. D., Canals, M., Saona, C. *et al.* (1998) Rigid gas permeable contact lenses surface roughness examined by interferential shifting phase and scanning electron microscopies. *Ophthal. Physiol. Opt.*, **18,** 75–82.

Meyers, W. E. (1997) The clinical implications of contact lens machinability. *Contact Lens Spectrum,* **12,** 36–40.

Morgan, P. B. and Efron, N. (2006) A decade of contact lens prescribing trends in the United Kingdom (1996–2005). *Cont Lens Anterior Eye,* **29,** 59-68.

Morgan, P. B. and Efron, N. (2008) The evolution of rigid contact lens prescribing. *Cont Lens Anterior Eye.*, **31,** 213-214.

Orssengo, G. J., Pye, D. C. and Ho, A. (1997a) Analysis of the colleting method of producing spherical surfaces in contact lens blanks using finite element and experimental methods. *Contact Lens Ant. Eye,* **20,** 41–48.

Orssengo, G. J., Pye, D. C. and Ho, A. (1997b) Analysis of the crimping method of producing toric surfaces in contact lens blanks using finite element and experimental methods. *Contact Lens Ant. Eye,* **20,** 49–55.

Orssengo, G. J., Pye, D. C. and Ho, A. (1997c) Variation in optic zone radii of a contact lens during manufacturing and the effects of temperature on this variation. *Contact Lens Ant. Eye,* **20,** 143–151.

Proctor, E. (1997) Contact lens manufacturing. In *Contact Lenses,* 4th edn (A. J. Phillips and L. Speedwell, eds), pp. 777–800, Oxford: Butterworth-Heinemann.

Proctor, E. and Efron, N. (1997) Radical changes to back optic zone radii of rigid gas permeable contact lenses. *Contact Lens Ant. Eye.*, **20,** 172.

Sanford, M. (1987) Crazing facts and opinions. *Contact Lens Forum,* **12**(7), 54.

Rigid lens optics

W Neil Charman

Introduction

Unlike soft lenses, which drape to fit the cornea so that on the eye the geometry of the back surface closely conforms to that of the anterior cornea, the back surface of a rigid lens maintains its shape. As a result, a tear lens of predictable form and power is generated between the contact lens and the cornea. The overall optical system producing the retinal image therefore effectively contains three elements: the rigid lens, the tear lens and the eye itself. We can imagine each of these elements as being separated from its neighbour by an infinitely thin film of air (Figure 14.1A). This chapter will largely be concerned with the role of the tear lens and the factors that influence its properties. Aberration will also be discussed. Questions of effectivity, spectacle magnification and related matters are addressed in Chapter 3.

Basic tear lens properties

The power of the tear lens, sometimes called the liquid, fluid or lacrimal lens, depends on the relative geometry of the optic zone of the back surface of the rigid lens and the anterior surface of the cornea. Figure 14.1B shows possible variations on the basic tear lens form. The tear lens may contribute negative, zero or positive power to the overall lens–eye system, depending on whether the fitting of the rigid lens is flat, in alignment or steep, respectively.

From a clinical perspective it is important to determine the likely magnitude of the power of the tear lens and how it varies as the back optic zone radius (BOZR) of the lens is changed. If r_1 and r_2 are the front optic zone radius (FOZR) and BOZR of the rigid lens and r_C is the radius of the anterior cornea, then the front and back radii of the tear lens are r_2 and r_C, respectively. With corneal lenses it is reasonable to consider that the thickness of the tear lens can be neglected, so that its power, F_T, will therefore be:

$$F_T = (n_T - 1)(1/r_2 - 1/r_C) = (n_T - 1)(r_C - r_2)/r_2 r_C \quad \text{(Equation 14.1)}$$

DOI: 10.1016/B978-0-7506-8869-7.00014-8

where n_T is the refractive index of the tears (1.336). Both r_2 and r_C will normally be about 8 mm. This gives, with adequate accuracy:

$$F_T \approx (1.336 - 1)(r_C - r_2)/(64.10^{-6})$$

where the radii are in metres. Setting, as an example, $r_C - r_2 = 0.05$ mm, we find:

$$F_T \approx (0.336) \cdot (0.05 \times 10^{-3})/64.10^{-6} \approx +0.25 \text{ D}$$

Thus, as an approximate rule of thumb, for a rigid lens the tear lens power increases by about +0.25 D for each 0.05 mm that the BOZR of the lens is steeper than the corneal radius. Correspondingly, on any cornea the back vertex power (BVP) of the rigid contact lens needs to be changed by −0.25 D for each 0.05 mm that the BOZR is made steeper, to compensate for the extra positive power of the liquid lens. If the lens BOZR is made flatter by 0.05 mm, the BVP needs to be changed by +0.25 D.

More exact calculation of F_T can, of course, be carried through using Equation 14.1. The approximation is less acceptable for corneas that are much steeper or flatter than the normal value of about 7.8 mm. This can be seen if we note that, for small changes δr_2 in r_2, we can write for the change, δF_T, in tear lens power:

$$\delta F_T = (\partial F_T/\partial r_2)\delta r_2 = -[(n_T - 1)/r_2^2]\delta r_2$$

That is, for a given change in r_2, the change in tear lens power is actually inversely proportional to r_2^2.

The tear lens during trial lens fits

Trial or diagnostic lenses are often used to find the BOZR that gives the required fit with a particular lens design – an overrefraction then being carried out to determine any additional power needed in combination with the trial lens used to give the patient clear vision. In this case the ordered lens power is simply the sum of the BVP of the trial lens and the overrefraction (assuming that the power of the latter is small enough for effectivity to be ignored; see Chapter 3). This is because the BOZR and corneal radii, r_2 and r_C, with the final lens will be exactly the same as with

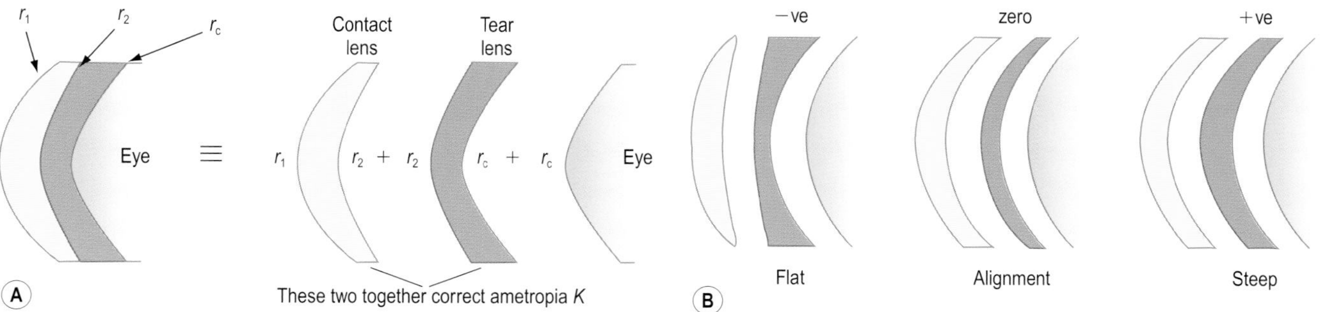

Figure 14.1 (A) The basic tear lens concept. Although exaggerated for clarity, the air gaps between the contact and tear lenses and tear lens and cornea are effectively negligible. See text for definitions of r_1, r_2 and r_C. (B) Geometry of the tear lens as a function of fit.

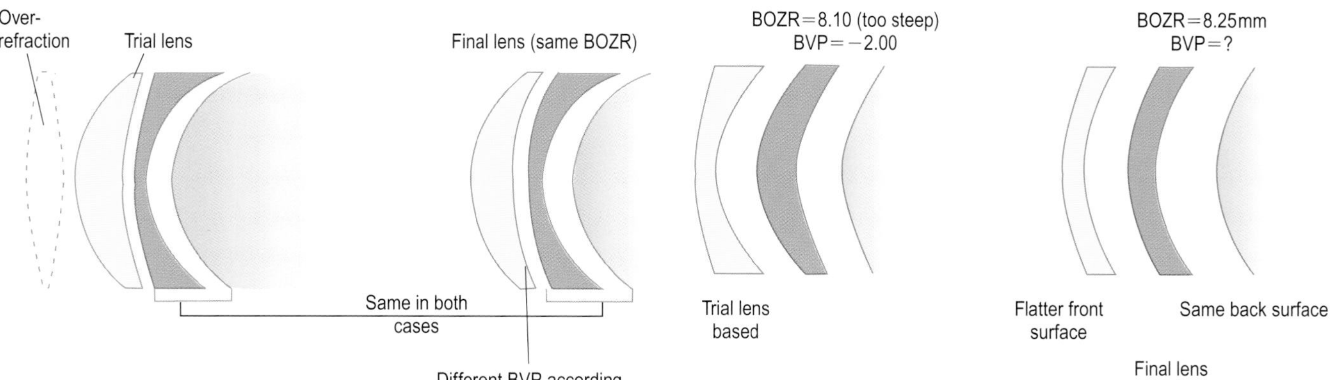

Figure 14.2 Geometry of the rigid lens and the tear lens when a trial lens with the same back optic zone radius (BOZR) as the final lens is used. BVP = back vertex power.

Figure 14.3 Change in tear lens geometry and required back vertex power (BVP) when the back optic zone radius (BOZR) of the ordered lens differs from that of the trial lens.

the trial lens, so that the tear lens has equal power in both cases (Figure 14.2).

Required BVP when the lens to be ordered has a different BOZR from the trial lens used

The situation may arise where a trial lens with a given BOZR is not available, in which case it may be necessary to order a lens with a BOZR that differs from that of the trial lens actually used. Since the BOZR, r_2, in the two cases differs, so also will the power of the tear lens, and this in turn will influence the required BVP of the ordered lens. This effect is best illustrated by an example (Figure 14.3).

Suppose that the trial lens giving a fit that is closest to that desired has a BOZR of 8.10 mm and a BVP of -3.00 D. With this lens, an overrefraction of +1.00 D is found. Consideration of fluorescein patterns and the corneal radius, however, suggests that trial lens fit is too steep and that the ordered lens should have a BOZR (r_2) = 8.25 mm. Qualitatively, it can be seen from Figure 14.3 that this flattens the front surface of the tear lens and hence tends to make its power less positive. To compensate for this, the final contact lens must have relatively more positive power. What is the required BVP for the ordered lens?

Evidently, taking into account the BVPs of the trial lens and the overrefraction, the ideal BVP for a lens of the original 8.10 mm BOZR would be:

$$F'_V = -3.00 + 1.00 = -2.00\ \text{D}$$

Thus light would leave the back surface of the correcting lens of 8.10 mm BOZR with a vergence of -2.00 D. The power of the anterior surface of the original tear lens (in air) is:

$$(1.336 - 1)/(8.10 \times 10^{-3}) = +41.48\ \text{D}$$

Using the general vergence equation,

$$L' - L = F$$

where L and L' are the object and image vergences and F is the surface power, we find that, after passing through the anterior surface of the tear lens, the vergence of the light would be:

$$-2.00 + 41.48 = +39.48\ \text{D}$$

If we assume that the tear lens has negligible thickness, this vergence incident upon the rear surface of the tear lens will correct the eye.

Now consider the ordered lens with a BOZR of 8.25 mm. Since the rear surface of the tear lens is unchanged, we again require that the vergence of the light leaving the anterior surface of the tear lens be +39.48 D. The power of the anterior surface of the new tear lens is:

$$(1.336 - 1)/(8.25 \times 10^{-3}) = +40.73\ \text{D}$$

Thus the vergence, L, incident upon the anterior surface of the tear lens must be:

$$L = L' - F = 39.48 - 40.73 = -1.25\ \text{D}$$

Since this vergence is provided by the correcting lens, the required BVP for the ordered lens of BOZR 8.25 mm is –1.25 D (as compared with the value of –2.00 D for a lens of BOZR 8.10 mm). This agrees well with our earlier rule of thumb, which suggests that, since the BOZR is 0.15 mm (or 3 × 0.05 mm) flatter, the required BVP must be +0.75 D (or 3 × 0.25 D) more positive than its original value of –2.00 D; i.e. the required BVP is –1.25 D, as also found by the more exact approach.

Calculation of required surface radii from a trial lens fit

Assuming that the BOZR that gives the desired fit has been determined by the use of trial lenses, it is of interest to determine what value of FOZR, r_1, is needed to give the required BVP, given values for the centre thickness and refractive index for the lens. Again, it is helpful to give an illustrative example to demonstrate the thick lens calculation involved.

Let us suppose that it is found that a good fit is achieved with a trial lens of BVP –7.00 D and a BOZR of 8.00 mm. The overrefraction is –1.00 D at a vertex distance of 13 mm. The lens index is 1.49 and its centre thickness is to be 0.30 mm.

We are justified in ignoring tear lens effects since these are identical for the initial and final lens. As the overrefraction is small, effectivity can be ignored and the required BVP for our final lens is –8.00 D.

The power of the back surface of the final lens is:

$$F_2 = (1 - 1.49)/(8.00 \times 10^{-3}) = -61.25\text{ D}$$

Since we require the emergent vergence at the back surface to be:

$$F'_V = L_2' = -8.00\text{ D}$$

the incident vergence at that surface, L_2, must be:

$$L_2 = L_2' - F_2 = -8.00 - (-61.25) = +53.25\text{ D}$$

But $L_2 = 1.49/l_2$, so that the object distance, l_2, for the second surface is:

$$l_2 = 1.49/L_2 = 1.49/(+53.25)\text{ m} = +27.98\text{ mm}$$

Thus, for a centre thickness of 0.30 mm, the image distance for the first surface is:

$$l_1' = 27.98 + 0.30 = 28.28\text{ mm}$$

and the corresponding image vergence is:

$$L_1' = 1.49/l_1' = 1.49/(28.28 \times 10^{-3}) = 52.69\text{ D}$$

As, for a distant object, the incident vergence at the first surface is zero, the exiting vergence L_1' must correspond to the power of the surface, that is:

$$F_1 = (1.49 - 1)/r_1 = 52.69\text{ D}$$

where r_1 is in metres. This gives r_1 = 9.30 mm. If a toric lens is required, the same process can be repeated in each principal meridian.

Neutralization of corneal astigmatism by a rigid lens of spherical power

We can see qualitatively that, in air, the astigmatism arising from a difference in the radii r_{C1} and r_{C2} in the two principal meridians of the anterior cornea is:

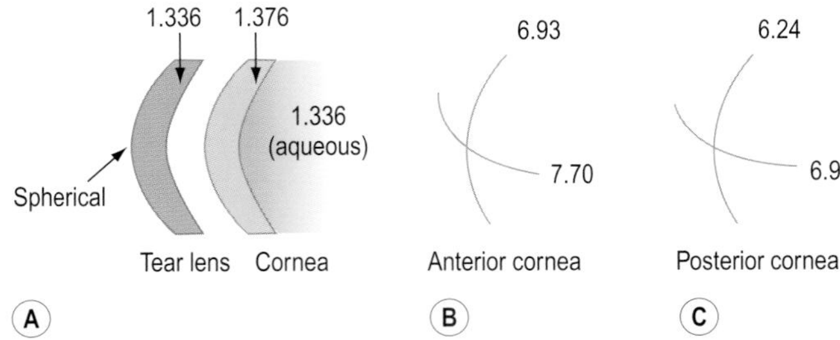

Figure 14.4 Situation with a spherical contact lens on an astigmatic cornea. (A) Basic lens geometry; (B) anterior corneal and posterior tear lens radii (mm); (C) posterior corneal radii.

$$(n_C - 1)(1/r_{C1} - 1/r_{C2})$$

where n_C is the corneal index. If, however, the anterior cornea is in contact with the tears rather than air, this astigmatism is reduced to:

$$(n_C - n_T)(1/r_{C1} - 1/r_{C2})$$

Taking n_C as 1.376 and n_T as 1.336, we see that the astigmatism is likely to be reduced by a factor:

$$(n_C - n_T)/(n_C - 1) = 0.040/0.036 \approx 0.1\times$$

In fact the situation is slightly more complex than this because of the contribution of the rear surface of the cornea to the overall corneal astigmatism, but this does not alter the basic conclusion that corneal astigmatism can be almost completely neutralized by the use of a spherical rigid lens. An example will illustrate this (Figure 14.4).

Suppose that the anterior surface of the cornea shows with-the-rule astigmatism, with:

$$r_{180} = 7.70\text{ mm, giving power}$$
$$F_{180} = (1.376 - 1)/(7.70 \times 10^{-3}) = 48.83\text{ D}$$

$$r_{90} = 6.93\text{ mm, giving power}$$
$$F_{90} = (1.376 - 1)/(6.93 \times 10^{-3}) = 54.26\text{ D}$$

Hence the astigmatism of the anterior surface of the cornea is:

$$F_{90} - F_{180} = 54.26 - 48.83 = 5.43\text{ DC (with-the-rule)}$$

Now suppose that the posterior corneal radii are 10% smaller than the anterior radii, i.e. r_{180} = 6.93 mm, and r_{90} = 6.24 mm, and that the refractive index of the aqueous humour is 1.336. The posterior meridional powers will be:

$$F_{180} = (1.336 - 1.376)/(6.93 \times 10^{-3}) = -5.77\text{ D}$$

$$F_{90} = (1.336 - 1.376)/(6.24 \times 10^{-3}) = -6.41\text{ D}$$

Thus the astigmatism of the posterior surface is:

$$F_{90} - F_{180} = -6.41 + 5.77 = -0.64\text{ DC}$$

The total uncorrected corneal astigmatism is thus slightly lower than that due to the anterior surface alone, i.e.:

$$5.43 - 0.64 = 4.79\text{ DC (with-the-rule)}$$

What is the effect of a spherical rigid contact lens? Since the lens itself and the anterior surface of the tear lens can only contribute spherical power, they do not affect the astigmatism. The powers of the posterior surface of the tear lens are:

$$F_{180} = (1 - 1.336)/(7.70 \times 10^{-3}) = -43.64\text{ D}$$

$$F_{90} = (1-1.336)/(6.93\times10^{-3}) = -48.48\text{ D}$$

$$\text{i.e. } F_{90} - F_{180} = -4.84\text{ DC}$$

When balanced against the astigmatism of the cornea, this leaves a mere 4.79 - 4.84 = -0.05 DC of uncorrected astigmatism of corneal origin, so that the original corneal astigmatism has been almost completely neutralized. Note that this does not depend in any way upon the refractive index of the correcting lens. Any residual astigmatism due to the crystalline lens will, of course, remain uncorrected. Very occasionally a patient may be encountered who has a spherical refractive error but non-zero corneal astigmatism. This therefore implies that the residual (lenticular) astigmatism is of opposite sign to the corneal astigmatism and that correcting the corneal astigmatism with a spherical rigid lens will leave the residual astigmatism manifest. In such cases a spherical soft lens will result in better visual acuity, since the failure of the soft lens to correct the corneal astigmatism will allow the balance between the corneal and lenticular astigmatism to be maintained.

Although the above discussion has concerned regular astigmatism, it is obvious that irregular astigmatism and, indeed, general corneal irregularity will similarly be masked by a spherical lens and its accompanying tear lens (see below).

It is, however, important to note that, although nominally a spherical rigid lens will neutralize any value of corneal astigmatism, the fitting relationship is likely to be unsatisfactory for corneal astigmatism greater than about 2.00 DC. Thus for higher levels of astigmatism some form of toroidal correction is required (see Chapter 17).

Excellent expositions of further rigid and soft lens calculations of this type, together with many numerical examples, are given by Ford and Stone (1997) and Douthwaite (2005).

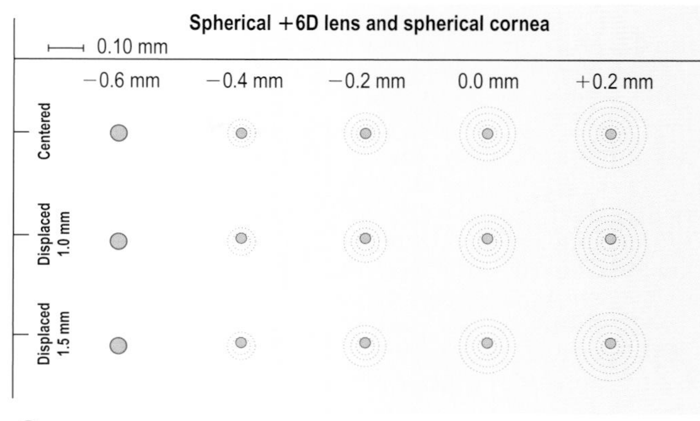

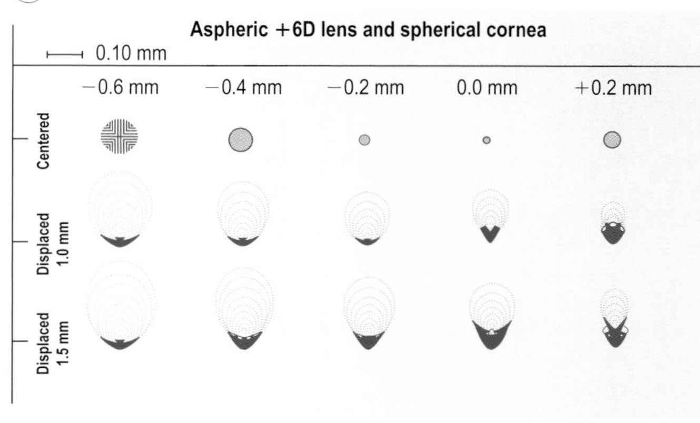

Figure 14.5 Spot diagrams for a +6.00 D lens combined with a spherical cornea, as a function of defocus and decentration. Lens displacements are 0 mm (top row), 1.0 mm (middle row) and 1.5 mm (bottom row). Each row shows various planes of focus. The gaussian image plane is at 0.0 mm and negative values correspond to movement of the image plane towards the cornea. (A) Spherical contact lens. (B) Rigid contact lens with an aspheric front surface (p = +0.6): the chosen p-value nearly eliminates spherical aberration, giving minimal blur in the gaussian image plane (0.0 mm). (Adapted from Atchison, D. A. (1995) Aberrations associated with rigid contact lenses. J. Opt. Soc. Am. A., 12, 2267–2273.)

Aberrations of rigid contact lenses

As in the case of soft lenses, the steep surface curvatures of rigid lenses mean that, if they remain well-centred, their major aberration in relation to foveal imagery ought to be spherical aberration (Westheimer, 1961). Early calculations by Campbell (1981) emphasized that it was the aberration of the combined lens–eye system that was of importance, rather than that of the lens alone in air: it appeared that the dominant factor was the form of the front surface of the lens, although amounts of spherical aberration were likely to be low. Cox (1990) went on to demonstrate that levels of spherical aberration only started to reduce significantly visual performance for pupils larger than 6 mm and when rigid lens powers were more positive than -3.00 D. Hammer and Holden (1994) broadly agreed with these results and pointed out that, for conicoidally aspheric lens surfaces, on-eye aberration became more positive as the p-value of the front surface was increased and, to a lesser extent, more negative as the p-value of the back surface was increased.

Atchison (1995) made the important point that, although a well-centred aspheric contact lens might reduce the overall spherical aberration with respect to a lens with spherical surfaces, this advantage could break down if the lens decentred by more than about 1 mm, when substantial amounts of coma and defocus could be introduced, depending upon the exact lens parameters involved. Image quality with a spherical lens is generally more robust against decentration. This is illustrated in Figure 14.5, which shows spot diagrams (i.e. retinal images of a point as calculated by ray optics) for the case of a +6.00 D lens and a 5 mm pupil. Various combinations of defocus and decentration are shown.

Relatively few earlier experimental studies explored the possible impact of the spherical aberration of rigid contact lenses on visual performance. Collins *et al.* (1992), however, found that when a group of 12 subjects was fitted with rigid lenses with front surface asphericities corresponding to p = 1.0 (sphere), 0.74 and 0.49 (flattening ellipsoids), both high- and low-contrast photopic visual acuities were statistically identical with all lenses. In mesopic conditions, when pupils were larger, low-contrast visual acuity was significantly worse with the p = 0.49 lenses, but only by one line. Interestingly, when asked which lens they preferred, all except three subjects chose the lenses with a spherical (p = 1.0) front surface. Those who chose the lenses with p = 0.74 had demonstrably better visual performance with them than with the other lenses. Thus, although the effects of rigid lens spherical aberration on visual performance at photopic levels were generally small, there was some evidence that asphericities that optimized vision for the individual were appreciated by the wearer.

More recent work using wavefront aberrometry has clarified some aspects of the effects of rigid lenses on the combined lens–eye aberration in individual patients.

As discussed earlier, the effect of a spherical rigid lens and the associated tear lens is to neutralize almost all of the eye's original corneal astigmatism (i.e. the cornea's second-order astigmatic wavefront errors). The residual astigmatism associated with the crystalline lens remains uncorrected, however. In broad terms, it can be seen that similar compensation is likely to occur for the other higher-order aberrations associated with the asymmetries and irregularities of the cornea (Griffiths *et al.*, 1998). The result is that, as far as the earlier parts of the contact lens–eye system are concerned, the original corneal aberrations become relatively unimportant and it is the aberrations associated with the anterior surface of the contact lens that dominate. However, that part of the original ocular wavefront aberration that was contributed by the crystalline lens will not be affected by the presence of the contact lens. Thus the overall wavefront aberration of the rigid contact lens–eye system will approximate to the sum of that due to the anterior surface of the contact lens and that due to the crystalline lens of the eye.

The impact of these rigid lens-induced changes will depend upon the balance between the contributions to the ocular wavefront aberration made by the cornea and the crystalline lens. How do these contributions compare? Intriguingly, recent studies confirm what had been suspected from earlier work (El Hage and Berny, 1973; Millodot and Sivak, 1979): in young adult eyes the aberrations of the cornea, particularly spherical aberration, tend to be of similar magnitude but opposite sign to those of the lens, so that the aberrations of the total eye are often smaller than those of its component parts (Artal *et al.*, 2002; Kelly *et al.*, 2004). However, the degree of balance between corneal and lenticular aberration varies between individuals and tends to deteriorate with age, largely as a result of increases in the wavefront errors of the crystalline lens. It appears likely that aberration-balancing occurs passively as a result of the basic optical design of the eye, rather than being an active process like emmetropization (Artal *et al.*, 2006).

The key point is that elimination of corneal aberrations by a suitable design of contact lens does not necessarily reduce the wavefront aberration of the complete contact lens–eye system. Practical measurements of aberrations with eyes wearing rigid lens support this conclusion (Lu *et al.*, 2003; Choi *et al.*, 2007). Contact lenses may either reduce or increase the higher-order wavefront aberration in comparison to that of the original eye. Those subjects whose aberrations are dominated by high levels of corneal aberration are likely to have reduced aberrations with rigid lens wear, whereas those with low initial levels of both corneal and total aberrations may suffer from an increase in aberrations during lens wear. Rigid lens wear is, then, likely to be helpful in reducing the effect of higher-order aberrations in corneal conditions such as keratoconus (Griffiths *et al.*, 1998; Dorronsorro *et al.*, 2003; Choi *et al.*, 2007).

It is important to note that contact lens wear does not simply introduce changes in spherical aberration, it also affects coma and other asymmetric aberrations, presumably as a result of factors such as the lack of rotational symmetry in the cornea and decentration of the contact lens. What is not clear at the present time is the longer-term effect of rigid lens wear on lens–eye aberrations. Gross corneal warpage has long been recognized as a possible problem of rigid-lens wear (Efron, 2004) and it may be that some corneal change occurs in all eyes. Associated aberrational changes may be small, however, due to the masking effect of the tear lens.

All recent authors (Hong *et al.*, 2001; Dorronsorro *et al.*, 2003; Lu *et al.*, 2003; Choi *et al.*, 2007) agree that aberrometry can provide a better understanding of the on-eye effects of rigid lenses on the vision of individual patients. Undoubtedly further studies will clarify the benefits of particular materials, lens designs and fitting philosophies in reducing aberration and increasing visual performance.

Other rigid lens effects

Certain optical effects occur when rigid lenses move during wear, or are distorted over time, via interactions between the lids, the lens and the cornea. Disturbing optical effects can also result from reflections off the lens edge or optical zone junctions. These phenomena are considered here.

Prismatic effects due to decentred or tilted lenses

Prismatic effects may arise as a result of the lens either decentring or tilting, the latter often being due to pressure from the upper lid. To a reasonable approximation, the corneal lens and the associated tear lens will both become decentred by the same amount with respect to the pupil centre, so that, applying the Prentice rule, $P = Fc$, where P dioptres is the prism power resulting from a decentration of c centimetres, and F is the combined dioptric power of the contact lens and tear lens. If, for example, $F = \pm 10$ D and there is 1 mm of lens decentration, a 1 dioptre prism can be induced. This will be of little importance if similar effects occur in both eyes – that is, if the correcting powers are similar and fitting has ensured that similar amounts of movement occur in the two eyes. Fuller discussions of prismatic effects are found in Ford and Stone (1997) and Douthwaite (2005).

Flexure effects with rigid corneal lenses

Although the basic assumption of this discussion has been that a spherically powered rigid lens remains so when placed on the eye, these lenses may flex on strongly toroidal corneas, particularly when the lenses are thin (Harris and Chu, 1972). This leads to a failure to correct the corneal astigmatism. Steps that may be taken to minimize flexure in such cases include fitting the BOZR as flat as possible and minimizing the back optic zone diameter. Flexure effects are difficult to predict and tend to vary as the lens moves on the eye: they are therefore best assessed empirically by direct objective and subjective determination of the effectiveness of the correction.

Visually disturbing effects with rigid lenses

A number of disturbing visual effects may arise with some designs of rigid lens (Figure 14.6). If the optic zone is small and the eye pupil is large, the outer zones of the pupil will

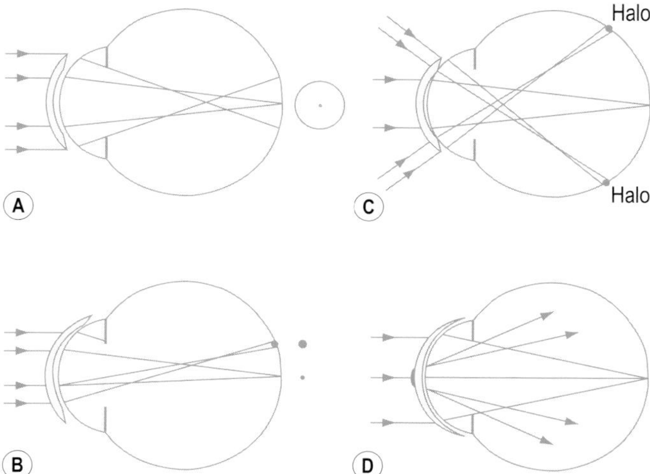

Figure 14.6 Possible disturbing effects arising with rigid lenses. (A) 'Haloes' arising from the optic zone being smaller than the dilated pupil. (B) Asymmetric retinal point images due to a high-riding lens. (C) Disturbance of vision in the peripheral field due to scattering and refraction at the lens edge. (D) Scattering from lens deposits.

be imperfectly corrected, leading to a 'halo' under dim lighting conditions. Similar effects may occur with smaller pupils if the lenses are badly decentred. In cases where the overall diameter of the lens is less than that of the cornea, discontinuities and flare light effects may arise in the peripheral field. Other disturbing effects may result from lens deposits or, in the case of scleral lenses, from bubbles.

Conclusion

From the purely optical point of view, spherical-powered rigid lenses have the merit of correcting modest amounts of corneal astigmatism as well as any spherical refractive errors. Since flexure effects are relatively slight their performance is, perhaps, more predictable than their soft lens counterparts.

References

Artal, A., Berrio, E., Guirao, A. *et al.* (2002) Contribution of the cornea and internal surfaces to the change in ocular aberrations with age. *J. Opt. Soc. Am. A.*, **19,** 137–143.

Artal, P., Benito, A. and Tabernero, J. (2006) The human eye is an example of robust optical design. *J. Vision,* **6,** 1–7.

Atchison, D. A. (1995) Aberrations associated with rigid contact lenses. *J. Opt. Soc. Am. A.*, **12,** 2267–2273.

Campbell, C. E. (1981) The effect of spherical aberration of contact lens to the wearer. *Am. J. Optom. Physiol. Opt.*, **58,** 212–217.

Choi, J., Wee, W.R., Lee, J.H. *et al.* (2007) Changes of ocular higher-order aberration in on- and off-eye of rigid and gas permeable contact lenses. *Optom. Vis. Sci.*, **84,** 42–51.

Collins, M. J., Brown, B., Atchison, D. A. *et al.* (1992) Tolerance to spherical aberration induced by rigid contact lenses. *Ophthal. Physiol. Opt.*, **12,** 24–28.

Cox, I. (1990) Theoretical calculation of the longitudinal spherical aberration of rigid and soft lenses. *Am. J. Optom. Physiol. Opt.*, **67,** 277–282.

Dorronsorro, C., Barberos, S., Llorente, L. *et al.* (2003) On-eye measurement of optical performance of rigid gas permeable contact lenses based on ocular and corneal aberrometry. *Optom. Vis. Sci.*, **80,** 115–125.

Douthwaite, W. A. (2005) *Contact Lens Optics and Lens Design.* 3rd edn, Oxford: Butterworth-Heinemann.

Efron, N. (2004) *Contact Lens Complications.* 2nd edn, pp. 187–197, Oxford: Butterworth-Heinemann.

El Hage, S .G. and Berny, F. (1973) Contribution of the crystalline lens to the spherical aberration of the eye. *J. Opt. Soc. Am.*, **63,** 205–211.

Ford, M. W. and Stone, J. (1997) Practical optics and computer design of contact lenses. In *Contact Lenses,* 4th edn (A. J. Phillips and L. Speedwell, eds), pp. 154–231, London: Butterworth-Heinemann.

Griffiths, M., Zahner, K., Collins, M., *et al.* (1998) Masking of irregular corneal topography with contact lenses. *Contact Lens Assoc. Ophthalmol. J.*, **24,** 76–81.

Hammer, R. M. and Holden, B. A. (1994) Spherical aberration of aspheric contact lenses on eye. *Optom. Vis. Sci.*, **71,** 522–528.

Harris, M. G. and Chu, C. S. (1972) The effect of contact lens thickness and corneal toricity on flexure and residual astigmatism. *Am. J. Optom. Physiol. Opt.*, **49,** 304–307.

Hong, X., Himebaugh, N. and Thibos, L. N. (2001) On-eye evaluation of optical performance of rigid and soft contact lenses. *Optom. Vis. Sci.*, **78,** 872–880.

Kelly, J. E., Mihashi, T., Howland, H. C. (2004) Compensation of corneal horizontal/vertical astigmatism, lateral coma, and spherical aberration by internal optics of the eye. *J. Vision,* **4,** 262–271.

Lu, F., Mao, X., Qu, J. *et al.* (2003) Monochromatic wavefront aberration in the human eye with contact lenses. *Optom. Vis. Sci.*, **80,** 135–141.

Millodot, M. and Sivak, J. (1979) Contribution of the cornea and lens to the spherical aberration of the eye. *Vision Res.*, **19,** 685–687.

Westheimer, G. (1961) Aberrations of contact lenses. *Am. J. Optom. Arch. Am. Acad. Optom.*, **38,** 445–448.

15 CHAPTER

Rigid lens measurement

Sudi Patel

Introduction

Contact lens laboratories employ a variety of methods to check the quality of rigid contact lenses during the manufacturing process. The physical, mechanical, optical and chemical properties are closely monitored until final dispatch. The manufacturer is responsible for fulfilling the contact lens order. The clinician must be satisfied that the lens received will safely fit the patient with the least amount of discomfort, and will fully correct vision.

As a result of technological advancements and increasing use of manufacturing automation over the past few years, which aim to guarantee lens reproducibility, there is a reduced need for routine contact lens checking by the clinician. However, certain core parameters of a finished rigid contact lens will need to be checked from time to time in order to identify individual lenses, determine the parameters of a previously 'unseen' lens, and check if any lens parameters have changed (e.g. due to lens warpage). These essential parameters are:

- radius of back surface (central optic and peripheral zones)
- diameter (central optic zone, overall diameter (OD))
- back vertex power
- thickness, central and peripheral
- edge profile
- surface quality
- surface wettability
- flexibility
- material
- tint.

Finished rigid lenses can be very flexible. These lenses must be handled with care, making sure that the product is checked in a free and natural state, and subjected to minimum external forces. There are numerous approved tests and procedures for checking each of the listed parameters. This chapter will concentrate on key techniques of immediate clinical relevance.

DOI: 10.1016/B978-0-7506-8869-7.00015-X

Surface radius

Radiuscope

The radiuscope (microspherometer) is the standard instrument for checking the back optic zone radius (BOZR) of a rigid lens (Figure 15.1).

The basic optical arrangement of the radiuscope for measuring a concave surface is shown in Figure 15.2. Rays from an illuminated target are focused on a point *A*. A travelling microscope is focused on this same point. The rays are directed towards the back surface of a rigid lens. For a spherical surface, a sharp, clear image of the target will be observed in two conditions – when the travelling microscope is focused on:

1. The back surface of the lens (*A*).
2. When the lens is moved away from the microscope and the incident rays are perpendicular to the surface.

For the second condition the reflected light again passes through point *A* and the distance *AB* is the BOZR of the lens. To reduce the effects of unwanted reflections, the lens front surface reflectivity is greatly reduced by immersing the lens in water. This optical arrangement, known as the 'Drysdale method', is employed in most contact lens radiuscopes. Using cross-shaped targets, the radiuscope can measure both spherical and toric surfaces. This technique is valuable not just for checking new lenses, but also for monitoring changes in lens shape due to flexure.

For aspheric surfaces, the measured BOZR is the radius over the chord diameter shown in Figure 15.2. By extending the size of the target, it is possible to focus on different parts of the reflected image and to detect non-spherical surfaces. This is not the best quantitative method for numerically evaluating an aspheric surface; nevertheless, it is useful as a quick check for regularity. Peripheral curves can be assessed in multicurve lenses by tilting the lens (Figure 15.2).

The device for holding the lens could inadvertently distort the lens and affect the regularity of lens surface and

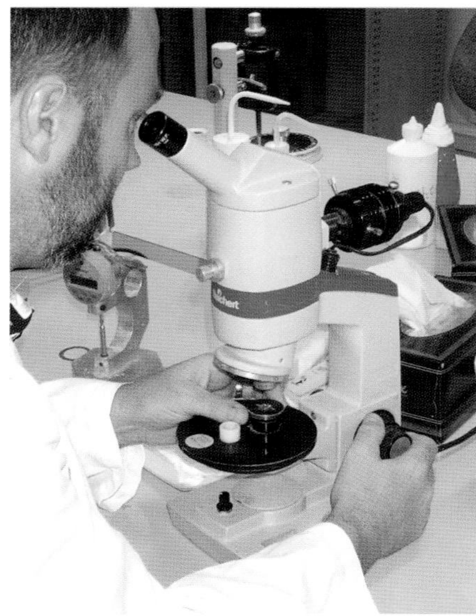

Figure 15.1 A radiuscope is used to measure lens surface curvature.

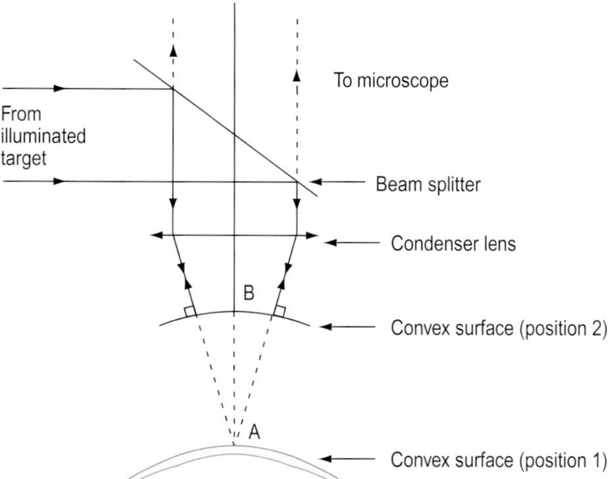

Figure 15.3 Basic optical arrangement of the radiuscope for measuring a convex (front) lens surface (Drysdale method).

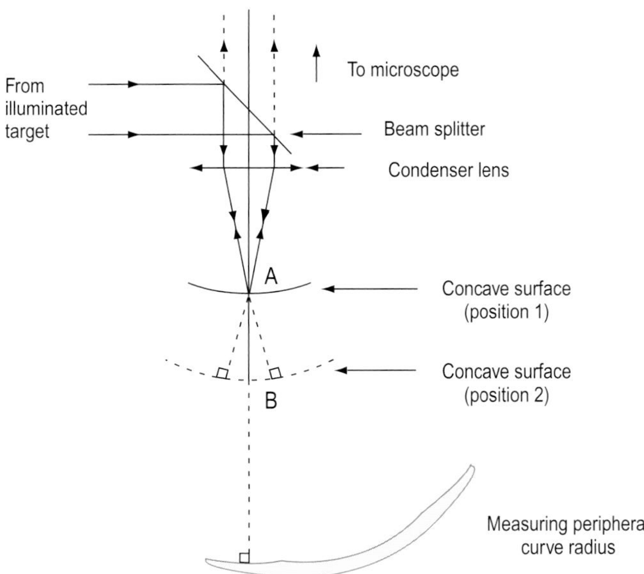

Figure 15.2 Basic optical arrangement of the radiuscope for measuring a concave (back) lens surface (Drysdale method).

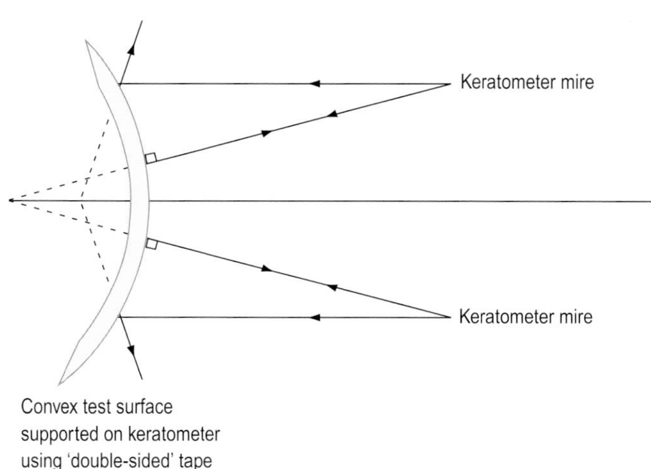

Figure 15.4 Use of the keratometer for checking the convex (front) surface of a rigid lens.

quality. This can cause the reflection to appear fuzzy, which will in turn affect radius measurement. McMonnies (1998) described a 'pressure-free' holder and manipulator to solve this problem. The radiuscope can also be used for checking the front surface of the lens, as shown in Figure 15.3.

Keratometer

Using a suitable lens holder (e.g. double-sided adhesive tape), the front surface of a rigid lens can be checked with a standard keratometer (Figure 15.4) or videokeratoscope. With the aid of a mirror and holder (e.g. in the form of a wet cell; see Chapter 8), the keratometer can be used to measure the curvature of the lens back surface (Figure 15.5). The specific instrument will need to be recalibrated for this purpose.

Some videokeratoscopes are not suited for lens back surface analysis because the inherent software package is designed for analysing convex surfaces only. Videokeratoscopes are ideal for checking aspheric front lens surfaces, with the lenses on or off the eye. Also, videokeratoscopes can be used to monitor lens front surface shape in cases of suspected lens flexure or dimensional instability.

To measure aspheric back surfaces Dietze *et al.* (2003) explored methods using a keratometer and found it can be efficiently used to verify the back vertex radius within its International Organization for Standardization tolerance

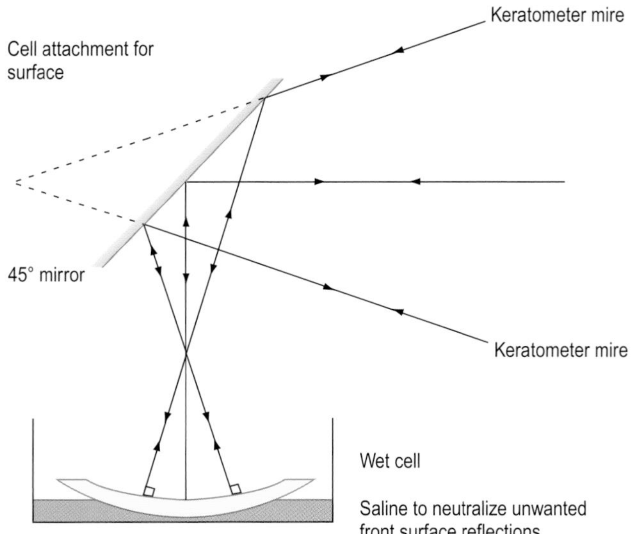

Figure 15.5 Use of the keratometer for checking the concave (back) surface of a rigid lens.

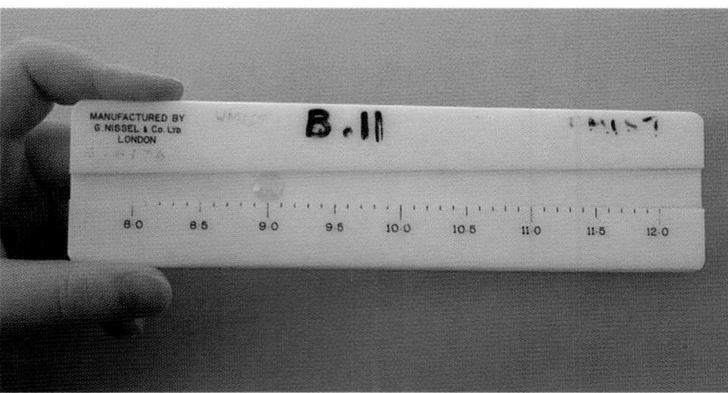

Figure 15.6 Checking rigid lens overall diameter with a V-gauge. The lens is inserted into the wide opening of the V-shaped groove on the right, and allowed to slide down to the left until the gauge becomes too narrow for the lens to slide any further. The total diameter of the lens is read off the scale that runs along the lower border of the groove. In this case, the lens has a diameter of 9.0 mm.

and the back surface asphericity within an eccentricity/*p*-value tolerance of ±0.1.

Optical interferometric techniques are arguably the most sensitive and critical means of checking steep surfaces such as contact lenses. For example, the Twyman–Green interferometer is of great value in qualitative and quantitative lens surface analysis. Unfortunately, interferometric methods are time-consuming, cumbersome and expensive, and as such are more suited for the laboratory than clinical practice (Biddles, 1969). Nevertheless, a standard stereomicroscope can be easily modified to produce a clinically viable interferometeric checking device suitable for both spherical and non-spherical contact lens surfaces (Garner, 1981).

Diameter

The OD of a rigid lens can be measured using a V-gauge. This is a triangular channel cut into a plastic strip with markings and numerical diameter values arranged in descending order of magnitude towards the apex of the triangle. In Figure 15.6, the lens is placed at the wide end of the strip and pushed gently along the strip until it becomes lightly wedged in the V-gauge. Care must be taken in making sure the V-gauge does not flex the lens. This would underestimate lens diameter. The OD is read off the precalibrated scale.

Projection systems or calibrated loupes (Figure 15.7) can be used for checking overall lens diameter or the diameter of intermediate zones. Magnification of 7× to 10× is sufficient. Port (1987) found that lens diameters measured using a V-gauge were more reproducible compared with using a projection system, and a tolerance limit of about 0.1 mm was possible. Projection systems are also useful for checking optical boundaries inside a contact lens, e.g. diameter of optical zones in multicurve lenses, quality of oval junctions in toric lenses and the segment in some bifocal designs.

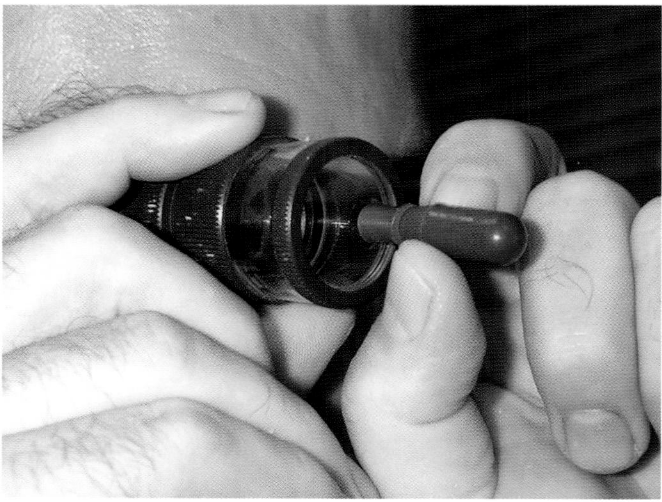

Figure 15.7 Checking rigid lens overall diameter with a calibrated loupe.

Back vertex power

In Chapter 8, it was noted that soft lens power can be checked *in vivo* by objective means by application of videotopography, optical wavefront analysis or refractometry. The same techniques can be applied to rigid lenses. The remainder of this section will concentrate on laboratory bench tests for rigid lens power checking.

Back vertex power is measured using a focimeter (Figure 15.8). Care must be taken to prevent flexure and damage to the lens. A flat plastic disc with a range of circular apertures is often used to support the delicate lens during focimetry.

A graduated rotating device is useful for checking toric lenses. The standard focimeter is calibrated for spectacle lenses placed at a specific location on the instrument-measuring stop. The physical limitations of the focimeter combined with the highly curved back surface of the lens cause the lens to rest in a position away from this location. This will result in a systematic error when reading off lens power. This error is significant especially when checking high-powered lenses. The particular focimeter should be

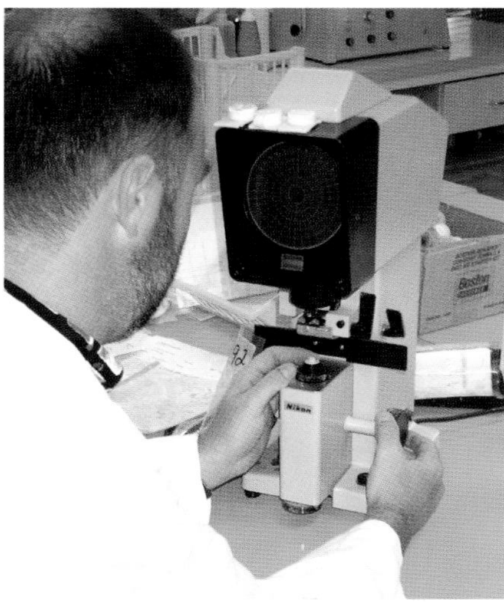

Figure 15.8 Vertically oriented focimeter used to measure lens power.

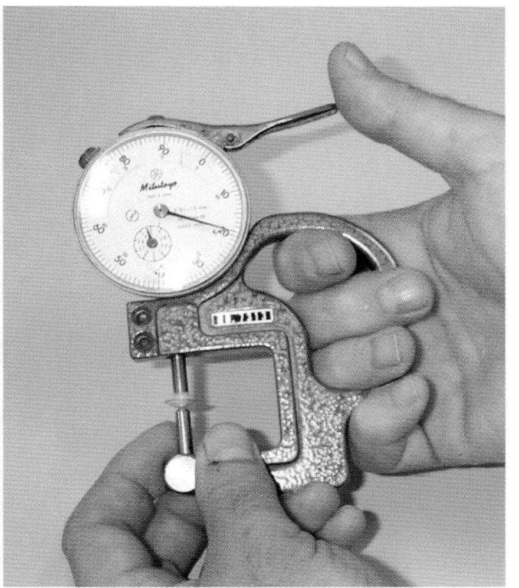

Figure 15.9 Measuring rigid lens thickness using a mechanical calliper.

recalibrated for contact lens checking; ideally, a dedicated focimeter should be set aside for the exclusive purpose of checking the powers of contact lenses. The focimeter is also used to measure the magnitude and direction of prismatic power in prism ballast and scleral lenses. In addition to the quantitative data obtained using this technique, the clarity of the viewed image formed by transmission through the contact lens can provide an indication of lens optical quality.

The optical configuration of most focimeters is such that lens power is checked by sampling over an aperture of approximately 4 mm diameter. In many advanced rigid lens designs (e.g. bifocal, multifocal and aspheric), there can be significant power variations within such a small zone and this will not be measured adequately by standard focimetry (Woods, 2003).

Reducing the aperture can help; however, in advanced optical designs, lens power variations are best checked using optical interferometric techniques such as the Twyman–Green interferometer. Optical wavefront analysis systems can be adapted to check the power distribution and aberration profile over the optical zone of finished lenses (see Chapter 14). These systems are destined to become both more practical and affordable and, as such, enter mainstream practice, allowing the clinician to check the power distribution delivered to the eye by the specific rigid lens *in vivo*.

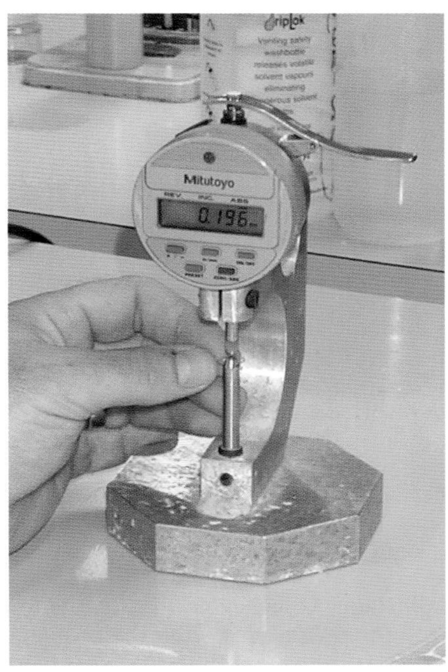

Figure 15.10 Measuring rigid lens thickness using an electromechanical gauge.

Thickness

Knowledge of lens centre thickness is required for calculation of gas transmissibility (Fatt and Ruben, 1994) and noting lens flexibility. The central and peripheral thickness can be measured using mechanical contact lens thickness callipers (Figure 15.9) or an electromechanical device (Figure 15.10). Most rigid lens radiuscopes include a micrometer suitable for thickness measurement. The contact probe may depress the surface; thus, the reading may be lower than expected.

A non-contact optical method can be used in one of two ways, as shown in Figure 15.11. Using a travelling microscope – by focusing on the back surface then the front – the apparent thickness, t, can be measured. Using the lens material refractive index (n_1), the true thickness is tn_1.

A modified optical pachymeter can be used, but this is time-consuming, cumbersome and subject to an operator learning curve (Guillon *et al.*, 1987). The Orbscan (Orbtek, Salt Lake City) corneal topographer and pachymeter operates by analysing the anterior and posterior boundaries of a corneal optical section as the incident slit scans over the cornea. The dedicated software quickly generates a two-dimensional pattern of corneal surface topography and

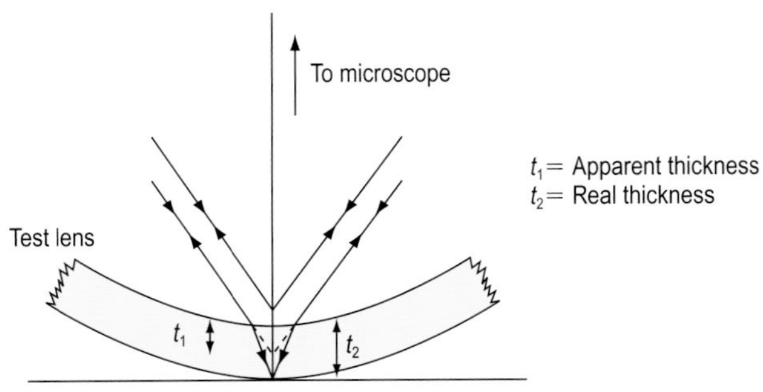

Figure 15.11 Measuring rigid lens thickness using an optical technique.

thickness distribution (Lattimore *et al.*, 1999). The Orbscan could be used to measure thickness variations within a contact lens.

Interferometric techniques are most useful in checking and quantifying the thickness distribution of aspheric or toric lenses. In prism-ballasted, truncated or bifocal lenses, interferometry offers a unique tool for identifying the quality of transition at the junction between adjacent portions of the lens.

Cross-polarizing filters used for checking stress patterns in spectacle lenses can also be used for assessing stress formations in rigid lenses.

Lens edge

Profile

The edge profile may be a key factor in the success or otherwise of a particular contact lens design. Rigid lens edge design and profile have a direct impact on lens comfort (LaHood, 1988). A well-formed smooth rounded edge is accepted by patients in terms of comfort, and departures from a comfortable edge profile can lead to discontinuation of lens wear. A sudden change in lens comfort could be attributed to surface scratches or chipping of the lens edge.

The edge profile of rigid lenses can be checked using a projection magnifier and graticule (Henry and Barr, 1990). It is of paramount importance to check the lens edge for any sharp regions or roughness and deal with the problem before dispensing to the patient. Caroline and Norman (1991), using a simple aid for microscopic examination of the lens edge (Figure 15.12), established five descriptive categories of rigid lens edge defects. The edge categories were 'square', 'thick', 'sharp', 'rolled inwards' and 'rolled outwards'.

Detecting and correcting lens edge defects should enhance both patient acceptance and confidence. Ehrmann and Schindhelm (1999) developed a sophisticated non-invasive lens edge profile analytical tool. A narrow infrared laser beam is directed on to the surface of the lens close to the edge. The incident angle is altered in a controlled manner to map the surface of the lens from front to back over the edge. A general profile of the boundary is established by monitoring the periphery at specific loci over the lens circumference. Thus, the edge profile can be graphically illustrated, mathematically analysed and checked for overall quality. If the circumferential analysis of the lens edge proves to be unacceptable the lens can either be returned to have the edge reworked or discarded.

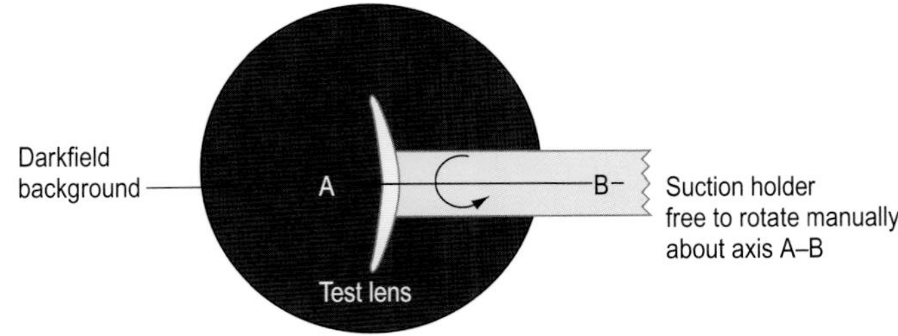

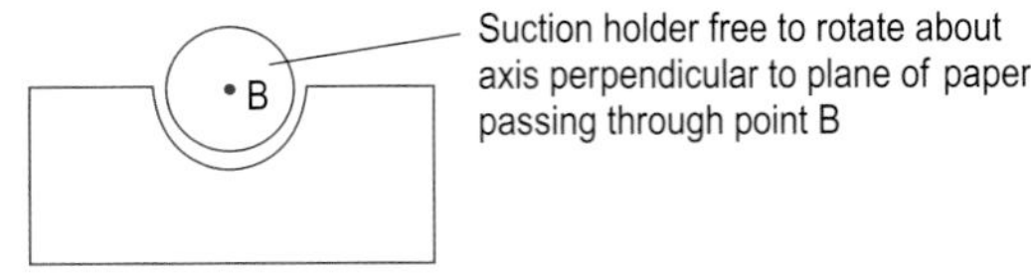

Figure 15.12 Lens edge profilometry.

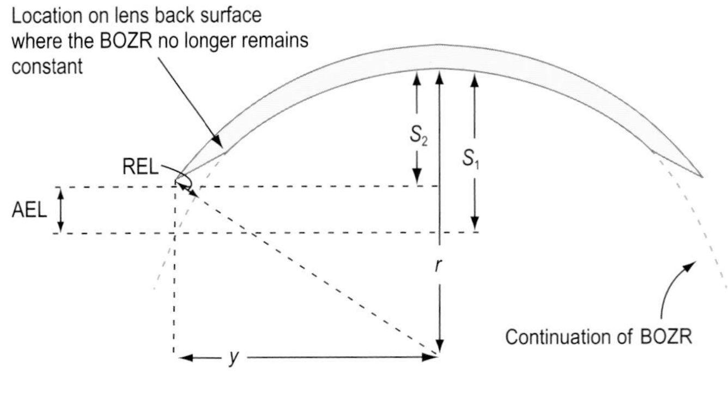

Figure 15.13 The form of the edge of a rigid lens can be defined in terms of either axial edge lift (AEL) or radial edge lift (REL). This nomenclature applies to all lens powers and designs. BOZR = back optic zone radius.

Edge lift

Certain lens-fitting philosophies are based on the concept of edge lift or clearance. Figure 15.13 summarizes the various parameters used to describe edge lift. Edge lift is the distance between a point on the edge of the lens back surface and the circular continuation of the back optic zone.

With reference to Figure 15.13, the edge lift can be calculated from the basic geometry of the lens surface as follows:

$$\text{REL} = \sqrt{\left[(r - s_2)^2 + y^2\right]} - r \qquad \text{(Equation 15.1)}$$

$$\text{AEL} = (s_1 - s_2), \text{ where } s_1 = r - \sqrt{(r^2 - y^2)} \qquad \text{(Equation 15.2)}$$

where REL is radial edge lift and AEL is axial edge lift. Measuring the overall sag of a finished lens, namely s_2, allows both the axial and radial edge lift to be derived. However, the error in both derivations is dependent upon errors in r and y. The likely magnitude of the final error can be estimated using partial differential equations for the two expressions. For example, consider a lens of BOZR 7.7 mm and OD 10 mm. If the respective errors in r, y and s_1 were ±0.015 mm, ±0.1 mm and ±0.01 mm, then it can be shown that the errors in REL and AEL would be ±0.053 mm and ±0.071 mm. These figures represent the precision in the determination of REL and AEL.

Alternatively, for AEL, the sag of a monocurve lens of identical BOZR and OD could be used to measure s_1 directly in an attempt to improve precision. The lens may be placed on a glass plate, and using a travelling microscope, s_2 could be measured (Pearson, 1990). The exact shape and dimensions of the lens edge profile will affect the estimation of edge lift.

Douthwaite and Hurst (1998) developed an attractive 'pillar and collar' device that avoids the physical problem caused by the lens edge but still uses a travelling microscope to measure s_2. The lens is supported with minimal effort - without physically touching the edge - as shown in Figure 15.13. The device could be easily adapted to assist, for example, in checking the angles of adjacent zones in multicurve lenses, or evaluating the transition in scleral lenses. The device could be extended to measure the apical height of the back central optical zone over more than one chord diameter. Such measurements could then be used to estimate the asphericity of continuous curve lenses as described elsewhere (see Chapter 8, Equation 8.4).

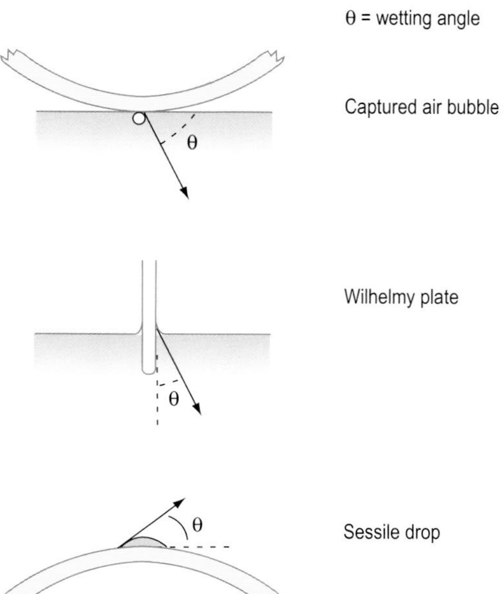

Figure 15.14 Techniques for assessing lens wetting angles.

Lens surface

Surface quality

The quality of the surface of a rigid lens can be evaluated using a projection microscope. Rigid lenses should be inspected for the presence of irregularities such as scratches, scuff marks and overpolishing, prior to lens dispatch. Scanning electron microscopy is a high-resolution method for checking the integrity of a lens surface but it is destructive. An optical interference phase microscope can be used as an easier, less expensive and non-destructive alternative (Merindano *et al.*, 1998).

Surface wetting

A stable uniform tear film over the surface of a rigid lens is required to maintain good stable vision. A surface with poor wetting characteristics will break up the pre-lens tear film, creating sources of light scatter, which will impair optical transmission and hence visual quality. High-oxygen-permeability (*Dk*) silicone-based lens materials have intrinsically poor wetting properties. The wettability of the surfaces of lenses made from these materials can be improved using a variety of manufacturing and chemical techniques. Lens surface wetting properties are measured using a variety of techniques, including the captured air bubble, Wilhelmy plate and sessile drop methods (Fatt, 1984) (Figure 15.14). The contact angle between the test surface and fluid can also be measured using laser-assisted techniques (Bush *et al.*, 1988).

These are laboratory procedures, and the clinical value of the data generated is questionable. Clinicians are interested in wetting *in vivo*, not *in vitro*. The friction from high-speed polishing may singe the surface and thus affect wettability. Chemical conditioning solutions may improve lens wettability *in vitro* (Knick and Huff, 1991) but not necessarily *in vivo*. Placing the lens on the eye and checking the stability of the pre-lens tear film using a tear break-up test is a useful *in vivo* clinical measure of lens wetting. The Keeler Tearscope can assess lens wettability quantitatively and allow the clinician to categorize the structure of the pre-lens tear film (Guillon *et al.*, 1995).

Flexibility

It is beneficial to make a rigid lens as thin as possible to improve comfort and maximize oxygen performance; however, thinner lenses tend to be more flexible (Harris *et al.*, 1982; Lydon and Guillon, 1984). Flexure affects lens performance *in vivo*; therefore, it is a parameter that needs to be monitored and controlled. The extent to which a strip of material will either extend or shorten when a force is applied to the material can be predicted using Young's modulus. This is a universally accepted method for quantifying lens materials; however, it does not help the clinician gauge how a finished lens will perform in relation to its thickness variation. Thin, rigid lenses made from high-*Dk* materials tend to flex after a short period of patient use. Also, spherical lenses fitted to toric corneas to neutralize corneal astigmatism can gradually assume a toric form that matches the corneal toricity, thus reducing the efficacy of the lens.

Fatt (1987) investigated the forces required to induce lens flexure by measuring the change in apical height of a finished lens as the diameter was reduced in a centripetal fashion. The lens was placed in an annular holder with a built-in mechanism to reduce the diameter of the annulus in a controlled manner while monitoring apical height. A relatively simple, clinically useful method for assessing lens flexibility and the effects of flexure on lens power has been described by Patel *et al.* (1988). Using a simple vertical-bracketing column supporting the lens (Figure 15.15), the change in diameter of the lens along a particular axis was measured using a travelling microscope as specific weights were added to the lens. The change in diameter was directly related to both lens material and power.

Material

There are many physicochemical techniques for identifying contact lens materials. The contact lens practitioner needs a quick, reproducible, non-destructive and non-hazardous way of identifying contact lens materials. This can be achieved by checking lens refractive index and/or specific gravity (SG).

Refractive index

Refractometers are commonly used to measure the refractive index of solids and liquids. In the case of solids, the sample material should have a flat surface, which is placed in contact with the refractometer measuring prism. A suitable contact fluid can be used to facilitate the measurement when the surface is irregular. It may not be desirable to place the contact fluid on the finished lens because it may prove difficult to remove. By placing the convex surface of the lens on to the measuring prism and applying gentle digital pressure, the surface will flatten slightly and create an area of contact sufficient for measurement. This has been attempted with success using a hand-held refractometer, with a precision of ±0.001 (Model N3000 Refractometer, Atago, Japan). Traditional polymethyl methacrylate has a relatively high refractive index of 1.49 whereas fluorosilicone acrylates tend to have refractive indices lower than 1.458. Many of the silicone acrylates and fluorosilicone acrylates have refractive indices between 1.458 and 1.469 (Tranoudis and Efron, 1998). Cross-checking the measured refractive index with published tables will help you identify the material of your lens. Most refractometers, as mentioned in Chapter 8, are prone to subjective errors. An automated refractometer suitable for contact lenses has been developed to overcome some of the difficulties associated with more tradional refractometers (Index Instruments, Huntingdon, UK).

Specific gravity

The SG of a material is a ratio defined as its density divided by the density of water (thus, the SG of water is unity). If a lens is placed in a saturated saline solution, it will float on condition that the SG of the lens is less than that of saturated saline (1.197). Adding distilled water to the saline reduces the SG, and the lens will sink when the SG falls below the SG of the lens material. By adding saturated saline to the solution the SG will gradually increase and the lens will start to float again. At this point, no more saline is added. The SG of the lens material is the same as the SG of the surrounding saline. Using a hygrometer, the SG of the saline - and hence that of the lens material - is measured, and the material is identified using a table. This simple technique, which is referred to as densitometry, is dependent upon ambient conditions and is limited by the available range of SG of the saturated immersion fluid (Arce *et al.*, 1999). Alternatively, the SG of the lens can be quickly estimated by placing the lens in a range of different strengths of either saline or calcium chloride solution (Refojo and Leong, 1984). Both are suitable immersion media for rigid lens material identification.

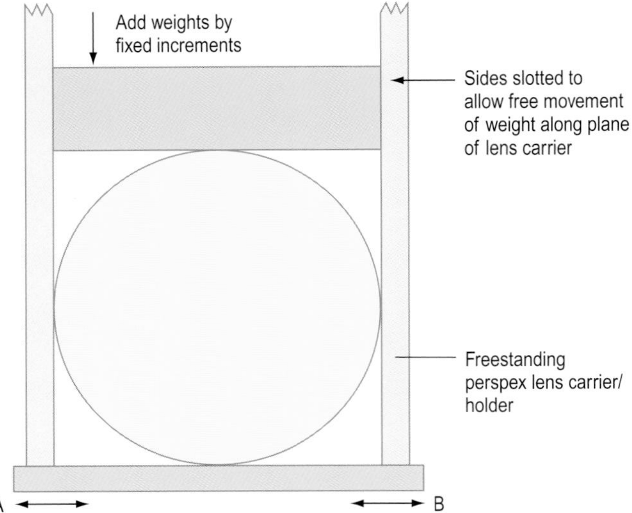

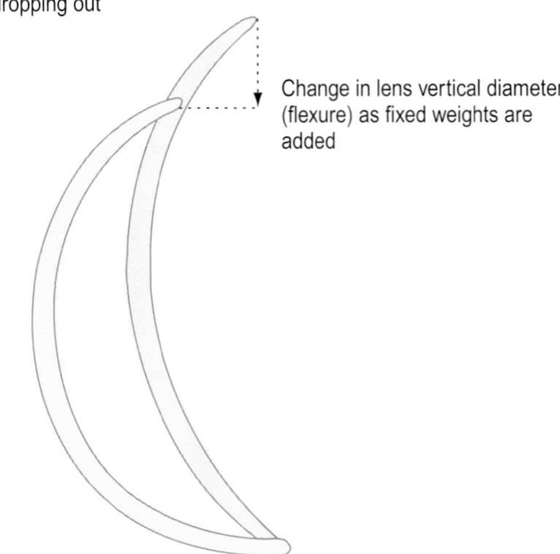

Figure 15.15 Apparatus for assessing the flexibility of a finished rigid lens.

Tint

There are several laboratory techniques, such as spectrophotometry, for checking and identifying optical tints. In practice, a simple qualitative check can be made using either a projection magnifier or observing the lens on the eye with a slit-lamp biomicroscope. Non-light-transmitting cosmetic lenses are best checked using a loupe or slit-lamp biomicroscope.

Conclusion

There are many simple tests that a clinician can incorporate in a routine practice environment. Details regarding reproducible measurements, tolerances, precision and features of the major contact lens-specific tests and instruments are noted in various British and international standards. It would appear that current tolerance limits for rigid lenses may allow the apical tear layer thickness to differ significantly from that intended but the edge fit may still be acceptable. While the full specifications of a rigid lens should be verified prior to its supply to a patient, it is particularly important to measure the BOZR and desirable to measure the BOZD, to ensure that resultant apical tear layer thickness is acceptable (Pearson, 2008). Rigid lens tolerances are summarized in Appendix B.

References

Arce, C. G., Schuman, P. D. and Schuman, W. P. S. (1999) Qualitative identification of RGP contact lens materials by densitometry. *Contact Lens Assoc. Ophthalmol. J.*, **25,** 204–208.

Biddles, B. J. (1969) A non-contacting interferometer for testing steeply curved surfaces. *Optica Acta,* **16,** 137–157.

Bush, J., Huff, J. W. and MacKeen, D. (1988) Laser-assisted contact angle measurements. *Am. J. Optom. Physiol. Opt.,* **65,** 722–728.

Caroline, P. J. and Norman, C. W. (1991) RGP edge analysis and modification. *Contact Lens Spectrum,* **6,** 39–49.

Dietze, H. H., Cox, M. J. and Douthwaite, W. A. (2003) Verification of aspheric contact lens back surfaces. *Optom. Vis. Sci.,* **80,** 596–605.

Douthwaite, W. A. and Hurst, M. A. (1998) Validating a 'pillar and collar' technique for measuring the edge lift of rigid contact lenses. *Optom. Vis. Sci.,* **75,** 208–216.

Ehrmann, K. E. and Schindhelm, K. (1999) A novel method to quantify the edge contour of RGP contact lenses. *Contact Lens Ant. Eye,* **22,** 19–25.

Fatt, I. (1984) Contact lens wettability. Myths, mysteries and realities. *Am. J. Optom. Physiol. Opt.,* **61,** 419–430.

Fatt, I. (1987) Flexure of hard contact lenses: An old problem with a new twist. *Contax,* September, pp. 12–16.

Fatt, I. and Ruben, C. M. (1994) A simple formula for calculating the harmonic average oxygen transmissibility of an optically powered RGP contact lens. *J. Br. Contact Lens Assoc.,* **17,** 115–118.

Garner, L. F. (1981) A simple interferometer for hard contact lenses. *Am. J. Optom. Physiol. Opt.,* **58,** 944–950.

Guillon, M., Crosbie-Walsh, J. and Brynes, D. (1987) Application of pachometry to the measurement of rigid contact lens edge profiles. *J. Br. Contact Lens Assoc.,* **10,** 16–22.

Guillon, M., Guillon, J-P., Shah, D. *et al.* (1995) In vivo wettability of high Dk RGP materials. *J. Br. Contact Lens Assoc.,* **18,** 9–15.

Harris, M. G., Kadoya, J., Nomura, J. A. *et al.* (1982) Flexure and residual astigmatism with Polycon and PMMA lenses on toric corneas. *Am. J. Optom. Physiol. Opt.,* **59,** 263–266.

Henry, V. A. and Barr, J. T. (1990) Verification, modification and care. *Contact Lens Spectrum,* **5,** 57–67.

Knick, P. D. and Huff, J. W. (1991) Effects of temperature and conditioning on contact lens wetting angles. *Contact Lens Assoc. Ophthalmol. J.,* **17,** 177–180.

LaHood, D. (1988) Edge shape and comfort of rigid lenses. *Am. J. Optom. Physiol. Opt.,* **65,** 613–618.

Lattimore, M. R., Kaupp, S., Schallhorn, S. *et al.* (1999) Orbscan pachymetry: implications of a repeated measures and diurnal variation analysis. *Ophthalmology,* **106,** 997–998.

Lydon, D. P. M. and Guillon, M. (1984) Effect of central thickness variation on the performance of RGP contact lenses. *Am. J. Optom. Physiol. Opt.,* **61,** 23–30.

McMonnies, C. W. (1998) Key factors for radiuscope measurement accuracy including an improved lens mounting design. *Int. Contact Lens Clin.,* **25,** 158–165.

Merindano, M. D., Canals, M., Saona, C. *et al.* (1998) Rigid gas permeable contact lens surface roughness examined by interferential shifting phase and scanning electron microscopies. *Ophthal. Physiol. Opt.,* **18,** 75–82.

Patel, S., Kinsey, A. C. E., Brown, R. A. *et al.* (1988) The influence of power and material on the flexibility of RGP lenses. *Optician,* March 4, pp. 39–42.

Pearson, R. M. (1990) Measurement of axial edge lift of rigid corneal lenses. *Clin. Exp. Optom.,* **73,** 172–177.

Pearson, R. M. (2008) Rigid gas permeable lens tolerance limits and their possible effect on mode of fit. *Clin. Exp. Optom.,* **91,** 379–384.

Port, M. J. A. (1987) Measurement of rigid lens diameters. *J. Br. Contact Lens Assoc.,* **10,** 23–26.

Refojo, M. F. and Leong, F. (1984) Identification of hard contact lenses by their specific gravity. *Int. Contact Lens Clin.,* **11,** 179–182.

Tranoudis, I. and Efron, N. (1998) Refractive index of rigid contact lens materials. *Contact Lens Ant. Eye,* **21,** 15–18.

Woods, C. A. (2003) Verification of the vertex powers of varifocal rigid contact lenses. *Cont. Lens Anterior Eye,* **26,** 181–187.

16 CHAPTER

Rigid lens design and fitting

Graeme Young

Introduction

Fitting rigid lenses is an improbable achievement. Essentially it involves constructing a complex three-dimensional structure to sit, without the aid of any supplementary adhesive, on a vertically inclined surface while being repeatedly dislodged by a covering structure. Fortunately, the task is made easier by a number of mitigating factors:

- The lids help to prevent the lens falling from the eye.
- The change in curvature at the limbal junction helps prevent sideways drift.
- The capillary forces in the pre-lens tear film are usually strong enough to hold the lens in place but weak enough to avoid adherence.

On the other hand, a number of factors can make rigid lens fitting difficult:

- No two eyes have precisely the same dimensions.
- The worse the refractive error, the less predictable the fit.
- Reflex tearing during adaptation can alter the lens fit.
- Rigid lenses can be very uncomfortable, no matter how good the fit.

The fit of a rigid lens is affected by a range of factors, many of which are not easily quantifiable, such as corneal and limbal anatomy, lid geometry and mechanics, and extraneous factors such as pterygia. As a result, many practitioners consider rigid lens fitting to be more of a craft than a science. There is, therefore, a wide variation in competence between practitioners, which primarily relates to experience. Practitioners new to rigid lens fitting can benefit greatly in the initial stages from being overseen by a more experienced colleague.

Ocular topography

A number of ocular dimensions are relevant to the selection of rigid lenses. These are summarized in Table 16.1, along with typical population variations. Precise measurement of each of these dimensions is not essential to successful rigid lens fitting; however, for a given patient, it is helpful to assess whether the eye is close to average or atypical, for instance, whether the corneal diameter is larger or smaller than average.

Cornea

The cornea is generally aspheric in shape and is frequently described as ellipsoid (Kiely *et al.*, 1982). In most cases, a corneal section can be approximated to a prolate ellipse; that is, one that gradually flattens towards the periphery. Conventional keratometers give readings corresponding to points approximately 1.5 mm either side of the corneal apex. Given that corneas with similar keratometer readings (K-readings) can show widely differing peripheral curvature (asphericity), keratometry alone does not always indicate the optimum rigid lens fit.

The degree of corneal asphericity is often expressed as either corneal eccentricity or corneal shape factor. With eccentricity (e) a spherical surface equals zero while a flattening ellipse equates to a positive value. Shape factor (SF) is a function of eccentricity, whereby:

$$SF = 1 - e^2$$

Using shape factor, a spherical surface equals 1.0, a flattening ellipse is <1.0, while a steepening ellipse is >1.0.

With-the-rule astigmatic corneas are steeper in the vertical meridian and are generally easier to fit than against-the-rule astigmatic corneas on which rigid lenses tend to show sideways decentration. With-the-rule astigmatic corneas often show greater corneal astigmatism in the inferior cornea compared to the superior cornea. As a rule of thumb, 1.00 D of corneal astigmatism corresponds to a difference in K-readings of approximately 0.2 mm. The peripheral cornea tends to show less toricity than the central cornea (Read *et al.*, 2006).

There is no correlation in the population between corneal asphericity and central corneal curvature (Guillon *et al.*, 1986). However, there is a correlation between K-readings and corneal diameter such that larger corneas tend to be flatter in curvature while smaller corneas tend to be steeper (Mandell, 1989). Also, there is a correlation between

DOI: 10.1016/B978-0-7506-8869-7.00016-1

Table 16.1 Ocular dimensions and typical population variations

	Mean (mm)	±2 SD (mm)
Flattest corneal curvature* – keratometry	7.85	7.35–8.35
Corneal shape factor*	0.85	0.55–1.15
Corneal diameter†	12.9	11.7–14.1
Horizontal visible iris diameter†	11.6	10.6–12.6
Palpebral aperture‡	10.1	7.9–12.3

SD = standard deviation.
* (Guillon *et al.*, 1986)
† (Martin and Holden, 1982)
‡ (Fonn *et al.*, 1996)

asphericity and the degree of myopia; higher myopes show less peripheral corneal flattening consistent with the longer axial length of the myopic eye (Carney *et al.*, 1997b).

The cornea is invariably larger in the horizontal meridian than in the vertical. It is not easy to measure the true diameter of the cornea due to the gradual change in transparency at the limbus. In practice, the width of the visible iris (horizontal visible iris diameter, HVID) is used as a gauge of corneal diameter. The HVID is approximately 1.2 mm smaller than the actual corneal diameter (Martin and Holden, 1982). Corneal diameter influences the choice of lens diameter. The typical variation in corneal diameter of 1.5 mm (Table 16.1) is mirrored by a similar typical variation in rigid lens diameter, that is, 8.30–9.80 mm.

Lids

The lower lid usually aligns with the lower limbus while the upper lid tends to cover the limbus and overlap by approximately 1 mm. Both of the eyelids help to position the lens high enough to cover the pupil and, in many cases, the lens is effectively passed from one lid to the other between blinks.

The maximum vertical distance between the lids (palpebral aperture) is generally measured prior to fitting. Smaller palpebral apertures tend to require smaller-diameter lenses; however, the relationship of the lids to the superior and inferior limbus is also relevant, and therefore there is no simple relationship between palpebral aperture and optimum lens diameter. Rigid lens wear itself can cause a reduction in palpebral aperture. Fonn *et al.* (1996) noted that the palpebral aperture in rigid lens wearers is, on average, 0.5 mm smaller than that in soft lens wearers.

When the upper lid is relatively high, the lens tends to decentre low and a large-diameter lens is often required to encourage the upper lid to grip the lens and hold it in place; this is known as lid attachment. A relatively low upper lid and narrow palpebral aperture tends to result in upwards decentration (Carney *et al.*, 1997a).

In cases where the lower lid is positioned higher than the limbus, a smaller lens may be required. On the other hand, when the lower lid is low or ineffective due to ectropion, a large-diameter lens is often required, again to encourage lid attachment.

There is a correlation between palpebral aperture and corneal diameter. Larger corneas, as well as being relatively flat, tend to be accompanied by a wider palpebral aperture.

Ethnic variations in ocular dimensions

Some ethnic variations in ocular topography have been noted in the literature. In the UK-resident Chinese population, corneas have been noted to be steeper and smaller and to show less corneal flattening than Caucasian eyes (Lam and Loran, 1991). This suggests a requirement for smaller rigid lenses showing less peripheral flattening for such patients. In a study of an American Japanese population, eyes were also found to show, on average, a smaller HVID but no difference in corneal curvature (Matsuda *et al.*, 1992). It is likely that environmental factors, such as nutrition, as well as ethnic differences influence corneal topography and probably account for the mean flattening in corneal curvature noted in the Japanese population over a 20-year period (Hirotsuji, 1990). As expected, oriental eyes tend to show a narrower palpebral aperture: on average, about 1.0 mm smaller than Caucasian eyes (Lam and Loran, 1991).

There is less information on ethnic variations in Afro-Caribbean populations, although there is some evidence that these corneas tend to be larger and flatter than corneas of Chinese or Japanese populations (Babalola and Szajnicht, 1960).

Forces acting on the rigid lens

A number of forces act on the rigid lens and have to be suitably balanced in order to achieve a satisfactory fit (Figure 16.1). The gravitational force of the lens and pre-lens tear film causes the lens to drop. The effect will be greater, and the lens less stable, the further forwards the centre of gravity lies. The centre of gravity is further forward in plus lenses compared with minus lenses (Figure 16.2). It is shifted posteriorly by increasing the diameter, steepening the back optic zone radius (BOZR), or decreasing the thickness of the lens. With both plus and minus lenses, the greatest shift and most effective stabilization are achieved through changing the lens diameter (Carney and Hill, 1987).

The lens is held in place by the capillary forces in the post-lens tear film and the surface tensional force in the tear meniscus at the lens edge. The capillary force increases with increasingly closer alignment of the lens and the cornea. The force is therefore greater with spherical corneas compared with astigmatic corneas. Figure 16.3 shows the change in apparent alignment with increasing astigmatism.

Surface tension forces act at the lens edge where the edge meniscus is not covered by the lid. There will be no surface tension where a meniscus is absent due to excessive edge clearance. This force can be increased by reducing edge clearance and edge thickness (Khorassani and Peterson, 1988).

Eyelid forces (primarily the upper lid) act to move the lens in a vertical direction during the blink. Between blinks, these forces help to stabilize the lens in the case of a lid attachment fit but have no effect in the case of an interpalpebral fit.

Rigid lens design

Back optic zone diameter

The back optic zone diameter (BOZD) is usually fixed for a given design in a given total diameter (TD) and is generally

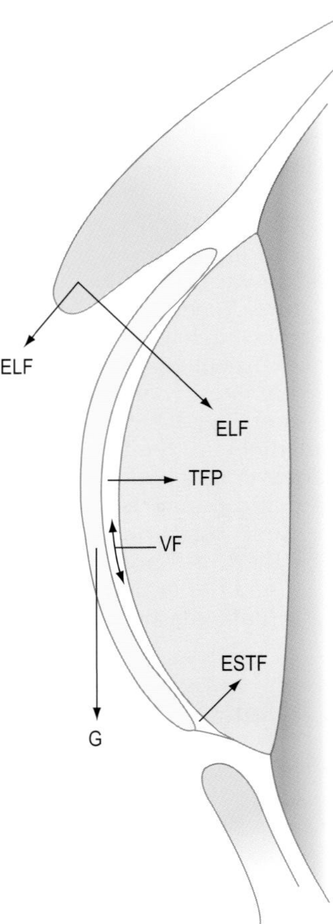

Figure 16.1 Forces acting on a lid-attached rigid lens. ELF = eyelid force; ESTF = edge surface tension force; G = gravity, TFP = tear fluid pressure; VF = viscous forces. (Adapted from Guillon, M., Sammons, W. A. (1994) Contact lens design. Chapter 5. In: Contact Lens Practice, Ed: Ruben, M. and Guillon, M. G. London, Chapman & Hall Medical, pp. 87–112.)

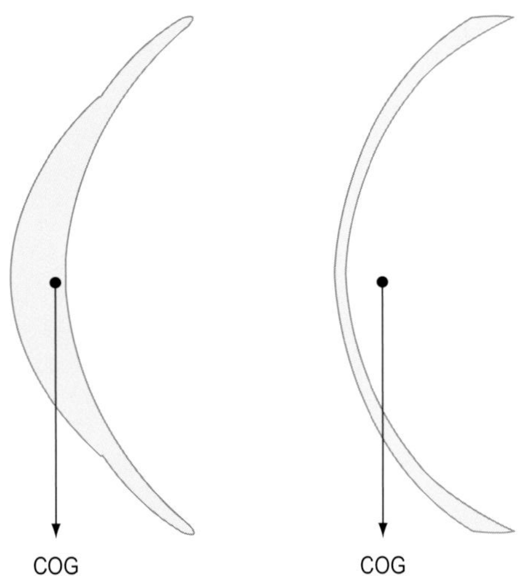

Figure 16.2 Rigid lens centre of gravity (COG) in a plus (left) and minus (right) power lens.

1–1.5 mm smaller than the TD. The BOZD should be large enough to cover the pupil in most conditions, including low illumination.

With toroidal corneas, using a smaller BOZD can increase the area of alignment and therefore improve the fit. However, if the BOZD is reduced while maintaining the same TD, this results in a wider periphery and flatter peripheral curves are required in order to maintain edge clearance.

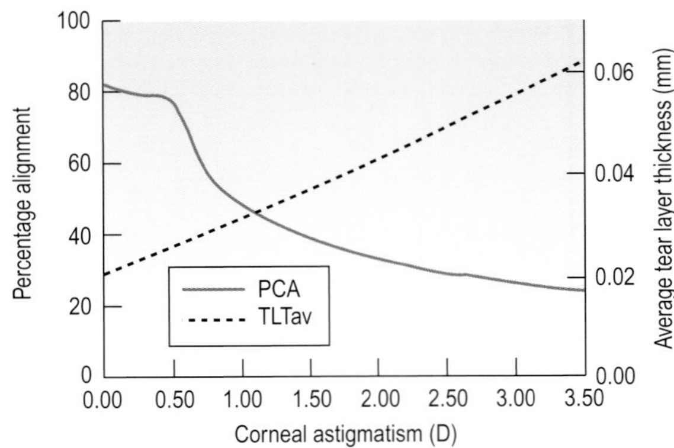

Figure 16.3 Apparent percentage corneal alignment (PCA) and average tear layer thickness (TLTav) with increasing corneal astigmatism.

If the BOZD is changed, it is usually necessary to change the BOZR in order to maintain a clinically equivalent fit. Reducing the BOZD without reducing the BOZR results in a sagittal depth that is more shallow and therefore a flatter fit. As a rule of thumb, an increase in BOZD of 0.5 mm requires an increase in BOZR of 0.05 mm.

Front optic zone diameter

The front optic zone diameter (FOZD) should be at least 0.5 mm larger than the BOZD. Except in low powers, most rigid lenses are lenticulated to reduce thickness and weight.

Lenses occasionally incorporate a negative carrier in order to encourage lid attachment and to centre the lens. A negative carrier is a peripheral zone that is thinner at the optic zone junction than the lens periphery. A positive carrier or tapered-edge design – where the peripheral zone is thicker at the optic zone junction than the lens periphery – is occasionally used to discourage lid attachment in a high-riding lens.

Centre thickness

If lenses are made too thin, not only is there a greater risk of breakage but the lenses tend to flex on astigmatic corneas, leaving residual astigmatism. Since flexure is a function of lens thickness, it is worse with low-minus-powered lenses. For a given family of materials flexure tends to increase with increasing *Dk*. It is therefore necessary to increase lens centre thickness with higher-*Dk* materials. Table 16.2 gives suggested centre thickness values for lenses of varying power.

Edge lift and edge clearance

Without a peripheral gap between the edge of the lens and the cornea, mechanical pressure leads to superficial corneal

Table 16.2 Suggested centre thicknesses

Lens power (D)	Centre thickness (mm)
−1.00	0.18
−2.00	0.17
−3.00	0.16
−4.00	0.15
≥−5.00	0.14

Add 0.02 mm for corneal astigmatism ≥2.00 D.

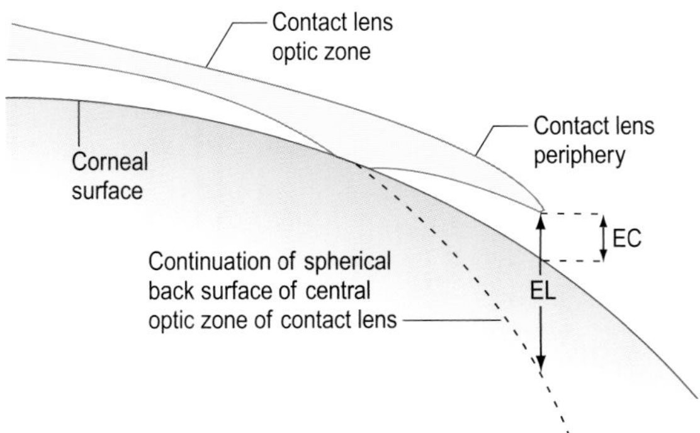

Figure 16.4 Axial edge lift (EL) and edge clearance (EC).

damage. Such a gap is also important for tear exchange and to enable lens removal using the lids. This gap is termed the edge clearance and can be specified axially or radially. A minimum axial edge clearance of 60–80 μm when the lens is centred is considered to be the optimal value (Atkinson, 1987).

While edge clearance relates to the lens and cornea, edge lift relates to the lens only (Figure 16.4).

Some rigid lens designs follow a concept of constant edge lift throughout the range of BOZRs; however, this tends to result in greater edge clearance at the flatter end of the range. A superior design is one that gives constant edge clearance for corneas of similar asphericity. Constant edge clearance designs based on those proposed by Guillon *et al.* (1983) are given in Appendix H.

Edge form

The shape of the lens edge is one of the most important factors in minimizing any discomfort. Poor edge rounding, in particular, can result in greater edge awareness by the upper eyelid. Good rounding of the front surface edge has been shown to be more important than rounding of the posterior edge (La Hood, 1988). This suggests that the interaction of the edge of the lens with the eyelid is more important in relation to comfort than the interaction with the cornea. Figure 16.5 shows examples of edge shapes.

Spherical versus aspheric designs

A wide variety of surface shapes have been used in rigid lenses. These can be broadly categorized as: spherical,

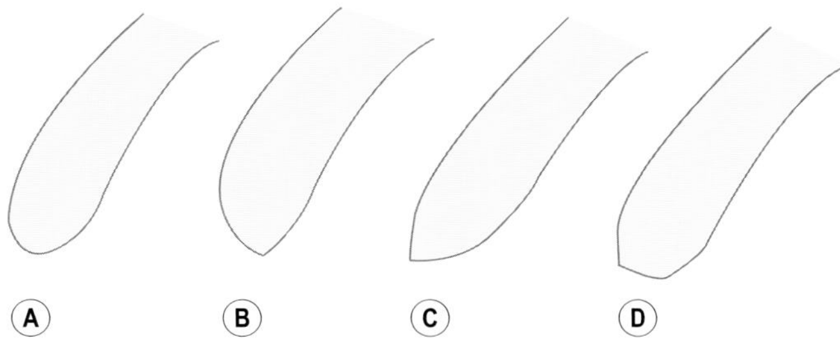

Figure 16.5 Rigid lens cross-sections showing variations in edge form. (A) Well-rounded edge; (B) sharp posterior edge; (C) sharp anterior edge; (D) flat edge.

Table 16.3 Advantages and disadvantages of aspheric versus spherical rigid lenses

	Spherical	Aspheric
Manufacture	Relatively easy	Easy with computer-controlled lathes Not easy with conventional lathes
Verification	Easy	Difficult
Induced astigmatism	None	Small amount with decentration
Presbyopic correction	None	Small amount
Corneal alignment	Adequate	Slightly greater
Edge clearance	Usually 80–120 μm	Usually 60–90 μm
Back surface junctions	Can be a problem if not blended	Rarely a problem
Thickness	Can be minimized by lens design	Thinner periphery possible
Comfort	Slight to moderate discomfort	Sometimes better due to reduced thickness and edge clearance

aspheric or a combination of the two, e.g. spherical centre with aspheric periphery. An aspheric back surface design is theoretically capable of providing better alignment to the cornea (which is aspheric), although there are a number of advantages and disadvantages to both types (Table 16.3).

Spherical designs

Spherical designs incorporating a spherical back optic zone with a number of flatter spherical peripheral zones are the most widely used and readily understood form of rigid lens. The peripheral zone is generally 1–2 mm in width and composed of one to four peripheral curves. Tricurve designs (i.e. a central curve plus two peripheral zones) are probably the most commonly used lens form. Bicurve designs are occasionally used with small lenses (e.g. <8.5 mm). Tetracurve and other multicurve designs are used with larger lenses or where a smoother transition is required between the peripheral zones.

The front surfaces of most spherical designs are bicurve, incorporating an optic zone slightly larger than the BOZD and a front-surface peripheral zone. The curvature of the optic zone is governed by the required lens power and that of the peripheral zone governed by the edge thickness, the power and FOZD of the lens; these parameters are invariably calculated by the manufacturing laboratory. Monocurve front-surface designs (single-cut) are occasionally used in small, low-power lenses but most lenses are lenticulated (i.e. made with a thinner peripheral zone) in order to reduce mass and overall thickness. Multicurve front-surface designs are occasionally used with higher-power lenses in order to reduce peripheral thickness.

Aspheric designs

From a mathematical point of view, the choice of spherical geometry is almost arbitrary since the sphere is merely one of an infinite number of conic sections. As noted earlier, few if any corneas are spherical in shape and therefore a spherical back surface is not the obvious choice. However, aspheric rigid lenses have two important disadvantages compared with spherical lenses: (1) they are more difficult to manufacture, particularly using conventional lathes; and (2) they cannot easily be checked using a radiuscope or keratometer. Nevertheless, they offer a number of advantages which arguably outweigh their disadvantages (Table 16.3).

The main advantages of aspheric designs relate to comfort. Aspheric designs tend to show less edge clearance and therefore induce less edge sensation from contact with the palpebral conjunctiva. Poor blending of back-surface junctions in spherical lenses can cause irritation on version when the lens moves off-centre and the peripheral zones come into contact with the cornea. This is generally avoided with aspheric lenses unless the periphery is poorly blended. The gradual flattening of aspheric lens surfaces results in a thinner periphery which may also help reduce edge sensation.

Optically, aspheric designs can both improve and degrade image quality. When not aligned with the visual axis, aspheric lenses will induce astigmatism. On the other hand, with higher-power lenses, aspheric optics can reduce spherical aberration. In myopic early presbyopes, the reduced minus power in the periphery of aspheric lenses can help with near vision and delay the need for a presbyopic correction.

Aspheric designs take different forms but these differences are usually so subtle as to be evident only from the product literature of the manufacturer. The simplest aspheric design is an elliptical shape selected to be close to, or slightly flatter than, the average cornea. More complex aspheric designs change their degree of flattening (or eccentricity) from centre to edge. Some designs are spherical in the centre, changing to aspheric geometry towards the periphery. Most aspheric designs incorporate a much flatter, often spherical, peripheral zone about 0.2 mm wide. This peripheral zone helps to avoid mechanical irritation when the lens decentres to the peripheral cornea.

PMMA versus RGP lens design

Given the risk of corneal exhaustion syndrome and other chronic hypoxic effects of the cornea, there is little or no justification for fitting polymethyl methacrylate (PMMA) lenses (Sweeney, 1992). However, it is useful to have an appreciation of differences in design between non-gas-permeable PMMA lenses and rigid gas-permeable (RGP) lenses so that, when PMMA lenses are being refitted, these differences can be taken into account. Because of the reliance on transfer of oxygen through the tears to the post-lens cornea, PMMA lens designs generally incorporate a wider and flatter periphery. This results in a narrower optic zone and greater edge clearance (Khorassani and Peterson, 1988). In comparison, RGP lens designs usually incorporate the following features:

- larger TD
- larger BOZD
- narrower periphery
- steeper peripheral curves (resulting in less edge clearance).

Trial fitting options

The conventional method of fitting rigid lenses is by way of reusable trial lenses, although other options such as empirical fitting can also be used. With the theoretical risk of transmission of prion disease by contact lenses the use of trial lenses has been questioned, although Hogan (2003) showed the chance of obtaining prion disease through contact lens use to be negligible.

Trial fitting set

Most rigid lens fitting is still undertaken using trial (or diagnostic) lens fitting sets in a range of BOZRs and TDs. A set of lenses in a given trial fitting set generally follows a single design concept, for instance, constant edge clearance.

Lenses in a standard trial fitting set are typically available in a single diameter and back vertex power (BVP) with a range of BOZRs in 0.1 mm steps; however, it is preferable to use fitting sets that have lenses available in two diameters (e.g. 9.2 and 9.8 mm). Examples of additional useful fitting sets include:

- Plus power, e.g. +3.00 D, smaller diameter.
- High minus, e.g. –8.00 D, larger diameter.
- Small diameter for interpalpebral fitting, e.g. 8.6 mm.
- Keratoconic, diameter varying with BOZR.

Sodium hypochlorite (Milton) in 20 000 ppm solution has been suggested as an effective method of disinfecting rigid trial lenses.

Empirical fitting

A high degree of success can be achieved by empirical fitting, i.e. ordering initial lenses based on keratometry and refraction. In one study, 91% of eyes were successfully fitted by this method (Back *et al.*, 1996).

Most contact lens laboratories will supply lenses on a per-case basis, that is, a fixed cost for an unlimited number of lens exchanges for a given patient until a final satisfactory fit is obtained. This is an attractive option, especially in avoiding concerns about cross-infection. Notwithstanding such concerns, there are occasions when most practitioners would wish to use this method, for example when wishing to fit a design not covered by an available fitting

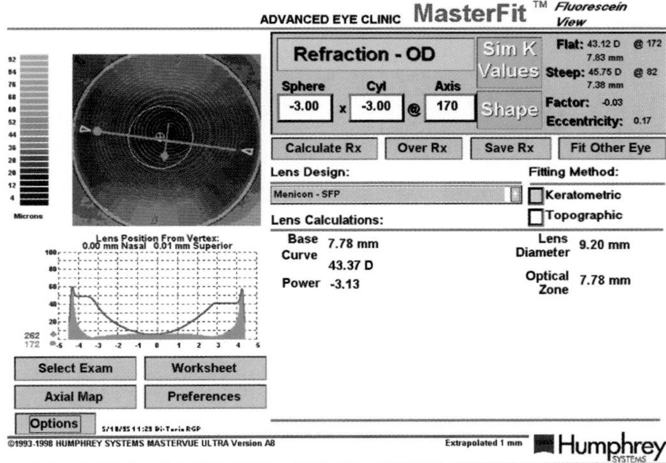

Figure 16.6 An example of videokeratoscope rigid lens fitting software.

set or when an initial trial fitting is simply not convenient for the patient.

Videokeratoscopic fitting

Most videokeratoscopy (VK) instruments incorporate rigid lens fitting software (Figure 16.6). This enables practitioners to model different rigid lenses designs on an accurate representation of the cornea of the patient (Caroline *et al.*, 1994). The fitting success rates are relatively low when relying solely on using the default settings of the VK instrument manufacturer, but can be relatively high (77–93%) when an experienced practitioner uses the software to select an appropriate lens (Jani and Szczotka, 2000).

Most VK instruments use a Placido disc image reflected from the cornea which is automatically measured and interpreted to produce corneal topography maps or videokeratograms. These maps can be presented as power maps or corneal contour maps. From the point of view of rigid lens fitting, contour maps are the most useful. Conventionally, steeper parts of the cornea are presented as 'hotter' colours, e.g. red, orange (see Chapter 4). With-the-rule astigmatism corneal maps show a vertically oriented 'bow-tie' pattern. Keratoconic corneas show a rapid change in colour (or curvature) near the corneal apex.

The main advantages of VK contour maps in rigid lens fitting are that they:

- Indicate whether the corneal apex is decentred.
- Show atypical corneal shapes, e.g. extremes of corneal asphericity.
- Allow the practitioner to monitor changes in corneal shape.
- Allow virtual trial fitting of rigid lenses.

There is an apparent trend for rigid lens fitting to be used more for specialist fits (Morgan and Efron, 2008), in which case VK contour maps are likely to prove increasingly useful. The obvious limitation of VK contour maps in trial lens fitting is that they fail to take into account the influence of the lids.

Table 16.4 Guidelines for the initial selection of a rigid lens

A. Selection of lens total diameter

HVID (mm)	Small PA <9.5 mm	Average >10.7 mm	Large PA
<11.2	8.2	8.6	9.2
11.2–11.6	8.6	9.2	9.6
11.6–12.0	9.2	9.6	10.0
>12.0	9.6	10.0	10.0

HVID = horizontal visible iris diameter; PA = palpebral aperture.

B. Selection of lens back optical zone radius (BOZR)

Lens diameter (mm)	BOZR (mm)	BVP (D)
8.2	K–0.05	S
8.6	K–0.05	S–0.25*
9.2	K–0.05	S–0.25*
9.6	K–0.05	S–0.25*
10.0	K	S

BVP = back vertex power; K = flattest K-reading; S = vertex-corrected sphere from minus-cylinder spectacle prescription.
* Add –0.25D.

Selection of initial lenses

Trial fitting set

The procedure for selecting an initial fitting of spherical lenses using a trial fitting set is as follows:

1. Select a lens diameter based on corneal diameter, palpebral aperture and lid configuration (Table 16.4).
2. Select the BOZR based on flattest keratometer (K) reading, adjusting the BOZR to be flatter or steeper than K depending on BOZD. Since relatively steep-fitting lenses are easier to visualize with fluorescein, err on the steep side.
3. If more than one power is available, select a lens power closest to the refraction of the patient.

Empirical fitting

The procedure for empirical fitting of spherical lenses is as follows:

1. Select a lens diameter based on corneal diameter, palpebral aperture and lid configuration (Table 16.4).
2. Select the BOZR based on flattest K-reading (K), adjusting the BOZR to be flatter or steeper than K depending on BOZD. Flatter radii tend to be used with larger BOZD and vice versa.
3. If the lens is an average diameter, select the BVP based on the sphere power from the refraction (minus cylinder form) corrected for vertex distance. With an average-diameter lens, no adjustment is necessary; however, an adjustment is necessary if the BOZR is steeper or flatter than K.

4. Order the lens and use this effectively as a trial fitting lens, being prepared to modify or reorder before dispensing.

Lens insertion, removal and settling

Lens insertion

Whether the initial lens is selected empirically, by VK or from a trial fitting set, it is necessary to assess the lens on the eye. With experienced rigid lens wearers, having the patient insert the lens enables the practitioner to assess the patient's technique. Some patients fall into bad habits such as licking lenses or inserting them on to the sclera. With new patients, it is preferable for the practitioner to insert the lenses rather than adding to the patient's anxiety.

Before inserting the first lens in new wearers, it is helpful to prepare the patient for some initial discomfort, to advise that this will recede and to suggest that any discomfort will be minimized by looking downwards. Anxiety may also be reduced by explaining that any discomfort will be to the eyelid rather than the eye itself, which will be unaffected. Applying wetting solution to the lens before insertion will tend to make the lens more comfortable and transfer more readily to the eye, but avoid applying more than a small drop as too much can make fluorescein assessment more difficult.

To minimize initial discomfort in new wearers the use of a topical anaesthetic has been advocated. By reducing reflex lacrimation it is possible that a more accurate assessment of lens fit may be made. Although still controversial, Bennett *et al.* (1998) showed that the use of a topical anaesthetic at the fitting and dispensing visits for first-time wearers of rigid lenses resulted in significantly fewer drop-outs, improved initial comfort and gave an enhanced perception of the adaptation process and greater overall satisfaction after 1 month of lens wear.

To insert a rigid lens:

1. Ask the patient to fixate a distant object to steady the eyes.
2. Place the lens on the index finger of the hand that will be holding the patient's bottom lid.
3. Hold the patient's top lid using the index finger or thumb of the other hand (Figure 16.7A). If this proves difficult, have the patient first look down until the lid is securely held.
4. Hold the bottom lid using the middle finger of the hand holding the lens (Figure 16.7B) and place the lens directly on to the centre of the cornea (Figure 16.7C).
5. Release the bottom lid but continue to hold the top lid and ask the patient to look down.
6. At this point, the lens is often quite comfortable. Warn the patient that once you let go of the lid, the patient will be more aware of the lens.

If the lens locates on to the sclera, the lens will probably not be uncomfortable. Have the patient look in the opposite direction to where the lens is located, e.g. upwards if the lens is located on the lower sclera. With two fingers, manipulate the lens towards the cornea using the lids (Figure 16.8). If this proves difficult, remove the lens using the patient's lids or a suction holder.

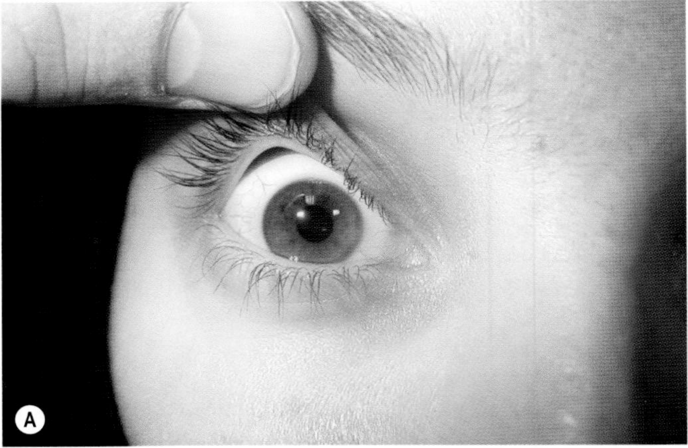

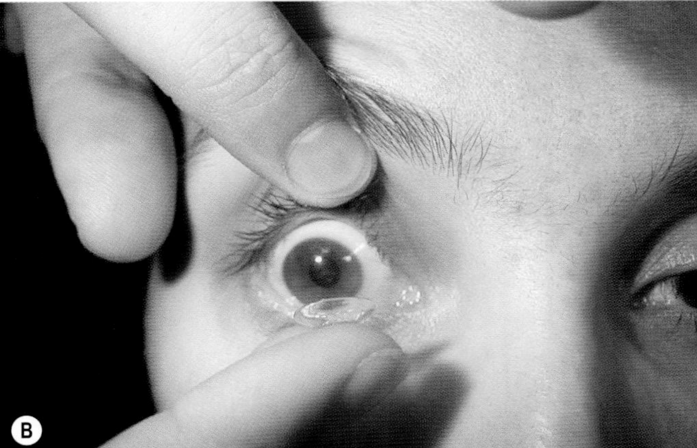

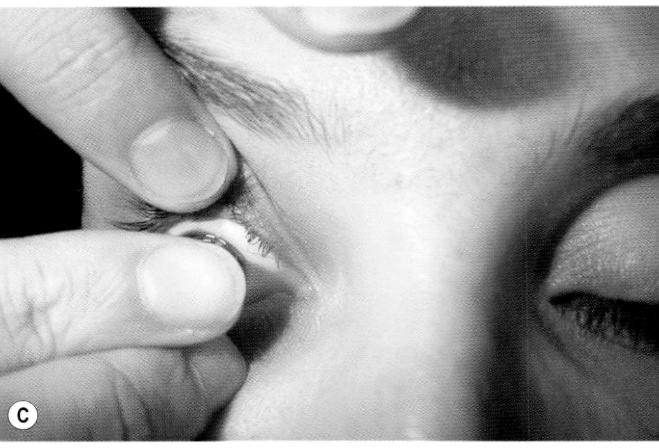

Figure 16.7 Inserting a rigid lens. (A) Direct the gaze of the patient straight ahead. Restrain the patient's upper eyelid with your left thumb or forefinger. (B) With the lens on the forefinger of your right hand, move the lens in close to the cornea, and retract the inferior eyelid with the middle finger. (C) Touch the lens to the centre of the cornea, then gently release the lids and ask the patient to blink gently.

Lens removal

To remove a rigid lens:

1. Place the index fingers of each hand on the lids of the patient above and below the centre of the lens (Figure 16.9A).
2. If necessary pull the lids apart in order to position the lid margins at the lens edges.

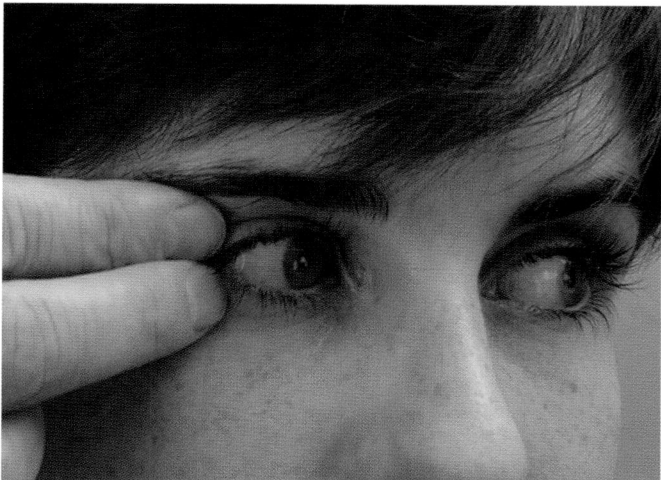

Figure 16.8 Repositioning a mislocated rigid lens.

3. Gently press the eyelid margins on to the eye and towards each other (Figure 16.9B).
4. The lens may then be grasped and removed (Figure 16.9C).

Settling time

With new wearers, the patient's initial reaction to rigid lenses is useful and can give an indication of how easily the individual will adapt to rigid lens wear. Clearly, those showing little or no lacrimation and who are able to move the eyes without apparent discomfort are the most promising candidates. In these cases, the lens fit can be assessed immediately. However, in most cases, it will be necessary to wait 5–10 min for any lacrimation to subside. This period can be used to discuss aspects of the process, such as costs and hygiene and to answer any questions.

In a few cases it may be some time before lacrimation subsides enough to allow examination. It is necessary, however, to consider other possible reasons for the discomfort. This might be due to a foreign body attached to the lens (the tears usually clear any loose foreign bodies) or, alternatively, the fit might be so poor as to be causing some mechanical trauma to the cornea or conjunctiva. Having ruled out other causes of discomfort, it might be necessary to give a longer settling period, e.g. 10–30 min. It is better that the patient does not leave the practice during this period.

Lens fit characteristics

Optimum lens fit

A well-fitting rigid lens will centre in such a way that the pupil is fully covered by the optic zone while the eye is open. The lens should position within the limbal boundary. In the case of a lid attachment fit, the lens edge will be positioned under the top lid, whereas with an interpalpebral fit, the lens will be positioned between the lids. Also, lenses are occasionally designed with thicker edges incorporating a negative carrier in order to encourage lid attachment and lens centration. The requirements of a well-fitting rigid lens are summarized in Table 16.5.

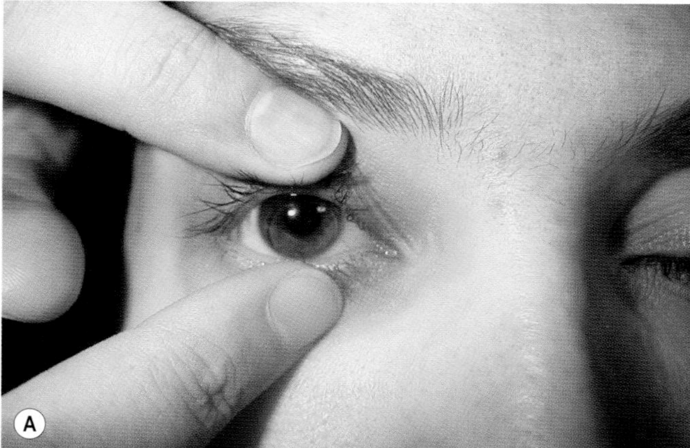

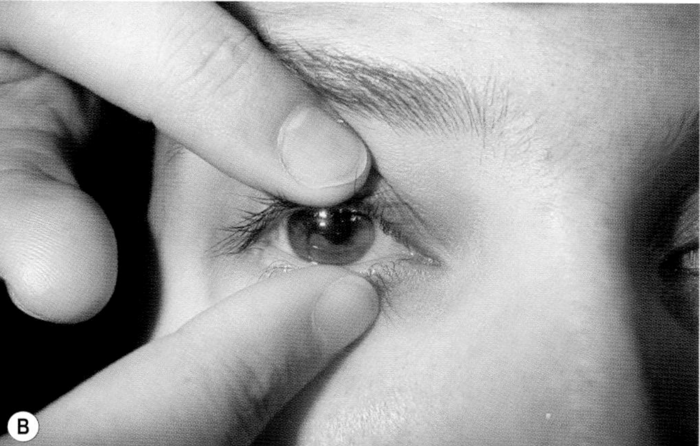

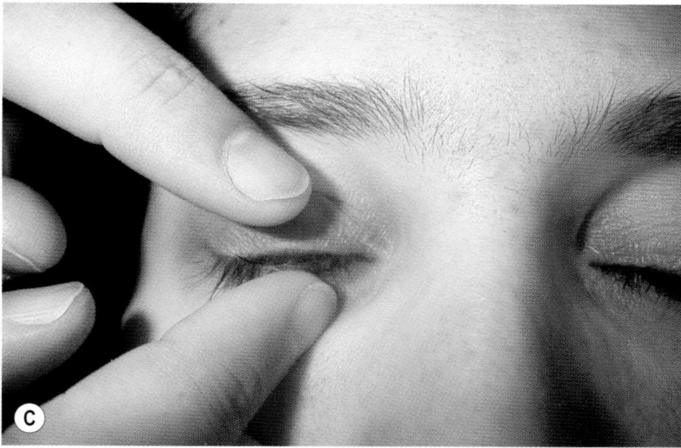

Figure 16.9 Removing a rigid lens. (A) Place the forefingers of each hand on the lids of the patient above and below the centre of the lens. (B) If necessary move the eyelids slightly apart in order to position the lid margins at the lens edges. Gently press the eyelid margins on to the eye and towards each other. (C) The lens may then be grasped and removed by the practitioner.

Satisfactory lens fit

A lens with less than optimum fitting may drift downwards between blinks, but not so fast as to disrupt vision or irritate the bottom lid or lower limbus. It will move vertically with a blink, being first pushed as far as the lower limbus and then lifted by the lid almost to the upper limbus. In the case of with-the-rule astigmatism, the lens will pivot along the horizontal meridian or, if there is apical clearance, at the

Table 16.5 Requirements of a well-fitting rigid lens

Requirement	Importance	Relevant rigid lens parameters
Comfort	Patient satisfaction	Edge thickness, Edge form Edge clearance Back surface junctions
Good centration	Corneal coverage Stable peripheral vision	Edge clearance BOZR Diameter
Movement on blink or version	Adequate post-lens lubrication Avoidance of lens adherence Supply of oxygen (low-*Dk* materials)	Diameter
Constant pupil coverage	Stable vision	BOZD
Adequate corneal alignment	Avoidance of excessive mechanical pressure	BOZR
Optimum edge clearance	Avoidance of mechanical disruption Comfort Avoidance of 3 and 9 o'clock staining	Peripheral curve radii Peripheral curve width

BOZR = back optical zone radius; BOZD = back optical zone diameter.

edge of the optic zone at the 3 and 9 o'clock corneal locations (Caroline *et al.*, 1994).

Assessment of lens fit

There is a temptation to assess rigid lens fitting purely in terms of whether the lens is steep or flat; however, this approach fails to consider other aspects of rigid lens fit. In particular, when new to rigid lens fitting, it is helpful to work through the following checklist of fitting characteristics:

- TD
- centration
- movement
- central fit
- edge clearance.

There is also a tendency to assess rigid lenses only in one position. However, during normal wear, rigid lenses move to all positions on the cornea and it is therefore necessary to assess the lens in a variety of positions, where necessary manipulating the lens through the lids to move it to different corneal locations. In particular, it is important to assess the peripheral fit of the lens when it decentres along the flattest meridian, e.g. at 3 and 9 o'clock in with-the-rule astigmatism.

Hand-held ultraviolet (UV)-illuminated magnifiers (Burton lamps) can be used for the assessment of rigid lens fit and have the advantage of allowing the patient to maintain normal head posture. This type of assessment is also relatively quick and allows the two eyes to be easily compared. On the other hand, the magnification is not good enough to evaluate some important aspects of fit, such as edge clearance. For this reason alone, slit-lamp evaluation is the method of choice for properly assessing rigid lens fit.

Some rigid lens materials contain a UV inhibitor that absorbs wavelengths corresponding to that emitted by Burton lamps, making fluorescein evaluation impossible. The blue filters on most slit lamps have a wider spectral range, which overcomes this problem.

White light assessment of fit

The position of the lens may change when fluorescein is added to the tear film. To avoid this confounding influence, the lens should first be assessed in white light prior to the instillation of fluorescein. It is necessary to ensure that the illumination setting of the slit-lamp biomicroscope is not so bright as to induce reflex tearing or an aversion reflex that could cause the patient to adjust lid position.

Diameter

The lens should appear to be the appropriate size for the eye. With a relatively small lens, problems will tend to arise from decentration. The lens may fail to cover the cornea through sitting high or resting on the bottom lid. It may also be less comfortable because of greater interaction between the upper lid margin and the lens edge. Alternatively, the lens may irritate the bottom lid by dropping between blinks.

Lenses that are larger than the palpebral aperture can result in problems through interacting with the bottom lid as well as the top lid. In some cases, the lens will be pushed into a high-riding position by occasional interaction with the bottom lid, while in other cases the lens may rest on the bottom lid.

Centration

The lens diameter may appear to be appropriate for the corneal diameter and palpebral aperture but nevertheless show some decentration. The position of the lens between blinks is important. Some decentration may be acceptable if the optic zone maintains pupil coverage, but this may also indicate poor central or peripheral fit. Flat-fitting lenses, for example, can show decentration in any direction, depending on factors such as lid position or tightness.

Movement

All rigid lenses, however steep, show some movement. The task, therefore, is to assess the extent, speed and direction of movement. This should be observed in normal primary gaze. Sluggish, limited postblink movement may indicate a relatively steep-fitting lens. Fast movement sometimes indicates a flat-fitting lens but may also be due to strong interaction with the top lid, perhaps due to excessive edge clearance.

In addition, it is sometimes useful to retract the lids and observe the lens moving under gravity alone. Hold the lids apart and manoeuvre the lens upwards. On releasing the lens, it should drop slowly. If the lens shows less movement without the influence of the lids, this would suggest excessive lid interaction. A true flat-fitting lens often shows downward movement in an arcuate direction.

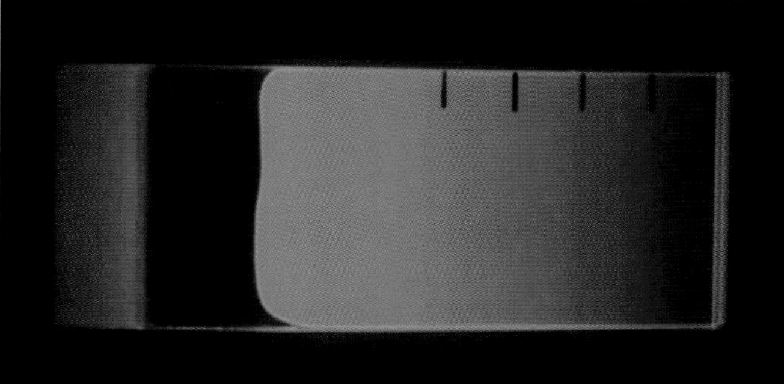

Figure 16.10 Fluorescein wedge. Two converging glass plates are filled with fluorescein; the plates are touching at the right side of the wedge.

Peripheral fit

Instances of markedly excessive edge clearance can be observed with white light. The peripheral tear meniscus may be absent, particularly in the steeper meridian. In severe cases, this results in bubbles forming behind the lens, which in turn can lead to dimple staining. Patients also tend to find such lenses uncomfortable due to excessive interaction with the sensitive lid margins.

Fluorescein assessment of fit

Interpretation of fluorescence

Fluorescein sodium is soluble in water. It absorbs most light in the blue part of the spectrum but most of its emitted light is in the yellow part of the spectrum with some in the green. The intensity of light emitted is governed by the concentration and pH of the solution, and, critically in rigid lens fitting, the thickness of the fluorescein sample. The effect of concentration and thickness of fluorescein can be analysed using wedges of fluorescein (Figure 16.10). At the thinner end of the wedge, fluorescein is not visible until a critical thickness of about 15 μm is reached. The intensity can be seen to increase towards the thicker end of the wedge until another critical thickness of about 60 μm is reached, beyond which the fluorescein is seen as a uniform bright yellow colour (Young, 1988).

In rigid lens fitting, the fluorescein pattern is a simple two-dimensional representation of a complex three-dimensional shape. This provides useful information about the relationship of the lens with the shape of the eye. Areas of tear pooling appear bright yellow. Where the tear layer is absent or extremely thin, there is no visible fluorescence and the area appears dark blue or black. Between these extremes, varying thicknesses of post-lens tear film are seen in varying intensities of yellow/green. Fluorescein therefore provides a contour map of the thickness of the tear film.

Fluorescein instillation

As noted earlier, excessive fluorescein will disrupt the lens fit and it is therefore best to instil a minimal amount, preferably from a fluorescein strip. Placing a drop of fluorescein on the superior sclera will maximize the length of time the dye remains in the eye. In particularly sensitive patients, the process can be simplified by touching the fluorescein strip against the front of the lens.

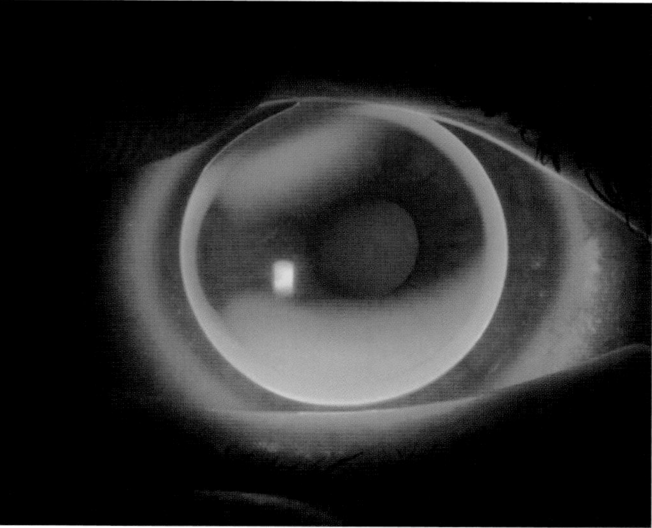

Figure 16.11 Assessing central fluorescein fit having centred the lens and retracted the top lid.

A thick fluorescein-stained pre-lens tear film may confound interpretation of the true post-lens fluorescein pattern (the object of interest), so it may be necessary to wait till this has dissipated before assessing the pattern.

Three primary annular regions of the fluorescein fit should be evaluated systematically: the central fit, peripheral fit and edge clearance. In the case of a tricurve lens, these three annular zones essentially correspond to the three back surface zones of the lens. It is important to note areas showing no fluorescence as well as those that do.

Central fit

If the lens is half covered by the top lid, or the lens is decentred, it may not be possible to observe the central fit without retracting the lid and repositioning the lens. This is achieved by gently holding the top and bottom lids with the index finger and thumb respectively (Figure 16.11). The lids can be used to manoeuvre the lens into a central position and also to pump extra fluorescein beneath the lens.

The fluorescein pattern for well-fitting lenses will vary according to corneal asphericity and astigmatism. As one would expect, spherical corneas show the simplest fluorescein patterns. The optimum fit is one that shows central alignment or just a trace of fluorescein indicating minimal central clearance.

With astigmatic corneas, in the steeper meridian the central fluorescein pattern will show increasing thickness towards the edge. The most recognizable fluorescein pattern is the 'dumbbell' pattern seen with spherical lenses on astigmatic corneas (Figure 16.11); however, the pattern varies according to the:

- Asphericity of the cornea (Figure 16.12).
- Amount of corneal astigmatism (Figure 16.13).
- Lens design.
- Fitting relationship, i.e. whether the lens is relatively steep or flat.

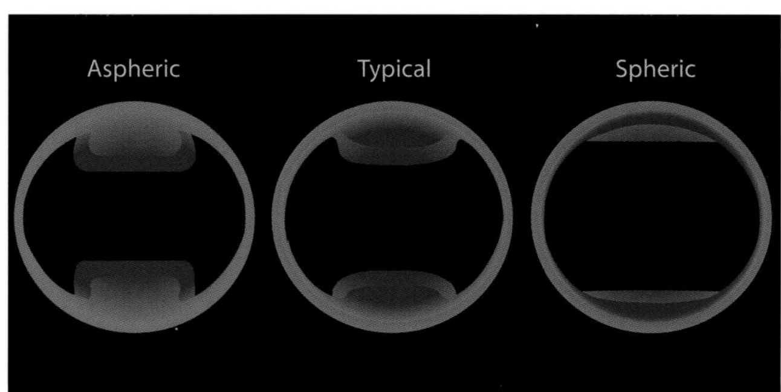

Figure 16.12 Typical fluorescein pattern with well-fitting lens on astigmatic (1.00 D) corneas of similar K-readings but varying corneal asphericity (corneal shape factors = 0.60, 0.85 and 1.10).

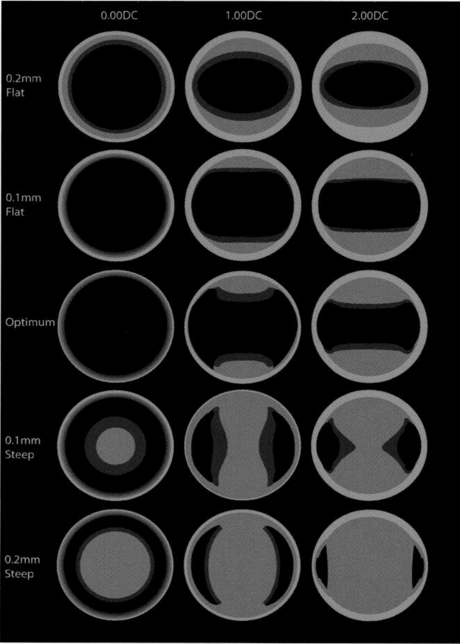

Figure 16.13 Fluorescein patterns of rigid lens of varying back optic zone radius on with-the-rule corneas of varying astigmatism.

With steep-fitting lenses, fluorescein assessment will show a central pool of fluorescein. This pool will appear brighter the steeper the fit. In extreme cases, an air bubble may be present.

With flat-fitting lenses, central touch will be visible as an area of dark blue or black. The flatter the fit, the smaller the area of touch. Fluorescein will be present in the mid-periphery and may be continuous with the peripheral band of fluorescein.

Mid peripheral fit

Spherical lenses, particularly on astigmatic eyes, make contact with the cornea at the edge of the optic zone. If the lens is poorly blended or makes contact at a sharp angle, it may be uncomfortable and cause epithelial disruption. If a narrow line of contact between optic zones can be seen upon lens inspection, it is likely that there is a sharp junction from poor blending. A band of contact corresponding to the first peripheral zone may indicate relatively steep peripheral curves and the need for peripheral lens flattening.

In the case of a flat-fitting lens, the mid peripheral band of fluorescein may merge with that of the central zone, even in the flattest meridian.

Edge fit

The width and the brightness of the peripheral band of fluorescein give an indication of the extent of edge clearance. Where the edge clearance is small, the tear film thickness may be less than the critical thickness above which the fluorescein appears a saturated yellow colour. This is generally less than the desired clearance of 80 μm or more. A less-than-bright yellow peripheral ring therefore indicates suboptimal edge clearance. This will be confirmed by an apparent break in the peripheral band of fluorescein when the lens decentres towards the limbus.

In the case of excessive edge clearance, bubbles may be seen forming under the lens periphery. The peripheral band may also be wider than expected and show the saturated yellow appearance over much of the peripheral band.

Overrefraction

Measuring the overrefraction during a rigid lens trial fitting not only helps to determine the final lens power but also gives an indication of whether the optimum fit has been obtained. An unexpected overrefraction suggests that either the lens is wrongly labelled or that the fit is not perfect. The steeper the lens fit, the more minus power will be required in order to compensate for a relatively plus-powered tear lens. Variable vision may indicate a decentred or flat-fitting and relatively mobile lens fit.

Rigid lens fitting problems

Decentration

Poor centration is more common with higher levels of astigmatism. In the case of with-the-rule astigmatism, the decentration tends to be upwards (Figure 16.14), while in the case of against-the-rule astigmatism, it tends to be sideways.

Decentration can be investigated as follows:

1. Check whether the central fit is relatively flat. A change in BOZR of 0.05 or 0.10 mm is unlikely to have much effect on centration; however, larger changes than this may make a critical difference.
2. Check that the edge clearance and edge thickness are not excessive and resulting in undue lid influence. In particular, this is often the case with a high-riding lens.
3. Assuming no fundamental errors in fit, the next approach is to consider an increase in overall diameter and optic zone diameter. The lens may still show some decentration but this is acceptable so long as there is pupil coverage by the optic zone.
4. If the decentration is deemed to be due to corneal astigmatism, consider refitting with a back surface toric design (see Chapter 17).

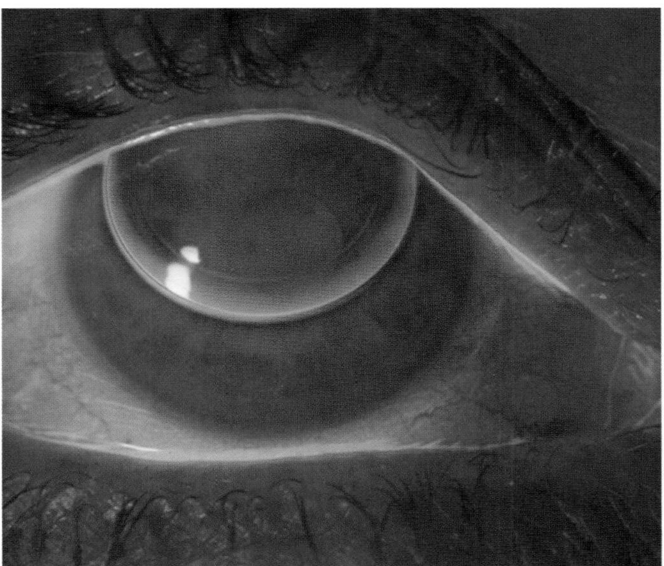

Figure 16.14 High-riding rigid lens.

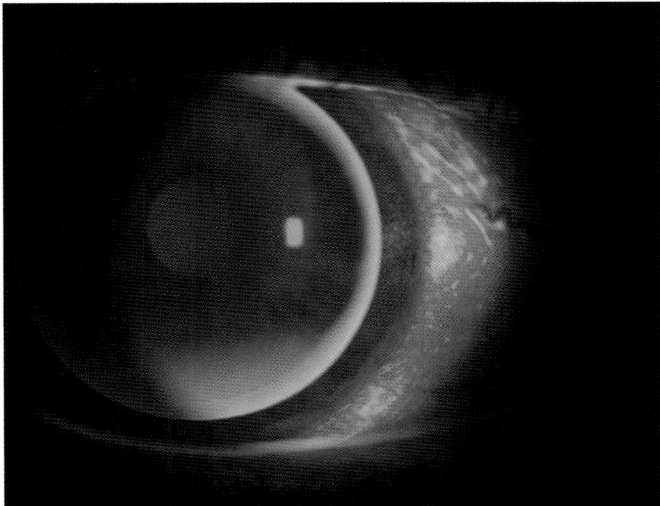

Figure 16.15 Mild 3 and 9 o'clock staining (shown here in the 3 o'clock location).

Peripheral corneal desiccation

The appearance of 3 and 9 o'clock corneal staining can arise due to either mechanical trauma or, more commonly, desiccation. The extent of staining does not correlate with patient symptoms (van der Worp *et al.*, 2009). Some minimal 3 and 9 o'clock desiccation staining is considered acceptable; however, coalescent or widespread staining can lead to vascularization, scarring and corneal thinning (dellen) – conditions that often require remedial attention. The characteristic appearance of 3 and 9 o'clock staining is a triangular shape delineating those areas not wetted by the action of the upper lid. The apex of the triangle corresponds to the location of the widest part of the lens (Figure 16.15). Research suggests that the incidence of 3 and 9 o'clock

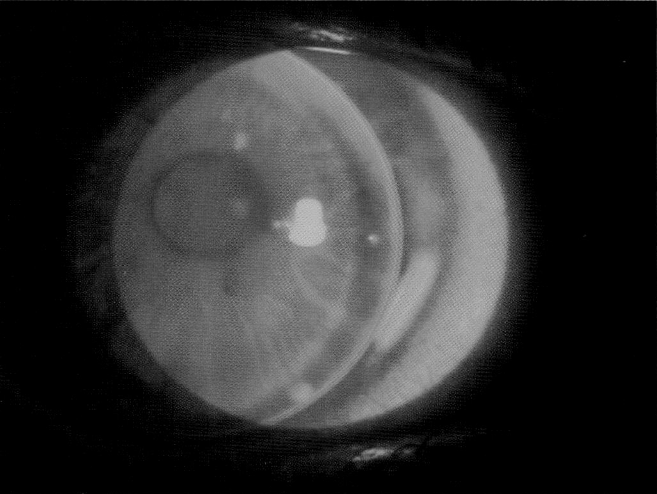

Figure 16.16 Poor edge clearance with a rigid lens with resultant confluent staining.

staining is lower with larger lenses (>9.5 mm) incorporating a moderately wide tear reservoir (Schnider *et al.*, 1997).

A number of factors can contribute to 3 and 9 o'clock desiccation staining:

- infrequent blinking
- poor tear quality
- inferior lens decentration
- excessive lid clearance due to lens edge clearance or edge thickness (Schnider *et al.*, 1996).

A diverse range of possible treatment options has been proposed to overcome this type of staining (van der Worp *et al.*, 2003). The following are the most useful options:

- Encourage blink awareness if the patient demonstrates partial or infrequent blinking.
- Modify the lens to reduce edge thickness.
- Blend the back surface junctions, if appropriate, to reduce edge clearance.
- Refinish the lens edge to reduce the diameter and therefore reduce edge clearance.
- Redesign the lens to reduce edge clearance.
- Increase the diameter, incorporating a wide peripheral band.
- Refit with soft lenses – this can be surprisingly successful even when tear film quality is a contributing factor.

Peripheral corneal mechanical trauma

Desiccation 3 and 9 o'clock staining can be mistaken for mechanically induced staining resulting from poor edge clearance. A lens may show adequate edge clearance when centred but exert mechanical pressure when decentred towards the limbus. On examination of the fluorescein fit, the staining coincides with an arcuate area of contact (Figure 16.16). This problem may be remedied as follows:

- Modify the existing lens to increase edge clearance, assuming that the lens periphery is thick enough.
- Redesign the lens with increased edge clearance.

Substantial changes in peripheral curve radii are required to effect a significant change in edge clearance (Young, 1998). For instance, with a 9.5 mm diameter tricurve design, flattening both peripheral curves by 0.25 mm is required to achieve a minimal significant change in edge clearance of about 10 μm.

Discomfort

The most common reason for discontinuing rigid lens wear is discomfort. The description of symptoms offered by (or elicited from) the patient can be helpful in determining the cause of the problem, such as whether the discomfort arises from the cornea, palpebral conjunctiva or lid margin; whether it arises from symptoms of dryness, edge sensation or mechanical pressure on the cornea; or whether it is connected with any particular activity or environment.

Possible modifications to rigid lens designs that might improve comfort include:

- Reblending the back surface optic zone transitions.
- Re-rounding and/or thinning the edges.
- Reducing edge clearance by reducing the TD.
- Increasing the TD.
- Refitting with an aspheric design.

The first three of the strategies described above can be undertaken by modifying an existing lens as opposed to making a new lens. Such modifications can be undertaken in the practice if suitable equipment is available; however, lens modification requires some skill (Phillips, 2007) and most practitioners prefer to instruct a lens laboratory to undertake such tasks.

If the problem can be alleviated by modification, redesign or some change in lens wearing habits, then clearly these steps should be followed. However, after taking such actions and allowing for a reasonable period of adaptation to rigid lens wear, some patients report that the discomfort remains unacceptable. Such patients may never adapt to comfortable rigid lens wear and other options should be considered, the obvious one being a change to soft lenses. Alternatively a hybrid lens design may be preferable in the case of an irregular cornea.

Poor or unstable vision

The accepted tolerances in rigid lens manufacture are relatively wide. Because errors in BOZR and BOZD as well as BVP affect the refractive correction, a rigid lens can be within tolerance but still under- or overcorrect by nearly 1.00 D. In this case, an overrefraction will bring the visual acuity back to normal. If, however, the vision quality is still poor, the following factors should be considered:

- poor surface wetting – if new, the lens may not have been sufficiently hydrated
- optical distortion – occasionally waves in the polymer or on the surface of the lens can disturb vision. These can be observed by cleaning the lens and looking through it with the naked eye
- surface scratches – can usually be polished out of the lens
- surface deposits – normally removable with a surface cleaner, particularly an abrasive surface cleaner.

Variable vision can arise either through inadequate pupil coverage (small BOZD or decentration) or poor surface quality (scratches, deposits or poor wetting).

Lens loss

Rigid lens wearers who do not have spare lenses are at a disadvantage compared with most soft lens wearers for whom the loss of an occasional disposable lens is not a problem. The repeated loss of a rigid lens may relate to the lens design. Tight lids combined with generous edge clearance can result in a lens being flipped out of the eye. Aside from optimizing the edge clearance, increasing the lens diameter can also help to make lenses more secure. In the case of significant corneal astigmatism, it may also be necessary to consider a back surface toric design.

Practitioners should be cognizant of the fact that reports of lost lenses may be due to the lens becoming mislocated and sometimes embedded beneath the upper eyelid, unknown to the patient. Numerous reports have appeared in the literature describing this phenomenon, the most astonishing being that of Kelly (1994), who described the case of a female patient who had reported losing numerous rigid lenses over a 3-month period. A mucus-coated pellet was eventually removed from beneath her upper eyelid: this comprised eight PMMA lenses and one rigid gas-permeable lens.

Conclusion

Although most lenses prescribed today are soft lenses, there is still a role for rigid lenses. Advances in lens material technology have enabled rigid lenses that interfere minimally with ocular physiology. In some cases of poor corneal optics, rigid lenses are the only optical solution short of keratoplasty. However, as has been demonstrated above, rigid lenses are far less forgiving than soft lenses in terms of fitting characteristics and comfort. Successful rigid lens fitting therefore demands patience, careful patient management and good skill levels on the part of the practitioner, coupled with perseverance and understanding on the part of the patient.

References

Atkinson, T. C. O. (1987) The development of the back surface design of rigid lenses. *Contax,* November, pp. 5–18.

Babalola, J. and Szajnicht, E. (1960) Ocular characteristics in West Africans and Europeans: A comparison of two groups. *Brit. J. Phy.s Opt.,* **17,** 27–35.

Back, A., Chong, M. S. and La Hood, D. (1996) Empirical fitting of RGP lenses. *Optom. Vis. Sci.,* **73,** S18.

Bennett, E. S., Smythe, J., Henry, V. A. *et al.* (1998) Effect of topical anesthetic use on initial patient satisfaction and overall success with rigid gas permeable contact lenses. *Optom. Vis. Sci.* **75,** 800–805.

Carney, L. G. and Hill, R. M. (1987) Centre of gravity of rigid lenses: some design considerations. *Int. Cont. Lens Clin.,* **14,** 431–435.

Carney, L. G., Mainstone, J. C., Carkeet, A. *et al.* (1997a) Rigid lens dynamics: Lid effects. *Contact Lens Assoc. Ophthalmol. J.,* **23,** 69–77.

Carney, L. G., Mainstone, J. C. and Henderson, B. A. (1997b) Corneal topography and myopia. A cross-sectional study. *Invest. Ophthalmol. Vis. Sci.,* **38,** 311–320.

Caroline, P. J., Andre, M. P. and Norman, C. W. (1994) Corneal topography and computerized contact lens-fitting moles. *Int. Cont Lens Clin.,* **21,** 185–195.

Fonn, D., Pritchard, N., Garnett, B. *et al.* (1996) Palpebral aperture sizes of rigid and soft contact lens wearers compared with nonwearers. *Optom. Vis. Sci.,* **73,** 211–214.

Guillon, M., Sammons, W. A. (1994) Contact lens design. Chapter 5. In: *Contact Lens Practice,* Ed: Ruben, M. and Guillon, M. G. London, Chapman & Hall Medical, pp. 87–112.

Guillon, M., Lydon, D. P. M. and Sammons, W. A. (1983) Designing rigid gas-permeable contact lenses using the edge clearance technique. *J. Br. Contact Lens Assoc.,* **6,** 19–25.

Guillon, M., Lydon, D. P. M. and Wilson, C. (1986) Corneal topography: a clinical model. *Ophthal. Physiol. Opt.,* **6,** 47–56.

Hirotsuji, I. (1990) The corneal base curve of the Japanese eye in 1990 – compared to 20 years ago. *J. Jap. Contact Lens Soc.,* **32,** 276–280.

Hogan, R. N. (2003) Potential for transmission of prion disease by contact lenses: an assessment of risk. *Eye Contact Lens,* **29,** S44–S48; discussion S57–59, S192–194.

Jani, B. R. and Szczotka, L. B. (2000) Efficiency and accuracy of two computerized topography software systems for fitting rigid gas-permeable contact lenses. *Contact Lens Assoc. Ophthalmol. J.,* **26,** 91–96.

Kelly J. M. (1994) Contact lens build-up (letter). *Optician,* **207,** 13.

Khorassani, A. A. and Peterson, J. E. (1988) Effects of peripheral curve width and radius changes on the retention forces measured for PMMA and Boston IV rigid lenses. *Int. Cont. Lens Clin.,* **15,** 311–315.

Kiely, P. M., Smith, G. and Carney, L. G. (1982) The mean shape of the human cornea. *Optica Acta,* **29,** 1027–1040.

La Hood, D. (1988) Edge shape and comfort of rigid lenses. *Am. J. Optom. Physiol. Opt.,* **65,** 613–618.

Lam, C. S. Y. and Loran, D. F. C. (1991) Designing contact lenses for oriental eyes. *J. Br. Contact Lens Assoc.,* **14,** 109–114.

Mandell, R. B. (1989) Contact Lens Practice, 4th edn., pp. 127–128, Springfield, IL: Charles C. Thomas.

Martin, D. K. and Holden, B. A. (1982) A new method for measuring the diameter of the in vivo human cornea. *Am. J. Optom. Physiol. Opt.,* **59,** 436–441.

Matsuda, L. M., Woldorff, C. L., Kame, R. T. *et al.* (1992) Clinical comparison of the corneal diameter and curvature in Asian eyes with those of the Caucasian eye. *Optom. Vis. Sci.,* **69,** 51–54.

Morgan, P. B. and Efron, N. (2008) The evolution of rigid contact lens prescribing. *Cont. Lens Anterior Eye,* **31,** 213–214.

Phillips, A. J. (2007) Modification procedures. In *Contact Lenses,* 5th edn. (A. J. Phillips and L. Speedwell, eds), pp. 563–575, London: Butterworth-Heinemann.

Read, S. A., Collins, M. J., Carney, L. G. *et al.* (2006) The topography of the central and peripheral cornea. *Inv. Ophthal. Vis. Sci.,* **47,** 1404–1414.

Schnider, C. M., Terry, R. L. and Holden, B. A. (1996) Effect of patient and lens performance characteristics on peripheral corneal desiccation. *J. Am. Optom. Ass.,* **67,** 144–150.

Schnider, C. M., Terry, R. L. and Holden, B. A. (1997) Effect of lens design on peripheral corneal desiccation. *J. Am. Optom. Assoc.,* **68,** 163–170.

Sweeney, D. F. (1992) Corneal exhaustion syndrome with long-term wear of contact lenses. *Optom. Vis. Sci.* **69,** 601–605.

van der Worp, E., De Brabander, J., Swarbrick, H. *et al.* (2003) Corneal desiccation in rigid contact lens wear: 3- and 9-o'clock staining. *Optom. Vis. Sci.,* **80,** 280–290.

van der Worp, E., de Brabander, J., Swarbrick, H. A. *et al.* (2009) Evaluation of signs and symptoms in 3- and 9-o'clock staining. *Optom. Vis. Sci.,* **86,** 260–265.

Young, G. (1988) Fluorescein in rigid lens fit evaluation. *Int. Cont. Lens Clin.,* **15,** 95–100.

Young, G. (1998) The effect of rigid lens design on fluorescein fit. *Cont. Lens and Ant. Eye* **21,** 41–46.

17 CHAPTER

Rigid toric lens design and fitting

Richard Lindsay

Introduction

The use of rigid toric lenses (in preference to rigid spherical lenses) is indicated under the following circumstances:

1. To improve the vision in cases where a lens employing spherical front and back optic zone radii is unable to provide adequate refractive correction.
2. To improve the physical fit in cases where a lens with a spherical back optic zone radius (BOZR) and spherical back peripheral zone radii fails to provide an adequate physical fit.

These two main uses of toroidal surfaces on contact lenses are not always distinct, such that occasionally a toric lens will be used for both physical and optical reasons. For example, when fitting an eye with both a high degree of residual astigmatism and a large amount of corneal toricity, a toric lens is required optically (to correct the residual astigmatism) as well as physically (to optimize the fit of the lens) (Lindsay, 1996).

Forms of toric lens

There are many varieties of rigid toric lens available to the practitioner. Most commonly, a lens will have both a toroidal back optic zone and peripheral zone. These lenses are generally used in attempting to obtain a good physical fit on a cornea that is too toroidal to allow a good fit with a lens having a spherical BOZR and spherical peripheral radii. Lenses with toroidal back optic and peripheral zones can be produced with or without a toroidal front optic surface. A lens that has a toroidal back optic zone and a toroidal front surface is said to have a bitoric construction. If the principal meridians are not parallel, then the lens is designated as having an oblique bitoric construction.

Occasionally, a rigid toric lens may be prescribed, consisting of a spherical back optic zone and a toroidal peripheral zone. This type of lens can also be produced with or without a toroidal front surface, the latter usually being the preferred option. Lenses with spherical back optic zones and toroidal peripheral zones are used as a means of attempting to improve the physical fit of a lens on an astigmatic cornea without the optical complications inherent in the use of lenses with toroidal back optic zones.

Very rarely, a rigid toric lens is produced with a toroidal back optic zone and a spherical peripheral zone, with the intention of improving the circulation of tears beneath the lens. However, when this is done, it is possible that the lens may become less stable with regard to resisting rotation. One limitation of employing a spherical periphery is that the peripheral radius must be greater than, or equal to, the flatter radius of the toroidal back central optic zone. Once again, this form of lens can be made with or without a toroidal front surface.

The only other rigid toric lens form consists of a spherical back optic zone and spherical peripheral zone combined with a toroidal front optic surface. This type of lens is required in the situation where there is significant residual (non-corneal) astigmatism but minimal corneal astigmatism. In this case, the residual astigmatism needs to be corrected by means of a toroidal front surface, with a spherical optic zone indicated for the back surface due to the negligible corneal astigmatism.

Criteria for use

Since rigid lenses with both spherical BOZR and peripheral radii are often used successfully on corneas with medium to high degrees of astigmatism, it is important to decide what degree of corneal astigmatism should indicate the use of toroidal back optic zones. In general, these lenses should only be used when a lens with a spherical BOZR cannot be made to fit successfully. It is rare to find that toroidal back optic zones are necessary unless the corneal astigmatism exceeds 2.50 D (i.e. the difference in the corneal radii, as measured with a keratometer, exceeds approximately 0.5 mm).

In cases of uncertainty (e.g. where the corneal astigmatism is between 2.00 and 3.00 D), a toroidal back optic zone would be used in preference to a spherical back surface curve in the following situations:

DOI: 10.1016/B978-0-7506-8869-7.00017-3

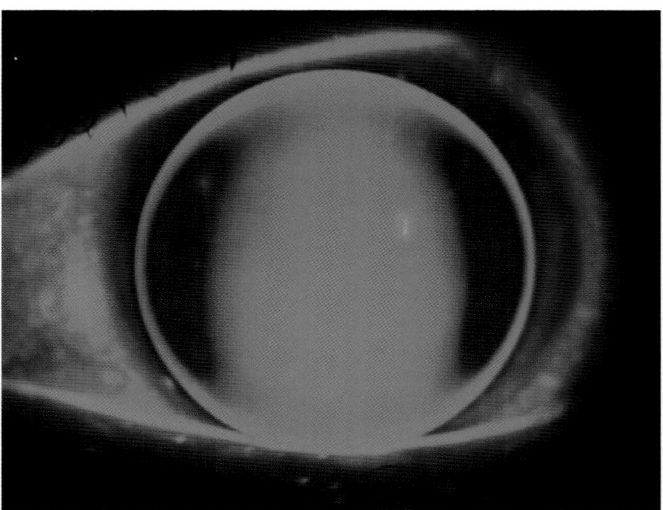

Figure 17.1 Left eye with high corneal astigmatism. Keratometer reading 8.19 mm along 176, 7.47 mm along 86. Fitting with spherical (7.70 mm) back optic zone radius reveals harsh bearing along the horizontal (flatter) meridian and poor centration.

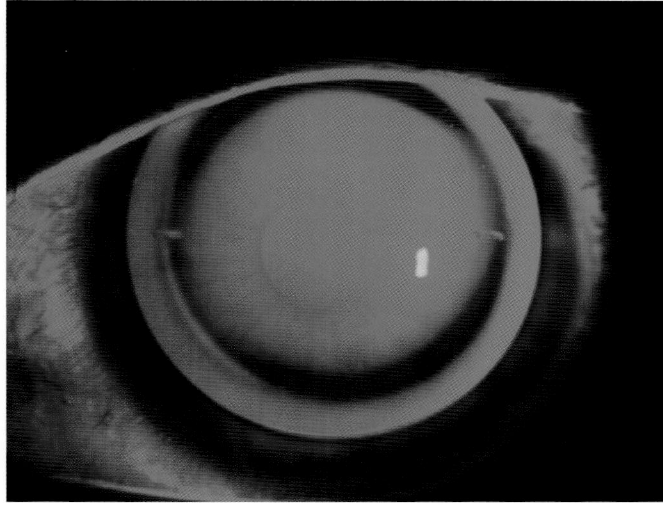

Figure 17.2 Same left eye as in Figure 17.1 wearing an alignment fitted rigid lens using a toroidal curve of back optic zone radius 8.15 × 7.50 mm.

- A spherical lens exhibits poor centration or excessive movement.
- Excessive lens flexure is noted with a spherical lens.
- Fluorescein patterns with a spherical lens reveal excessive bearing along the flatter corneal meridian, regardless of the BOZR that is fitted.
- Significant 3 and 9 o'clock staining occurs with a spherical lens.
- There is marked corneal distortion and spectacle blur upon removal of the spherical lens from the eye. This occurs as a result of poor alignment between the spherical lens and the toric cornea, with the spherical lens subsequently having a moulding effect on the toric cornea.
- There is significant residual astigmatism. In this case, a spherical back surface may provide an adequate fit; however, a toric back surface is utilized to stabilize the lens and prevent rotation, due to the presence of the correction for the residual astigmatism on the front surface of the lens.

A great deal depends on factors other than corneal astigmatism. Lid positions and tension are important. In a case of high with-the-rule corneal astigmatism – and a low, loose lower lid – a toroidal back optic zone may be needed to obtain a good physical fit and centration. But a similar eye with a firm, high lower lid may well be successfully fitted using a lens with spherical back surface curves.

The majority of cases of corneal astigmatism are found with the steeper corneal curve in the vertical meridian (with-the-rule). If an attempt is made to fit such an eye with a spherical BOZR, the lens often exhibits harsh bearing along the flatter (horizontal) meridian of the cornea and poor centration, causing physical discomfort and/or poor vision. Such an example is illustrated in Figure 17.1. If the same eye is fitted using a lens with toroidal back optic and peripheral curves, then the physical fit and centration are usually much improved (Figure 17.2).

The presence of against-the-rule corneal astigmatism usually necessitates the use of a toroidal back optic zone earlier than would be required with an equivalent amount of with-the-rule corneal astigmatism. This is due to the tendency for rigid spherical lenses to decentre laterally on corneas with even just moderate amounts (1.50–2.00 D) of against-the-rule astigmatism.

Design considerations

Although rigid lenses in general may be successfully fitted with either apical clearance or apical contact, it is generally more satisfactory to fit lenses with toroidal back optic zones in or near alignment. The physical fit, as denoted by the fluorescein pattern, will be similar to that seen with a well-fitted spherical lens in alignment to a cornea devoid of clinically significant astigmatism.

A toric lens aligning too closely to the cornea can lead to poor tear interchange. Consequently, it is advisable to use a toroidal back optic zone with the steeper radius fitted slightly flatter (longer radius) than the corresponding corneal radius so as to assist the interchange of tears. The flatter radius will generally be fitted 'on K' or else slightly steeper than its corresponding corneal radius.

Consider the type of physical fitting which might be derived from keratometer readings:

Keratometry reading: 7.90 mm (42.72 D) along 180
7.35 mm (45.91 D) along 90

Prescribed lens: C3 toric $\bigg/\dfrac{7.85}{7.40}$:7.50$\bigg/\dfrac{8.45}{8.00}$:8.50$\bigg/\dfrac{9.25}{8.80}$:9.50

The back optic zone radii should always be chosen such that there is at least a 0.3 mm meridional difference in radii (or 1.50 D difference if the BOZR are specified in dioptres). Otherwise, the toroidal BOZR may not position properly on the toroidal cornea, leading to lens rotation and possible visual disturbance, depending on the type of toric lens design. (Note that BOZR indicates back optic zone radius for a spherical surface and back optic zone radii for a toroidal surface.)

The peripheral radii are usually chosen to reflect the type of peripheral fit preferred by the practitioner concerned.

Each meridian is considered separately, and the peripheral fittings in the two principal meridians are selected to provide the same difference between back optic and peripheral radii most commonly used by the practitioner in fitting spherical corneas. In addition, the peripheral curves will usually have the same degree of toricity as the BOZR. For example, if a practitioner usually specifies the secondary curve 0.9 mm flatter than the BOZR for a spherical lens, then for a lens with toroidal BOZR of 7.90/7.40, the secondary curve ordered would be 8.80/8.30.

For lenses with a spherical back optic zone and a toroidal peripheral zone, the peripheral curve region should be as large as possible to increase the likelihood of alignment with the toric cornea. These lenses are usually fitted fairly small to minimize meridional sag differences and slightly steeper centrally than the flatter corneal meridian to achieve a compromise fit. The meridional difference in the peripheral curves should be at least 0.6 mm to help minimize lens rotation (Ruston, 1999).

A typical case might be as follows:

Keratometry reading: 7.90 mm (42.72 D) along 180
7.30 mm (46.23 D) along 90
BOZR chosen: 7.70 mm
BOZD chosen: 6.50 mm
TD chosen: 9.50 mm
Prescribed lens:

$$C4/7.70{:}6.50\Big/\frac{8.50}{7.90}{:}7.50\Big/\frac{9.20}{8.60}{:}8.50\Big/\frac{10.00}{9.40}{:}9.50$$

While this type of lens can be very useful in certain cases where a fully spherical lens is not adequate, the toroidal peripheral zones are, at best, only an attempt at compromise. They usually rotate more than lenses with all toroidal back surface curves, and the steeper peripheral radii occasionally end up in close proximity to the flatter corneal meridian, thus causing slight corneal abuse.

Optical considerations

The calculations involved in determining the necessary radii and power of these lenses are quite straightforward and the complexity of this topic is often exaggerated. It is important, however, that the fundamentals of the optics of contact lenses are understood if some of the complications of toroidal optic surfaces on corneal lenses are to be appreciated.

To help understand and perform some of the calculations needed in toric lens work, the reader is referred to Chapter 14 and also to Douthwaite (1995).

Refraction

Calculating the back vertex powers (BVPs) for a rigid lens with toroidal back optic zone is undoubtedly a more complex task than determining the BVP for a spherical lens, and yet the two processes involve the same basic principles. For spherical lenses, the power of the contact lens in air plus the power of the tear lens in air should add up to the ocular refraction. With toric lenses, the same rule applies, but here the two separate meridians must be considered.

Example 1: Calculating the back vertex power for a rigid lens with a toroidal back optic zone

Spectacle refraction (vertex distance ignored):
$+2.50/-3.00 \times 180$

(Note that the effect of the vertex distance must be taken into account if this distance is great or if the refractive power in either meridian exceeds 4.00 D.)

Keratometry reading: 8.04 mm (42.00 D) along 180
7.50 mm (45.00 D) along 90′

A rigid spherical trial lens with BOZR 7.95 mm and BVP +1.00 D is placed on the cornea. Refraction with this lens *in situ* gives +1.00 DS (no residual astigmatism) and 6/6 acuity. Note that the over-refraction is usually best performed over a spherical trial contact lens aligned along the flattest meridian of the cornea and only one over-refraction is required to calculate both BVPs.

Based on the keratometry readings, BOZR of 8.00 mm and 7.55 mm are chosen to fit the horizontal and vertical meridians respectively.

The power determination is now performed in the same way as with a rigid spherical lens, except that two meridians need to be considered instead of one. The BVP that needs to be ordered (BVP_{CL}) is calculated by taking into account the BVP of the trial lens (BVP_{trial}) and the overrefraction (OR) and then using the formula:

$$BVP_{CL} = BVP_{trial} + OR.$$

For a spherical lens, if the BOZR of the trial lens is different from the BOZR to be ordered, then, when determining the BVP_{CL}, it is necessary to take into account the change in tear lens power that will occur as a result of changing the BOZR.

Based on a tear lens refractive index of 1.336, this change in tear lens power is given by the formula:

$$\left(\frac{336}{BOZR_{final}} - \frac{336}{BOZR_{trial}}\right)$$

where $BOZR_{final}$ is the BOZR that has been chosen for the lens to be ordered and $BOZR_{trial}$ is the BOZR of the trial lens.

It can be approximated that, for every 0.05 mm decrease in BOZR, −0.25 D must be added to the BVP of the contact lens. Likewise, +0.25 D must be added to the BVP of the contact lens for every 0.05 mm increase in BOZR. This approximation only holds for relatively small differences in BOZR and, if in doubt, it is safer to use the above formula.

Given that the BOZR is being changed from that used for the fitting, the BVP that needs to be ordered (BVP_{CL}) is given by:

$$BVP_{CL} = BVP_{trial} + OR - \left(\frac{336}{BOZR_{final}} - \frac{336}{BOZR_{trial}}\right)$$

When calculating the BVPs for a rigid toric lens based on fitting with a spherical trial lens, there will be a change to the trial lens BOZR in at least one meridian. In this example, the back optic zone radii to be ordered are both different from the trial lens BOZR and so it will be necessary to allow for the change in tear lens power in both meridians.

$$\text{Along 180,}\quad BVP_{CL} = +1.00 + 1.00 - \left(\frac{336}{8.00} - \frac{336}{7.95}\right) = +2.25\text{ D}$$

$$\text{Along 90,}\quad BVP_{CL} = +1.00 + 1.00 - \left(\frac{336}{7.55} - \frac{336}{7.95}\right) = -0.25\text{ D}$$

(When calculating BVP, values are rounded off to the nearest 0.25 D.)

Final prescription (Rx) of lens:
BOZR 8.00 mm along 180 +2.25 D
BOZR 7.55 mm along 90 −0.25 D

Alternatively, the BVPs of the contact lens can be calculated empirically, firstly by using the required BOZR and the keratometry reading of the patient to calculate the tear lens power (BVP_{tears}) and then using the formula:

$$BVP_{CL} = \text{ocular refraction} - BVP_{tears}$$

to calculate the BVPs along both meridians.

The power of the tear lens is obtained from the following formula:

$$BVP_{tears} = \left(\frac{336}{BOZR} - \frac{336}{K}\right)$$

where K is the corneal front surface radius of curvature (in millimetres) along that respective meridian.

Once again, it can be approximated (for very small differences) that there is 0.25 D of tear lens power for every 0.05 mm difference between the BOZR and the corneal front surface radius of curvature.

Along 180,

$$BVP_{tears} = \left(\frac{336}{8.00} - \frac{336}{8.04}\right) \sim +0.25\text{ D}$$

$$BVP_{CL} = +2.50 - 0.25 = +2.25\text{ D}$$

Along 90,

$$BVP_{tears} = \left(\frac{336}{7.55} - \frac{336}{7.50}\right) \sim -0.25\text{ D}$$

$$BVP_{CL} = -0.50 - (-0.25) = -0.25\text{ D}$$

While the empirical method is probably simpler, clinical experience would suggest that more accurate results are usually obtained when the BVP is calculated based on a refraction over a trial lens.

Residual astigmatism

The term ‘residual astigmatism’ is often used loosely and is frequently confused with induced astigmatism or corneal astigmatism. Residual astigmatism has been defined in various ways (Goldberg, 1964), including the simplistic definition of residual astigmatism as the component of the spectacle (ocular) astigmatism that is not due to the cornea. In the context of rigid lens fitting, a better definition would be: residual astigmatism is the astigmatic component of a lens required to correct fully an eye wearing a spherical powered rigid contact lens with a spherical BOZR.

Example 2: Calculating the back vertex power for a rigid lens with a toroidal back optic zone when there is residual astigmatism present.

Spectacle refraction (vertex distance ignored):

$+2.50/-2.00 \times 180$

Keratometry reading: 8.04 mm (42.00 D) along 180
7.50 mm (45.00 D) along 90′

A rigid spherical trial lens with BOZR 7.95 mm and BVP +1.00 D is placed on the cornea. Refraction with this lens *in situ* gives +2.00/–1.00 × 90 and 6/6 acuity.

Based on the keratometry readings, BOZR of 8.00 mm and 7.55 mm are chosen to fit the horizontal and vertical meridians respectively.

In this case, residual astigmatism is equal to –1.00 DC × 90. If the patient is to be given the best possible vision it is necessary to incorporate the correction for this residual cylinder into the BVP to be ordered.

The method for determining the BVPs is the same as used in the previous example.

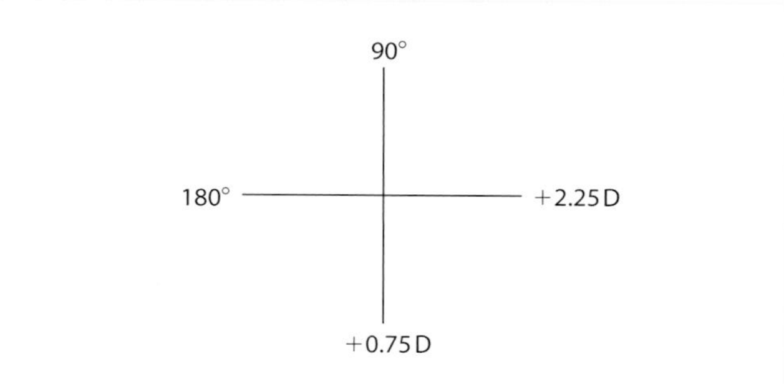

Figure 17.3 Meridional powers required in example 2. This shows the powers and directions as they will be measured by the contact lens laboratory.

$$\text{Along 180, } BVP_{CL} = +1.00 + \mathbf{1.00} - \left(\frac{336}{8.00} - \frac{336}{7.95}\right) = +2.25\text{ D}$$

$$\text{Along 90, } BVP_{CL} = +1.00 + \mathbf{2.00} - \left(\frac{336}{7.55} - \frac{336}{7.95}\right) = +0.75\text{ D}$$

The values for the over-refraction are in bold to emphasize the fact that there is residual astigmatism present in this case.

Final Rx of lens:

BOZR 8.00 mm along 180 +2.25 D
BOZR 7.55 mm along 90 +0.75 D

In examples 1 and 2, the powers specified are the BVPs of the toric lens in the appropriate meridians. These are the powers read by the laboratory when checking the lens on a focimeter (vertometer).

It is frequently useful, in considering bitoric lenses, to draw a representation of meridional powers to ensure that simple errors in confusing axes and meridians are not made. Such a power cross is shown in Figure 17.3.

Sometimes, the axis of the residual astigmatism does not correspond exactly with one of the principal meridians of curvature of the cornea. If the difference between the axes of the spectacle refraction and the principal meridians of the cornea is marginal (less than 20°), one can assume that the axes of the spectacle refraction over the lens *do* correspond with the principal meridians of corneal curvature. By doing this, the need for any complex oblique cylinder calculations is obviated and the resulting error in the power calculations is usually not significant (Lindsay, 1996). If there is a large difference between the cylinder axis of the ocular refraction and the axis of the corneal astigmatism, then an oblique bitoric lens (where the principal meridians of the toroidal front and back surfaces are not parallel) will be required.

Induced astigmatism

Induced astigmatism is the astigmatic effect created in the contact lens/tear lens system by the toroidal back optic zone bounding two surfaces of different refractive index, namely the lens (refractive index 1.41–1.49 depending on the material) and the tears (refractive index 1.336). As a general rule, rigid lenses with refractive indices lower than 1.458 are made from fluorosilicone acrylates; lenses with refractive indices in the range 1.458–1.469 are made from either fluorosilicone acrylates or silicone acrylates;

and lenses with refractive indices greater than 1.469 are made from silicone acrylates (Tranoudis and Efron, 1998).

Consider the lens designed in example 1 with back surface toric curves of 8.00 mm and 7.55 mm. Assuming a refractive index of 1.47 for the lens material, the surface powers of these curves in air are −58.75/−62.25, giving a back surface cylinder of −3.50 DC × 180. On the eye, where the back surface rests against the tear layer ($n = 1.336$), the powers of the back surface interface are now −16.75/−17.75 respectively and the back surface cylinder in tear fluid is −1.00 DC × 180. This 1.00 D back surface cylinder ('induced astigmatism') must be compensated by generating a +1.00 D cylinder axis 180 on the front surface (Sarver *et al.*, 1985).

The front surface cylinder correction for the induced astigmatism is automatically incorporated into the lens prescription when the practitioner calculates the BVPs for the rigid toric lens. Once again, consider the lens designed in Example 1. If a refractive index of 1.47 for the lens material and a lens centre thickness of 0.25 mm is assumed, the required front surface powers (calculated using thick lens formulae) based on BOZR of 8.00 and 7.55 mm and BVP of +2.25 and −0.25 D would be +60.37/+61.35 respectively. Specification of the appropriate BOZR and BVP therefore results in the front surface incorporating the required compensating cylinder of +1.00 DC × 180.

A quick way to calculate the induced astigmatism is to use the appropriate radii considered with the change from the rigid lens to the tears. That is:

$$\text{Power of the RGP lens/tear boundary} = \frac{1000(1.336 - 1.47)}{r} = \frac{-134}{r}$$

where r = radius (in millimeters) and the refractive index of the rigid lens material is assumed to be equal to 1.47.

By subtracting the values found of $-134/r$ for one principal meridian from the other, the value for the induced astigmatism may be obtained directly. With rigid lens materials of refractive index not equal to 1.47, the figure of $-134/r$ no longer applies: for example, a refractive index of 1.45 would yield a figure of $114/r$ for determining the surface power at the lens/tear boundary.

Spherical power equivalent ('compensated') bitoric lenses

These are lenses that, like spherical lenses, do not correct for any residual astigmatism (Sarver, 1963). They are bitoric because the front surface contains a cylinder solely for the correction of the induced astigmatism. The lens designed in Example 1 would be characterized as a compensated bitoric lens.

A compensated bitoric can be thought of as a lens designed to correct all of the refractive cylinder created due to the corneal toricity (Lowther, 1990). If the corneal toricity is equal to the spectacle astigmatism, when a compensated bitoric is placed on the cornea the cylinder will be fully corrected.

A compensated bitoric lens can rotate on the eye without visual disturbance because the effect of the rotation is counteracted by an equal change in the cylinder power of the tear lens.

Cylindrical power equivalent toric lenses

All other types of rigid toric lenses come under this classification, and the unifying feature of these lenses is that they incorporate a correction for residual astigmatism. This type of lens can be further categorized as follows.

Alignment bitoric lenses

These are also known as parallel bitoric lenses. Both the front and back surfaces are toroidal. The front surface incorporates correction for residual astigmatism as well as for the induced astigmatism. In addition, the axes of the spectacle refraction over the lens correspond with the principal meridians of corneal curvature, so the correction for the residual astigmatism will be along one of the principal meridians of the lens (hence the name 'alignment bitoric'). As such, the use of the term 'alignment bitoric' here should not be confused with alignment in regard to lens fitting. The lens specified in Example 2 was an alignment bitoric lens.

Back surface toric lenses

These lenses have a toroidal back surface but a spherical front surface. The design principle is similar to that for alignment bitorics. As with alignment bitorics, the front surface incorporates correction for residual astigmatism as well as for the induced astigmatism and the axes of the spectacle refraction over the lens correspond with the principal meridians of corneal curvature, so the correction for the residual astigmatism is along one of the principal meridians of the lens.

In the case of a back surface toric lens, however, the correction for the residual astigmatism is equal and opposite to the correction for the induced astigmatism. Hence the two required cylindrical corrections cancel each other out, meaning that the front surface can be left spherical.

Very occasionally a case of induced and residual astigmatism cancelling out one another is encountered in practice, as in the following example.

Example 3: Spectacle refraction (vertex distance ignored):

+3.00/−4.00 × 180

Keratometry reading: 8.04 mm (42.00 D) along 180
7.50 mm (45.00 D) along 90'

A rigid spherical trial lens with BOZR 7.95 mm and BVP +1.00 D is placed on the cornea. Refraction with this lens *in situ* gives +1.50/−1.00 × 180 and 6/6 acuity. Hence there is residual astigmatism present, namely −1.00 DC × 180.

Based on the keratometry readings, BOZR of 8.00 mm and 7.55 mm are chosen to fit the horizontal and vertical meridians respectively.

The induced astigmatism can be determined using the method described previously of calculating the change in power of the RGP lens/tear boundary. By subtracting the values found of $-134/r$ for one principal meridian from the other (assuming a lens refractive index of 1.47), the value for the induced astigmatism is obtained.

$$\text{Induced astigmatism} = \frac{-134}{8.00} - \frac{-134}{7.55} = +1.00\ \text{D}$$

The induced astigmatism, expressed in negative cylinder form, will always have the same axis as the corneal astigmatism . Hence, the induced back surface cylinder here is −1.00 DC × 180.

The correction for the residual astigmatism is –1.00 DC × 180, so the residual astigmatism and the induced astigmatism should cancel each other out. This can be confirmed by calculation of the BVPs and the front and back surface powers of the lens (assuming a lens centre thickness of 0.25 mm).

Along 180,

$$\text{BVP}_{\text{CL}} = +1.00 + 1.50 + \left(\frac{336}{7.95} - \frac{336}{8.00}\right) = +2.75\ \text{D}$$

$$\text{Back surface power of the contact lens} = \frac{1000(1-1.47)}{+8.00} = -58.75\ \text{D}$$

$$\text{Front surface power of the contact lens} = +60.86\ \text{D}$$

Along 90,

$$\text{BVP}_{\text{CL}} = +1.00 + 0.50 + \left(\frac{336}{7.95} - \frac{336}{7.55}\right) = -0.75\ \text{D}$$

$$\text{Back surface power of the contact lens} = \frac{1000(1-1.47)}{+7.55} = -62.25\ \text{D}$$

$$\text{Front surface power of the contact lens} = +60.86$$

The front surface is spherical (same power along both principal meridians) so the residual and induced astigmatism have indeed cancelled each other out. (When calculating surface powers, for clinical purposes a difference in power of ≤0.12 D between the principal meridians constitutes a spherical surface.)

A back surface toric design is only possible if the correction for the residual astigmatism is equal and opposite to the correction for the induced astigmatism. A back surface toric design is therefore only worth considering if the ocular astigmatism of the patient is greater than the corneal astigmatism (Meyler and Ruston, 1995). The residual astigmatism must also then be of a magnitude whereby it will be neutralized by the resultant induced astigmatism. The likelihood of both of these requirements being met is low, so only in a small percentage of cases will a back surface toric design be appropriate. Indeed, in most cases the induced astigmatism usually exaggerates the effect of the residual astigmatism.

Front surface toric lenses

Residual astigmatism frequently needs to be corrected in cases where the patient is fitted well, physically, with a lens utilizing a spherical back optic zone. Such a lens therefore requires a toroidal front surface, but lens rotation must be avoided, otherwise visual disturbance will result. When the corneal astigmatism is less than 2.00 D, a toric back surface will not generally prevent lens rotation and so other forms of lens stabilization, such as prism ballast or truncation, are required.

Prism ballast is the most commonly used method of lens stabilization for rigid lenses that have toroidal front surfaces combined with spherical back optic zones. With prism ballasting, the lens is prescribed in the normal manner with the addition of between 1 and 3Δ. When ordering the lens, practitioners assume that the weight or prism ballast orients the lens in a certain fixed position on the cornea and order the cylinder axis with respect to this position. To avoid recording the prism base position as 'down along 90' or 'down along 100', its actual location is recorded as being at 270 or 280 respectively.

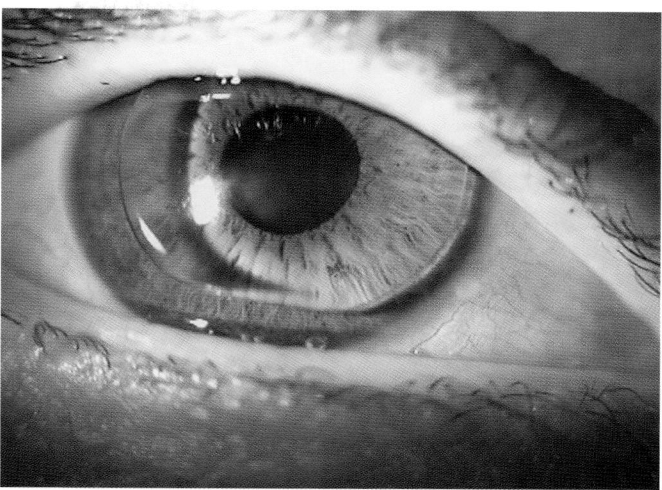

Figure 17.4 A prism-ballasted rigid toric lens with single truncation. This often proves very successful in preventing unwanted rotation.

Prism ballast may also be used in combination with a toroidal back surface where a patient's corneal astigmatism is too small (<2.00 D) to maintain the proper position of a bitoric lens but large enough (>1.00 D) to cause a front toric lens to become unstable (Gonce and Kastl, 1994).

Truncations can also be added to front surface toric lenses if prism ballasting is insufficient to stabilize the lens. The usual method of designing a truncation for a prism-ballasted lens is to prescribe the lens in the normal way with the addition of the front surface cylinder at the correct angle relative to the estimated or observed position of the prism base. The relationship of the lower lid to the edge of the lens is observed and a truncation is then cut to align with the lower lid (Figure 17.4).

Prism ballasting can often cause rigid lenses to sit inferiorly, causing patients to experience symptoms of discomfort and flare. Truncations can also be uncomfortable for the patient and they are not always successful in preventing lens rotation. Consequently, a soft toric contact lens is generally preferred to a rigid toric contact lens when fitting patients who have significant residual astigmatism but negligible corneal astigmatism.

Oblique bitoric lenses

As with alignment bitoric lenses, oblique bitoric lenses have a toroidal front and back surface. With oblique bitorics, however, the principal meridians of the toroidal back and front surfaces are not parallel, due to a difference between the axes of the spectacle refraction and the principal meridians of corneal curvature. The specification and manufacture of these type of lenses are very difficult. One solution is to use a fitting set of lenses, all of which have a toroidal back optic zone and a spherical front surface. A refraction is performed over the appropriate trial lens and then the oblique cylinder obtained from this refraction is incorporated on to the front surface of the lens. These lenses are rarely prescribed.

Effect of lens rotation

With all cylindrical power equivalent bitoric lenses, some visual disturbance will occur with rotation as the lenses

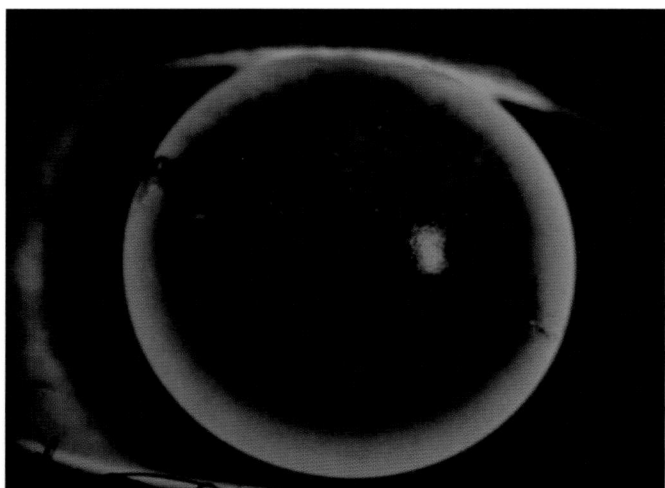

Figure 17.5 A right lens with a toroidal back optic zone fitted in alignment. Keratometer reading is 8.13 mm along 160 and 7.62 mm along 70. Lens back optic zone radius 8.10 × 7.70 mm. The 8.10 meridian is marked with grease pencil and can be seen aligning well with the 160 meridian. There is no significant rotation, thus permitting accurate correction of residual astigmatism, as well as induced astigmatism, with a front surface cylinder.

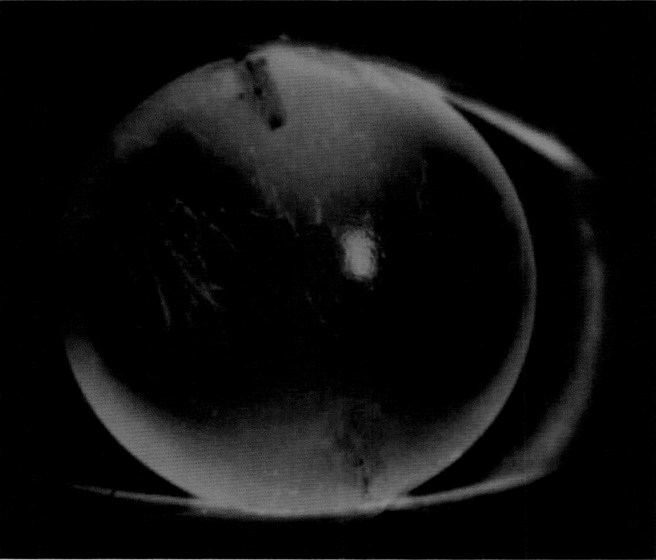

Figure 17.6 Same right eye as in Figure 17.5. Lens back optic zone radius 8.05 × 7.75 with 8.05 meridian marked with grease pencil. This should be located along the 160 meridian, but, as shown, this lens rotates badly, thus permitting only the accurate correction of induced astigmatism with a front surface cylinder.

incorporate a correction for residual astigmatism and the axis of correction for the residual astigmatism remains fixed in relation to the eye.

This limitation on rotation is important, for when residual astigmatism is of a low degree from a clinical standpoint, then it is not worthwhile incorporating its correction with that for the induced astigmatism. If, however, the residual astigmatism is clinically significant, then it is worth incorporating provided that lens rotation can be kept to a minimum (Figures 17.5 and 17.6).

With lenses incorporating a toroidal back surface, rotation is generally not a problem due to the stabilizing effect of the toric back surface on the toric cornea (provided there is sufficient corneal toricity).

Conclusions

Advances in soft toric lens technology have resulted in it being the predominant and preferred method of correcting astigmatism, especially when considering the increased chair time required to arrive at a successful rigid toric lens fitting. Nevertheless, there will be occasions when one of the more sophisticated rigid toric lenses is required for a given patient. In fact there is an apparent trend for rigid lenses to be used more for specialist fits, such as sophisticated toric designs, multifocals and orthokeratology (Morgan and Efron, 2008). Blackmore *et al.* (2006) surveyed diplomates of the American Academy of Optometry, most of whom considered that back surface toric and bitoric rigid lenses are easy to design and fit. Some practitioners, however, may choose to refer especially challenging cases to a colleague who takes a special interest in rigid toric lens fitting and who has the necessary repertoire of custom-designed trial lens sets. Notwithstanding that possibility, the utility of this chapter is that it provides an overview of the optical considerations and possible lens designs for the various forms of complex astigmatic correction that can sometimes present in practice.

References

Blackmore, K., Bachand, N., Bennett, E. S. *et al.* (2006) Gas permeable toric use and applications: survey of Section on Cornea and Contact Lens Diplomates of the American Academy of Optometry. *Optometry,* **77,** 17–22.

Douthwaite, W. A. (1995) *Contact Lens Optics and Lens Design.* Oxford: Butterworth-Heinemann.

Goldberg, J. B. (1964) The correction of residual astigmatism with corneal contact lenses. *Br. J. Physiol. Opt.,* **21,** 169–174.

Gonce, M. A. and Kastl, P. R. (1994) Bi-rigid toric contact lens with prism fitting in rare cases of moderate corneal and residual astigmatism. *Contact Lens Assoc. Ophthal. J.,* **20,** 176–178.

Lindsay, R. G. (1996) Rigid toric gas-permeable contact lenses: Indications, fitting principles and prescription calculations. *Practical Optometry,* **7,** 218–224.

Lowther, G. E. (1990) Toric RGPs: Should they be used more often? *Int. Contact Lens Clin.,* **17,** 260–261.

Meyler, J. and Ruston, D. (1995) Toric RGP contact lenses made easy. *Optician,* **209** (5504), 30–35.

Morgan, P. B. and Efron, N. (2008) The evolution of rigid contact lens prescribing. *Cont. Lens Anterior Eye,* **31,** 213–214.

Ruston, D. (1999) The challenge of fitting astigmatic eyes: rigid gas-permeable toric lenses. *Contact Lens Ant. Eye (suppl),* **22,** S2–S13.

Sarver, M. D. (1963) A toric base corneal contact lens with spherical power effect. *J. Am. Optom. Assoc.,* **34,** 1136–1137.

Sarver, M. D., Kame, R. T. and Williams, C. E. (1985) A bitoric gas permeable hard contact lens with spherical power effect. *J. Am. Optom. Assoc.,* **56,** 184–189.

Tranoudis, I. and Efron, N. (1998) Refractive index of rigid contact lens materials. *Contact Lens Ant. Eye,* **21,** 15–18.

CHAPTER 18

Rigid lens care systems

Philip B Morgan

Introduction

This chapter reviews the care systems used with rigid contact lenses. Of course, many of the general principles of contact lens care, such as the rationale for lens cleaning and disinfection, regulatory control of the contact lens care industry and various approaches to comparing the efficacy of different solutions, have already been discussed in Chapter 11 and will not be repeated here.

Disinfection and wetting solutions

Traditionally, rigid lens products were preserved with benzalkonium chloride, thiomersal and chlorhexidine. However, there is some evidence that sufficient levels of chlorhexidine or benzalkonium chloride can bind to the surface of a rigid lens, leading to a toxic reaction at the ocular surface after lens insertion (Rosenthal *et al.*, 1986). More recent products have seen a move away from these preservative agents or, as in the case of the Boston Advance product, a reduction in chlorhexidine concentration compared with previous care solutions. Also, polyhexanide (more traditionally part of soft lens disinfectant products) has been introduced as a second preservative in rigid lens solutions (Table 18.1). For example, Total Care (Advanced Medical Optics) contains polyhexanide of concentration 5 parts per million (Figure 18.1).

Multipurpose solutions for cleaning and disinfecting rigid gas-permeable lenses have replaced single-purpose solutions, but there are few reports of the efficacy of these multipurpose solutions, or of the effects of storage conditions on their disinfecting capacities. Boost *et al.* (2006) showed that multipurpose solutions for rigid lenses lose activity over the 3 months' recommended time of use but remain satisfactory for use. Disinfecting capacity reduced more quickly when stored in the refrigerator.

In addition to their role in lens disinfection, most rigid lens storage solutions also act to wet or to condition the lens. This role is principally to act as a lubricant, affording a degree of protection to the cornea and lid margins when the lens is inserted. The cushioning effect minimizes discomfort at insertion. The secondary effects of successful lens wetting are that the lens surface is, firstly, rendered hydrophilic to aid a stable prelens tear film, and secondly, made more biocompatible, which might reduce protein deposition.

Various agents are incorporated into rigid lens solutions to aid surface conditioning. Polyvinyl alcohol is a positively charged polymer which is attracted to the negatively charged surface of lenses containing methacrylic acid to provide a more wettable lens (Walker, 1997). Another agent which is used to increase wettability is the viscosity agent hydroxyethylcellulose. In addition to a preservative and conditioning/wetting agents, rigid lens care solutions contain buffering agents to maintain a stable pH, and chelating agents to increase antimicrobial action and assist in lens cleaning.

Cleaning solutions

Some rigid lenses are cleaned with a separate solution to the disinfectant and wetting product, whereas others follow many of the soft lens care systems and are multipurpose products. Separate rigid lens cleaning solutions can be more intensive than their soft lens equivalents because there is less opportunity for the solution to enter the lens material, with the subsequent possibility of toxic reaction. For example, Total Care Daily Cleaner (Advanced Medical Optics) contains three cleaning agents and Boston Advance cleaner (Bausch & Lomb) contains a silica suspension of microscopic beads which act like a gentle polish on the lens; this is beneficial with deposits such as denatured proteins which can otherwise be difficult to remove. This cleaner also contains an alcohol base which assists in removing lipid-type spoilation.

Protein removal solutions

Protein removal is arguably more important with rigid lenses than with soft lenses, in view of the fact that most soft lenses prescribed today are replaced more regularly than rigid lenses. With few exceptions, protein removal

DOI: 10.1016/B978-0-7506-8869-7.00018-5

Table 18.1 Constituents of rigid lens disinfecting solutions

Company	Product	Preservative (ppm)	Surfactant/conditioner/viscosity agents
Alcon	Unique pH	Polidronium chloride (11)	Poloxamine HP-Guar
Advanced Medical Optics	Total Care	Polyhexanide (5)	Hydroxyethyl cellulose
Bausch & Lomb	Boston Advance	Polyhexanide (5) Chlorhexidine (30)	Polyquaternium 10 Polyvinyl alcohol Derivatized polyethylene glycol Cellulose viscosifier
Bausch & Lomb	Boston Simplus	Polyhexanide (5) Chlorhexidine (30)	Poloxamine Hydroxypropyl methylcellulose
Sauflon	Delta Plus	Polyhexanide (1)	Poloxamer

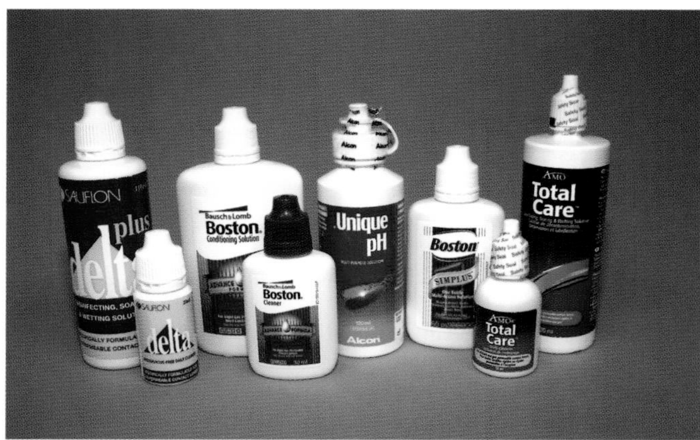

Figure 18.1 Most care systems for rigid lenses comprise a soaking/wetting solution and a separate daily cleaner.

systems that were originally designed for use with soft lenses can also be used with rigid lenses. The frequency with which patients should be advised to use protein removal systems, and how such systems should be applied to the lenses, will vary depending on the lens material and the strength of the active ingredient in the protein removal system. Advice on these issues should be obtained from the manufacturer.

Individual patient factors will also have an impact on the way protein removal systems should be applied. Patients who display a propensity for depositing protein on lenses, and who wear their lenses more frequently and for longer periods of time, may need to treat their lenses more regularly. Typical frequencies of usage of protein removal systems vary from weekly to monthly.

Disinfection of trial lens sets

Proper application of the standard lens care protocols described in this chapter will be efficacious at killing most bacteria, viruses, fungi and protozoa, especially those known to cause infection in the eye. However, certain infectious agents have more recently been identified that are apparently resistant to current soft and rigid lens care regimens. Of particular concern at the present time is a proteinaceous vector known as a prion – a chameleon-like infectious agent that exists in different strains which have distinct biological properties and can alter when the disease for which it is responsible crosses the species barrier. It has been suggested by health authorities in the UK that there is a remote theoretical risk of transmission of variant Creutzfeldt–Jacob disease (vCJD) between humans, via transfer of bodily tissues and fluids such as tears.

An extension of the above argument leads to the conclusion that vCJD could theoretically be transmitted from an infected individual to another person via a trial contact lens contaminated with the offending prion. Although such transmission is theoretically possible, it remains highly improbable (Armstrong, 2006). In the light of this the following guidance was given: 'wherever practicable, a contact lens or ophthalmic device that comes into contact with the ocular surface should not be used on more than one patient, as to do so may expose patients to unnecessary risk through the transmission of disease' (Anonymous, 2008).

Excellent success rates in fitting rigid lenses empirically (i.e. the lens is ordered based on measures of refraction and ocular dimensions) have been demonstrated. However, it is recognized that in certain cases, particularly where there is disease or abnormality of the lid, cornea or ocular surface, special complex diagnostic contact lenses may be necessary for a successful clinical outcome. These lenses may need to be reused. An obvious case is keratoconus, as a practitioner who fits patients with this condition may have access to a number of trial fitting sets, each representing a different design philosophy.

Where empirical fitting is impracticable suitable items should be decontaminated using a recognized method. Comoy *et al.* (2003) found Menicon Progent and Menicon MeniLAB (0.4 and 0.5% sodium hypochlorite respectively) decreased the infectivity of prions retained on the surface of experimentally contaminated lenses by a factor of at least 10 million. Current advice, however, is to use a readily available sodium hypochlorite 2% solution (20 000 ppm available chlorine), such as is sold for household use, and to follow the procedure below (Anonymous, 1999):

1. The item to be decontaminated should not be allowed to dry following use.
2. It should be cleaned in the usual manner.
3. It should then be soaked in the sodium hypochlorite solution for 1 hour.

4. It should be removed from the solution and residual solution shaken off.
5. It should then be thoroughly rinsed with sterile normal saline solution, or freshly boiled water at room temperature.
6. It should then be disinfected using the normal procedure (this is because sodium hypochlorite is not effective against spores and cysts of certain organisms).

The item may then be safely reused. Macalister and Buckley (2002) concluded that sodium hypochlorite does not appear to distort rigid lenses; however, it may not be used on soft lenses.

Conclusions

Multipurpose care systems are becoming the norm for the maintenance of rigid contact lenses. Because rigid lenses typically have a life span in excess of 6 months, occasional use of protein removal systems may be required. The reuse of rigid trial lenses to determine the best lens fit should be minimized because of the remote theoretical risk of transmission of diseases by agents such as prions, which are resistant to conventional antimicrobial methods. Sodium hypochlorite solution is an effective rigid lens disinfecting solution with antiprion activity.

References

Armstrong, R. A. (2006) Creutzfeldt–Jakob disease and vision. *Clin. Exp. Optom.*, **89,** 3–9.

Boost, M., Cho, P. and Lai, S. (2006) Efficacy of multipurpose solutions for rigid gas permeable lenses. *Ophthalmic Physiol. Opt.*, **26,** 468–475.

Anonymous (1999) Guidance on the re-use of contact lenses and ophthalmic devices. London: College of Optometrists.

Anonymous (2008) Guidance on Infection Control. London: College of Optometrists.

Comoy, E., Bonnevalle, C., Métais, A. *et al.* (2003) Disinfection of gas-permeable contact lenses against prions. *J. Fr. Ophtalmol.*, **26,** 233–239.

Macalister, G. O. and Buckley, R. J. (2002) The risk of transmission of variant Creutzfeldt–Jakob disease via contact lenses and ophthalmic devices. *Cont. Lens Anterior Eye,* **25,** 104–136.

Rosenthal, P., Chou, M. H., Salamone, J. C. *et al.* (1986) Quantitative analysis of chlorhexidine gluconate and benzalkonium chloride adsorption on silicone/acrylate polymers. *Contact Lens Assoc. Ophthalmol. J.*, **12,** 43–50.

Walker, J. (1997) New developments in RGP lens care. *Optician,* **213**(5583), 16–19.

PART: IV

Lens replacement modalities

CHAPTER 19

Unplanned lens replacement

Nathan Efron

Introduction

Prior to the soft lens era, a single pair of haptic or rigid lenses were typically used by a patient for many years. This generally did not pose a problem because these lenses were made of glass or solid plastic (polymethyl methacrylate, or PMMA), and had surfaces that were chemically inert. Thus, such lenses could be cleaned, disinfected and stored with appropriate solutions. Any surface damage could be rectified by repolishing the surface. In this way, such lenses could last beyond a decade. In essence, all lenses of this era were prescribed to be used until there was a clear clinical indication for replacing the lenses with a new pair.

Soft contact lenses have a more reactive surface, and because they have a modulus that is much lower than rigid lenses, are more susceptible to damage. Furthermore, any damage to the surface or edge of the lens cannot be repaired because a hydrated soft lens cannot be repolished. Although these factors would seem to indicate the desirability of regular soft lens replacement, the high cost of soft lenses throughout the 1970s and much of the 1980s precluded such, so strategies were devised to prolong lens life for as long as possible. The norm during this period was to prescribe soft lenses in the same way that rigid lenses were being prescribed - that is, for the patient to keep using the same pair of lenses until they became damaged or lost, were too uncomfortable to wear, resulted in a noticeable deterioration of vision or induced ocular pathology that was either self-diagnosed or detected during an eye examination. Some patients were known to use the same pair of lenses for up to 7 years. Indeed, it was even possible to take out insurance policies against the risk of lens loss or damage.

All of this changed with the introduction of planned lens replacement schemes and disposable lenses in the late 1980s. This concept rapidly became established and it is now universally accepted that contact lenses must be replaced regularly. In fact, a recent survey of international prescribing trends conducted by Morgan *et al.* (2009) revealed that, across 27 countries, unplanned replacement represented only 1% of all soft contact lens fits, and was 0% in 12 countries. The practice of regular lens replacement is more variable with rigid lenses, with only 46% of rigid lenses being prescribed in this way (Morgan *et al.*, 2009).

There are currently no indications for non-planned replacement of either soft or rigid lenses. This raises the question of why a virtually obsolete, non-indicated practice should even be considered in a 21st-century contact lens textbook. Perhaps more than anything else, this chapter will serve as a reminder of the reason why it is considered necessary to replace lenses on a regular basis. In that context, this chapter will review long-term changes in the lens and eye that can occur if lenses are not regularly replaced.

Long-term changes in lenses that are not replaced on a planned basis

Lens deterioration over time manifests in a variety of ways and is attributable to many factors. Lenses become deposited, irreversibly lose water, suffer surface damage and crazing and can become contaminated during storage. Each of these factors will be considered in turn.

Lens deposits

The extent of lens deposition increases over time (Figure 19.1) (Gellatly *et al.*, 1988). Numerous factors, many of which are interactive, are involved in the formation of deposits on the front or back surface of contact lenses. These factors include lens wear modality (daily or continuous wear), the bulk chemical composition of the lens, lens water content, the physicochemical nature of the lens surface (such as ionicity), the chemical composition of lens maintenance solutions, the adequacy of lens maintenance procedures (a measure of patient compliance), hand contamination, proximity to environmental pollutants and intrinsic properties of the tears of the patient (Tighe *et al.*, 1991; Maissa *et al.*, 1998). The most common tear-derived components of lens deposits are proteins (Jones *et al.*, 1997), which cannot be detected under normal conditions. A

DOI: 10.1016/B978-0-7506-8869-7.00019-7

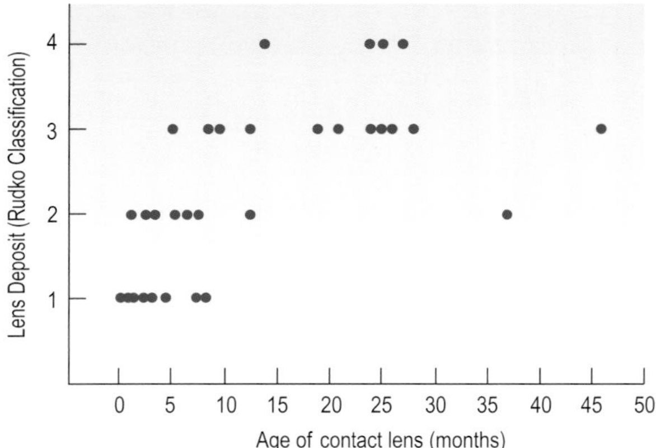

Figure 19.1 Relation between lens deposition (determined using the Rudko classification system) on non-replacement hydroxyethyl methacrylate (HEMA) lenses versus lens age (months). (Adapted from Gellatly, K. W., Brennan, N. A. and Efron, N. (1988) Visual decrement with deposit accumulation on HEMA contact lenses. Am. J. Optom. Physiol. Opt., 65, 937–941.)

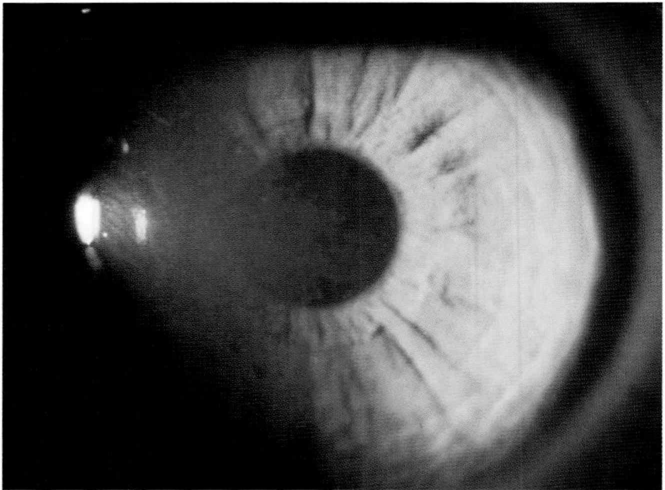

Figure 19.3 Film of protein on a soft lens worn on a non-replacement basis.

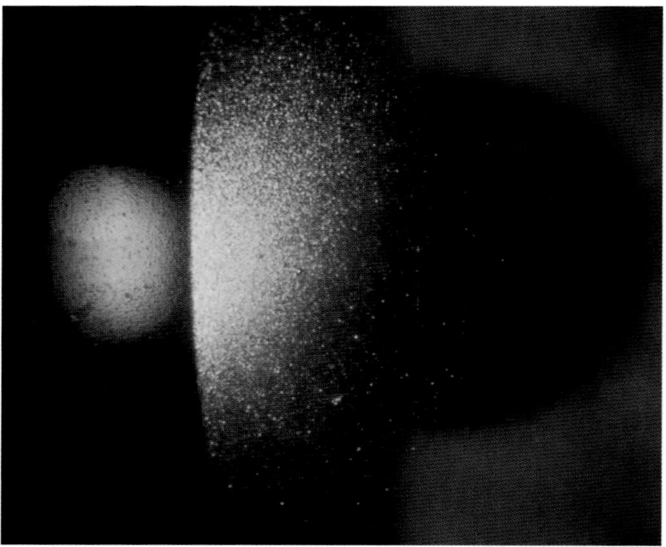

Figure 19.2 Protein haze on a rigid lens worn on a non-replacement basis. (Courtesy of Bausch & Lomb Photo Library (www.bausch.com).)

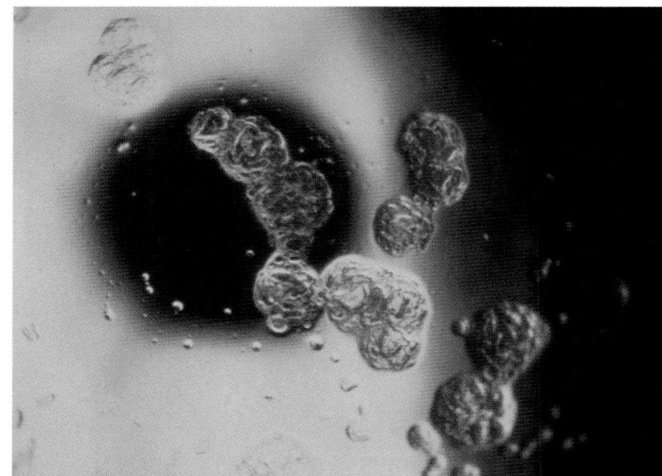

Figure 19.4 'Jelly bumps' on a soft lens worn on a non-replacement basis.

heavy deposition of protein can manifest as a general lens haze on the surface of both rigid lenses (Figure 19.2) and soft lenses (Figure 19.3), and extensive lipid formation can appear as a clear smear or smudge on the lens surface.

Visible soft lens deposits take months or years to form, and are thus only encountered in patients wearing lenses on a non-planned replacement basis. The most common form of visible deposition that is derived from the tear film is known as 'jelly bumps' or 'mulberry deposits', which consist of various layered combinations of mucus, lipid, protein and sometimes calcium (Figure 19.4). Barnacle-like calcium carbonate deposits, which are also derived from the tear film, can project anteriorly and be a source of discomfort (Figure 19.5). Iron deposits, which contaminate the lens from exogenous sources, appear as small red-orange spots or rings and form when iron particles become embedded in the lens and oxidize to form ferrous salts (Figure 19.6). These were often seen in patients who frequently commute on trains or trams, as there is a high

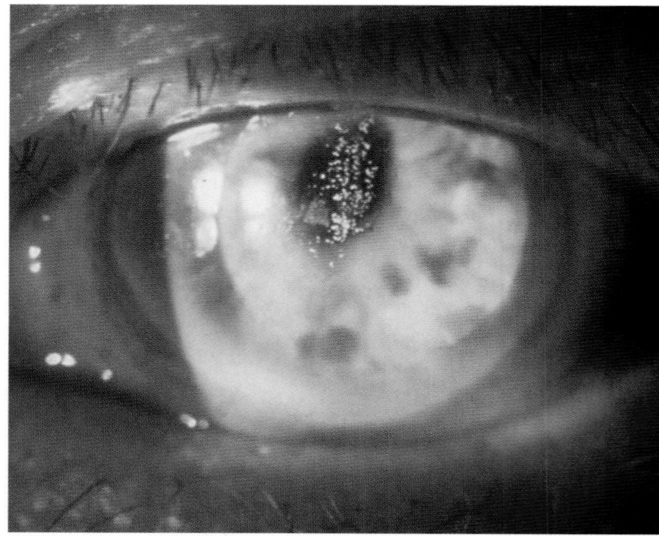

Figure 19.5 Calcium deposits on a soft lens worn on a non-replacement basis.

probability of fine iron particles – which are thrown into the air as the vehicle moves along the steel tracks – coming to rest on the lens surface. Deposits such as those described above are rarely seen on rigid lenses because of the inability of contaminants to become embedded in the lens surface.

It is clear that proteins and lipids from the tears can deposit on soft lenses, and to a lesser extent on rigid lenses, within minutes of insertion (Jones *et al.*, 1997); however, such deposits are thought to be innocuous over periods of less than 1 month. Lipid is easily removed with surfactant cleaning. A small amount of protein deposition may even be beneficial to the eye, as long as it does not become denatured, because the protein forms a natural biocompatible lens coating (Sack *et al.*, 1987). Although these rapidly forming deposits cannot be seen and do not generally compromise vision or comfort, they can reduce lens surface wettability (Jones *et al*, 1996).

Long-term protein deposition can be problematic because, in time, it can become denatured and thus no longer 'recognized' by the eye, leading to an adverse immunological reaction (Sack *et al.*, 1987). Lens surface protein can also absorb, and concentrate, preservatives and other active ingredients in contact lens care solutions, which may be released back into the eye in noxious concentrations, leading to toxic reactions. The physical presence of excess deposits can also cause direct mechanical insult to the anterior eye.

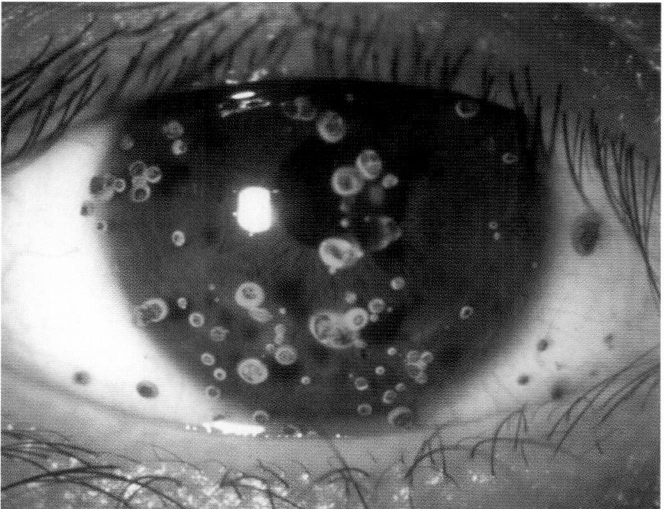

Figure 19.6 Iron deposits on a soft lens worn on a non-replacement basis.

Soft lenses can also become discoloured over extended time periods (many months or years). The cause may be intrinsic or extrinsic. High levels of melanin can lead to a brown discoloration. Nicotine can become absorbed into the lenses of patients who smoke or spend time in a smoky environment, leading to an orange-brown discoloration. Exposure to mercury can lead to a black/grey discoloration. Extreme lens discoloration can be cosmetically unsightly to an onlooker.

Irreversible water loss

Morgan and Efron (2000) noted a significant lens ageing effect whereby the pre-insertion lens water content decreased significantly over a 28-day cycle for four soft lens types evaluated (Figure 19.7). This ageing process is different from the well-known phenomenon of lens dehydration over the course of a number of hours throughout a day. Although this irreversible water loss was only monitored for 28 days, the trend clearly indicated that water loss would continue well beyond this timeframe, albeit at a progressively slower rate.

It is clear that a combination of physical and/or physiological factors caused a reduction in water content of the hydrogel lenses examined by Morgan and Efron (2000). It follows that some change to the lens appears to have caused a progressive reduction in water uptake by the lens each night during storage, in what amounts to a 'lens ageing' effect. The most likely explanation for this ageing effect is that lens spoilation acts either to displace water from the lens or alters the nature of the lens material in such a way that less water is absorbed by the lens. Some significant intersubject differences in lens dehydration were observed;

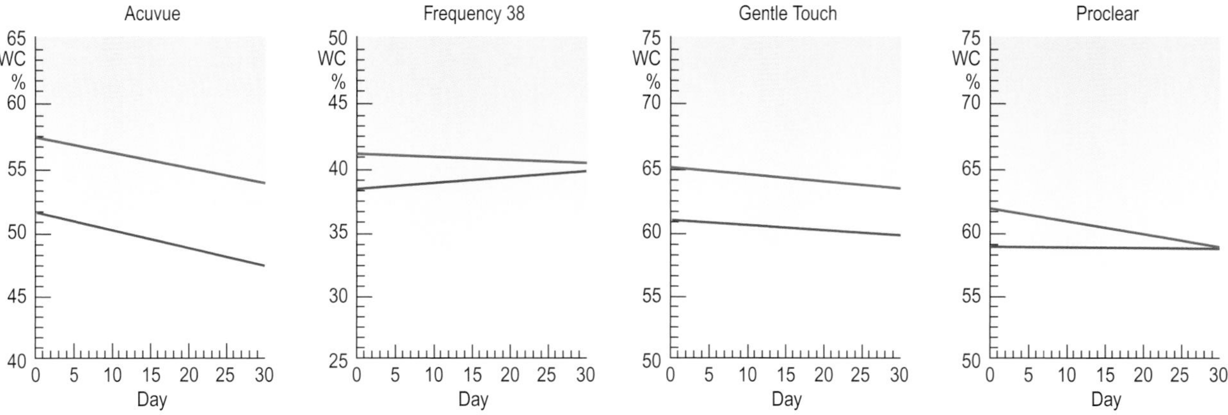

Figure 19.7 Relation between pre-insertion water content (WC: red regression line) and post-removal water content (blue regression line) versus time for the Acuvue, Frequency 38, Gentle Touch and Proclear lenses. The ageing effect is indicated by the decrease in pre-insertion water content over time. (Adapted from Morgan, P. B. and Efron, N. (2000) Hydrogel contact lens ageing. Contact Lens Assoc. Ophthalmol. J., 26, 85–90.)

the range of daily dehydration for the group of 6 subjects investigated by Morgan and Efron (2000) was 1.67–5.91% for all lenses for all days. These differences may relate to intersubject difference in ocular physiology.

One of the most important clinical ramifications of this phenomenon is that there is an associated loss of oxygen performance with dehydration of hydrogel lenses (Efron and Morgan, 1999). Thus, the corneas of patients wearing hydrogel lenses on a non-replacement basis will be more prone to hypoxic complications over time.

Surface damage and crazing

All soft lenses are manufactured with a shelf-life, which primarily indicates how long the lens can be guaranteed to be sterile. In addition, there is the possibility of natural polymer degradation over time, whereby clinically relevant changes could be noticed after about 5 years from the time of manufacture.

It is self-evident that physical trauma can lead to a variety of lens defects. If a defect is obvious – such as a large piece of the lens breaking off – then the patient will typically notice this and discard the lens. If such a defect is not noticed, discomfort on insertion will normally alert the wearer to this problem. However, small defects may not be noticed, which is potentially problematic because such defects can compromise ocular integrity at a subclinical level (Efron and Veys, 1992).

Rigid lenses can develop fine surface scratches over time (Figure 19.8), necessitating lens polishing, or fine splits (Figure 19.9), requiring lens replacement. Another ageing problem with rigid lenses is the development of crazing; that is, the appearance of interconnecting surface cracks that can extend deep into the lens (Figure 19.10). Crazing predisposes the lens to the development of secondary deposits, and the lens can become uncomfortable due to the crazing and/or the existence of deposits (Lembach *et al.*, 1988). Crazing can also be due to problems occurring during manufacture (McLauchlin and Schoessler, 1987).

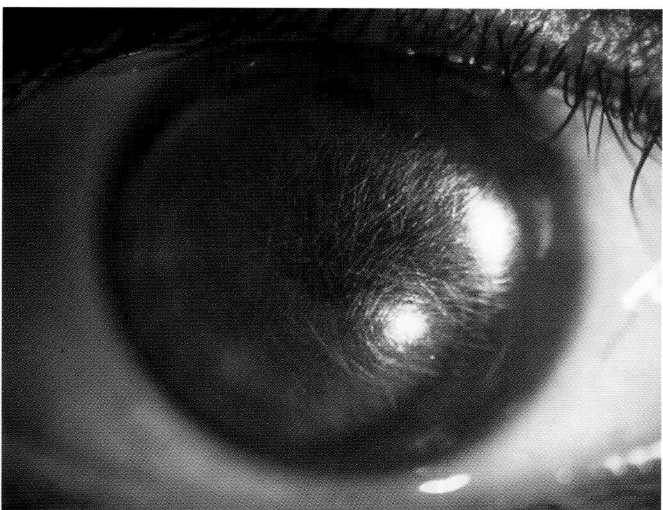

Figure 19.8 Scratches on the surface of a rigid lens worn on a non-replacement basis.

Storage contamination

For a variety of reasons, patients may suspend lens wear for extended periods of time, for reasons such as not wearing lenses when unwell or when travelling. Also, for a variety of lifestyle reasons, some patients only wear lenses very occasionally. The potential for contamination of the lens and storage case during such periods is potentially problematic. In particular, some contact lens storage solutions are inefficacious at killing fungi, which have a propensity for invading the lens matrix and destroying lenses in storage (Figure 19.11) (Wilson and Ahearn, 1986). Stringent measures need to be enforced for the preservation of lenses during long-term storage, such as regular cleaning and disinfection and the use of storage solutions known to be highly efficacious at killing all forms of microorganisms.

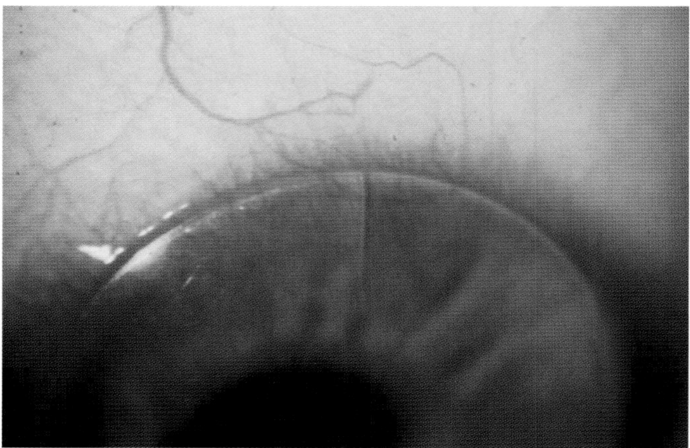

Figure 19.9 Fine split at the edge of a rigid lens worn on a non-replacement basis.

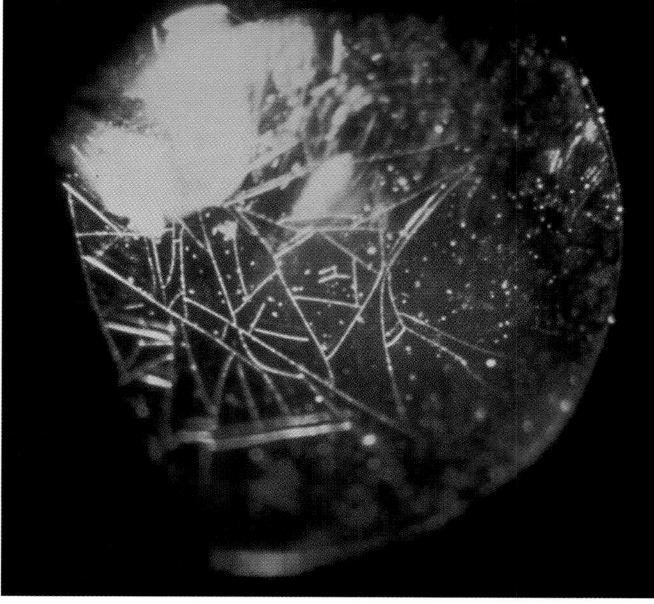

Figure 19.10 Crazing on the surface of a rigid lens worn on a non-replacement basis.

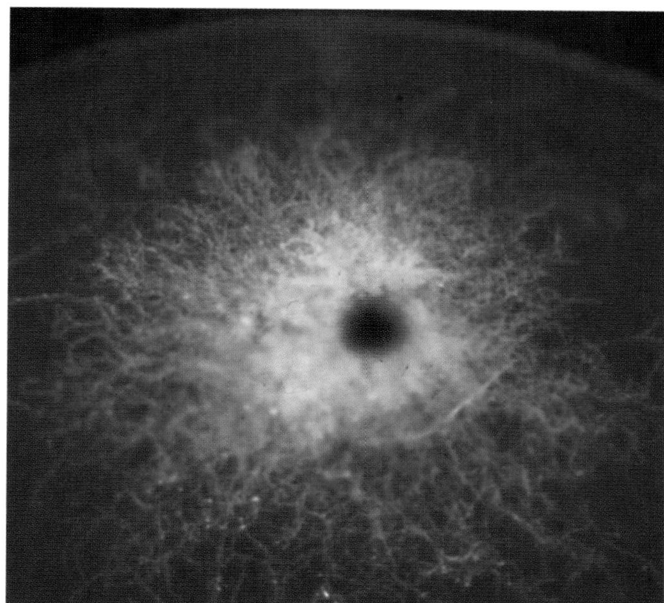

Figure 19.11 Fungal growth within the matrix of a non-replacement soft lens following long-term storage in a solution of low antifungal efficacy.

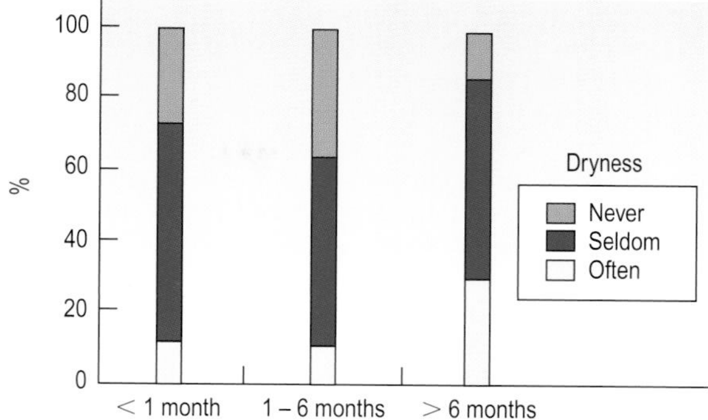

Figure 19.12 Frequency of the symptom of dryness for non-replacement hydroxyethyl methacrylate (HEMA) lenses, categorized by lens age. (Adapted from Brennan, N. A. and Efron, N. (1989) Symptomatology of HEMA contact lens wear. Optom. Vis. Sci. 1989, 66, 834–838.)

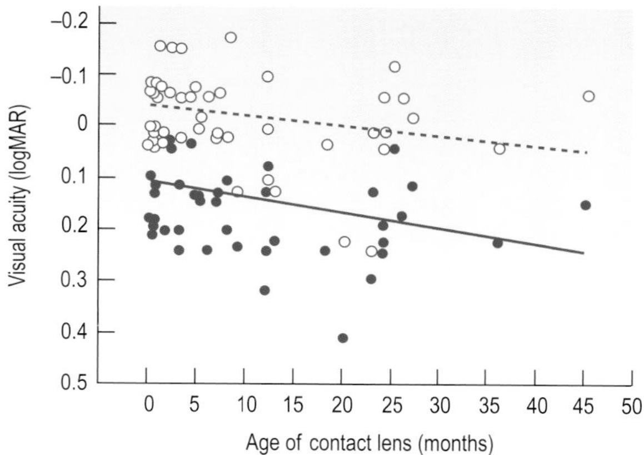

Figure 19.13 Relation between high-contrast visual acuity (logMAR) (open circles and dotted line) and low-contrast visual acuity (logMAR) (closed circles and continuous line) during wear of non-replacement hydroxyethyl methacrylate (HEMA) lenses versus lens age (months). (Adapted from Gellatly, K. W., Brennan, N. A. and Efron, N. (1988) Visual decrement with deposit accumulation on HEMA contact lenses. Am. J. Optom. Physiol. Opt., 65, 937–941.)

Ocular ramifications of non-planned lens replacement

Primary indicators of long-term lens degradation include symptoms of discomfort and reduced vision, and signs associated with adverse ocular reactions.

Discomfort

As indicated above, numerous factors can lead to lenses becoming less comfortable over time; these include the existence of microscopic lens defects, physical trauma and/or immunological reaction due to lens deposition, and progressive hypoxic effects due to lens ageing. In a retrospective study of nearly 2000 2-weekly and non-planned replacement daily-wear patients, Poggio and Abelson (1993) found a higher rate of symptoms in the non-planned replacement group.

Brennan and Efron (1989) surveyed the symptoms experienced by 104 patients wearing hydroxyethyl methacrylate (HEMA) lenses that were not being replaced on a planned basis. They found a clear and statistically significant association between the symptom of dryness and age of the lenses. Of those patients whose lenses were older than 6 months, 31% often experienced dryness, whereas only 12% of patients whose lenses were less than 6 months old experienced this symptom (Figure 19.12).

Reduced vision

The loss of vision associated with deposit accumulation on HEMA contact lenses was assessed by Gellatly *et al.* (1988) in 51 patients presenting consecutively to a large clinic. Both high- and low-contrast visual acuity decreased with increased deposition and with lens age. As a general rule, unacceptable vision loss and deposit formation occurred after 12 months or 4000 hours of lens wear (Figure 19.13).

Ocular surface pathology

Numerous authors have reported that patients using non-planned lens replacement systems suffer from a higher incidence of adverse ocular reactions compared with patients using planned replacement lenses. While planned replacement lenses are made of similar materials, and have a similar design, as lenses supplied on a non-planned replacement basis, the minimization of lens surface deposition on frequently replaced lenses has a significant effect on reducing complication rates (Nilsson, 1997).

Pritchard *et al.* (1996) observed that there was significantly more clinically relevant corneal staining and conjunctival injection, as well as a higher incidence of infiltrates and lens deposits, in patients using lenses on a non-planned replacement basis. Additionally, the overall satisfaction of patients wearing non-planned replacement lenses decreased over time. Conventional soft lenses worn on a daily-wear basis increase the goblet cell count, possibly due to deposit build-up, in the inferior bulbar conjunctiva. This problem does not appear to occur with disposable lens wear. Indeed, there is a direct correlation between the length of wear of a soft contact lens and an irritative goblet cell response (Conner *et al.*, 1997). Poggio and Abelson (1993), in a retrospective study of nearly 2000 2-weekly and conventional daily-wear patients, found a significantly lower prevalence of complications in the planned replacement group for corneal abrasions, oedema and superficial punctate keratitis. Furthermore, patients wearing planned replacement lenses had a lower rate of symptoms.

Soon after their introduction on to the market, disposable lenses were recognized as an effective management strategy for specific complications of lens wear such as contact lens-associated papillary conjunctivitis, sterile infiltrative keratitis and bulbar hyperaemia (see Chapter 40). Papillary conjunctivitis especially has been shown to decrease with more frequent lens replacement – typically 1 month or less (Porazinski and Donshik, 1999). Disposable lenses of a thin, medium-water content design have been suggested as an effective management option for superior epithelial arcuate lesions (Jones and Jones, 1995).

Nilsson and Montan (1994) retrospectively evaluated contact lens-associated keratitis with stromal involvement and concluded that patients wearing lenses on a 2-weekly disposable basis had a significantly lower incidence of keratitis – about one-third the rate – than patients wearing daily-wear soft lenses on a non-planned replacement basis. Similarly, Marshall *et al.* (1992) found the complication rate for disposable lens wearers to be about one-third of that for those who wore lenses on a non-planned replacement basis.

Although many disposable hydrogel lenses are made from ionic lens materials that accumulate tear protein rapidly, the protein does not denature significantly prior to replacement. Against this, any protein may provide binding opportunities for bacteria. Planned replacement is a proven strategy for minimizing the potential adverse effects relating to these phenomena.

Conclusions

In view of the low cost and ready availability of disposable soft lenses in virtually all possible parameters, there is no justification today for prescribing lenses on a non-planned replacement basis. If lenses are prescribed in such a way, the requirements for thorough patient education, the frequency and intensity of patient care and the costs involved will generally be far in excess of those required for patients using planned lens replacement systems.

References

Brennan, N. A. and Efron, N. (1989) Symptomatology of HEMA contact lens wear. *Optom. Vis. Sci.* **66**, 834–838.

Conner, C., Campbell, J. and Steel, S. (1997) The effects of disposable daily wear contact lenses on goblet cell count. *Contact Lens Assoc Ophthalmol. J.*, **23**, 37–39.

Efron, N. and Morgan, P. B. (1999) Hydrogel contact lens dehydration and oxygen transmissibility. *Contact Lens Assoc. Ophthalmol. J.*, **25**, 148–151.

Efron, N. and Veys, J. (1992) Defects in disposable contact lenses can compromise ocular integrity. *Int. Contact Lens Clin.*, **19**, 8–18.

Gellatly, K. W., Brennan, N. A. and Efron, N. (1988) Visual decrement with deposit accumulation on HEMA contact lenses. *Am. J. Optom. Physiol. Opt.*, **65**, 937–941.

Jones, L. and Jones, D. (1995) Photofile part 3 – superior epithelial arcuate lesions. *Optician*, **209**(5500), 32–33.

Jones, L., Franklin, V. and Evans, K. (1996) Spoilation and clinical performance of monthly vs three monthly group II disposable contact lenses. *Optom. Vis. Sci.*, **73**, 16–21.

Jones, L. W., Evans, K., Sariri, R. *et al.* (1997) Lipid and protein deposition of *N*-vinyl pyrrolidone containing group II and group IV frequent replacement contact lenses. *Contact Lens Assoc. Ophthalmol. J.*, **23**, 122–126.

Lembach, R. G., McLaughlin, R. and Barr, J. T. (1988) Crazing in a rigid gas permeable contact lens. *Contact Lens Assoc. Ophthalmol. J.*, **14**, 38–41.

Maissa, C., Franklin, V., Guillon, M. *et al.* (1998) Influence of contact lens material surface characteristics and replacement frequency on protein and lipid deposition. *Optom. Vis. Sci.*, **75**, 697–705.

Marshall, E., Begley, C. and Nguyen, C. (1992) Frequency of complications among wearers of disposable and conventional soft contact lenses. *Int. Contact Lens Clin.*, **19**, 55–60.

McLauchlin, R. G. and Schoessler, J. (1987) Manufacturing defect in a rigid gas-permeable lens. *Int. Eye Care*, **14**, 167.

Morgan, P. B. and Efron, N. (2000) Hydrogel contact lens ageing. *Contact Lens Assoc. Ophthalmol. J.*, **26**, 85–90.

Morgan, P. B., Woods, C. A., Tranoudis, I. G. *et al.* (2009) International contact lens prescribing in 2008. *Contact Lens Spectrum*, **24**, 28–32.

Nilsson, S. (1997) Ten years of disposable lenses – a review of benefits and risks. *Contact Lens Ant. Eye*, **20**, 119–128.

Nilsson, S. and Montan, P. (1994) The hospitalised cases of contact lens induced keratitis in Sweden and their relation to lens type and wear schedule: results of a three-year retrospective study. *Contact Lens Assoc. Ophthalmol. J.*, **20**, 97–101.

Poggio, E. and Abelson, M. (1993) Complications and symptoms with disposable daily wear contact lenses and conventional soft daily wear contact lenses. *Contact Lens Assoc. Ophthalmol. J.*, **19**, 95–102.

Porazinski, A. and Donshik, P. (1999) Giant papillary conjunctivitis in frequent replacement contact lens wearers: a retrospective study. *Contact Lens Assoc. Ophthalmol. J.*, **25**, 142–147.

Pritchard, N., Fonn, D. and Weed, K. (1996) Ocular and subjective responses to frequent replacement of daily wear soft contact lenses. *Contact Lens Assoc. Ophthalmol. J.*, **22**, 53–59.

Sack, R., Jones, B., Antignani, A. *et al.* (1987) Specificity and biological activity of the protein deposited on the hydrogel surface. *Invest. Ophthalmol. Vis. Sci.*, **28**, 842–849.

Tighe, B., Bright, A. and Franklin, V. (1991) Extrinsic factors in soft contact lens spoilation. *J. Br. Contact Lens Assoc.*, **14**, 195–200.

Wilson, L. A. and Ahearn, D. G. (1986) Association of fungi with extended-wear soft contact lenses. *Am. J. Ophthalmol.*, **101**, 434–436.

CHAPTER 20

Daily soft lens replacement

Nathan Efron

Introduction

Daily disposable lenses are one of the two versions of true, single-use-only, disposable lenses – the other being disposable extended-wear lenses.

Daily disposable lenses were first available in 1994. The Premier daily disposable lens was launched in the UK (later this was sold to Bausch & Lomb) and Johnson & Johnson released the 1-Day Acuvue daily disposable lens into western regions of the USA around the same time (Meyler and Ruston, 2006). In the UK, daily disposable lenses gained rapid acceptance, accounting for 28% of all soft lenses prescribed by 1998, and increasing further to 47% by 2008 (Morgan *et al.*, 2009) (Figure 20.1).

Three brands of daily disposable hydrogel lenses became established into major contact lens markets from the mid-1990s: Soflens one-day (Bausch & Lomb; Figure 20.2), Focus Dailies (CIBA Vision; Figure 20.3) and 1-Day Acuvue (Johnson & Johnson; Figure 20.4). Since then, numerous brands of daily disposable hydrogel lenses have entered the market, and in 2009, 16 brands of spherical, four brands of toric, one brand of multifocal and one brand of cosmetic coloured daily disposable hydrogel lens were available in the UK (Kerr and Ruston, 2009).

In 2009, Johnson & Johnson and Sauflon introduced the first daily disposable lenses on to the market made of silicone hydrogel materials; these lenses are known as TruEye (Figure 20.5) and Clariti, respectively. Details of all daily disposable contact lenses on the market in 2009 are presented in Table 20.1.

Unlike 2-weekly and monthly replacement lenses, which dominate the prescribing habits of many practitioners worldwide, usage varies widely among the western contact lens markets. For example, in Denmark, practitioners prescribed 64% of all wearers with daily disposables lenses, a value that rises to 87% if only daily-wear spherical soft lenses are considered. In fact, the high use of daily disposable lenses and the relatively low use of silicone hydrogels for daily wear in Denmark make it the contact lens market that is most disparate from the global average. Daily disposable lenses account for less than 10% of lenses prescribed in markets such as Canada, China and the Netherlands (Morgan *et al.*, 2009). Global average distribution of fitting by lens type is shown in Figure 20.6.

Patterns of wear

The influence of contact lens type on wearing frequency was investigated by Efron and Morgan (2009). All daily-wear lenses were categorized into three groups: rigid, soft daily disposable and 'soft other'. The latter group comprises all reusable (non-daily disposable) soft lenses. The proportion of all fits in relation to the number of days lenses are worn each week is shown in Figure 20.7 for each of these three categories. For rigid and 'soft other' lenses, there is an increasing proportion of fits being used for a greater number of days each week; this distribution is more sharply skewed in respect of rigid lens wearers. The distribution for daily disposable lens wearers appears to be bimodal, with peak wearing frequencies at 2 and 7 days per week. Soft daily disposable lenses are worn, on average, 3.5 ± 2.0 days per week. If part-time and full-time wear is defined as lenses being worn 1–3 and 4–7 days per week, respectively, 40% of those fitted with daily disposable lenses wear lenses full-time versus 91% of those using 'other soft' lenses.

The bimodal distribution of daily disposable lens wearing frequency may reflect two distinct approaches to lens wear. The peak around 1–3 days per week self-evidently represents those using daily disposable lenses on a part-time basis. Indeed, daily disposable lenses are a logical choice for part-time wear because of increased convenience and enhanced safety, as discussed below. Full-time wear of daily disposable lenses is an expensive option compared with full-time wear of 2-weekly or monthly disposable lenses, and those who wear daily disposable lenses full-time (wearing lenses 4–7 days per week) have presumably determined that the enhanced safety and convenience of this approach are worth the higher cost.

The health and lifestyle benefits of daily disposable lenses are clearly reflected in many aspects of the prescribing patterns of this lens type in the UK (Efron and Morgan, 2008). Practitioners in the UK now prescribe this modality to a significant proportion of new and existing patients. The

DOI: 10.1016/B978-0-7506-8869-7.00020-3

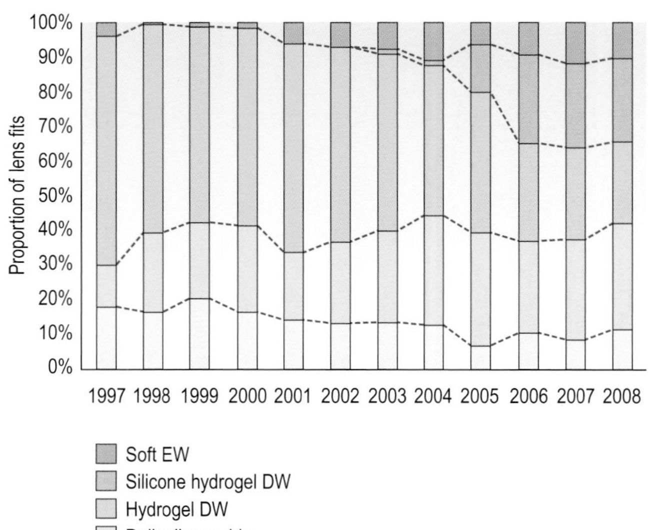

Figure 20.1 Proportion of contact lens fits in the UK between 1997 and 2008. EW = extended wear; DW = daily wear.

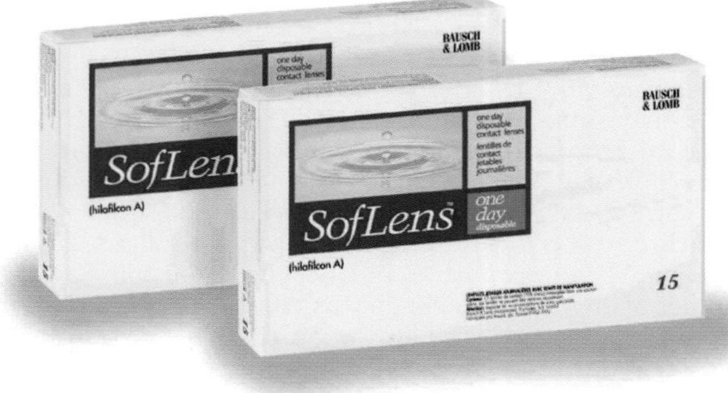

Figure 20.2 SofLens one-day daily disposable contact lens. (Courtesy of Bausch & Lomb Photo Library (www.bausch.com).)

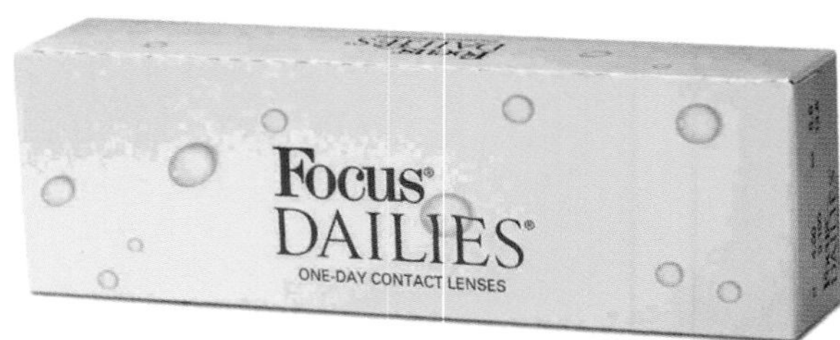

Figure 20.3 Focus Dailies daily disposable contact lens. (Courtesy of CIBA Vision.)

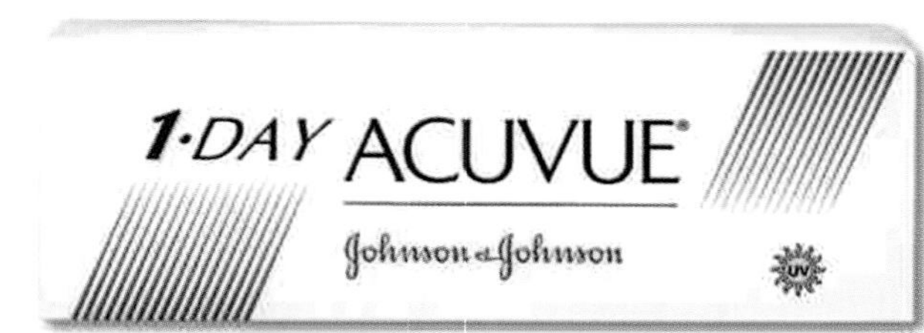

Figure 20.4 1-Day Acuvue daily disposable contact lens. (Courtesy of Johnson and Johnson.)

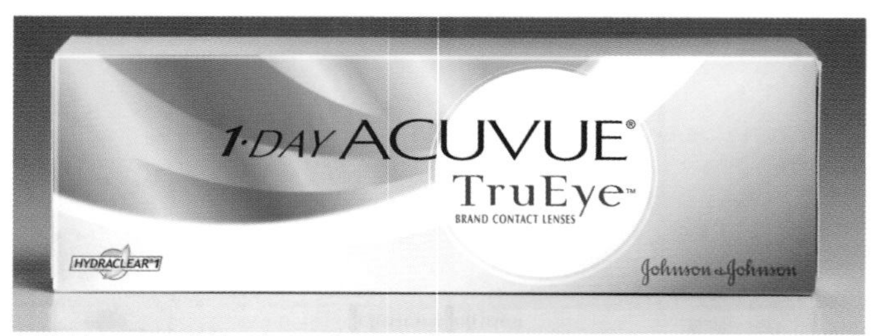

Figure 20.5 Acuvue TruEye daily disposable contact lens. (Courtesy of Johnson and Johnson.)

higher proportion of males fitted with daily disposable lenses and the substantial use of this lens type on a part-time basis are probably related, in that daily disposable lenses are widely promoted for use during sport (ostensibly a part-time activity), and a higher proportion of males in the UK engage in sporting activities (Rowe *et al.*, 2004).

In 2007, the proportion of spherical, toric and multifocal designs, and monovision modalities prescribed as daily disposable soft lenses represented 41%, 22%, 37% and 46%, respectively, of all soft lenses prescribed in those categories (Efron and Morgan, 2008). These data indicate that daily disposable lenses have gained wide acceptance across all categories, making this lens type a viable option for almost any refractive requirement, notwithstanding the reduced choice of designs and parameters compared with other soft lens replacement modalities.

Clinical benefits

If the clinical benefits of planned replacement are accepted, then it would seem logical to change lenses as often as possible. Solomon *et al.* (1996) reported that daily disposable lens wearers had fewer symptoms, fewer deposits, better vision, fewer tarsal abnormalities, fewer ocular complications and better overall satisfaction than patients using conventional lenses. Jones *et al.* (1996) found that lens comfort, subjective symptoms (i.e. dryness, soreness, scratchiness) and vision were significantly better with daily disposable lenses compared to the previously used lens replacement modality (42% of patients were using monthly or fortnightly replacement). Hamano *et al.* (1994) observed a 4.9% incidence of complications for daily disposable lens wearers

Table 20.1 Daily disposable contact lenses

Lens brand	Manufacturer	Material	Water content (%)	BOZR (mm)	Diameter (mm)
Spherical – hydrogel					
SofLens Daily Disposable	Bausch & Lomb	Hilafilcon B II 2	59	8.6	14.2
Focus Dailies AquaComfort Plus	CIBA Vision	Nelfilcon A II 2	69	8.7	14.0
Focus Dailies All Day Comfort	CIBA Vision	Nelfilcon A II 2	69	8.6	13.8
Focus Dailies Basic	CIBA Vision	Nelfilcon A II 2	69	8.6	13.8
Clear 1-day	ClearLab	Hioxifilcon A II 2	58	8.7	14.2
BioMedics 1 Day	CooperVision	Ocufilcon B IV 2	52	8.7	14.2
Proclear 1 Day	CooperVision	Omafilcon A II 2	60	8.7	14.2
FreshCare Daily	David Thomas	Methafilcon A IV 1	58	8.7	14.3
1-Day Acuvue	Johnson & Johnson	Etafilcon A IV 2	58	8.5, 9.0	14.2
1-Day Acuvue Moist	Johnson & Johnson	Etafilcon A IV 2	58	8.5, 9.0	14.2
Daysoft UV 58	Provis	Filcon A II 1	58	8.6	14.2
Daysoft UV 72	Provis	Filcon A II 2	72	8.6	14.2
New Day	Sauflon	Methafilcon A 2	58	8.7	14.3
Safegel 1 Day	Safilens	Filcon IV 1	60	8.6	14.1
Bioclear	Sauflon	Filcon IV 1	56	8.6	14.1
Penta Daily	Scotlens	Methafilcon A IV 1	58	8.7	14.3
Spherical – silicone hydrogel					
1-Day Acuvue TruEye	Johnson & Johnson	Narafilcon A I 4	54	8.5, 9.0	14.2
Clariti 1 day	Sauflon	Filcon II 3	56	8.6	14.1
Toric – hydrogel					
Focus Dailies Toric All Day Comfort	CIBA Vision	Nelfilcon A II 2	69	8.6	14.2
BioMedics 1 Day Toric	CooperVision	Ocufilcon D IV 1	55	8.7	14.5
1-Day Acuvue for Astigmatism	Johnson & Johnson	Etafilcon A IV 2	58	8.5	14.5
Soflens Daily Disposable Toric for Astigmatism	Bausch & Lomb	Hilafilcon B	59	8.6	14.2
Multifocal – hydrogel					
Focus Dailies Progressive All Day Comfort	CIBA Vision	Nelfilcon A II 2	69	8.6	13.8
Cosmetic – hydrogel					
FreshLook One-Day*	CIBA Vision	Nelfilcon A II 2	69	8.6	13.8

BOZR = back optical zone radius.
* Available in blue, green, grey and hazel.

compared with 8.5% for conventional daily-wear soft lens wearers. In a comparison of 2-weekly versus daily disposability, Sindt (2000) noted that, at the very least, patients wearing single-use lenses benefited from greater convenience and comfort.

The obvious advantage offered by daily lens disposal is a fresh, sterile pair of lenses for wear each day. If cost and parameter availability were not limiting factors, then it could be argued that all daily-wear soft lens patients should be using this modality.

Advantages from the perspective of practitioners

Specific advantages of daily disposable lenses from the standpoint of the practitioner include the following:

- Less patient education time is required (virtually no advice needs to be given about lens care).
- The absence of a lens storage case from the regime is beneficial given the role that a lens case can play

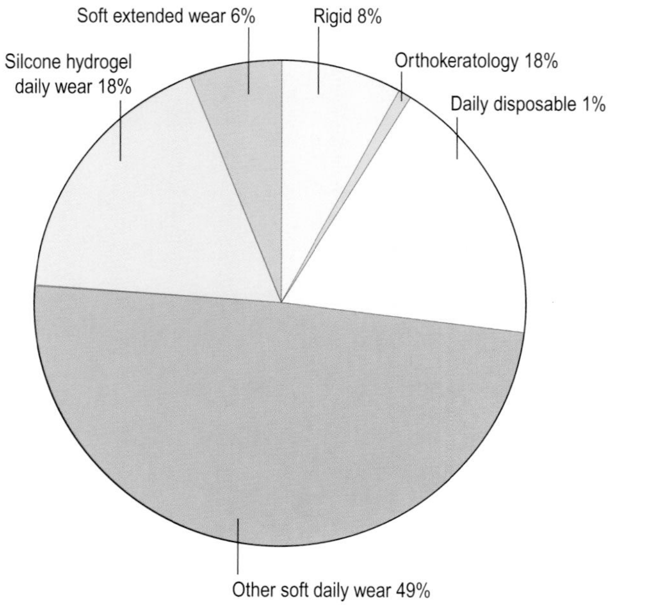

Soft extended wear 6%
Rigid 8%
Silcone hydrogel daily wear 18%
Orthokeratology 18%
Daily disposable 1%
Other soft daily wear 49%

Figure 20.6 The percentage of daily disposable lenses as a proportion of all soft contact lenses prescribed in different nations in 2008.

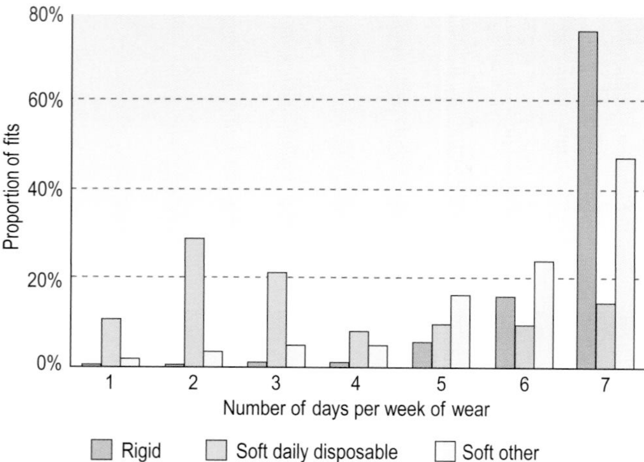

Figure 20.7 Proportion of rigid, daily disposable soft, and all other soft lenses that are worn for between 1 and 7 days per week.

in the development of ocular infection (Clark *et al.*, 1994).

- Less professional 'chair time' is required because there are no problems relating to lens care solutions (e.g. toxicity or sensitivity reactions) or to patient non-compliance with the use of lens care systems. Patient non-compliance with lens care regimens is a major cause of ocular compromise with non-daily-replacement lenses (Claydon and Efron, 1994).
- Less ancillary staff time is required because there is no need for discussions and sales relating to lens care products.
- There are no disputes concerning wearing frequency (e.g. some patients might argue that a lens designed for monthly replacement, but only worn once a week, can last for 3 months).
- Daily disposability is more hygienic for intermittent wearers, as long-term storage problems are eliminated, making daily disposability the replacement modality of choice for such patients.

Advantages from the perspective of lens wearers

Advantages of daily disposable lenses from the perspective of lens wearers include:

- There is no need to be concerned with lens care systems (although it is desirable for daily disposable lens wearers to have a supply of sterile saline or multipurpose solution for lens rinsing if there is discomfort during, or soon after, lens insertion).
- There are no anxieties about lost or damaged lenses.
- Daily disposable lenses are convenient and compact for travel; there is no need to carry bulky lens care solutions.
- Daily disposable lenses are highly cost-effective in that lens wear is directly linked to lens cost (unlike, say, monthly disposable lenses that may be worn only a few times during the month).
- Daily disposable lenses are excellent for monovision correction of presbyopia, as it is easy to alternate between various lens combinations (e.g. two distance lenses versus monovision, depending on the need; see Chapter 25).
- Daily disposable lenses are easy to discard ('any time, any place, without a case').
- Compliance is easier because there are fewer instructions to remember.

Since daily disposable contact lenses eliminate the need for cleaning and disinfection, they should be strongly considered as a contact lens treatment option for children. Walline *et al.* (2004) demonstrated that 8–11-year-old children are able to care for daily disposable contact lenses independently and wear them successfully.

Disadvantages

Potential disadvantages of daily disposable lenses include the following:

- New daily disposable lens wearers who have not previously worn other lens types – and have thus never been instructed in lens care – may adopt unwise practices through ignorance (e.g. storing a lens overnight in tap water).
- Because of the low unit cost of lenses, patients may think it is all right to give lenses to friends to try.

Comfort enhancement strategies

A number of strategies have been adopted by different manufacturers to enhance the comfort of daily disposable lenses. CIBA Vision has modified Dailies All Day Comfort lenses to include additional, non-functional, polyvinyl

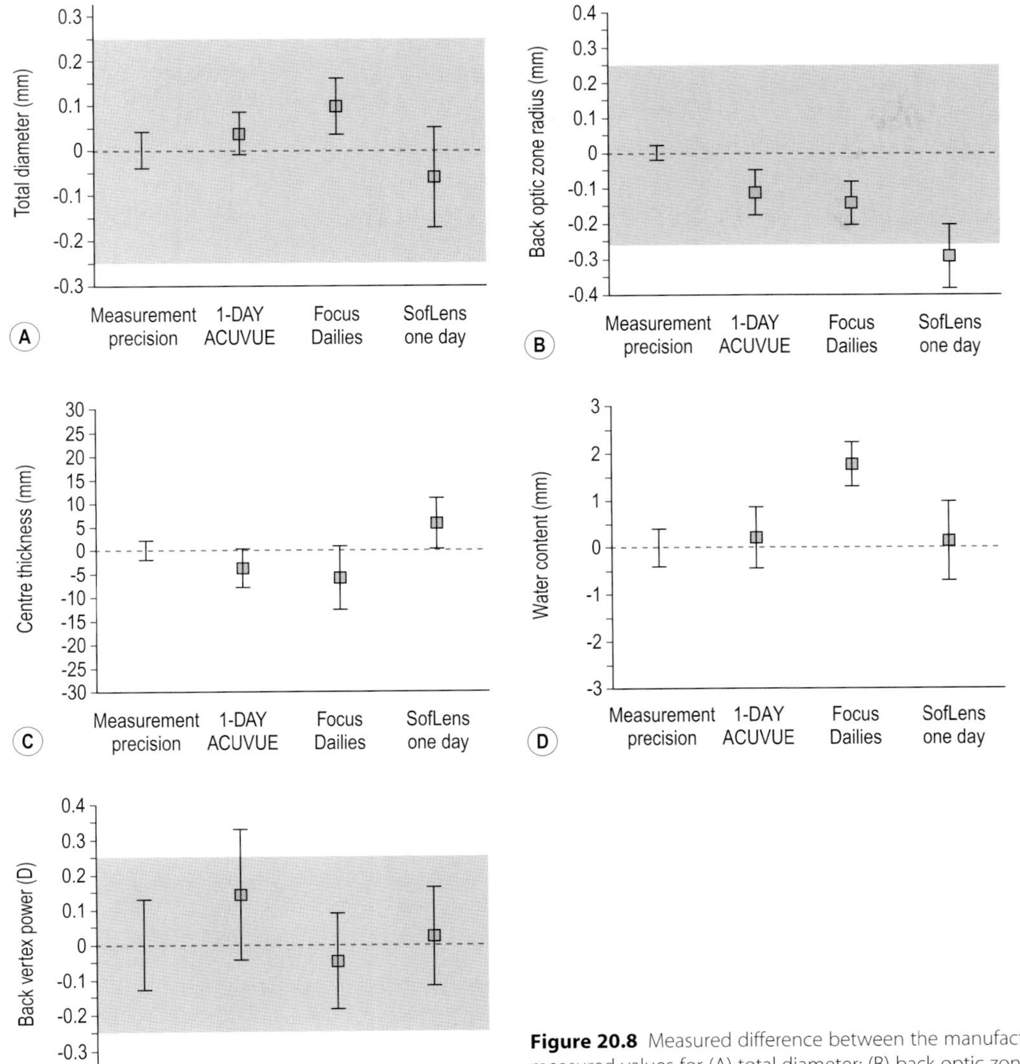

Figure 20.8 Measured difference between the manufacturers' specification and the mean of the measured values for (A) total diameter; (B) back optic zone radius; (C) centre thickness; (D) water content; and (E) back vertex power. Error bars are mean ± standard deviation. The vertical extent of the shaded areas indicate the tolerance allowed under ISO8321-2 (1995). There is no ISO tolerance for water content.

alcohol (PVA). PVA is a successful tear film stabilizer and is widely used in comfort drops. According to Peterson *et al.* (2006), release of additional non-functionalized PVA appears to enhance comfortable contact lens wear. Dailies with AquaComfort Plus contain hypromellose (short for hydroxypropyl methylcellulose, or HPMC), polyethylene glycol (PEG) and dual-molecular-weight PVA, as comfort-enhancing agents.

Vistakon have incorporated proprietary wetting agents into their daily disposable lenses. Acuvue Moist contains Lacreon, and Acuvue TruEye contains Hydraclear, although the detailed chemical formulations of these agents are not in the public domain.

The use of daily disposable lenses has been shown to be an effective strategy for managing allergy-suffering contact lens wearers. Hayes *et al.* (2003) monitored subjective comfort and slit-lamp findings with daily disposable contact lenses in a population of allergy sufferers during periods when allergen levels were elevated. Sixty-seven per cent of subjects agreed that the daily disposable lenses provided improved comfort when compared to the lenses they wore prior to the study, versus 18% agreeing that the new pair of habitual lenses provided improved comfort. The daily disposable lenses also resulted in a greater improvement in slit-lamp findings from baseline than new habitual lenses.

Manufacturing reliability

Efron *et al.* (1999) examined 150 −3.00 D lenses of each of the first three brands of daily disposable lenses on the market, and reported an overall high degree of accuracy and reproducibility (Figure 20.8). They found that, with one inconsequential exception, all measured parameters of all three lens types examined fell well within clinically acceptable limits for providing wearers of these lenses with consistent vision and fit.

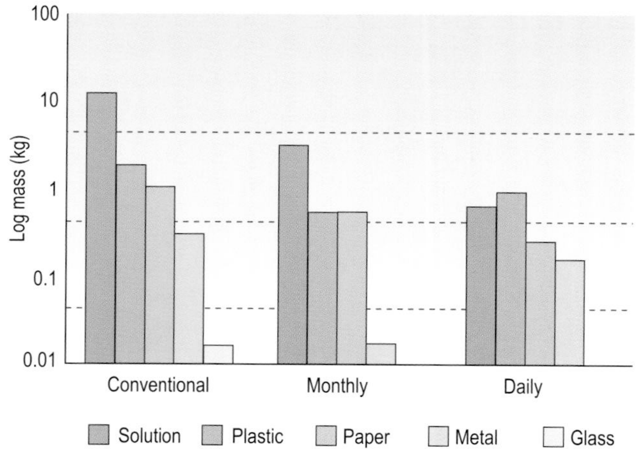

Figure 20.9 Annual wastage involved in the use of unplanned, monthly and daily replacement systems.

Each of the currently marketed daily disposable soft lenses is only available in a single diameter. However, diameter is an important parameter in relation to optimizing lens fit. Young (2008) measured the diameters of 13 designs of daily disposable lenses at room and eye temperature. He observed that lenses labelled 14.2 mm ranged in diameter from 13.5 to 14.1 mm when measured at eye temperature. The three lenses showing the greatest shrinkage when raised to eye temperature were all Food and Drug Administration group IV lenses. Young (2008) concluded that comparing labelled diameters is unhelpful, and in some cases misleading, for predicting the on-eye performance of current daily disposable soft lenses.

Environmental impact

Concerns that daily disposability will have a greater adverse environmental impact compared with other replacement modalities – with respect to disposal of the lenses and associated packaging – have been dispelled by Morgan *et al.* (2003). These authors measured the annual wastage involved in the use of unplanned, monthly and daily replacement systems. Specifically, the amount of waste glass, plastic, metal and paper was determined (solutions were ignored because they have a negligible environmental impact) (Figure 20.9). Of the three replacement systems studied, unplanned lens replacement was found to have the highest environmental impact and monthly lens replacement had the lowest environmental impact. It is possible that the levels of wastage in contact lens manufacture might be more significant than those incurred by consumers. From a wider perspective, the environmental impact of wastage in the use of contact lenses and care systems by consumers pales into insignificance when considered against major sources of world environmental pollution (e.g. road construction, general domestic wastage).

Limitations to more general acceptance

Notwithstanding their current popularity, there appear to be four main reasons why daily disposable lenses are not even more widely used:

1. Parameter and material limitations. This factor is diminishing as volumes increase and more manufacturers launch daily disposable lenses in wider power ranges, with toric, multifocal, cosmetically coloured and silicone hydrogel lenses available.
2. Practitioner concerns about patient non-compliance. Compliance is always likely to be a problem to some extent. For example, between 10–13% of patients reuse daily disposable lenses (Qureshi et al., 1998; Dumbleton et al., 2009). With all contact lens wear, thorough initial and ongoing patient education to promote compliance is essential.
3. Practitioner concerns about non-optical-practice lens supply. The topic of non-optical practice supply is considered in Chapter 21 as part of a discussion of practice management issues.
4. Patient concerns about the cost of full-time wear. Daily disposable lenses are the preferred choice in part-time wear, where the cost is lower. As noted above, the distribution of daily disposable lens wear is bimodal, with peaks at 2 days and 7 days per week of wear. Clearly many patients value the convenience over cost in full-time wear.

Corneal infiltrative events and keratitis

Sankaridurg *et al.* (2003) evaluated the type and incidence of adverse events seen with daily disposable hydrogel contact lens wear compared with a control (spectacle) group over 12 months. Asymptomatic infiltrates were seen in both contact lens and spectacle groups, at 20.5 events versus 11.3 events per 100 eyes per year of wear, respectively. No significant events were seen with the spectacle group. With the contact lens group, the type and incidence of significant events per 100 eyes per year of lens wear were: corneal peripheral ulcer, 2.5 events; infiltrative keratitis, 1.5 events; and papillary conjunctivitis, 1 event. The incidence of both significant and non-significant events was greater with the contact lens group ($P < 0.05$). A greater number of subjects were lost to follow-up or permanently discontinued from the contact lens group relative to the spectacle group (33% versus 17%, $P = 0.002$). Lens-related problems such as dryness, discomfort and difficulty with insertion and removal accounted for 27% of discontinuations from the contact lens group.

Efron *et al.* (2005) examined the distribution of corneal infiltrative events (CIEs) of all levels of severity in symptomatic contact lens wearers presenting to a hospital emergency clinic. Figure 20.10 shows the distribution of CIEs in patients wearing daily disposable hydrogel lenses versus all other forms of daily hydrogel lens wear. CIEs tended to occur more towards the lens periphery in those wearing daily-wear hydrogel lenses and more towards the lens centre in those wearing daily disposable hydrogel lenses.

Efron *et al.* (2005) suggested that the disproportionately greater number of corneal infiltrates occurring in the periphery of those using daily-wear hydrogel lenses is related to the typical methods adopted by patients for manually cleaning soft lenses. The two classic techniques used to clean contact lenses with solutions are: (1) to place the lens on the palm of one hand and rub the lens in a circular motion with the index finger of the other hand; and (2) to rub the lens between the index finger and thumb

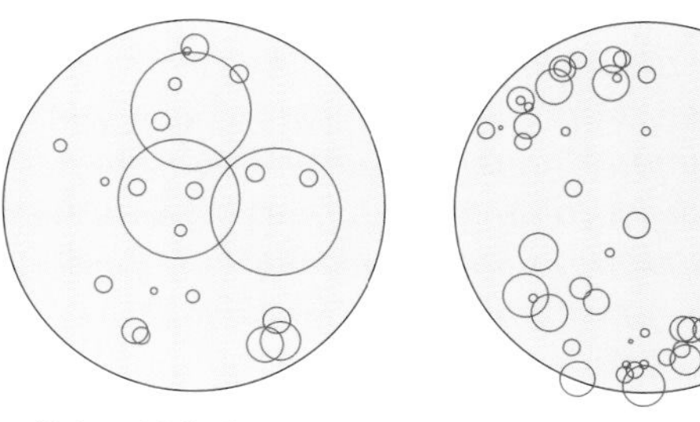

Figure 20.10 Distribution and size of corneal infiltrative events (blue circles) in patients wearing daily disposable hydrogel lenses versus all other forms of daily hydrogel lens wear. The two large black circles represent corneas (right eye representation).

(Stein *et al.*, 2002). In both cases, there is a tendency for the cleaning effect to be concentrated towards the centre of the lens, which leads to a higher concentration of deposits, such as denatured proteins, in the lens periphery compared to the more thoroughly cleaned lens centre (Heiler *et al.*, 1991). Lens deposits can compromise corneal integrity in a number of ways, such as: having a direct mechanical effect; harbouring environmental antigens and causing an immunological reaction in the adjacent cornea; or harbouring microorganisms and inducing an infection in the underlying cornea. Excess deposits in the lens periphery resulting in these forms of compromise in the peripheral cornea could account for the distribution of infiltrates observed in patients wearing daily-wear hydrogel lenses in this study.

Given the above arguments, it would be expected that daily-wear hydrogel daily disposable lenses - which are discarded after each use and never manually cleaned - would be associated with a random distribution of infiltrates. However, a disproportionately greater number of infiltrates were observed towards the centre of the corneas of patients wearing such lenses. Efron *et al.* (2005) suggested that this may relate to patterns of lens contamination from the fingers of patients at the time of lens insertion. That is, prior to lens insertion, patients typically 'fish' the lens from the blister pack with the forefinger, which is placed on or near the centre of the lens as it is removed. Thus, there is a greater propensity for contamination of the centre of the lens, and for such contaminants to be transferred directly to the centre of the cornea upon lens insertion.

Radford *et al.* (2009) reported that, compared with planned-replacement soft lenses, daily disposable lenses significantly reduced the risk of toxic/hypersensitivity and metabolic disorders. However, one particular lens brand was associated with a 2.7× increased risks of sterile keratitis, a 2.2× increased risk of mechanical disorders and a tendency for patients to have lens removal difficulties.

There are reports of *Acanthamoeba* keratitis in patients who reuse daily disposable contact lenses. Diagnosis can be difficult to make but should still be considered in all patients who wear contact lenses, including daily disposable lenses (Niyadurupola and Illingworth, 2006). A case of a *Pseudomonas* corneal ulcer has been documented in a fully compliant occasional user of daily disposable lenses (Munneke *et al.*, 2006). The lenses were not overworn, reused or slept in - all risk factors for corneal infection.

Dart *et al.* (2008) reported that, compared with planned-replacement soft lenses, the risk of microbial keratitis was increased 1.56× with daily disposable contact lenses and differed between different lens brands. However, the risk of vision loss with daily disposable lenses was less than for planned-replacement soft lenses and no daily disposable lens users lost vision to the level 6/12.

Two studies have determined the incidence of microbial keratitis with daily disposable lenses. Morgan *et al.* (2005) reported an incidence of 4.9 and 6.4 cases of severe (microbial) keratitis per 10 000 wearers per year with daily disposable hydrogel lenses and 'other' hydrogel lenses, respectively. Stapleton *et al.* (2008) reported an incidence of 2.0 and 1.9 cases of microbial keratitis per 10 000 wearers per year with daily disposable hydrogel lenses and 'other' hydrogel lenses, respectively. However, in patients who occasionally slept overnight in daily disposable hydrogel lenses, the incidence of microbial keratitis increased to 4.2 cases per 10 000 wearers per year. These reports suggest that, for daily lens wear, daily disposability does not appreciably reduce the risk of microbial keratitis compared with planned lens replacement protocols.

Conclusions

It is likely that all lenses prescribed in the future will be 'single-use' products, such as daily disposable or extended-wear lenses. However, patients who wear daily disposable contact lenses should be reminded that the benefits of this modality of contact lens are only possible if the lenses are worn once and thrown away.

Acknowledgements

The author wishes to thank Trevor Rowley, Bausch & Lomb, CooperVision, CIBA Vision, Biocompatibles Hydron, Lunelle and Vistakon for providing photographs.

References

Clark, G., Harkins, L., Munro, F. *et al.* (1994) Microbial contamination of cases used for storing contact lenses. *J. Infec.*, **28**, 293–304.

Claydon, B. and Efron, N. (1994) Non-compliance in contact lens wear. *Ophthal. Physiol. Opt.*, **14**, 356–364.

Dart, J. K., Radford, C. F., Minassian, D. *et al.* (2008) Risk factors for microbial keratitis with contemporary contact lenses: a case-control study. *Ophthalmology*, **115**, 1647–1654.

Dumbleton, K. A., Richter, D., Woods, C. A. (2009) Patient and practitioner compliance with silicone hydrogel and daily disposable lens replacement in the USA and Canada. Paper presented at the Annual Meeting of the American Academy of Optometry, Orlando, Florida, USA. November 11–14.

Efron, N. and Morgan, P. B. (2008) Prescribing daily disposable contact lenses in the UK. *Cont. Lens Anterior Eye*, **31**, 107–108.

Efron, N. and Morgan, P. B. (2009) How often are contact lenses worn? *Cont. Lens Anterior Eye*, **32**, 35–36.

Efron, N., Morgan, P. B. and Morgan, S. L. (1999) Accuracy and reproducibility of one day disposable contact lenses. *Int. Contact Lens Clin.*, **26**, 168–173.

Efron, N., Morgan, P. B., Hill, E. A. *et al.* (2005) The size, location and clinical severity of corneal infiltrative events associated with contact lens wear. *Optom. Vis. Sci.*, **82**, 519–527.

Hamano, H., Watanabe, K., Hamano, T., *et al.* (1994) A study of the complications induced by conventional and disposable contact lenses. *Contact Lens Assoc. Ophthalmol. J.,* **20,** 103–108.

Hayes, V. Y., Schnider, C. M. and Veys, J. (2003) An evaluation of 1-day disposable contact lens wear in a population of allergy sufferers. *Cont. Lens Anterior Eye,* **26,** 85–93.

Heiler, D. J., Gambacorta-Hoffman, S., Groemminger, S. F. *et al.* (1991) The concentric distribution of protein on patient-worn hydrogel lenses. *Contact Lens Assoc. Ophthalmol. J.,* **17,** 249–251.

Jones, L., Jones, D., Langley, C. *et al.* (1996) Subjective responses of 100 consecutive patients to daily disposables. *Optician,* **211**(5536), 28–32.

Kerr, C. and Ruston, D. (2009*) The ACLM Contact Lens Year Book 2009.* Wiltshire: The Association of Contact Lens Manufacturers. pp. 19–20.

Meyler, J. and Ruston D. (2006) The world's first daily disposables. *Optician,* **231**(6053), 12.

Morgan, S. L., Morgan, P. B. and Efron, N. (2003) Environmental impact of three replacement modalities of soft contact lens wear. *Contact Lens Anterior Eye,* **26,** 43–46.

Morgan, P. B., Efron, N., Hill, E. A. *et al.* (2005) Incidence of keratitis of varying severity among contact lens wearers. *Br. J. Ophthalmol.,* **89,** 430–436.

Morgan, P. B., Woods, C. A., Tranoudis, I. G. *et al.* (2009) International contact lens prescribing in 2008. *Contact Lens Spectrum,* **24**(2), 28–32.

Munneke, R., Lash, S. C. and Prendiville, C. (2006) A case of a pseudomonas corneal ulcer in an occasional use daily disposable contact lens wearer. *Eye Contact Lens,* **32,** 94–95.

Niyadurupola, N. and Illingworth, C. D. (2006) Acanthamoeba keratitis associated with misuse of daily disposable contact lenses. *Cont. Lens Anterior Eye,* **29,** 269–271.

Peterson, R. C., Wolffsohn, J. S., Nick, J. *et al.* (2006) Clinical performance of daily disposable soft contact lenses using sustained release technology. *Cont. Lens Anterior Eye,* **29,** 127–134.

Qureshi, S., Forrest, I. and Lee, R. (1998) Patient compliance. *Optician,* **216**(5671), 32–36.

Radford, C. F., Minassian, D., Dart, J. K. *et al.* (2009) Risk factors for non-ulcerative contact lens complications in an ophthalmic accident and emergency department: a case-control study. *Ophthalmology,* **116,** 385–392.

Rowe, N., Beasley, N. and Adams, R. (2004) Sport, physical activity and health: future prospects for improving the health of the nation. *In: Driving up participation: the challenge for sport.* London: Sport England, p. 14–26.

Sankaridurg, P. R., Sweeney, D. F., Holden, B. A. *et al.* (2003) Comparison of adverse events with daily disposable hydrogels and spectacle wear: results from a 12-month prospective clinical trial. *Ophthalmology,* **110,** 2327–2334.

Sindt, C. (2000) Daily disposable versus two-week disposable lenses. *Contact Lens Spectrum* **14**(5), 33–38.

Solomon, O., Freeman, M., Boshnik, E., *et al.* (1996) A 3-year prospective study of the clinical performance of daily disposable contact lenses compared with frequent replacement, and conventional daily wear contact lenses. *Contact Lens Assoc. Ophthalmol. J.,* **22,** 250–257.

Stapleton, F., Keay, L., Edwards, K. *et al.* (2008) The incidence of contact lens-related microbial keratitis in Australia. *Ophthalmology,* **115,** 1655–1662.

Stein, H. A., Slatt, B. J., Stein, R. M. *et al.* (2002) Care systems for soft lenses. In: *Fitting Guide for Rigid and Soft Contact Lenses: A Practical Approach,* pp. 127–142, St Louis, MO: Mosby.

Walline, J. J., Long, S. and Zadnik, K. (2004) Daily disposable contact lens wear in myopic children. *Optom. Vis. Sci.,* **81,** 255–259.

Young, G. (2008) Daily disposable soft lens diameters. *Optician,* **235**(March), 24–26.

CHAPTER 21

Planned soft lens replacement

Joe Tanner

Introduction

Despite the widespread use of contact lenses that are prescribed on a planned replacement basis, there are no internationally consistent definitions for this or related terms. In this book, 'planned replacement' refers to lens replacement at intervals from 1 day to 12 months and, therefore, includes all 'disposable lenses', which are defined as lenses replaced at least monthly. This nomenclature is presented in Table 21.1.

The first disposable lenses were released internationally in the late 1980s (Figure 21.1). The acceptance of disposability by practitioners and patients has been one of the most significant changes in the contact lens market, as shown in Figure 21.2. By 2006, UK practitioners were fitting 99% of their new soft lens patients with disposable lenses, compared with 61% 10 years before (Morgan and Efron, 2006).

The Acuvue lens (Johnson & Johnson) was initially packaged in plastic boxes, but this was soon replaced by cardboard boxes for reasons of reduced cost and packaging efficiency (to enable storage of the maximum number of lenses per unit volume). The NewVues lens (CIBA Vision) was originally supplied in glass vials, but this was soon changed to blister packs for the same reasons. The form of packaging initially used for the SeeQuence lens (Bausch & Lomb) is now adopted by virtually all disposable lens manufacturers. Products replaced at least monthly have invariably been designed, packaged and promoted for replacement at specific intervals. However, this applies less for lenses replaced 3-monthly, and is almost never the case for lenses offered for biannual and annual replacement; such lenses are usually conventional lenses packaged in vials (Figure 21.3), and many of these lenses were developed prior to widespread use of planned replacement.

Planned replacement has been shown to be clinically useful for extended-wear applications, and since their advent in 1998 silicone hydrogel soft lenses for both extended and daily wear have been marketed on a planned replacement basis. Discussion of planned lens replacement in this chapter will be confined to lenses intended to be used on a daily-wear basis (i.e. lenses that are not worn overnight) for at least a week. The specific issue of planned replacement of continuous-wear lenses is dealt with in Chapter 26 and daily disposable lenses are specifically covered in Chapter 20.

Advantages of planned replacement

The rationale for the planned replacement of soft contact lenses is simple: cleaner lenses should produce fewer adverse ocular effects. A significant proportion of clinical problems relating to the wear of soft contact lenses can be attributed to deposition on the lens surface with tear-derived substances. Contact lens deposits result in reduced acuity, comfort and wettability and increased inflammatory complications such as papillary conjunctivitis and acute red eye (Jones *et al.*, 2000). All soft contact lenses suffer gradual spoilation from the environment and tear film components over time. Daily cleaning and periodic protein removal can slow this rate of deposition but not prevent its occurrence. By ensuring that soft lenses are replaced at a suitable predetermined interval, one of the most enduring medical management axioms – that of prevention being better than cure – is brought to bear. In practice, patients who replace lenses regularly report fewer symptoms and exhibit fewer physiological changes in most instances (Marshall *et al.*, 1992; Poggio and Abelson, 1993; Nilsson and Montan, 1994; Pritchard *et al.*, 1996; Nilsson, 1997; Porazinski and Donshik, 1999), compared with patients who do not replace lenses regularly.

Long-term adverse changes in contact lenses and in the anterior eye when lenses are not replaced on a planned basis were discussed in Chapter 19. As well, specific benefits arise from the use of planned replacement lenses (Ehlers *et al.*, 2003); these are so compelling that any decision not to prescribe soft lenses on this basis requires special justification, such as parameter and/or design unavailability, and should be a comparatively rare event.

The principal benefits of planned replacement lenses – further to the avoidance of problems experienced with unplanned lens replacement as discussed in Chapter 19 – are outlined below.

DOI: 10.1016/B978-0-7506-8869-7.00021-5

Table 21.1 Proposed nomenclature for discussing lens replacement*

Planned replacement daily-wear lenses						
Disposable			**Non-disposable**			
Daily	Weekly	2-weekly	Monthly	3-monthly	6-monthly	Yearly

* Unplanned replacement refers to lenses that are prescribed to be worn until they are lost or damaged, or until they begin to compromise vision, comfort or ocular health.

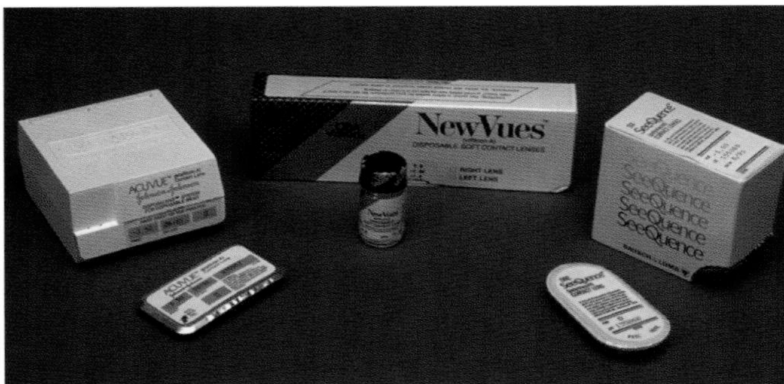

Figure 21.1 The first disposable lenses released on to the international market in the late 1980s. Left: The Acuvue lens (Courtesy of Johnson & Johnson). Centre: NewVues lens (Courtesy of CIBA Vision). Right: SeeQuence lens (Courtesy of Bausch & Lomb).

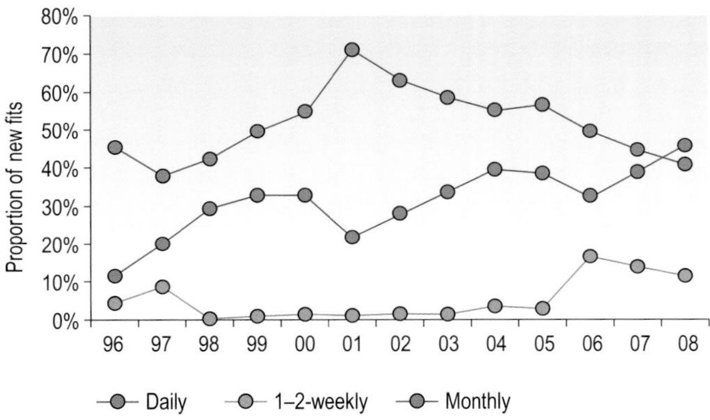

Figure 21.2 Proportion of new fits by replacement frequency.

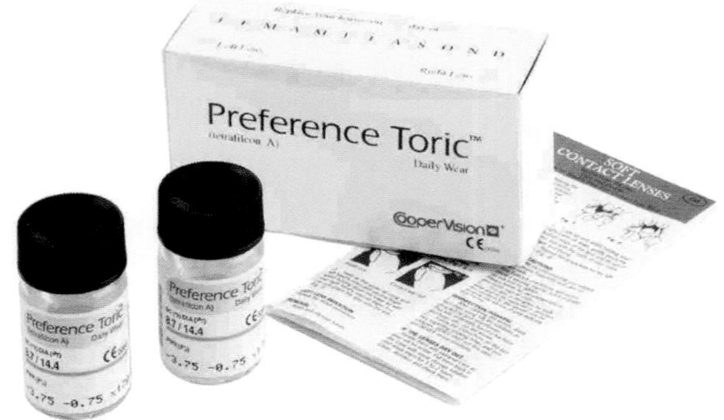

Figure 21.3 Example of a non-disposable planned replacement lens. This lens is replaced 3-monthly.

Use of higher-water-content hydrogel materials

There are two strategies for improving the oxygen transmissibility (*Dk/t*) of contact lenses made from conventional hydrogel materials – reduce the lens thickness profile and/or increase the lens water content. An analysis of these options by Brennan *et al.* (1991) demonstrated that, particularly in higher powers, the latter strategy is more effective at improving corneal oxygenation. However, lenses made from higher-water-content materials generally have lower elastic moduli and therefore reduced durability than their lower-water-content counterparts. High-water-content materials, particularly those with an ionic surface chemistry, also attract tear film deposits such as jelly bumps and protein at a faster rate (Jones, 1990).

As a result of the above factors, the life expectancy of lenses made from higher-water-content materials is limited to approximately 6 months on average (Jones *et al.*, 1996). If a planned replacement system is used, then the issues of durability and especially deposit resistance become less significant. Planned lens replacement therefore provides a rationale for the use of medium- to high-water-content materials.

Use of silicone hydrogel materials

Silicone hydrogel lenses (Figure 21.4) tend to have lower water contents and may accumulate surface deposits of significantly different type and quantity to conventional hydrogels (Jones *et al.*, 2003). Although the amount of protein spoilation on these materials tends to be lower, the proportion which is denatured and therefore potentially a cause of contact lens-associated papillary conjunctivitis may be higher. Lipid deposition tends to be greater with silicone hydrogels (Cheung et al., 2007). Planned replacement is therefore still the preferred appropriate strategy for these materials.

Simple lens care regimes

While the need to clean and disinfect multiuse soft lenses is self-evident, a powerful argument for prolonging the life of lenses with elaborate lens care systems emerged in the early days of soft lenses because of their relatively high cost of production. By the start of the 1980s, soft lenses were becoming the preferred option in many countries. To achieve the then lens life norm of at least a year, a minimum of three lens care product types were needed. Daily cleaners were used to remove loose deposits and microorganisms from the lens surface; disinfecting solutions were used to kill any remaining microorganisms; and protein removal tablets were used to reduce the build-up of tear proteins on the lens surface. The ongoing cost of these products was often found to be more than that of the contact lenses themselves.

Planned replacement lenses (excluding daily disposable lenses) still need high standards of lens care to ensure safe wear, but the shorter replacement cycles allow some scope for simplification. It should not be necessary to deproteinize lenses changed at least monthly. In cases where lens surface spoilation is a problem with monthly replacement, shortening the replacement interval to 2 weeks or even

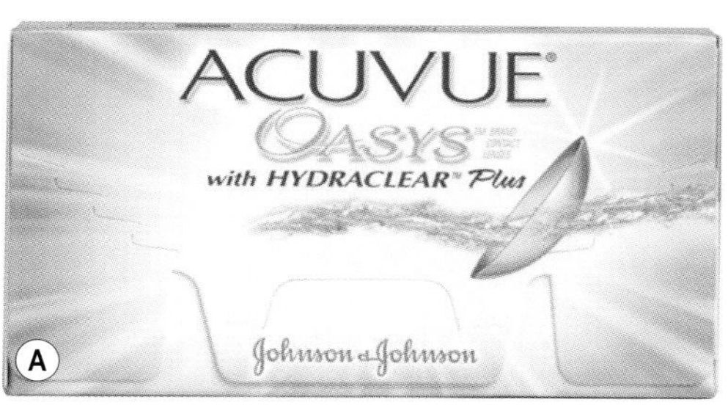

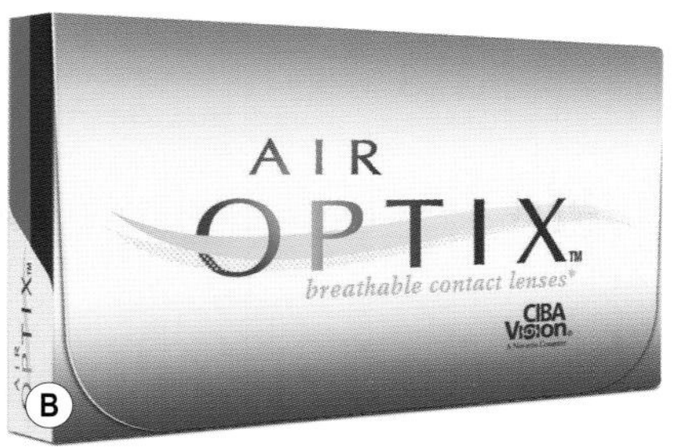

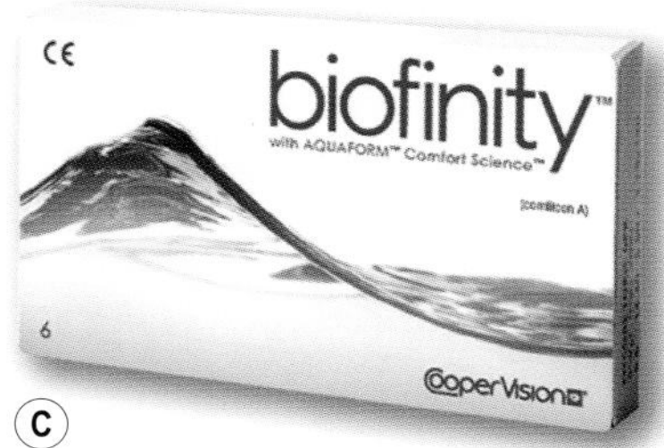

Figure 21.4 Examples of silicone hydrogel lenses. (A) Acuvue Oasys. (B) AirOptix. (C) Biofinity.

Table 21.2 Functional contact lens care for daily-wear soft lenses used for different replacement intervals

Frequency of lens replacement	Daily cleaning	Rinsing	Disinfecting	Protein removal
Daily	×	✓	×	×
Weekly	✓	✓	✓	×
Two-weekly	✓	✓	✓	×
Monthly	✓	✓	✓	×
Three-monthly	✓	✓	✓	?
Six-monthly or more	✓	✓	✓	✓

1 day is likely to be a superior option – at least in terms of patient convenience and therefore compliance – than adding a protein removal step to the care regime.

Table 21.2 outlines the typical functional steps that need to be carried out in the care of lenses replaced at different intervals.

While mechanical daily cleaning, rinsing and disinfection are still essential in the care of 2-weekly and monthly replacement lenses, in most cases these functions can be effectively achieved with a single lens care product, namely a multipurpose solution (Franklin, 1997) (see Chapter 11).

Typical lens care systems that are used for different planned replacement intervals are listed in Table 21.3.

As the replacement interval increases, the need for a separate protein removal step becomes more likely, although the inclusion of a sequestering agent in multipurpose solutions has been shown to obviate the need for this (Edwards, 1998).

Table 21.3 Typical lens care systems for daily-wear soft lenses used for different replacement intervals

Frequency of lens replacement	Typical lens care regime
Daily	Saline/multipurpose solution for rinsing
Weekly	Multipurpose solution
Two-weekly	Multipurpose solution
Monthly	Multipurpose solution
Three-monthly	Multipurpose solution (possibly with protein removal) or Hydrogen peroxide with separate daily cleaner (possibly with protein removal)
Six-monthly or more	Hydrogen peroxide with separate daily cleaner and protein removal

Ready availability of replacement lenses

Lenses replaced weekly, fortnightly or monthly are normally supplied in packs of three or six. It follows that the loss or damage of a lens should not, in most cases, be an inconvenience to a patient wearing disposable lenses. Practices fitting disposable lenses are also likely to have numerous trial lenses, and even stocks of the more popular parameters, on the premises, which enables rapid replacement if lens loss or damage occurs.

Enhanced compliance with aftercare schedules

Planned replacement protocols require patients to return at regular intervals for fresh lenses. Aftercare visits can be scheduled to coincide with lens collection, which is a further benefit of prescribing this modality. However, regular repurchasing does not necessarily imply compliance with the wearing schedule (Claydon and Efron, 1994).

Single-use trial lenses

In the case of disposable lenses, new diagnostic or trial lenses are used with each patient, and disposed of thereafter. This eliminates the risk of cross-infection from a previous wearer of the lens. It also has the advantage of eliminating the time-consuming chore of trial lens cleaning, disinfection and storage.

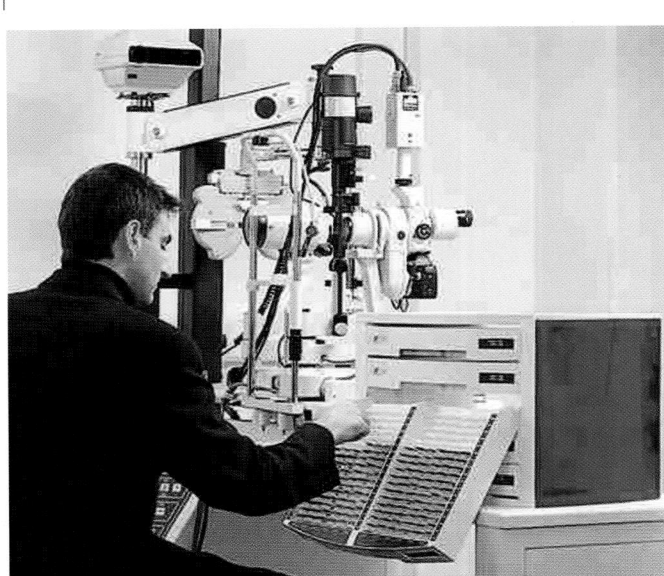

Figure 21.5 The availability of single-use diagnostic lenses allows for accurate trialling and eliminates the risk of cross-infection.

Trial lens fitting with accurate prescription

With the ready availability of a comprehensive stock of trial lenses (Figure 21.5), it is nearly always possible to undertake a lens-wearing trial on a prospective disposable lens patient with the required lens parameters, especially with respect to lens power.

This will, of course, allow for the most realistic subjective impression of lens wear and allow the practitioner to assess the fit of what is likely to be the final lens specification in many instances. For certain specialist fittings, such as presbyopia, trial fitting is more meaningful if the appropriate lens powers for the refractive condition of the patient are used.

Lens parameters easy to change

By the very nature of planned replacement, it is straightforward to modify the prescription of a patient, particularly with respect to changes in refractive error. From a practice management viewpoint, it is advisable to carry out the annual aftercare appointment before dispensing the next supply of lenses for the patient. Any alteration in lens power can then be made without the need to exchange unwanted lenses.

Potential disadvantages of planned replacement

There are probably no clinical disadvantages in prescribing planned, as opposed to unplanned, replacement lenses. However, there are some points to bear in mind that may have negative implications.

Patient non-compliance

Soon after the introduction of disposable lenses into the market, Matthews *et al.* (1992) reported a higher level of complications with disposable daily-wear lenses than with 'conventional' lenses not replaced on a planned basis. This was attributed to poor lens hygiene, the use of relatively inefficacious disinfecting systems such as chlorine, patient non-compliance and lens type. The first disposable lens on the market – Acuvue (Johnson & Johnson) – was originally promoted as an extended-wear lens, and many problems could be traced to non-compliance relating to overnight lens wear. These issues have now been largely solved; Acuvue lenses are used primarily for daily wear, and chlorine solutions are no longer marketed.

Although it can now be assumed that the use of planned replacement lenses and simple lens care products (e.g. multipurpose solutions) enhances patient compliance (Claydon *et al.*, 1996), the potential for patient non-compliance is ever present, and practitioners should be constantly alert to this potential problem (see Chapter 42).

Nilsson (1997) suggested that because disposable lenses are discarded so often, patients and practitioners can become complacent about lens care. Daily cleaning and disinfection remain a vital part of safe lens wear for any reusable lens, regardless of replacement frequency. Since the available parameters of disposable lenses, as opposed to prescription or custom lenses, are limited, practitioners may also be guilty of 'sloppy fitting' (Nilsson, 1997). It has also been suggested that disposable lens wearers may seek to solve a problem, which would otherwise be in need of professional attention, by simply changing the lens (Gasson and Morris, 1992).

It may be difficult to manage infrequent lens wearers via a planned replacement system simply because the rates of lens spoilation will be lower and more variable compared with that in full-time wearers. Also, compliance with the recommended replacement schedule may become problematic if the lenses are discarded at irregular intervals (Saitou *et al.*, 2005). For part-time wearers, therefore, daily disposable lenses are the preferred choice.

Provided lens fitting, aftercare and patient education are of a good standard, there are no compelling reasons for avoiding planned replacement, as long as the required parameters are available.

Quality and reproducibility issues

Efron and Veys (1992) observed small defects in all types of disposable lenses and suggested that these can cause complications. With any lens replaced at least monthly, it is not practical for each lens to be inspected, either prior to insertion or in the eye of the patient. For planned replacement to be successful it is a requirement that lenses are sufficiently consistent in quality such that the patient will not notice any change in comfort, fit or visual acuity from lens to lens. Certainly, the various types of moulding systems used to produce most disposable lenses are developed on the principle of building quality into the product, as the traditional manual methods previously used by manufacturers to examine conventional lenses would not be cost-effective with a mass-produced lens.

Wider quality issues are also important when the patient is using many lenses each year. Consistency of packaging and labelling are of great significance when the patient is supplied with unopened packages. If patients find that some blister packs are empty, dry or contain more than one lens, their confidence in the product is likely to be reduced.

Notwithstanding the above considerations, the recent literature is free of descriptions of complications attributable to poor disposable lens quality; nevertheless, patients should be advised to inspect visually all lenses prior to insertion and discard any lenses exhibiting surface or edge defects, or lenses that are persistently uncomfortable, cause significant eye redness or provide poor vision.

Practitioners can be reassured that the processes used to manufacture disposable lenses result in consistent lens parameters. Young *et al.* (1999) evaluated eight frequent replacement lenses and found reproducibility to be good for power, base curve and centre thickness, and acceptable for total diameter. The same researchers found adequate reproducibility of frequent replacement soft toric lenses (Young *et al.*, 2001).

Determining the appropriate lens replacement frequency

The ideal replacement frequency would be one selected on the basis of the rate of lens spoilation of each patient, and would be such that comfort and vision do not deteriorate throughout the life of the lens. This rate will depend upon the lens material and the tear film quality of the patient (Bleshoy *et al.*, 1994). In general, a high-water-content ionic material (Food and Drug Administration (FDA) group IV) requires at least monthly replacement, and a high-water-content non-ionic material (FDA group II) requires 3-monthly replacement. These are guidelines only, as individual patient variation can have a significant impact. Later work by Guillon *et al.* (1995) concluded that monthly or more frequent replacement ensures consistent performance over the period of use of the lens in terms of subjective comfort and visual performance for FDA group I and group IV lenses. Jones *et al.* (2003) and Keith *et al.* (2003) described the deposition characteristics of silicone hydrogel materials. Generally these materials show less protein and greater lipid deposition than conventional hydrogels.

In practice, it is not straightforward to identify the ideal lens replacement frequency for a given patient. Instead, an appropriate replacement interval can be chosen from one of the standard replacement intervals formulated for various products by contact lens manufacturers. Such a decision is made after consideration of the desired pattern of wear and contact lens history of the patient. For example, excessive lens deposition observed with a monthly lens replacement regimen may necessitate changing to a 2-weekly or even daily replacement regimen. It is advisable for legal and practical reasons to use the replacement interval(s) for a given lens recommended by the manufacturer as a maximum.

Practice management issues relating to planned soft lens replacement

As the use of planned lens replacement has become the norm, practitioners have had to introduce new systems for tracking and managing lens stocks, delivering lenses and solutions to patients, sending recall reminders and arranging aftercare visits. New approaches to financial management have also been devised. In many instances, these new approaches have necessitated a closer working relationship between practitioners and manufacturers.

Lens delivery systems

Two main methods for managing the implementation of planned lens replacement systems have evolved – manufacturer-driven systems and practice-driven systems.

Manufacturer-driven systems

This approach is perhaps more common in the UK than elsewhere. The names of new patients are registered with the manufacturer by the practice along with relevant prescription details. Depending on the lens type, there may also be an option to select a frequency of lens delivery to the practice; for example, monthly replacement lenses may be supplied to the practice in 3- or 6-month quantities. Once the patient is registered, fresh supplies of lenses will be automatically dispatched to the practice until countermanded by the practice.

Manufacturers have, in some cases, branded their systems to promote the service provided. The main benefit to practices is reduced administration. Simple computer programs run the systems, and the arrival of a new supply of lenses for a given patient acts as a trigger for the practice to recall that particular lens wearer.

In the UK, such systems complement the method by which many patients pay for frequent replacement lenses – namely, monthly direct payment from their bank account to the practice's account. In this way, both payment and regular lens supply are automated and compliance with the designated replacement schedule is encouraged. This practice is much less common in other countries, however.

Some manufacturers have expanded their service to include direct delivery of lenses and lens care products (so-called 'bundling') to the home address of the patient (Figure 21.6).

The increased convenience afforded by this approach is promoted as a means of retaining the custom of the patient for replacement lenses, given the growth of non-practice sources of supply such as direct mail and the internet (see below).

Practice-driven systems

If a manufacturer-driven system is not employed, an in-house system is required to ensure the timely purchase of replacement lenses and recall of patients. With larger patient bases, the amount of stock involved can soon

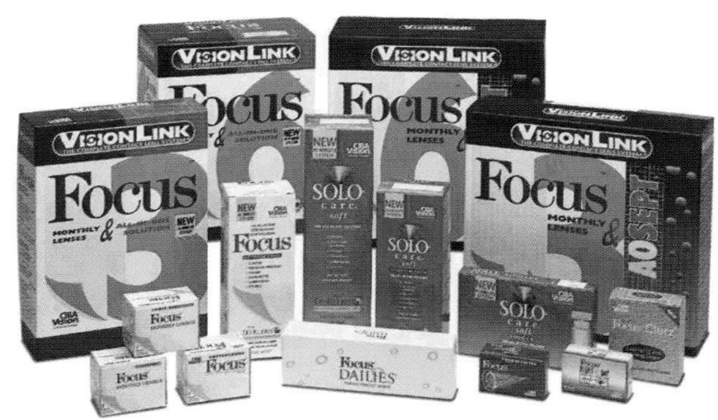

Figure 21.6 Planned replacement enables practices to provide lenses and lens care products in a convenient bundle.

Table 21.4 Parameter availability for commonly available disposable daily-wear lenses (excludes private labels and alternative branding of the same lens, and lenses primarily intended for extended wear)

Lens type	Diameters (mm)	Base curves (mm)	Powers (D)
Two-weekly and monthly sphere	14.00–14.50	8.20–9.30	+10.00 to −16.00
Two-weekly and monthly toric	14.00–14.60	8.30–9.20	+8.50 to −11.00 DS −0.75 to −5.75 DC Axes 10 to 180 in 5° steps
Two-weekly and monthly bi/multifocal	14.00–14.50	8.30–8.90	+6.00 to −9.00 Adds to +3.50
Two-weekly and monthly tint	14.00–14.50	8.60–8.90	+6.00 to −8.00

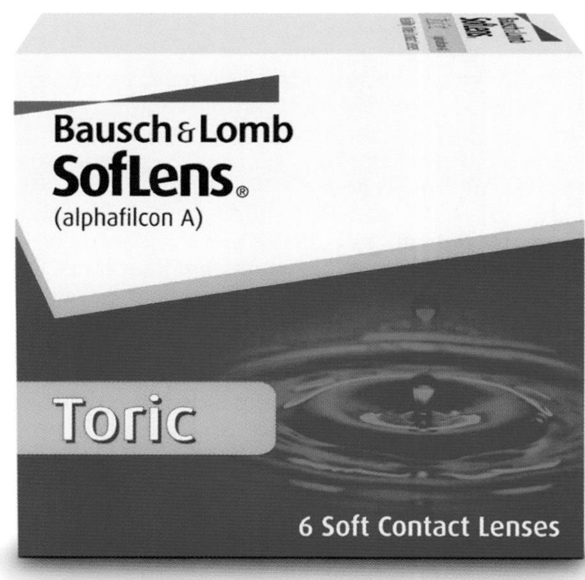

Figure 21.7 An example of a disposable toric lens which has become available since the mid-1990s.

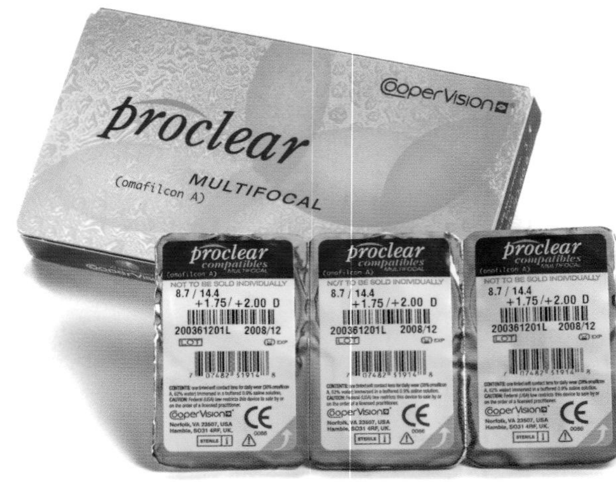

Figure 21.8 The concept of planned replacement has been expanded to include lenses for presbyopic patients.

become quite large and adequate storage space is often an issue. On the other hand, bulk purchasing may allow practices to secure preferential terms from suppliers. A practice operating its own system is also in complete control of the process and less vulnerable to any manufacturer supply problems.

Lenses available for planned replacement

It is possible to fit a substantial majority of soft lens patients with lenses replaced at least monthly (Table 21.4).

The principal lens types – such as spherical, toric (Figure 21.7), multifocal (Figure 21.8) and tinted – are available in several alternative replacement frequencies.

Patients for whom the desired lens replacement is unavailable are now mainly restricted to those with extreme prescriptions. Patients needing a lens diameter that is smaller than usual, say 13.50 mm, are also less easily fitted with the current range of disposable lenses, most of which are at least 14.00 mm total diameter. However, 3-monthly replacement potentially allows manufacturers to offer custom or prescription lenses, so that even outlying parameter requirements can be met in many cases.

Practice logistics

There is no doubt that planned replacement, particularly when practised with disposable lenses, can generate a considerable extra workload in a practice. The main issues are stock levels, patient aftercare and recall, and payment.

As an example, a practice with 500 patients using 2-weekly disposable lenses will handle over 4000 six-packs of lenses per annum, ignoring new fits, or over 80 lens packs per week on average. Five hundred patients will also require 500–1000 aftercare appointments, depending on the preference of the practitioner. This is perhaps as much as 30% of annual available chair time. If patients collect their supplies quarterly, practice staff will deal with nearly 40 collections per week.

Assuming the above level of activity, a reasonable stock, or inventory, of lenses will need to be kept in the practice to ensure good service to patients, and such stocks can consume a considerable amount of space (Figure 21.9).

There are several approaches to deciding what levels of stock to maintain. The simplest involves keeping a few

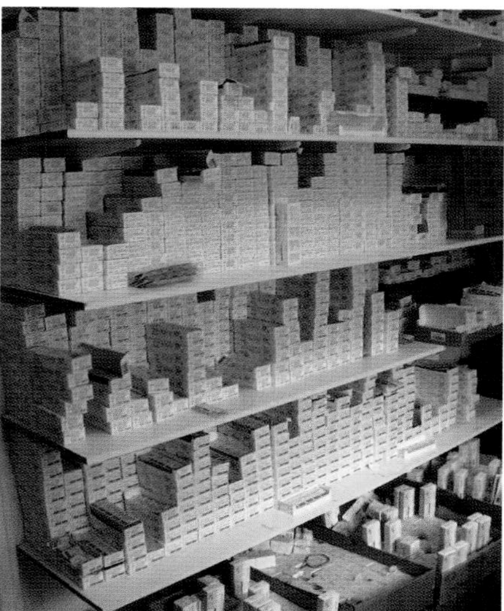

Figure 21.9 Practices with large patient bases will need to manage, and find space for, extensive stocks of planned replacement lenses.

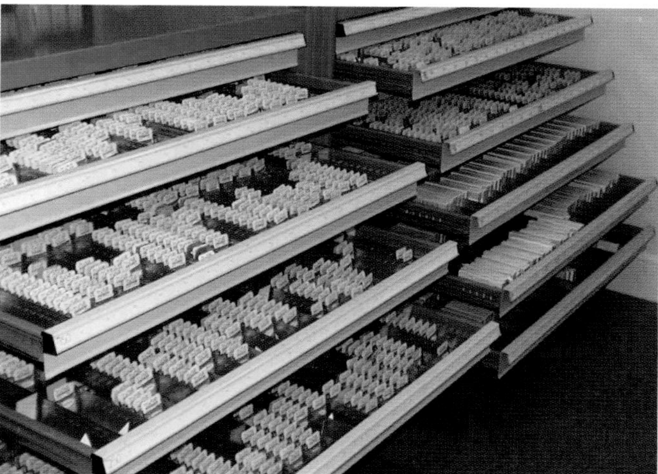

Figure 21.10 Diagnostic lenses allow for convenient and accurate fitting assessment.

boxes of each parameter or stock kept unit (SKU). As next-day delivery is often available, large numbers of lenses do not need to be stocked, although several spherical disposable lens brands have parameter ranges of over 100 SKUs. Practices may wish to weight their stock towards the more commonly occurring prescriptions, such as the range from −1.00 to −5.00 D. With very large patient bases, it may be helpful to consult with suppliers, who can advise on an appropriate in-practice stock holding based on statistical stock models used to manage their own inventory.

Practices that are computerized may wish to model their stock on the actual prescriptions of their patient base. This approach can be tied in with the aftercare recall system. Due allowance needs to be made for unpredictable purchasing patterns, which can arise, for example, ahead of holiday periods. As well as holding sufficient stock for purchase, an adequate number of trial or diagnostic lenses are needed for ongoing fitting (Figure 21.10).

Cost to the patient

Morgan *et al.* (1999) constructed a cost per wear (CPW) model to assist practitioners and patients in considering the cost implications of various lens replacement frequencies, tailored to the wearing habits of individual patients. The CPW is a simple calculation of the total cost of lenses (and solutions for non-daily lens replacement) over a 12-month period divided by an estimate of the number of days lenses will be worn over 12 months. Although unplanned replacement lenses proved to be the cheapest option, for the full-time wearer, the difference in CPW between unplanned replacement and monthly replacement lenses was small. For part-time wearers, daily disposable lenses were usually cheaper than monthly replacement lenses (Morgan *et al.*, 1999).

Financial management

The clinical benefits of planned replacement have been described above. It would be remiss not to mention the commercial benefits that this modality also delivers. Patients changing their lenses regularly, particularly if wearing disposable lenses, will generate a more predictable practice cash flow.

Contact lenses are often promoted as 'practice builders' since they usually require more practice visits and a more detailed appreciation by the patient of the professional skills required to maintain successful wear. This encourages greater loyalty than for spectacle-wearing patients. By reducing complications and increasing patient satisfaction, frequently replaced lenses further enhance the business benefits of developing a large base of contact lens wearers.

Alternative supply routes

The issue of non-optical-practice supply now affects virtually all contact lens types, although disposable lenses are particularly susceptible to third-party distribution given the brand awareness that many of these products have with the public. In the USA, the Fairness to Contact Lens Consumers Act (2004) is intended to allow contact lens wearers the freedom to shop around for their contact lens supplies.

The critical issue here is that it is in the public interest to have a system of lens supply that guarantees the ongoing preservation of the ocular health of lens wearers. A system that provides no disincentives to patients to continue to purchase lenses for many years without having their eyes examined poses a significant public health risk.

Notwithstanding the role of regulatory authorities in discharging their responsibilities for public health and safety, there are strategies that practitioners can employ to retain control of lens supply and to link this to patient care. Fee splitting – where materials are charged at relatively low mark-ups on cost, and these charges are separated from professional fees – helps demonstrate to patients that most of the cost involved in wearing contact lenses is attributed to the professional time involved. Home delivery plans, perhaps operated on behalf of the practice by a supplier, enable practitioners to match the perceived convenience of mail order and internet supply companies. Large practices or group practices may be able to come to an arrangement with manufacturers so that lenses and solutions supplied by that manufacturer are 'rebranded' prior to delivery. The rebranding (or so-called 'own-labelling' or 'private labelling') facilitates an association of the products with the practice and thereby serves to enhance patient loyalty. However, as the lens specifications cannot be altered, it is relatively straightforward to determine the original brand and therefore purchase the original brand elsewhere if the patient desires.

Conclusions

Planned replacement, especially in the form of disposable soft lenses, has transformed contact lens practice over the past two decades. This approach is clearly justified in terms of clinical performance, increased convenience and practice profitability. It is likely that planned soft lens replacement will continue to dominate prescribing habits into the future.

Acknowledgements

The author wishes to thank Trevor Rowley, Bausch & Lomb, CooperVision, CIBA Vision and Johnson & Johnson Vision Care for providing photographs, and Phil Morgan for supplying information on the UK market.

References

Bleshoy, H., Guillon, M. and Shah, D. (1994) Influence of contact lens material surface characteristics on replacement frequency. *Int. Contact Lens Clin.*, **21,** 82–94.

Brennan, N., Efron, N., Weissman, B. *et al.* (1991) Clinical application of the oxygen transmissibility of powered contact lenses. *Contact Lens Assoc. Ophthalmol. J.*, **17,** 169–172.

Cheung, S. W., Cho, P., Chan, B. *et al.* (2007) A comparative study of biweekly disposable contact lenses: silicone hydrogel versus hydrogel. *Clin. Exp. Optom.*, **90,** 124–131.

Claydon, B. and Efron, N. (1994) Non-compliance in contact lens wear. *Ophthal. Physiol. Opt.*, **14,** 356–364.

Claydon, B. E., Efron, N. and Woods, C. (1996) A prospective study of non-compliance in contact lens wear. *J. Br. Contact Lens Assoc.*, **19,** 133–140.

Edwards, K. (1998) Lens care with frequent replacement lenses. *Optician,* **215**(5641), 32–34.

Efron, N. and Veys, J. (1992) Defects in disposable contact lenses can compromise ocular integrity. *Int. Contact Lens Clin.*, **19,** 8–18.

Ehlers, W. H., Donshik, P. C. and Suchecki, J. K. (2003) Disposable and frequent replacement contact lenses. *Ophthalmol. Clin. North Am.*, **16,** 341–352.

Franklin, V. (1997) Cleaning efficacy of single-purpose surfactant cleaners and multi-purpose solutions. *Contact Lens Ant. Eye,* **20,** 63–68.

Gasson, A. and Morris, J. (1992) *The Contact Lens Manual – A Practical Fitting Guide,* Oxford: Butterworth-Heinemann.

Guillon, M., Guillon, J. P., Shah, D. *et al.* (1995) Visual performance stability of planned replacement daily wear contact lenses. *Contactologia,* **17,** 118–130.

Jones, L. (1990) Daily wear high water content lenses – continued. *Optician,* **199**(5240), 15–23.

Jones, L., Woods, C., Efron, N. (1996) Life expectancy of rigid gas permeable and high water content contact lenses. *Contact Lens Assoc. Ophthalmol. J.*, **22,** 258–261.

Jones, L., Mann, A., Evans, K. *et al.* (2000) An in vivo comparison of the kinetics of protein and lipid deposition on group II and group IV frequent-replacement contact lenses. *Optom. Vis. Sci.*, **77,** 503–510.

Jones, L., Senchyna, M., Glasier, M.-A. *et al.* (2003) Lysozyme and lipid deposition on silicone hydrogel contact lens materials. *Eye & Contact Lens,* **29,** S75–S79.

Keith, D., Christensen, M., Barry, J. *et al.* (2003) Determination of the lysozyme deposit curve in soft contact lenses. *Eye & Contact Lens,* **29,** 79–82.

Marshall, E., Begley, C. and Nguyen, C. (1992) Frequency of complications among wearers of disposable and conventional soft contact lenses. *Int. Contact Lens Clin.*, **19,** 55–60.

Matthews, T., Frazer, D., Minassian, E. *et al.* (1992) Risks of keratitis and patterns of use with disposable contact lenses. *Arch. Ophthalmol.*, **110,** 1559–1562.

Morgan, P. B. and Efron, N. (2006) A decade of contact lens prescribing trends in the United Kingdom (1996–2005). *Cont. Lens Ant. Eye,* **29,** 59–68.

Morgan, S. L., Morgan, P. B. and Efron, N. (1999) 'Cost per wear' as a model for the comparison of contact lens prices. *Optom. Vis. Sci.*, **76,** S165.

Nilsson, S. (1997) Ten years of disposable lenses – a review of benefits and risks. *Contact Lens Ant. Eye,* **20,** 119–128.

Nilsson, S. and Montan, P. (1994) The hospitalised cases of contact lens induced keratitis in Sweden and their relation to lens type and wear schedule: results of a three-year retrospective study. *Contact Lens Assoc. Ophthalmol. J.*, **20,** 97–101.

Poggio, E. and Abelson, M. (1993) Complications and symptoms with disposable daily wear contact lenses and conventional soft daily wear contact lenses. *Contact Lens Assoc. Ophthalmol. J.*, **19,** 95–102.

Porazinski, A. and Donshik, P. (1999) Giant papillary conjunctivitis in frequent replacement contact lens wearers: a retrospective study. *Contact Lens Assoc. Ophthalmol. J.*, **25,** 142–147.

Pritchard, N., Fonn, D. and Weed, K. (1996) Ocular and subjective responses to frequent replacement of daily wear soft contact lenses. *Contact Lens Assoc. Ophthalmol. J.*, **22,** 53–59.

Saitou, H., Kato, Y., Nishizaki, R. *et al.* (2005) An investigation of the actual conditions of use of daily-disposable soft contact lenses and two-week disposable soft contact lenses. *Eye Contact Lens,* **31,** 225–230.

Young, G., Lewis, Y., Coleman, S. *et al.* (1999) Process capability measurement of frequent replacement spherical soft contact lenses. *Contact Lens Ant. Eye,* **22,** 127–135.

Young, G., Lewis, Y., Coleman, S. *et al.* (2001) Process capability measurement of frequent replacement toric soft contact lenses. *Contact Lens Ant. Eye,* **24,** 25–33.

CHAPTER 22

Planned rigid lens replacement

Craig A Woods

Introduction

The perceived advantages of rigid lenses, compared to soft lenses, include increased corneal oxygenation (Efron and Ang, 1990), longer life expectancy (Atkinson and Port, 1989), reduced risk of microbial keratitis (Dart *et al.*, 2008; Stapleton *et al.*, 2008), fewer toxic/allergic complications (Hamano *et al.*, 1988) and superior vision in cases of corneal astigmatism. Many clinicians believe that rigid lenses should be considered the lens of first choice (Dart *et al.*, 1991).

It has been shown that, as soft lenses age, their physical and clinical performance deteriorates, resulting in reduced comfort (Poggio and Abelson, 1993), reduced vision (Gellatly *et al.*, 1988) and decreased wettability (Guillon *et al.*, 1992). This has resulted in the wide acceptance of planned replacement for soft contact lenses (Jones, 1994).

The concept of planned replacement for soft contact lenses is well established and the benefits of regular replacement of soft contact lenses are covered in Chapter 21. The effect of regularly replacing soft lenses generally has been to reduce the adverse effects of lens ageing. The incidence of many adverse ocular effects can also be reduced significantly. Additionally, it has been possible to use lens materials and lens designs that might not have been appropriate for unplanned lens replacement (e.g. due to reduced durability and increased tendency to spoilation). It is reasonable to suppose, therefore, that regular replacement of rigid lenses might give rise to similar benefits.

Life expectancy of rigid contact lenses

The perception might be that rigid lenses have a longer life than soft contact lenses. Due to their negligible water content and high modulus of elasticity, rigid materials lend themselves well to prolonged life. The method of manufacturing (lathe cutting) is relatively labour-intensive and costly compared to that of manufacturing disposable soft lenses, which raises questions of the cost-effectiveness of regular rigid lens replacement.

The literature reports a wide range for the life expectancy for rigid lenses. Atkinson and Port (1989) concluded that they last between 2 and 3 years and Yokota *et al.* (1992) estimated the life of rigid lenses to be between 5 and 10 years. Both of these reports reflect the clinical opinions of the authors with limited evidence-based data. Jones *et al.* (1996) analysed data from 600 patients and were able to show that the life expectancy of rigid lenses was related to the material's oxygen permeability (*Dk*). The mean life expectancy of rigid lenses was found to be 20 ± 17 months for low-*Dk* materials, 16 ± 13 months for mid-*Dk* materials, and 9 ± 8 months for high-*Dk* materials (Figure 22.1).

In the same study, the life expectancy of high-water-content soft lenses was found to be 6 ± 5 months. This compared well to other published data (Jones, 1990), which also established an expected lifespan for high-water-content soft lenses of about 6 months.

All contact lenses should have sufficient oxygen transmissibility (*Dk*/*t*) to maintain near-normal corneal metabolism. A *Dk*/*t* of 24 Barrer/cm is required from a lens worn on a daily-wear basis, for an average cornea (Holden and Mertz, 1984). High-*Dk* materials have been shown to result in reduced hypoxia and hypercapnia (Efron and Ang, 1990), reduced stromal acidosis (Polse *et al.*, 1992), a lower overall complication rate (Hamano *et al.*, 1988) and reduced binding of *Pseudomonas aeruginosa* to the corneal surface (Imayasu *et al.*, 1994). The conclusion from these studies is that, from a physiological standpoint, contact lenses should be made from high-*Dk* materials wherever possible.

The study by Jones *et al.* (1996) demonstrated that lenses manufactured from higher-*Dk* materials have a reduced life expectancy when compared to lower-*Dk* materials. This is not unexpected, since lenses made from high-*Dk* materials are less mechanically stable (i.e. subject to warpage) and more prone to surface scratching (Tranoudis and Efron, 1996) than lenses made from low-*Dk* materials. Figure 22.1 indicates that lenses manufactured from materials with nominally quoted uncorrected *Dk* values of ≥90 Barrer should last approximately 9 months, compared with 20 months for lenses with a *Dk* of ≤40 Barrer.

All contact lenses demonstrate a deterioration in performance with age. While this has been clearly demonstrated with soft lenses (Poggio and Abelson, 1993), studies of rigid lenses also show a gradual deterioration in wettability (Guillon *et al.*, 1995), visual performance (Jones *et al.*,

DOI: 10.1016/B978-0-7506-8869-7.00022-7

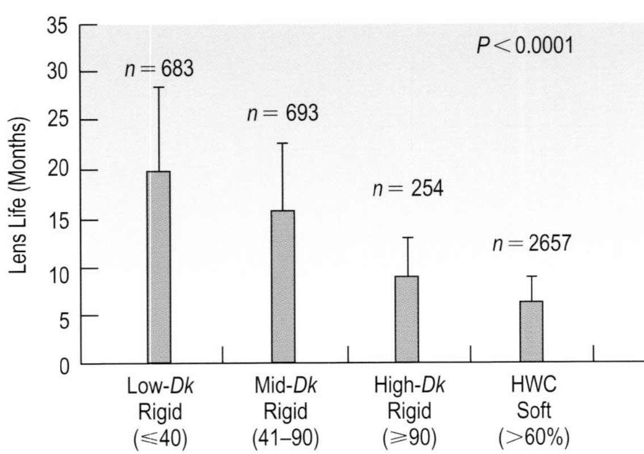

Figure 22.1 Mean lens life for various contact lens materials. Ranges for low-, mid- and high-*Dk* materials are shown in brackets. HWC = high-water-content materials.

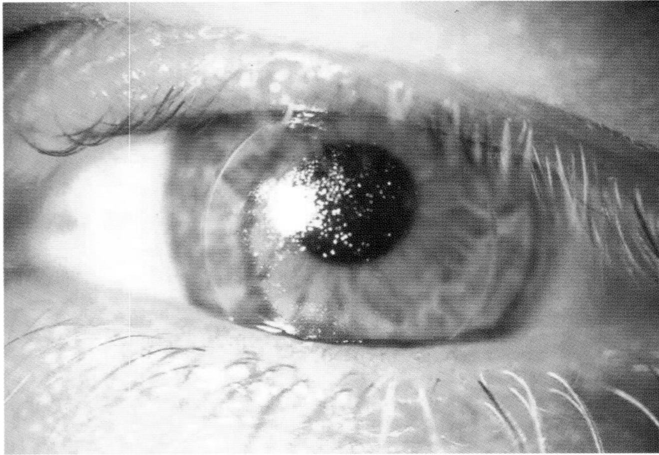

Figure 22.2 Rigid lens surface displaying the effects of overpolishing.

1995) and an increase in surface scratching and deposition (Allary *et al.*, 1989; Guillon *et al.*, 1995; Jones *et al.*, 1995), irrespective of *Dk* or material type.

It was common with PMMA materials to 'prolong' the life of the lens by repolishing the lens surfaces. Some clinicians believe that repolishing techniques can also be applied to prolong the life of rigid lenses; however, caution should always be exercised with this procedure as overpolishing can lead to reduced surface wettability and ultimately result in reduced comfort and visual performance (Grohe *et al.*, 1988) (Figure 22.2).

Regular replacement of rigid lenses

The concept of regular replacement of rigid lenses was first considered by Grohe in 1992. He concluded that the major problem with the introduction of such systems would be the increased cost to the patient with little obvious benefit (Grohe, 1992). However, if it is accepted that: (1) higher-*Dk* materials should be fitted for clinical reasons; (2) such lenses have a reduced life expectancy; and (3) all lenses show a deterioration in performance with age, then the planned replacement of high-*Dk* rigid lenses would appear to be a logical modality for practitioners and patients to adopt. The benefits of such a schedule have been demonstrated for lenses worn on a daily-wear basis (Guillon *et al.*, 1995) (Table 22.1). Allary *et al.* (1989) reported that surface scratching and deposition on rigid lenses increase with lens age; however, this study was not controlled or designed to investigate lens ageing, and their comments were an aside to the actual purpose of their study.

Grohe (1992) considered the above issues and expressed concern that rigid contact lens disposability might be introduced for marketing rather than clinical reasons. Hannon (1990) expressed the view that there were tremendous benefits in regularly replacing rigid lenses from a marketing point of view, and that patients would find the concept acceptable.

It could be reasonably argued that, with the success of soft disposable lenses and that disposability being now associated with improvements and advancement in technology, rigid lens improvements and changes may not be easy to convey unless they are associated with 'disposability'. Introducing such a concept for rigid lenses is potentially important in order to allow rigid lens wearers to perceive equivalent benefits from their lens-wearing experience. Offering planned replacement of rigid lenses purely as a marketing tool may, at the very least, encourage existing rigid lens wearers to stay with rigid lenses.

Advantages of regular replacement of rigid lenses

Woods and Efron (1996a, b) investigated the effects of planned replacement of rigid lenses on the integrity of the lens and the anterior ocular structures. In a masked, controlled and randomized experiment, these authors compared a group of subjects using rigid lenses on a planned replacement basis with a control group of subjects who were not scheduled to replace their rigid lenses over a 12-month period. This investigation was performed on subjects wearing rigid contact lenses on a daily-wear basis (Woods and Efron, 1996a) and subjects wearing their lenses on an extended-wear basis (Woods and Efron, 1996b).

Daily wear

For the subjects wearing the lenses on a daily-wear basis, planned replacement was shown to reduce the grade for:

- Corneal staining within 12 months of commencing the study.
- The extent of limbal hyperaemia over time.
- The extent of tarsal conjunctival changes over time (Woods and Efron, 1996a).

Regarding the condition of the lenses, planned replacement reduced:

- Surface drying within 9 months of commencing the study (Figure 22.3).
- Surface scratching within 9 months of commencing the study (Figure 22.4).
- Mucus coating within 12 months of commencing the study.
- Surface deposition within 12 months of commencing the study (Woods and Efron, 1996a).

Table 22.1 Time scale for the development of adverse changes to various parameters of the contact lens and eye during rigid lens wear

Parameter	Time span for effect on parameter	Mode of wear	Reference source
Life expectancy	5–10 years	Daily wear	Yokota *et al.*, 1992
Life expectancy	2–3 years	Daily wear	Atkinson and Port, 1989
Life expectancy*	20 months	Daily wear	Jones *et al.*, 1996
Life expectancy†	16 months	Daily wear	Jones *et al.*, 1996
Corneal staining	12 months	Daily and extended wear	Woods and Efron, 1996a
Conjunctival staining	12 months	Extended wear	Woods and Efron, 1996b
Limbal hyperaemia	12 months	Daily wear	Woods and Efron, 1996a
Mucus coating	12 months	Daily and extended wear	Woods and Efron, 1996a
Surface deposition	12 months	Daily wear	Woods and Efron, 1996a
Tarsal changes	12 months	Daily wear	Woods and Efron, 1996a
Life expectancy‡	9 months	Daily wear	Jones *et al.*, 1996
Surface drying	9 months	Daily wear	Woods and Efron, 1996a
Surface scratching	9 months	Daily and extended wear	Woods and Efron, 1996a
Surface wetting	9 months	Daily wear	Woods and Efron, 1996a
Lens binding	6 months	Extended wear	Woods and Efron, 1996b
Surface deposition	6 months	Daily wear	Guillon *et al.*, 1995
Surface wetting	6 months	Daily wear	Guillon *et al.*, 1995

* Low-*Dk* materials.
† Mid-*Dk* materials.
‡ High-*Dk* materials.

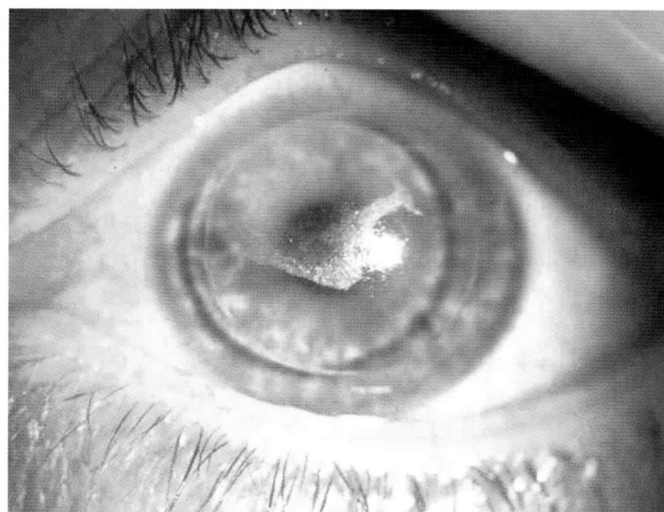

Figure 22.3 Rigid lens with a non-wetting surface.

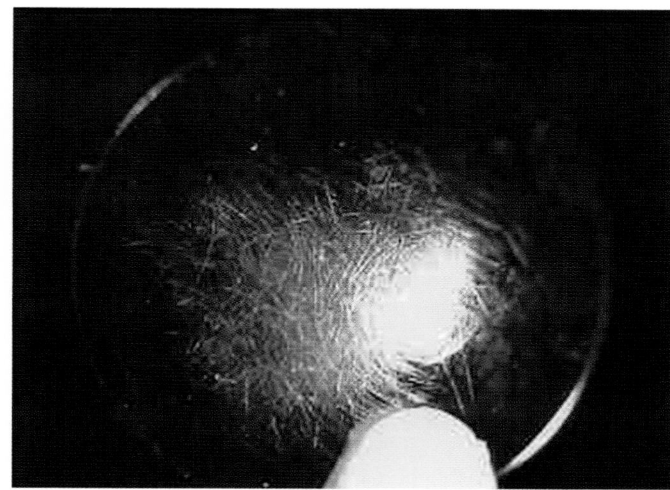

Figure 22.4 Rigid lens with a scratched surface.

Conventionally worn daily-wear rigid lenses demonstrated a significant reduction in lens thickness over time (Woods and Efron, 1999); this is attributed to the rubbing action causing an erosion of material from the lens centre.

Extended wear

For subjects using the lenses on an extended-wear basis, planned replacement significantly reduced:

- The grade for corneal staining over time (Woods and Efron, 1996b).
- The grade for conjunctival staining over time (Woods and Efron, 1996b).
- The measured immunoglobulin E levels in the tear film over time (Woods, 1997).

Planned replacement did not prevent a significant increase in tarsal conjunctival changes in the extended-wear group.

Subjects not in the planned lens replacement group displayed a significant increase in myopia and a reduction in high-contrast acuity.

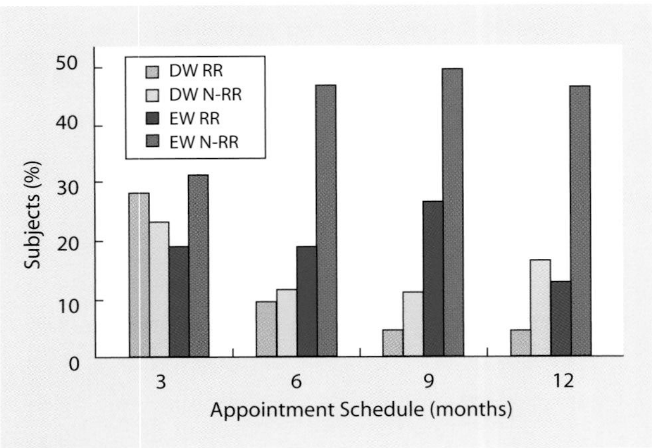

Figure 22.5 Percentage of subjects reporting lens binding. DW RR = daily-wear regular replacement; DW N-RR = daily-wear non-regular replacement; EW RR = extended-wear regular replacement; EW N-RR = extended-wear non-regular replacement.

Regarding the condition of the lenses, planned replacement reduced the grade for:

- Mucus coating over time.
- Surface scratches over time (Woods and Efron, 1996b).

Lens binding

In their studies, Woods and Efron (1996c) observed that lens binding occurred in both the daily-wear groups and the extended-wear groups of subjects. The occurrence of binding was monitored both subjectively and objectively. Subjective binding assessment appeared to be a reliable indicator as to the occurrence of this phenomenon, whilst objective assessment appeared to provide less reliable results. Regular replacement of lenses worn on an extended-wear basis significantly reduced the level of subjectively reported lens binding compared to that reported for the unplanned replacement group. A low incidence of lens binding was shown to occur with daily wear of rigid lenses, irrespective of whether lenses are regularly replaced or not (Figure 22.5).

Optimum replacement schedule

With very little published in the literature to demonstrate the time course of occurrence of adverse events in the eye and lens during rigid contact lens wear (Table 22.1), it is difficult to formulate a clinical criterion for the ideal rigid lens replacement frequency. This criterion can be determined using clinical data, or it can be based on a theoretical model. Both of these approaches are presented below.

Clinical data

The data of Guillon *et al.* (1995) suggest that a measurable reduction in surface wettability and increase in surface deposit formation occurs with rigid lenses after 6 months of use. The data of Woods and Efron (1996a, b) suggest that those changes occur after a longer period of wear; that is, clinically significant changes do not appear to occur until after about 9 months. Furthermore, a recommended frequency of replacement should not exceed the life expectancy of any form of rigid lens, which is 9 months. It is reasonable to assume, therefore, that an optimum replacement frequency for rigid lenses would be less than 9 months. In conclusion, therefore, a recommendation to replace rigid lenses every 6 months would seem reasonable, based on the argument that: (1) lenses should be replaced before any adverse ocular or lens surface changes would be expected to occur; and (2) this is an easy-to-remember calendar-based frequency that would facilitate patient and practitioner compliance.

Theoretical model

An alternative approach to formulating a recommended replacement frequency for rigid lenses would be to estimate the theoretical ideal replacement schedule using the lifespan and optimum replacement frequency of high-water-content soft lenses as a guide. High-water-content soft lenses have been shown to have an average lifespan of 6 months (Jones, 1990; Jones *et al.*, 1996). The optimum replacement frequency for planned replacement soft lenses could be considered to be between 2 weeks and 3 months (Guillon *et al.*, 1992). A simple ratio of lifespan to optimum replacement frequency could act as a guide to determine how frequently to replace the rigid lenses. Jones *et al.* (1996) established that the lifespan of rigid lenses made from high-*Dk* materials is on average 9 months, which is 50% greater than that for high-water-content soft lenses (6 months). The ideal theoretical rigid lens replacement frequency would therefore be 50% more than the range of the optimal soft lens replacement frequencies, that is, between 0.75 and 4.5 months.

Planned replacement schemes available

As is the case with soft contact lenses, manufacturers and practitioners had to be prepared to embrace the concept of planned rigid replacement if this modality was to succeed. Planned replacement of soft lenses required manufacturer-driven schemes to be adopted by practitioners as an accepted standard of practice. The same situation might have been thought to apply to rigid lenses; however, rigid lenses generally are produced by a large number of relatively small prescription or specialist laboratories. It would be unreasonable to expect all of these manufacturers to develop a universal approach to the question of planned rigid lens replacement. As a consequence, any manufacturer-driven rigid lens replacement schemes are likely to be diverse, which can potentially create confusion among practitioners. Nevertheless, some rigid lens planned replacement schemes exist and the results from a 2008 international fitting survey (Morgan *et al.*, 2009) suggest the concept appears to have been put into practice in many countries; indeed, in 11 of the 19 countries surveyed, 40% or more rigid lenses were prescribed using planned replacement schemes. The results from 16 countries are shown in Figure 22.6. The replacement frequency built into such planned replacement schemes appears to be calendar-driven; that is, based on 3-, 6- or 12-month lens replacement cycles.

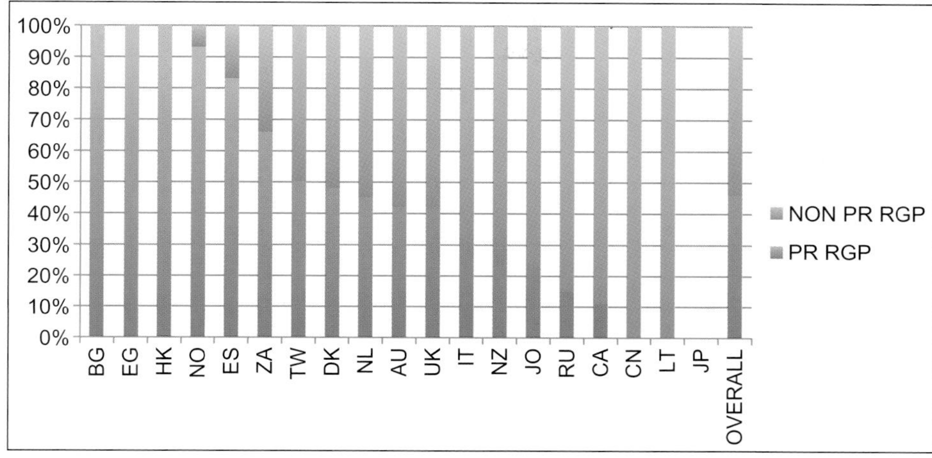

Figure 22.6 The distribution of planned replacement rigid lenses prescribed in 15 countries in 2008. Country codes: ES = Spain; ZA = South Africa; HK = Hong Kong; JO = Jordan; TW = Taiwan; PT = Portugal; NO = Norway; RU = Russia; UK = United Kingdom; IT = Italy; NL = Netherlands; SI = Slovenia; CA = Canada; AU = Australia; NZ = New Zealand.

Conclusions

The planned replacement of rigid contact lenses has been shown to be clinically beneficial, in terms of maintenance of the integrity of the surface of the contact lens and preservation of ocular health (Woods and Efron, 1996a, b, c). These benefits have been demonstrated to apply to patients wearing rigid lenses on daily and extended-wear regimens. Based on the limited amount of information available, it is concluded that optimum ocular physiology will be realized by fitting lenses made from high-*Dk* materials that are designed to be replaced every 6 months. Recent data also appear to suggest that practitioners are embracing planned replacement of rigid lenses as they have done for soft lenses.

References

Allary, J. C., Mapstone, V., Guillon, J. P. *et al.* (1989) Rigid gas permeable lens surface evaluation. *J. Br. Contact Lens Assoc.*, **12,** 18–19.

Atkinson, K. W. and Port, M. J. A. (1989) Patient management and instruction. In *Contact Lenses,* 4th edn (A. J. Phillips and L. Speedwell, eds), pp. 282–312, London: Butterworth-Heinemann.

Dart, J. K. G., Stapleton, F. and Minassin, D. (1991) Contact lenses and other risk factors in microbial keratitis. *Lancet,* **338,** 650–653.

Dart J. K., Radford C. F., Minassian D. (2008) Risk factors for microbial keratitis with contemporary contact lenses: a case-control study. *Ophthalmology.* **115**(10):1647–1654, 1654.e1-3. Epub 2008 Jul 2.

Efron, N. and Ang, J. H. B. (1990) Corneal hypoxia and hypercapnia during contact lens wear. *Optom. Vis. Sci.*, **67,** 512–521.

Gellatly, K. W., Brennan, N. A. and Efron, N. (1988) Visual decrement with deposit accumulation on HEMA contact lenses. *Am. J. Optom. Physiol. Opt.*, **65,** 937–941.

Grohe, R. M. (1992) Disposable RGPs check out the merits. *Contact Lens Spectrum,* **7,** 47–48.

Grohe, R. M., Caroline, P. J. and Norman, C. W. (1988) The role of in-office modifications for RGP surface defects. *Contact Lens Spectrum,* **3,** 52–60.

Guillon, M., Allary, J. C., Guillon, J. P. *et al.* (1992) Clinical management of regular replacement: Part I. Selection of replacement frequency. *Int. Contact Lens Clin.*, **19,** 104–120.

Guillon, M., Guillon, J. P., Shah, D. *et al.* (1995) In vivo wettability of high *Dk* RGP materials. *J. Br. Contact Lens Assoc.*, **18,** 9–15.

Hamano, H., Hamano, T., Iwasaki, N. *et al.* (1988) Clinical evaluation of various contact lenses from the incidence of complications. *J. Br. Contact Lens Assoc.*, **11,** 25–30.

Hannon, F. (1990) Annual replacement of high *Dk* RGP's? Why not? *Eyecare Business,* **5,** 78–79.

Holden, B. A. and Mertz, G. W. (1984) Critical oxygen levels to avoid corneal edema for daily and extended wear contact lenses. *Invest. Ophthalmol. Vis. Sci.*, **25,** 1161–1167.

Imayasu, M., Petroll, W. M., Jester, J. V. *et al.* (1994) The relation between contact lens oxygen transmissibility and binding of *Pseudomonas aeruginosa* to the cornea after overnight wear. *Opthalmology,* **101,** 371–388.

Jones, L. (1990) Daily wear of high water content lenses. Part 3. *Optician,* **199**(5240), 15–23.

Jones, L. (1994) Disposable contact lenses: A review. *J. Br. Contact Lens Assoc.*, **17,** 43–49.

Jones, L., Langley, C. and Jones, D. (1995) A comparative evaluation of two aspheric RGP contact lenses. *Optician,* **210**(5526), 28–36.

Jones, L., Woods, C. A. and Efron, N. (1996) Life expectancy of rigid gas permeable and high water content contact lenses. *Contact Lens Assoc. Ophthalmol. J.*, **22,** 258–261.

Morgan, P. B., Woods, C. A., Tranoudis, I. G. *et al.* (2009) International contact lens prescribing in 2008. *Contact Lens Spectrum,* **24,** 28–32.

Poggio, E. and Abelson, M. (1993) Complications and symptoms with disposable daily wear and conventional soft daily wear. *Contact Lens Assoc. Ophthalmol. J.*, **19,** 95–102.

Polse, K. A., Rivera, R., Gan, C. *et al.* (1992) Contact lens wear affects corneal pH: Implications and new directions for contact lens research. *J. Br. Contact Lens Assoc.*, **15,** 171–177.

Stapleton F., Keay L., Edwards K. (2008) The incidence of contact lens-related microbial keratitis in Australia. *Ophthalmology.* **115**(10):1655–1662. Epub 2008 Jun 5.

Tranoudis, I. and Efron, N (1996) Scratch resistance of rigid contact lens materials. *Ophthal. Physiol. Opt.*, **16,** 303–309.

Woods, C. A. (1997) The benefits of planned replacement of rigid gas permeable contact lenses. PhD thesis, University of Manchester Institute of Science and Technology, Manchester, UK.

Woods, C. A. and Efron, N. (1996a) Regular replacement of daily-wear rigid gas-permeable contact lenses. *J. Br. Contact Lens Assoc.*, **19,** 83–89.

Woods, C. A. and Efron, N. (1996b) Regular replacement of extended wear rigid gas permeable contact lenses. *Contact Lens Assoc. Ophthalmol. J.*, **22,** 172–178.

Woods, C. A. and Efron, N. (1996c) Regular replacement of rigid contact lenses alleviates binding to the cornea. *Int. Contact Lens Clin.*, **23,** 13–18.

Woods, C. A. and Efron, N. (1999) The parameter stability of a high *Dk* rigid lens material. *Contact Lens Ant. Eye,* **22,** 14–18.

Yokota, M., Goshima, T. and Itoh, S. (1992) The effect of polymer structure on durability of high *Dk* gas-permeable materials. *J. Br. Contact Lens Assoc.*, **15,** 125–129.

PART: V

Special lenses and fitting considerations

CHAPTER 23

Scleral lenses

Kenneth W Pullum

Introduction

Scleral contact lenses are generally perceived as being cumbersome, difficult to fit and problematic. However, rigid gas-permeable (RGP) materials have enabled predictable and straightforward scleral lens fitting methods, creating opportunities for effective, non-surgical visual rehabilitation at all levels of pathology. The uniquely valuable role offers respite from the problems caused by other lens types or can be the only option when a successful visual outcome is most needed. The aim of this chapter is not to provide an indepth coverage of clinical techniques, but rather a broad overview, so that the practitioner can be aware of what to expect should a scleral lens wearer seek advice.

To meet a clinical definition of a scleral lens, the diameter must be large enough to have a scleral bearing surface with optic zone clearance extending just beyond the limbus (Figure 23.1). Assuming a corneal diameter of 12 mm, a minimum annular limbal clearance of 1 mm and a minimum annular scleral bearing surface of 1 mm, the very smallest possible diameter is 16 mm for an eye of normal dimensions. Lenses of less than 16 mm have a role to play, but it is confusing to put them in the category of a scleral lens. At the other end of the range, impression lenses could be greater than 25 mm if necessary, but 23 mm is a more normal diameter for a 'full-diameter' scleral lens.

Advantages and disadvantages of scleral lenses

Contrary to popular belief, the large size and bearing surface provide many positive benefits. Close alignment between the corneal surface and the lens is not necessary, therefore a scleral contact lens can be successful with virtually any corneal topography (Kok and Visser, 1992). They are surprisingly comfortable for the unadapted eye because there is no eyelid–lens edge interaction, foreign bodies behind lenses are not a problem, and there is no localized exposure due to disrupted blinking.

Generally, the end point to the fitting process is well defined and quickly reached, and an extensive power range is possible without excessive mobility. Insertion may be easier for less dextrous patients, because the lens is not balanced on one finger but held between the thumb and a finger. Maintenance is straightforward as dry storage is generally satisfactory even with gas-permeable materials. Polishing or resurfacing is possible.

For a balanced view it is also necessary to appreciate the drawbacks. Production is labour-intensive compared to most other lens types. The large size can be intimidating, and there may be a feeling and appearance of excessive bulkiness. Even if skilfully fitted, corneal oxygenation is reduced, and the visual performance is not always as good as with a smaller corneal lens in cases of keratoconus, although Salam *et al.* (2005) showed that scleral lenses are not necessarily optically inferior to corneal lenses. Decentration in the vertical meridian can cause significant prismatic effects, especially if only one eye is wearing a lens. However, the reason for scleral lens fitting is not usually to enhance the vision compared to corneal lenses, but to provide respite from other problems.

Indications for scleral lenses

Provided there is a sound underlying indication for contact lens management, scleral lenses are indicated when they can be applied to beneficial effect (Schein *et al.*, 1990; Visser, 1990; Kok and Visser, 1992; Foss *et al.*, 1994; Pullum *et al.*, 2005; Pullum and Buckley, 2007; Jacobs, 2008). The main indication is optical correction of an irregular corneal surface (Visser *et al.*, 2007a).

An analysis of 888 consecutive patients (1353 eyes) who were continuing scleral lens wear at their most recent aftercare appointment was carried out at a dedicated clinic at Moorfields Eye Hospital, London; the percentages for each indication are shown in Figure 23.2. A total of 61.6% (824 eyes) were for keratoconus or other primary corneal ectasia (PCE), and 20.5% (274 eyes) were for corneal transplant, most of which were keratoconus-indicated. Retention of a precorneal fluid reservoir for various ocular surface disorders constituted 10.7% (143 eyes), high myopia or aphakia combined 4.1% (55 eyes) and ptosis props 1.8% (18 eyes).

DOI: 10.1016/B978-0-7506-8869-7.00023-9

Ocular surface disorders where scleral lenses might be beneficial include Terrien's marginal degeneration (Cotter and Rosenthal, 1998), Stevens–Johnson syndrome (Fine *et al.*, 2003), pellucid marginal degeneration (Looi *et al.*, 2002), ocular cicatricial pemphigoid and persistent corneal epithelial defects (Rosenthal *et al.*, 2000). Their use may reduce the rate of epithelial defect recurrence in stem cell-deficient and neurotrophic corneas (Rosenthal and Cotter, 2003). Margolis *et al.* (2007) have also reported on their use in advanced atopic keratoconjunctivitis.

Moderate ametropia rarely warrants scleral lens fitting as first choice, but should be considered if there are intractable problems with corneal or hydrogel lenses. There is an indication for recreational or occupational reasons when extra stability is required, sometimes for water sports, or to cater for dusty environments. Many people were issued with scleral lenses before the use of corneal and hydrogel lenses became widespread: they are mostly elderly, but some have every intention of continuing lens wear. They may not be receptive to refitting with corneal or hydrogel lenses, nor do they need to be if any sequelae do not represent a threat to their vision for the duration of their expected lifespan.

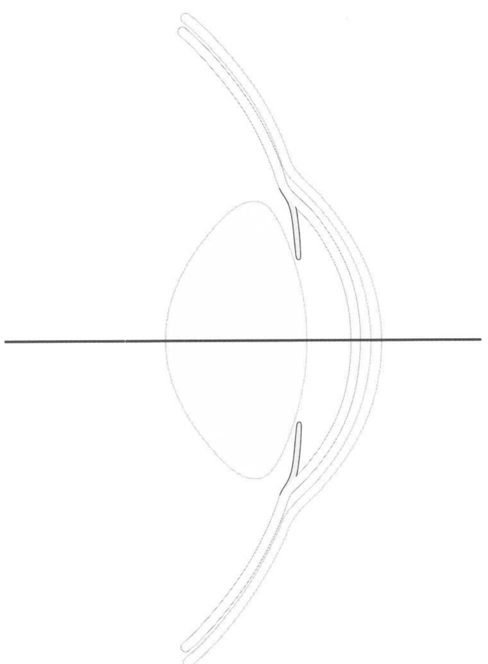

Figure 23.1 Scleral zone alignment with optic zone clearance extending just beyond the limbus.

Fitting principles

Initially scleral lenses were made from glass (from 1888 until the 1940s), then in polymethyl methacrylate (PMMA); however, the introduction of RGP materials brought renewed interest in the fitting of scleral lenses (Ezekiel, 1983; Pullum 1987; Lyons *et al.*, 1989; Ruben and Benjamin, 1985; Schein *et al.*, 1990). Scleral lenses can be fitted either from preformed sets or by impression moulding.

Non-ventilated preformed scleral lenses

The term 'sealed' has been widely used to describe a lens without a fenestration. However, the same word can also mean there is no or minimal tear exchange under the scleral zone, or that the lens retains an air-free precorneal fluid reservoir. There may be a significant tear exchange or even admission of air bubbles into the precorneal fluid reservoir via unintentional scleral zone channels if a non-fenestrated lens is imperfectly aligned with the sclera. To clarify for the remainder of this text, 'non-ventilated' rather than 'sealed' is used to describe a lens designed with no intentional means of tear exchange, such as a fenestration.

The increased corneal oxygenation available with RGP materials avoids the need for fenestrations (Pullum *et al.*, 1990, 1991; Pullum and Stapleton, 1997), thereby reducing the problem of air bubbles admitted to the precorneal fluid reservoir. The reservoir acts as an effective cushion, therefore settling on the globe is reduced, and the effect is more

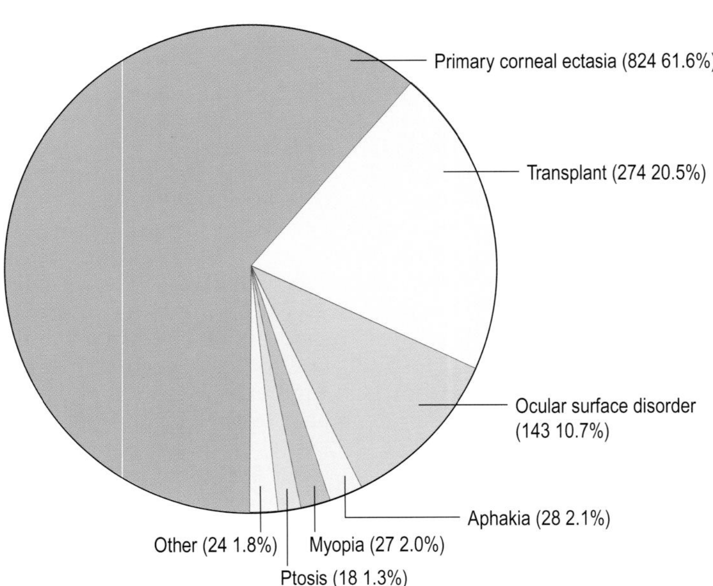

Figure 23.2 Indications for contact lens management of patients attending Moorfields Eye Hospital 2000–2007. A total of 888 patients (1353 eyes) were studied.

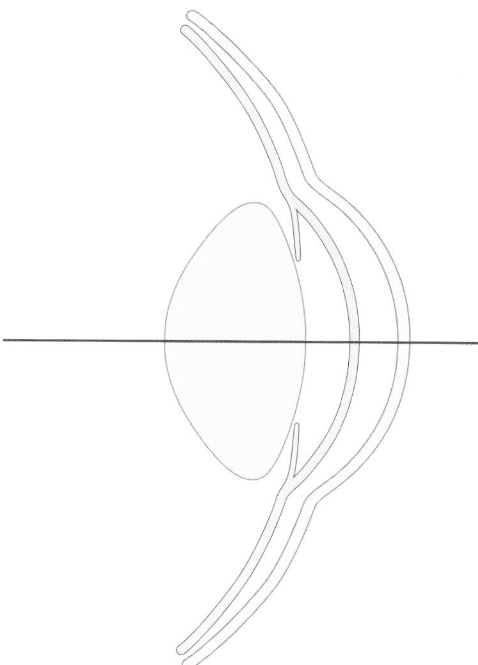

Figure 23.3 Steep scleral zone causing vaulting and increased optic zone clearance with an unchanged back optic zone radius.

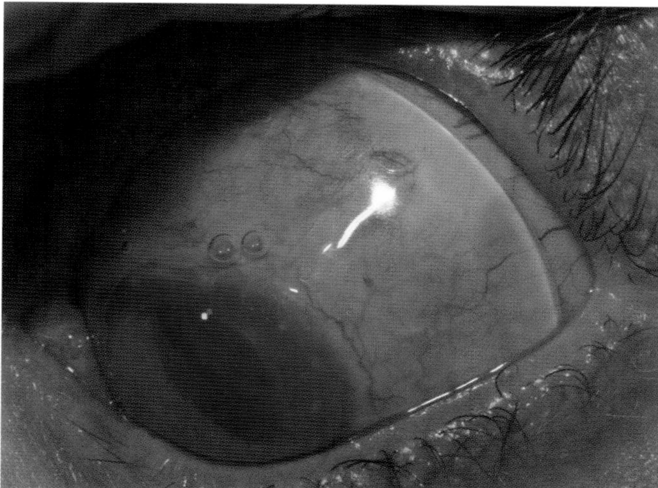

Figure 23.4 Preformed rigid gas-permeable scleral *in situ* illustrating a steep scleral zone. Fluorescein is seen extending beyond the limbus, although not excessively. However, the peripheral conjunctival blood vessels beneath the lens are occluded, giving a blanched appearance. The pathology is corneal transplant which has been complicated by secondary glaucoma. A bleb just above the limbus is visible. Although somewhat steep on the sclera, this was deemed preferable to changing to a flatter fitting, which could compress more on the bleb following any settling back.

predictable, giving increased latitude reaching an end point in the fitting process. Consequently, many more eyes can be fitted with coaxial preformed designs than was ever possible with PMMA (Ramero-Rangel *et al.*, 2000).

A detailed description of the fitting process is beyond the scope of this chapter, but it is appropriate to outline the principles. More indepth accounts can be found in two recent texts (Pullum, 2005, 2007).

The scleral zone

The objective in non-ventilated RGP scleral lens fitting is to achieve corneal clearance extending far enough into the scleral zone to avoid compression of the limbus with optimum scleral alignment over the broadest possible area, as previously shown in Figure 23.1. Perfect alignment to the sclera is not crucial, and nor is it possible, as it is not conveniently spherical or symmetrical about its axis. There should be minimal occlusion of the conjunctival blood vessels, but sufficient sealing on the sclera to prevent introduction of air bubbles into the precorneal fluid reservoir.

The back optic zone radius (BOZR), back optic zone diameter (BOZD) and back scleral radius (BSR) influence the optic zone clearance. If the BSR is too steep, the lens may vault the whole anterior eye from its periphery, occluding the peripheral conjunctival vessels if excessive, as illustrated in Figures 23.3 and 23.4.

If the BSR is too flat, the scleral zone stands off the globe, and may occlude the mid peripheral conjunctival vessels, as seen in Figures 23.5 and 23.6.

The back scleral size (BSS) has a less predictable impact. A larger diameter lens may impinge on peripheral scleral nodules, e.g. the medial and lateral recti muscle insertion points. If so, the lens vaults from the periphery, giving a similar appearance to that with a steep BSR. The optic should be displaced 1–1.5 mm if the diameter is greater than

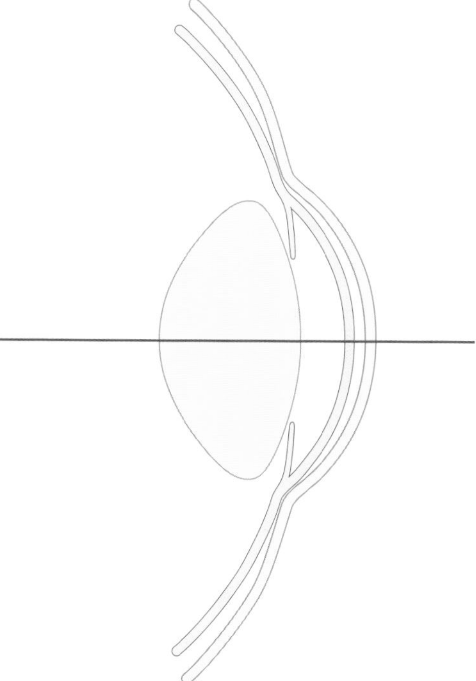

Figure 23.5 Flat scleral zone with a reduced annular scleral bearing surface just outside the limbus, but no change to the apical clearance.

20 mm. This reduces the width of the nasal scleral zone, improving centration and preventing the edge impinging on the inner canthus on nasal gaze movements.

Optic zone sagittal depth and optic zone projection

The optic zone sagittal depth (OZS), and hence the corneal clearance, is determined by varying the BOZR and BOZD in combination. Modern designs blend the optic zone–scleral zone junction so that it is barely perceptible, or include an aspheric transition zone. The primary BOZD remains at the junction between the continuation of the BOZR and the BSR. Alternatively, progressive increments in the projection of the optic zone (OZP) from the extrapolation of the BSR, but without reference to the BOZR or BOZD, can be used to determine the optimum apical clearance (Figure 23.7).

For an indication of the OZP scale, the range for most normal corneas is 1.0–2.0 mm compared to a rare highly globic corneal profile which may require up to 5.0 mm (Figure 23.8). Figure 23.9 shows a non-ventilated RGP scleral lens *in situ* with a glancing contact on the same eye. Even an eye with such a protrusive corneal profile is quite often straightforward when fitting a non-ventilated RGP scleral lens.

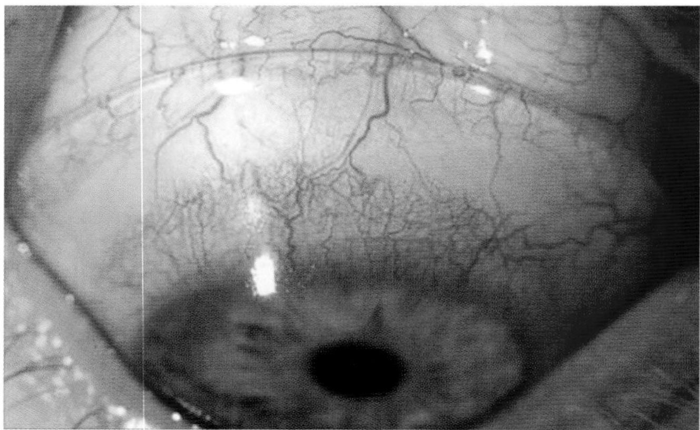

Figure 23.6 Preformed rigid gas-permeable scleral *in situ* illustrating a flat scleral zone. Conjunctival vessel blanching is clearly seen in the mid-periphery. The annular scleral compression zone causes a marked unsightly congestion between the blanched region and the limbus, which may lead to an increased risk of corneal vascularization in a predisposed eye.

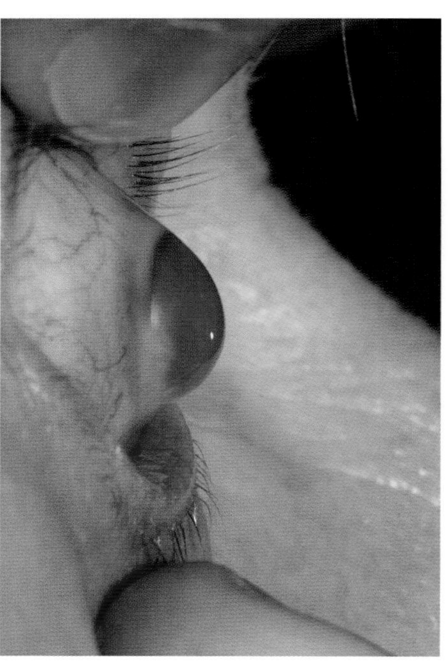

Figure 23.8 Spectacular, but rare, keratoglobus. This case was also diagnosed as Terrien's marginal degeneration, typified by circumferential opacification at the limbus, but the impact on the visual function and the management options are the same irrespective of the name given to the condition.

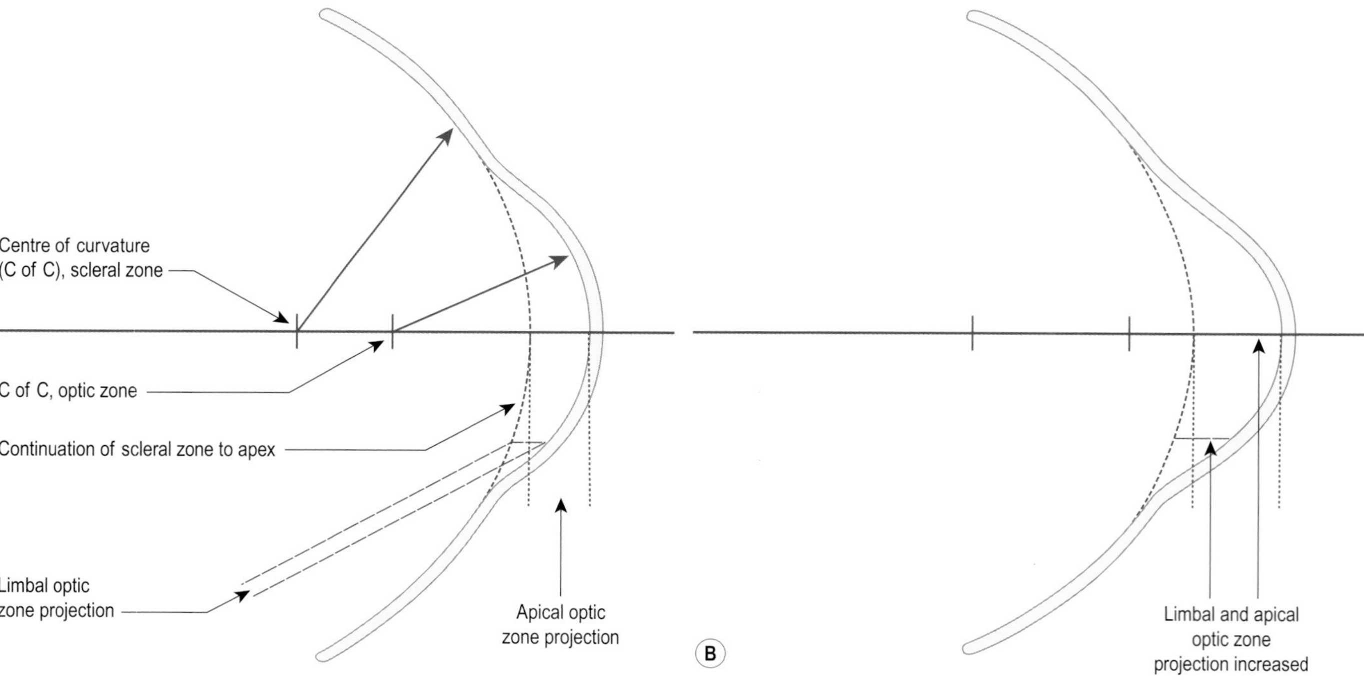

Figure 23.7 (A) Optic zone projection (OZP). (B) Increased apical and limbal OZP.

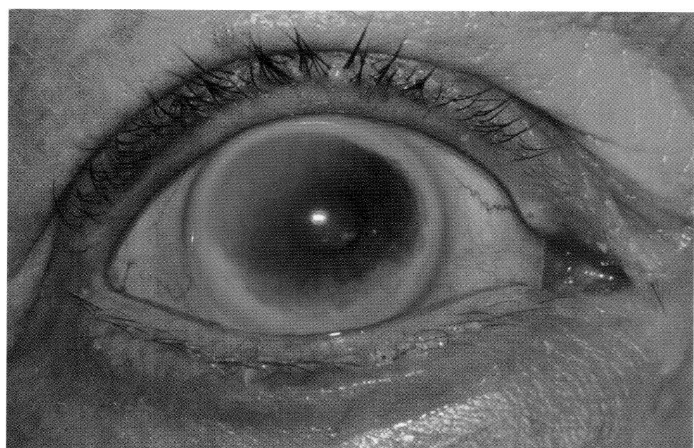

Figure 23.9 Preformed rigid gas-permeable scleral lens *in situ* on the same eye as shown in Figure 23.8, illustrating a glancing apical contact zone but limbal clearance.

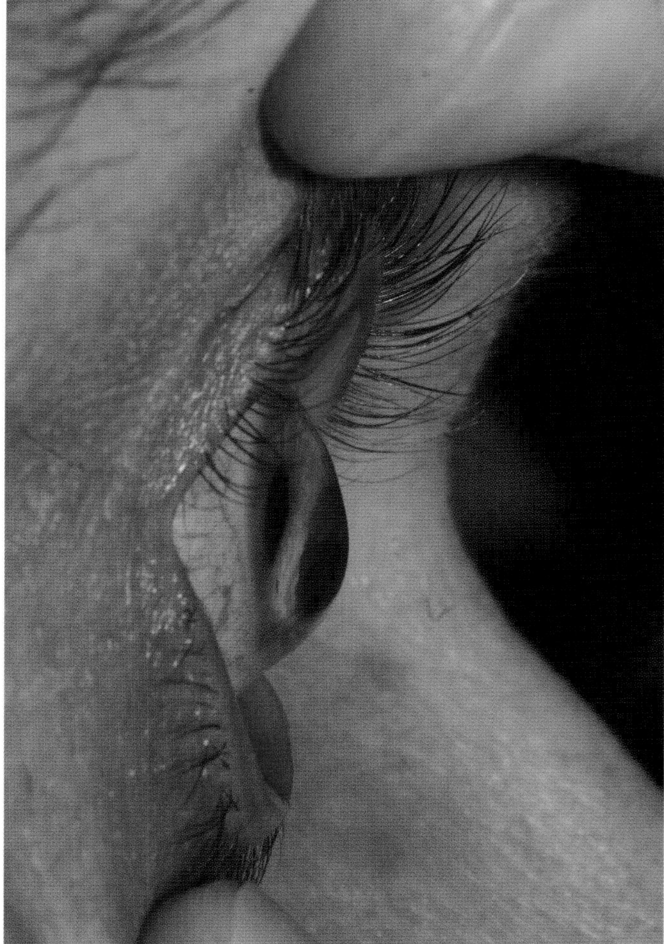

Figure 23.10 Moderately advanced keratoconus with a downwardly decentred apex.

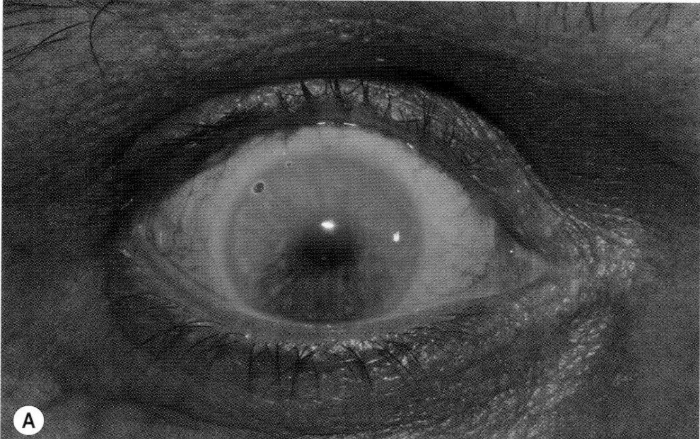

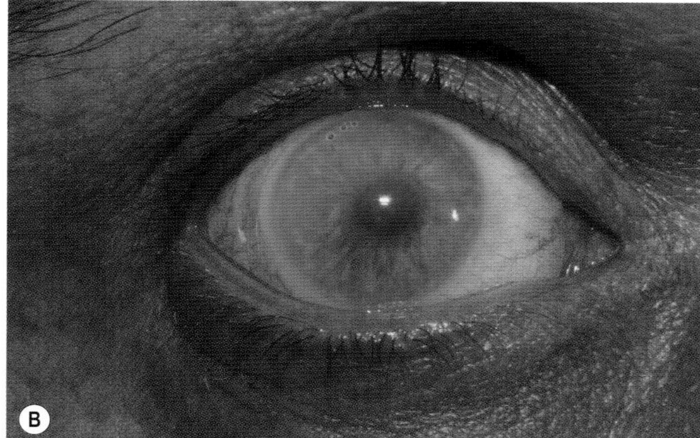

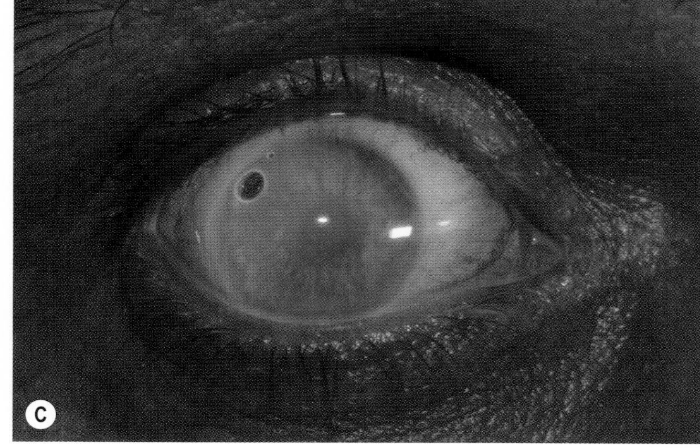

Figure 23.11 Preformed rigid gas-permeable scleral lenses *in situ* on the same eye as shown in Figure 23.10. (A) The apical contact could be described as compressive. (B) Lens with an apical optic zone progression increment of 0.25 mm to give glancing contact. (C) Lens with an apical optic zone progression increment of 0.5 mm to give corneal clearance.

Between 0.20 and 0.30 mm is a suitable OZS or OZP increment for non-ventilated lenses, and 0.25 ± 0.1 mm an optimal apical clearance. Pachymetry is not necessary as the depth of the precorneal fluid reservoir is estimated accurately enough in comparison to the corneal thickness. 0.25 mm is considerably greater than a typical clearance for a fenestrated lens, where anything over 0.1 mm at the apex would admit air bubbles crossing the visual axis. Figure 23.10 shows an eye with moderate keratoconus. The same eye is fitted with scleral lenses to illustrate corneal contact (Figure 23.11A), the effect of an OZP increment of 0.25 mm giving glancing contact (Figure 23.11B) and the effect of an OZP increment of a further 0.25 mm giving corneal clearance (Figure 23.11C).

If air bubbles do become trapped in the precorneal fluid reservoir, refitting a lens with reduced apical clearance, if there is scope, tends to shift the bubbles towards the periphery. Fitting with a flatter BSR may improve scleral zone sealing by moving the bearing surface closer to the limbus, which is the most symmetrical region of the sclera. Reducing the diameter may have the same effect. If still unsuccessful, an eye impression may be necessary to improve alignment on the sclera.

Non-coaxial scleral lenses

Toroidal lenses

If a non-ventilated coaxial RGP lens is impossible to fit because the sclera is insufficiently symmetrical, toroidal scleral zone designs and impression RGP lenses are available (see below). The fitting objectives are similar to those for non-ventilated coaxial lenses, i.e. optimal scleral zone alignment and a precorneal fluid reservoir extending 1–2 mm beyond the limbus. A toroidal design remains an approximation to the scleral topography but may be a closer match to typical scleral contours than a coaxial design, hence may improve centration and sealing on the sclera. Toric scleral lenses have been shown to return rapidly to their original position after rotation (Visser *et al.*, 2006). Wearing time, comfort, visual quality and overall satisfaction may be improved when back-surface toric designs are used compared to spherical ones (Visser *et al.*, 2007b).

Impression moulding

An impression lens has by definition the best possible alignment, but requires development of different skills on the part of both the clinician and the manufacturer (Pullum, 1987; Lyons *et al.*, 1989; Pullum *et al.*, 1989). Unlike with PMMA, an RGP scleral lens cannot be produced by heat moulding as the materials are not thermoplastic, but an optimally fitting PMMA lens can be duplicated in an RGP material.

Fenestrated lenses

A means of ventilation is a prerequisite for a PMMA scleral lens to facilitate some tear exchange. Most commonly this is done with a fenestration; however, slots, truncations and channels have also been used (Pullum and Trodd, 1984a). Compared to fitting a non-ventilated lens, fenestrated scleral lens fitting represents a major undertaking, but there are indications for trying, for example, if there are intractable difficulties inserting a non-ventilated lens air-free. Some fenestrated PMMA scleral lenses are used by established wearers and some are still being issued for new cases. If there is a satisfactory wearing schedule, and acceptable sequelae, the best option may be to leave well alone. If unacceptable, an RGP scleral lens could be offered, either by refitting a non-ventilated design, or, if necessary, by duplicating the existing shape. However, the wearer may have had the same lens for many years, and could have a distinct preference for his/her 'old friend'. In particular, the author's observation is that a corneal contact zone with a PMMA lens that has been well tolerated could be less comfortable if the original shape is duplicated in an RGP material, probably due to the increased coefficient of surface friction with RGP materials.

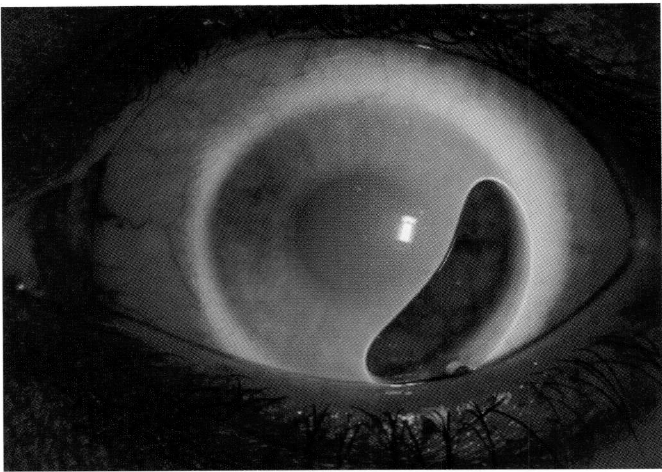

Figure 23.12 Typical shape and size of bubble beneath a fenestrated scleral lens.

Bubbles trapped in the precorneal fluid reservoir are almost unavoidable with fenestrated lenses, hence the fit of the lens is in part determined by their appearance. If the bubble crosses the visual axis, the vision is disrupted. A crescent-shaped bubble extending approximately one-third of the corneal diameter, but restricted to the limbus, is considered optimal (Figure 23.12).

If the lens settles back on the globe, which it usually does, the apical clearance is reduced. If initially there was optimal clearance, just avoiding a bubble, after a few minutes there may be an unacceptable contact zone. If the corneal topography is not regular, which is the case in the majority of cases needing scleral lenses, the depth of the precorneal fluid reservoir is not uniform. The lens therefore fits too close in places as well as there being bubbles in the precorneal fluid reservoir. An impression at the starting point helps to reduce these problems as the scleral-bearing surface is maximized, and the optic zone is fabricated according to the individual topography.

Modification

It is likely that a currently worn fenestrated PMMA lens was originally fitted from an eye impression. The practitioner should never attempt to modify an existing impression lens but should make adjustments to a new shell pressed over a dental stone cast of the original lens. Alternatively another eye impression should be taken to start again from the beginning. Modification of an RGP scleral lens, other than a power change carried out by a competent laboratory, should not be attempted as the outcome is far from predictable, and it is impossible to restore a lens to its original condition.

Ordering scleral lenses

For a preformed scleral lens of 'traditional' style, the practitioner should specify the BOZR, the primary BOZD, the

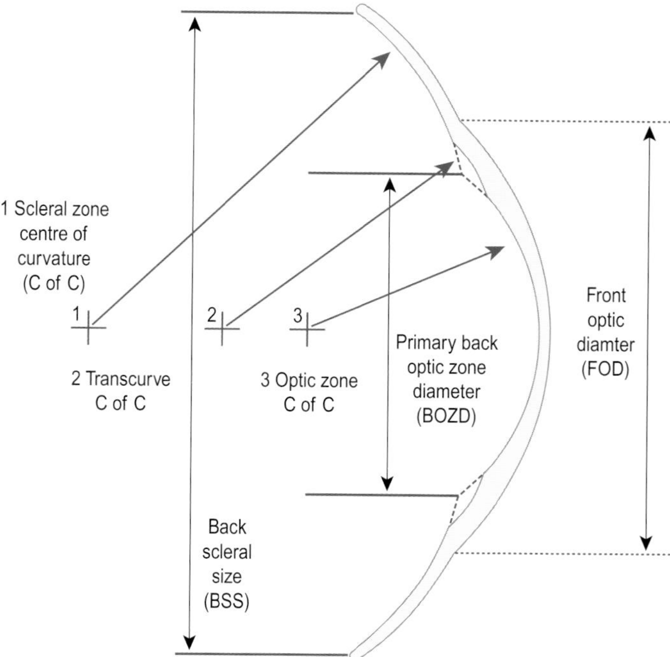

Figure 23.13 Preformed scleral lens parameters.

BSR, the optic zone displacement (D) in mm, the BSS, which is independent of the thickness and the BVP. A transition curve to blend the optic–scleral junction is usually required, but the manufacturer should be left to select the optimum design. Figure 23.13 illustrates the parameters of a scleral lens. Wide-angle lenses are probably the most widely used integrated scleral zone/optic zone lenses and have been available, unchanged from their original design, for over 50 years. The BOZD is a function of the BOZR and the BSR, so specification requires just the BOZR, BSR, BSS, D and BVP.

For non-ventilated RGP scleral lenses, it has become more usual for manufacturers to have their own ordering system, which should be followed to avoid errors. Usually, this entails stating the optimum lens used from the diagnostic fitting set, and details of the over-refraction, with any departures from the trial set parameters described.

A cast of an impression or preferably a cast from which a moulded lens can be made can be sent to a competent laboratory. The BSS can be indicated by drawing a line on the cast. If the requirement is for a PMMA lens, the manufacturer should be given full freedom to produce the back surface. The optic zone is fabricated by grinding diamond-coated spherical stones on to the back surface of the shell, the optimum reached by a skilled trial-and-error process. A power formula must be provided, i.e. the result of a refraction over a scleral lens or a limbal diameter corneal lens of known BOZR and BVP. The manufacturer can then make the appropriate power allowance for the difference between that BOZR and that of the final lens. For a non-ventilated impression RGP lens, a specialist manufacturer would need a fitted PMMA shell or a cast of the shell in order to duplicate the lens in an RGP material.

Lens hygiene and maintenance

Storage

Dry storage is normal for PMMA scleral lenses, and in the author's opinion, also satisfactory for RGP sclerals. Wet storage may enhance surface wetting in some cases, in which case hydrogel lens multifunctional solutions are preferable to the more viscous rigid lens soaking solutions.

Cleaning and conditioning

There being very little tear exchange with non-ventilated RGP scleral lenses, viscous solutions to condition the back surface remain in contact with the cornea for long periods and they may lead to accumulative sensitivity to the preservatives. A non-preserved cleaner, rather than a conditioning solution, which is rinsed off with non-preserved saline prior to insertion may be preferable.

Saline for filling non-ventilated RGP scleral lenses

Non-preserved saline is necessary for filling non-ventilated RGP scleral lenses prior to insertion, because the solution is retained in contact with the cornea for the duration of wear. Some wearers become sensitive to multidose saline, in which case preservative-free unit dose preparations are necessary. Aerosol saline tends to be too gassy for this application.

Rewetting

If lenses need refreshing during the day, soft lens multipurpose solutions may be beneficial. The cleaning action is not as powerful as dedicated cleaners, but rinsing from the surface prior to reinsertion is a quick process compared to the use of a cleaning agent.

Problems and complications with scleral lens wear

Discomfort

Some degree of discomfort from any contact lens cannot always be completely eliminated. With scleral lenses it can be a consequence of apical corneal contact zones, limbal occlusion, an ill-fitting scleral zone or an early symptom of corneal hypoxia.

Bubbles

Elimination of air bubbles behind the lens is also not always possible, especially when the depth of the precorneal reservoir is not uniform. They may enter via non-aligned scleral zone sectors, but rarely disappear without removing and reinserting the lens. Lining the inside surface of the lens with a non-preserved viscous eye drop prior to inserting helps to reduce the problem. Bubbles entering the precorneal fluid reservoir via fenestrations sometimes

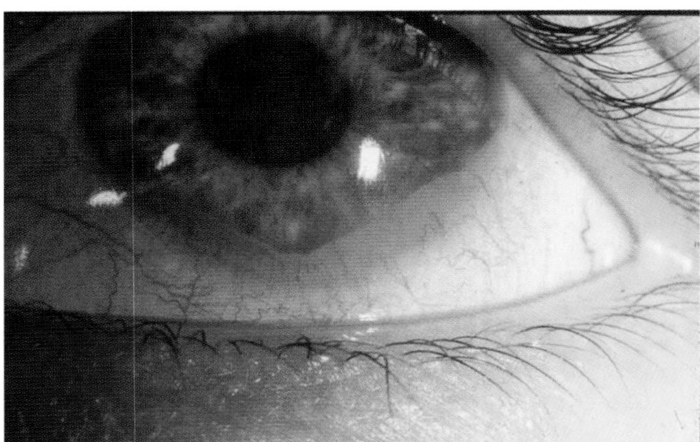

Figure 23.14 Conjunctival displacement over the limbus is a common minor problem. It can be unsightly, but normality is restored immediately after removal of the lens.

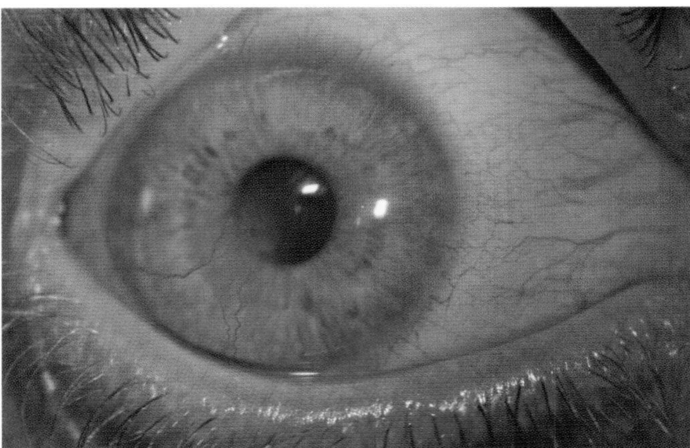

Figure 23.15 Neovascularization after 5 years' rigid gas-permeable scleral lens wear. The indication for fitting was optical irregularities consequent to herpes simplex, so it is possible that the vessel growth was partly hypoxia and partly due to the disease process.

cause clicking sounds which can be very annoying. Instilling a viscous eye drop just at the site of the fenestration may offer a solution for a short period.

Accumulation of mucus

Scleral lenses sometimes generate oversecretion of mucus which is trapped in the precorneal space. It can be globular or fine particulate matter. This is more of a problem with non-ventilated RGP lenses as there is some flushing action through a fenestration. Removal and reinsertion with fresh saline are necessary, and lining the back surface with a non-preserved viscosity agent appears to give an improvement in some cases. Instillation of mucolytic drops such as acetylcysteine before reinsertion may be considered.

Conjunctival blanching and hyperaemia

If localized, conjunctival blanching and adjacent hyperaemia may indicate compressive contact on the scleral zone. The limbus should be watched carefully for early signs of limbal vessel engorgement, which may be the precursor of corneal vascularization, but otherwise some hyperaemia is not a threat and may be impossible to alleviate.

Conjunctival displacement over the limbus

Displacement of the conjunctival flap over the limbus and peripheral cornea can occur, in particular with non-ventilated RGP scleral lenses, if there is insufficient limbal clearance (Figure 23.14). It does not cause a serious problem as reversal takes place on removal of the lens, but wearers notice it when looking in a mirror.

Degradation of the surface

RGP materials are subject to spoilation and deposition. Polishing is possible, but this can only be carried out a limited number of times before the optic quality is lost. Resurfacing is also possible provided there is sufficient substance. There is much to be said for issuing a new lens before attempting to polish or resurface one that is currently worn.

Infection

Infection does not appear to be a common problem with scleral lenses. Cleaning can be carried out effectively both prior to storage and insertion. A dry, clean case is a hygienic environment and unfavourable for bacteria replication.

Giant papillary conjunctivitis

Upper tarsal plate changes are seen sometimes with long-term scleral contact lens wear, but do not often appear to cause the typical discomfort described by soft lens wearers. This is presumably because there is no tarsal plate–lens edge interaction, and deposits are easily cleaned from rigid lens surfaces. The issue is clouded as atopy is a common coexisting pathology in keratoconus.

Hypoxia

The corneal response to scleral lens wear has greatly improved with the introduction of gas-permeable materials (Bleshoy and Pullum, 1988; Pullum *et al.*, 1990, 1991). Corneal thickness changes are demonstrably less (Mountford *et al.*, 1994; Pullum and Stapleton, 1997). Hypoxia and consequent corneal vascularization have been significantly reduced. This means that, with the use of modern materials, overnight wear of scleral lenses can be considered (Rosenthal *et al.*, 2000; Tappin *et al.*, 2001; Smith *et al.*, 2004).

Neovascularization

Corneal vascularization is the long-term effect of chronic corneal oedema (Figure 23.15). Corneal vessels do not necessarily cause a major visual loss, but have a tendency to leak lipid, and can cause a dense opacity. Sudden-onset visual loss can occur even if the vessels are apparently quite fine in calibre. Some absorption is possible after a time, but the rate is slower for older patients. There have been some cases when PMMA scleral lens-induced vascularization has been reversed on refitting with RGP scleral lenses, leaving only ghost vessels (Tan *et al.*, 1995).

Some vessel ingrowth may be an acceptable complication if the visual indication for scleral lens wear is strong, and especially if the alternative management options are likely to be worse. The main concern is that any hypoxic changes may be sight-threatening: complacency must be avoided, but overstating the threat is not productive if there is a significant benefit from continued wear. It is possible that vascularization is self-limiting if compensating for an oxygen deficit. A small amount of vascularization is not sight-threatening if, after the anticipated rate of progress, based on the existing extent of the vessels and assuming the same rate of progress, the vessels do not cross the visual axis within the patient's expected lifespan.

Neovascularization in keratoconus

It must be recognized, however, that a bed of corneal vessels may increase the risk of later corneal transplant rejection. This is especially the case when the apex is eccentric, requiring a larger donor cornea which is in closer proximity to the limbal arcades. Careful monitoring and liaison with the ophthalmologist who may carry out future surgery are clearly essential.

Conclusion

Today's requirement for scleral lenses constitutes the smallest of all contact lens types, but their applications are often when other lens types are unsuccessful, or when the patient may face the alternative of potentially hazardous ocular surgery. It is vital to preserve clinical fitting skills as effectively as possible to avoid discredit due to too many unsatisfactory results. A relatively small number of practitioners need to be actively involved but those who may not wish to undertake the work personally can still be familiar with the application of scleral lenses so that suitable patients are recognized and referred for fitting.

Acknowledgement

The author is indebted to Moorfields and Oxford Eye Hospitals for support over many years during the development of modern clinical scleral contact lens practice.

References

Bleshoy, H. and Pullum, K. W. (1988) Corneal response to gas permeable impression scleral lenses. *J. Br. Contact Lens Assoc.*, **11**, 31–34.

Cotter, M. and Rosenthal, P. (1998) Scleral contact lenses. *J. Am. Optom. Assoc.*, **69**, 33–40.

Ezekiel, D. (1983) Gas permeable haptic lenses. *J. Br. Contact Lens Assoc.*, **6**, 158–161.

Fine, P., Savrinski, G. and Millodot, M. (2003) Contact lens management of a case of Stevens–Johnson syndrome: a case report. *Optometry*, **74**, 659–664.

Foss, A. J. E., Trodd, T. C. and Dart, J. K. G. (1994) Current indications for scleral contact lenses. *Contact Lens Assoc. Ophthalmol. J.*, **20**, 115–118.

Jacobs, D. S. (2008) Update on scleral lenses. *Curr. Opin. Ophthalmol.*, **19**, 298–301.

Kok, J. H. C. and Visser, R. (1992) Treatment of ocular surface disorders and dry eyes with high gas-permeable scleral lenses. *Cornea*, **11**, 518–522.

Looi, A. L., Lim, L. and Tan, D. T. (2002) Visual rehabilitation with new-age rigid gas-permeable scleral contact lenses – a case series. *Ann. Acad. Med. Singapore*, **31**, 234–237.

Lyons, C. J., Buckley, R. J., Pullum, K. W. *et al.* (1989) Development of the gas-permeable impression-moulded scleral contact lens. A preliminary report. *Acta Ophthalmol.*, **67**(Suppl. 192), 162–164.

Margolis, R., Thakrar, V. and Perez, V. L. (2007) Role of rigid gas-permeable scleral contact lenses in the management of advanced atopic keratoconjunctivitis. *Cornea*, **26**, 1032–1034.

Mountford, J., Carkeet, N. and Carney, L. (1994) Corneal thickness changes during scleral lens wear: Effect of gas permeability. *Int. Contact Lens Clin.*, **21**, 19–21.

Pullum, K. W. (1987) Feasibility study for the production of gas permeable scleral lenses using ocular impression techniques. *Trans. Br. Contact Lens Assoc. Annual Clinical Conference.*

Pullum, K. W. (2005) Chapter 33: Scleral lenses. In *Clinical Contact Lens Practice* (E. S. Bennett and B. A. Weismann, eds), pp. 629–648, Philadelphia: Lippincott, Williams and Wilkins.

Pullum, K. W. (2007) Chapter 15: Scleral Contact Lenses. In *Contact Lenses*, 5th edn.(A.J. Phillips and L. Speedwell, eds.), pp. 333–353, Oxford: Elsevier.

Pullum, K. W. and Buckley, R. J. (2007) Therapeutic and ocular surface indications for scleral contact lenses. *The Ocular Surface Journal*, **5**, 41–50.

Pullum, K. W. and Stapleton, F. J. (1997) Scleral lens induced corneal swelling: what is the effect of varying *Dk* and lens thickness? *Contact Lens Assoc. Ophthalmol. J.*, **23**, 259–263.

Pullum, K. W. and Trodd, T. C. (1984a) Development of slotted scleral lenses. *J. Br. Contact Lens Assoc.*, **7**, 28–38 and 92–97.

Pullum, K. W. and Trodd, T. C. (1984b) The modern concept of scleral lens practice. *J. Br. Contact Lens. Assoc.*, **7**, 169–178.

Pullum, K. W., Parker, J. H. and Hobley, A. J. (1989) Development of gas permeable impression scleral lenses. The Josef Dallos Award Lecture, Part One. Transactions of the BCLA Conference. *J. Br. Contact Lens Assoc.*, **13**, 77–81.

Pullum, K. W., Hobley, A. J. and Parker, J. H. (1990) Dallos award lecture part two. Hypoxic corneal changes following sealed gas permeable impression scleral lens wear. *J. Br. Contact Lens Assoc.*, **13**, 83–87.

Pullum, K. W., Hobley, A. J. and Davison, C. (1991) 100 + *Dk*: Does thickness make much difference? *J. Br. Contact Lens Assoc.*, **6**, 158–161.

Pullum, K. W., Whiting, M. A. and Buckley, R. J. (2005) Scleral contact lenses: The expanding role. *Cornea*, **24**, 269–277.

Ramero-Rangel, T., Stavrou, P., Cotter, J. M. *et al.* (2000) Gas-permeable scleral contact lens therapy in ocular surface disease. *Am. J. Ophthalmol.*, **130**, 25–32.

Rosenthal, P. and Cotter, J. (2003) The Boston Scleral Lens in the management of severe ocular surface disease. *Ophthalmol Clin. North Am.,* **16,** 89–93.

Rosenthal, P., Cotter, J. M. and Baum, J. (2000) Treatment of persistent corneal epithelial defect with extended wear of a fluid-ventilated gas-permeable scleral contact lens. *Am. J. Ophthalmol.,* **130,** 33–41.

Ruben, C. M. and Benjamin, W. J. (1985) Scleral contact lenses: preliminary report on oxygen-permeable materials. *Contact Lens,* **13,** 5–10.

Salam, A., Melia, B. and Singh, A. J. (2005) Scleral contact lenses are not optically inferior to corneal lenses. *Br. J. Ophthalmol.,* **89,** 1662–1663.

Schein, O. D., Rosenthal, P. and Ducharme, C. (1990) A gas-permeable scleral contact lens for visual rehabilitation. *Am. J. Ophthalmol.,* **109,** 318–322.

Smith, G. T. H., Mireskandari, K. and Pullum, K. W. (2004) Corneal swelling with overnight wear of scleral contact lenses. *Cornea,* **23,** 29–34.

Tan, D. T. H., Pullum, K. W. and Buckley, R. J. (1995) Medical applications of scleral contact lenses: 2. Gas-permeable scleral contact lenses. *Cornea,* **14,** 130–137.

Tappin, M. J., Pullum, K. W. and Buckley, R. J. (2001) Scleral contact lenses for overnight wear in the management of ocular surface disorders. *Eye,* **15,** 168–172.

Visser, R. (1990) Een nieuwe toekomst hoogzuurtofdoorlatende scleralenzen bij verschillende pathologie. *Nederlands Tijdschrift voor Optometrie en Contactologie,* **3,** 10–14.

Visser, E. S., Visser, R. and van Lier, H. J. (2006) Advantages of toric scleral lenses. *Optom. Vis. Sci.,* **83,** 233–236.

Visser, E. S., Visser, R., van Lier, H. J. *et al.* (2007a) Modern scleral lenses part I: clinical features. *Eye Contact Lens,* **33,** 13–20.

Visser, E. S., Visser, R., van Lier, H. J. *et al.* (2007b) Modern scleral lenses part II: patient satisfaction. *Eye Contact Lens.* **33,** 21–25.

CHAPTER 24

Tinted lenses

Nathan Efron and Suzanne Efron

Introduction

Eye colour is universally recognized as an important and defining natural physical characteristic of the body human, and a contact lens is an effective vehicle for modifying or enhancing this appearance for those who wish to do so. More importantly, tints can be applied to contact lenses to help normalize the appearance of disfigured eyes and help improve vision in diseased eyes.

Tints have been applied to all forms of contact lenses since their invention over a century ago. In his original treatise in 1888, Fick clearly recognized the potential prosthetic benefits of contact lenses upon which opaque iris patterns and black pupils could be painted (Efron and Pearson, 1988). The inventor of the corneal lens, Kevin Tuohy, attempted to tint lenses, and Otto Wichterle, the inventor of the soft lens, was awarded two patents describing processes for tinting hydroxyethyl methacrylate (HEMA) lenses. This chapter describes the various applications of tinted lenses and current technology used for lens tinting.

Basic options

An important initial consideration in deciding on the most appropriate tinted lens for a given patient is whether to use a rigid or soft lens. A particular lens type may be indicated for clinical reasons; for example, a rigid lens would be required in the case of a sighted eye with corneal distortion.

An advantage of rigid lenses is that it is possible to paint unique designs and so effect a realistic iris appearance in terms of a more precise match of colour and iris features. However, full corneal coverage is not possible, and rigid lenses move on the eye. These effects can be minimized by fitting slightly tight, large-diameter lenses. In general, rigid lenses are best suited for prosthetic use. In certain cases of extensive ocular disfiguration, painted haptic lenses may give the best result. Soft lenses have the advantage of offering full corneal coverage and stability on the eye, and are thus particularly suited for cosmetic use.

The applied tint can be translucent or opaque. The resulting lens may be wholly translucent if translucent tints alone are applied, semiopaque if opaque tints have been used on portions of the lens and completely opaque if opaque tints have been applied across the entire lens surface. A translucent tint allows certain wavelengths of light to pass through, thus effecting a colour change. Light passing through such a tint, and reflecting back off the iris, will be further modified such that the cosmetic effect is a combination of the colour of the translucent tint and iris. Translucent tints can therefore be said to enhance or modify natural iris colours. This effect is only successful with relatively light-coloured irides.

Opaque tints can substantially or completely block the passage of light. A coloured pattern can be applied over a totally opaque base to effect a complete change of eye colour, while at the same time, for example, masking out underlying iris disfigurations. Thus, the primary cosmetic application of opaque tints is to change the colour of dark irides or have the prosthetic effect of restoring a normal appearance to a disfigured eye.

Tinted lens designs and applications

Translucent and opaque tints are applied to rigid or soft lenses for a variety of reasons, which are outlined below.

Handling tints

Handling tints – which are also known as 'lens visibility tints' or 'locator tints' – are incorporated into soft lenses so that these lenses can be easily seen in the lens case or on a domestic surface if accidentally dropped (Figure 24.1). Such tints are very light (between 5 and 15% absorption) and do not alter iris colour; however, they make the lens slightly more visible on the eye by virtue of the handling tint being noticable where the lens edge impinges over the sclera. Handling tints do not affect vision or colour perception. Some wearers find lens handling difficult as even with the pale handling tint the lenses can be hard to see. In those

DOI: 10.1016/B978-0-7506-8869-7.00024-0

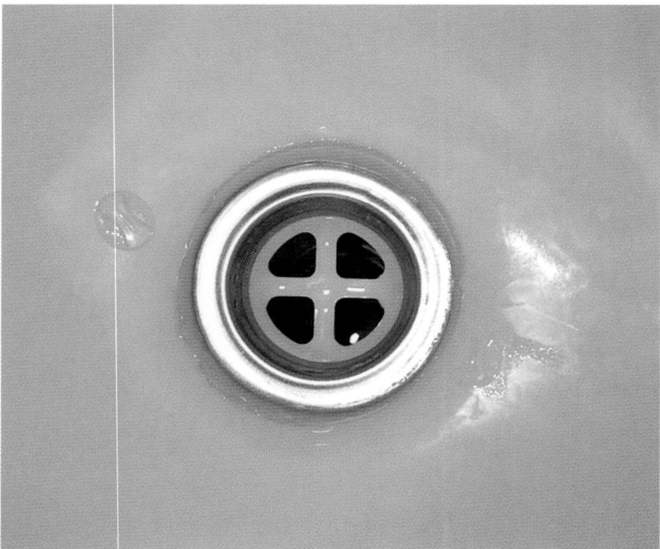

Figure 24.1 Lenses dropped in a bathroom sink. The lens with the handling tint can be clearly seen at the half-past-nine position with respect to the drain hole, about 10 mm from the edge of the drain-plate. The lens without the handling tint is far less visible; its right-hand edge can just be detected at the 4 o'clock position, about 10 mm from the edge of the drain-plate.

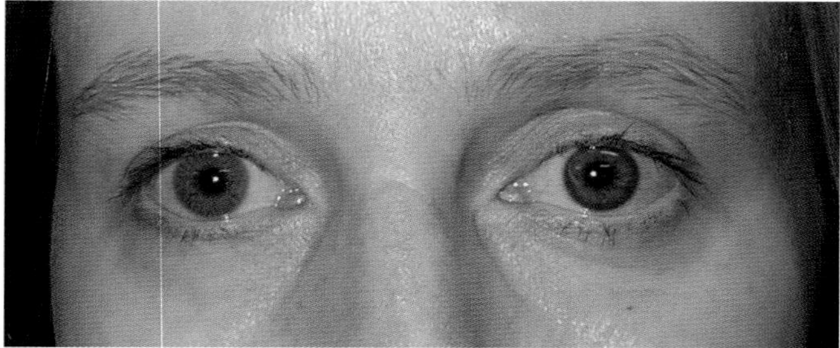

Figure 24.2 Stunning cosmetic effect created by a lens with a blue dot matrix tint in the right eye of a patient with identical irides in the right and left eyes (there is no lens in the left eye).

cases a cosmetic tinted lens may be fitted to enable easier handling.

Cosmetic tinted lenses

A cosmetic tinted lens can be defined as a lens that is designed to beautify an otherwise normal appearance. This can amount to enhancing eye colour with translucent tints, modifying eye colour with a combination of translucent and opaque tints or completely changing eye colour with opaque tints. Cosmetic tinted lenses are considered to be a fashion accessory, and as such they are often worn by emmetropes. Indeed, most tinted lenses are produced for their cosmetic effect (Figure 24.2). The most frequently used tints are aquamarine, blue, green and amber. As is the case with handling tints, cosmetic tints do not appreciably affect vision or colour perception (Tan *et al.*, 1987), although patients may report an initial transient effect. The light transmission through cosmetic tinted lenses is usually in the range 75–85% (Harris *et al.*, 1999).

A recently introduced concept in cosmetic lenses is the iris-enhancing ring. This is aimed at the Asian wearer, whose average horizontal visible iris diameter is 11.2 mm. The outer diameter of the limbal ring of the 1-Day Acuvue Define lens is 12.5 mm, thus enlarging the appearance of the eyes (Figure 24.3).

Prosthetic tinted lenses

A prosthetic tinted lens can be defined as a lens that is designed to normalize an otherwise abnormal appearance. Providing the patient does not have unreasonable expectations the lenses are generally satisfactory in terms of wearing time, comfort and colour (Cole and Vogt, 2006). Typical cases for which such lenses are indicated include aftermath of trauma, ocular disease and congenital abnormalities (Figure 24.4).

Visible deformities of the anterior ocular structures – in particular the cornea, iris and crystalline lens – can be effectively masked using opaque tints (Key and Mobley, 1987). Specific tinting configurations can be tailored for different circumstances (Figure 24.5); examples include:

- A painted iris and clear pupil for a sighted eye with a disfigured iris.
- A painted iris and opaque pupil for a non-sighted eye.
- A clear iris and opaque pupil for a non-sighted eye with a dense cataract.

Therapeutic tinted lenses

A therapeutic tinted lens can be defined as a lens that is designed to treat an underlying defect or disease. Primary therapeutic applications of contact lenses include reducing excessive photophobia and glare due to aniridia (Figure 24.5), eliminating monocular polyopia due to trauma, eliminating binocular diplopia in squint (in cases where surgical and optical intervention is not viable or contraindicated) and variable nystagmus (Astin, 1998).

Several studies have show that red tinted contact lenses may be useful in relieving the photophobia associated with a number of cone disorders, including achromatopsia (Zeltzer, 1979; Park and Sunness, 2004; Schornack *et al.*, 2007). The dark-tinted glasses with side-shields and floppy hats usually used to manage these conditions are very conspicuous and can cause marked psychological morbidity in children. Rajak *et al.* (2006) fitted children with 70% brown contact lenses and observed marked improvements in their quality of life. Similar dark brown tinted lenses were shown to help patients with Bothnia dystrophy (Jonsson *et al.*, 2007), a variant of retinitis pigmentosa.

There are often secondary therapeutic benefits of tinted lenses designed for prosthetic use. These include the following examples: a lens with an opaque pupil masking a cataract but also eliminating disturbing light in a near-blind eye; a rigid lens with an opaque iris pattern fitted to a distorted cornea in a sighted eye also having the effect of improving vision by neutralizing corneal optics and the incorporation of appropriate lens power to correct vision; and a lens with an opaque iris pattern to mask aniridia in a sighted eye also reducing glare.

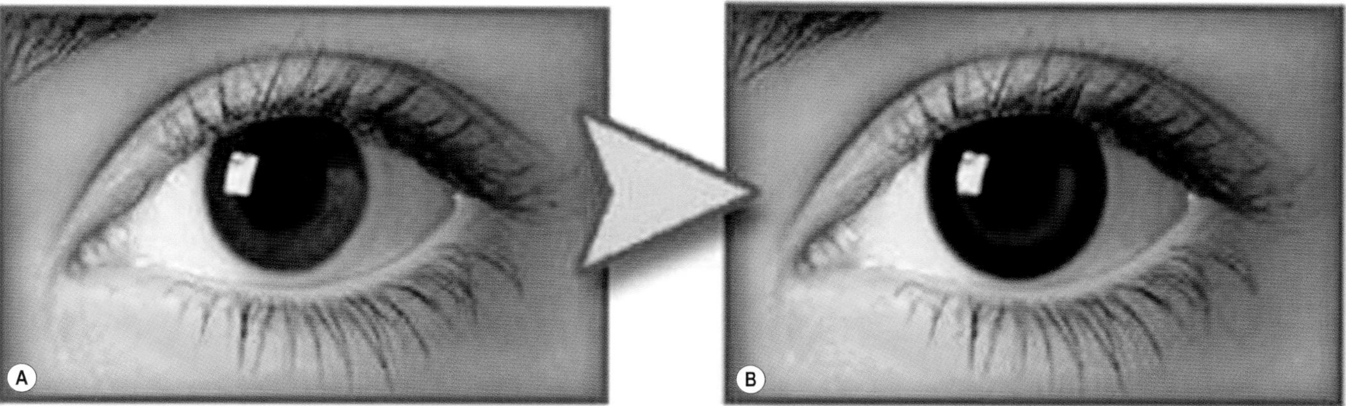

Figure 24.3 Eye without (A) and with (B) a lens with iris enhancing ring.

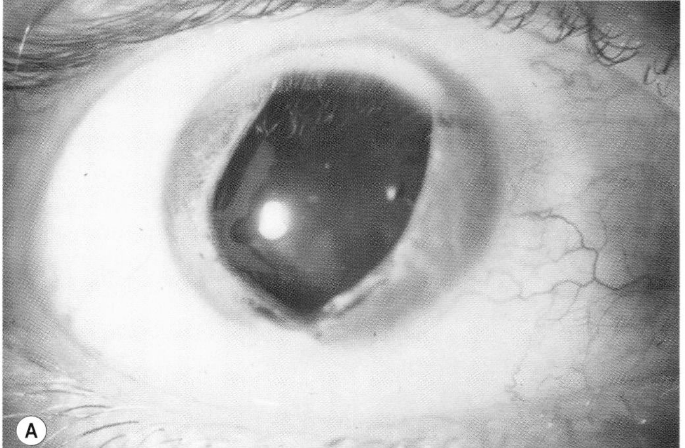

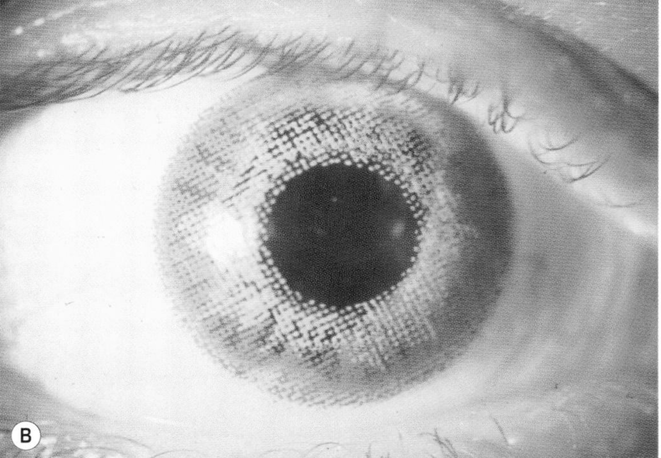

Figure 24.4 (A) Trauma has resulted in partial aniridia, giving rise to an unsightly appearance and excess glare. (B) An opaque dot matrix print soft lens offers the prosthetic advantage of an improved appearance and the therapeutic benefit of reducing excess glare.

Opaque contact lenses have been used for occlusion therapy in amblyopia (Eustis and Chamberlain, 1996) and prosthetic lenses have also been trialled for this purpose. The degree of penalization can be varied with different iris print patterns and opaque pupil sizes. Peripheral fusion can be preserved with some lenses (Collins *et al.*, 2008).

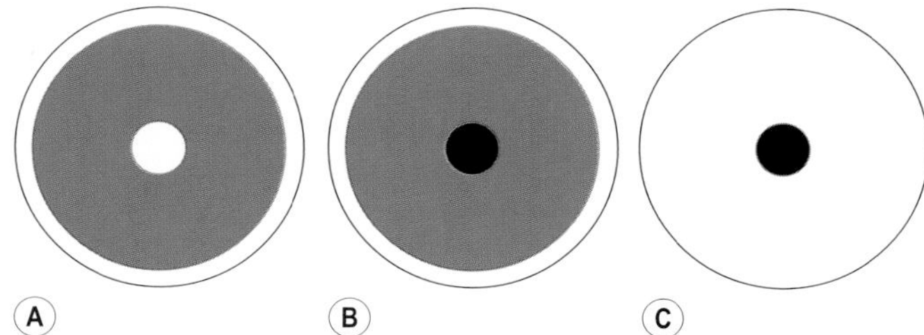

Figure 24.5 Three basic lens tint configurations for combined prosthetic/therapeutic effects. (A) Clear pupil and opaque iris; (B) opaque pupil and opaque iris; (C) opaque pupil only.

Performance-enhancing tinted lenses

Colour vision

Monocular prescription of red tinted lenses to enhance colour vision in colour-defective patients has long been advocated; however, their use is controversial. X-Chrom lenses have a dark red pupil, the diameter of which may be varied to suit individual needs. One eye receives a different luminance and chromatic signal from the other eye and through a process of retinal rivalry a wider range of colours apparently can be interpreted.

Swarbrick *et al.* (2001) showed the ChromaGen lens significantly reduced Ishihara error rates, particularly for deutan subjects, but had no significant effect on Farnsworth lantern test performance. There are medicolegal implications in prescribing these lenses to enable patients to pass the colour vision tests required in occupations with colour vision-related restrictions.

Dyslexia

Various tinted lenses have been devised to cure dyslexia and to alleviate migraine. These can also technically be described as therapeutic applications, although in most cases improvements are attributed to a placebo effect rather than a true therapeutic effect.

Sport

Sport-tinted contact lenses have become available to athletes in an attempt to improve performance by enhancing

Table 24.1 Ultraviolet (UV) blocking characteristics of a range of soft contact lenses

Lenses	Manufacturer	Material	UV blocker	Centre thickness (mm)	UV transmittance (%)	Protection factor*
1-Day Acuvue Moist	Johnson & Johnson	Etafilcon A	Yes	0.06	16.08 ± 0.58	6.22
Focus Dailies	CIBA Vision	Nelfilcon A	No	0.10	55.96 ± 0.19	1.79
SofLens 1-day disposables	Bausch & Lomb	Hilafilcon A	No	0.17	58.29 ± 1.03	1.72
Acuvue Advance	Johnson & Johnson	Galyfilcon A	Yes	0.07	9.98 ± 0.26	10.02
Acuvue Oasys	Johnson & Johnson	Senofilcon A	Yes	0.02–0.05	8.36 ± 0.28	11.96
Night & Day	CIBA Vision	Lotrafilcon A	No	0.08	54.47 ± 0.94	1.84
02 Optix	CIBA Vision	Lotrafilcon B	No	0.08	50.31 ± 0.79	1.99
PureVision	Bausch & Lomb	Balafilcon A	No	0.09	38.18 ± 1.55	2.62

* Protection factor $= 1/T_\lambda$ where T is the percentage transmittance of UV in a given waveband.
(Adapted from Moore and Ferreira, 2006)

contrast. Two shades are suggested for different sports. An amber tint is suggested for fast-moving ball sports such as football, rugby, tennis and baseball. A grey-green tint is suggested for golf, running and training. The Amber and Gray-Green Nike Maxsight lenses have 50% and 36% visible light transmission, respectively.

Although there may be statistically significant differences in contrast when sport-tinted contact lenses are worn, there does not appear to be evidence that the lenses provide any clinically significant difference when considering contrast enhancement (Porisch, 2007; Cerviño *et al.*, 2008). However, the results of one study (Erickson *et al.*, 2009) claimed that the Maxsight Amber and Gray-Green lenses provide better contrast discrimination in bright sunlight, better contrast discrimination when alternating between bright and shaded target conditions, better speed of visual recovery in bright sunlight and better overall visual performance in bright and shaded target conditions compared with clear lenses. These lenses are currently not in production.

Prophylactic tints

The purpose of a prophylactic tint is to prevent injury or disease of the eye. The primary prophylactic application of tinted lenses is protection from excess ultraviolet (UV) light. Lenses with UV protection tints may be beneficial to lens wearers who are frequently exposed to UV radiation, such as those who:

- Pursue an active outdoors lifestyle, especially near snow, sand and sea.
- Work outdoors (such as professional tennis players).
- Use photosensitizing drugs.
- Are often exposed to artificial UV sources during work or recreation.
- Are aphakic.

Some argue that everyone can benefit from UV tints to prevent chronic ocular damage. Non-tinted lenses and lenses with standard cosmetic tints transmit light down to 230 nm and thus do not provide acceptable UV protection (Tønnesen *et al.*, 1997; Harris *et al.*, 1999). Lenses with special UV tints were found by Harris *et al.* (1999) to block light lower than about 350 nm from entering the eye, thus affording the desired protective effect.

The UV transmittance characteristics of a range of daily disposable and silicone hydrogel contact lenses are shown in Table 24.1. Those contact lenses not incorporating an UV-blocking monomer do show some attenuation of the UV spectrum and can therefore also serve to reduce the amount of UV incident at the anterior ocular surface (Moore and Ferreira, 2006).

Patients must, however, be warned of the limitations of UV-tinted contact lenses. For example, solar keratitis can occur in exposed regions of the cornea in UV-tinted rigid lens wearers, and the conjunctiva is susceptible to solar damage in both soft and rigid lens wearers. Accordingly, patients should be advised to wear UV-protecting sunglasses or goggles during prolonged periods of UV exposure, and to protect exposed regions of skin in extreme conditions. Contact lenses may be the only form of UV protection possible in situations where spectacles cannot be worn, for example for sports such as surfing.

Theatric tinted lenses

Lenses can be designed and tinted – typically with opaque agents – to create dramatic or theatrical effects. Such lenses are also known as 'costume' or 'party' lenses. Effects such as wolf eyes (Figure 24.6), national flags, hearts, stars and smiley faces can be created, and some companies market afocal lenses specifically for this purpose.

Although these lenses are viewed as a fashion accessory, potential users must be advised to have a thorough initial eye examination to check that their eyes are suitable for wearing contact lenses, and that the fit is satisfactory. Regular aftercare examinations are also recommended. Users should also be warned that such lenses should never be shared with anyone else because: (1) the contact lenses may not fit, or be contraindicated, in another person; and (2) there is a danger of cross-contamination and infection (Johns and O'Day, 1988; Steinemann *et al.*, 2003; Connell *et al.*, 2004; Lee *et al.*, 2007).

Opaque lenses with clear pupils may also cause changes in corneal topography during wear, which can take up

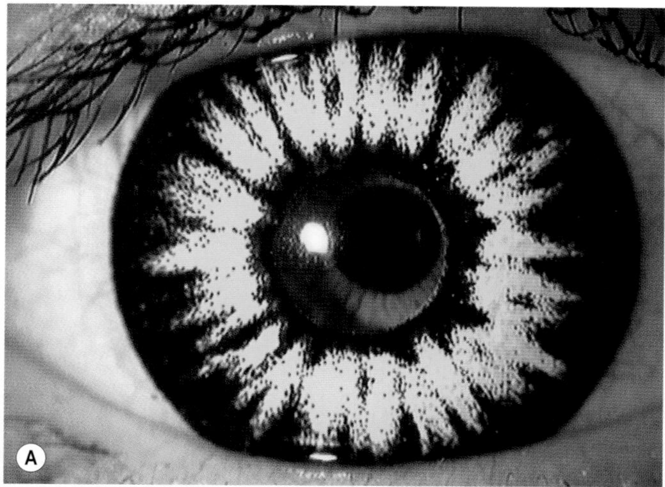
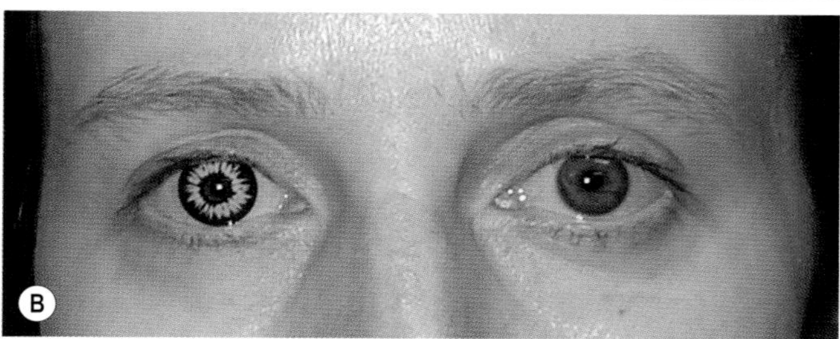

Figure 24.6 Theatric 'wolf-eye' lens. (A) The clear pupil of the lens featured here is slightly decentred with respect to the natural pupil. (B) Viewed at arms length, the 'wolf-eye' lens is seen in the right eye of a patient with identical irides in the right and left eyes (there is no lens in the left eye). The yellow tint contains fluorescent dyes so that the lens glows in the dark under ultraviolet radiation.

to 150 minutes to recover. Wearers of such lenses need to be made aware of the potential for reduced visual performance, both during lens wear and for several hours after lens wear (Voetz *et al.*, 2004).

Identification tints

Lens buttons are colour-coded with light tints by some manufacturers who supply a wide range of products so as to facilitate correct product identification at the lens fabrication stage. Tints are sometimes used as lens identification imprints and toric lens axis location marks.

Manufacture

A vast array of ingenious chemical processes and manufacturing techniques has been devised for tinting contact lenses (Meshel and Smith-Kimura, 1996). Concepts have been variously 'borrowed' from industries as diverse as fabric dying, map-making, leather decorating, paper printing, photography and lithography. A vast patent literature protects the proprietary interests of many of those who have devised the various processes. The general principles underlying some of the key techniques for producing translucent, opaque and combination tints are outlined below.

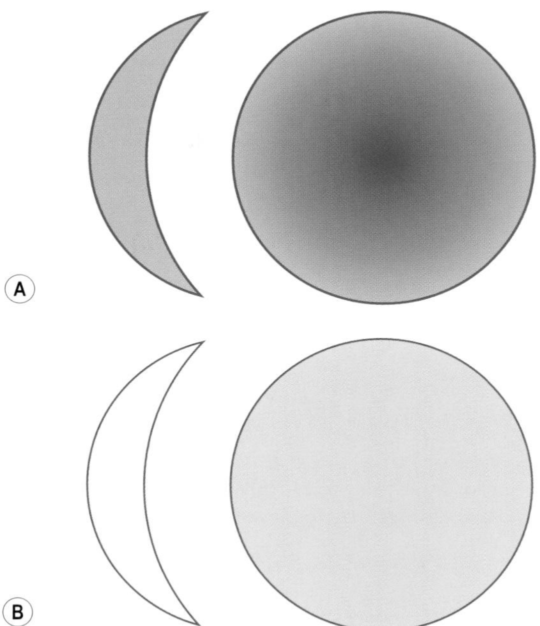

Figure 24.7 Effects of tint process on lens appearance. (A) Dye dispersion tinting of a plus-powered lens can result in greater tint density towards the lens centre. (B) Vat dye and chemical bond tint processes result in an even tint distribution across the lens.

Translucent tints

Translucent tints can be created using four basic techniques – dye dispersion tinting, vat dye tinting, chemical bond tinting and printing.

Dye dispersion tinting

This method is used primarily to tint rigid lenses. A dye or pigment is mixed into the polymer matrix by adding the dye to the monomer mixture prior to polymerization, or by adding the dye to the polymer and then mixing to disperse the colour. This results in an evenly distributed, stable dye. The disadvantages of this process are:

- It is not possible to vary the distribution of tint across the lens (e.g. to create a clear pupil).
- The density of tint is proportional to lens thickness (Figure 24.7).
- This process is unsuitable for soft lenses because the dye, which is non-water-soluble, can leach out from the polymer during hydration.

Vat dye tinting

This process is suitable for soft lens tinting. The finished contact lens is soaked in a water-soluble dye for a fixed amount of time and at a specified temperature. The lens is then exposed to air, rendering the dye insoluble and trapped within the lens matrix. Because the dye only enters the lens surface to a depth of about 10 μm, the lens will appear to have a uniform tint across its entirety, the intensity of which will be independent of optical power (see Figure 24.8). The dye is held in position by strong absorptive forces, resulting

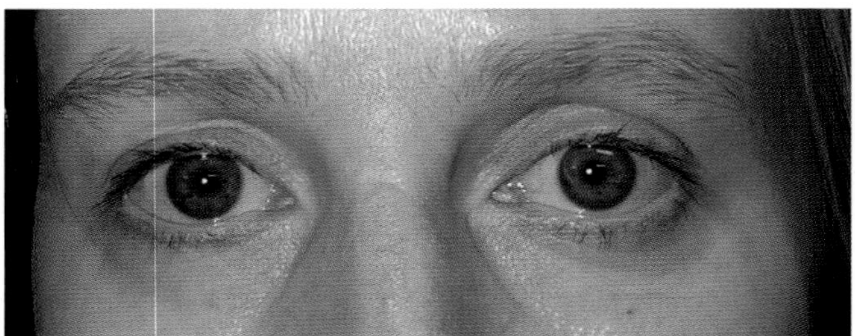

Figure 24.8 Subtle cosmetic effect created by a light aqua chemical bond tint in the right eye of a patient with identical irides in the right and left eyes (there is no lens in the left eye).

in a stable, permanent tint (Lutzi *et al.*, 1985). The dye can only be extracted by the use of powerful solvents. This technique can be used for tinting prosthetic silicone hydrogel lenses.

Chemical bond tinting

In this process, a strong covalent chemical bond is formed between the dye chromophore and the polymer. The technique involves soaking the lens in a dye solution, in the presence of a catalyst, for a fixed time at a specified temperature. The lens then needs to be put through a series of extraction processes to remove any residual unreacted agents. The result, as with vat dye tinting, is a stable, uniform tint (Figure 24.8).

Printing

Dye can be placed on the lens surface in a controlled manner using a printing process similar to that used for ink printing on paper. In this way, realistic iris patterns containing many colour elements can be applied, and the pupil region can be kept clear.

Opaque tints

Opaque tints can be applied using dot matrix printing, laminate constructions and opaque backing.

Dot matrix printing

This technique involves applying a matrix pattern of small opaque dots to the front surface of the lens (Figure 24.9). The dots are created by bonding an opaquing agent, such as titanium dioxide, and a colouring agent, which may be a pigment or dye, to the lens surface. A binding polymer, such as diisocyanate, is used to form a strong chemical bond between the opaque tinted agent and the lens surface. The final cosmetic effect will be a combination of dot matrix pattern and reflections from the natural iris between the opaque matrix dots (Figure 24.10).

Laminate constructions

An opaque tinted iris pattern can be incorporated within the lens using a laminate construction. An iris pattern is painted, using opaque dyes and tints, on to the surface of an unhydrated HEMA button which has been lathed to the curvature of the intended finished lens. A second pouring of HEMA over the top of this pattern is effected. Once set, the laminate button is lathed to create the finished lens form, which is then hydrated in the usual way. The advantage of this process is that the painted features are encapsulated, and therefore protected, within the lens. The disadvantages are that the lens is thicker, thus reducing oxygen transmissibility, and the tensile properties of the lens are altered, which can affect fitting characteristics (Figure 24.11).

A variation of laminate construction is known as 'sandwich technology'. The top and bottom layers of clear HEMA are co-polymerized with a thin middle layer of coloured non-toxic pigments, allowing the composite button to be lathed and then hydrated into an ultrathin lens design. An alternative approach is to use non-coloured opaquing agents to create an iris pattern in the centre of the two HEMA buttons, and then tinting the top HEMA section to create the desired cosmetic coloration.

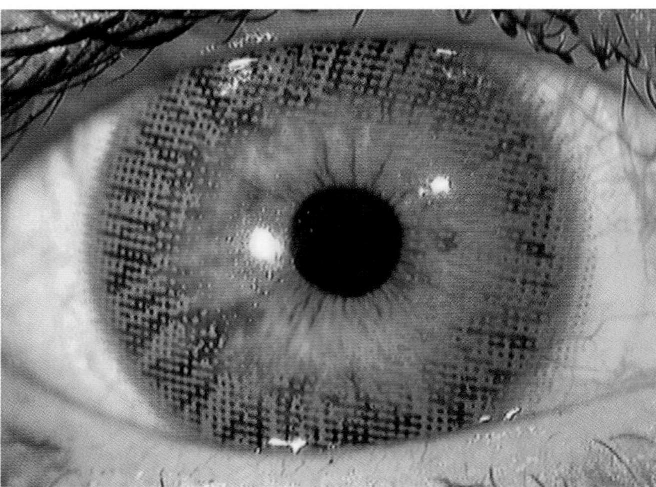

Figure 24.9 Lens with a matrix of opaque blue dots (the appearance of this lens at arms length can be seen in Figure 24.2).

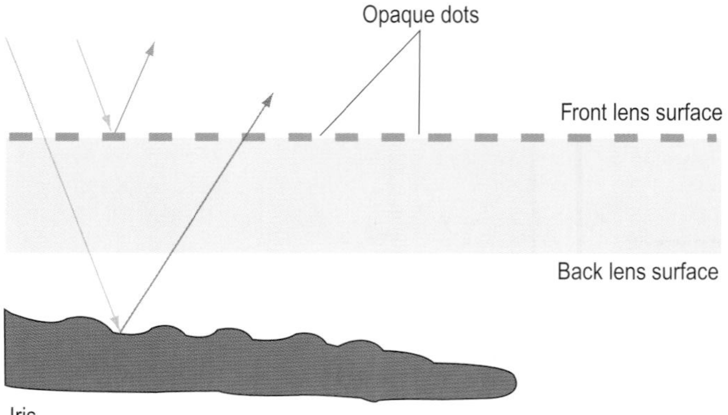

Figure 24.10 The cosmetic appearance of a dot matrix lens will result from a combination of the colour of the dots on the lens surface and the natural colour of the underlying iris.

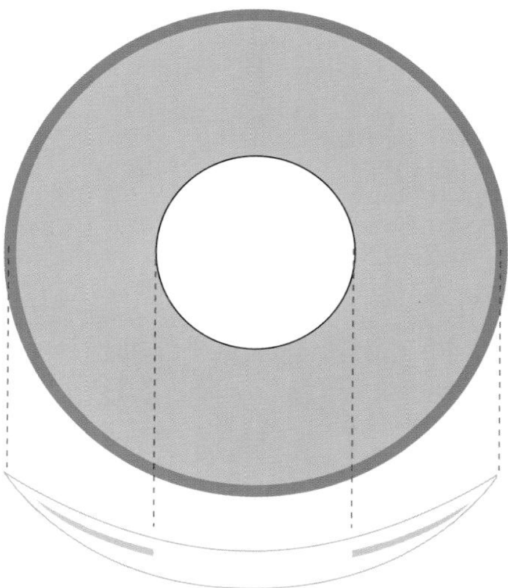

Figure 24.11 Laminate tinted lens construction, whereby the opaque iris tint is essentially encapsulated within the centre of the lens. The laminate is absent from the pupillary region and lens periphery.

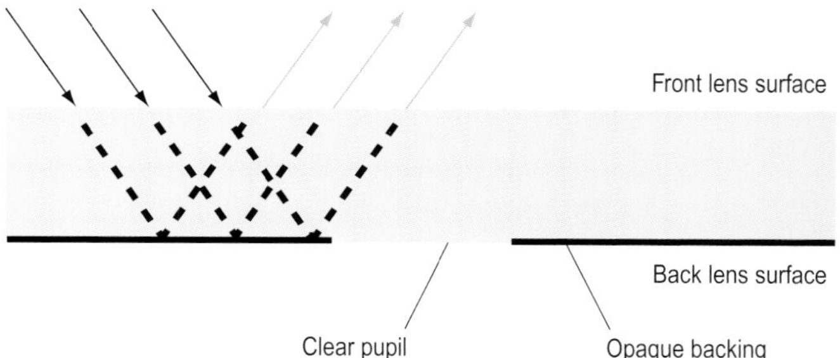

Figure 24.12 Light reflects off an opaque backing and returns through the tinted body of the lens, giving the iris a coloured appearance.

Figure 24.13 Four basic combinations of cosmetic tint.

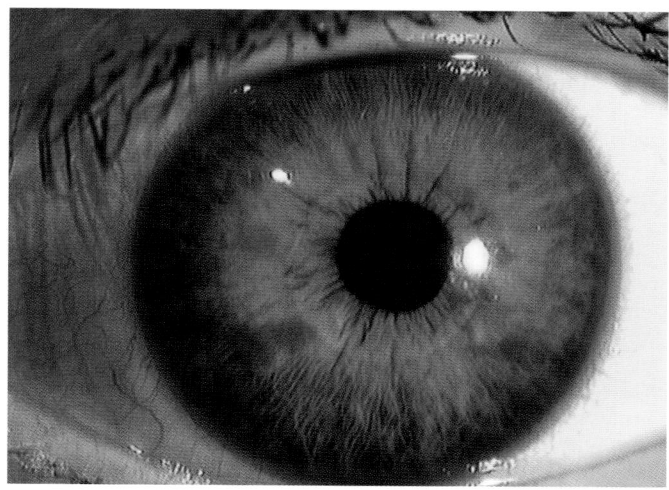

Figure 24.14 Blue tint with a clear pupil. Here in bright light, the natural pupil is much smaller than the tint-free pupillary zone of the lens, giving rise to an imperfect but acceptable cosmetic effect of a heterochromic iris with a large blue outer zone (from the tinted lens) and small hazel inner zone (from the natural iris).

Opaque backing

The matrix of a lens can be tinted with a translucent dye, and an iris pattern and black pupil are applied to the back surface of the lens using opaque paints. In this way, the entire back surface of the lens is rendered opaque; light reflects off the opaque layer and the coloured appearance is created from the translucent tint in the lens body (Figure 24.12).

Clinical considerations

The distribution of tint and method of manufacture of tinted lenses have certain clinical ramifications of which the practitioner needs to be aware. These considerations are outlined below.

Tint distribution

Selective distribution of a tint across the surface of lenses designed for cosmetic use allows four basic combinations (Figure 24.13). The variables are: (1) whether or not to leave a 1.5 mm band clear of tint around the lens edge; and (2) whether or not to have a clear pupil. A full tint covering the pupil appears more natural, but this creates a small but constant tinting effect on vision. A clear pupil eliminates the visual effect but introduces problems of obtaining good alignment and size-matching between the clear pupillary zone of the lens and the natural pupil of the eye, which of course will vary with ambient lighting (Figure 24.14). Tints that extend to the edge of the lens are cosmetically unsatisfactory because they are visible against the white sclera at the limbus.

Lens fitting

The procedures for fitting tinted lenses may differ from those employed for fitting non-tinted lenses. Tinted rigid lenses need to be of a large diameter so as to cover as much of the cornea as possible and to minimize lens movement. Tinted soft lenses are also best fitted marginally steeper than non-tinted lenses to reduce lens movement. A full appreciation of the cosmetic effect of tinted lenses is gained by viewing the lenses in the eyes (using a mirror in the case of the patient) in environments that the patient anticipates being in – that is, both inside under artificial light and outside in natural light.

Lens maintenance

Chlorine-based disinfecting solutions can cause some lens fading (Brazeau, 1989). All other lens care products appear to be innocuous in this regard, including hydrogen peroxide disinfecting solutions (Janoff, 1988) and alcohol-based daily cleaning surfactant solutions (Lowther, 1987). Intensive cleaners that employ acids, bases and oxidizing agents could cause tint fading, and so should not be used on tinted lenses.

Oxygen transmissibility

Although tinting using laminate construction reduces oxygen transmissibility by increasing lens thickness, the other tint processes described above do not appear to affect lens oxygen performance (Benjamin and Rasmussen, 1986).

Visual effects

Patients who wear opaque lenses with a clear pupil sometimes complain of haze or a veiling effect in their peripheral vision. This is due to a slight restriction of the visual field during the wear of such lenses. The phenomenon is more noticeable if the lens becomes decentred. Spraul *et al.* (1998) have demonstrated measurable visual impairment when wearing such lenses, and advise against wearing them when driving. Their finding is backed up by Albarrán Diego *et al.* (2001), who showed tinted lenses also affected static perimetry results, but not colour vision (Farnsworth-Munsell 100-hue colour test) or contrast sensitivity (Vistech 6000). Others have found colour-tinted contact lenses are associated with a reduction of contrast sensitivity function (Ozkagnici *et al.*, 2003) due to an increase in ocular higher-order aberrations (Hiraoka *et al.*, 2009).

Replacement frequency

Tinted lenses are now available in daily disposable, weekly, fortnightly, monthly and for unplanned replacement modalities. The choice of replacement frequency is governed by many factors (see Chapters 19–22). Whilst a hand-painted prosthetic lens cannot be supplied on a frequent replacement basis, where lenses are fitted for a medical reason they are likely to be worn regularly so should be replaced as frequently as possible. The majority of cosmetic tinted soft lenses are only worn occasionally. Daily disposable tinted lenses are the most convenient way of avoiding problems of compliance with intermittent use of reusable lenses.

Care of multiple pairs

Some fashion-conscious patients may possess numerous pairs of lenses of different tint designs. Such patients should be advised to mark their lens cases to avoid repeated opening, thus reducing the risk of contaminating stored lenses. Advice should be given to the patient concerning long-term lens storage, such as the desirability of periodic lens cleaning even if the lenses have not been worn.

Lens deposits

Although disposable tinted lenses are available, some products, such as theatric lenses, are more expensive and retained for long periods of time. Long-term lens maintenance therefore becomes an important issue. Some tinting processes can alter the lens surface charge. This could facilitate increased protein deposition (Lowther, 1987), the consequences of which may be decreased vision and comfort, sensations of dryness, susceptibility to adverse eye reactions, lens distortion and alterations to lens fitting characteristics.

Discomfort and dryness

Tinting processes can alter lens surface chemistry, which in turn can reduce surface wettability and lead to symptoms of dryness (Daniels and Mariscotti, 1989). Slight irregularities caused by surface tints may render tinted lenses slightly less comfortable than equivalent non-tinted lenses (Steffen and Barr, 1993). Ocular lubricants can help alleviate these sensations.

Conclusions

The utility of contact lenses has been extended considerably as the result of the development of innovative tinting procedures, so that almost any desired effect can be achieved. Tinted lenses therefore constitute an important vehicle for satisfying the cosmetic, prosthetic, therapeutic and prophylactic needs of patients. However, they remain a niche area of lens fitting as cosmetic soft lenses were prescribed in 4–8% of soft lens fits between 1997 and 2001, but have declined in use and in 2008 accounted for only 2% of soft lens fits (Morgan and Efron, 2009).

References

Albarrán Diego, C., Montés-Micó, R., Pons, A. M. *et al.* (2001) Influence of the luminance level on visual performance with a disposable soft cosmetic tinted contact lens. *Ophthalmic Physiol Opt.*, **21**, 411–419.

Astin, C. L. K. (1998) The use of occluding tinted contact lenses. *Contact Lens Assoc. Ophthalmol. J.*, **24**, 125–127.

Benjamin, W. and Rasmussen, M. (1986) EOPs of tinted lenses. *Contact Lens Spectrum*, **1**, 12–16.

Brazeau, D. (1989) Preliminary study of Opt-tab system on Softcolor lenses from CIBA. *Can. J. Optom.*, **51**, 26–27.

Cerviño, A., Gonzalez-Meijome, J. M., Linhares, J. M. *et al.* (2008) Effect of sport-tinted contact lenses for contrast enhancement on retinal straylight measurements. *Ophthalmic Physiol. Opt.*, **28,** 151–156.

Cole, C. J. and Vogt, U. (2006) Medical uses of cosmetic colored contact lenses. *Eye Contact Lens,* **32,** 203–206.

Collins, R. S., McChesney, M. E., McCluer, C. A. *et al.* (2008) Occlusion properties of prosthetic contact lenses for the treatment of amblyopia. *J. Am. Assoc. Pediatric. Ophthalmol. Strab.*, **12,** 565–568.

Connell, B. J., Tullo, A., Morgan, P. B. *et al.* (2004) *Pseudomonas aeruginosa* microbial keratitis secondary to cosmetic coloured contact lens wear. *Br. J. Ophthalmol.*, **88,** 1603–1604.

Daniels, K. and Mariscotti, C. (1989) Clinical evaluation of dot matrix hydrogel tinted lenses. *Contact Lens Spectrum,* **4,** 69–71.

Efron, N. and Pearson, R. M. (1988) Centenary celebration of Fick's *Eine Contactbrille. Arch. Ophthalmol.*, **106,** 1370–1377.

Erickson, G. B., Horn, F. C., Barney, T. *et al.* (2009) Visual performance with sport-tinted contact lenses in natural sunlight. *Optom. Vis. Sci.*, **86,** 509–516.

Eustis, H. S. and Chamberlain, D. (1996) Treatment for amblyopia: results using occlusive contact lens. *J. Pediatr. Ophthalmol. Strabismus.*, **33,** 319–322.

Harris, M. G., Haririfar, M. and Hirano, K. Y. (1999) Transmittance of tinted and UV-blocking disposable contact lenses. *Optom. Vis. Sci.*, **76,** 177–180.

Hiraoka, T., Ishii, Y., Okamoto, F. *et al.* (2009) Influence of cosmetically tinted soft contact lenses on higher-order wavefront aberrations and visual performance. *Graefes Arch. Clin. Exp. Ophthalmol.*, **247,** 225–233.

Janoff, L. (1988) The effect of thirty cycles of hydrogen peroxide disinfection on CIBA Softcolor lenses. *Int. Contact Lens Clin.*, **15,** 155–164.

Johns, K. and O'Day, D. (1988) *Pseudomonas* corneal ulcer associated with colored cosmetic contact lenses in an emmetropic individual. *Am. J. Ophthalmol.*, **105,** 210.

Jonsson, A. C., Burstedt, M. S., Golovleva, I. *et al.* (2007) Tinted contact lenses in Bothnia dystrophy. *Acta Ophthalmol. Scand.*, **85,** 534–539.

Key, J. and Mobley, C. (1987) Cosmetic hydrogel lenses for therapeutic uses. *Contact Lens Forum,* **4,** 18–22.

Lee, J. S., Hahn, T. W., Choi, S. H., *et al.* (2007) *Acanthamoeba* keratitis related to cosmetic contact lenses. *Clin. Experiment. Ophthalmol.*, **35,** 775–777.

Lowther, G. (1987) A review of transparent hydrogel tinted lenses. *Contax,* March, 6–9.

Lutzi, F., Chou, B. and Egan, D. (1985) Tinted hydrogel lenses permanency of tint. *Am. J. Optom. Physiol. Opt.*, **62,** 329–333.

Meshel, L. G. and Smith-Kimura, P. (1996) The full spectrum of contact lens tinting. *Ophthalmol. Clin. N. Am.*, **9,** 117–127.

Moore, L. and Ferreira, J. T. (2006) Ultraviolet (UV) transmittance characteristics of daily disposable and silicone hydrogel contact lenses. *Cont. Lens Anterior Eye,* **29,** 115–122.

Morgan, P. B. and Efron, N. (2009) Patterns of fitting cosmetically tinted contact lenses. *Cont. Lens Anterior Eye,* **32,** 207–208.

Ozkagnici, A., Zengin, N., Kamiş, O. *et al.* (2003) Do daily wear opaquely tinted hydrogel soft contact lenses affect contrast sensitivity function at one meter? *Eye Contact Lens,* **29,** 48–49.

Park, W. L. and Sunness, J. S. (2004) Red contact lenses for alleviation of photophobia in patients with cone disorders. *Am. J. Ophthalmol.*, **137,** 774–775.

Porisch, E. (2007) Football players' contrast sensitivity comparison when wearing amber sport-tinted or clear contact lenses. *Optometry,* **78,** 232–235.

Rajak, S. N., Currie, A. D., Dubois, V. J. *et al.* (2006) Tinted contact lenses as an alternative management for photophobia in stationary cone dystrophies in children. *J. Am. Assoc. Pediatric. Ophthalmol. Strab.*, **10,** 336–339.

Schornack, M. M., Brown, W. L. and Siemsen, D. W. (2007) The use of tinted contact lenses in the management of achromatopsia. *Optometry,* **78,** 17–22.

Spraul, C. W., Roth, H. J. G., Gäckle, A. *et al.* (1998) Influence of special effect contact lenses (*Crazy Lenses*®) on visual function. *Contact Lens Assoc. Ophthalmol. J.*, **24,** 29–32.

Steffen, R. B. and Barr, J. T. (1993) Clear versus opaque soft contact lenses: initial comfort comparison. *Int. Contact Lens Clin.*, **20,** 184–186.

Steinemann, T. L., Pinninti, U., Szczotka, L. B. *et al.* (2003) Ocular complications associated with the use of cosmetic contact lenses from unlicensed vendors. *Eye Contact Lens,* **29,** 196–200.

Swarbrick, H. A., Nguyen, P., Nguyen, T. *et al.* (2001) The ChromaGen contact lens system: colour vision test results and subjective responses. *Ophthalmic Physiol. Opt.*, **21,** 182–196.

Tan, A., Ting, L. and Wildsoet, C. (1987) Colour vision and tinted contact lenses. *Clin. Exp. Optom.*, **70,** 78–81.

Tønnesen, H., Mathiesen, S. S. and Karlsen, J. (1997) Ultraviolet transmittance of monthly replacement lenses on the Scandinavian market. *Int. Contact Lens Clin.*, **24,** 123–127.

Voetz, S. C., Collins, M. J. and Lingelbach, B. (2004) Recovery of corneal topography and vision following opaque-tinted contact lens wear. *Eye Contact Lens,* **30,** 111–117.

Zeltzer, H. I. (1979) Use of modified X-Chrom for relief of light dazzlement and color blindness of a rod monochromat. *J. Am. Optom. Assoc.*, **50,** 813–818.

Presbyopia

John Meyler

Introduction

One of the more challenging areas within contact lens practice is fitting presbyopic patients with contact lenses so as to allow them to fulfil the majority of their visual requirements. The availability of newer designs, single-use disposable trial lenses and lens designs in silicone hydrogel and high-permeability rigid lens materials means there is little restriction to the modality of wear or physiological compromise when attempting to correct presbyopia with contact lenses. This should result in a higher rate of prescribing by practitioners of contact lenses for presbyopic patients.

With the presbyopic population growing in size at an ever-increasing rate along with the prepresbyopic contact lens-wearing population, practitioners can expect to see a rise in the number of presbyopic patients attending for this form of lens fitting, which should now be considered as an integral, routine part of contact lens practice.

The options for the correction of presbyopia to both existing and new contact lens wearers include:

- Distance-powered contact lenses and near reading spectacles.
- Monovision.
- Bifocal contact lenses:
  - Simultaneous vision contact lenses.
  - Alternating vision contact lenses.

The contact lens options for presbyopic correction are shown in Figure 25.1 with some examples of different brands available.

Each option has advantages and disadvantages, which vary with the lens type, fitting approach used and the degree of presbyopia present. A systematic approach to lens selection can be used depending on the stage of presbyopia, as shown in Table 25.1 (Christie and Beertren, 2007).

Distance-powered contact lenses combined with near reading spectacles may be the simplest and least expensive option. However, it does not address the problem for the patient who does not wish to wear spectacles, and it may even demotivate an existing lens wearer. Nevertheless, the quality and stability of vision in this mode of correction are such that it may prove to give the best optical correction when compared to bifocal or monovision contact lenses.

Patient selection

Patient motivation plays an important role in any form of contact lens fitting. However, this motivation is often restricted to those patients who are aware of the various contact lens options, which they are then keen to explore further. Perhaps more important is informed choice based on the advantages and disadvantages of the various options available, as the majority of patients are not aware that contact lenses are a possibility for the correction of presbyopia. This more 'proactive' approach may result in lower success rates but inevitably, to a larger contact lens patient base. Back *et al.* (1989) have shown that a significant proportion of an unselected presbyopic population can achieve success with simultaneous-vision bifocal contact lenses.

Caution should prevail when considering patients with compromised binocular vision, amblyopia, distance acuity of less than 6/12 or exacting critical vision needs for either distance or near vision. High- and low-contrast visual acuity charts (Figure 25.2) give more information about acuity. In particular, the difference in low-contrast acuity between spectacles and contact lenses may give some indication of possible success.

It is more important, however, to have access to trial lenses to obtain an idea of potential success for any particular type of bifocal lens or fitting technique based on both patient subjective feedback and objective measurement. As with any contact lens pre-assessment, careful attention should be paid to tear quality and quantity, which are often reduced in this age group, as well as eyelid tone and position. When getting started with this form of lens fitting, it may help to start with selecting patients that are generally accepted as being 'better' candidates versus choosing those who might be considered as 'more challenging' to fit successfully. Table 25.2 summarizes the different patient types when considering monovision fitting, simultaneous vision and alternating vision fitting (Bennett, 2007).

DOI: 10.1016/B978-0-7506-8869-7.00025-2

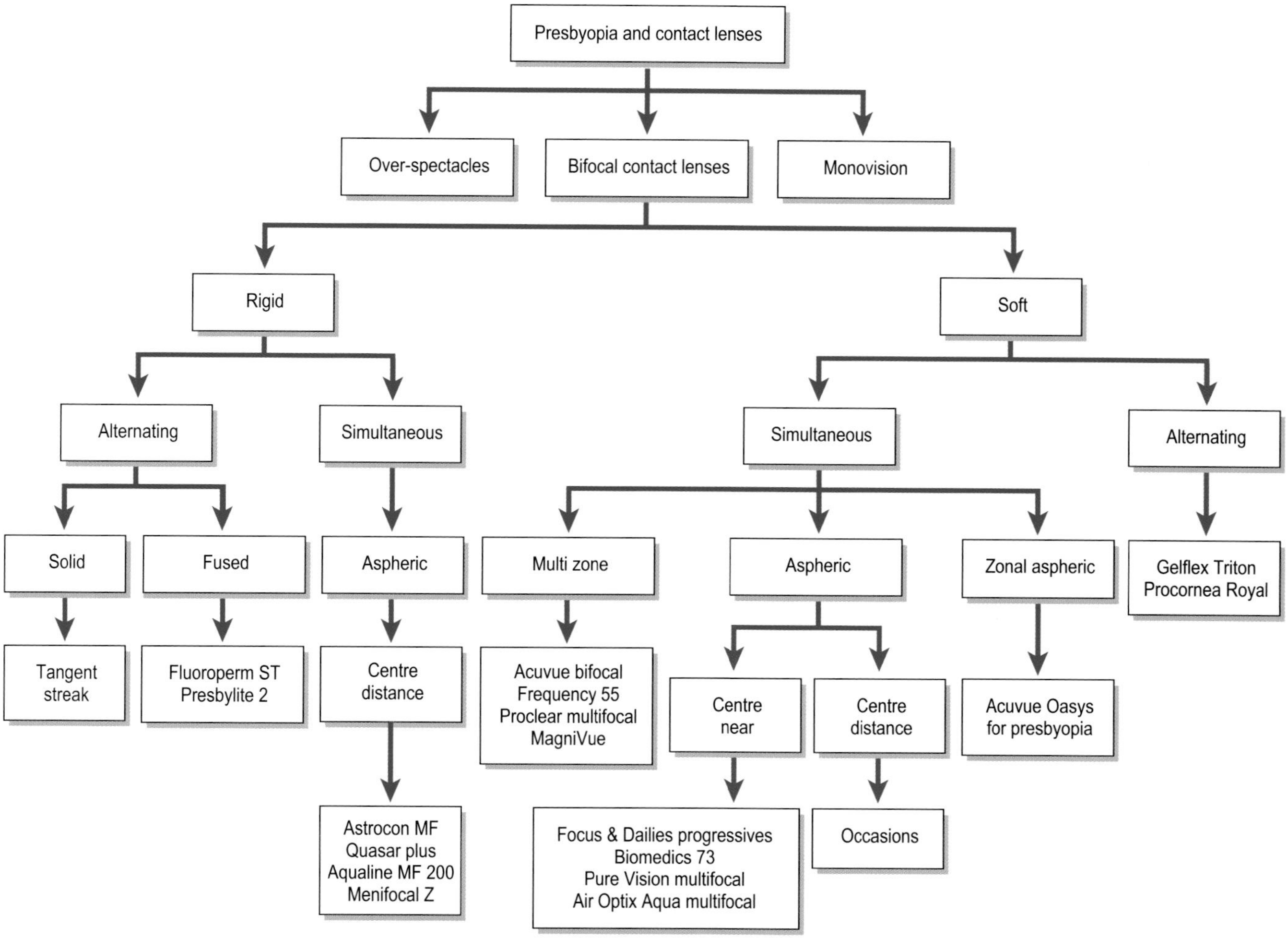

- Presbyopia and contact lenses
  - Over-spectacles
  - Bifocal contact lenses
    - Rigid
      - Alternating
        - Solid
          - Tangent streak
        - Fused
          - Fluoroperm ST Presbylite 2
      - Simultaneous
        - Aspheric
          - Centre distance
            - Astrocon MF, Quasar plus, Aqualine MF 200, Menifocal Z
    - Soft
      - Simultaneous
        - Multi zone
          - Acuvue bifocal, Frequency 55, Proclear multifocal, MagniVue
        - Aspheric
          - Centre near
            - Focus & Dailies progressives, Biomedics 73, Pure Vision multifocal, Air Optix Aqua multifocal
          - Centre distance
            - Occasions
        - Zonal aspheric
          - Acuvue Oasys for presbyopia
      - Alternating
        - Gelflex Triton, Procornea Royal
  - Monovision

Figure 25.1 Contact lens options for presbyopia correction with some examples of various brands.

Table 25.1 Fitting approach depending on degree of presbyopia

Emerging presbyope (up to +1.00 DS)
Simultaneous: full correction in both eyes
Monovision: distance and full near
Mid-presbyope (+1.25 DS to +2.00 DS)
Simultaneous: full correction to both eyes
Translating: full correction to both eyes (do not overcorrect add)
Monovision: distance and full near
Late presbyope (+2.25 DS to +3.00 DS)
Translating: full correction to both eyes
Simultaneous: modified monovision; enhanced monovision
Monovision: distance and partial near; consider top-up spectacles to provide additional plus
(Adapted from Christie and Beertren, 2007)

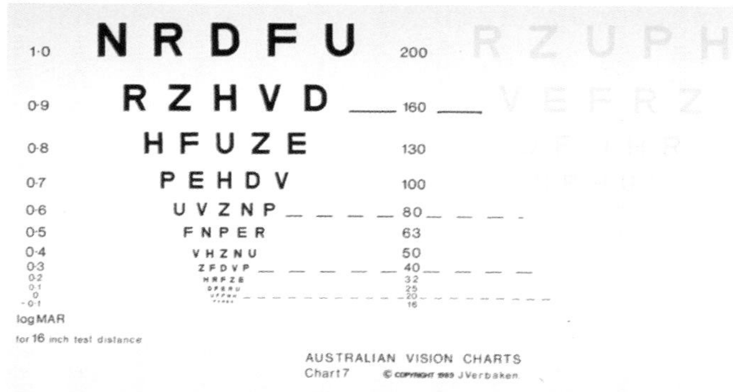

Figure 25.2 High- and low-contrast visual acuity chart. (Modified from Bennett, E. S. (2007) Bifocal and multifocal contact lenses. In Contact Lenses, 5th edn (A. J. Phillips and L. Speedwell, eds) pp. 311–331, Oxford: Butterworth-Heinemann.)

Patient expectations

It is important that patients are given realistic expectations about the likely level of vision, as with any type of vision correction for presbyopia. It is necessary to ensure that patients fully understand the basis of presbyopia and their

Table 25.2 Patient selection for presbyopic contact lens correction

	Patient selection		
	Monovision	**Simultaneous**	**Alternating**
Good candidates (getting started)	Significant refractive error Reading positions other than standard downward gaze Current contact lens wearers Motivated and realistic expectations	Existing soft lens wearers who are emerging presbyopes Moderate intermediate-vision requirements Spherical or near-spherical refractive errors Willing to accept some compromise in distance vision	Early and advanced presbyopes Lower lid above, tangent to, or no more than 1 mm below the limbus Myopic or low hyperopic powers Normal to large palpebral apertures Normal to tight lid tension
More challenging candidates (experience required)	Emmetropes, previously uncorrected hyperopes, low myopes Concentrated specific visual needs Dry-eye symptoms or clinical signs High visual demands and expectations	Do not desire any compromise in distance vision Moderate hyperopic refractive correction Emmetropic or near-emmetropic distance refractive error Would benefit from a toric correction Small pupil size (<3 mm)	High hyperopes Small palpebral apertures Loose lower lids

(Modified from Bennett, E. S., 2007 Bifocal and multifocal contact lenses. In Contact Lenses, 5th edn (A. J. Phillips and L. Speedwell, eds) pp. 311–331, Oxford: Butterworth-Heinemann)

expectations should be set out in a positive but informative manner. This involves discussing the benefits of combined distance/near correction without the need for spectacles (less head movement, no peripheral distortion) as well as likely differences between the visual performance of monovision, simultaneous-vision or alternating-vision lenses. When compared to spectacles or single-vision contact lenses, visual decrements may be noticed, such as reductions in visual acuity (especially in low luminance) and stereopsis, and reduced intermediate vision depending on the type of lens fitted. It should also be explained to the patient that it is quite normal for fitting to require more than one appointment in order to try out alternative lens powers and fitting approaches.

Initial measurements

Measurement of the ocular dominance or sighting preference is useful in establishing which eye to correct for distance vision during monovision fitting or while making adjustments during simultaneous lens fitting. Ocular dominance can be determined using preferential looking tests or alternatively by the +2.00 D test. The former is carried out by sitting opposite the patient and asking the patient to look through a hole in a piece of card at an open eye of the practitioner. Whichever eye the patient lines up with the open eye of the practitioner is the dominant one. The latter test involves placing the best binocular distance refraction in the trial frame and, while patients look at the lowest line they can read, a +2.00 D lens is placed alternatively in front of each eye. Patients indicate when the vision is clearest. If the +2.00 D lens is in front of the left eye when the image is reported as clearest then the right eye is considered as distance-dominant, and vice versa. It has been found that unsuccessful wearers became successful after switching near and distance corrections contrary to the dominance as measured by traditional methods, but rarely contrary to the +2.00 D test (Michaud *et al.*, 1995). Historically, pupil size measurements were useful when fitting biconcentric designs; however, this procedure is less relevant with more recent designs. Nevertheless, larger pupils can be more challenging when fitting alternating-vision lenses and smaller pupils may be less successful when fitting simultaneous-vision lenses.

Monovision

Monovision is the correction of one eye with the required distance refractive power and the other eye with the required near refractive power. This approach is based upon the principle that the visual system can alternate central suppression between the two eyes when viewing is alternating between distance and near targets. The degree of interocular blur suppression, which varies between patients, may be linked to the final success of monovision. Essentially all forms of soft and rigid contact lenses can be used for monovision corrections, whether spherical or toric. The more recent availability of silicone hydrogel materials, some of which can reduce lens-related dryness symptoms in this age group, is also helpful when fitting monovision.

With monovision correction, there is only a slight reduction in performance in distance acuity tests when compared with spectacle correction, and no significant difference in acuity results at near (Back *et al.*, 1992). Distance and near stereopsis is compromised with monovision but the degree of reduction is patient-specific and may or may not result in failure with this method of fitting. Contrast loss and difficulty in suppressing bright images against dark backgrounds (e.g. car headlights) while wearing monovision may also contribute to poor tolerance (Schor *et al.*, 1987). Glare when driving at night is the most common complaint and this should be discussed with the potential monovision wearer during the initial fitting assessment. Despite such compromises, monovision has high patient acceptance with success rates varying from 67% to 86% (Koetting and Castellano, 1984; Back *et al.*, 1989; Collins *et al.*, 1994). Monovision causes minimal compromise in near visual acuity performance in all illumination conditions; thus, this type of fitting option should be considered for presbyopic patients with strong near-vision demands. However, when critical or sustained tasks requiring good distance binocularity predominate, it is advisable to avoid monovision or to consider supplementary correction.

General principles of monovision fitting

No single predictive test exists to identify successful monovision patients, so systematic trial and error is the best approach. However, the initial impression of the patient can be an important indicator of likely success. The more usual fitting approach is to fit the dominant eye with the distance vision-correcting lens and the non-dominant eye with the near vision-correcting lens (Jain *et al.*, 1996; Maldonado-Codina *et al.*, 1997). It is important to correct any astigmatism equal to or greater than 0.75 D in either or both eyes; uncorrected astigmatism can result in reduced visual performance, asthenopic symptoms and poor tolerance. Binocular visual acuity similar to that achieved with the spectacle correction – with no significant reduction in stereopsis or contrast sensitivity – is usually a good sign of likely success.

Some patients require spectacles for deficiencies with monovision to wear 'over' their monovision contact lens correction. For example, there may be a requirement for extra minus correction over the near correcting lens/eye and plano over their distance correcting lens to give full binocular vision and optimal distance acuity for night driving, especially when higher reading additions are required. The degree of interocular blur suppression, which varies between individuals, may be linked to the final success of monovison.

Partial monovision

In general, the acceptance and therefore success of monovision falls as the reading add increases (Schor *et al.*, 1987; Erikson, 1988). With reading adds over +2.50 D at low levels of illumination or with near-threshold stimuli, visual performance of monovision wearers is reduced (Johannsdottir and Stelmach, 2001). As the indicated add exceeds +2.00 D, tolerance can often be improved if a reduced reading addition is given. The patient may need supplementary glasses for small print, a different pair of supplementary glasses for driving or a secondary distance-correcting contact lens. This form of monovision is ideal for social users whose near-vision demands will be lower than that of full-time wearers. Partial monovision may also be a useful strategy for patients who have greater intermediate-vision needs.

Enhanced monovision

Enhanced monovision – which is considered by some to be a modified monovision fitting approach – involves fitting one eye with a bifocal lens and the other with a single-vision lens. A variety of options exist. The most frequent approach involves fitting the dominant eye with a single-vision distance lens (spherical or toric) and the non-dominant eye with a bifocal lens. This improves binocular summation and offers some level of stereoacuity to the monovision wearer who is experiencing increasing blur with a higher reading add. Alternatively, the same approach can be used when fitting patients who require sharper distance vision than bilateral simultaneous vision can offer. The bifocal lens in the non-dominant eye usually needs more bias for near vision. This modification can be achieved effectively by increasing the distance power of the bifocal lens by + 0.50 D to + 0.75 D.

Other enhanced monovision options include:

- A single-vision near lens in the dominant eye to improve near vision and a distance-bias bifocal lens in the non-dominant eye.
- A single-vision lens with slightly excess plus power in the dominant eye and an intermediate-bias bifocal lens in the non-dominant eye.

A summary of the different problem-solving approaches for monovision fitting is shown in Figure 25.3.

Monovision remains an effective approach for presbyopic patients and offers less objective visual compromise in high- and low-contrast visual environments than simultaneous-vision lenses. However, a study by Dutoit *et al.* (2000) has shown that adapted monovision wearers rated many aspects of subjective vision performance – such as distance vision in good and poor lighting, driving at night and depth perception – to be superior with simultaneous-vision bifocal contact lenses. Near vision in poor lighting was rated higher during monovision wear. Subjects with no previous experience of presbyopic contact lens correction preferred monovision when compared to bifocal correction (58% versus 42% if excluding spectacle lens preference).

Modified monovision

Modified monovision involves adjusting the refractive power of the lens or selecting alternative lens designs for each eye to improve distance vision deliberately in one eye, at the expense of near performance in that eye, while improving near vision in the other. This can be achieved by increasing minus power/decreasing plus power on the dominant eye to enhance distance vision while decreasing minus power/increasing plus power in the non-dominant eye. A similar bias can be obtained by using different add powers in each – the lower-add power being fitted to the dominant eye to improve distance vision. Similarly, one eye may be fitted with a centre distance simultaneous design and the other with a centre near design lens. More recently lens designs are available that use this modified-monovision approach automatically when fitting presbyopic patients (see below).

Bifocal and multifocal contact lenses

Bifocal and multifocal contact lenses can be simultaneous- or alternating-vision designs. Simultaneous designs generally require the lens to be relatively stable on the eye and will be associated with some form of visual compromise because objects at both distance and near are imaged simultaneously on the retina. Alternating-vision bifocal lenses require significant lens movement so that the distance and near portions of the lens can be positioned over the pupil by interaction with the lids.

Recent comparative studies have concluded that multifocal contact lenses perform better, in many different forms of visual measurements, than monovision correction (Rajagopalan *et al.*, 2006; Richdale *et al.*, 2006; Bennett, 2008;

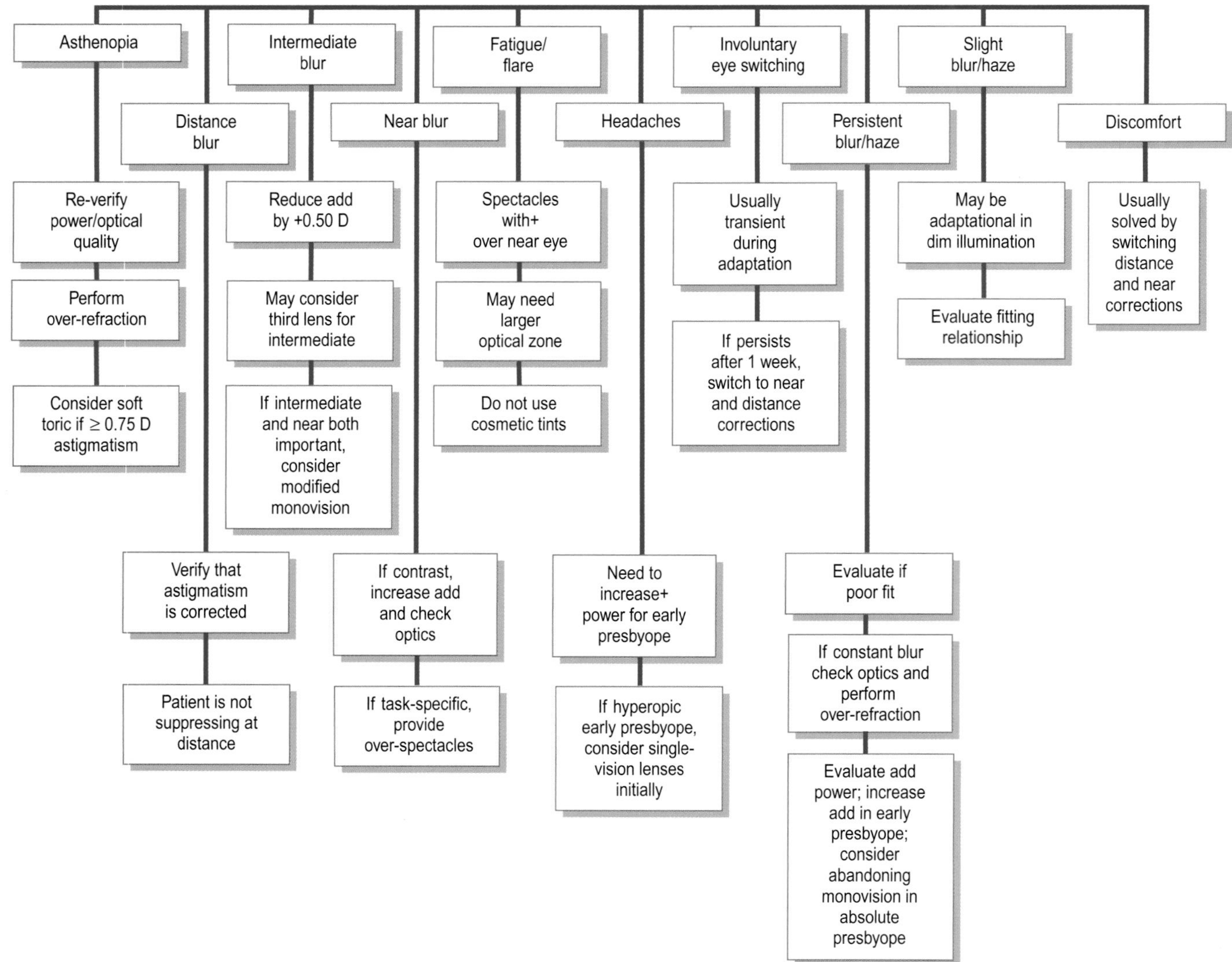

Figure 25.3 Problem-solving approaches for monovision fitting. (Adapted from Bennett, E. S., Jurkus, J. M. and Schwartz, C. A. (2000) Bifocal contact lenses. In Clinical Manual of Contact Lenses, 2nd edn (E. S. Bennett and V. A. Henry, eds), pp. 410–449, J. B. Lippincott Co.)

Gupta *et al.*, 2009). However, Chu *et al.* (2009) reported that multifocal contact lens wearers were significantly less satisfied with aspects of their vision during nighttime than daytime driving, particularly regarding disturbances from glare and haloes.

Simultaneous-vision designs

A variety of simultaneous lens designs are available in both rigid and soft materials. The availability of single-use disposable soft trial lenses and empirically ordered individually based aspheric rigid lenses has resulted in an increased prescribing of this form of lens correction; however, in 2008, only 19% of contact lens wearers over 45 years of age received soft or rigid multifocal corrections (Morgan and Efron, 2009).

In simultaneous-vision designs, the distance and near correction zones are both positioned in front of the pupil in every direction of gaze so that light from either a distant or near object passes through both zones. As fixation is directed to either a distant or a near object, one zone produces a focused image while the other produces a blurred image that overlaps the same retinal elements as the focused one (Benjamin and Borish, 1994) (Figure 25.4).

The placing of simultaneous images on the retina by any optical system relies on the visual system being able to select the clearer picture and to ignore the out-of-focus image, whether a distant or near object is being viewed.

The spread of light from the defocused image reduces the contrast of the focused image (Borish, 1988). As a result, the fitting of a simultaneous-vision lens is likely to result in a reduction in image quality in comparison with that resulting from a single-vision correction. The extent of contrast loss will depend upon the relative amounts of in-focus to out-of-focus light striking the retina. If equal contrast is to be achieved for both near and far viewing, the refractive system should allow approximate equality of the areas of the two portions of the lens transmitting to the pupil. Lens performance may be affected by many factors, which include pupil size, lens design and centration of optics relative to the pupil. The theoretical retinal intensity of different lens designs and the effect of variations in pupil size can be investigated by measuring their modular transfer function (Young *et al.*, 1990).

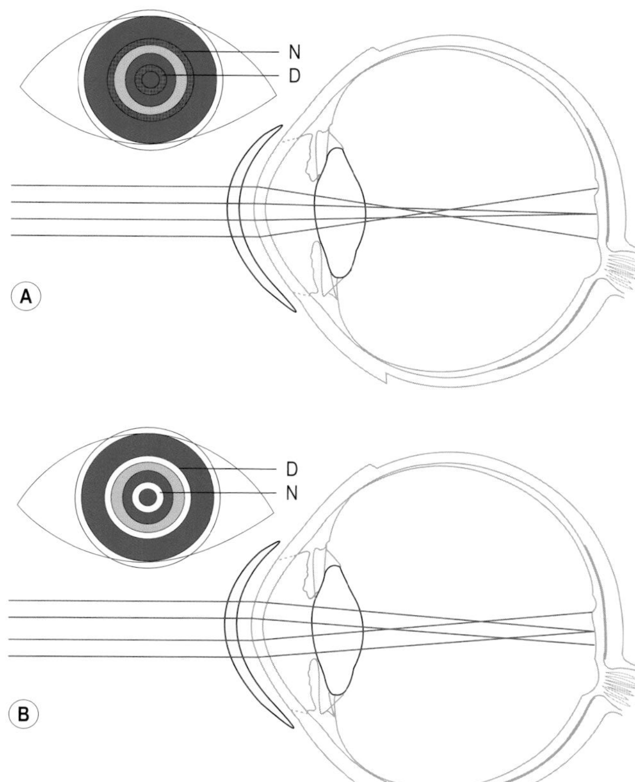

Figure 25.4 Principle of simultaneous vision design. (A) Centre-distance design. (B) Centre-near design. D = distance; N = near.

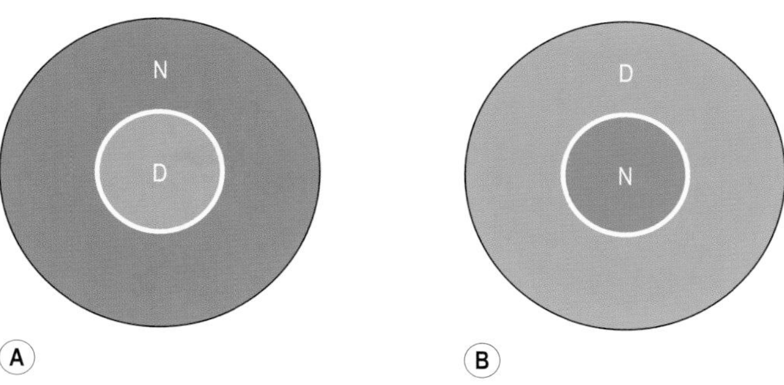

Figure 25.5 (A) Biconcentric centre-distance design. (B) Biconcentric centre-near design. D = distance; N = near.

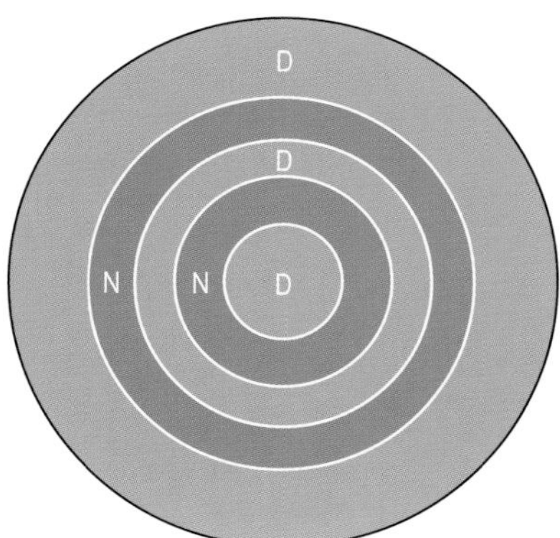

Figure 25.6 Multizone concentric centre-distance design. D = distance; N = near.

Regardless of the different optical principles and designs available, large well-controlled independent studies are required to determine whether patient acceptance is more successful with any one design. Comparing patient acceptance success rates from different studies is difficult due to differences in success criteria, patient profile and length of study. A study by Situ *et al.* (2003) showed that exisiting successful monovison wearers could be successfully fitted with bifocal contact lenses and that after a 6-month period 68% preferred bifocal lenses compared to a 25% preference for monovision.

Biconcentric designs

Early soft and rigid simultaneous-vision bifocal lenses were biconcentric in design, consisting of two discrete zones of distance and near power. A centre-distance design has the central portion of the optical zone for distance vision, which is surrounded by an area containing the near power (Figure 25.5A).

The ratio split between light forming the distance image to that forming the near image can be controlled for a given pupil size by altering the diameter of the central segment. As the pupil is a dynamic structure, a fundamental concern with such a design is its dependency on the pupil size. The near pupil reaction means that, as a near object is brought into view, proportionally less of the pupil allows light in from the near zone of the centre-distance design. In addition, as the eye ages, the pupil naturally decreases in size, resulting in less light from the near portion of the lens and a reduction in near-vision quality. In low luminance levels, the pupil naturally dilates, resulting in more light proportionally from the near zone and a reduction in the quality of distance vision.

In centre-near designs, the optical principle is the same as for the centre-distance lens, although reversed so that the central portion of the lens focuses the light from close objects and this is surrounded by a distance-powered area (Figure 25.5B). The design remains pupil-dependent; therefore, in bright conditions giving pupil constriction, distance vision becomes progressively less clear. Biconcentric designs in both soft and rigid materials are still available but are now used less frequently due to the availability of more advanced, easier-to-fit designs and single-use disposable lenses.

Multizone concentric designs

A consequence of the above discussion is that benefits should be possible if the dependency of lens function on pupil size could be minimized, especially in relation to different lighting conditions. One approach is to increase the number of concentric zones, and to power these zones alternatively for distance and near vision. This concept has been employed in a centre-distance multizone design consisting of five alternating distance and near-powered zones (Figure 25.6).

The width and spacing of the zones are based on the variation of pupil size in different illuminations within the presbyopic population. Theoretically, this lens design favours distance vision in extreme high and low lighting conditions and provides a more equal ratio of light division

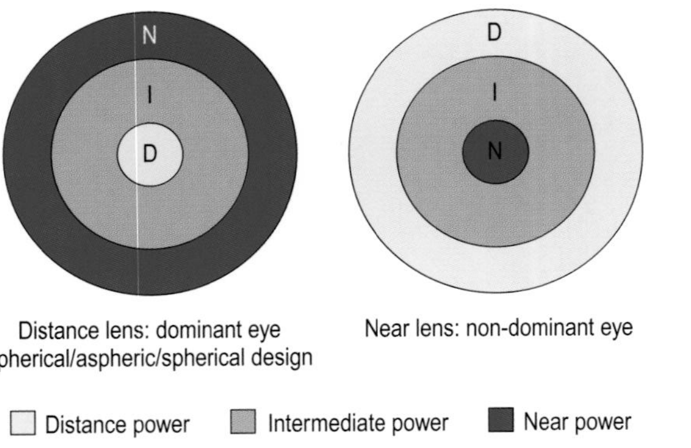

Figure 25.7 Multizone concentric modified monovision design.

in ambient illumination conditions (Meyler and Veys, 1999). The multiple-ring configuration is designed to provide vision that is more specific to the available lighting conditions. Transition curves between the concentric zones are such that the zones are not readily visible on the slit-lamp biomicroscope.

Modified monovision multizone concentric designs

These lens designs use a modified monovision approach in that the lens used for the dominant eye is a centre-distance lens design whilst the lens for the other eye is centre-near in design. Lens designs can use aspheric surfaces, spherical surfaces or a combination of both with unique zone sizes to produce two complementary but inverse-geometry lenses (Figure 25.7). Each lens is a multifocal and the intention is that binocular summation will still occur, providing acceptable vision at all distances under binocular conditions. This type of lens design results in a modified monovison approach with the first pair of lenses trialled.

Diffractive designs

Diffractive bifocal contact lenses use refraction to correct distance vision and a combination of refraction and diffraction to correct near vision. This is achieved by a diffractive 'zone plate' on the back surface of the lens, which is able to split the incident light passing through into two discrete focal points. This is achieved by etching individual facets ('echelettes') in a concentric ring pattern on to the posterior lens surface (Figure 25.8).

The diffractive rings are visible under high magnification on the slit-lamp biomicroscope; they are more easily seen with the aid of fluorescein (Figure 25.9A).

The diffractive ring pattern can also be appreciated by examining an image obtained using the Ho quality optical analyser, which is a modified Focault knife-edge test (Williams, 1998) (Figure 25.9B). The individual facets are only 2–3 μm deep and therefore will not traumatize the epithelium.

As with any simultaneous-vision lens, incident light is divided between the distance and near foci so that the intensities of these images are reduced and the images are superimposed on each other, resulting in a reduction in retinal image quality. In addition, approximately 20% of incident light is lost to higher orders of diffraction, leaving 40% of light to make up each image (Benjamin and Borish,

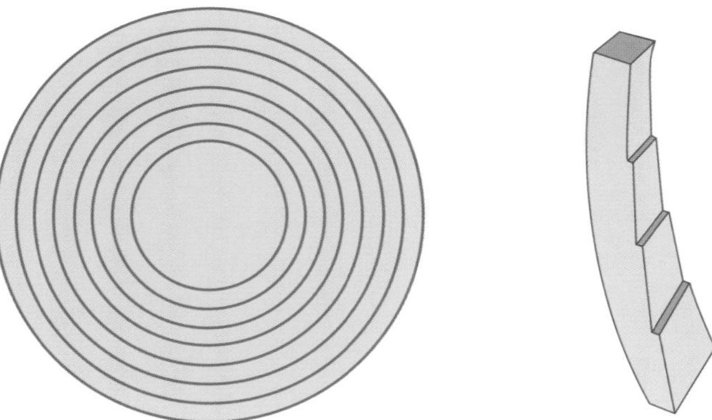

Figure 25.8 Diffractive design. Left: concentric design of facets. Right: each facet is 3 μm deep.

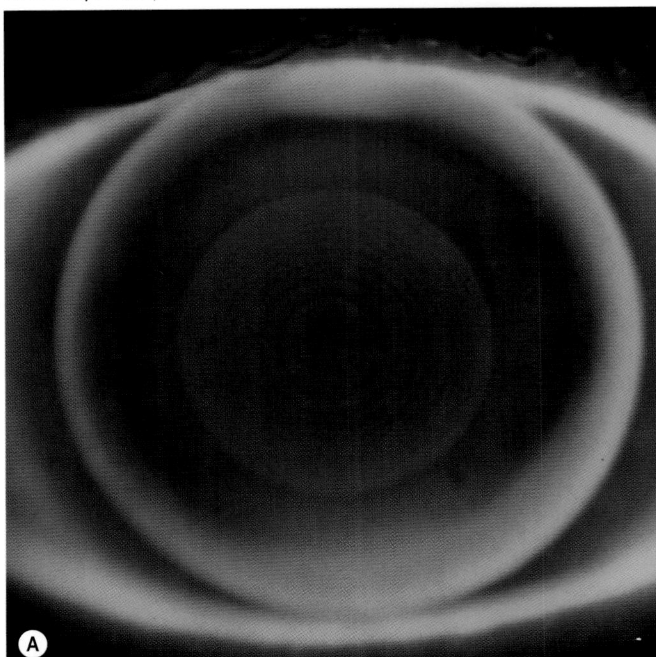

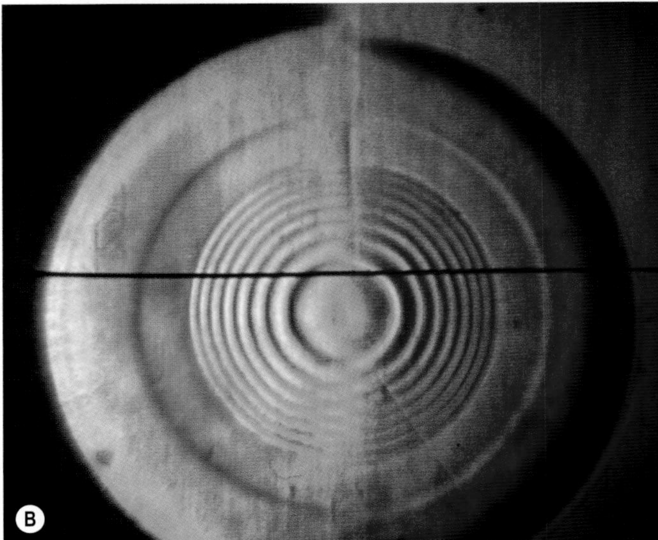

Figure 25.9 Diffractive design contact lens. (A) Diffractive rings visible on a slit-lamp biomicroscope with the aid of fluorescein. (B) Diffractive rings visible on a Ho quality optical analyser.

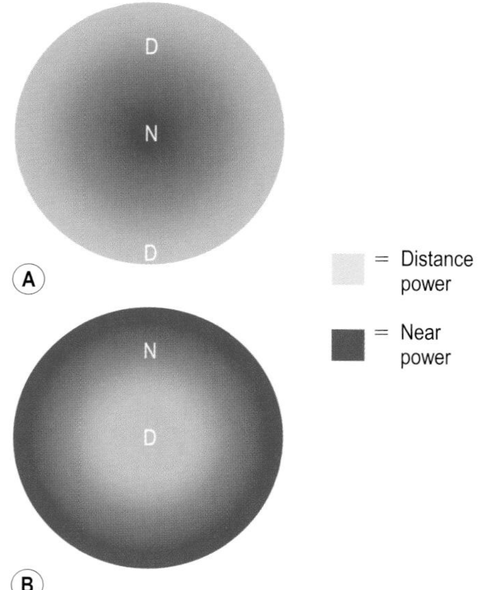

Figure 25.10 (A) Front surface aspheric centre-near design. (B) Back surface aspheric centre-distance design.

1994). This may explain the greater reduction in low-contrast acuities with such lenses when compared to monovision correction (Harris *et al.*, 1992). Diffractive lenses are largely independent of pupil size (Young *et al.*, 1990); however, like aspheric designs, they are dependent on lens centration. This design was available in both soft and rigid materials but neither product is now available.

Aspheric designs

With aspheric designs the refractive power gradually changes from the geometric centre of the lens to the more peripheral area of the optic zone. Such lenses are best described as 'multifocal' due to the progression of powers, but can also be considered as a type of concentric design as the power distributions are concentric around the centre of the lens. By the nature of their design, lens function will vary with changes in pupil size. This will lead to variations in distance and near-vision image contrast similar to that described previously for biconcentric designs.

Power distribution is produced by the use of a continuous aspheric surface of fixed or variable eccentricity. As with biconcentric designs, aspheric lens designs can be subdivided according to whether the power distribution is most plus (least minus) centrally, resulting in a centre-near design (Figure 25.10A), or most minus (least plus) centrally resulting in a centre-distance design (Figure 25.10B).

Both options are available in soft and rigid materials.

Back surface aspheric designs

Back surface aspheric designs result in power changes from the central distance correction to that required for near vision by inducing positive spherical aberration. The greater the eccentricity (or rate of flattening), the higher the reading power in relation to distance power. However, the higher the reading addition, the more likely that distance vision will be affected adversely, especially in low-contrast and/or low-light conditions. Current back surface centre distance aspheric soft lenses are therefore recommended for early presbyopia only (up to +1.25 D).

In soft lenses, the aspheric back surface will not normally have any significant impact on fit but in rigid lenses the back surface geometry may depart significantly from corneal topography with the 'higher-eccentricity' designs. This is due to rapidly flattening back surface aspheric geometry. Such lenses will need to be fitted fairly steep to allow for appropriate lens centration (Edwards, 2000). Back surface aspheric rigid lens designs can now be based on corneal topography and ocular prescription to create an individual lens design for correcting presbyopia (Woods *et al.*, 1999). The aim is to modify the combined optical system of the lens, tears and cornea to provide a predictable varifocal effect.

Front surface aspheric designs

Front surface soft aspheric designs promote negative spherical aberration, resulting in decreasing plus power from the geometric centre of the lens. This in essence creates a centre-near design. The aspheric curve is calculated to limit the spherical aberrations of the eye and, if necessary, of the lens itself. The improvement of retinal image quality and increase in depth of focus can be effective at correcting the early presbyopic patient (up to +1.50 D). Apart from the visual demands of the presbyopic patient, it would also be expected that visual performance would depend upon the interaction of the optical characteristics of the particular lens design with the aberrations of the eyes of the wearer. Consequently, variations in ocular aberration between individuals may explain in part why lenses of this type meet the needs of some wearers but not others (Plakitsi and Charman, 1995). As presbyopia increases, correcting the spherical aberration of the wearer alone will not be sufficient and the front surface curve must have a greater degree of asphericity to allow more plus refractive power within the optical system. This often involves more complex surface geometry of varying eccentricity to allow stabilized distance and near power zones within a specified area.

Theoretical variation in image contrast with the different designs is summarized in Figure 25.11.

Zonal aspheric design

This approach is designed to allow balanced vision at all distances and synergistically combines the benefits of multizone spherical and aspheric designs. The resulting lens has a zonal aspheric front surface designed to leverage the eyes' natural depth of clear focus. It is available with three different add powers (low, mid and high) which cover measured near additions from +0.75 D to +2.50 D. The power profile and zone distribution for each of the add powers have been optimized for the normal physiological change in pupil size with age as well as illumination changes (Figure 25.12). The lens has an aspheric back surface to optimize centration and an easy-to-follow, clinically validated fitting guide which allows optimal initial lens selection and effective lens adjustments if required.

Lens fitting

Initial lens power selection and optimal adjustments will vary with each individual lens type; however, the distance power of the bifocal lens will most often be based on the vertex distance-corrected best sphere prescription. Front surface aspheric lenses, however, may be designed so that

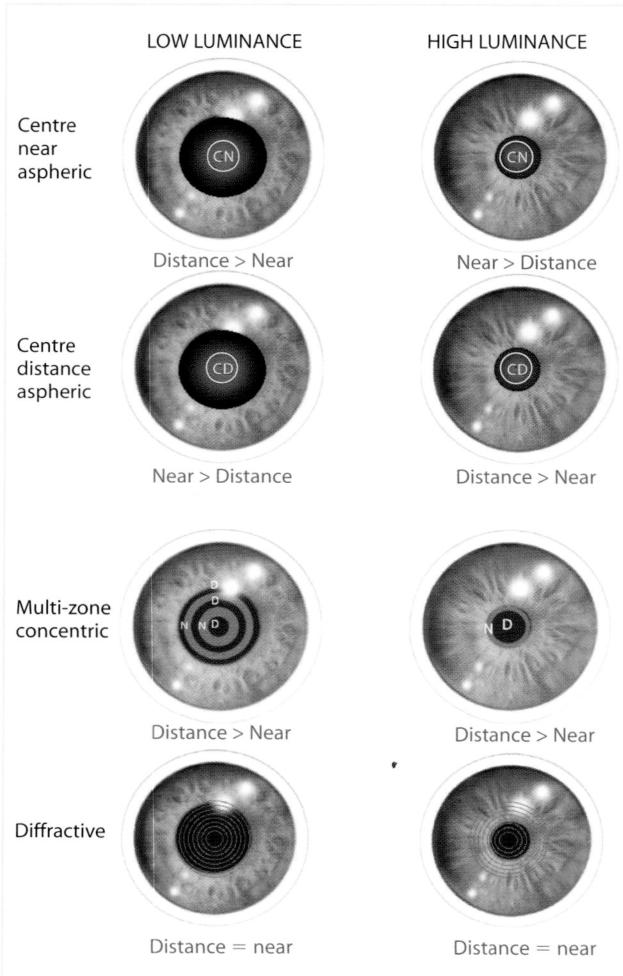

Figure 25.11 Variation of image contrast in low and high luminance with different lens designs.

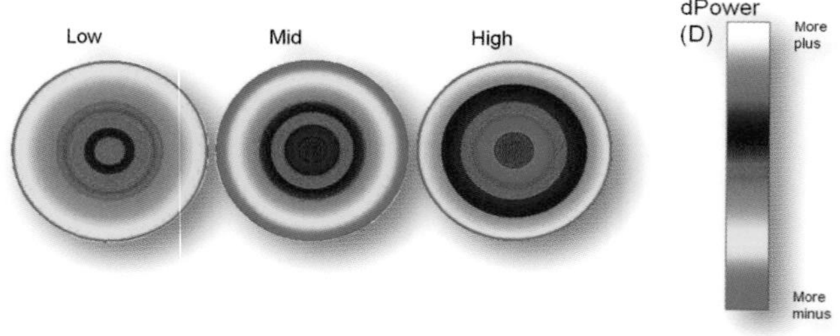

Figure 25.12 Zonal aspheric design.

lens power is based on the total reading power or a value midway between the distance and near power. Always refer to the manufacturers' fitting advice which is specific for that particular lens design.

Refractive end-points are more difficult to determine when wearing a simultaneous-vision correction in each eye, and therefore the lens power selected should always be based on a current refraction. The refraction should also be carefully binocularly balanced.

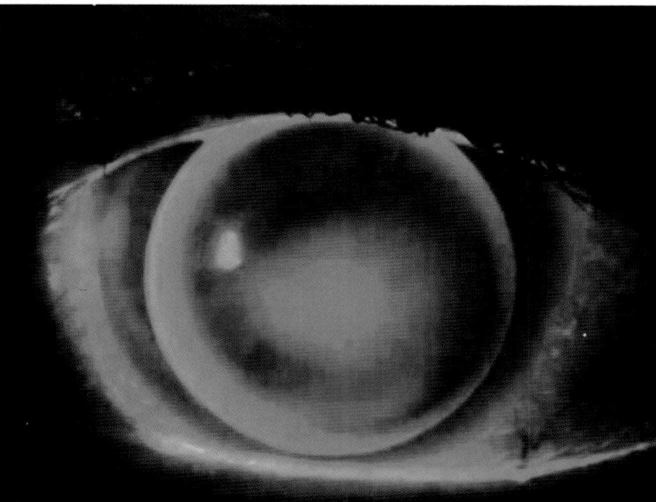

Figure 25.13 Fluorescein pattern of high-eccentricity back surface aspheric design showing central apical clearance and mid peripheral alignment.

The fit of a soft lens should meet the normal criteria used for single-vision soft lens fitting, as outlined in Chapter 9; however, good lens centration and minimal movement are especially critical in allowing optimal vision performance with bifocal lenses. This is even more important if fitting an aspheric lens design, as decentration may result in induced higher-order aberrations (Efron *et al.*, 2008).

Back surface aspheric rigid lens designs are usually fitted 0.5–0.8 mm steeper than the cornea to give the desired optical effect and to obtain the required centration. Although this may sound excessively steep, the rapidly flattening aspheric back surface should result in a fluorescein pattern that shows a small central area of apical clearance surrounded by a wide area of mid peripheral alignment (Figure 25.13).

Near performance will benefit, with this lens type, from lens translation during downward gaze.

Lens adjustments

The most common problem that the practitioner has to address with simultaneous lens fitting is poor visual performance for either distance vision or near vision, or both. The first step is to confirm lens fitting and end-point over-refraction. Although the most effective adjustment options may vary with the lens design being used, most designs are sensitive to 0.25 D adjustments to the distance lens power, which can have a profound effect on distance or near visual performance. Lens power adjustments are best investigated by using –0.25 D twirls/flippers or trial lenses during binocular vision in ambient illumination or the illumination where problems are being experienced by the wearer. The use of phoropters should be avoided during overrefraction as the resulting light reduction will increase pupil size and alter optical performance. Any distance minus-power adjustment should only be made if it has been demonstrated to make a significant impact on distance visual acuity (i.e. half to one line of Snellen visual acuity) combined with a subjective improvement. Small additional minus-power adjustments can be shown to the dominant eye first whilst investigating distance-vision improvement,

Table 25.3 Adjustment options for improving distance vision during simultaneous-vision fitting

Add additional minus to distance lens power
Show more minus power in −0.25 D steps to the dominant eye first or to both eyes if necessary
Ensure significant improvement to distance-vision performance (subjective and objective)
Ensure near vision remains unchanged or acceptable
Only continue to add additional minus power if further improvement is confirmed while near-vision performance is maintained
Reduce reading add power
If parameter range allows, reduce reading add power in one or both eyes
Alter back surface fitting relationship
Some rigid lens designs require alternative fitting to achieve a change in power gradient over the pupil area and the necessary distance vision improvement
Explore modified monovision
Push extra minus in dominant eye and extra plus power in non-dominant eye
Decrease reading add by one step in the dominant eye
Try centre-near design in one eye and centre-distance in the other
Explore enhanced monovision
Trial single-vision distance lens in dominant eye and near-bias bifocal in the other

Table 25.4 Adjustment options for improving near vision during simultaneous-vision fitting

Add additional plus to distance lens power
Show more plus power in +0.25 D steps to the non-dominant eye first or both eyes if necessary
Ensure significant improvement to near-vision performance (subjective and objective)
Ensure distance vision remains unchanged or acceptable
Adding extra lens power to non-dominant eye alone may reduce the risk of reducing distance vision performance while improving near vision
Alter back surface fitting relationship
Some rigid lens designs require alternative fitting to achieve the change in power gradient over the pupil area and the necessary near-vision improvement
Explore modified monovision
Push extra minus in dominant eye and extra plus power in non-dominant eye
Increase reading add by one step in the non-dominant eye
Try centre-near design in one eye and centre-distance in the other
Explore enhanced monovision
Trial single-vision near lens in dominant eye and distance-bias bifocal in the other

or to both eyes at the same time. The former approach may lessen the risk of reducing near-vision performance whilst improving distance vision. In addition, if the parameter range allows, distance vision may be improved by reducing the reading addition by one step in the dominant or both eyes (Key *et al.*, 1996). Adjustment options are summarized in Tables 25.3 and 25.4.

Alternating (translating)-vision designs

The majority of alternating designs are available as rigid gas-permeable lenses due to challenges in soft lenses translating effectively. However in recent years a number of soft alternating-vision designs have become available. Both soft and rigid gas-permeable designs have distance and near powered portions, set out in a similar way to that observed in a bifocal spectacle lens. During primary gaze the distance portion of the contact lens is positioned over the pupil. When gaze is directed downwards during reading, the near portion translates upwards to allow near-vision correction (Figure 25.14A, B).

Segment position and lens translation are the keys to success, and the lower lid has an important role in positioning and stabilizing the lens against the globe. The position of the lower lid should be no lower than the inferior limbus, otherwise translation is less effective and often inadequate (Figure 25.14C). Upper-lid movement also plays an important role in lens translation, as the upward movement of the lower lid is restricted to about 0.8 mm (Borish and Perrigin, 1987). It may be more challenging to fit patients with ambient pupil sizes greater than 3 mm, as the segment has to be positioned lower to avoid the pupil margin and consequently requires greater translation to achieve adequate pupil coverage of the near portion.

General principles of lens designs

The two distinct portions that make up an alternating lens may be either fused or solid segments, and a range of alternative shapes are available (Figure 25.15).

Lens stability, position and translation can be controlled by introducing prism on to the lens, truncating the lens, or both. A more recent alternating soft lens design uses prism and dynamic stabilization to orient the lens correctly and is available as a toric option. Regardless of lens design, the success of alternating-vision contact lenses is made possible by adequate lower-lid tone, which facilitates upward translation of the lens during downgaze. This positions the near portion of the lens over the pupil and allows near vision. The truncated edge should be finished in such a way as to encourage comfortable effective translation and minimize the risk of the lens slipping beneath the lower lid.

Solid design

As the name suggests, these designs can be cut from a single piece of material and the segment shape and design can vary (Figure 25.15). If the optical centres of the distance and near portion do not coincide, image jump will occur with downgaze, and lenses of 3.00 D or greater frequently result in intolerable diplopia for the wearer. For this reason, it is better to avoid solid construction lenses in these powers unless using a monocentric design. In these designs optical centres of both distance and near portions of the lens are coincident, which produces a straight-top segment bifocal contact lens with the same properties as an 'executive' bifocal spectacle lens. Triangular-shaped segments are also available, which makes the design more independent of

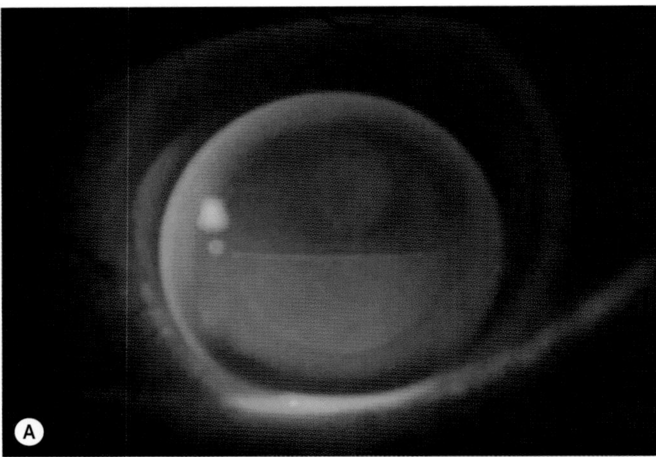

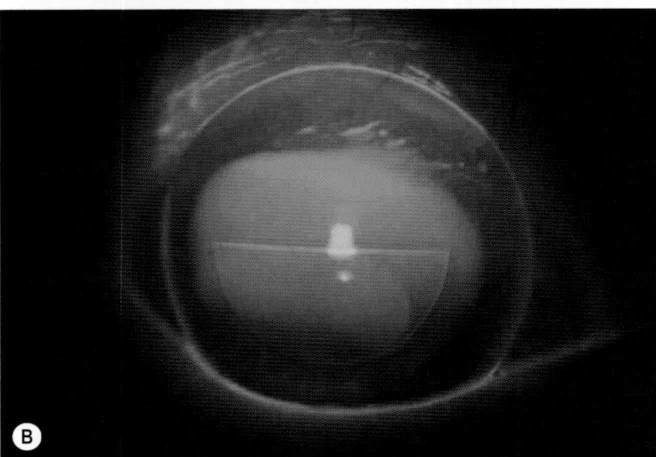

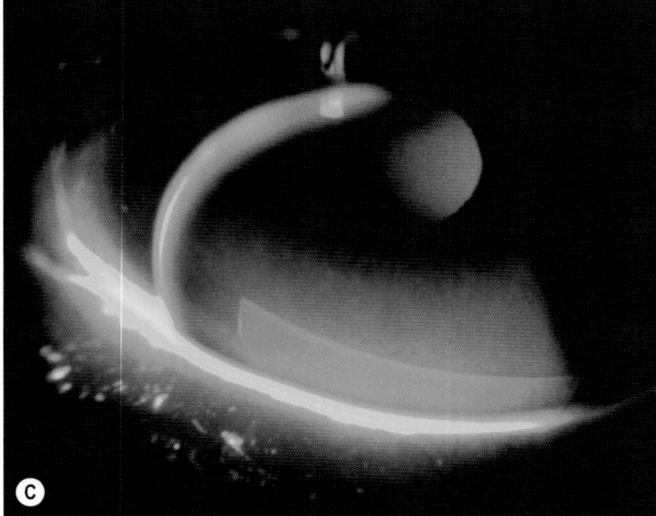

Figure 25.14 (A) Segment positioned in primary position of gaze. (B) Segment positioned over pupil in downgaze due to successful lens translation. (C) In another patient, segment positioned poorly due to failure of the lower lid to translate the lens upwards.

pupil diameter compared to straight-top bifocals, and often less translation is required to allow effective near correction. The design is also more forgiving if the lens rotates out of position when compared to straight-top designs (Figure 25.16).

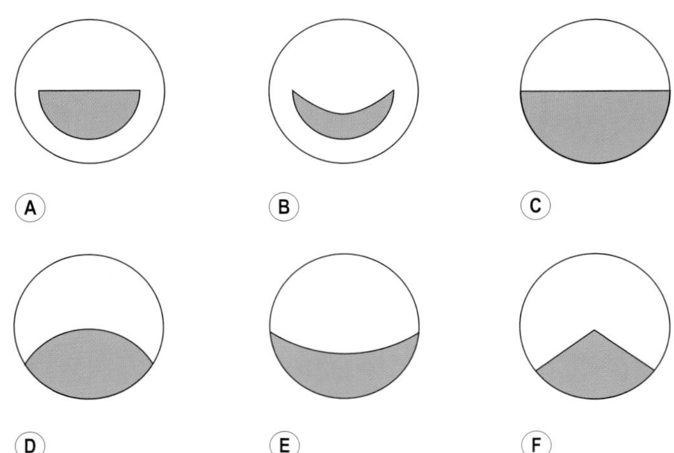

Figure 25.15 Bifocal segment shapes. Fused: A = straight top; B = crescent. Solid one-piece: C = straight top; D = reversed crescent; E = crescent; F = triangular.

Fused design

Fused-segment rigid lenses use a fused insert of higher refractive index than the rest of the lens to generate the add power, while the front surface curvature remains continuous. There is minimal image jump and blanks are supplied to laboratories allowing individual lens specifications to be made to order, including more complex front and back surface geometries. Care must be taken not to fit these lenses with the segment position too high as this increases the risk of reflections being noticed from the top of the segment (Ruston and Meyler, 1995). The fused segment is fluorescent, allowing easy observation using a Burton lamp.

Lens fitting

Alternating lenses are generally fitted on alignment or with minimal apical corneal touch. The truncation should rest on the lower lid. The lens should have a vertical diameter at least 2 mm smaller than the horizontal visible iris diameter; this encourages the required inferior centration and rapid recovery of lens position following blink as well as upward movement during depressed gaze. Translation over the corneal surface is more likely if there is unimpeded vertical movement, so a steep-fitting approach should be avoided. In general, a lens fitted too steeply will tend to rotate nasally (Figure 25.17) and shows poor translation, unlike a flat lens fit, which rotates temporally and decentres.

Most alternating bifocal contact lenses are fitted so that the segment is positioned in line with the inferior pupil margin during primary gaze in ambient illumination. Alternatively, some solid designs are such that the segment should be fitted higher to occupy approximately 20% of the pupil area (Figure 25.18).

More importantly, the near segment should occupy at least 75% of the pupil diameter during depressed gaze to allow adequate near vision. An exception is when fitting fused rigid lens designs, as the segment position should be positioned approximately 0.4–0.7 mm below the pupil margin when observed under slit-lamp illumination. This minimizes light reflections from the segment line interfering with distance vision performance. As a general rule, it is best to err on setting the segment top slightly

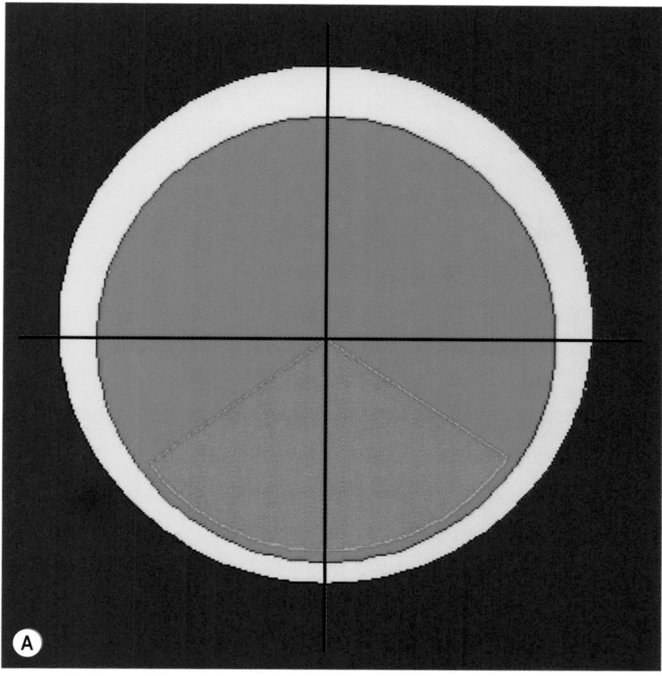

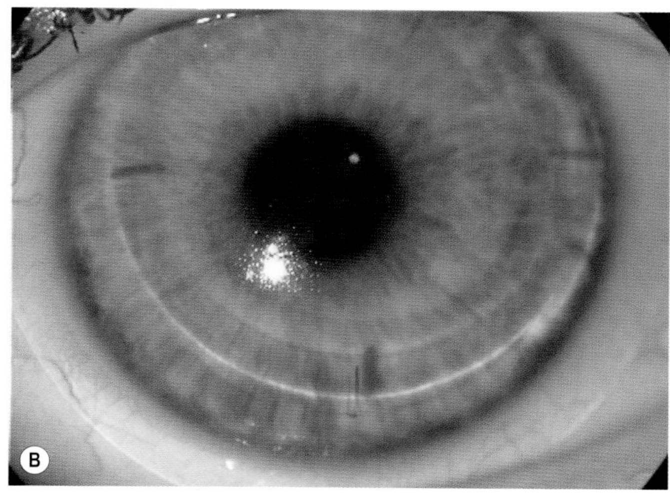

Figure 25.16 (A) Triangle-shape segment design. (B) Triangle-shape segment in primary position of gaze.

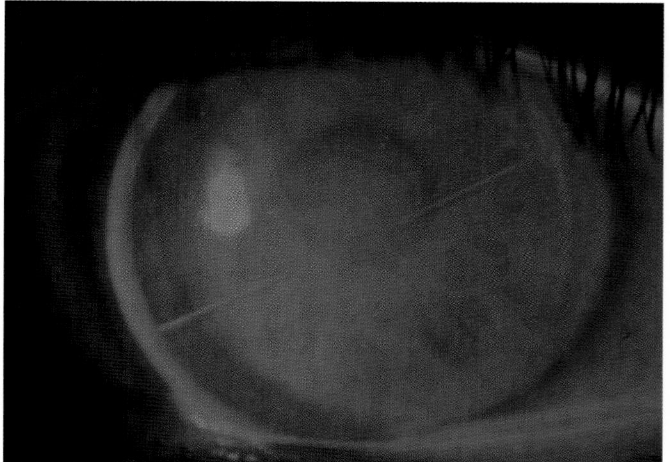

Figure 25.17 Nasal rotation resulting from steep-fitting lens.

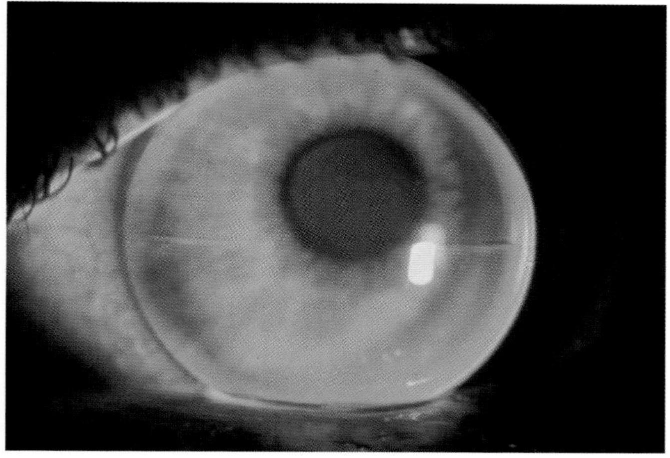

Figure 25.18 Ideal segment line position of a straight-top solid design for distance vision.

high as this can subsequently be lowered by increasing truncation (Gasson and Morris, 1998). A near-horizontal segment line position is preferred; however, a small amount of nasal rotation is acceptable because the natural convergence of the eyes at near helps offset this rotation (Edwards, 1999).

Observing segment positions under slit-lamp illumination can be deceptive due to the resultant pupil miosis. A better assessment can be made using an ophthalmoscope focused on the lens surface. If an optimal alignment fit shows significant rotation away from the desired position, the lens can be reordered with prism offset by the angle through which the lens mislocates to compensate for the rotation. For example, if the lens persists in rotating by 15° nasally in the right eye, ordering the prism base at 285° rather than 270° orients the lens correctly. Increasing the amount of prism can also be useful in reducing superior centration. Discomfort and adequate oxygen delivery (mainly due to lens thickness) are still challenges for soft alternating designs.

Conclusions

The key to meeting the visual needs of a presbyopic patient is the development of an awareness of the different fitting approaches and bifocal lens designs, and the associated advantages and disadvantages of each (Table 25.5).

It is equally important to gain an appreciation of the personality, occupation and previous lens-wearing history (if

Table 25.5 Advantages and disadvantages of lens fitting options for presbyopia correction

Advantages	Disadvantages
Monovision	
Least complicated method for correcting presbyopia	Significant reduction in stereopsis (especially at near); however patient-dependent
Binocular high-contrast visual acuity less compromised when compared to spectacle correction	Unsuitable for monocular patients or those with significant amblyopia (6/12 or worse)
Easy to trial	Loss of contrast sensitivity
Less expensive than bifocal options	Reduced intermediate correction as reading add increases
Large range of lens designs/materials to choose from	Reduced binocular summation
No additional fitting sets required	Headlight glare can be difficult to tolerate
Patients quickly accept or reject technique	
Simultaneous vision	
Available in both rigid and soft designs	Visual adaptation required by patient
Vision in all directions of gaze	Contrast loss always occurs, especially in low luminance
Stereoscopic vision maintained	Optical performance can depend on pupil size (varies with design)
No rotational stability required	Lens centration more critical
Usually more comfortable than alternating designs	High-contrast acuity usually one Snellen line less than spectacle/single-vision correction
Available as single-use soft disposable trial and prescription lenses	More difficult to establish refractive end-point during overrefraction
Easier to fit than alternating designs	
Alternating vision	
Distance and near acuity comparable to spectacle correction	Fitting more complex
Minimal reduction in stereopsis	Performance gaze-dependent
Minimal reduction in contrast	Intermediate correction not always an option Lid position and tightness critical to success

any) of the patient. Presbyopia correction is often perceived by practitioners as being complicated to fit, with limited success rates; however, there are now more lens options than ever to offer our presbyopic patients. No correction option for presbyopia (including spectacles) is without some compromise and the lack of a 'perfect' contact lens option should not discourage practitioners from fitting this ever-increasing patient base. New simultaneous designs with improved optical performance and fitting approcah are now relatively easy to fit, supported further by the availability of single-use diagnostic trial lenses that allow effective trials to help eliminate failures prior to dispensing. Daily disposable bifocal lenses are also available for patients, offering even greater levels of convenience. There are multifocal lens designs available in both silicone hydrogel and high-permeability rigid lens materials which may enable continuous wear of the lenses (Lakkis *et al*., 2006).

If the initial lens powers selected fail to provide adequate visual performance, alternative fitting approaches, such as enhanced and modified monovision, can be explored. Key fitting tips are summarized in Table 25.6.

Alternating lens designs can be added to the lens choice to offer patients bifocal correction if more exacting visual performance is required. In addition, the simplicity of monovision remains an effective solution for many presbyopic patients. It is recommended that practitioners select and use two to three alternative lens designs so that a sound clinical approach can be developed and used with confidence.

Table 25.6 Clinical pearls for presbyopia fitting

Set realistic expectations upfront. Success is what is right for the patient and remember the 20/happy rule	Always assess vision performance with both eyes open. Let patient trial lens performance at home and work and have the patient return in a week for follow-up assessment
Decide your clinical strategy with each patient and avoid trying different designs based on the same optical principle. Consider different approaches, including modified monovision and enhanced monovision	Avoid phoropters for overrefraction. Trial frame or flippers are best and look for an improvement in overall vision. Use the Snellen letter chart only to record visual acuity for legal purposes and as a benchmark for future lens changes
Study and follow the manufacturer's fitting advice for any one particular design of lens, as they all differ slightly in design characteristics and optimal fitting	Always look for the optimal balance between near and distance vision that meets the patient's visual needs

(Adapted from Christie and Beertren, 2007)

Acknowledgements

The author would like to acknowledge Eric Papas for his constructive input to the content of this chapter.

References

Back, A., Holden, B. A. and Hine, N. A. (1989) Correction of presbyopia with contact lenses: comparative success rates with three systems. *Optom. Vis. Sci.,* **66,** 518–525.

Back, A., Grant, T. and Hine, N. (1992) Comparative visual performance of three comparative contact lens corrections. *Optom. Vis. Sci.,* **69,** 474–480.

Benjamin, W. J. and Borish, I. M. (1994) Presbyopia and the influence of aging on prescription of contact lenses. In *Contact Lens Practice* (M. Ruben and M. Guillon, eds), pp. 763–828, London: Chapman & Hall.

Bennett, E. S., (2007) Bifocal and multifocal contact lenses. In *Contact Lenses,* 5th edn (A. J. Phillips and L. Speedwell, eds) pp. 311–331, Oxford: Butterworth-Heinemann.

Bennett E. S. (2008) Contact lens correction of presbyopia. *Clin. Exp. Optom.,* **91,** 265–278.

Bennett, E. S., Jurkus, J. M. and Schwartz, C. A. (2000) Bifocal contact lenses. In *Clinical Manual of Contact Lenses,* 2nd edn (E. S. Bennett and V. A. Henry, eds), pp. 410–449, Philadelphia, PA: J. B. Lippincott.

Borish, I. M. (1988) Pupil dependency of bifocal contact lenses. *Am. J. Optom. Physiol. Opt.,* **65,** 417–423.

Borish, I. M. and Perrigin, D. (1987) Relative movement of lower lid and line of sight from distant to near fixation. *Am. J. Optom. Physiol. Opt.,* **64,** 881–887.

Christie, C and Beertren, R. (2007) The correction of presbyopia with contact lenses. *Optom. In. Pract.,* **8,** 19–30.

Chu, B. S., Wood, J. M. and Collins, M. J. (2009) Effect of presbyopic vision corrections on perceptions of driving difficulty. *Eye Contact Lens,* **35,** 133–143.

Collins, M., Goode, A. and Tait, A. (1994) Monovision: the patient's perspective. *Clin. Exp. Optom.,* **77,** 69–75.

Dutoit, R., Situ, P., Simpson, T. *et al.* (2000) Results of a one year clinical trial comparing monovision and bifocal contact lenses. *Optom. Vis. Sci.,* **77,** S18.

Edwards, K. (1999) Contact lens problem solving: bifocal contact lenses. *Optician,* **218**(5721), 26–32.

Edwards, K. (2000) Progressive power contact lens problem-solving. *Optician,* **219**(5749), 16–20.

Efron, S., Efron, N. and Morgan, P. B. (2008) Optical and visual performance of aspheric soft contact lenses. *Optom. Vis. Sci.,* **85,** 201–210.

Erikson, P. (1988) Potential range of clear vision in monovision. *J. Am. Opt. Assoc.,* **59,** 203–205.

Gasson, A. and Morris, J. (1998) Bifocal lenses for presbyopia. In *The Contact Lens Manual,* 2nd edn, pp. 261–277, London: Butterworth-Heinemann.

Gupta, N., Naroo, S. A. and Wolffsohn, J. S. (2009) Visual comparison of multifocal contact lens to monovision. *Optom. Vis. Sci.* **86,** 98–105.

Harris, M., Sheedy, J. and Gan, C. (1992) Vision and task performance with monovision and bifocal contact lenses. *Optom. Vis. Sci.,* **69,** 609–614.

Jain, S., Arora, I. and Azar, D. T. (1996) Success of monovision in presbyopes: review of the literature and potential applications to refractive surgery. *Surv. Ophthalmol.,* **40,** 491–499.

Johannsdottir, K. R. and Stelmach, L. B. (2001) Monovision: a Review of the Scientific Literature. *Optom. Vis. Sci.,* **78,** 646–651.

Key, J., Morris, K. and Mobley, C. (1996) Prospective clinical evaluation of Sunsoft multifocal contact lens. *Contact Lens Assoc. Ophthalmol. J.,* **22,** 179–184.

Koetting, R. and Castellano, C. F. (1984) Successful fitting of the monovision patient. *Contacto,* **28,** 24–26.

Lakkis, C., Goldenberg, S. A. and Woods, C. A. (2006) Investigation of the performance of the Menifocal Z gas-permeable bifocal contact lens during continuous wear. *Optom. Vis. Sci.,* **82,** 1022–1029.

Maldonado-Codina, C., Meyler, J. and Morgan, P. M. (1997) Monovision revisited. *Optician,* **214**(5608), 23–28.

Meyler, J. and Veys, J. (1999) A new 'pupil-intelligent' lens for presbyopic correction. *Optician,* **217**(5687), 18–23.

Michaud, L., Tchang, J. P., Baril, C. *et al.* (1995) New perspectives in monovision: a study comparing aspheric with disposable lenses. *Int. Contact Lens Clin.,* **22,** 203–208.

Morgan, P. B. and Efron, N. (2009) Contact lens correction of presbyopia. *Contact Lens Ant. Eye,* **32,** 191–192.

Plakitsi, A. and Charman, W. N. (1995) Comparison of the depths of focus with the naked eye with three types of presbyopic contact lens correction. *J. Br. Contact Lens Assoc.,* **18,** 119–125.

Rajagopalan, A. S., Bennett, E. S. and Lakshminarayanan, V. (2006) Visual performance of subjects wearing presbyopic contact lenses. *Optom. Vis. Sci.,* **83,** 611–615.

Richdale, K., Mitchell, G. L. and Zadnik, K. (2006) Comparison of multifocal and monovision soft contact lens corrections in patients with low-astigmatic presbyopia. *Optom. Vis. Sci.,* **83,** 266–273.

Ruston, D. M. and Meyler, J. (1995) How to fit alternating vision RGP bifocals. Part 2: the Fluoroperm ST bifocal. *Optometry Today,* 23 November, pp. 27–31.

Schor, C., Landsman, L. and Erickson, P. (1987) Ocular dominance and the interocular suppression of blur in monovision. *Am. J. Optom.,* **64,** 723–730.

Situ, P., du Toit, R., Fonn, D. *et al.* (2003) Successful monovision contact lens wearers refitted with bifocal contact lenses. *Eye Contact Lens,* **29,** 181–184.

Williams, L. (1998) Advanced techniques and instrumentation. Lecture 9.1. In *The IACLE Contact Lens Course.* Module 9 (D. Fonn, ed.), pp. 59–60. Sydney: International Association of Contact Lens Educators.

Woods, C., Ruston, D., Hough, T. *et al.* (1999) Clinical performance of an innovative back surface multifocal contact lens in correcting presbyopia. *Contact Lens Assoc. Ophthalmol. J.,* **25,** 176–181.

Young, G., Grey, C. and Papas, E. (1990) Simultaneous vision bifocal contact lenses: a comparative assessment of the in vitro optical performance. *Optom. Vis. Sci.,* **67,** 339–345.

Continuous wear

Noel A Brennan and M-L Chantal Coles

Introduction

Practitioners and researchers have long sought to develop a lens that can be worn on an extended-wear basis. The term 'extended wear' has generally been applied to describe wear of contact lenses for periods in excess of 24 h between removal, including sleep with the lenses on eye and regular, planned removal of the lenses. The term 'continuous wear' was originally used to describe prolonged wear of unspecified duration, but was discarded during the early 1980s because prolonged wear was considered to be an unachievable goal. In the late 1990s, 'continuous wear' was reintroduced as a term to describe intended lens wear of up to 30 days between removals, consigning the term 'extended wear' to periods of up to 7 uninterrupted days.

The demand for more convenient forms of optical correction has increased over the years. Numerous marketing surveys have revealed the desire of the majority of the contact lens-wearing population for extended or continuous wear. Various factors influence this desire: convenience, a sense of vulnerability, particularly in patients with higher refractive errors, relief from tedious maintenance and handling procedures, and vocational and lifestyle issues. The widespread interest in refractive surgery since the 1980s underscores the appeal of a longer-term solution to refractive error. Marketing surveys agree that the recommendation of the practitioner is critical in determining the choice of correction. The industry, practitioners and patients alike have therefore keenly sought the development of a safe and effective continuous-wear contact lens.

For a detailed history of extended wear the reader is referred to Brennan and Coles (1997). Analysis of the early ventures in extended wear provides important clues as to the pitfalls with this wearing style. The current status of extended wear and its current format can be traced to the prominent aspects of this history.

Experiences with extended wear

The earliest report of extended wear appears to be a 1957 description of a non-compliant patient wearing a polymethyl methacrylate (PMMA) contact lens continuously for 3 months. Details of a planned clinical trial were published in 1965, reporting on 50 patients wearing PMMA on a continuous-wear basis over a 7-year period. Although such lenses have since proven to be unsuitable for extended wear, the absence of long-term complications in these reports is noteworthy, and indicative of the resilience of the eye to sleeping in contact lenses.

Conventional soft extended wear

The original soft lenses, designed for long-term repeated usage, are now referred to as 'conventional' or 'unplanned-replacement' hydrogel lenses to distinguish them from 'frequent-replacement' or 'disposable' lenses. In this chapter, the term 'traditional' soft lens materials will also be used when referring to these original hydrogels, to distinguish them from silicone hydrogel contact lens materials (see below). Soft hydrophilic lenses were introduced around the world in the late 1960s and early 1970s as a result of the pioneering work of Wichterle. These lenses were very well received by the public, principally due to the comfort afforded. Contact lens sales promptly soared. But the inconvenience of caring for the lenses and the need to insert and remove the lenses on a daily basis led to increased experimentation with extended periods of wear.

Early reports focused on the use of prolonged periods of wear for therapeutic use, particularly in aphakia. Perceived advantages included alleviation of the possible risks associated with removal and handling of lenses from diseased eyes and relief for patients with limited dexterity. Studies of soft lens extended wear for cosmetic use soon appeared with encouraging results. Following approval by the US Food and Drug Administration (FDA) for cosmetic extended wear in 1981, a large proportion of contact lens prescriptions, particularly in the USA, were written for this purpose. An intense and exciting period of research followed in which many of the problems in achieving successful extended contact lens wear were identified.

The reports of early clinical experiences with hydrogel extended-wear lenses are too numerous to review here, but even a cursory review shows dramatic variation in quoted

DOI: 10.1016/B978-0-7506-8869-7.00026-4

success rates. Such differences appeared to depend upon patient selection, the type of lenses fitted, fitting approach (tight or loose), diligence of follow-up and criteria used by investigators in assessing the severity of adverse reactions and in the categorization of success. For example, the study of Lamer (1983) reports a success rate as high as 81% following 3 years' extended wear compared to 48% reported by Binder (1983). Variation in study design remains a common problem in modern evaluation of continuous-wear success.

Despite the apparently low success rate, the retrospective study of Binder (1983) provides good insight to the success of these trials. This article reviewed over 1000 patients entered into a number of FDA regulatory studies of extended-wear lenses, with intended wearing times of 2–4 weeks. As noted above, nearly half (48.5%) of patients 'survived' extended wear with only minor problems, for 3½ years. Almost a third (31.3%) of the subjects who discontinued did so prior to beginning extended wear, and 16.2% were lost to follow-up, leaving only 4% who were known to discontinue for lens-related reasons during more than 3 years of extended wear. Of the discontinuations, 14.5% found lens comfort inadequate, and 12% experienced ocular complications. The frequency of individual complications was as follows: injection 3.7%, abrasion 1.6%, conjunctivitis 1.4%, papillary conjunctivitis 1.4%, neovascularization 1.1%, dry eye, epithelial staining and oedema, all less than 1%, and infections 0.2%.

It should be remembered that these trailblazing studies were performed with thick hydrogel lenses, which provided oxygen transmissibility (Dk/t) levels that were later deemed inadequate to maintain short- and long-term physiological integrity of the cornea. The period between lens removal was also up to 6 months in many of the early studies, and more recent research has deemed this to be unsafe. By modern standards, these lenses and their usage were grossly inappropriate for extended wear. Their relative success was therefore quite astounding and provided considerable scope for optimism that relatively minor adjustments to the lens parameters would provide a safe effective correction. Nonetheless, the expectations for these early lenses were high; the rate of discontinuations along with an emerging picture of severe complications due to infectious keratitis prompted studies of alternative materials for extended wear.

Non-hydrophilic materials

The high oxygen permeability of silicone elastomer led to interest in using this material for extended contact lens wear. In the late 1970s, a number of fitting trials were undertaken. Unfortunately, the hydrophobic nature of the lens surface resulted in poor wetting and surface deposition (Figure 26.1). The highly elastic nature of the material and resistance of the material to water permeation also brought about lens binding. These factors prevented the success of this material except for limited use in paediatric and aphakic fitting.

Towards the mid-1980s, rigid gas-permeable materials became a popular alternative to traditional hydrogels for extended wear, the principal attraction being a higher Dk/t without the adverse properties of silicone elastomer. Other perceived advantages of rigid lenses over traditional soft lenses include a higher rate of tear exchange beneath these lenses, less corneal coverage and a more inert lens surface.

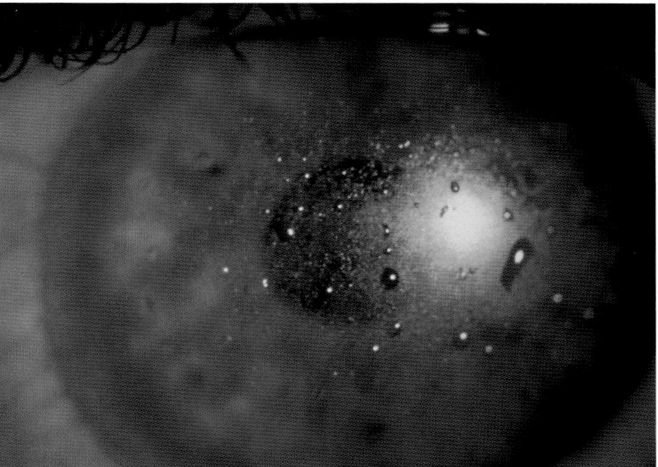

Figure 26.1 A silicone elastomer lens displaying poor wetting.

Preclinical evaluations demonstrated that rigid lenses produced fewer oxygen-related physiological changes, such as corneal oedema, than traditional soft lenses. A considerable body of literature provided evidence for successful extended wear in patients using these lenses (Maehara and Kastl, 1994); however, there remained a range of limitations inherent with rigid lenses. These lenses induce a greater degree of initial discomfort than hydrogels, including complications largely unseen with hydrogels, such as 3 and 9 o'clock staining, corneal distortion and lens binding. Other complications found with hydrogels, such as infiltrative keratitis, papillary conjunctivitis and infectious keratitis, were not eliminated. Most practitioners have been unwilling to devote the additional time required to achieve a suitable fit and deal with patient complaints of discomfort, so rigid lens correction of refractive errors in extended wear has become a subspecialty. Overnight wear of rigid lenses to achieve temporary reversal of refractive errors, known as orthokeratology, maintains a fervent, if specialized, approach and has become a mainstream research topic in the field of contact lens wear (Chapter 34).

Disposable soft lenses

Frequent-replacement lenses offer a range of advantages in increasing extended-wear success. Practitioners perceived the most significant problem with conventional hydrogel lenses to be the build-up of surface deposits and associated complications, such as papillary conjunctivitis (Orsborn and Zantos, 1989). Frequent replacement restricts exposure of the eye to accumulated aged or denatured protein, which seems to act as an antigen in inducing inflammatory reactions such as papillary conjunctivitis and infiltrative keratitis. Control of deposit build-up by frequent replacement has the further advantage of reducing patient symptoms related to vision and comfort.

While reducing exposure of the eye to lens deposition is the outstanding advantage of disposable lenses, the regular provision of fresh, clean lenses also showed promise in other areas. There was hope that frequent lens replacement would lead to fewer bacteria being introduced to the eye, thereby reducing the risk of infectious keratitis during extended wear. In regard to lens maintenance, disposability offers simplification of cleaning procedures, easier lens fitting and replacement, and may serve to enhance patient compliance.

Efficiencies of manufacture brought low-cost disposable lenses to the US market in 1987. The concept was well received and replacement of lenses every day to every 2 weeks to 1 month is now the most common wearing pattern around the world (Morgan *et al.*, 2009). In practice, the benefits with respect to ocular physiology, symptomatology and convenience are compelling and it seems that forever more frequent replacement will be the preferred model for all forms of lens wear, including extended wear.

Clinical studies have certainly confirmed that frequent replacement reduces the occurrence of papillary conjunctivitis during extended wear (Boswall *et al.*, 1993). However, the condition is not entirely eliminated: a significant incidence of papillary conjunctivitis remains during extended wear with replacement intervals of 2 weeks or greater.

There have been divergent reports on the relative incidence of non-infectious corneal infiltrative conditions with conventional versus disposable lens wear. In part, this may relate to the various schemes that have been advanced for the classification of contact lens-related infiltrative conditions. For example, the condition referred to as contact lens-related acute red eye seems to be reduced with increasing frequency of lens replacement (Kotow *et al.*, 1987). However, Cutter *et al.* (1996) found an increased prevalence of focal stromal infiltrates with overlying fluorescein staining with disposable lenses, an effect which was amplified in extended wear.

Frequent contact lens replacement has also failed to achieve the desired impact on the rate of infectious keratitis in contact lens wear. Indeed, confusion created by study designs and diagnostic criteria initially suggested a higher rate of infection with disposable lenses compared to conventional lenses; a number of studies have since shown that the rate is essentially equivalent between disposable and conventional lens usage, but remains higher with extended wear. Despite the significant advantages offered by disposability, the failure to reduce the rate of corneal infection meant that extended wear of contact lenses was again considered unfavourably in most countries by the mid-1990s.

Silicone-containing hydrogel contact lenses

In the late 1990s, silicone hydrogel contact lenses were introduced to the market. The details of the advances incorporated in these materials are presented in Chapter 5. In short, high Dk/t and good handling characteristics of silicone are combined with the flexibility and comfort of hydrophilic materials. Considerable advances in technology over previously manufactured lenses were required to combine these two ostensibly incompatible materials, not the least of which was new technology to produce a wettable, deposit-resistant surface. The early lenses used plasma surface coatings but later generations of lenses managed to circumvent the need for this additional manufacturing step.

Clinical research has demonstrated that silicone hydrogel lenses provide substantial improvement over hydrogel lenses for extended and continuous wear, by producing fewer microcysts, limbal injection, bulbar injection, striae and endothelial blebs (Covey *et al.*, 2001; Brennan *et al.*, 2002; Inagaki *et al.*, 2003; Radford *et al.*, 2009). These benefits arise from the lowered resistance of the lenses to oxygen flow. Silicone hydrogel lenses may also, on occasion, provide the added benefits of less corneal staining, subjective dryness and discomfort, and better handling, due to properties such as hydration, modulus, surface and design characteristics.

The advantages of silicone hydrogel lenses were quickly recognized and some countries such as Australia, which had previously shunned extended wear, enthusiastically adopted this new approach. Other countries such as the USA and the UK, following failure of the extended-wear foray of the 1980s, were more cautious in approach. By 2008, the rate of extended-wear prescribing in these countries seems to have stabilized at around 10–15% of all soft lenses prescribed (Morgan *et al.*, 2009).

As the first decade of the 21st century drew to a close, it had become apparent that, although the increased corneal oxygenation accorded by silicone hydrogel lenses reduced the incidence of severe keratitis compared to hydrogel lenses for overnight wear, the risk of keratitis was still greater than for open-eye lens wear. As a result, continued growth in the use of silicone hydrogel lenses for continuous wear ceased and the industry consolidated by concentrating on promoting silicone hydrogel lenses for daily-wear use. Nonetheless, many practitioners continued to provide silicone hydrogel lenses for continuous wear based on their positive personal experiences and lessons learnt from the industry's previous tribulations with the modality.

Mechanisms of adverse effects in extended wear

The application of a contact lens to the eye brings with it a number of potentially adverse responses. This is the case whether the lens is worn on a daily-wear or extended-wear basis. A detailed discussion of adverse events with contact lens wear is provided in Chapter 40. Some specific events are more prevalent during extended wear and these are presented below. The main feature of this discussion is to analyse the mechanisms of the ocular changes and to review risk factors and strategies to minimize these effects. Table 26.1 summarizes the major risk factors and options for dealing with these problems. Other issues common to daily-wear contact lenses, such as corneal staining, discomfort and the symptom of dryness, remain important in extended wear, but are dealt with elsewhere in this book.

Acute physiological effects

When worn during eye closure, traditional hydrogel lenses induce corneal oedema, observable clinically on awakening as striae and folds (Figure 26.2). The effects persist for some time following eye opening, and in some cases, throughout the day. In some circumstances, visual disturbance, in the form of haze and blur, is noted. Although the acute effects on corneal oedema resolve rapidly, wearing a traditional hydrogel contact lens in extended wear produces a recurring pattern of oedema during the night followed by partial resolution during the day (Holden *et al.*, 1983). Chronic exposure to this unfavourable environment is considered to be detrimental to long-term corneal health.

The short-term corneal oedema response has been the gold standard by which the physiological threat of a lens to the eye is assessed. Understanding factors influencing

Table 26.1 Risk factors for infectious and physiological changes identified in clinical and epidemiological studies

Risk factor	Remedy
Modifiable risk factors	
Long periods between removal	Reduce duration of extended wear
Tightly fitting lenses	Fit more mobile lenses
Long periods between lens replacement	Fit disposable lenses of greater replacement frequency
Low oxygen permeability	Fit silicone hydrogel lenses
Hot climates	Advise patients that care and maintenance are critical when travelling to/living in warmer climates
Poor care and maintenance	Fit disposable lenses and counsel patients
Sleeping in lenses	Sleep less in lenses or fit silicone hydrogel lenses
Smoking	Advise patients of increased risks
Non-modifiable risk factors	
Non-professional workers	Use discretion in prescribing
Diabetes	Advise patients of increased risks
Male gender	Use discretion in prescribing

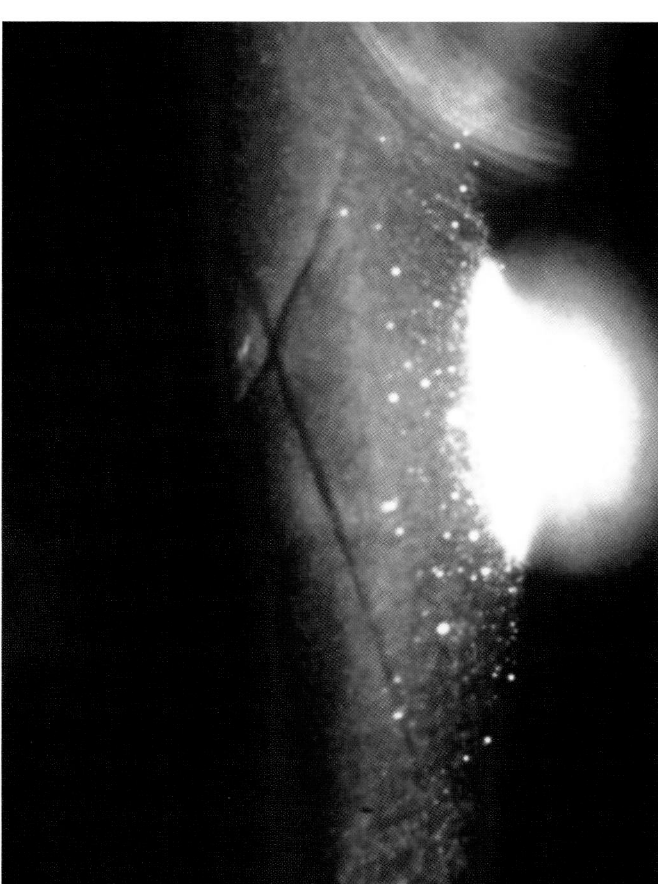

Figure 26.2 Folds observed in the posterior stroma following overnight wear of lenses of low to medium *Dk/t*.

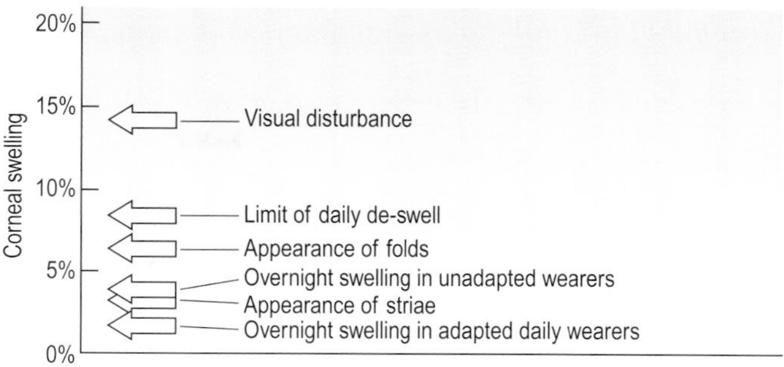

Figure 26.3 Guide for assessing the impact of oedema in extended wear.

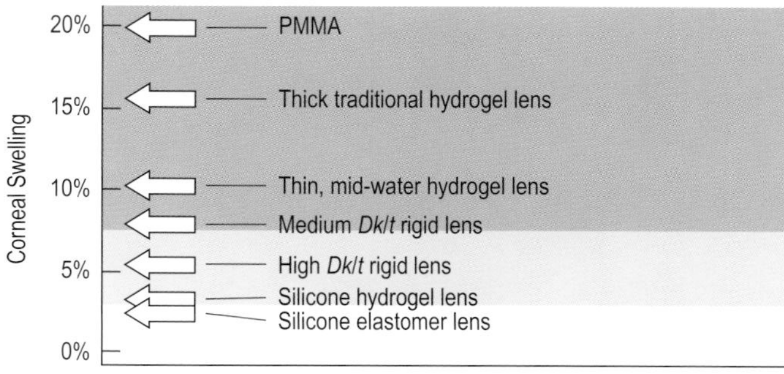

Figure 26.4 Representative overnight corneal swelling in response to different lens types. PMMA = polymethacryl methacrylate.

this response potentially enables the practitioner to avert long-term adverse physiological effects. Interpretation of corneal swelling data relies on comprehension of the expression of measurement, and some standards against which this can be compared. Typically, corneal oedema is expressed as a percentage swelling from baseline corneal thickness, which is usually judged to be the thickness of the cornea prior to sleep.

Since the cornea that is unadapted to contact lens wear swells by approximately 4% centrally overnight, this value has been suggested as a criterion for the safe maximum level of oedema in response to overnight contact lens wear (Holden *et al.*, 1983). Figure 26.3 plots this value against some of the yardsticks for evaluating oedema effects, and Figure 26.4 gives the average corneal swelling for a range of different lens types.

These values are for central corneal swelling, but the cornea does not swell uniformly. Figures 26.5–26.7 plot the topographical corneal swelling for three different lens types.

In each circumstance, the temporal and nasal mid peripheral cornea swell more than the central cornea. It is apparent from Figures 26.4 and 26.7 that silicone hydrogel lenses provide near-normal levels of oxygen to the cornea during sleep, whereas other common lens types fail to do this. Given the ability of silicone hydrogel lenses to meet the needs of the cornea in this regard, other previously suggested criteria for acceptable levels of overnight oedema should be abandoned.

Not all corneas exhibit the same baseline thickness, and not all corneas swell by the same amount in either relative or absolute terms. Figure 26.8 plots the absolute change in corneal thickness at two separate occasions versus the base-

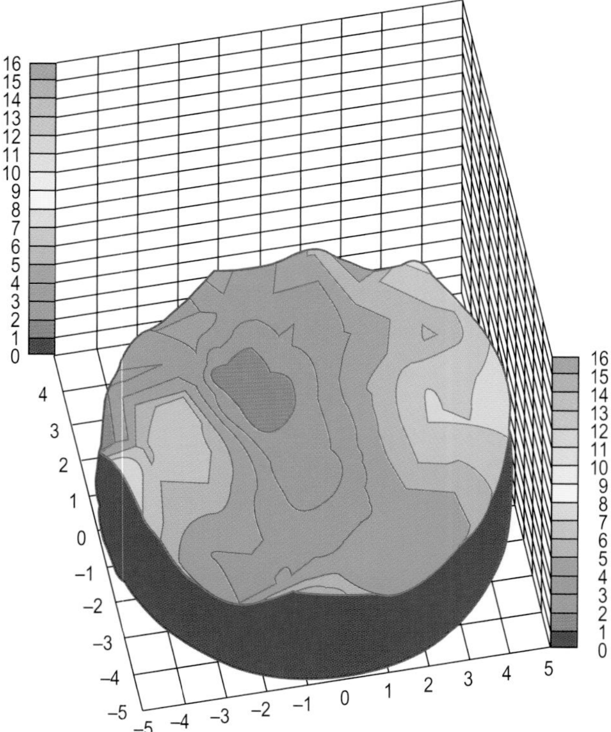

Figure 26.5 Three-dimensional representation of average topographical corneal oedema response to wear of silicone elastomer lenses under closed-eye conditions. To the right is the nasal direction, and the closer region is the inferior cornea.

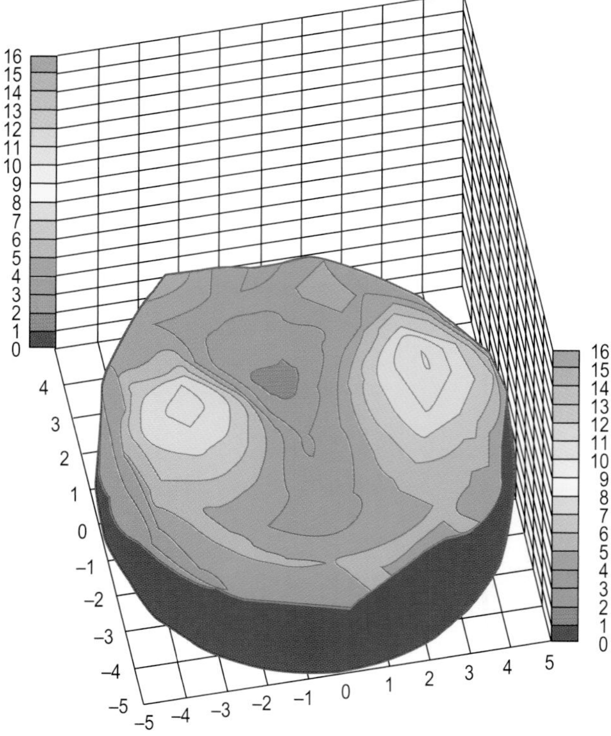

Figure 26.6 Three-dimensional representation of average topographical corneal oedema response to wear of silicone hydrogel contact lenses under closed-eye conditions. To the right is the nasal direction, and the closer region is the inferior cornea.

line central thickness for 15 subjects wearing thin, medium-water, traditional hydrogel lenses.

This graph demonstrates intersubject variability in both baseline thickness and the extent of swelling. While variation in swelling between subjects is probably determined by a complex combination of anatomical and functional factors – such as endothelial cell density – one additional prominent feature seems to be the level of adaptation to contact lens wear. The cornea of a subject adapted to daily wear of traditional hydrogel lenses swells by 2% less than observed in an unadapted wearer, with adapted extended wearers swelling less by a further 1% (Cox *et al.*, 1990). The relative roles of adaptation versus residual swelling in this effect are open to some interpretation. Nonetheless, this observation may in part explain some of the variation in different reports for mean swelling results to the same stimulus. For example, estimates of the closed-eye swelling response in the absence of a contact lens vary between 1.0% and 5.5%, a result that can be traced in part to the adaptation levels of the subjects. The criterion for the maximum acceptable level of overnight corneal swelling should be viewed in the context of this finding.

Another important corollary to the finding of high intersubject variability in corneal swelling is the question of how this impacts on long-term wear. One study has shown that subjects prone to higher amounts of oedema are more likely to discontinue lens wear and experience adverse ocular findings (Solomon, 1996). Another study found no effect, in that subjects experiencing infiltrative keratitis show the same degree of swelling as subjects without complications (Stapleton *et al.*, 1998). An opposite argument can be put – that the cornea adapted to extended wear, which shows the least amount of swelling, has a reduced metabolic rate and thus has less healing capacity and lower reserves for defences against potential threats. Thus, the patient with a cornea that shows a high degree of swelling may be intolerant to contact lens wear, but at the same time may be more resilient to threats against corneal health. Further research is needed to resolve this question.

The role of hypoxia

The principal factor causing corneal swelling during overnight lens wear is hypoxia (Holden and Mertz, 1984). A decrease in oxygen concentration within the corneal epithelium leads to anaerobic metabolism, of which the principal byproduct is lactate. Accumulation of lactate within the stroma leads to an osmotic pressure gradient into the cornea and also has the effect of lowering pH. Temperature, tear osmolarity and tear pH may also vary under the closed eye but such variances contribute only a small amount of the overall oedema response.

One way of assessing the oxygen flow through a contact lens is by measurement of its Dk/t (see Chapter 5). This laboratory-derived figure gives an *in vitro* indication of the likely impact of a lens on the eye and has become an industry standard. Certainly, the amount of swelling that occurs in a cornea can be approximately related to the Dk/t of the lens (Figure 26.9).

Holden and Mertz (1984) have established a criterion for Dk/t of 87 Barrer/cm to avoid excess oedema during overnight wear. There have been attempts in the interim to

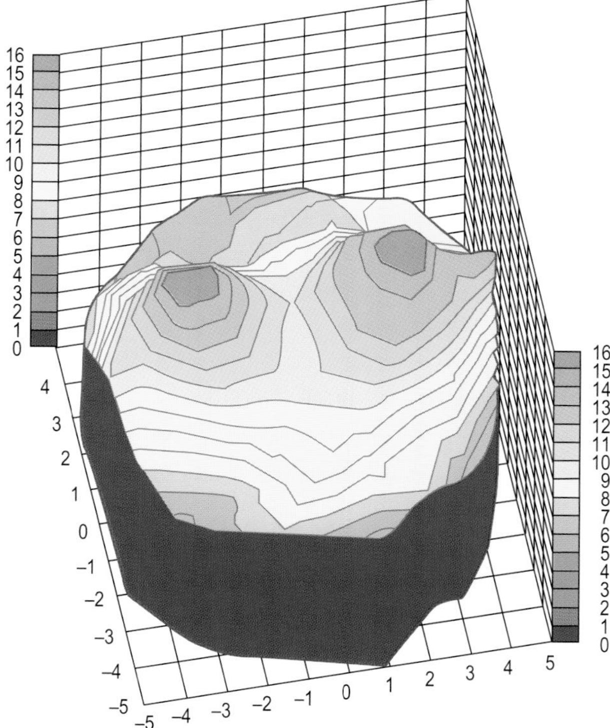

Figure 26.7 Three-dimensional representation of average topographical corneal oedema response to wear of mid-water traditional hydrogel lens under closed-eye conditions. To the right is the nasal direction, and the closer region is the inferior cornea.

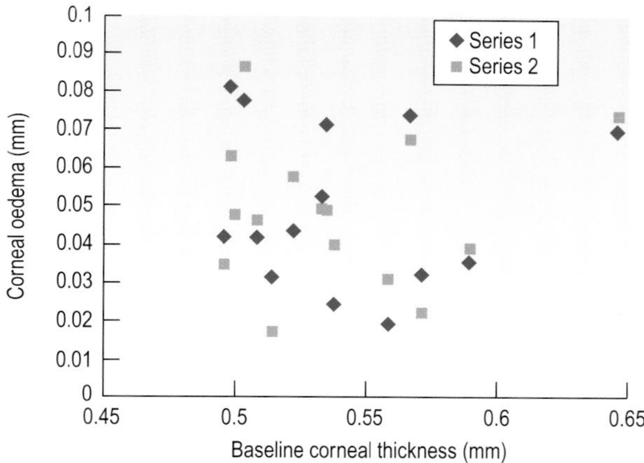

Figure 26.8 Overnight central corneal swelling of 15 subjects on two occasions (Series 1 and 2) with wear of a mid-water traditional hydrogel lens. Individual baseline thickness variability is demonstrated by variation along the *x*-axis, and individual swelling differences are shown by the variation along the *y*-axis.

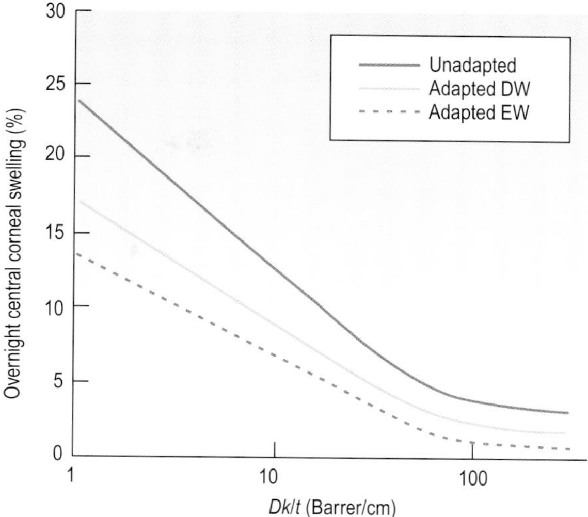

Figure 26.9 Variation in overnight corneal swelling with wear of lenses of various *Dk/t* values for different levels of adaptation to daily lens wear (DW) and extended lens wear (EW).

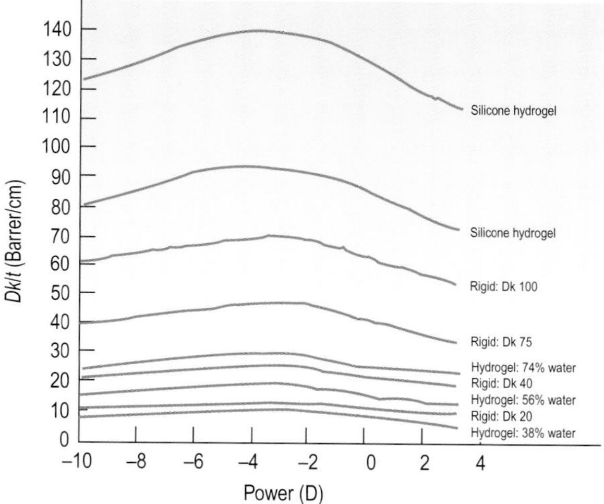

Figure 26.10 Variation in *Dk/t* versus power for various lens types.

instate alternate values, but there seems to be limited scientific basis to this rewriting of history. Figure 26.10 gives a graphical demonstration of the variation in Dk/t for different lens materials manufactured at minimum practical thickness for various powers.

It is clear that hydrogel materials fall considerably short of the Holden–Mertz criterion. Silicone hydrogel and some rigid lenses meet the desired level. However, the use of Dk/t values as a concept falls short of providing a simple index by which the negative impact of a lens can be assessed. For example, doubling the Dk/t does not double the amount of oxygen available.

Consumption values provide a more meaningful index of the corneal oxygen supply since these are direct linear estimates of the volume of oxygen metabolized and of the energy thereby delivered (Brennan, 2005). Figure 26.11 plots a mathematically derived relationship between consumption and the anterior corneal oxygen tension.

Comparison with Dk/t values and known swelling at these values enables further estimates of corneal swelling for various closed-eye oxygen tensions. This information is illustrated in Figure 26.12. Table 26.2 presents data for consumption values for various lens types under closed-eye conditions. It is evident that there are decreasing returns in overall consumption for increasing values of Dk/t.

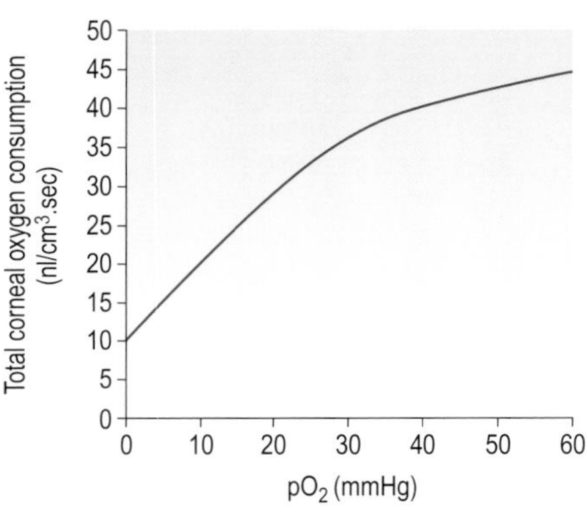

Figure 26.11 Variation in corneal oxygen consumption versus anterior corneal oxygen tension.

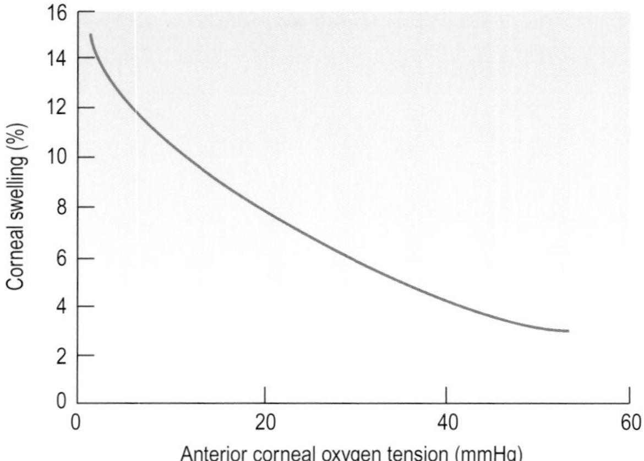

Figure 26.12 Variation in overnight corneal swelling versus anterior corneal oxygen tension.

Table 26.2 Oxygen consumption estimates for various lens types assuming minimum practical thickness for –3.00 D lenses during closed-eye wear

Lens type	Oxygen consumption (nl/cm³/s)
Low-water-content traditional hydrogel lens	21
Medium-water-content traditional hydrogel lens	30
High-water-content traditional hydrogel lens	31
Rigid lens: *Dk** 25	32
Rigid lens: *Dk* 50	40
Rigid lens: *Dk* 100	43
Silicone hydrogel: *Dk* 110	44
Silicone hydrogel: *Dk* 140	44
Silicone elastomer lens	45
No lens	45

* Barrer.

Although corneal oedema is the most-studied short-term response to closed-eye contact lens wear, two other acute effects are worthy of note – limbal hyperaemia and endothelial blebs. The extent of both limbal hyperaemia (Papas *et al.*, 1997) and endothelial blebs (Inagaki *et al.*, 2003; Brennan *et al.*, 2008) has been associated with oxygenation, and both conditions are reduced when lenses of high *Dk/t* are worn. The amount of limbal hyperaemia (Figure 26.13) may have clinical consequences (in that inflammatory episodes of the cornea are often associated with limbal hyperaemia), but the endothelial bleb response seems to be clinically inconsequential.

Chronic physiological changes

Over the years, researchers have diligently assembled an inventory of structural and functional changes in the anterior eye as a result of long-term extended contact lens wear. Many of these findings might be considered as harmless changes of physiological interest rather than clinically relevant pathological effects. The former category includes phenomena that are characterized by:

- A non-inflammatory nature.
- A lack of threat to vision.
- An absence of significance, unknown significance or limited significance when detected at a low level.

Long-term physiological changes have a modest impact on the rate of patient discontinuation from extended wear. It should be noted that these changes are not necessarily restricted to extended wear, and many of them are equally prevalent in daily wear. However, the presence of these changes may be indicative of a compromise to normal ocular function and thus may leave the eye more susceptible to other pathology, and to poor recovery following eye disease.

The following is a non-exhaustive list of changes that have been observed in humans during extended wear:

- Altered epithelial oxygen consumption.
- Altered epithelial cell size.
- Altered epithelial cell sloughing rate.
- Altered epithelial permeability.
- Increased epithelial fragility.
- Epithelial thinning.
- Microcystic oedema (Figure 26.14).
- Excess corneal staining (Figure 26.15).
- Stromal thinning.
- Stromal neovascularization (Figure 26.16).
- Endothelial polymegethism (Figure 26.17).
- Altered corneal shape.
- Reduced corneal sensitivity.
- Limbal injection.
- Eye redness.

There have also been studies that have documented alterations to the concentration of a wide range of aspects of tear composition, including cell types, protein levels and inflammatory components, and also altered ocular microbiota. Even corneal exhaustion – a syndrome characterized by lens intolerance, endothelial polymegethism and ongoing changes in corneal refraction and astigmatism – may be considered a severe physiological imbalance rather than a pathological state. Furthermore, animal studies have revealed

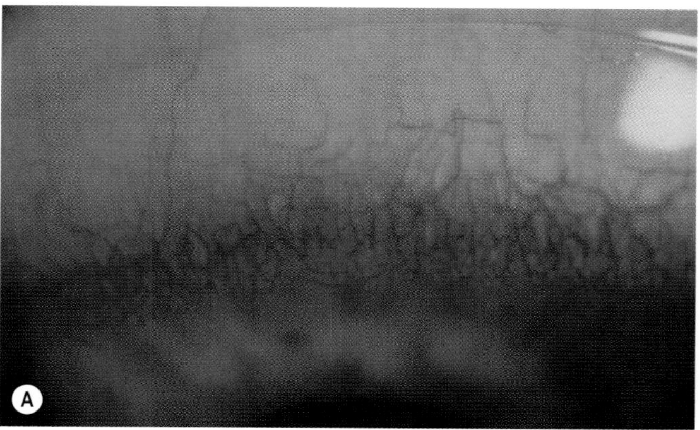

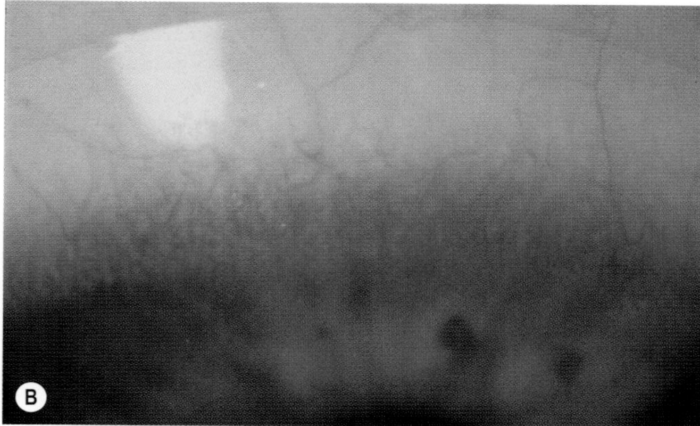

Figure 26.13 Demonstration of the effect of hypoxia on limbal hyperaemia. (A) Grade 2.2 limbal hyperaemia is evident in this patient wearing a 38% water content hydroxyethyl methacrylate (HEMA) contact lens in one eye. (B) The same patient is wearing a high-*Dk/t* silicone hydrogel contact lens in the other eye; the extent of limbal hyperaemia (grade 1.0) is much less than that in the eye wearing the HEMA lens.

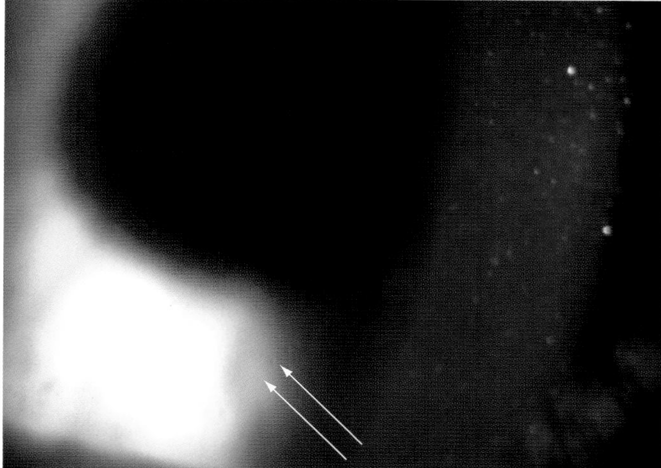

Figure 26.14 Two microcysts (arrows) can be observed at the lower pupil margin, to the left of the optic section in which extensive tear debris is highlighted.

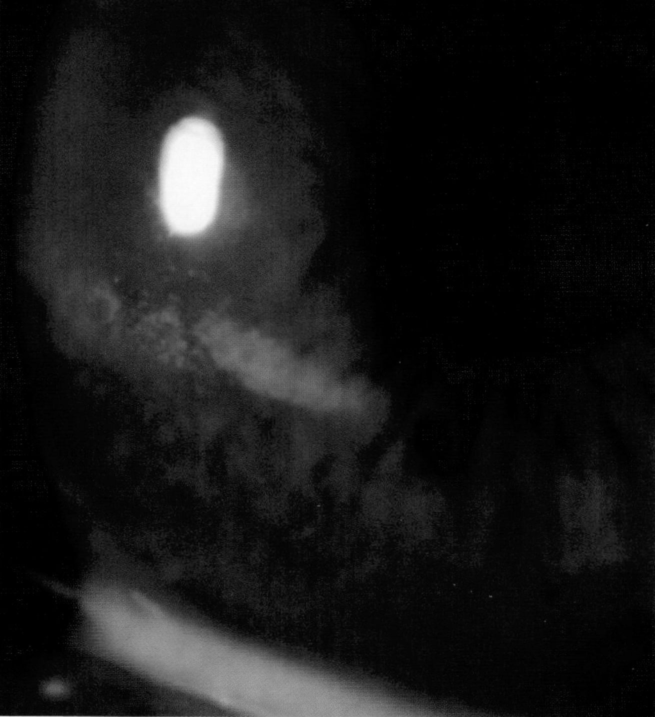

Figure 26.15 Contact lens-induced corneal staining.

changes in epithelial mitoses, adhesion, cellular junctional integrity, healing and cellular reserves of glycogen.

Hypoxia during closed-eye lens wear has been definitively linked to a great number of these corneal physiological changes. For example, the link between *Dk/t* and epithelial microcysts has been established in clinical trials. Evidence linking corneal neovascularization and endothelial polymegethism to chronic hypoxia is circumstantial but has widespread acceptance. Animal studies link hypoxia and low-*Dk/t* contact lenses with slower epithelial healing following injury, bacterial binding to the intact cornea and episodes of corneal infection.

The main template for managing long-term physiological problems with contact lens wear was the landmark 'Gothenburg study' by Holden *et al.* (1985). These authors investigated the effects of 5 years of unilateral extended wear in a sample of 27 patients using the contralateral eyes as a control. The physiological markers under study included epithelial oxygen uptake, epithelial thickness, epithelial microcysts, acute stromal oedema, chronic stromal thinning, endothelial polymegethism, and limbal and bulbar conjunctival hyperaemia. The cornea of the lens-wearing eye showed a 15% reduction in oxygen consumption, a 6% reduction in epithelial thickness, a 2.3% reduction in stromal thickness and a 22% increase in endothelial polymegethism. Epithelial metabolism recovered 1 month after wear, but the stromal and endothelial changes persisted for over 6 months. Patients with thinner corneas, higher endothelial cell densities and lower endothelial polymegethism before commencing lens wear showed fewer effects from contact lens wear. The study demonstrated that adverse physiological responses could be minimized by fitting lenses that were more regularly removed

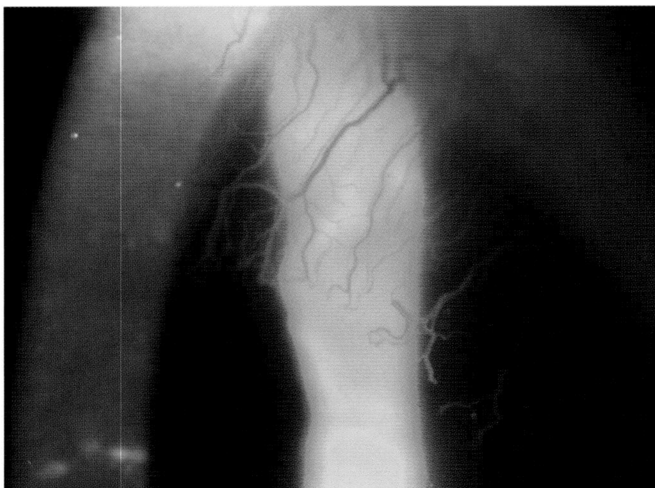

Figure 26.16 Hypoxia during contact lens wear is implicated in causing vascularization of the peripheral cornea.

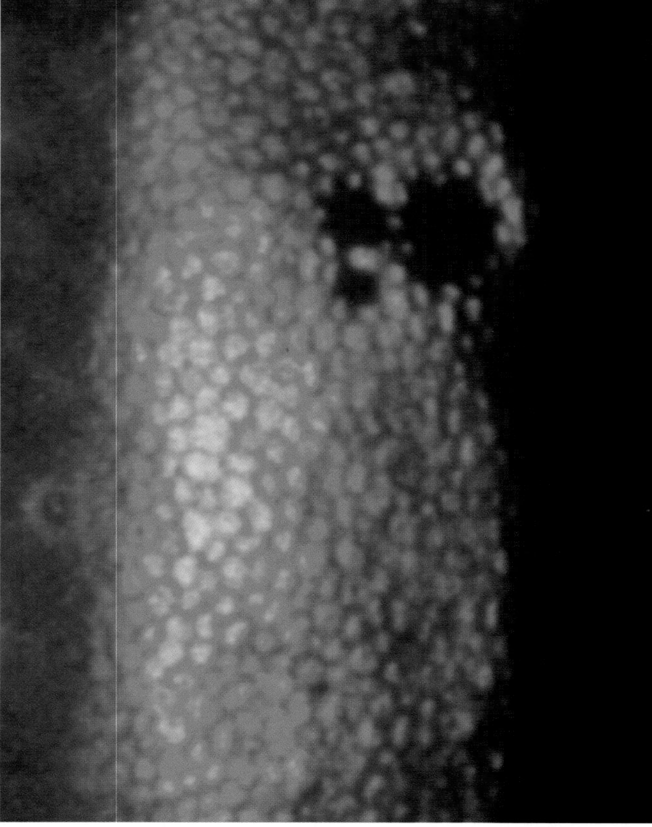

Figure 26.17 Specular reflection of the endothelium following extended wear of a traditional hydrogel lens, showing moderate polymegethism and general disruption as evidenced by the bright and dark patches.

from the eye, more frequently replaced, more mobile on the eye and were more permeable to oxygen. To some extent, these objectives have been met by silicone hydrogel lenses. In particular, their high oxygen transmissibility has largely relegated major corneal physiological change during contact lens wear to the position of a historical curiosity.

Mechanical effects

Rigid materials provide a range of positive effects when used for lens manufacture. These can include a stable front surface with accompanying optical benefits. The rigidity of the lens and the difference in shape between the posterior surface of the lens and the anterior cornea mean that a mismatch of shape occurs. This maintains a certain degree of tear pooling under the lens. With the blink there is a greater exchange of tears, which has the beneficial effect of flushing debris and bacteria away from the corneal surface and enhancing corneal oxygenation.

Notwithstanding the advantages described above, many problems arise because of the stiffness and size of rigid lenses. Discomfort is the principal reason for discontinuation with rigid lenses. Larger flexible lenses, which provide less interaction between the lid and lens edge, provide greater comfort, at least initially. Lens rigidity and size also play an important role in complications such as 3 and 9 o'clock corneal staining. Air bubbles beneath the lens can be trapped against the cornea, producing an effect known as 'dimple veiling'. Pressure from the eyelid during sleep and settling of the lens can lead to close alignment of the posterior lens profile and the cornea, resulting in a depletion of the postlens tear film and ultimately in lens binding, corneal distortion and lens edge imprint in the cornea.

Soft lenses contrast with rigid materials in that they drape across the cornea and thus show a high degree of conformity to corneal shape. This has the effect of minimizing postlens tear film thickness. The thinness of the postlens tear layer, along with the size of the lens and small amounts of lateral movement during the blink, limits the extent of tear exchange beneath soft lenses. During sleep, in particular, the lenses may become immobile, trapping a stagnant tear layer at the corneal surface. It may take more than a few minutes following eye opening for lenses to recover mobility, although binding does not occur to the same extent as observed with rigid lenses. Lack of tear exchange means that sloughed cells, metabolic byproducts, trapped incidental tear debris and bacteria may be kept in contact with the corneal surface, presenting the opportunity for inflammatory and infectious conditions.

Direct pressure from soft lenses may play a role in the formation of some epithelial defects, which manifest as fluorescein staining. In particular, superior epithelial arcuate lesions (SEALs) may be induced by physical interaction of the lens surface with the superior region of the cornea (Figure 26.18). There is some evidence that these lesions occur more commonly where lid pressure is greater, such as in Asian eyes, thereby increasing the physical effect of the lens. The mechanical properties of silicone hydrogel lenses have also directed attention to the issue of translucent postlens debris, sometimes referred to as 'mucin balls' (Figure 26.19). Although present with traditional hydrogel materials, these phenomena occur frequently with silicone hydrogel lenses. The bodies appear to form as a result of shear forces related to material stiffness and perhaps specific surface properties of the lenses. This debris has not been specifically associated with adverse reactions and the effects appear limited to minor indentations of the epithelial surface.

Surface friction and lens edge rubbing can lead to palpebral conjunctival changes, including hyperaemia and oedema. In association with possible antigenic effects of lens deposition, this can also lead to the condition of contact lens-associated papillary conjunctivitis (CLPC: Figure 26.20). Traditional hydrogel lenses and, to a lesser extent, rigid lenses are also associated with the development of CLPC. More is presented on this condition below.

Non-infectious inflammatory events

While infectious keratitis is most often cited as the reason for failure of extended wear in the 1980s, the high incidence of non-infectious inflammatory events probably contributed strongly to practitioner aversion to this mode of wear. Although these events are not sight-threatening, they constitute a sufficiently acute response to cause interruption or even termination of extended lens wear. Corneal inflammation is characterized by the migration and accumulation of inflammatory cells into the epithelial and anterior stromal space; such events are collectively termed 'corneal infiltrative events' (CIEs).

There has recently been a significant shift in thinking in relation to the clinical evaluation of CIEs (Efron and Morgan, 2006a). In particular, there has been a shift away from the approach of classifying CIEs into various subtypes, such as the so-called contact lens-associated acute red eye and contact lens peripheral ulcer (Sweeney *et al.*, 2003). The new approach is to consider all CIEs as part of a disease continuum, and to make clinical decisions based upon an overall assessment of the severity of the condition (Efron and Morgan, 2006a). The reason for this shift in approach is that there is so much overlap in the clinical presentations of the various supposed subtypes of CIE that clinical decision making based on such schemes is virtually impossible (Efron and Morgan, 2006b).

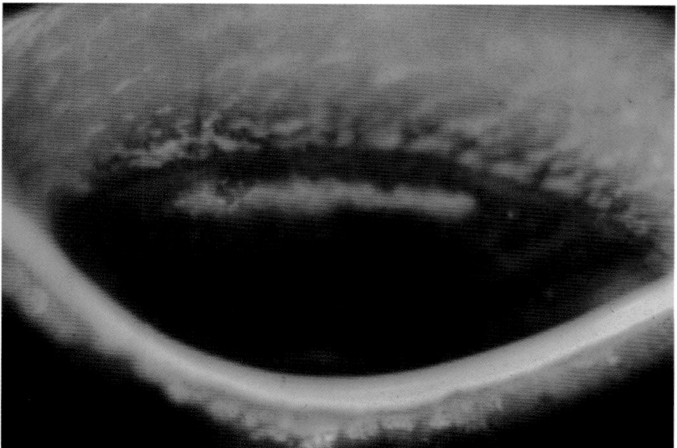

Figure 26.18 Superior arcuate epithelial lesions may occur during wear of both traditional hydrogels and silicone hydrogel contact lenses in extended wear. (Courtesy of Bausch & Lomb Photo Library (www.bausch.com).)

The simple reality is that, in the early stages of symptomatic CIE, it is not possible to tell whether the condition is indeed a non-infectious CIE or an early-stage microbial keratitis. The previous approach of attempting to classify a CIE as a contact lens-associated acute red eye and contact lens peripheral ulcer was potentially dangerous, because the typical supposed clinical advice attached to such diagnoses was 'wait and see'. There are a number of recorded cases in the literature where this 'wait and see' approach was adopted, and the condition developed into a serious microbial keratitis (Sweeney *et al.*, 2003). Thus, a non-infectious CIE is a condition that can only be labelled as such towards the end of the natural history of the disease process. From a clinical perspective, if a contact lens wearer presents with ocular discomfort and an infiltrative event is observed in the cornea, the condition must be considered to be a potential case of microbial keratitis, and managed accordingly.

CLPC was possibly the major hindrance to successful extended wear with early hydrogel lenses. This is a chronic inflammatory reaction of the palpebral conjunctiva, resembling vernal conjunctivitis but directly related to contact lens wear (see Chapter 40 for more details). CLPC is observed in patients wearing both conventional hydrogel and silicone hydrogel extended-wear lenses (Fonn *et al.*, 2002).

Superior limbic keratoconjunctivitis was an infrequent adverse reaction to hydrogel lens extended wear in the early 1980s. It was characterized by inflammation of the superior cornea with infiltrates and pannus (see Chapter

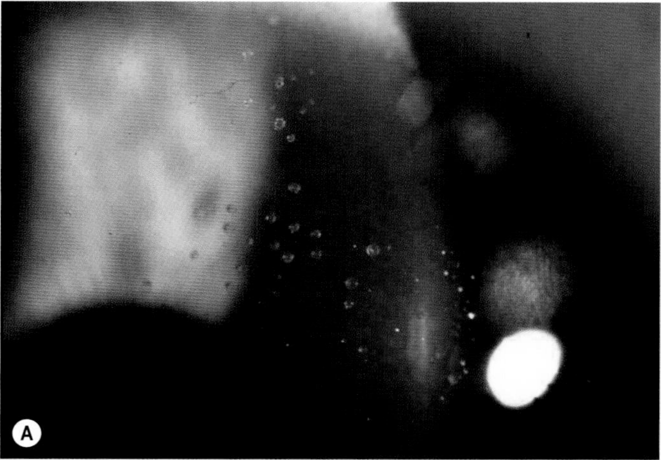

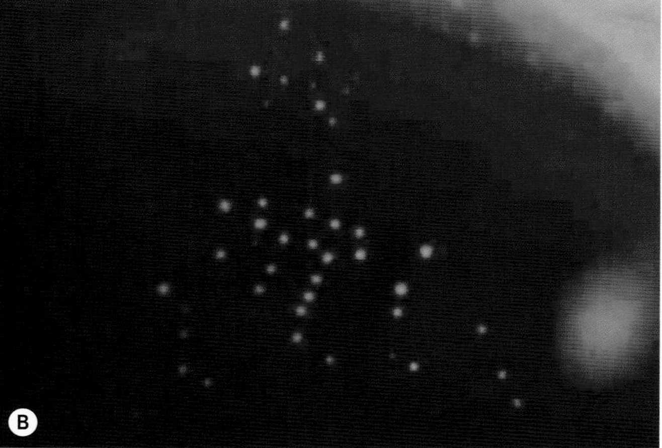

Figure 26.19 Translucent spheroidal postlens debris, referred to as 'mucin balls', is a common slit-lamp finding with silicone hydrogen lens wear. (A) Mucin balls observed behind the lens. (B) After lens removal, most of the mucin balls are washed away, but some remain. Fluorescein stains the remaining mucin balls, and fills epithelial indentations created by the mucin balls that were subsequently washed away.

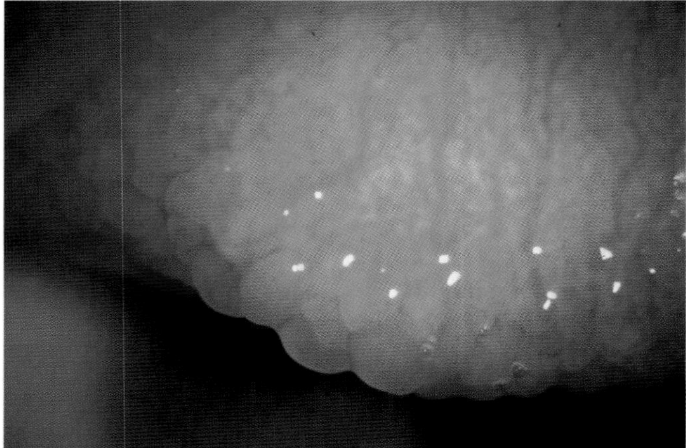

Figure 26.20 Both mechanical and hypersensitivity responses to lens deposits can lead to contact lens-related papillary conjunctivitis.

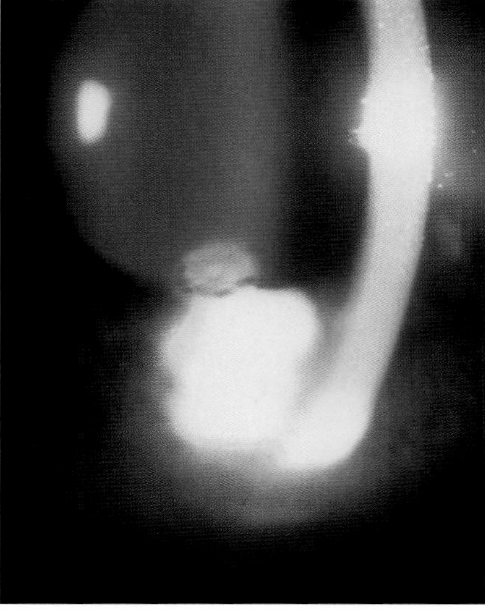

Figure 26.21 Microbial keratitis is the most concerning feature of extended contact lens wear. This picture shows a *Pseudomonas* infection.

40). The reaction appeared to be largely due to an allergic response to thimerosal preservatives used in older lens maintenance systems. The advent of hydrogen peroxide and later non-thimerosal-based, multipurpose solutions seems to have largely eliminated this problem.

Infectious corneal ulceration

Infectious corneal ulceration occurs with higher frequency in contact lens wearers (Figure 26.21) than non-lens-wearers. The infection can lead to tissue necrosis and massive inflammation. *Pseudomonas* and *Serratia* species are the more commonly isolated bacteria from infectious corneal ulcers in extended-wear patients. In tropical regions, fungi may be a more common pathogen. Although viral and chlamydial keratoconjunctivitis occurs in contact lens wearers, it is not typically associated with the use of the lenses. Microbial keratitis causes severe pain, photophobia and distress, and in some cases vision loss. These problems were sensationalized by the lay press with early hydrogel extended wear. Numerous cases of legal action were initiated. The reported success of the early trials in the light of later reports of a raised incidence of infectious keratitis with extended wear is not surprising given the rarity of infection. Despite this low incidence, the large number of people adopting extended wear led to a disturbingly high frequency of hospital admissions with contact lens-related infections. The problem came to the attention of authorities who described it as a 'significant, preventable, public health problem'.

A major epidemiological study, sponsored by the Contact Lens Institute in the USA, determined that the incidence of clinically diagnosed infectious keratitis for daily-wear and extended-wear traditional hydrogel lenses was approximately 4 and 20, respectively, per 10 000 wearers per year (Poggio *et al.*, 1989). Subsequent studies have confirmed that extended wear entails a higher relative risk than daily wear of traditional hydrogel materials, whether worn in disposable or conventional mode (Cheng *et al.*, 1999). Re-examination of the methods of various epidemiological studies has highlighted a certain amount of confusion in the estimates of relative risk and incidence of contact lens-related corneal infections. However, the case reports and epidemiological studies identified a number of risk factors for keratitis. These included handling of lenses, duration of uninterrupted wear, poor lens care and maintenance, smoking, gender and socioeconomic group.

Lens *Dk*/*t* was not specifically identified as a risk factor in the early epidemiological studies because all these reports involved the use of lenses that are relatively impermeable to oxygen (*Dk*/*t* 30 Barrer/cm). It was hoped that the introduction of silicone hydrogel lenses for continuous wear would be accompanied by a reduced risk of infection. Epidemiological studies showed that the incidence of microbial keratitis associated with continuous wear of silicone hydrogel lenses remains close to 20 per 10 000 wearers per year and that the risk remains several times higher than that with daily wear of any lens type (Morgan *et al.*, 2005; Schein *et al.*, 2005; Stapleton *et al.*, 2008). In short, high-*Dk/t* lenses did not prove to be the saviour of continuous wear.

Clinical extended-wear practice

Is extended wear safe?

Community and professional opinion determined that the rate and relative risk of microbial keratitis with continuous wear quoted above were unacceptable in 1989. Despite the publication of similar figures with silicone hydrogel lenses, continuous wear of silicone hydrogel lenses continued to be pursued. Are there additional considerations that might have made a difference to prescribing rates with silicone hydrogel lenses?

There is a reasonable basis for arguing that the concern over the rate of infection with traditional hydrogel extended wear has been overstated and that the risk–benefit equation has not been adequately addressed (Brennan and Coles,

1997). Furthermore, our understanding of the risk factors for infection has increased because of the publicity and studies surrounding these adverse events, with the result that better education of practitioners and patients can minimize the threat to vision. In this circumstance, an infection rate with silicone hydrogel lenses that matches that with traditional hydrogels may be reasonable considering the benefits that extended wear offers in terms of improving other aspects of ocular health (e.g. eliminating pathology relating to hypoxia) and patient convenience.

Studies investigating contact lens-related infection have used a clinical case definition, and commonly fewer than half of the cases yield positive cultures. Furthermore, those that yield a negative culture or were not cultured are known to be associated with less impact on visual outcome. Figure 26.22 illustrates the culture status of ocular infections quoted in various publications and the proportion of these that can be attributed to vision loss with extended wear of contact lenses.

Vision loss of two lines of acuity or more occurs in only 10–20% of patients with microbial keratitis (Nilsson and Montan, 1994; Cheng *et al.*, 1999). This places the rate of vision loss at about 1 in 2500 to 1 in 5000 per annum. On a comparable basis, refractive surgery is some 10 times more likely to lead to substantial vision loss over a decade (Figure 26.23). The dangers of extended wear seem difficult to reconcile with the public acceptance of procedures such as refractive surgery.

Another commonly used argument against extended wear is that the risk of suffering a microbial keratitis is higher than that with daily wear. However, daily wear is not a risk-free venture. The relative risk of corneal infection from daily wear of contact lenses is about 60–80 times that of members of western society without any predisposing factors. Sleeping in contact lenses adds a further risk, but only five times that of daily wear.

History has taught us some important techniques for avoiding detrimental outcomes with extended wear. One of the important factors identified by early epidemiological studies was the increased risk associated with longer periods of uninterrupted wear. For this reason, the recommended wearing time for extended wear was reduced to 7 days in the USA in 1989. Adopting this conservative approach is likely to maintain safer extended wear. Other experts advocated that decreased handling by patients – who remove lenses from the eye less frequently – leads to decreased complications, and therefore recommend 30 days between lens removal dates with silicone hydrogel lenses. In addition to the avoidance of the risk factors mentioned above, the accurate diagnosis of corneal infection, a conservative approach to care, the instigation of timely treatment, and improved patient and practitioner education together mean that infections are more likely to be diagnosed and treated expeditiously, leading to less vision loss.

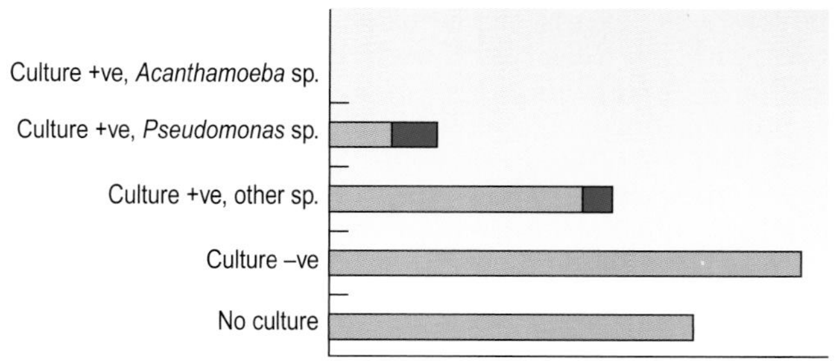

Figure 26.22 Relative rates of different culture results to suspected corneal infections. The dark blue section details those that are likely to cause substantial vision loss.

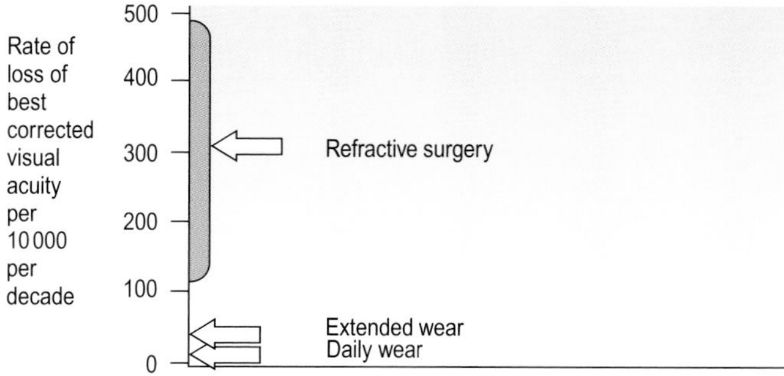

Figure 26.23 Projected rate of substantial vision loss for various refractive options over a 10-year period.

Application of continuous wear in practice

Incorporating continuous wear into contact lens practice should be a proactive management decision. A number of systems should to be set in place, involving support staff, documentation and emergency precautions. In particular, the practitioner should provide the patient with a document disclosing fully the risks of continuous wear, and informed consent should be obtained from the patient. Although it is not necessary to purchase additional equipment, practitioners should obtain grading scales to assess the severity of ocular complications of extended lens wear. Practitioners may also wish to adopt a scoring system for assessing the severity of CIEs (Aasuri *et al.*, 2003). Twenty-four-hour access to care is also considered mandatory by many experts.

The current standard for continuous wear is to fit a highly permeable lens, most specifically a silicone hydrogel lens, or in certain circumstances a rigid lens. Fitting patients with traditional hydrogel materials for continuous wear is considered inappropriate and practitioners are strongly advised against this.

A most important component of continuous-wear practice is the diagnosis and management of adverse events. Below is a discussion on the significant adverse events that may be observed during continuous wear, and a management plan for dealing with these problems.

Managing extended-wear complications

Success in continuous-wear practice relies on a number of factors, the most important of which is diagnosing and managing adverse reactions. Details of the pathogenesis

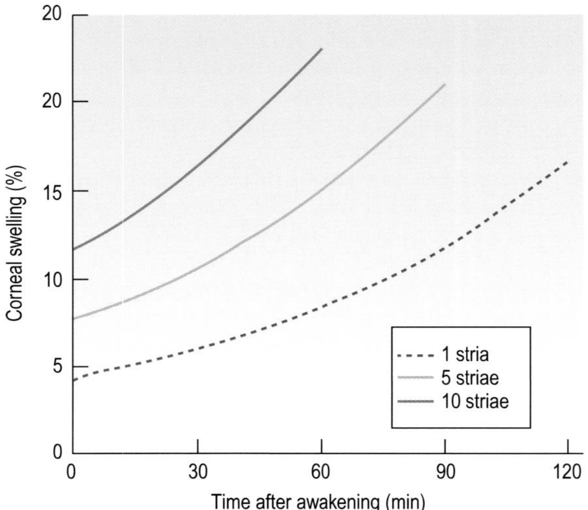

Figure 26.24 Likely overnight oedema for a specific number of visible striae at a given time after eye opening.

and risk factors are presented above. The following sections provide details of symptomatology, signs, differential diagnosis and a management plan. One of the encouraging features of this list is that the number of serious adverse events likely with continuous wear is small.

Acute responses

There is widespread belief that the individual with chronic oedema is at risk of developing further complications and ultimately failure with continuous wear. Certainly, an individual wearing a contact lens that provides a higher mean swelling in the population is more likely to suffer from hypoxic complications. Oedema assessment is difficult in practice without the aid of an optical pachymeter, an Orbscan instrument or an ultrasonic pachymeter, and few contact lens practices have ready access to such equipment. An alternative method of assessing the oedema level is by observing striae and endothelial folds. Figure 26.24 plots the likely amount of overnight oedema present when striae are observed at a given time after awakening, based upon projections from known levels of striae with oedema, and studies examining the rate of corneal deswelling.

Chronic physiological stress

The likelihood of chronic physiological stress can be predicted from the short-term oedema response to lens wear. However, as mentioned above, it is sometimes difficult to make an assessment of the oedema by examination later in the day. Evaluation of the extent of limbal hyperaemia is another technique by which the oxygenation can be assessed, although this response is not specific to hypoxia.

One suitable method for assessing chronic hypoxia is to evaluate the epithelial microcyst response. It is important to note that microcysts are considerably smaller than vacuoles and mucin balls, which are commonly confused with microcysts. Observation is best achieved by looking in marginal retroillumination with the focus at the level of the tear film such that small particles within the tears can be observed. During the blink, the small particles that do not move should be examined closely for reversed illumination. Once identified, the total number of microcysts in the cornea should be estimated. With a lens of adequate oxygen transmissibility, there should be no more than 10 microcysts present.

Another suitable method to assess long-term physiological compromise is endothelial evaluation. Chronic hypoxic stress is associated with altered endothelial regularity, and regular examination of the endothelium allows a practitioner to grade successfully different levels of anomaly (which must be related to patient age). Grade 2 endothelial irregularity in a patient under 30 years of age may be a precursor to further adverse corneal changes. Signs indicating the presence of chronic physiological stress should be managed by refitting with a silicone hydrogel lens.

Microbial keratitis

Infectious ulcerative keratitis consists of invasion and colonization of the corneal epithelial and stromal tissue by a pathogenic microorganism. This problem is the only condition associated with continuous wear that is a serious threat to vision and the long-term health of the eye.

Symptomatically, the patient is aware of rapidly developing irritation, which quickly progresses to severe pain, both within the eye and around the periorbital region. Photophobia and reflex lacrimation are present, and aversion to light is particularly strong. On removal of the contact lens, the pain does not subside. The intensity of the pain leads the patient to seek assistance, possibly at a medical clinic or at an emergency room. On presentation, the patient will be in obvious distress. Ocular examination shows the ulcer as an epithelial defect with underlying stromal infiltrate. Small or large regions of the cornea may be involved, and the surrounding conjunctiva will be red and inflamed. There may be obvious mucopurulent discharge. As the disease progresses, the anterior chamber may become involved. Aqueous flare may be observed, and a hypopyon can form in very severe cases.

As discussed previously, in the early stages of the disease process, microbial keratitis can be confused with other non-infectious CIEs. Because of the potential for an adverse outcome, practitioners are advised to adopt the conservative approach of considering all such conditions as infectious until proven otherwise. In advanced stages, microbial keratitis is typically characterized by intense pain and photophobia that do not resolve with lens removal. The extent of pain is such that the patient frequently presents to the emergency room with a wet towel covering the eye. Other key features evident with a severe infection are the presence of epithelial defect, greater likelihood of discharge and corneal infiltrates. The presence of anterior-chamber reaction or mucopurulent discharge in association with these other signs should be treated as pathognomonic of an infectious corneal condition.

All eyes with suspected microbial keratitis should be cultured and receive immediate medical treatment. The patient may need to be hospitalized. The condition should be assumed to be a Gram-negative bacterial infection, and hourly application of antibiosis should be instigated. Nine out of 10 ulcers diagnosed as infectious resolve without serious loss of vision, but the key to this successful outcome is the speed with which treatment is instigated.

Papillary conjunctivitis

This common contact lens complication involves invasion of the palpebral conjunctiva by inflammatory cells, including mast cells, eosinophils and basophils. It can occur with any type of lens wear but will be more common in extended wear of hydrogel lenses.

The patient reports gradual onset of itchy eyes, awareness of excessive lens movement, lens deposition, lacrimation and possibly a stringy discharge. These signs will also be evident to the practitioner. On lid eversion, the most pronounced effect will be enlarged conjunctival papillae across the tarsal conjunctival plate.

Early treatment of the condition with a mast cell stabilizer may enable the patient to continue with extended or continuous wear. If the treatment is unsuccessful, reversion to daily wear may be necessary. Use of daily disposable lenses is a useful alternative. The condition will resolve over a period of weeks without any consequence to vision.

Superior epithelial arcuate lesions

SEALs present as regions of corneal epithelial abrasion which, as the name suggests, are located in the superior region of the cornea under the top lid. The stain is regularly punctate but may coalesce and takes on an arcuate shape, parallel to the limbus. The borders of the region of staining may be slightly raised. Occasionally there may be a diffuse infiltrate underlying the lesion. The condition may be more prevalent in Asian eyes.

Patients may be unaware of the problem and sometimes present with the condition at a routine follow-up examination. Others may report discomfort consisting of lens awareness and foreign-body sensation. The condition is self-limiting and will subside following lens removal. It is inadvisable to allow a patient with SEALs to continue with continuous wear using the offending lens type. Refitting with a lens of different geometry or lower modulus will often solve the problem. Discontinuing continuous wear is recommended if a change of lens type fails to resolve the inflammation.

Conclusions

While continuous contact lens wear remains attractive to the population, ongoing concerns about microbial keratitis mean this modality should be approached with caution. Practitioners contemplating a continuous-wear practice should carefully plan their management of lens wearers with this risk in mind. Silicone-containing hydrogel contact lenses should preferentially be used for continuous wear because of their high Dk/t and associated benefits for corneal health.

References

Aasuri, M. K., Venkata, N. and Kumar, V. M. (2003) Differential diagnosis of microbial keratitis and contact lens-induced peripheral ulcer. *Eye Contact Lens,* **29**(1 Suppl), S60–S62.

Binder, P. S. (1983) Myopic extended wear with the Hydrocurve II soft contact lens. *Ophthalmology,* **90,** 623–626.

Boswall, G. J., Ehlers, W. H., Luistro, A. *et al.* (1993) A comparison of conventional and disposable extended wear contact lenses. *Contact Lens Assoc. Ophthalmol. J.,* **19,** 158–165.

Brennan, N. A. (2005) Beyond flux: total corneal oxygen consumption as an index of corneal oxygenation during contact lens wear. *Optom. Vis. Sci.,* **82,** 467–472.

Brennan, N. A. and Coles, M-L. C. (1997) Extended wear in perspective. *Optom. Vis. Sci.,* **74,** 609–623.

Brennan, N. A., Coles, M. L. C., Levy, B. *et al.* (2002) One-Year prospective clinical trial of balafilcon A (PureVision) silicone-hydrogel contact lenses used on a 30-Day continuous wear schedule. *Ophthalmol.,* **109,** 1172–1177.

Brennan, N. A., Coles, M. L., Connor, H. R. *et al.,* (2008) Short-term corneal endothelial response to wear of silicone-hydrogel contact lenses in East Asian eyes. *Eye Contact Lens,* **34,** 317–321.

Cheng, K. H., Leung, S. L., Hoekman, H. W. *et al.* (1999) Incidence of contact-lens-associated microbial keratitis and its related morbidity. *Lancet,* **354,** 181–185.

Covey, M., Sweeney, D. F., Terry, R. *et al.* (2001) Hypoxic effects on the anterior eye of high-*Dk* soft contact lens wearers are negligible. *Optom. Vis. Sci.,* **78,** 95–99.

Cox, I., Zantos, S. G. and Orsborn, G. N. (1990) The overnight corneal swelling responses of non-wear, daily wear, and extended wear soft lens patients. *Int. Contact Lens Clin.,* **17,** 134–137.

Cutter, G. R., Chalmers, R. L. and Roseman, M. (1996) The clinical presentation, prevalence, and risk factors of focal corneal infiltrates in soft contact lens wearers. *Contact Lens Assoc. Ophthalmol. J.,* **22,** 30–36.

Efron, N. and Morgan, P. B. (2006a) Can subtypes of contact lens-associated corneal infiltrative events be clinically differentiated? *Cornea,* **25,** 540–544.

Efron, N. and Morgan, P. B. (2006b) Rethinking contact lens associated keratitis. *Clin. Exp. Optom.,* **89,** 280–298.

Fonn, D., MacDonald, K. E., Richter, D. *et al.* (2002) The ocular response to extended wear of a high *Dk* silicone hydrogel contact lens. *Clin. Exp. Optom.,* **85,** 176–182.

Holden, B. A. and Mertz, G. W. (1984) Critical oxygen levels to avoid corneal edema for daily and extended wear contact lenses. *Invest. Ophthalmol. Vis. Sci.,* **25,** 1161–1167.

Holden, B. A., Mertz, G. W. and McNally, J. J. (1983) Corneal swelling response to contact lenses worn under extended wear conditions. *Invest. Ophthalmol. Vis. Sci.,* **24,** 218–226.

Holden, B. A., Sweeney, D. F., Vannas, A. *et al.* (1985) Effects of long-term extended contact lens wear on the human cornea. *Invest. Ophthalmol. Vis. Sci.,* **26,** 1489–1501.

Inagaki, Y., Akahori, A., Sugimoto, K. *et al.* (2003) Comparison of corneal endothelial bleb formation and disappearance processes between rigid gas-permeable and soft contact lenses in three classes of *Dk*/l. *Eye Contact Lens,* **29,** 234–237.

Kotow, M., Holden, B. A. and Grant, T. (1987) The value of regular replacement of low water content contact lenses for extended wear. *J. Am. Optom. Assoc.,* **58,** 461–464.

Lamer, L. (1983) Extended wear contact lenses for myopes. A follow-up study of 400 cases. *Ophthalmology,* **90,** 156–161.

Maehara, J. R. and Kastl, P. R. (1994) Rigid gas permeable extended wear. *Contact Lens Assoc. Ophthalmol. J.,* **20,** 139–143.

Morgan, P. B., Efron, N., Hill, E. A. *et al.* (2005) Incidence of keratitis of varying severity among contact lens wearers. *Br. J. Ophthalmol.,* **89,** 430–436.

Morgan, P. B., Woods, C. A., Tranoudis, I. G. *et al.* (2009) International contact lens prescribing in 2008. *Contact Lens Spectrum,* **24**(2), 28–32.

Nilsson, S. E. G. and Montan, P. G. (1994) The annualized incidence of contact lens induced keratitis in Sweden and its relation to lens type and wear schedule: results of a 3-month prospective study. *Contact Lens Assoc. Ophthalmol. J.* **20,** 225–230.

Orsborn, G. N. and Zantos, S. G. (1989) Practitioner survey: management of dry-eye symptoms in soft lens wearers. *Contact Lens Spectrum,* **4,** 23–26.

Papas, E. B., Vajdic, C. M., Austen, R. *et al.* (1997) High-oxygen-transmissibility soft contact lenses do not induce limbal hyperaemia. *Curr. Eye Res.,* **16,** 942–948.

Poggio, E. C., Glynn, R. K., Schein, O. D. *et al.* (1989) The incidence of ulcerative keratitis among users of daily-wear and extended-wear soft contact lenses. *N. Eng. J. Med.,* **321,** 779–783.

Radford, C. F., Minassian, D., Dart, J. K. *et al.* (2009) Risk factors for nonulcerative contact lens complications in an ophthalmic accident and emergency department: a case-control study. *Ophthalmology,* **116,** 385–392.

Schein, O. D., McNally, J. J., Katz, J. *et al.* (2005) The incidence of microbial keratitis among wearers of a 30-day silicone hydrogel extended-wear contact lens. *Ophthalmology,* **112,** 2172–2179.

Solomon, O. D. (1996) Corneal stress test for extended wear. *Contact Lens Assoc. Ophthalmol. J.,* **22,** 75–78.

Stapleton, F., Lakshmi, K. R., Kumar, S. *et al.* (1998) Overnight corneal swelling in symptomatic and asymptomatic contact lens wearers. *Contact Lens Assoc. Ophthalmol. J.,* **24,** 169–174.

Stapleton, F., Keay, L., Edwards, K. *et al.* (2008) The incidence of contact lens-related microbial keratitis in Australia. *Ophthalmology,* **115,** 1655–1662.

Sweeney, D. F., Jalbert, I., Covey, M. *et al.* (2003) Clinical characterization of corneal infiltrative events observed with soft contact lens wear. *Cornea,* **22,** 435–442.

CHAPTER 27

Sport

Nathan Efron

Introduction

Sport and recreation are often cited as the reason for seeking contact lenses. Frequent-replacement lenses, and even daily disposable lenses, are now available in silicone hydrogel materials in powers that will correct almost all potential wearers. As a result, many of the problems encountered by sportspersons wishing to wear contact lenses in the past can now be overcome.

With modern contact lens technology, there is no reason why an ametropic sportsperson cannot compete with a normally sighted opponent on an equal basis from the standpoint of visual function. This chapter presents an overview of factors that should be considered when prescribing contact lenses for those participating in various sports (Figure 27.1).

Deciding on the best form of correction

The primary vision correction options are: soft contact lenses, rigid contact lenses, orthokeratology, refractive surgery or spectacles. Scleral lenses are sometimes prescribed, but usually only in very demanding circumstances; they will therefore not be considered in detail in this section (see Chapter 23).

Refractive surgery

Refractive surgery represents the most radical alternative. The benefits are that no correction needs to be worn for sport; problems of lens loss, lens movement and lens maintenance are all avoided. Whilst it might seem an obvious solution, laser correction is not without potential drawbacks. Corneal haze and regression can lead to less than perfect visual acuity. There is also potential for flap damage in patients who have had laser *in situ* keratomileusis (LASIK). Tetz *et al.* (2007) reported on a case where the left eye of a 39-year-old man was struck by the finger of a friend while the two were practising karate, resulting in loss of the flap, which occurred 3 years and 5 months after LASIK. Booth and Koch (2003) noted that a 38-year-old man sustained a dislocated flap after being struck in the left eye with a football more than 30 months after uneventful LASIK. These cases illustrate the need for LASIK patients to wear protective eyewear when participating in contact sports.

A comparison of the key features of the primary options for vision correction for sport is presented in Table 27.1.

Do contact lenses enhance sporting performance?

Some clinicians have offered the anecdotal opinion that, compared to spectacles, contact lenses enhance visual skills of the ametropic sportsperson; however, properly controlled clinical trials do not support these claims. Schnider *et al.* (1993) applied a battery of tests (including measurement of high- and low-contrast visual acuity, assessment of lens fit and subjective assessment of visual performance) to ametropic athletes wearing their spectacle correction versus low-water-content soft contact lenses. The authors found that, although contact lenses did not offer a measurable advantage over spectacles in terms of visual performance under these testing conditions, the psychological advantages were significant, and in this way contact lenses may enhance overall sports-oriented visual performance.

There have been suggestions that specially tinted contact lenses can enhance sporting performance. For example, Erickson *et al.* (2009) have demonstrated that Maxsight Amber lenses (50% visible light transmission) and Gray-Green lenses (36% visible light transmission) provide better contrast discrimination in bright sunlight, better contrast discrimination when alternating between bright and shaded target conditions, better speed of visual recovery in bright sunlight and better overall visual performance in bright and shaded target conditions compared with clear lenses. However, the extent to which these visual performance attributes translate to enhanced sport performance is less clear (Porisch, 2007). The prescription of performance-enhancing tinted contact lenses for sport is discussed further in Chapter 24.

DOI: 10.1016/B978-0-7506-8869-7.00027-6

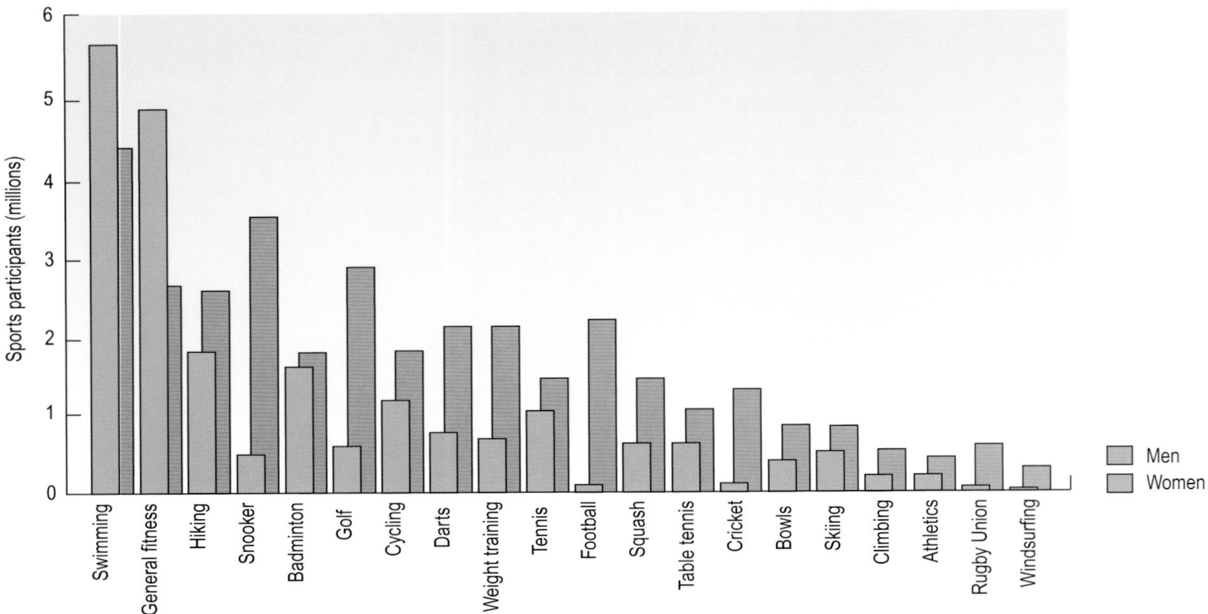

Figure 27.1 Number of men and women participating in the 20 most popular sports in the UK.

Environmental and physical constraints

The choice of contact lens for use in a given sport must be made with reference to the length of time that it takes to play the sport, the environment in which it is played and the general physical demands of the sport. The majority of sports are completed within 2 hours, which equates to a total period of lens wear of 4 hours, allowing for pre- and post-match activity during which lens insertion and removal would be impractical and/or undesirable. Even when these factors are understood, the lens of first choice may not be obvious. The most appropriate lens is sometimes only determined by trial and error.

Environmental conditions

Contact lens wear is often associated with signs and symptoms of ocular dryness. These drying effects can be exacerbated by certain environmental factors, such as low humidity, wind and visual tasks. Ousler *et al.* (2008) found that wearing silicone hydrogel contact lenses may provide greater relief of subjective ocular discomfort in adverse environmental conditions than that afforded by both the habitual lenses of contact lens wearers or with no contact lens wear. Sports are played in almost every environment. Climatic conditions play a role in disease severity and causative organism in contact lens-related microbial keratitis and therefore have implications for practitioners involved in contact lens care of wearers who may be engaging in sporting activities in the tropics (Stapleton *et al.*, 2007). The following environmental conditions are considered since they will directly affect the choice of lens for the sportsperson.

Cold

Many sports take place in cold environments, typically in close proximity to ice and snow. Because of the intrinsic temperature of the eye and tear film (33°C), contact lenses cannot freeze up in the eye. In an extensive survey of 105 contact lens wearers who were frequently engaged in cold-weather sports, Socks (1983) found no evidence of eye injury or disease. 'Eye redness' was the most common complaint of rigid lens wearers; soft lens wearers most frequently complained of slightly reduced vision. Large-diameter, medium-water-content or silicone hydrogel soft lenses may provide the best results in cold conditions.

Altitude

The ability of oxygen to reach the cornea through a contact lens, which is a key prerequisite to sustain good ocular health during lens wear, is a function of the oxygen transmissibility of the contact lens and the partial pressure of oxygen in the atmosphere. This argument is particularly relevant to sports which are played at altitude. The partial pressure of oxygen in the atmosphere decreases with altitude, which effectively means that the tolerance of the eye to a lens of given oxygen performance will decrease with increasing altitude. In addition, temperature falls about 10°C per 1500 m increase in altitude to a minimum of −50°C; the effects of extreme cold on the cornea were dealt with in the previous section. There appears to be a significant connection between the level of available oxygen during contact lens wear and improved patient symptoms of comfort, including dryness (Dillehay, 2007). In view of the rarified oxygen atmosphere at high altitude, and the length of time lenses may be worn, high-oxygen-performance silicone hydrogel lenses are indicated.

Table 27.1 Comparison of different forms of vision correction for the sportsperson

Characteristic	Soft lenses	Rigid lenses	Orthokeratology	Spectacles lenses	Refractive surgery
Field of view	Full	Full	Full	Restricted	Full
Stability of vision (post-blink)	Excellent	Good	Excellent	Excellent	Excellent
Glare	None	In low light	None	None	Some post-surgery
Glare protection tint possible	Cosmetic only	No	No	Yes	N/A
Ultraviolet protection possible	Yes	Yes	No	Yes	N/A
Initial comfort	Good	Poor	Fair	Good	Fair
Long-term comfort	Good	Good	Excellent	Good	Excellent
Adaptation required	Very little	Yes	Yes	Sometimes	N/A
Suitability for intermittent use	Yes	Not usually	No	Yes	No
Disposability viable	Yes	No	N/A	No	N/A
Risk of loss	Low	Moderate	N/A	Low	N/A
Risk of dislodgement during wear	Low	Moderate	Nil	High	N/A
Risk of damage during wear	Low	Low	Nil	High	Moderate (LASIK flap mislocation)
Risk of damage with handling	High	Low	Low	Low	N/A
Ease of care	Simple (nil for daily disposable)	Simple	Simple	Simple	N/A
Initial cost	Low	Moderate	High	Moderate	High
Ongoing costs	High	Moderate	Moderate	Nil	Nil
Cost to correct astigmatism	High	Low	Only limited correction possible	Low	High
Bifocal correction possible	Compromise	Very difficult	No	Yes	Monovision
Use in rain	Good	Good	Excellent	Poor	Excellent
Susceptibility to fog up	No	No	No	Yes	No
Susceptibility to dirt up	No	No	No	Yes	No
Risk of complication	Low	Negligible	Low	None	Moderate

LASIK, laser *in situ* keratomileusis; N/A, not applicable.

Dirt and dust

Rigid contact lenses are prone to trap debris beneath the lens and are clearly contraindicated in dirty and dusty environments. Also, dirty and dusty sporting environments are typically associated with intense physical activity and a greater risk of dislodging the lens, which are further factors contraindicating the use of rigid lenses. Large-diameter soft lenses are the lens of first choice in such environments. Lens water content and oxygen transmissibility are less critical factors. Orthokeratology has a distinct advantage in such environments, in that the lenses are not present in the eyes to trap dirt or dust, or to become dislodged.

Aquatic environments

Aquatic sports are defined here as those that take place immediately above or in water, but generally not deeper than 2 m. Edmunds (1992) has suggested that sportspersons engaged in aquatic activities be advised of the following strategies for avoiding lens loss and preserving eye health:

- Close eyes on impact with water.
- Do not open eyes fully when under water; instead, squint and maintain a head position in the direction of gaze.
- Upon surfacing, gently wipe water from closed lids before opening eyes.
- Irrigate eyes with fresh saline upon leaving the water.
- Remove and disinfect lenses shortly thereafter.

Contact lens wear is known to increase the risk of infection slightly, and the use of lenses in aquatic environments must be considered as an additional risk factor. Choo *et al.* (2005) found that wearing a hydrophilic lens while swimming in a chlorinated pool allows accumulation of microbial organisms on or in the lens, in both hydrogel and silicone hydrogel materials. However, infections are rare, and the risk of lens-related eye disease can be reduced to almost zero if lenses are removed, cleaned and disinfected in the prescribed manner soon after leaving the water. Ideally daily disposable lenses can be worn and then discarded.

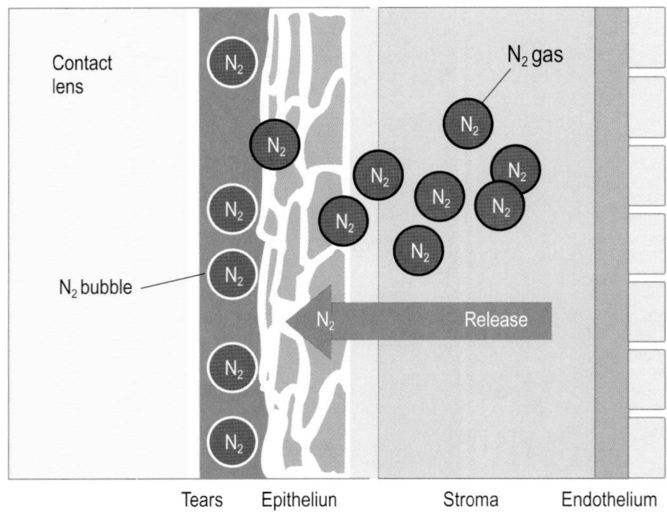

Figure 27.2 Nitrogen gas (N_2) forms in the cornea during decompression but cannot vent through the lens due to the relatively low nitrogen permeability of rigid lenses.

Larger lenses provide the greatest on-eye stability, which is of particular benefit when engaged in dynamic water sports (Banks and Edwards, 1987). Goggles worn over contact lenses, in the same way as worn by a non-lens wearer, will ensure good vision, help preserve ocular health and help reduce lens loss.

Subaquatic environments

Various authors advocate the use of both rigid lenses (Holland, 1993) and soft lenses (Bennett, 1985) for scuba diving. All seem to agree that the use of contact lenses with a standard face mask is preferred to the use of prescription face masks. As a result of the increased physical pressure experienced during deep dives, inert atmospheric gases, in particular nitrogen, dissolve in body tissues. As the diver returns to the surface slowly, these gases are released and become trapped as minute bubbles beneath the lens (Holland, 1993). This problem is especially acute with rigid lenses because of the extremely low permeability of rigid lens materials to nitrogen; the nitrogen gas cannot escape by permeating through the lens (Figure 27.2). This phenomenon can be alleviated by fitting lenses of very high gas permeability and encouraging the diver to concentrate on blinking. Brown and Siegel (1997) concluded there are no compelling reasons to change lens types in patients who are already fully adapted lens wearers. Nevertheless, silicone hydrogel lenses are the modality of choice.

Ultraviolet light

Sporting activities conducted on water, sand or snow will result in the sportsperson being exposed to excessive ultraviolet (UV) radiation, which can cause skin sunburn and solar keratitis in the short term, and cataracts (Taylor *et al.*, 1988) and pterygia (Hill and Maske, 1989) in the long term. Thus, contact lenses with UV protection tints are indicated (Cullen *et al.*, 1989). It must be recognized, however, that such lenses will not prevent excessive and potentially damaging UV light from reaching those parts of the external eye that are not covered by the lens, such as exposed parts of the cornea (in rigid lens wearers) and the bulbar conjunctiva. The use of goggles with UV-absorbing tints, to be worn over UV-absorbing contact lenses, constitutes an extra precaution for periods when the mask is removed. Skiers should be reminded also to apply UV protection creams to the remaining exposed skin on the face and neck. In surfing, where use of goggles may not be appropriate, a UV-absorbing contact lens will at least afford some protection.

Physical conditions

Special consideration needs to be given to ametropic sportspersons to facilitate their full participation in sports characterized by extreme body movement, body contact, airflow and gravitational forces. Eye, head or even general body protection is often mandatory for the sportsperson subjected to such physical extremes.

Extreme body movements

Stability of a contact lens in the eye is essential for the sportsperson participating in activities that involve extreme body movements. Spectacles and sunglasses may be unsuitable or even banned in many of these sports. Rigid lenses are contraindicated in view of the high risk of dislodgement during the sports action. Large-diameter soft lenses provide the greatest stability when excessive eye, head and body movements are involved. The lens should centre well and display minimal movement. Slightly thicker lenses resist folding up in the eye.

Body contact

The same considerations as above apply here, along with the additional factor of physical contact. Those participating in full-body contact sports can be subjected to excessive body shock and jarring, and there is also the possibility of direct physical insult to the face and eyes. The obvious extreme example is boxing; most authorities governing this sport (such as the British Boxing Board of Control) ban the use of contact lenses. The governing bodies of many body contact sports encourage the wearing of eye and face protection via the use of helmets and masks. In sports where this is optional, the contact lens-wearing sportsperson is advised to wear such protection to preclude accidental dislodgement of the lens through direct physical contact to the eyes by an opponent. In such situations, large-diameter soft lenses offer greatest stability, and rigid lenses are contraindicated. Daily disposable lenses are preferred as it is possible to have many spare replacement lenses available in the event of lens loss (see Chapter 20).

Airflow

Significant airflow over the eyes typically occurs in the course of speed sports, such as luge or motor cycle racing. The most extreme conditions of airflow over the eyes are experienced by parachutists during freefall, which can last up to 60 seconds. Airflow over the eyes can reach up to 290 km/h. Although contact lenses afford some mechanical protection for the eyes during freefall, they will not provide complete relief from the rapid and constant airflow or from flying debris and particles in the air (Gauvreau, 1976). It is preferable for ametropic parachutists to wear contact lenses beneath protective goggles. To avoid lens dehydration resulting from rapid airflow over the eyes, sportspersons should be advised about good blinking behaviour and should be fitted with large-diameter, silicone hydrogel content lenses. High-water-content hydrogel lenses are contraindicated.

Gravitational forces

Aerobatic pilots can be subjected to gravitational forces between +6 g and –3 g. Participants in luge, bobsleigh, motor car and motor cycle racing are generally subjected to lower g-forces - typically less than +2 g. Brennan and Girvin (1985) fitted volunteer pilots with 50% and 75% water content soft lenses and subjected them to downward (z) g-forces. Lenses displaced 1.50 mm downwards in response to +4 Gz and 1.75 mm downwards in response to +6 Gz; tightly fitted lenses remained central regardless of g-forces. Dennis *et al.* (1989) observed that positive forces of up to +9 Gz caused rigid lenses to decentre downwards with a maximum decentration of 2–3 mm, without adversely affecting vision. In view of this evidence, a sportsperson who is likely to be subjected to significant g-forces may find that a large tight-fitting soft lens provides maximum stability with minimum interference to visual performance. It is estimated that 10% of sports involve the body being subjected to intermittent forces greater than +1 g.

General considerations

The following points are of particular relevance to the prescription and aftercare management of those involved in sport:

- For young sportspersons participating in outdoor sports, prescribe minimum plus power (remember that an exact correction based on a 6 m test distance will result in 0.17 D excess plus power, which could be problematic in time-critical acuity-dependant activities).
- Silicone hydrogel lenses worn on an extended-wear basis are indicated for sportspersons who participate in endurance events such as rally car driving, ocean racing and mountaineering, which are typically spread over weeks and months.
- In view of the known post-blink visual degradation of about 100 ms with soft lenses (Ridder and Tomlinson, 1991), spectacles are preferred to contact lenses when critical static visual acuity is the fundamental requisite for optimum performance, especially in time-limited events (such as archery and shooting).
- The choice of correction for combination sports may involve considerable compromise if there is no pause between component events (e.g. triathlon, Nordic biathlon and Nordic combined). Conversely, various forms of correction may be used when events are spread out over many days (e.g. decathlon and modern pentathlon).
- Practitioners should be familiar with details of the particular sport or sports in which the lens wearer is participating so that the visual demands involved can be appreciated and appropriate advice offered.
- Most sports have seasonal cycles: mid-seasonal contact lens fitting or alteration should be avoided as this could provide an unnecessary distraction. For routine care, the best time is immediately following the conclusion of the season.
- Athletes often come into contact with grip resin, grease, tape dressings and ointments which are toxic to the eye and highly irritative, as well as dirt, soil or general contaminants; thus, hygiene and general compliance must be emphasized.
- The coach of a contact lens wearer should have full knowledge of the type of lenses being worn, insertion and removal techniques, the limitations of the particular lens type, the care system used, and any special constraints on lens wear, and should maintain a supply kit of lenses and solutions.
- Since contact lenses will not shield the eye from potential trauma, the usual protective eyewear or headgear used in a given sport should also be used by contact lens-wearing sportspersons.
- Effective glare relief can be provided by sunglasses (to be worn in addition to the contact lenses) and sunshades or visors. In exceptional cases where the wearing of sunglasses is not possible - such as water sports - very dark tinted lenses (70% absorption) can provide some relief (Edmunds, 1992).
- In general, presbyopic sportspersons are less often engaged in sports that are physically demanding such as rugby or football, and may be involved in sports such as golf that require attention to near tasks like recording and reading strategy notes (Carlson, 1990). Monovision is generally contraindicated, and a spectacle overcorrection is often the best option.
- Ametropic referees are subject to the same environmental extremes and visual demands as the competitions they are adjudicating. Three main factors will govern the choice of vision correction for the ametropic referee:
    1. age - in particular, whether or not the referee is presbyopic
    2. orientation - a spectacle correction may be more suited to a static official (e.g. gymnastics) and a contact lens correction to a dynamic official (e.g. wrestling)
    3. field of vision - a static referee of a sport that is played out over a wide field of view relative to the viewing position (e.g. tennis) may prefer contact lenses.

Conclusions

Both soft and rigid contact lenses are capable of affording optimal visual function for sport. Relatively tight, large-diameter, silicone hydrogel lenses will provide the greatest in-eye stability, which appears to be an important prerequisite for the majority of sports. For certain specific activities where visual acuity is critical, such as shooting, archery and darts, spectacles may be the best option. Successful contact lens correction for sporting activities requires patience, perseverance and understanding. The reward for finding the right solution is the knowledge that the sportsperson is not hampered by ametropia and is capable of performing to his or her maximum visual capabilities.

References

Banks, L. D. and Edwards, G. L. (1987) To swim or not to swim. A remedy for patients prone to losing lenses while taking a dip. *Contact Lens Spectrum,* **6,** 46–48.

Bennett, Q. M. (1985) Contact lenses for diving. *Aust. J. Optom.,* **68,** 25–26.

Booth, M. A. and Koch, D. D. (2003) Late laser in situ keratomileusis flap dislocation caused by a thrown football. *J. Cataract Refract. Surg.,* **29,** 2032–2033.

Brennan, D. H. and Girvin, J. K. (1985) The flight acceptability of soft contact lenses: an environmental trial. *Av. Space Environ. Med.,* **56,** 43–48.

Brown, M. S. and Siegel, I. M. (1997) Cornea–contact lens interaction in the aquatic environment. *Contact Lens Assoc. Ophthalmol. J.,* **23,** 237–242.

Carlson, N. J. (1990) Contacts and golf: More presbyopic options. *Contact Lens Forum,* **14,** 16.

Choo, J., Vuu, K., Bergenske, P. *et al.* (2005) Bacterial populations on silicone hydrogel and hydrogel contact lenses after swimming in a chlorinated pool. *Optom. Vis. Sci.,* **82,** 134–137.

Cullen, A. P., Dumbleton, K. A. and Chou, B. R. (1989) Contact lenses and acute exposure to ultraviolet radiation. *Optom. Vis. Sci.,* **66,** 407–411.

Dennis, R. J., Woessner, W. M., Miller, R. E. *et al.* (1989). The effect of fluctuating +Gz exposure on rigid gas permeable contact lenses *Optom. Vis. Sci. (Suppl.),* **66,** 167.

Dillehay, S. M. (2007) Does the level of available oxygen impact comfort in contact lens wear?: A review of the literature. *Eye Contact Lens,* **33,** 148–155.

Edmunds, F. R. (1992) Contact lenses and sports. In *Sportsvision Program* (F. R. Edmunds, ed.) pp. 1–33, New York: Bausch & Lomb Incorporated.

Erickson, G. B., Horn, F. C., Barney, T. *et al.* (2009) Visual performance with sport-tinted contact lenses in natural sunlight. *Optom. Vis. Sci.,* **86,** 509–516.

Gauvreau, D. K. (1976) Effects of wearing Bausch & Lomb Soflens while skydiving. *Am. J. Optom. Physiol. Opt.,* **53,** 236–240.

Hill, J. C. and Maske, R. (1989) Pathogenesis of pterygium. *Eye,* **3,** 218–226.

Holland, R. (1993) Rigid contact lenses for scuba diving. *SportsVision,* **9,** 13–21.

Ousler, G. W. 3rd, Anderson, R. T. and Osborn, K. E. (2008) The effect of senofilcon A contact lenses compared to habitual contact lenses on ocular discomfort during exposure to a controlled adverse environment. *Curr. Med. Res. Opin.,* **24,** 335–341.

Porisch, E. (2007) Football players' contrast sensitivity comparison when wearing amber sport-tinted or clear contact lenses. *Optometry,* **78,** 232–235.

Ridder, W. H. and Tomlinson, A. (1991) Blink-induced, temporal variations in contrast sensitivity. *Int. Contact Lens Clin.,* **18,** 231–237.

Schnider, C. M., Coffey, B. M. and Reichow, A. R. (1993) Comparison of contact lenses versus spectacles for sports oriented vision performance. *Invest. Ophthalmol. Vis. Sci. (Suppl.),* **34,** 1005.

Socks, J. F. (1983). Use of contact lenses for cold weather activities. Results of a survey. *Int. Contact Lens Clin.,* **10,** 82–91.

Stapleton, F., Keay, L. J., Sanfilippo, P. G. *et al.* (2007) Relationship between climate, disease severity, and causative organism for contact lens-associated microbial keratitis in Australia. *Am. J. Ophthalmol.,* **144,** 690–698.

Taylor, H. R., West, S. K., Rosenthal, F. S. *et al.* (1988). Effect of ultraviolet radiation on cataract formation. *N. Eng. J. Med.,* **319,** 1429–1433.

Tetz, M., Werner, L., Müller, M. *et al.* (2007) Late traumatic LASIK flap loss during contact sport. *J. Cataract Refract. Surg.,* **33,** 1332–1335.

CHAPTER 28

Keratoconus

Karla Zadnik and Joseph T Barr

Introduction

Keratoconus is a progressive, asymmetric, non-inflammatory disease of the cornea characterized by steepening and distortion, apical thinning and central scarring (Krachmer *et al.*, 1984). These corneal changes lead to a mild to marked decrease in vision secondary to high irregular astigmatism and, frequently, central corneal scarring. There are several characteristic biomicroscopic corneal signs, which become more prevalent as the disease progresses (Krachmer *et al.*, 1984; Zadnik *et al.*, 1996, 2000). These include an inferiorly displaced, thinned protrusion of the cornea (Figure 28.1), corneal thinning over the apex of the cone (Figure 28.2), Vogt's striae in the posterior stroma (Figure 28.3), scars in Bowman's layer (Figure 28.4) and Fleischer's ring, a deposition of iron in the corneal epithelium at the base of the cone (Figure 28.5).

The aetiology of keratoconus is unknown. Atopic disease, eye rubbing, inheritance, and contact lens wear are commonly associated with keratoconus (Macsai *et al.*, 1990).

Demographics of keratoconus

Estimates of the prevalence of keratoconus vary from 4 to 108 per 100 000 population (Hofstetter, 1959; Duke-Elder and Leigh, 1965). The high estimate of Hofstetter (1959) is based on keratoscopy results alone and probably includes non-keratoconic cases of high or irregular astigmatism. In a population-based study over a period of 48 years (1935–1982) in Olmsted County, Minnesota, USA, Kennedy *et al.* (1986) found an average annual incidence of 2 per 100 000 and a prevalence rate of 54.5 per 100 000 population. There is no clear gender-specific predilection for the disease. Significant differences between men and women include a greater likelihood of a family history of keratoconus and significantly more keratoconus-related symptoms among women with the disease (Fink *et al.*, 2005).

Management options

Management of keratoconus varies with disease severity (Table 28.1). Non-surgical options are the primary method of patient management in keratoconus. Because the corneal curvature changes in keratoconus result in myopia and astigmatism (with rare exception), patients require some type of visual correction from the earliest stages of the disease. The visual correction often precedes the formal keratoconus diagnosis.

Although the visual disturbances in keratoconus may be managed with spectacles or soft lenses early in the disease process, rigid lenses are the treatment of choice for the irregular astigmatism associated with disease progression (Zadnik *et al.*, 1998). The essential choice is spectacles versus rigid lenses.

Spectacle correction

Most practitioners rely on spectacles in the early course of the disease. Limitations on spectacle correction in keratoconus include:

- High amounts of corneal toricity and resultant refractive astigmatism, the correction of which is not tolerable in spectacle form.

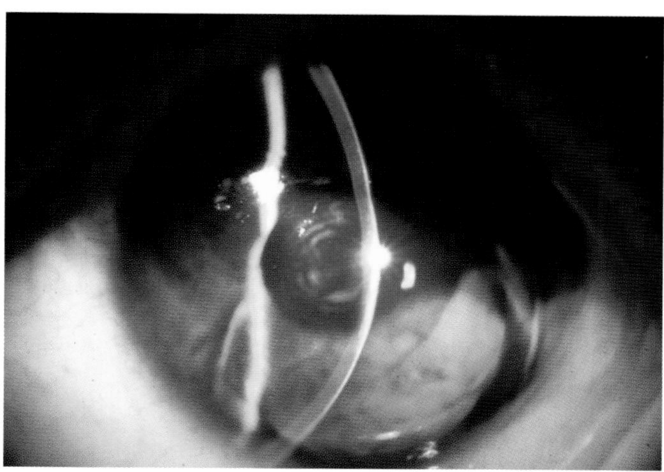

Figure 28.1 Inferiorly displaced, thinned protrusion of the cornea in a keratoconic eye.

DOI: 10.1016/B978-0-7506-8869-7.00028-8

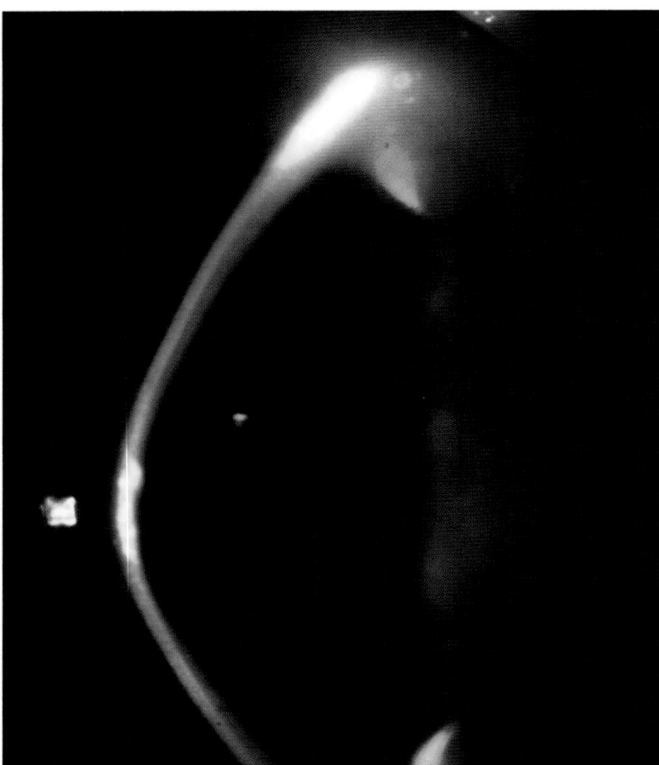

Figure 28.2 Corneal thinning over the apex of the cone in a keratoconic eye.

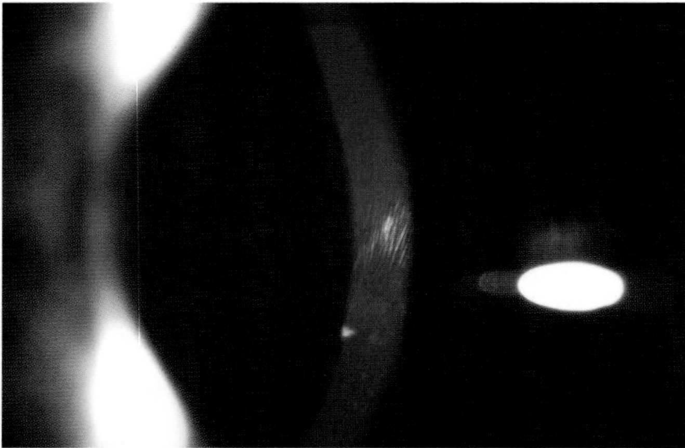

Figure 28.3 Vogt's striae in the posterior stroma of a keratoconic eye.

- Changing refractive error, either diurnally or from week to week, for which spectacles cannot be adequately prescribed.
- Inadequacy of visual acuity with spectacles because of uncorrected irregular astigmatism.
- Anisometropia present as a result of the asymmetric nature of the disease.

Even given these problems, however, spectacles are the first form of optical management of the disease, especially in its early stages, and can provide surprisingly good visual acuity (Zadnik *et al.*, 1996). Visual acuity measurement and subjective refraction are reasonably repeatable (Davis *et al.*, 1998). Contact lenses typically can correct irregular astigmatism and improve visual acuity beyond the level of spectacles but should be reserved for those patients in whom spectacles are no longer adequate because rigid contact lens wear has been associated with corneal scarring (Zadnik *et al.*, 2005).

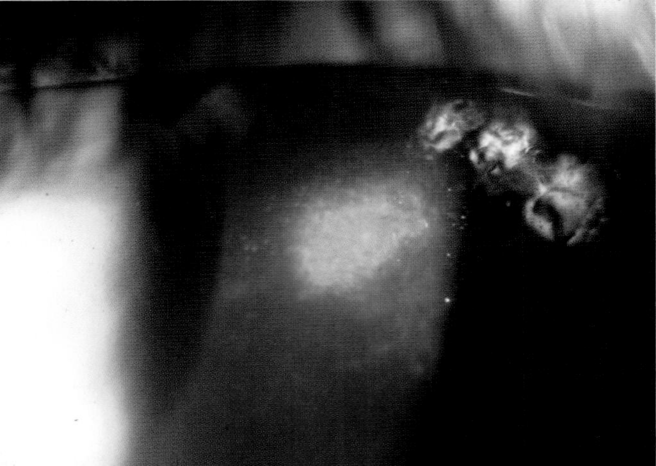

Figure 28.4 Corneal scars in Bowman's layer in a keratoconic eye. (Adapted fom Edrington, T. B., Barr, J. T., Zadnik, K. et al. (1996) Standardized rigid contact lens fitting protocol for keratoconus. Optom. Vis. Sci., 73, 369–375.)

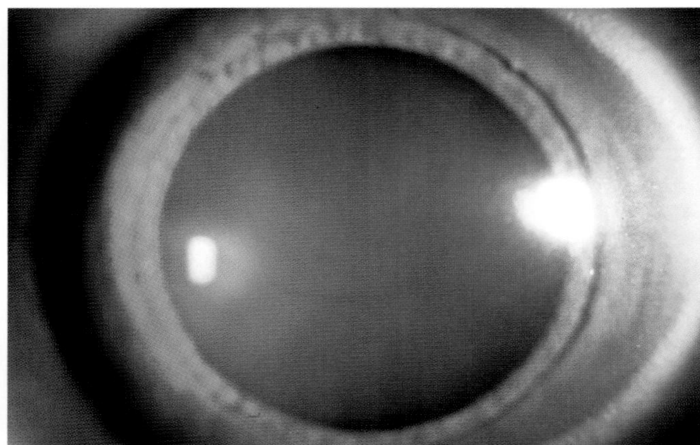

Figure 28.5 Fleischer's ring in a keratoconic eye.

Table 28.1 Management options for keratoconus

Disease severity	Non-surgical	Surgical
Early	Spectacles Soft toric lenses	Riboflavin/ultraviolet A therapy
Moderate	Rigid gas-permeable lenses Hybrid lenses Piggyback lenses	Intacs
Advanced	Semiscleral Scleral lenses	Lamellar keratoplasty Penetrating keratoplasty

Soft lenses

Hydrogel lenses are usually unsuitable, especially in cases of more advanced keratoconus, because they essentially

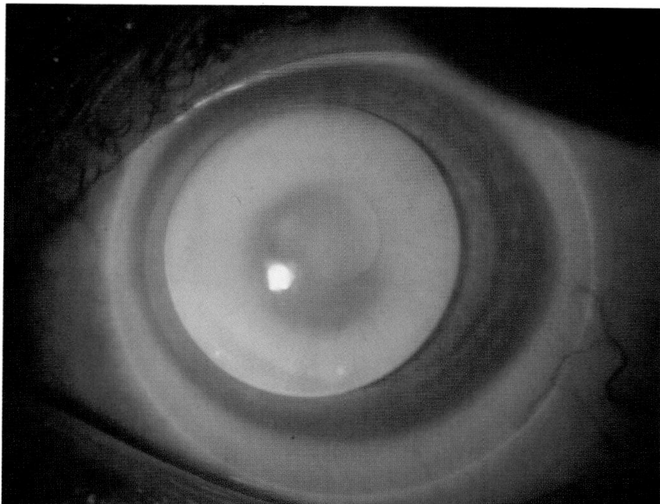

Figure 28.6 Piggyback combination fit enhanced with the use of fluorescein. A rigid lens is sitting on a large-diameter soft bandage lens.

drape over the cornea and faithfully transfer the distorted surface topography of the keratoconic cornea to the lens surface, typically resulting in poor vision. Silicone hydrogel lenses are now available in designs which may be marginally more suitable for keratoconus correction. The lenses have a modulus of elasticity which is greater than that for hydrogel lenses, therefore they may not drape on the cornea as much and provide for more stable vision.

Occasionally in later stages of the disease, when comfort is reduced or a stable fit can no longer be achieved, soft lenses may be used in conjunction with rigid lenses in a 'piggyback' combination lens design (Figure 28.6). Hypoxia complications are likely to occur when attempting this type of fit using a hydrogel lens; however, the availability of silicone hydrogel and hyperoxygen-transmissible rigid materials makes these dual-lens systems a viable option (O'Donnell and Maldonado-Codina, 2004).

Although they have only played a small role up to now, the future of keratoconus correction may well lie with soft lenses. It has been recognized that, even with the best rigid lens designs, there can still be significant uncorrected higher-order aberrations which lead to poor acuity. Decentration and movement of rigid lenses and the irregularity of the posterior corneal surface are the main sources of these residual aberrations. Developing corrections that more completely correct these aberrations may lead to improved visual performance in keratoconus (Marsack *et al.*, 2007). With their greater stability on the eye, soft lenses are more likely to be able to achieve this goal. Attempts have been made using custom wavefront-guided soft lenses (Chen *et al.*, 2007; Marsack *et al.*, 2008); however, more research needs to be undertaken before this could become a mainstream fitting option.

Hybrid lenses

Hybrid lenses have a rigid central zone and an outer 'skirt' of soft lens material. They tend to be more stable on the eye than a rigid lens alone and have better comfort as there is less lid interaction.

SoftPerm lenses (CIBA Vision) have been used in patients with keratoconus; however, their success is limited by concerns of lens damage, especially related to separation at the junction, and by the risk of peripheral corneal neovascularization, which occurs in around 25% of wearers (Chung *et al.*, 2001; Ozkurt *et al.*, 2007). The SynergEyes KC lens has been shown to allow significantly more oxygen to reach the central cornea during wear than the SoftPerm lens (Pilskalns *et al.*, 2007), although both lenses have low-permeability hydrogel 'skirts'. The water contents of the SoftPerm and SynergEyes KC lenses are 25% and 27%, respectively. Nevertheless, practitioners should attempt the fitting of a hybrid lens for patients who are otherwise unable to tolerate rigid gas-permeable contact lenses before referring for penetrating keratoplasty (Nau, 2008).

Rigid contact lens correction

Rigid contact lenses, both before and since the introduction of gas-permeable materials, have been the mainstay of the optical management of keratoconus. These lenses, which are manufactured in a large variety of unique designs, effectively resurface the irregular cornea and allow the intervening fluid lens to correct the corneal astigmatism adequately in most cases.

Certainly, a rigid contact lens allows for a far more uniform refracting surface than the irregular astigmatic surface of the keratoconic cornea. Local irregularities of the stained epithelium are filled in by the tears behind the rigid lens. However, the lacrimal lens only eliminates about 90% of the astigmatic error of the cornea due to the index difference between the tears and cornea (see Chapter 17). Corneal scarring and epithelial staining diffuse light and result in worse low-contrast visual acuity (Zadnik *et al.*, 2000). The rigid lens may also further distort the cornea.

Scleral lenses

In advanced disease, it may not be possible to achieve a sufficiently stable lens fit with a traditional rigid lens. Due to their larger size, better centration and stability may be achieved with scleral lenses, thus avoiding the need for surgery. The fitting of scleral lenses is covered in Chapter 23.

Surgical management

A promising breakthrough in the treatment of keratoconus is the use of riboflavin and ultraviolet-A to induce collagen cross-linking, which has a dampening effect on progressive disease (Wollensak *et al.*, 2003; Raiskup-Wolf *et al.*, 2008). If used early in the disease it might mean patients do not progress to needing penetrating keratoplasty.

Patients are generally referred for penetrating keratoplasty when they can no longer tolerate contact lenses or when contact lenses provide inadequate vision. Poor vision with contact lenses is often accompanied by apical corneal scarring, but vision can be compromised even with optimal contact lens correction and no corneal scarring. With concerted effort, the vast majority of patients initially referred for corneal transplants can be successfully refitted with contact lenses without surgery, yielding improved visual acuity and contact lens wearing time (Smiddy *et al.*, 1988).

Surgical procedures other than penetrating keratoplasty have been used for keratoconus, including Intacs segments

Table 28.2 Keratoconus contact lens designs and trial lens sets

Material	Lens design	Diameter (mm)	Optic zone (mm)	Peripheral curvatures (mm)
Rigid	Soper	8.5	7.0	7.5/0.25, 8.4/0.1, 9.1/0.2, 13.0/0.2
Rigid	McGuire	8.6 9.1 9.5	6.0 6.5 7.0	SCR = BCR + 0.5 mm TCR = BCR + 1.5 mm PCR = BCR + 4.5 mm, similar for all diameters
Rigid	Rose K	8.7	Varies with aspheric base curve	
Rigid	CLEK (Edrington *et al.*, 1996)	8.6	6.5	8.5 SCR, 11.5 PCR/0.2
Hybrid	SoftPerm	14.3 with 8.0 styrene rigid central portion		
Hybrid	SynergEyes KC	14.5 with 8.4 Paragon HDS rigid central portion		Skirt curvature: steep, medium or flat
Soft	Flexlens Tricurve design Harrison design Piggy Back	 14.0 15.0 14.5	 Note: for all these lenses, CT = 0.40 to 0.28 for correcting irregular astigmatism 10.2 mm cut out for rigid lens	
Silicone hydrogel	KeraSoft 3	14.0, 14.5, 15.0		

SCR = secondary curve radius; BCR = base curve radius; PCR = peripheral curve radius; TCR = tertiary curve radius; CT = centre thickness.

(Colin and Malet, 2007; Kymionis *et al.*, 2007) and lamellar keratoplasty (Tan *et al.*, 2006).

Most suitable rigid lens types

Although rigid lenses often position over the apex of the displaced ectatic area, they eliminate the difficulties associated with this displacement by also superimposing the visual axis. Rigid lens fitting in keratoconus is, however, by no means simple. Numerous lenses are often required, even for an initial fitting, and achieving an adequate cornea–lens fitting relationship with reasonable vision becomes more difficult as the disease progresses. Although most practitioners who fit a large variety of keratoconus patients have their preferences for lens design (Voss and Liberatore, 1962; Hall, 1963; Gould, 1970; Soper and Jarrett, 1972; Gasset and Lobo, 1975; Mackie, 1977; Caroline *et al.*, 1978; Mobilia and Foster, 1979; Korb *et al.*, 1982; Maguen *et al.*, 1983; Raber, 1983; Lembach and Keates, 1984; Cohen and Parlato, 1986; Rosenthal, 1986; Kastl, 1987), most practising clinicians still find each keratoconus patient a trial-and-error experience. Some common lens designs are summarized in Table 28.2.

Refitting is often required at relatively frequent intervals.

Virtually all literature reports on contact lens fitting in keratoconus are anecdotal in the sense that they represent retrospective data on a clinical population of keratoconus patients. Nonetheless, these studies provide information on the large variety of lens types that have been utilized successfully in the management of keratoconus, although success rates must be viewed with some scepticism because of lack of control subjects, possible bias in patients selected for fitting and varying definitions of what constitutes a successful contact lens fitting in a keratoconus patient (Table 28.3).

Table 28.3 Summary of studies on rigid lens correction in keratoconus

Author(s), year	Number of eyes	Number of patients	Lens type
Retrospective studies			
Gould, 1970	Not stated	44	PMMA
Soper and Jarrett, 1972	178	Not stated	Soper Cone
Gasset and Lobo, 1975	60	43	Dura-T
Mobilia and Foster, 1979	96	56	Polycon
Raber, 1983	23	19	CAB Soper Cone
Lembach and Keates, 1984	22	20	Silcon aspheric
Cohen and Parlato, 1986	123	Not stated	Polycon II
Kastl, 1987	83	64	PMMA, CAB
Edrington *et al.*, 1999	808	808	Any
Prospective studies			
Korb *et al.*, 1982	14	7	Polycon
Maguen *et al.*, 1983	31	17	Polycon

PMMA = polymethyl methacrylate; CAB = cellulose acetate butyrate.

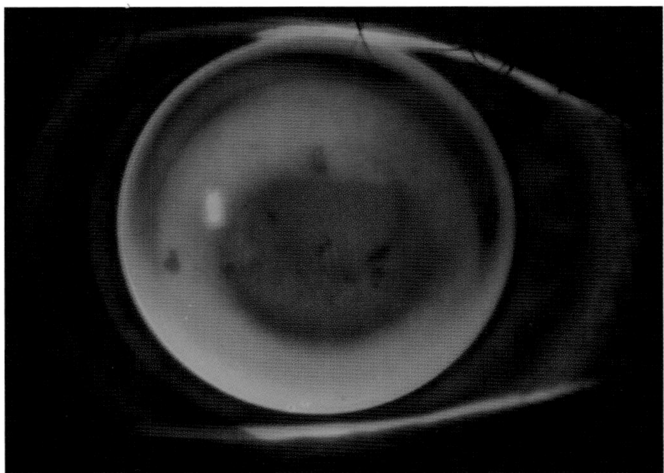

Figure 28.7 Fluorescein pattern on a keratoconic cornea showing apical bearing, with primary lens support on the apex of the cornea.

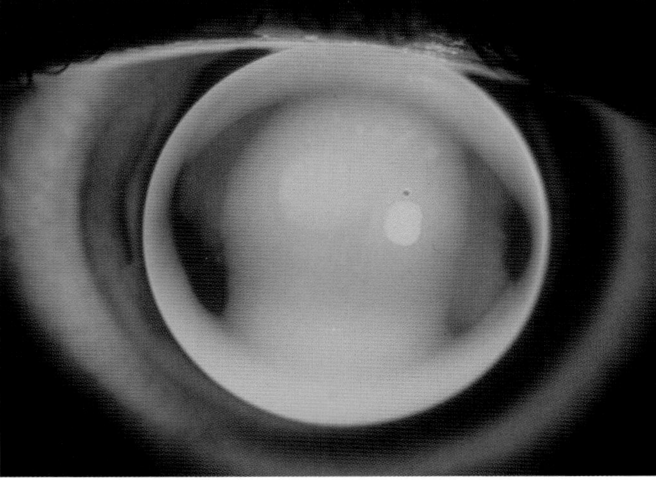

Figure 28.8 Fluorescein pattern on a keratoconic cornea showing apical clearance, with lens support and bearing directed off the apex and on to the paracentral cornea.

The studies outlined in Table 28.3 report variable success rates, although most are of the order of 80%, judged in some cases by the absence of adverse corneal physiological effects and in others by usable visual acuity or acceptable wearing time and comfort. By and large, it seems that whatever lens a particular clinician becomes comfortable with and adept at using works well in the hands of that clinician.

Fitting philosophies and fluorescein patterns

The major rigid lens fitting techniques in keratoconus, as succinctly described by Korb *et al.* (1982), are:

- Apical bearing, with primary lens support on the apex of the cornea (Figure 28.7), where the central optic zone of the lens actually touches or bears on the central corneal epithelium (Hall, 1963).
- Apical clearance, with lens support and bearing directed off the apex and on to the paracentral cornea (Figure 28.8), with clearance of the apex of the cornea (Voss and Liberatore, 1962).
- Divided support or three-point touch, with lens support and bearing shared between the corneal apex and the paracentral cornea (Figure 28.9).

Typically, an apical bearing fit is the easiest to achieve in keratoconus. Almost all rigid contact lenses touch the apex of the cone unless steps are taken to alleviate the bearing or to clear the corneal apex. In three-point touch – although possibly viewed as a variant of apical touch – the objective is to minimize the touch on the corneal apex by steepening the lens centrally and allowing the peripheral cornea to show areas of light touch, thereby theoretically minimizing trauma to all areas of the cornea. The major disadvantage of apical touch is the possibility of epithelial trauma and the inducement of corneal scarring. The advantages of apical touch include the possibility of superior acuity (Krachmer *et al.*, 1984; Sorbara *et al.*, 2000), although other studies have not borne out this observation (Zadnik and Mutti, 1987). In fact, the Collaborative Longitudinal Evaluation of Keratoconus (CLEK) study reported superior vision with steep-fitting rigid lenses (Zadnik *et al.*, 2005).

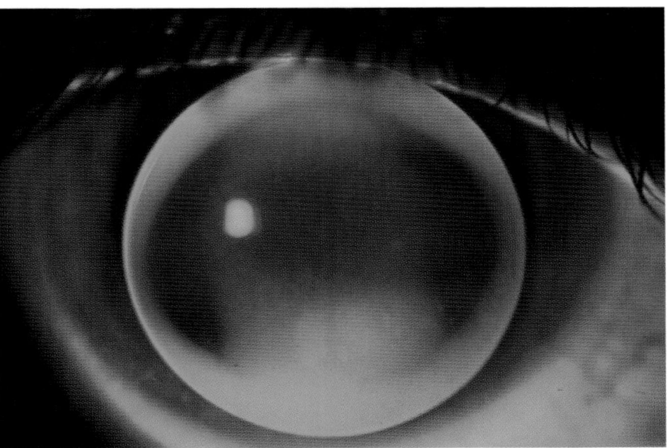

Figure 28.9 Fluorescein pattern on a keratoconic cornea showing divided support or three-point touch, with lens support and bearing shared between the corneal apex and the paracentral cornea.

In lenses fitted with an apical clearance technique, trauma to the central cornea and epithelium is presumably minimized. Lens wearing time may be lessened relative to lenses supported more by the central cornea, but rigorous, well-controlled studies have not been performed to verify this.

Apical touch versus apical clearance

One study has addressed the issues concerning the best fitting technique for keratoconus. Korb *et al.* (1982) performed a fitting study on 14 eyes of 7 keratoconus patients that conformed to a rigorous set of entry criteria. These authors 'semirandomized' the eyes to either a large flat or small steep lens (i.e. in half the patients the more severely affected eye was fitted with the flat lens and in the other half the less diseased eye was fitted with the flat lens). Within a 12-month period, 4 of the 7 eyes fitted with the flat-fitting method developed corneal scarring. Within the same period of time, none of the eyes fitted steep developed any scarring. Potential confounding variables that were not discussed included the influence of contact lens diameter,

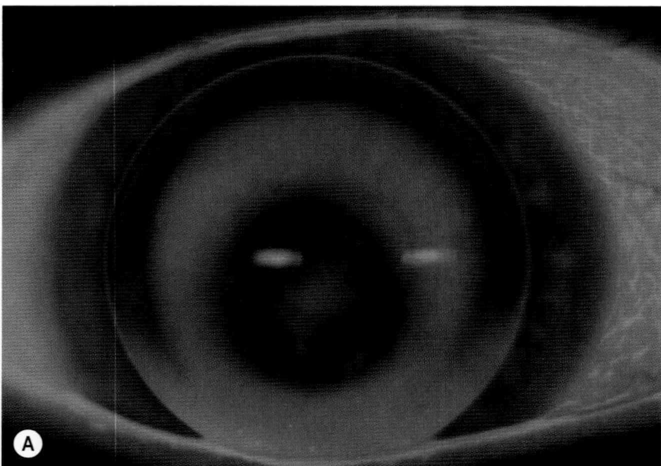

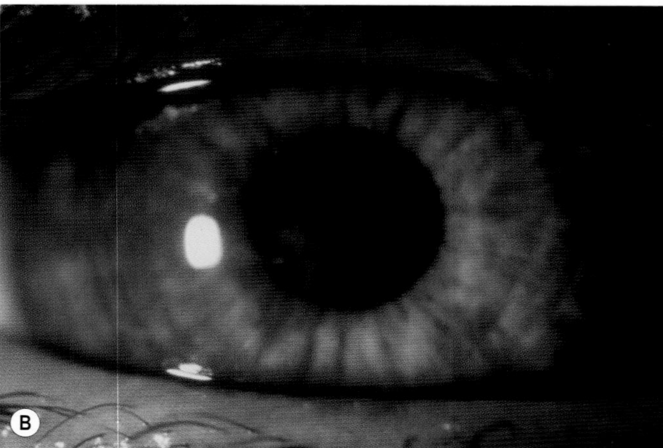

Figure 28.10 (A) This keratoconic patient had been fitted with a lens that was fitted too flat and created heavy central bearing. (B) The lens may have caused heavy scarring, which can be observed in the same proximity as the lens bearing.

the possibility of differential wearing time and the potential for increased corneal staining with the silicone acrylate material used, relative to other polymers. Nonetheless, this study still introduces the possibility that the current standard of care – wherein the corneal apex typically supports some of the weight of the contact lens across the cornea (Zadnik *et al.*, 1996, 2005) – may, in fact, result in some proportion of the corneal scarring observed in keratoconus (Figure 28.10).

It is clear that the ophthalmic community, at least in the USA, has not embraced the findings of Korb *et al.* (1982). There were 808 rigid contact lens-wearing patients at the start of a large study conducted by the authors of this chapter – the CLEK study. Clinician-reported, qualitative assessment of the apical fitting relationships of the habitual rigid contact lenses of these presenting patients revealed that 95 eyes (11.8%) were wearing lenses displaying apical clearance and that 713 eyes (88.2%) were wearing lenses displaying apical touch (Edrington *et al.*, 1999).

Lens fitting protocols

Contact lens fitting in keratoconus is difficult to specify. The cornea with keratoconus can vary with respect to any combination of the following factors:

- Cone position.
- Cone size.
- Degree of induced myopia.
- Amount of corneal toricity.
- Steepness of keratometric readings.
- Corneal topography.
- Disease progression with respect to both degree and rate.
- Contact lens-corrected visual acuity.
- Contact lens tolerance.

As such, a single recipe that applies to the fitting of all keratoconus patients cannot be written, but fitting advice is often helpful. Many rigid contact lens laboratories will loan trial lens sets to practitioners.

The contact lens practitioner needs to be extraordinarily creative in his or her lens design for keratoconus. The objective is to provide adequate vision with acceptable corneal tissue tolerance for an adequate number of hours of wear per day. Several fitting sets should be available for trial fitting (Korb *et al.*, 1982; Mandell, 1988; Edrington *et al.*, 1996). Smaller-diameter lenses (≤8.6 mm) can be used to achieve an apical clearance or a three-point touch fluorescein pattern, if such a fit is appropriate for a given cornea. Larger-diameter lenses (≥9.2 mm) lend themselves well to three-point touch or apical touch fitting methods and can be helpful in an inferiorly displaced cone. The choice of fitting philosophy and, therefore, lens choice, is often one of necessity. Although the practitioner may intend to fit a lens so that it clears the corneal apex, good comfort and vision may be better achieved with a lens that lightly touches the central cornea. On other keratoconic corneas, the apical clearance fitting pattern may be easily achieved.

Aspheric lenses, such as VFL II and Ellip-See-Con, among others, have been used successfully and are described in great detail by other authors (Lembach and Keates, 1984; Bennett, 1986). These lenses generally are fitted steep in relation to corneal curvature, and lens diameter is dependent on the base curve–eccentricity value relationship of the lens (i.e. if the eccentricity value of a given lens needs to be increased, then the base curve would be ordered steeper with a smaller overall diameter, to maintain proper edge lift) (Bennett, 1986).

In both diagnostic fitting and evaluating the fit of a dispensed lens, the malleability of the keratoconic cornea is important. Any rigid lens placed on a keratoconic cornea should be allowed to equilibrate on the eye for a minimum of 10–20 min. Often, dispensed lenses fit differently (either more or less successfully) at a 1-week follow-up visit than they do initially.

Diagnostic lenses with known peripheral curve systems must be used. If a decision needs to be made about altering the specified peripheral curves, it is better to err on the shorter radii of curvature (steep) side. This allows the practitioner to modify the peripheral system of the lens in the clinic by flattening the curves.

The capacity to undertake in-house modification of keratoconus lenses is imperative. In addition to peripheral curve modification, as mentioned above, edges frequently require small or moderate modifications. Peripheral curves frequently have to be blended to a greater degree than as supplied by the laboratory. Keratoconus patients often have difficulty with their responses during subjective over-refractions, and diagnostic lenses may have a different optical power than the final power ordered; thus, small, in-house additions of minus power may be necessary.

The retinoscope is a valuable tool both for diagnosing keratoconus and for managing this condition with rigid contact lenses. In attempting to overrefract a patient whose sensitivity to blur may be in the 1.00–2.00 D range, time, effort and frustration can often be minimized by first performing a retinoscopic overrefraction. Retinoscopy may be slightly more difficult to perform compared to a non-keratoconic eye, especially in advanced keratoconus, because of the appearance of spurious reflexes resulting from the aberrated corneal optics.

Refitting the successful keratoconus patient should be initiated with great restraint. The keratoconus patient who wears lenses 14 hours per day without discomfort and has good vision but would like 2 h more of wearing time is probably not a good candidate for refitting. Neither is the patient who has 6/7.5 acuity but complains of inadequate vision. The known decrements in vision in keratoconus are not typically eliminated in full with rigid contact lens correction.

Painstaking, up-to-date records should be maintained on each lens of a keratoconic patient. Modifications that have been performed on each lens should also be carefully documented, to facilitate rapid and efficient duplication in the event of a lost or damaged lens.

Rigid lens fitting procedure

Keratometry

Although keratometric readings may be of limited use in fitting keratoconus patients, they can assist in initial trial lens selection and in documenting disease progression. The keratometric range should be extended as necessary (Mandell, 1988). If the cornea of the patient is steeper than 52.00 D (i.e. off the keratometer's scale) in either meridian, the range of the keratometer will need to be extended as follows:

- Insert the supplied +1.25 D lens to the keratometer target (objective side).
- The readings with the +1.25 D lens in place should be converted to true values.
- If the cornea of the patient is off the scale of the keratometer in either meridian with the +1.25 D lens in place, steps 1–2 above should be repeated with the +2.25 D lens in place, and the keratometer drum reading must again be converted to the true reading.
- If the cornea of the patient is off the scale of the keratometer in either meridian with the +2.25 D lens in place, the keratometric reading in that meridian is recorded as '>68.30 D'.

Refraction

Careful refraction is mandatory. Patients with keratoconus often have unpredictably good best-corrected visual acuity. High amounts of cylinder, frequently at an increasingly oblique axis, are sometimes found. Retinoscopic and keratometric results are an excellent starting point for determining the subjective refraction. Careful refinement of cylinder axis and avoidance of over-minusing are necessary. Accurate refraction provides a baseline best visual acuity without contact lenses, which serves as a reference point for expected contact lens-corrected acuity. Contact lens-corrected acuity should be at least as good as that achieved with spectacles. Subjective refraction results can be prescribed, either as back-up spectacles for patients who wear contact lenses, or as the primary mode of correction for patients who cannot wear contact lenses (Zadnik *et al.*, 1996).

Trial lens fitting

A trial lens fitting is vital in fitting rigid lenses on patients with keratoconus. There is no 'formula' approach for predicting a proper lens fit. The initial trial lens should be chosen with a base curve that either splits the two keratometric readings or is slightly steeper than the average corneal curvature. If the patient has never worn contact lenses, instillation of a topical corneal anaesthetic may be helpful in obtaining an accurate visual acuity measurement and assessment of the fluorescein pattern without excessive tearing.

Fluorescein pattern analysis

The ideal keratoconic fluorescein pattern will be determined by the lens design chosen. The central pattern will depend on which of the contact lens fitting methods outlined above has been chosen. The peripheral curve should be flat enough to enable a reservoir of tears to collect without allowing excessive edge lift and lens dislocation. This combination aids in tear interchange and movement.

To analyse the fit, the fluorescein pattern should be divided into two areas – the central portion, including the entire area under the optic zone, and the peripheral zone. Each area should be analysed separately. The location and amount of bearing should be observed. As progressively steeper base curves are applied to the cornea, the fluorescein pattern may not change appreciably from lens to lens if the base curve change between lenses applied is relatively small. If there is central bearing, the lens should be steepened, assuming that an apical clearance pattern is desired (Korb *et al.*, 1982).

If pooling in the periphery is absent, the peripheral curves should be flatter. If there is insufficient lens movement and excessive bearing in the area of the secondary curve, then the secondary curve is too steep, preventing lens movement. Absence of fluorescein in the secondary or peripheral area can be due to the peripheral lens 'seal-off'. Horizontally, edge lift may be just adequate, while inferiorly, edge lift may be on the high end of acceptable. The presence of any air bubbles under the lens should be carefully noted as to location, size and persistence. A central air bubble may mean that the lens is too steep. Paracentral air bubbles, on the other hand, may mean that the optic zone is too large. A good rule of thumb is for the back optic zone diameter approximately to equal the back optic zone radius. Small optic zones on the steepest lenses may unfortunately result in flare to achieve the best fit.

The position of the corneal apex relative to the trial lens should be determined. Generally, the more inferior the apex, the larger the total diameter of the lens required for centration. A low-riding lens may be too flat or too small. In attempting to fit a larger lens, a lid attachment fit is desirable; however, the peripheral system must be flat enough to prevent paracentral seal-off, which would result in decreased lens movement and inadequate tear exchange.

Each trial lens should be allowed to settle on the eye for an appropriate amount of time (approximately 20 min) prior to evaluation. Keratoconic corneas are very pliable, and in the case of a previous wearer of flat lenses, for example, the degree of corneal moulding can be marked.

Successive trial lens overrefractions should be compared, and the total power of each system should be approximately equal. This is important for evaluating the consistency of the diagnostic lenses, their optical performance on the eye and the consistency of the patient's responses during subjective overrefraction.

Once an adequate fit is achieved, a manufacturing laboratory must be chosen that will make the lens according to specifications. Some laboratories have a standard keratoconic lens design, but these lenses are often too steep in the periphery. If the ordered lens differs from the diagnostic trial lens, in-house or laboratory modification will be necessary. It is extremely important that an individual trial lens set be manufactured according to specifications to ensure a standardization factor for comparison, both during fitting and as a check against ordered lenses. A rigid lens material of medium *Dk* (12–60 Barrer) is recommended. This allows ample lens oxygen transmissibility and makes the lens less prone to warpage and dryness.

CLEK study fitting protocol

The CLEK study group has published a standardized protocol for fitting keratoconus patients based on sagittal height (Edrington *et al.*, 1996). Parameters for the CLEK diagnostic keratoconus fitting set were determined as follows:

- Base curve radii were selected to encompass the corneal sagittal heights for mild to moderate keratoconus patients. Increments of 0.05 mm were chosen to increase the fitting sensitivity.
- Contact lens powers were selected to provide low-minus overrefractions for the majority of mild to moderate keratoconus patients.
- The overall diameter was set at 8.6 mm to provide an interpalpebral fit in which the lens is positioned over the apex of the conical area of the cornea.
- The optic zone diameter was standardized at 6.5 mm to minimize areas of tear pooling and debris accumulation under the optic zone of the lens.
- The secondary curve radius ranged from 8.00 to 8.25 mm in order to obtain average peripheral clearance. Corneal curvatures beyond the cone are similar to corneal curvatures of non-keratoconus patients. Therefore, secondary curve radii appropriate for non-keratoconus rigid contact lens fitting are indicated.
- The peripheral or third curve radius for the tricurve fitting lenses was set at 11.00 mm with a width of 0.2 mm. This curve was selected not only to be a fitting curve but also to start the posterior edge treatment.
- Centre thicknesses were calculated such that an edge thickness of approximately 0.10 mm was maintained for each trial lens. Centre thicknesses are greater than cosmetic rigid lenses of similar power because of the flatter secondary curve-to-base curve relationship.
- Diagnostic lenses were fabricated in polymethyl methacrylate (PMMA). This material was chosen because of its machinability, dimensional stability, durability and low cost. Lenses for patients can be manufactured in any rigid lens material.

To fit these lenses, it is necessary to determine the steep keratometry reading, convert it to millimetres, and refer to Table 28.4 for selection of the initial trial lens from the CLEK study diagnostic contact lens set. For example:

Keratometry readings:48.50/51.50 @ 115
Steep keratometry value:50.00 D = 6.55 mm
Select initial trial lens:6.55 mm base curve

The initial trial lens is applied to the eye of the patient and allowed to settle for 10 min prior to analysis of the fluorescein pattern. If the initial trial lens was judged to be flat, the next higher-numbered (steeper) trial lens is applied to the eye for fluorescein pattern evaluation. This procedure is repeated until a definite apical clearance pattern is achieved. Therefore, the end-point of the contact lens fitting procedure is the flattest lens in the trial lens set that exhibits a definite apical clearance fluorescein pattern such that the sagittal depth of the base curve chord diameter is greater than the sagittal depth of the cornea for the same chord diameter. The base curve radius of this lens is referred to as the 'first definite apical clearance lens'.

If the initial trial lens is judged to be steep centrally, the next lower-numbered (flatter) trial lens in Table 28.4 is applied to the cornea for fluorescein pattern evaluation. This procedure is repeated until a definite apical touch or a three-point touch is achieved (Edrington *et al.*, 1998).

Criteria for referral for evaluation for keratoplasty

Patients are generally referred for penetrating keratoplasty when they can no longer tolerate their contact lenses or when their contact lenses provide inadequate vision. Poor vision with contact lenses is often accompanied by apical corneal scarring, but vision can be compromised even with optimal contact lens correction and no corneal scarring. With concerted effort, the vast majority of patients initially referred for corneal transplants can be successfully refitted without surgery, yielding improved visual acuity and contact lens wearing time (Belin *et al.*, 1988; Fowler *et al.*, 1988; Smiddy *et al.*, 1988).

On average, 10–20% of keratoconus patients will need surgery (Kennedy *et al.*, 1986; Smiddy *et al.*, 1988; Zadnik *et al.*, 1998). Surgery is the accepted therapy when:

- Contact lenses provide adequate vision but cannot be tolerated.
- Contact lenses can be tolerated but do not provide adequate acuity.
- The cone extends so far towards the limbus that further progression may make corneal transplantation difficult.

Krachmer *et al.* (1984) state that the first two reasons cited above are more common, with the third occurring rarely. Keratoplasty for keratoconus is highly successful because the peripheral cornea is usually normal (Figure 28.11).

Table 28.4 Collaborative Longitudinal Evaluation of Keratoconus (CLEK) study keratoconus diagnostic lens set (Edrington *et al.*, 1996). All diagnostic contact lenses are polymethyl methacrylate (PMMA) with a third curve radius of 11.00 mm and a third curve width of 0.2 mm. The lenses are lightly blended, and the centre thickness is 0.13 mm (Adapter from Edrington, T. B., Barr, J. T., Zadnik, K. et al., 1996 Standardized rigid contact lens fitting protocol for keratoconus. Optom. Vis. Sci., 73, 369–375.)

Lens number	Inside sagittal depth under optic zone (mm)	Base curve mm (D)	Power (D)	Overall diameter/optic zone diameter (mm)	Secondary curve radius (mm)
1	0.704	7.85 (42.99)	–3.00	8.6/6.5	8.25
2	0.709	7.80 (43.27)	–4.00	8.6/6.5	8.25
3	0.714	7.75 (43.55)	–3.00	8.6/6.5	8.25
4	0.719	7.70 (43.83)	–4.00	8.6/6.5	8.25
5	0.725	7.65 (44.12)	–3.00	8.6/6.5	8.25
6	0.730	7.60 (44.41)	–4.00	8.6/6.5	8.25
7	0.735	7.55 (44.70)	–5.00	8.6/6.5	8.25
8	0.741	7.50 (45.00)	–4.00	8.6/6.5	8.25
9	0.746	7.45 (45.30)	–5.00	8.6/6.5	8.25
10	0.752	7.40 (45.61)	–6.00	8.6/6.5	8.25
11	0.757	7.35 (45.92)	–4.00	8.6/6.5	8.25
12	0.763	7.30 (46.23)	–5.00	8.6/6.5	8.25
13	0.769	7.25 (46.55)	–6.00	8.6/6.5	8.25
14	0.775	7.20 (46.87)	–5.00	8.6/6.5	8.25
15	0.781	7.15 (47.20)	–6.00	8.6/6.5	8.25
16	0.787	7.10 (47.54)	–7.00	8.6/6.5	8.25
17	0.794	7.05 (47.87)	–5.00	8.6/6.5	8.25
18	0.800	7.00 (48.21)	–6.00	8.6/6.5	8.25
19	0.807	6.95 (48.56)	–7.00	8.6/6.5	8.25
20	0.813	6.90 (48.91)	–6.00	8.6/6.5	8.25
21	0.820	6.85 (49.27)	–7.00	8.6/6.5	8.25
22	0.827	6.80 (49.63)	–8.00	8.6/6.5	8.25
23	0.834	6.75 (50.00)	–6.00	8.6/6.5	8.25
24	0.842	6.70 (50.37)	–7.00	8.6/6.5	8.25
25	0.848	6.65 (50.75)	–8.00	8.6/6.5	8.25
26	0.856	6.60 (51.14)	–6.00	8.6/6.5	8.00
27	0.865	6.55 (51.53)	–7.00	8.6/6.5	8.00
28	0.870	6.50 (51.92)	–8.00	8.6/6.5	8.00
29	0.879	6.45 (52.33)	–7.00	8.6/6.5	8.00
30	0.886	6.40 (52.73)	–8.00	8.6/6.5	8.00
31	0.895	6.35 (53.15)	–9.00	8.6/6.5	8.00
32	0.903	6.30 (53.57)	–7.00	8.6/6.5	8.00

Several authors have examined the contact lens and surgical histories of their keratoconus patients to determine what proportion of patients referred for corneal surgery are unable to be fitted with contact lenses. Smiddy *et al.* (1988) reported that fewer than 13% of 115 consecutive keratoconus patients could not be fitted with contact lenses. A total of 56% of pre-keratoplasty eyes needed more than three contact lenses over a 5-year period. In all, 60% of 88 postoperative eyes needed to wear contact lenses for best vision.

Keratoplasty can be delayed or avoided by using contact lenses. This was true in 69% of selected patients followed by Smiddy *et al.* (1988) for an average of 5 years. This was also true for 95% of the 64 patients followed for up to 20 years by Kastl (1987). Belin *et al.* (1988) and Fowler *et al.* (1988) were able to refit 29 of 33 patients originally classified as surgical candidates, with 85% achieving visual acuity of at least 6/9. These studies underscore the importance of rigid contact lens correction in keratoconus for patients who never proceed to surgical intervention, in

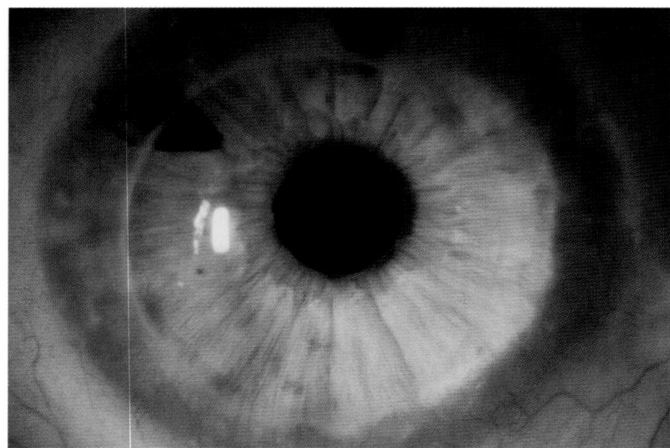

Figure 28.11 A penetrating keratoplasty performed for keratoconus.

patients thought to be surgical candidates, and in postoperative cases.

It is important that keratoconus patients be counselled adequately about the unknown aetiology of keratoconus, that its course is somewhat unpredictable and that it does not cause absolute blindness. Even early on, patients are often concerned about the possibility of corneal surgery, and they should know that the chances of that are as low as 1 in 10, that surgery is very successful (Sutton *et al*., 2008) and that ongoing care – both pre- and/or postsurgically – is the key to managing keratoconus.

Conclusion

Keratoconus is both a frustrating and fascinating disease. To treat it, the contact lens practitioner utilizes both the most scientific and the most artistic aspects of his or her profession. Keratoconus can require routine refractive error correction, the most subtle anterior-segment disease detection, complicated contact lens correction and surgical applications, within its typical course. This chapter defines aspects common to the disease; eye care practitioners caring for keratoconus patients can debate the range of its presentation.

Reference

Belin, M. W., Fowler, W. G. and Chambers, W. A. (1988) Keratoconus. Evaluation of recent trends in the surgical and nonsurgical correction of keratoconus. *Ophthalmology,* **95,** 335–339.

Bennett, E. S. (1986) Keratoconus. In *Rigid Gas Permeable Contact Lenses* (E. S. Bennett and R. M. Grohe, eds), pp. 297–394, New York: Professional Press Books.

Caroline, P. J., McGuire, J. R. and Doughman, D. J. (1978) Preliminary report on a new contact lens design for keratoconus. *Contact Intraoc. Lens Med. J.,* **4,** 69–73.

Chen, M., Sabesan, R., Ahmad, K. *et al.* (2007) Correcting anterior corneal aberration and variability of lens movements in keratoconic eyes with back-surface customized soft contact lenses. *Opt. Lett.,* **32,** 3203–3205.

Chung, C. W., Santim, R., Heng, W. J. *et al.* (2001) Use of SoftPerm contact lenses when rigid gas permeable lenses fail. *Contact Lens Assoc. Ophthalmol. J.,* **27,** 202–208.

Cohen, E. J. and Parlato, C. J. (1986) Fitting Polycon lenses in keratoconus. *Int. Ophthalmol. Clin.,* **26,** 111–117.

Colin, J. and Malet, F. J. (2007) Intacs for the correction of keratoconus: two-year follow-up. *J. Cat. Ref. Surg.,* **33,** 69–74.

Davis, L. J., Schechtman, K. B., Begley, C. G. *et al.* (1998) The CLEK Study Group. Repeatability of refraction and corrected visual acuity in keratoconus. *Optom. Vis. Sci.,* **75,** 887–896.

Duke-Elder, S. and Leigh, A. G. (1965) Keratoconus, Ch7, Part C(v). In *Diseases of the Outer Eye,* **Vol. 8,** Part 2. In *Systems of Ophthalmology* (S. Duke-Elder, ed.), pp. 964–976, London: Henry Kimpton.

Edrington, T. B., Barr, J. T., Zadnik, K. *et al.* (1996) Standardized rigid contact lens fitting protocol for keratoconus. *Optom. Vis. Sci.,* **73,** 369–375.

Edrington, T. B., Szczotka, L. B., Begley, C. G. *et al.* (1998) Repeatability and agreement of two corneal-curvature assessments in keratoconus: keratometry and the first definite apical clearance lens (FDACL). *Cornea,* **17,** 267–277.

Edrington, T. B., Szczotka, L. B., Barr, J. T. *et al.* (1999) Rigid contact lens fitting relationships in keratoconus. *Optom. Vis. Sci.,* **76,** 692–699.

Fink, B. A., Wagner, H., Steger-May, K., *et al.* (2005) Differences in keratoconus as a function of gender. *Am. J. Ophthalmol.,* **140,** 459–468.

Fowler, W. C., Belin, M. W. and Chambers, W. A. (1988) Contact lenses in the visual correction of keratoconus. *Contact Lens Assoc. Ophthalmol. J.,* **14,** 203–206.

Gasset, A. R. and Lobo, L. (1975) Dura-T semiflexible lenses for keratoconus. *Ann. Ophthalmol.,* **7,** 1353–1357.

Gould, H. E. (1970) Management of keratoconus with corneal and scleral lenses. *Am. J. Ophthalmol.,* **70,** 624–629.

Hall, K. G. C. (1963) A comprehensive study of keratoconus. *Br. J. Physiol. Opt.,* **20,** 215–256.

Hofstetter, H. W. (1959) A keratoscopic survey of 13,395 eyes. *Am. J. Optom. Arch. Am. Acad. Optom.,* **36,** 3–11.

Kastl, P. R. (1987) A 20-year retrospective study of the use of contact lenses in keratoconus. *Contact Lens Assoc. Ophthalmol. J.,* **13,** 102–104.

Kennedy, R. H., Bourne, W. M. and Dyer, J. A. (1986) A 48-year clinical and epidemiologic study of keratoconus. *Am. J. Ophthalmol.,* **101,** 267–273.

Korb, D. R., Finnemore, V. M. and Herman, J. P. (1982) Apical changes and scarring in keratoconus as related to contact lens fitting techniques. *J. Am. Optom. Assoc.,* **53,** 199–205.

Krachmer, J. H., Feder, R. S. and Belin, M. W. (1984) Keratoconus and related noninflammatory corneal thinning disorders. *Surv. Ophthalmol.,* **28,** 293–322.

Kymionis, G. D., Siganos, C. S., Tsiklis, N. S., *et al.* (2007) Long-term follow-up of Intacs in keratoconus. *Am. J. Ophthalmol.,* **143,** 236–244.

Lembach, R. G. and Keates, R. H. (1984) Aspheric silicone lenses for keratoconus. *Contact Lens Assoc. Ophthalmol. J.,* **10,** 323–325.

Mackie, I. (1977) Management of keratoconus with hard corneal lenses. The lens lid attachment technique. *Trans. Ophthalmol. Soc. U.K.,* **97,** 131–135.

Macsai, M. S., Varley, G. A. and Krachmer, J. H. (1990) Development of keratoconus after contact lens wear. Patient characteristics. *Arch. Ophthalmol.,* **108,** 534–538.

Maguen, E., Espinosa, G., Rosner, I. R. *et al.* (1983) Long-term wear of Polycon contact lenses in keratoconus. *Contact Lens Assoc. Ophthalmol. J.,* **9,** 57–59.

Mandell, R. B. (1988) Keratoconus. In *Contact Lens Practice,* 4th edn (R. B. Mandell, ed.), pp. 732–751, Springfield, IL: Charles C. Thomas.

Marsack, J. D., Parker, K. E., Pesudovs, K. *et al.* (2007) Uncorrected wavefront error and visual performance during RGP wear in keratoconus. *Optom. Vis. Sci.,* **84,** 463–470.

Marsack, J. D., Parker, K. E. and Applegate, R. A. (2008) Performance of wavefront-guided soft lenses in three keratoconus subjects. *Optom. Vis. Sci.,* **85,** E1172–1178.

Mobilia, E. F. and Foster, C. S. (1979) A one-year trial of Polycon lenses in the correction of keratoconus. *Contact Intraoc. Lens Med. J.,* **5,** 37–42.

Nau, A. C. (2008) A comparison of synergeyes versus traditional rigid gas permeable lens designs for patients with irregular corneas. *Eye Contact Lens,* **34,** 198–200.

O'Donnell, C. and Maldonado-Codina, C. (2004) A hyper-*Dk* piggyback contact lens system for keratoconus. *Eye Contact Lens,* **30,** 44–48.

Ozkurt, Y., Oral, Y., Karaman, A. *et al.* (2007) A retrospective case series: use of SoftPerm contact lenses in patients with keratoconus. *Eye Contact Lens,* **33,** 103–105.

Pilskalns, B., Fink, B. A. and Hill, R. M. (2007) Oxygen demands with hybrid contact lenses. *Optom. Vis. Sci.,* **84,** 334–342.

Raber, I. M. (1983) Use of CAB Soper Cone contact lenses in keratoconus. *Contact Lens Assoc. Ophthalmol. J.,* **9,** 237–240.

Raiskup-Wolf, F., Hoyer, A., Spoerl, E. *et al.* (2008) Collagen crosslinking with riboflavin and ultraviolet-A light in keratoconus: long-term results. *J. Cataract Refract. Surg.,* **34,** 796–801.

Rosenthal, P. (1986) The Boston lens and the management of keratoconus. *Int. Ophthalmol. Clin.,* **26,** 101–109.

Smiddy, W. E., Hamburg, T. R., Kracher, G. P. *et al.* (1988) Keratoconus. Contact lens or keratoplasty? *Ophthalmology,* **95,** 487–492.

Soper, J. W. and Jarrett, A. (1972) Results of a systematic approach to fitting keratoconus and corneal transplants. *Contact Lens Med. Bull.,* **5,** 50–59.

Sorbara, L., Chong, T., and Fonn, D. (2000) Visual acuity, lens flexure, and residual astigmatism of keratoconic eyes as a function of back optic zone radius of rigid lenses. (2000) *Cont. Lens Ant. Eye,* **23,** 48–52.

Sutton, G., Hodge, C. and McGhee, C. N. (2008) Rapid visual recovery after penetrating keratoplasty for keratoconus. *Clin. Experiment. Ophthalmol.,* **36,** 725–730.

Tan, B. U., Purcell, T. L., Torres, L. F., *et al.* (2006) New surgical approaches to the management of keratoconus and post-LASIK ectasia. *Trans. Am. Ophthalmol. Soc.,* **104,** 212–220.

Voss, E. H. and Liberatore, J. C. (1962) Fitting the apex of keratoconus. *Contacto,* **6,** 212–214.

Wollensak, G., Spoerl, E. and Seiler, T. (2003) Riboflavin/ultraviolet-A-induced collagen crosslinking for the treatment of keratoconus. *Am. J. Ophthalmol.,* **135,** 620–627.

Zadnik, K. and Mutti, D. O. (1987) Contact lens fitting relation and visual acuity in keratoconus. *Am. J. Optom. Physiol. Opt.,* **64,** 698–702.

Zadnik, K., Gordon, M. O., Barr, J. T. *et al.* (1996) Biomicroscopic signs and disease severity in keratoconus. *Cornea,* **15,** 139–146.

Zadnik, K., Barr, J. T., Edrington, T. B. *et al.* (1998) Baseline findings in the Collaborative Longitudinal Evaluation of Keratoconus (CLEK) Study. *Invest. Ophthalmol. Vis. Sci.,* **39,** 2537–2546.

Zadnik, K., Barr, J. T., Edrington, T. B. *et al.* (2000) Corneal scarring and vision in keratoconus – A baseline report from the Collaborative Longitudinal Evaluation of Keratoconus (CLEK) Study. *Cornea,* **19,** 804–812.

Zadnik, K., Barr, J. T., Edrington, T. B. *et al.* (2005) Comparison of flat and steep rigid contact lens fitting methods in keratoconus. *Optom. Vis. Sci,.* **82,** 1014–1021.

High ametropia

Joseph T Barr

Introduction

Care for the highly ametropic patient is one of the most challenging and yet one of the most rewarding aspects of contact lens practice. The most common indications for this care are high myopia, high corneal toricity and thus high astigmatism, and adult and paediatric aphakia. This is especially true in cases of unilateral high ametropia, resulting in high anisometropia and possibly aniseikonia. These cases are challenging due to the high lens centre thickness of plus lenses and high edge thickness for minus lenses, the need for lenticularization, and centre of mass difficulties, as well as the fact that these eyes often have pathological changes. These pathological changes include degenerative myopia, cataract surgery and increased risk of retinal detachment.

Highly hyperopic and aphakic patients benefit from decreased need for head turning, better peripheral vision, elimination of blind areas in their field of view with spectacles ('jack-in-the-box'), but they have less magnification in contact lens wear as compared to spectacles. These patients also have a larger image size with spectacles but prefer contact lenses due to the field-of-vision benefits. Highly myopic patients benefit from the increased magnification (less minification) as compared to spectacles (see Chapter 3). These high myopes have significantly improved visual acuity as a result. The highly astigmatic patient benefits from contact lenses as compared to spectacles primarily as a result of the elimination of aniseikonia.

All of these patients benefit from improved cosmesis as compared to thick, unsightly spectacle lenses. This factor, coupled with the superior visual performance overall compared with spectacles, generally means that the highly ametropic patient will be strongly motivated to persevere during the initial adaptation phase of lens wear (Astin, 1999).

Lens materials for high ametropia

Just like the thick spectacles high ametropes seek to avoid, their contact lenses are also likely to be relatively thick. This produces challenges for lens design and oxygen transmission to the cornea. High ametropia usually requires the use of custom-made lenses to produce the power and base curves necessary. The practitioner may choose from any of the following material types:

- High-water-content soft lenses (may be used with close monitoring).
- Silicone elastomer lenses (often wet poorly, can be hard to remove).
- Silicone hydrogel lenses (high transmissibility).
- Rigid lenses (give the best tear flow).

Silicone elastomer

The use of silicone elastomer lenses has not become widespread; however, they have a place in fitting aphakic and other high-plus patients. Silicone lenses are typically 11.3–12.5 mm in diameter and are fitted with base curve near or only slightly flatter than K.

Silicone hydrogel

Silicone hydrogel lenses have been available for some years for ametropia between +8.00 and −12.00 DS. The vast majority of lens wearers are potentially able to benefit from the increased oxygen that they provide. Unfortunately, it is precisely those with the highest amounts of ametropia, who would have the most to gain, that were not covered by the power ranges available.

Developing a silicone hydrogel material for the speciality contact lens industry has not been a straightforward proposition. First-generation lens materials were all developed for cast moulding and many required surface treatment. There were various obstacles to overcome before producing a silicone hydrogel material in button form that could be processed into a contact lens (Tapper, 2006):

- The lathing of silicone hydrogel materials is made difficult by the inclusion of a silicone component, as such materials are relatively soft. The lathe turning of these softer materials to produce lenses with

DOI: 10.1016/B978-0-7506-8869-7.00029-X

Table 29.1 Silicone hydrogels for custom fitting

Brand name	Manufacturer	Material name	Water content (%)	Oxygen permeability (Barrers)	Modulus (MPa)	Method of manufacture	Power range
Air Optix Individual	CIBA Vision	Sifilcon A II4	32	82	1.1	Lathe	+20.00 to –20.00 DS
Nissel Silicone Hydrogel	Cantor & Nissel	Filcon II 1	38	115	0.26	Lathe	+30.00 to –30.00 DS
Silicone Hydrogel	Ultravision CLPL	Definitive Filcon II 3	74	60	0.27	Lathe	+45.00 to –45.00 DS

acceptable optical quality requires the highest-performing machine platforms currently available.
- Commercial constraints: companies have invested heavily in developing these materials and considerable knowledge has been derived from these activities, with any significant breakthroughs being carefully protected by the enforcement of patents.
- High raw material costs.

There are currently three silicone hydrogel lenses available on the UK market that can be made in custom designs. Their properties are shown in Table 29.1. All the lenses are manufactured by lathing and are recommended for daily wear only. Although the transmissibility of the Define material (*Dk* 60) is not as high as other available silicone hydrogels, this still allows the criteria of Holden and Mertz (1984) for daily wear to be fulfilled in a wider range of designs than can currently be achieved with conventional hydrogels (Young and Tapper, 2008).

These lenses should therefore provide relief from the hypoxia that has been inherent with low-*Dk* soft lenses and allow better comfort and planned replacement of lenses compared to rigid materials. Silicone hydrogel high-plus lenses are fitted like soft contact lenses.

Principles of high-power lens design

The main aim when designing high-powered lenses is to reduce the mid peripheral thickness of minus lenses, or the centre thickness of plus lenses, and at the same time to ensure that the optic zone is of sufficient diameter and centred on the pupil. These principles apply equally to soft and rigid lenses.

High-plus

High-plus rigid lenses, unless they are of very small diameter (8.5 mm or less) and steep fit, must be made in regular (parallel) carrier form or minus (edge thicker than junction) carrier form (Figure 29.1). Lenticular lenses are thinner, have less mass and centre better than non-lenticular designs. Typically these lenses are 9.0–10.5 mm in diameter. Regular carrier designs are better for lens positioning between the eyelids. Minus carrier lenses are better for lid attachment fitting (Figure 29.2). The smaller the front optic zone diameter, the thinner the lens. The front optic zone diameter may be equal to, larger than or smaller than the back optic zone diameter. Typically the front optic zone diameter is 7.0–8.0 mm in diameter, and the back optic zone is designed as needed for fitting. Junction thickness for lenticular rigid plus lenses should be thin enough to minimize lens thickness but thick enough to allow adequate lens strength (about 0.15 mm). Regular carrier unfinished edge thickness is typically 0.10–0.12 mm and minus carrier unfinished edge thickness is typically approximately 0.2 mm. Lenticular (front peripheral) radii range from approximately 0.2 mm flatter than the posterior secondary curve (regular carrier) to 3.0 mm flatter than the posterior secondary curve (minus carrier) (Polse, 1988).

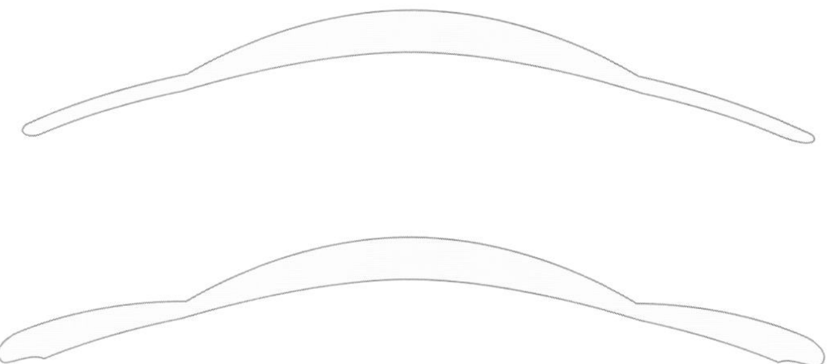

Figure 29.1 Lenticular lens designs. Top: regular (parallel) carrier. Bottom: minus carrier.

Even with a lenticulated front surface, the centre of gravity of a rigid lens is relatively anterior and may cause the lens to drop excessively. This can sometimes be solved by fitting a rigid lens of unusually large diameter, e.g. the Apex lens design has a diameter of up to 12.5 mm. Not only is centration improved, there is less movement and handling may be easier (Gasson and Morris, 2003).

Aphakia

Fortunately, adult aphakia is now rare due to the high success rate of intraocular lenses. However, in some cases, such as aniridia, chronic uveitis and glaucoma, contact lenses may be indicated.

If extended wear is desired to minimize frequent lens handling, lenses of maximum oxygen transmissibility are recommended. These patients may, with proper monitoring, wear their lenses for a month at a time, if the benefits outweigh the risks. High-water-content soft contact lenses may be preferred for comfort over rigid ones, particularly in monocular aphakia, and should be selected to maximize oxygen transmissibility for extended wear. Low-water-content lenses are not used, because the risk of

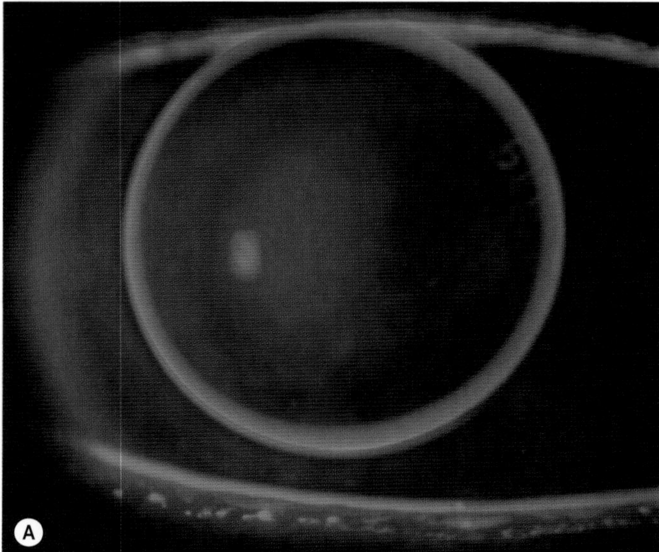

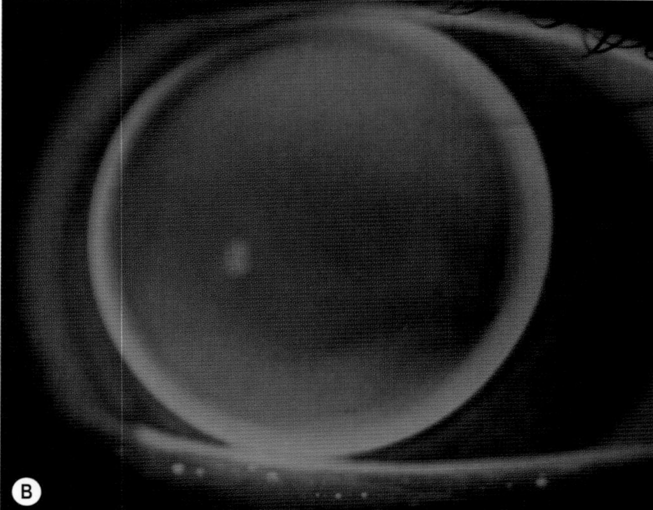

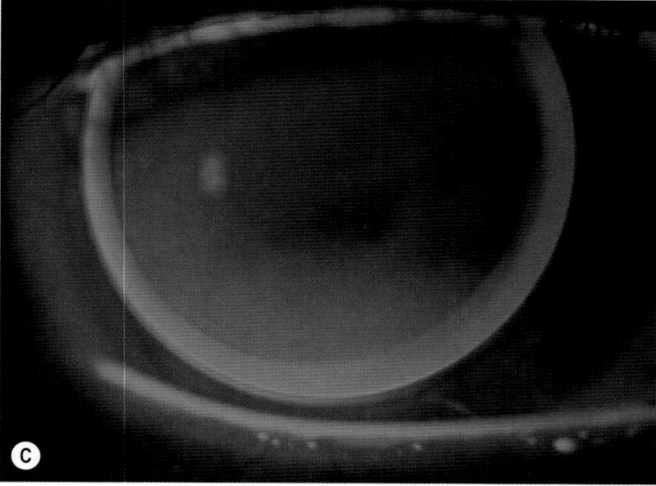

Figure 29.2 Fluorescein patterns for high-plus rigid lenses. (A) 7.5 mm diameter, +13.00 D lens, positioning temporally. (B) 9.5 mm diameter, +12.00 D lens, positioning temporally. (C) 9.5 mm diameter, +15.00 D lens, with position governed by upper lid.

hypoxic problems is high (interestingly, the aphakic eye may swell less than an unoperated eye; Holden *et al.*, 1982). Handling typically will be difficult in bilateral aphakic patients due to poor uncorrected vision and reduced manual dexterity in the elderly. Some aphakes may prefer to handle soft lenses due to their large size, and some may prefer rigid lenses because of their stiffness.

Residual astigmatism and reading additions for near work can be corrected in spectacles to be worn over the contact lenses.

Patients with conjunctival filtering blebs should be monitored closely and contact lenses should not impinge on these blebs excessively. Preferably, topical ocular medication is instilled before and after lens wear and only under close supervision during contact lens wear.

The correction of paediatric aphakia is dealt with in detail in Chapter 30.

High-minus

A rigid contact lens of –10.00 D would have an unfinished edge thickness of approximately 0.32–0.35 mm if the diameter is 8.8–9.6 mm. Because unfinished edge thickness for best comfort and lens stability should be approximately 0.10 mm, lenticularization of high-minus lenses is very important. This can be performed by CN bevelling, grinding the excess edge thickness by hand in a diamond-impregnated cone-shaped tool, and then polishing this area. Preferably, the laboratory will use a computer numeric-controlled lathe to cut a steeper anterior lenticular radius to obtain the proper edge thickness.

Typical front optic zone diameters range from 7.2 mm (8.8 mm lens diameter) to 7.8 mm (9.6 mm lens diameter) and are about 0.2 mm larger than the back optic zone. The lenticular radius may be cut flatter for a smaller front optic zone or steeper for a larger front optic zone. The latter design will result in higher mid peripheral thickness. The higher the power – with the same front optic zone – the thicker will be this mid peripheral area (Figure 29.3). This may complicate the fit and cause discomfort if the lens does not attach to the upper eyelid. Greater mid peripheral thickness may also cause a high-riding lens to ride even higher. Mid peripheral thickness can be reduced with proper polishing or advanced multicurve computer-controlled anterior-surface lathing (Figure 29.4) (Moore and Mandell, 1989).

High astigmatism

High astigmatism is typically caused by high corneal toricity. Custom soft toric contact lenses are available in high powers. Of course, the higher the cylinder power in the lens, the more a given degree of unwanted lens rotation will cause blur. If rigid lenses are not desirable, for example in dusty environments, soft toric lenses may be preferred. Oblique astigmatism is difficult to manage with soft toric contact lenses. The higher the corneal toricity, the better the orientation stability with rigid bitoric lenses. Against-the-rule toric corneas are difficult to fit with spherical rigid lenses due to poor lateral lens centration, unlike with-the-rule corneas where the upper eyelid can help position the lens properly. Bitoric rigid lenses may be fitted with toric base curves that are slightly less toric than the corneal toricity. The spherical power effect bitoric lens (where the

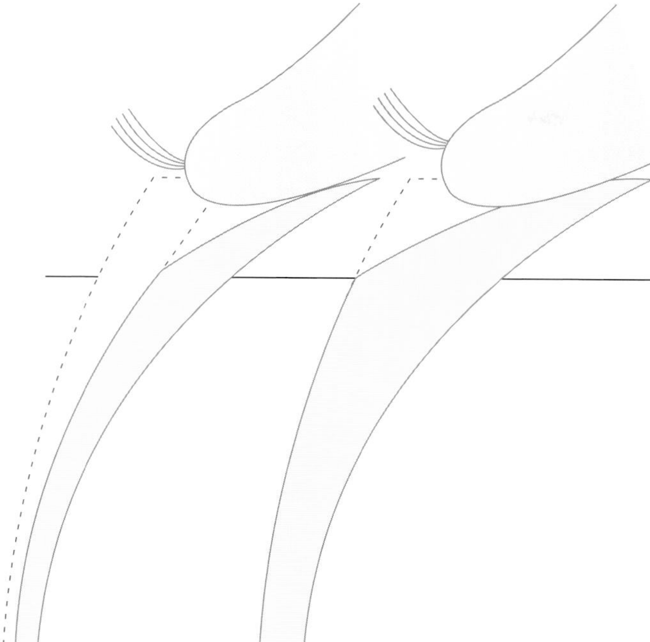

Figure 29.3 Low-minus power lens (left) with same front optic zone diameter as high-minus power lens (right). Junction thickness (horizontal straight line) is greater for the high-minus power lens.

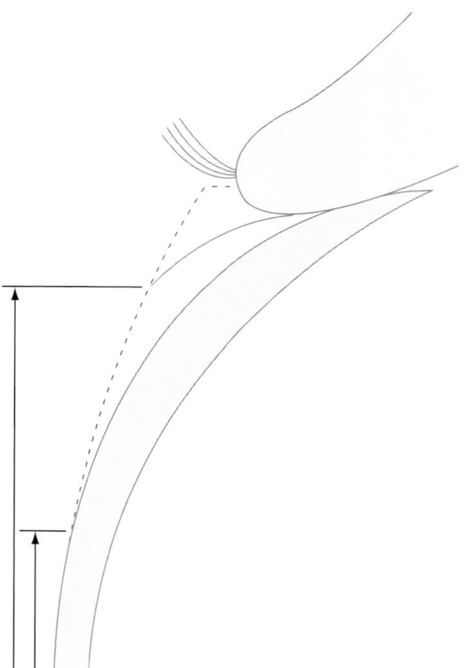

Figure 29.4 Optimized high-minus power lens design.

base curve toricity in dioptres equals power difference in dioptres) may rotate somewhat off-axis without causing residual astigmatism. Highly toric rigid lens designs – up to 11.00 D of base curve toricity and cylinder power – are possible.

Another option occasionally used for irregular astigmatism, such as keratoconus, is a very thick soft contact lens. Such a lens will minimize the irregular astigmatism and correct most of the spherical component of the refractive error; the residual refractive error is corrected with spectacles. The drawback of this approach is such lenses will generally have a very low oxygen transmissibility.

Fitting challenges

Blinking can result in excessive movement of high-plus rigid contact lenses, although more stability and less decentration can be achieved if lenticular designs are used. Soft lenses will generally be more stable in the eye.

Both high-plus and high-minus rigid lenses may tend to drop on the cornea to a low-riding position. This will result in peripheral corneal staining, as well as discomfort and possibly poor vision. Both lens types have high mass compared to low-power lenses, with the high-minus lens actually having more mass than a plus lens of equivalent power and diameter, due to the increased thickness around the lens periphery. This is complicated by the centre of mass differences. The minus lens has a centre of mass further behind the lens posterior surface (Carney *et al.*, 1987), which causes better centration forces for the minus lens and poorer fitting (dropping) of the plus lens. Lenticularization of both designs will assist in fitting and a minus carrier design on a plus lens can help the upper lid to hold the lens up, much like a high-minus lens that is held in place by the upper eyelid.

Lens positioning problems may be solved with 'piggy-back' fitting. Most commonly used in keratoconus, this system employs a soft spherical lens (typically a disposable lens in low-minus power) with a rigid lens fitting over it. A special soft lens with a cut-out central portion (depression in the front surface) is available. A rigid lens that is 0.5 mm smaller than the cut-out portion of the soft lens is fitted over this soft lens. Scleral lenses, manufactured from high-oxygen-permeability rigid materials, are always an option for the high ametrope (see Chapter 23).

Of course, for high ametropia, contact lens power may only partially compensate for the ametropia and the residual refractive error may be corrected with spectacles – especially residual astigmatism and presbyopic correction.

Low vision

One unique and rarely used contact lens application is the Galilean telescope system. For example a –30.00 D contact lens can be used in conjunction with a +20.00 D spectacle lens at a 17 mm vertex distance to obtain 1.5× magnification. With a 40 mm spectacle eye size, field of view is limited to 68° with this system (Mandell, 1988).

Conclusions

Best care for highly ametropic patients demands that the practitioner understand:

- Unique examination necessities, especially for paediatric patients.
- Lens design options, especially lenticular forms.
- Lens material options.
- The interaction between lens design and fitting of high-powered lenses.

- Magnification properties of high-power lenses.
- Contact lens treatment options.

By working in collaboration with a custom lens laboratory, practitioners should be able to find an appropriate contact lens solution for most cases of high ametropia.

References

Astin, C. L. K. (1999) Contact lens fitting in high degree myopia. *Contact Lens Ant. Eye,* **22,** S14–S19.

Carney, L. G., Barr, J. T. and Hill, R. M. (1987) The most important point in contact lens design. *Optician,* **94**(5126), 40–42.

Gasson A. and Morris J. (2003) Corneal lens fitting. In *The Contact Lens Manual: A Practical Guide to Fitting.* (A. Gasson and J. Morris), 3rd edn., p. 409. Boston: Elsevier Health Sciences.

Holden, B. A. and Mertz, G. W. (1984) Critical oxygen levels to avoid corneal edema for daily and extended wear contact lenses. *Invest. Ophthalmol. Vis. Sci.,* **25,** 1161–1167.

Holden, B. A., Polse, K. A. and Mertz, G. (1982) Effects of cataract surgery on corneal function. *Invest. Ophthalmol. Vis. Sci.,* **22,** 343–350.

Mandell, R. B. (1988) Low Vision. Ch. 28 In *Contact Lens Practice* 4th Ed. (R. B. Mandell, ed.) pp. 770–784, Springfield, IL: Thomas Publishing.

Moore, C. F. and Mandell, R. B. (1989) The design of high minus contact lenses. *Contact Lens Spectrum,* **11,** 43–47.

Polse, K. A. (1988) Aphakia. Ch. 27 In *Contact Lens Practice* 4th Ed. (R. B. Mandell, ed.) pp. 732–769, Springfield, IL: Thomas Publishing.

Tapper, T. (2006) Lathe cut silicone hydrogels. *Global Contact,* **46,** 28–29.

Young, R. and Tapper, T. (2008) A new silicone hydrogel for custom lens manufacturing. *Global Contact,* **49,** 30–33.

CHAPTER 30

Paediatric fitting

Cindy Tromans

Introduction

The contact lens practitioner is a key member of a multi-disciplinary team involving paediatric ophthalmologists, optometrists and orthoptists concerned with ocular health and visual development of the child. Fitting babies, infants and children with contact lenses is a challenging yet rewarding area of clinical contact lens practice. Contact lenses play an important role in the correction of complex refractive errors in the paediatric population (Davies, 1998), the management of binocular vision anomalies and for therapeutic and prosthetic purposes.

Indications

Aphakia

One of the most common indicators for paediatric contact lens fitting is aphakia resulting from the surgical removal of the crystalline lens in congenital cataract. The incidence of congenital cataract (Figure 30.1) is reported as being 2.1 per 10 000 live births and 7.7 per 10 000 at 4 years of age (Taylor, 1998). Of these cases around 40% and 50%, respectively, have unilateral cataracts. Aphakia can also result from lens subluxation, as seen in Marfan's syndrome, or ectopia lentis. Trauma to the eye may result in the immediate loss of the crystalline lens or subsequent development of traumatic cataract, which may require surgical intervention.

Refractive management of bilateral aphakia can be achieved with spectacles (Figure 30.2). However, the drawbacks of aphakic spectacles include the weight of the lenses and difficulty in achieving good frame fit in babies and young infants. In addition, the maximum power of lenses is restricted, even in lenticulated form, to around +26.00 D.

Figure 30.3 shows a 3-week-old bilateral aphake wearing high-water-content hydrogel contact lenses of around +35.00 D power.

In cases of unilateral cataract, contact lens correction is essential for managing the resultant anisometropia.

Surgery for congenital cataract is usually performed within the first 6 weeks of life, and so it is vital to be aware of the rapid changes in the ocular dimensions that occur within the first few months of life. The average radius of curvature in a newborn is around 6.90 mm and this will flatten rapidly in the first 6 months of life (Inagaki, 1986). Axial length will increase rapidly from around 17.00 mm in neonates to 21.00 mm within the first 6 months of life and then more slowly during infancy and childhood (Larsen, 1971). These changes cause a 'myopic shift', with the aphakic correction decreasing from +35.00 to +20.00 D in the first few years of life. However, eyes with congenital cataract can have associated disorders such as persistent hypoplastic primary vitreous and microphthalmos, which require steeper-radii lenses and powers in excess of +50.00 D.

Average fittings of a high-water-content hydrogel lens based upon age, corneal radius and diameter are shown in Table 30.1.

Since infants in the early stages of visual development require a focal length of around 30–50 cm to see a face, the power of the selected contact is usually 2–3 D greater than the ocular refraction. This overcorrection should be reduced at 18 months to 2 years when the toddler becomes more aware of distant objects. A reading correction or bifocals can be prescribed from around 3–4 years of age when the child starts preschool education.

Pseudophakia

The use of intraocular lenses (IOLs) in the management of congenital cataract is increasing in infants (Zwaan *et al.*, 1998), with IOL implantation being carried out in infants at around 6 weeks of age. The aim of IOL implantation at this early age is to alleviate the need for contact lenses or aphakic glasses when the eye is fully grown. Typically, the young eye will be left 6–10 D undercorrected with the implant to compensate for the 'myopic shift', although significant prediction error can occur when calculating IOL power in paediatric cataract surgery (Tromans *et al.*, 2001). The resultant refractive error can then be corrected with a contact lens in the early months, with a 2 D overcorrection, gradually reducing lens power until the eye reaches an emmetropic state.

DOI: 10.1016/B978-0-7506-8869-7.00030-6

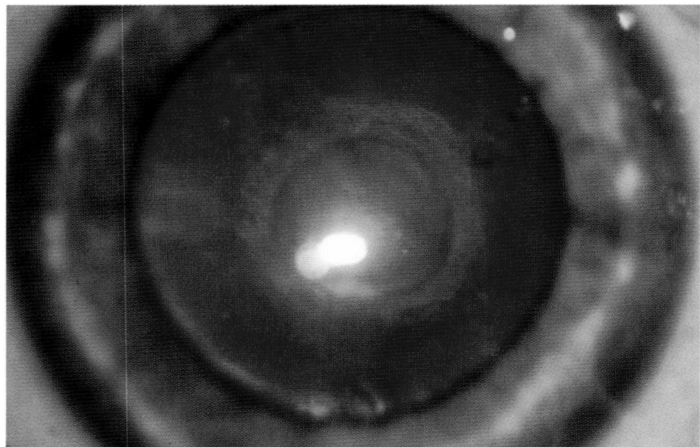

Figure 30.1 Congenital cataract.

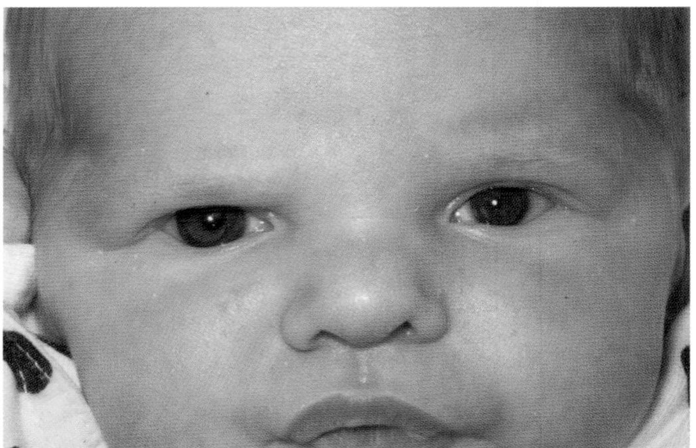

Figure 30.3 A 3-week-old bilateral aphake wearing high-powered soft lenses of around +35.00 D.

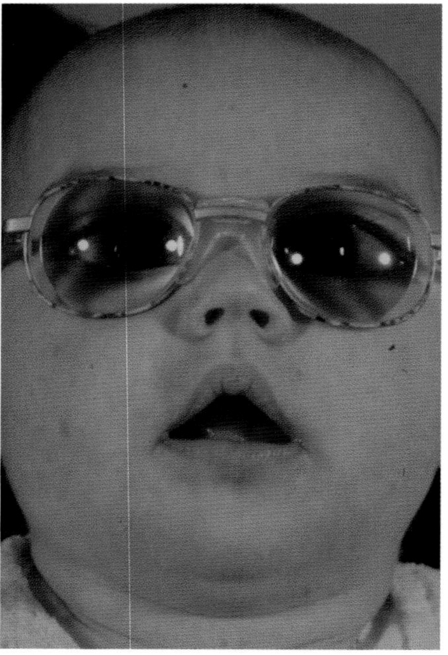

Figure 30.2 An 8-month-old bilateral aphake wearing her spectacle correction.

Table 30.1 Estimated hydrogel lens specifications based on age for an aphakic eye of normal size. These lenses would form the basis of a paediatric aphakic diagnostic fitting set

Age (months)	BOZR (mm)	TD (mm)	Power (D)
1	7.00	12.00	+35.00
2	7.20	12.50	+32.00
3	7.50	13.00	+30.00
6	7.80	13.50	+25.00
12	8.10	13.50	+20.00

BOZR = back zone optic radius; TD = total diameter.

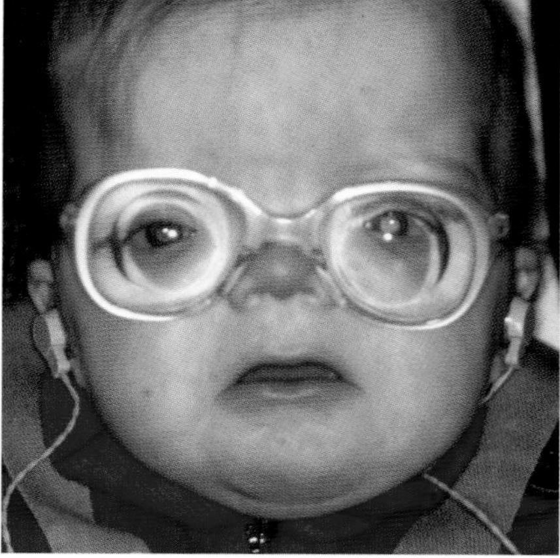

Figure 30.4 An infant with a high myopia in association with a craniofacial anomaly.

Myopia

Myopia in infants and young children is not uncommon and correction with spectacles is the accepted practice. However, in high myopia, spectacles have the disadvantage of reducing the retinal image size, inducing peripheral distortion and reducing the effective visual field (especially with lenticulated lenses). Contact lens correction is warranted where spectacle correction is problematic or normal visual development is threatened. High myopia (>10 D) may be present from birth and is related to a number of ocular and systemic disorders (Jensen, 1997). Also high myopia is associated with craniofacial anomalies, which can make the wearing of spectacles difficult (Figure 30.4).

The myopic eye is larger than normal and tends to have a flatter than average corneal radius and larger corneal diameter. Adult-sized lenses can often be used in young infants and children. Myopia can also result from buphthalmos where the corneal diameter is much larger than normal (>12.5 mm) and so requires a flatter and larger lens.

Contact lenses in unilateral high myopia have been shown to be more satisfactory than spectacle lenses in the

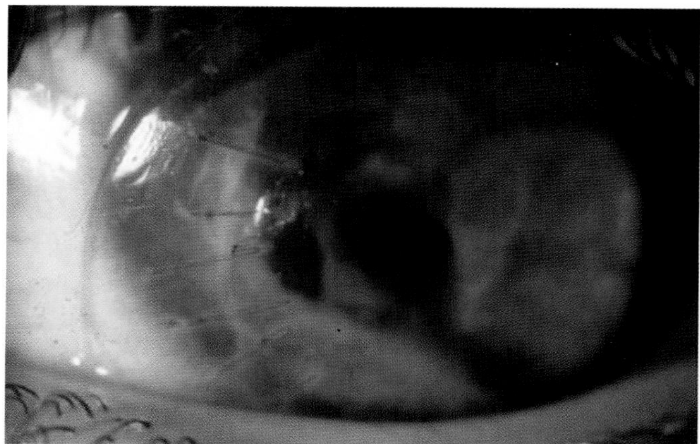

Figure 30.5 An aphakic eye, following trauma and a full-thickness corneal laceration, fitted with a hydrogel toric contact lens.

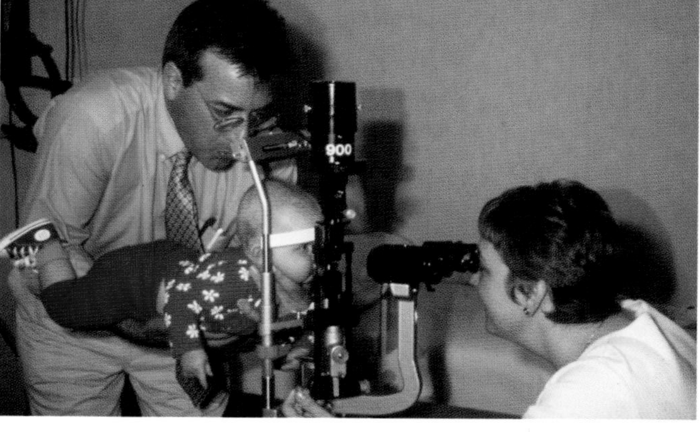

Figure 30.6 The 'flying baby' technique of child support during ophthalmic examination.

management of amblyopia in regard to cosmesis, comfort and treatment compliance (Mets and Price, 1981).

Ocular motility disorders

Contact lenses can be useful in the management of ocular motility disorders (Evans, 2006). Some uses include:

- Aniseikonia induced by anisometropia exceeding 6 D.
- Accommodative esotropia (older children).
- Nystagmus.
- Occlusion.

Irregular astigmatism

Irregular astigmatism derived from primary corneal ectasia is extremely rare in childhood. Most causes of corneal irregularity are secondary in nature, for example, following corneal infection or laceration (Figure 30.5). Neutralization of irregular astigmatism is important during the visual development period to prevent deprivational amblyopia. The optimum form of contact lens correction here is a rigid gas-permeable lens, although sometimes, if the irregularity is less severe, a toric soft lens may suffice.

Tinted and prosthetic lenses

The aim of this type of contact lens in paediatric use is to enhance visual performance by reducing the effect of photophobia or improving the cosmesis of the child by camouflaging an ocular defect. The most common reasons for fitting these lenses in childhood are:

- albinism
- aniridia
- achromatopsia
- iris defects, e.g. coloboma
- nanophthalmos or microphthalmos
- corneal anomalies, e.g. sclerocornea or Peter's anomaly.

The fitting of these lenses is described in more detail in Chapter 24.

Therapeutic lenses

Silicone hydrogel lenses have been shown to be safe and efficacious for continuous-wear therapeutic use in children (Benoriene and Vogt, 2006). Therapeutic contact lens use in the paediatric population is similar to adult use and is used mainly for the relief of pain, promotion of corneal healing and protection of the cornea. An example of their use is reported by Maycock *et al.* (2008), where two cases of upper-eyelid entropion secondary to neonatal conjunctivitis resolved spontaneously following the insertion of bandage contact lenses. Previously early surgical intervention was advocated to correct the eyelid abnormality and prevent any permanent corneal scarring and visual loss. The fitting of therapeutic lenses is described in more detail in Chapter 31.

Ocular response to lens wear

Walline *et al.* (2007) assessed the ocular response to contact lens wear in 8–12-year-old children and 13–17-year-old teenagers. Subjects returned for biomicroscopy examination at 1 week, 1 month and 3 months after lens dispensing. The presence of conjunctival staining increased from 7% of the subjects at baseline to 20% of the subjects at 3 months, but the changes were similar between children and teens. No other biomicroscopy signs increased significantly over the 3-month period. These findings suggest that contact lenses are a safe option for young children and can be routinely offered as a vision correction option, even for those as young as 8 years old.

Examination techniques

Anterior-segment examination

As with the adult patient, examination of the anterior segment is an important aspect of contact lens fitting and aftercare. A very simple method to determine the presence of corneal staining or ulceration is to use an ultraviolet lamp with fluorescein to determine the location and extent of the lesion. In babies, a major slit lamp can be used with the 'flying baby' technique (Figure 30.6) and in infants and

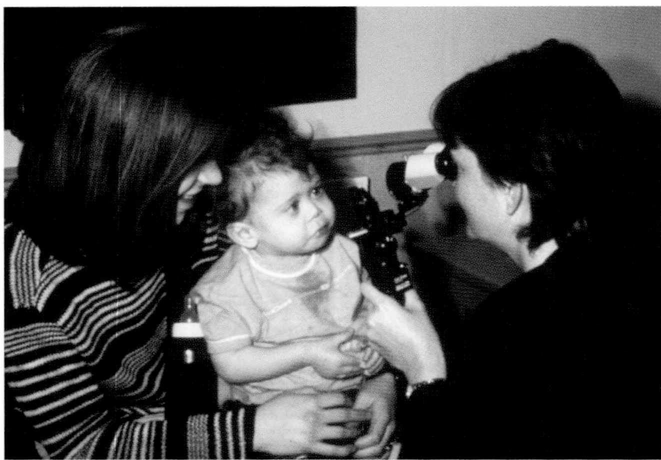

Figure 30.7 Examination of the eye of a child with a hand-held slit lamp.

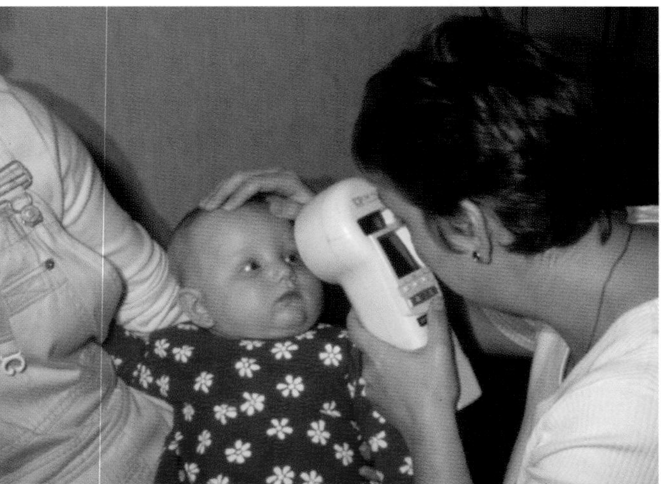

Figure 30.8 Use of a hand-held autokeratometer on a baby.

young children a hand-held slit lamp (Figure 30.7) can be used to examine the anterior segment in more detail. Older children, from 3 or 4 years of age, can usually sit at a slit lamp, kneeling on a chair and grasping the headrest support bars.

Keratometry

A hand-held automated keratometer can be used to determine the corneal radius of curvature in young infants and children too young to sit at a conventional keratometer (Figure 30.8).

Refraction

Determination of the refractive error or a contact lens overrefraction is performed with retinoscopy using hand-held lenses or a paediatric trial frame in an older child. The use of a cylcoplegic drug is recommended in those children with normal accommodative function. It is useful sometimes to dilate the pupil in aphakes or pseudophakes where there is a small or displaced pupil or where significant media opacity is apparent, e.g. posterior capsular thickening.

Biometry

Prior to cataract surgery, the axial length of the eye can be measured with ultrasound and the corneal radius of curvature by keratometry. These measurements can be used to determine the power of the contact lens required postoperatively by using an IOL calculation formula, e.g. Holladay, which can determine the ocular power at the corneal plane postsurgery. This is particularly useful as it allows more or less correct specifications to be ordered, which alleviates the need for many lenses to be used at the initial fitting and allows for fewer lenses to be kept in stock.

Lens selection

Hydrogel lenses

Hydrogel lenses are the most frequently used lens types in paediatric contact lens fitting. High-water-content lenses are usually selected as they can be worn for continuous or daily wear. Daily wear should be considered where possible to reduce the risk of infection as oxygen transmission can be reduced through high-powered lenses such as those used to correct aphakia (Amaya *et al.*, 1990). However, as babies and young children sleep during the daytime, the lenses can remain in the eye during these periods.

Lenses are usually fitted according to age or based on keratometry readings and corneal diameter.

The advantages of soft lenses are as follows:

- Custom-made in a range of radii, overall size, power and water content.
- Initially comfortable for the child.
- Parents tend to be less apprehensive about inserting a hydrogel lens into the eye of a baby or young child.

The disadvantages of soft lenses are as follows:

- they do not correct significant corneal astigmatism
- insertion can be difficult, especially for minus lenses, where there is considerable lid squeezing or a very small palpebral aperture
- hydrogel lenses are prone to dehydration – babies have relatively dry eyes due to low blink rate
- there may be frequent lens loss due to eye rubbing and dehydration.

Silicone hydrogel lenses

Silicone hydrogel lenses were initially not available in the range of base curves, diameters and powers that are required for fitting complex refractive error in young eyes. However, now that bespoke silicone hydrogels are available there has been an increase in the use of this lens type in paediatric contact lens practice. The use of custom-made silicone hydrogel lenses is discussed further in Chapter 29.

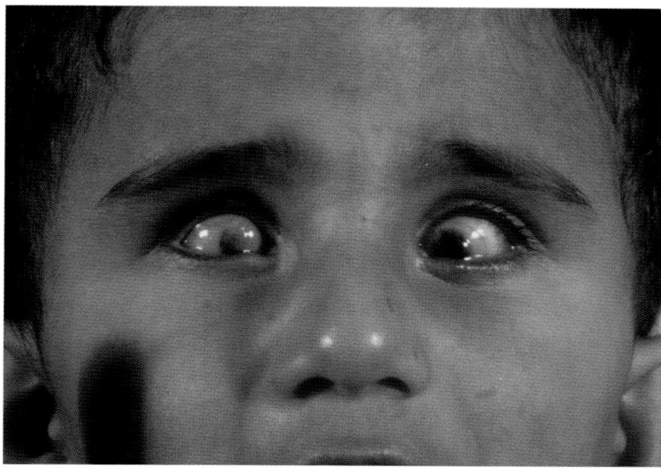

Figure 30.9 A silicone rubber lens fitted to the left aphakic eye of an infant with microcornea; a soft lens had failed due to lens dehydration.

Silicone rubber lenses

Silicone rubber lenses are often used in the correction of refractive errors in babies and young children, and are particularly useful where there is frequent lens loss or a dry ocular surface (Figure 30.9). The lens fit can be checked using fluorescein and ultraviolet light. A period of settling, for example 30 minutes, is required (Visser, 1997).

Silicone rubber lenses have the following advantages:

- Very high oxygen permeability.
- Not susceptible to dehydration on the eye.
- Less susceptible to damage.
- Not easily rubbed out.
- Easier to insert than hydrogel lens due to increased rigidity.

Silicone rubber lenses have the following disadvantages:

- Range of parameters and availability are limited.
- Need to be fitted precisely and require more chair time due to longer settling periods.
- Negative pressure effects can cause adhesion to the cornea if the lens is too tight.
- Surface coating degenerates, so lenses have a relatively short life span.
- More expensive than hydrogel and rigid lenses.

Rigid lenses

The development of automated hand-held keratometry and rigid lens design has led to the increased use of rigid lenses for paediatric use. They have been successfully used for the management of aphakia in infants and can be fitted without the need for general anaesthesia (Amos *et al.*, 1992) and for correcting high myopia and irregular astigmatism following corneal scarring and trauma (Shaughnessy *et al.*, 2001).

Rigid lenses have the following advantages:

- Available in a large range of materials and parameters.
- Correct corneal astigmatism.
- Durable.
- Rigidity can help ease insertion and removal.

Rigid lenses have the following disadvantages:

- Not usually suitable for continuous wear.
- Parents/carers can be more apprehensive about inserting rigid lenses.
- There is a risk of abrasion if insertion is difficult.
- Initial discomfort may be a problem in older children.

Rigid lenses are now available in hyperoxygen-permeable materials, designs and powers suitable for the treatment of paediatric aphakia and seem to provide adequate corneal oxygenation so that they can be used on a 1-week extended-wear basis (Saltarelli, 2008).

Handling of lenses

A modified technique for insertion and removal is required in the young eye and this technique is shown in Figure 30.10.

Some general points to consider when handling contact lenses in babies and young children are as follows:

- Lenses are easier to insert and remove with the child lying down on a firm, flat surface, e.g. examination couch.
- Babies can be swaddled in a blanket to make handling easier.
- It is far easier to learn how to handle lenses on a young infant than on a more active baby or toddler. It is therefore important to encourage parents and carers to undertake lens handling from the outset of lens fitting.
- Parents/carers should be advised to keep to regular times for handling, so that it becomes accepted as part of daily routine.
- If handling is difficult in young infants, lenses can always be inserted or removed during sleep.
- Handling often becomes more difficult from 18 months onward. Bilateral aphakes can start to use spectacles at this point and anisometropes can use a spectacle correction when occluded.
- Co-operation may be extremely limited in children aged between 2 and 5 years when fitting lenses for the first time. Spectacles may have to suffice in this age if the benefits of contact lenses are outweighed by the distress caused to the child by handling.

Common aftercare problems

In addition to lens fitting and handling problems, some other common problems include:

- Red or sticky eye – this can be due to numerous causes, including tight-fitting lens, infection, inflammation or allergic reaction. Parents/carers should be instructed to remove the lens immediately and seek urgent advice from a contact lens practitioner or ophthalmologist.
- Neovascularization – especially where thick hydrogel lenses have been used for continuous wear. Consider refitting with rigid or silicone hydrogel lenses.

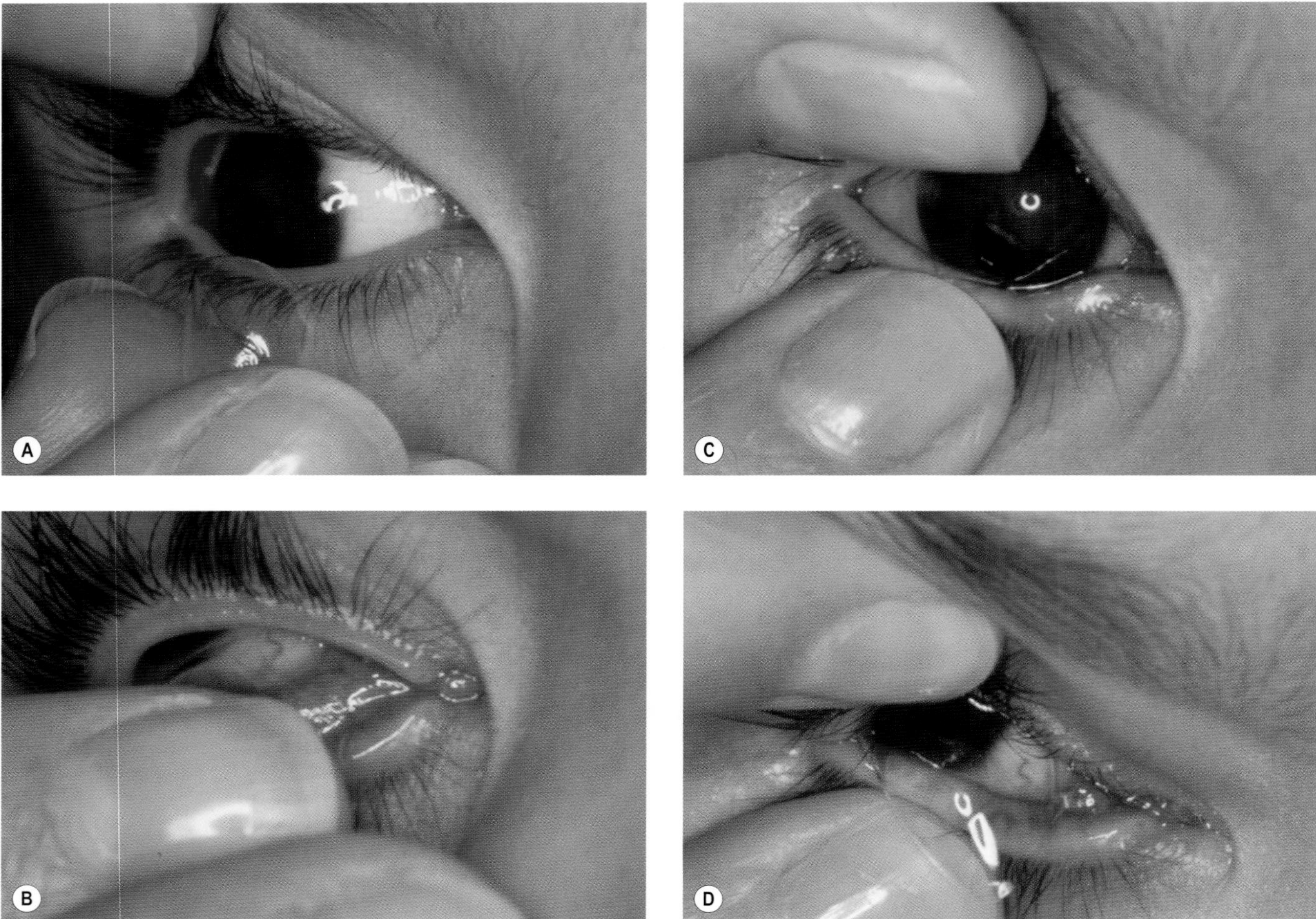

Figure 30.10 Paediatric contact lens insertion technique. (A) Hold the lens and upper lid prior to lens insertion. (B) The lens is inserted into the eye with the forefinger. (C) Positioning of fingers on the upper and lower lids prior to removal. (D) The lens is removed by applying gentle pressure and squeezing lids together.

- Papillary conjunctivitis – eye rubbing is often a sign of ocular irritation due to an allergy to care solutions or protein deposition on lenses. Management is similar to adult patients (see Chapter 40).
- Glaucoma – infant aphakes have a 25% risk of developing glaucoma (Johnson and Keech, 1996). Intraocular pressure can be measured on babies and young children with a hand-held non-contact tonometer, e.g. Pulsair, and this is advised at each visit.
- Other coexisting ophthalmic disease – regular fundoscopy should be performed by the contact lens practitioner or ophthalmologist to exclude the presence of, for example, retinal detachment, which is associated with high myopia and Marfan's syndrome.

Acknowledgement

The author would like to thank the Department of Ophthalmic Imaging at Manchester Royal Hospital for the production of the illustrations used in this chapter.

References

Amaya, L. G., Speedwell, L. and Taylor, D. (1990) Contact lenses for infant aphakia. *Br. J. Ophthalmol.,* **74,** 150–154.

Amos, C., Lambert, S. and Ward, M. (1992) Rigid gas permeable correction of aphakia following congenital cataract removal during infancy. *J. Pediatr. Ophthalmol. Strabismus,* **26,** 290–295.

Benoriene, J. and Vogt, U. (2006) Therapeutic use of silicone hydrogel lenses in children. *Eye Contact Lens,* **32,** 104–108.

Davies, L. (1998) Complex refractive errors in pediatric patients: cause, management, and criteria for success. *Optom. Vis. Sci.,* **75,** 493–499.

Evans, B. J. (2006) Orthoptic indications for contact lens wear. *Contact Lens Ant. Eye,* **29,** 175–181.

Inagaki, Y. (1986) The rapid change in corneal curvature in the neonatal period and infancy. *Arch. Ophthalmol.,* **104,** 1026–1027.

Jensen, H. (1997) Refraction and refractive errors. In *Paediatric Ophthalmology* (D. Taylor, ed.), pp 62–69, Oxford: Blackwell Science.

Johnson, C. P. and Keech, R. K. (1996) Prevalence of glaucoma after surgery for PHPV and infantile cataracts. *J. Pediatr. Ophthalmol. Strabismus,* **33,** 14–17.

Larsen, J. S. (1971) The sagittal growth of the eye: IV: Ultrasonic measurement of the axial length of the eye from birth to puberty. *Acta Ophthalmol.,* **49,** 873–886.

Maycock, N. J., Sahu, D. N., Mota, P. M. *et al.* (2008) Conservative management of upper eyelid entropion. *J. Pediatr. Ophthalmol. Strabismus,* **45,** 377–378.

Mets, M. and Price, R. L. (1981) Contact lenses in the management of myopic anisometropic amblyopia. *Am. J. Ophthalmol.,* **91,** 484–489.

Saltarelli, D. P. (2008) Hyper oxygen-permeable rigid contact lenses as an alternative for the treatment of pediatric aphakia. *Eye Contact Lens,* **34,** 84–93.

Shaughnessy, M. P., Ellis, F. J., Jeffery, A. R. *et al.* (2001) Rigid gas-permeable contact lenses are a safe and effective means of treating refractive anomalies in the paediatric population. *Contact Lens Assoc. Ophthalmol. J.,* **27,** 195–201.

Taylor, D. (1998) The Doyne Lecture. Congenital Cataract: the history, the nature and the practice. *Eye,* **12,** 9–36.

Tromans, C., Haigh, P. M., Biswas, S. *et al.* (2001) Accuracy of intraocular lens power calculation in paediatric cataract surgery. *Br. J. Ophthalmol.,* **85,** 939–941.

Visser, E. S. (1997) The silicone rubber contact lens: clinical indications and fitting technique. *Contact Lens Anterior Eye.* **20,** S19–25.

Walline, J. J., Jones, L. A., Rah, M. J. *et al.* (2007) Contact Lenses in Pediatrics (CLIP) Study: chair time and ocular health. *Optom. Vis. Sci.,* **84,** 896–902.

Zwaan, J., Mullaney P. B., Awad, A *et al.* (1998) Pediatric intraocular lens implantation. *Ophthalmology,* **105,** 112–119.

31 CHAPTER

Therapeutic applications

Roger J Buckley

Introduction

The therapeutic use of contact lenses goes back to the 1880s when Eugene Kalt (1861–1941) fitted a case of keratoconus. Since then, all types of contact lenses have been used as therapeutic aids. However, the term 'therapeutic contact lens' has become for many people synonymous with a soft plano 'bandage' lens. This is a misapprehension which should be dispelled by this chapter.

Indications

A contact lens may be fitted therapeutically for the relief of pain or discomfort, to assist the healing of injured or diseased ocular tissue or to improve vision in the case of unusual or distorted corneal shapes. Sometimes a therapeutic lens simultaneously addresses more than one clinical problem; it may in addition be used to correct a refractive error.

Unusual or distorted corneal shape

Congenital or developmental abnormalities of corneal topography, such as primary corneal ectasia (e.g. keratoconus and keratoglobus) and cornea plana (Figure 31.1), typically result in visual loss that can only be corrected with rigid forms of contact lenses – either corneal or scleral.

These conditions are rare but the patient is usually highly motivated to wear such lenses. Surgical treatment of severe keratoconus and keratoglobus may be technically difficult and, in the case of corneal transplantation, despite procedural advances such as deep anterior lamellar keratoplasty (DALK), there is still a risk of allograft rejection which can compromise the final outcome of the operation. Other newer procedures, such as the implantation of Intacs, with or without laser intervention, have not yet become generally accepted or their role clearly defined. Contact lens management, if successful, is nearly always to be preferred. Optimal visual correction can generally be provided and the lenses can be changed in design and power as the underlying condition and other ocular factors evolve.

DOI: 10.1016/B978-0-7506-8869-7.00031-8

Relief of pain

Corneal epithelial pain can be severe and disabling. A simple corneal abrasion usually heals quickly and needs no help from the clinician, but a persistent or recurrent epithelial failure may benefit from the fitting of a soft bandage lens of either hydrogel or silicone hydrogel material, which acts as a mechanical barrier between the injured corneal surface and the lid. Brilakis and Deutsch (2000) have described the use of a soft bandage lens in combination with topical anaesthesia to relieve pain following photorefractive keratectomy.

Recurrent erosion syndrome

Minor trauma to the cornea may predispose to this condition. Very often, corneal epithelial basement membrane dystrophy (such as Cogan's microcystic dystrophy or map-dot-fingerprint dystrophy) is found to be present; this is a bilateral condition, so both eyes should always be carefully examined. The eye with the erosion often becomes acutely painful when the eyes are opened during the night or when waking, for at that time tear production is minimal and friction maximal, so that the lid margin pulls on the unstable patch of epithelium, sometimes causing epithelial disruption. A contact lens, interposed between cornea and lid, can reduce the friction (Williams and Buckley, 1985; Liu and Buckley, 1996).

Corneal dystrophies involving the epithelium

Epithelial basement membrane dystrophy is by far the most common epithelial dystrophy, but other dystrophies that can involve the corneal epithelium also cause pain or discomfort that can be relieved with soft lenses. They include Reis–Bücklers' dystrophy, Meesman's dystrophy, lattice dystrophy, and Fuchs' dystrophy, in the last of which the failing corneal endothelium cannot prevent stromal oedema and bullous change in the epithelium (Andrew and Woodward, 1989). Thygeson's superficial punctate keratopathy is not recognized as a dystrophy but is appropriately considered here; this condition can sometimes be managed

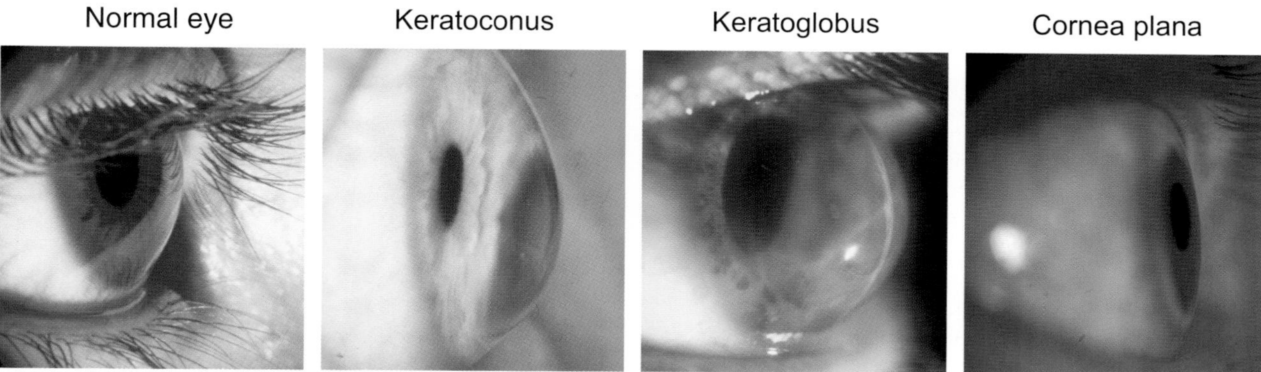

Figure 31.1 Unusual corneal shapes.

successfully with hydrogel lenses (Forstot and Binder, 1979), although weak topical steroid is a more usual form of management.

Filamentary keratitis

A 'wet' form of filamentary keratitis sometimes occurs without tear volume deficiency in herpes simplex keratitis, recurrent erosion, dystonia and in Theodore's superior limbic keratoconjunctivitis. This condition often responds well to the use of hydrogel lenses (Bloomfield *et al.*, 1973). The more usual 'dry' form of filamentary keratopathy occurs in tear deficiency, although contact lenses have little part to play in the management of this form of the disease. Scleral lenses have however been used successfully in 'dry' filamentary keratitis.

Corneal degenerations involving the epithelium

Conditions such as Salzmann's nodular degeneration, rosacea keratopathy and atopic keratoconjunctivitis - with or without ectasia - can sometimes be so uncomfortable that a therapeutic contact lens is indicated. Such a lens will probably also have visual improvement potential. Concurrent conjunctival disease and tear abnormality may well benefit from the use of a scleral lens.

Corneal trauma or surgery that has depleted endothelial functional reserves can lead to epithelial bullous keratopathy, the discomfort of which is often amenable to management with hydrogel or silicone hydrogel lenses. In some cases, a corneal transplant will subsequently provide a cure. Formerly this meant a full-thickness procedure but recently a method of replacing the endothelium, Descemet's stripping endothelial keratoplasty (DSEK), has been described and is gaining acceptance. A combination of phototherapeutic keratectomy and therapeutic contact lens wear for a limited period has been proposed in cases of bullous keratopathy not suitable for corneal transplantation (Lin *et al.*, 2001). Anterior stromal puncture is a low-cost alternative; however, it carries the risk of corneal perforation.

Chemical injuries

Much has been written about the use of contact lenses in the management of chemical injuries, especially alkali burns (Figure 31.2).

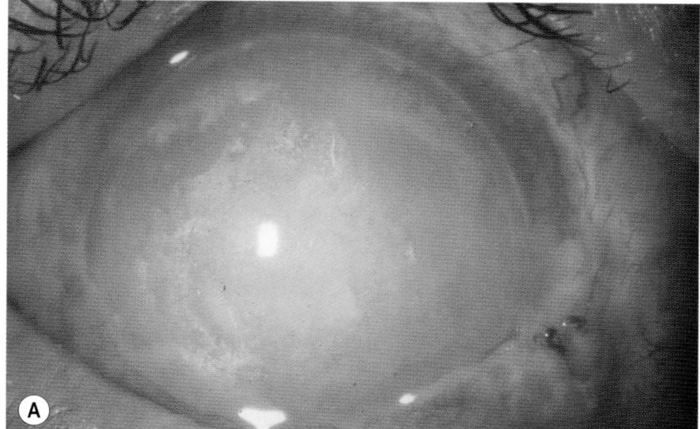

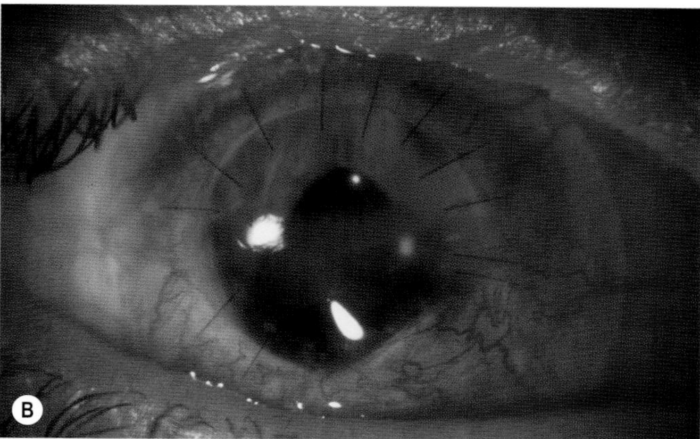

Figure 31.2 A 21-year-old woman suffered a sodium hydroxide chemical burn to the right eye. (A) After surgery (tenonplasty) a 12 mm diameter polymethyl methacrylate (PMMA) lens was glued to the cornea for 1 year (pictured here), after which a perforating keratoplasty was performed. (B) A high-water-content soft bandage lens was worn for 6 months to cover a persistent epithelial defect. The cornea remained clear and re-epithelialized.

However, research into the role of the limbal stem cell origin of the corneal epithelium has shown that contact lens coverage of the chronic epithelial defect cannot prevent the colonization of the cornea by conjunctivally derived epithelial cells. There are, however, some situations in which a contact lens can assist healing, supported by topical medications, although very close supervision is required.

Cicatricial conjunctivitis

It is clear that no type of contact lens can prevent conjunctival shrinkage. However, a scleral lens or ring can be used to support the fornices during the healing process following mucous membrane transplantation. More usually, contact lenses are fitted to protect the cornea from the hostile environment created by the disease (see below).

Tear deficiency

Tear deficiency is usually managed with the use of tear supplement drops and lubricating ointments, and sometimes the lacrimal puncta or canaliculi are deliberately blocked. Contact lenses are less often used. At one time it was thought that a high-water-content hydrogel lens could help to rehydrate a dry eye, but this is not possible as the lack of tears causes such a lens to dry and fall out of the eye. Silicone hydrogel (low-water-content) lenses are generally more successful in an abnormally dry ocular environment. The lens of choice is often a scleral lens, which covers the entire exposed surface of the eye, maintains a precorneal fluid reservoir and limits the evaporation of tears from the ocular surface.

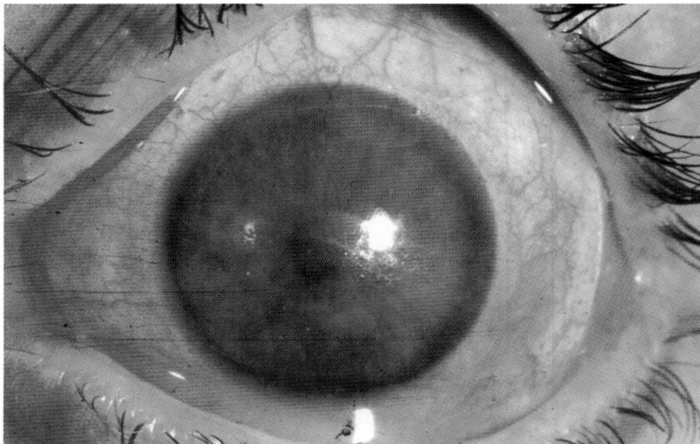

Figure 31.3 Severe Stevens–Johnson disease. The eye is fitted with a sealed gas-permeable scleral lens giving full corneal fluid coverage to maintain long-term hydration. There is extensive corneal neovascularization, which is not contact lens-induced but part of the disease process that was present before embarking on scleral lens fitting.

Protection from lids and environment

If the lids are deficient (e.g. congenitally or following trauma or surgery) or immobile (e.g. following seventh-nerve palsy), the eye is exposed and dry. The corneal epithelium becomes eroded and undergoes dysplasia, and blood vessels will invade the previously clear stroma, unless protection can be given. Possibilities include a temporary or permanent tarsorrhaphy, temporary paralysis of the levator palpebrae superioris muscle using botulinum toxin and the use of therapeutic contact lenses.

The lids themselves may constitute the challenge. They may be inturned (entropic), so that the lashes touch the globe (trichiasis), or the tarsal conjunctiva - especially the area adjacent to the lid margin - may be keratinized. Both situations are found in chronic cicatrizing disease, such as Stevens-Johnson disease (Figure 31.3) and cicatricial pemphigoid, and following chemical injury.

Keratinization without entropion is a feature of atopic keratoconjunctivitis. Most soft lenses will not survive in this type of environment, rapidly becoming decentred and often falling out of the eye. There is a place for corneal lenses here, especially lenses of large (limbal) diameter, but the first choice will often be a scleral lens.

When the cornea is insensitive, as occurs in trigeminal anaesthesia - such as following surgery for acoustic neuroma (Figure 31.4) and in herpes zoster involving the ophthalmic division - the condition of neurotrophic keratitis is commonly seen and great care must be taken when fitting contact lenses. The danger is that the reduced sensation will fail to alert the patient to complications such as retained foreign body, epithelial erosion and infection.

Patients with neuroparalytic keratopathy, that is, corneal disease secondary to exposure, for example in severe proptosis or ectropion, or resulting from facial nerve palsy, are initially best managed with lid taping, tarsorrhaphy or botulinum toxin-induced ptosis. There is sometimes a role for therapeutic contact lenses.

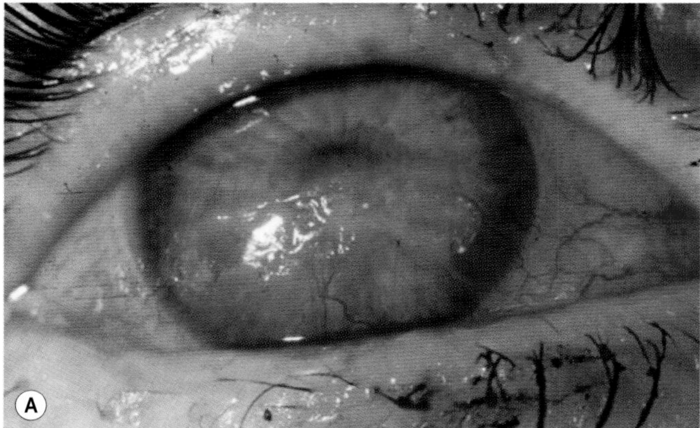

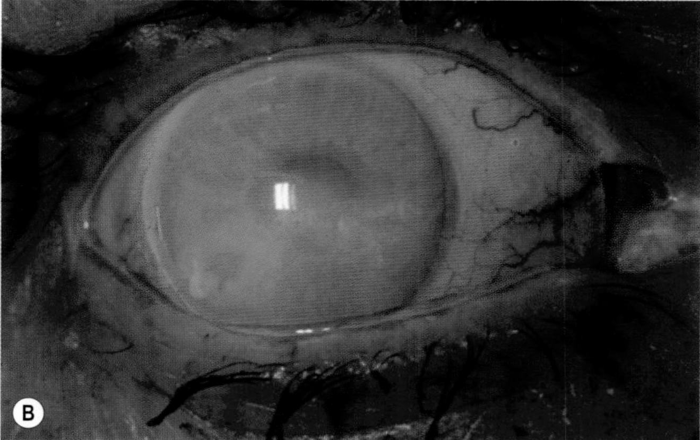

Figure 31.4 Severe exposure keratitis consequent to loss of lid closure function following an acoustic neuroma. (A) Viewed in white light without the lens, a severe exposure keratitis and neovascularization are evident. (B) A sealed gas-permeable scleral lens was prescribed for overnight wear. The precorneal fluid reservoir extends just beyond the limbus on the temporal side, and slightly further on the nasal side, providing an environment to enhance healing and maintain corneal hydration. The cosmetic appearance is improved by replacement of the highly irregular cornea with a smooth lens front surface and regular light reflex. The lens itself is barely visible: the edge can just be seen at the inner canthus.

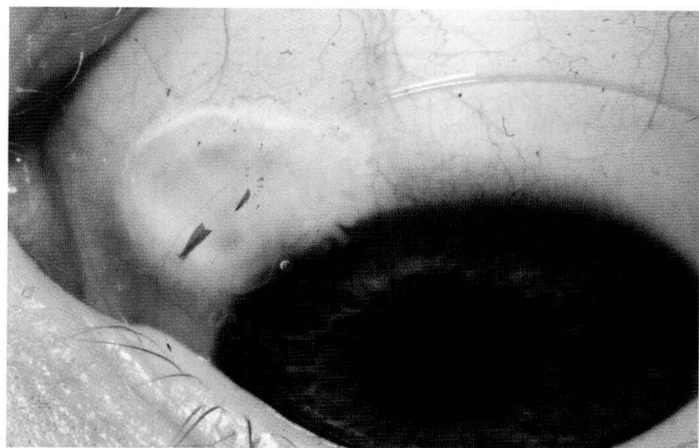

Figure 31.5 A leaking drainage bleb fitted with a large-diameter hydrogel lens in an attempt to form a seal. Even at 20 mm diameter, the lens was not large enough to cover the bleb fully, but was just functional as the perforation of the bleb was in proximity to the limbus.

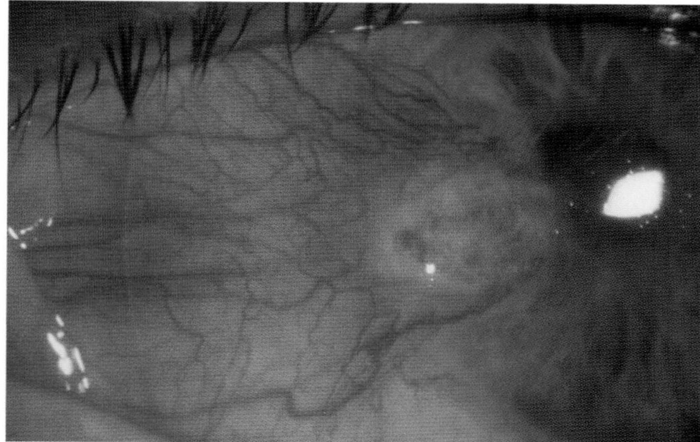

Figure 31.6 Corneal melting after perforating trauma with loss of sutures and wound leakage. The cornea was sealed with histo-acryl tissue glue and fitted with a large-diameter (20.5 mm) high-water-content (76.5%) soft bandage lens. The glue spontaneously dislodged after 10 days and the bandage lens was removed.

Maintenance of a precorneal tear reservoir

Where the eye cannot support a coherent tear film - for example, when a mucus abnormality or epithelial dysplasia renders the normally hydrophilic ocular surface hydrophobic - a precorneal tear reservoir can be created with the aid of a scleral lens with full corneal and limbal clearance. A sealed lens may be needed in order to retain the reservoir, in which case a gas-permeable material is used and the lens is filled with normal saline before being placed on the eye (see Chapter 23).

Following trauma or surgery

Persistent or recurrent epithelial defects may heal more rapidly following the application of a soft (hydrogel or silicone hydrogel) bandage lens. A small aqueous leak following surgery (Figure 31.5) or trauma (Figure 31.6) can often be sealed with such a lens; if the anterior chamber is shallow or absent, a slightly flat lens will be needed, and this will have to be changed for a steeper lens as the chamber reforms and the cornea steepens.

Shoham *et al.* (2000) have successfully used a custom-made 17.5 mm diameter 78% water content bandage lens to arrest leakage from trabeculectomy filtration blebs. Corneal transplant problems such as loosening sutures or slippage of the donor disc are usually best dealt with by further surgery, for example suture removal and/or resuturing. In such situations, contact lenses are unlikely to have more than a temporary role (for example, the relief of discomfort while arrangements are made for surgical intervention).

Following spontaneous perforation

Management of corneal perforation from acute hydrops may be attempted with bandage contact lens placement. A flat anterior chamber may reform within 24 hours (Yeh and Smith, 2008). Forooghian *et al.* (2006) reported on their success with a bandage lens following perforation in a patient with pellucid marginal degeneration.

Lens types

It should be recalled that all types of contact lens have therapeutic uses.

Soft hydrogel and silicone hydrogel lenses

When considering the fitting of a bandage lens, it is necessary to define or predict its probable pattern of use. The relevant considerations are:

- Whether extended wear is necessary.
- Whether the patient (or, failing the patient, a relative or friend) can be taught to handle, or at least to remove, the lens.
- The likely duration of therapeutic lens management.
- Whether the patient lives within practical travelling distance of the clinic or hospital.
- Whether the necessary topical medications are available unpreserved.
- Whether the risks of hypoxia, mechanical trauma and infection are outweighed by the perceived benefits of therapeutic lens wear.

Some hospital departments keep sets of bandage lenses - custom-made from high-water-content materials - in various radii and diameters. Others use commercially available lenses such as omafilcon A (Proclear, CooperVision, Fareham, UK) or daily disposable lenses of a number of types (Rubinstein, 1995; Bouchard and Trimble, 1996; Srur and Dattas, 1997). Silicone hydrogel lenses have an important therapeutic role because of their very high gas permeability, which minimizes the induced hypoxic and hypercapnic stress (Lim *et al.*, 2001). Their relatively low water content is an advantage where hydration of the lens by the tear film is problematic, for example in aqueous tear deficiency.

Comparison studies have been carried out between hydrogel and silicone hydrogel lenses in some therapeutic applications. Silicone hydrogel lens use has been shown to be a safe and effective alternative to conventional contact lenses for the treatment of bullous keratopathy (Lim and

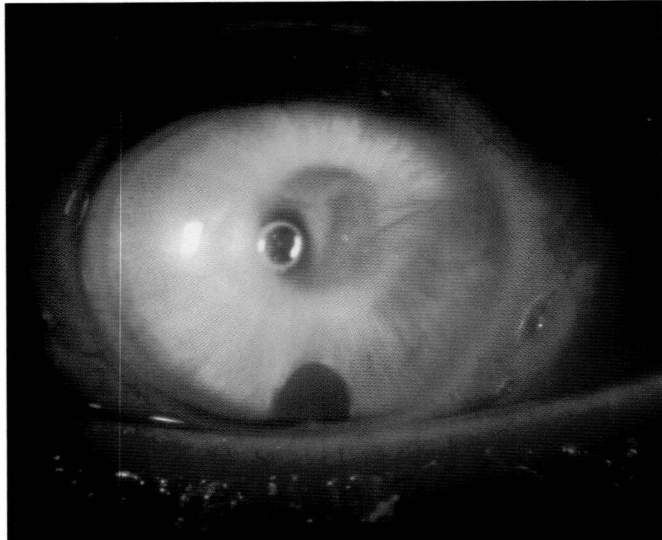

Figure 31.7 A large (20.5 mm diameter) soft bandage lens fitted to relieve pain in a 27-year-old man with Marfan's syndrome following ethylenediamine tetraacetic acid (EDTA) treatment. After numerous eye operations (cataract extraction, ablatio retinae, vitreous oil procedures), a painful band keratopathy formed, and a trophic ulcer was present.

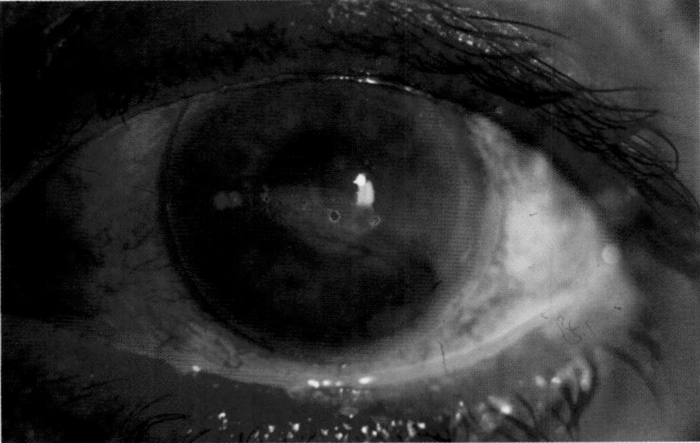

Figure 31.8 A large limbal diameter rigid lens has been fitted to protect a neurotrophic corneal lesion in the early stages of the healing process.

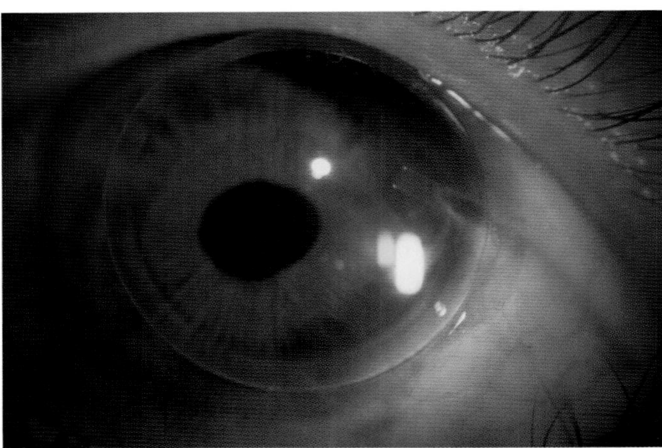

Figure 31.9 Rigid lens fitted to a buphthalmic eye.

Vogt, 2006). When fitting eyes after laser-assisted subepithelial keratomileusis (LASEK), the corneal epithelial status was statistically better in the eyes with a silicone hydrogel bandage contact lens 5 days after surgery compared to a hydrogel lens (Gil-Cazorla *et al.*, 2008a). No difference was found between the performance of two different silicone hydrogel lenses, except for comfort (Gil-Cazorla *et al.*, 2008b).

When fitting any soft lens, it is important to cover all areas requiring cover, and to aim for a little movement on blinking. There must be no compression of the limbal vessels (Figure 31.7).

Rigid lenses

Rigid lenses are frequently used for a combination of optical and therapeutic indications. Though of less than corneal diameter, they may provide enough cover to protect the cornea from abnormal lashes, keratinized lid margins and other hostile factors. Sometimes lenses of large diameters are used (Figure 31.8).

Figure 31.9 shows a rigid lens that has been fitted to a highly myopic (–10.00 D) buphthalmic eye of a 29-year-old male; a drainage tube can be seen entering the anterior chamber from the right of the image.

In ectatic conditions, such as keratoconus, keratoglobus and pellucid marginal degeneration (together constituting primary corneal ectasia), the cornea may become highly astigmatic, necessitating the fitting of a rigid bitoric lens. Such a case is demonstrated in Figure 31.10. A deep crescent-shaped corneal scar extends from the 4 o'clock to the 8 o'clock position. The scar is present at the level of Descemet's membrane and deep stroma, in the upper region of the zone of corneal thinning (Figure 31.10A). The vertically oval image of the perfectly circular Placido rings (Figure 31.10B) indicates against-the-rule astigmatism, and the closeness of the inferior rings indicates a very steep corneal profile due to ectatic bulging of the zone of corneal thinning. The bitoric rigid lens (Figure 31.10C) affords good vision. The fluorescein pattern is typical of such conditions (Figure 31.10D); the inferior ectatic corneal protrusion can be seen to bear against the lens.

Scleral lenses

Scleral lenses have a host of therapeutic roles (Tan *et al.*, 1995; Romero-Rangel *et al.*, 2000; Pullum and Buckley, 2007). Their advantages include the following:

- There need be no corneal contact whatsoever.
- Any eye shape can be fitted.
- Complete protection of the cornea and bulbar conjunctiva is provided.
- Sealed fits are possible, using gas-permeable materials, which simplifies the fitting process and minimizes 'settling back'.
- Using gas-permeable materials, overnight wear is possible.

At one time the fitting, and especially the ventilation, of scleral lenses required much practical experience. With the advent of gas-permeable scleral lenses, sealed fits have become the norm and so less skill is required. So many medical and therapeutic indications have been

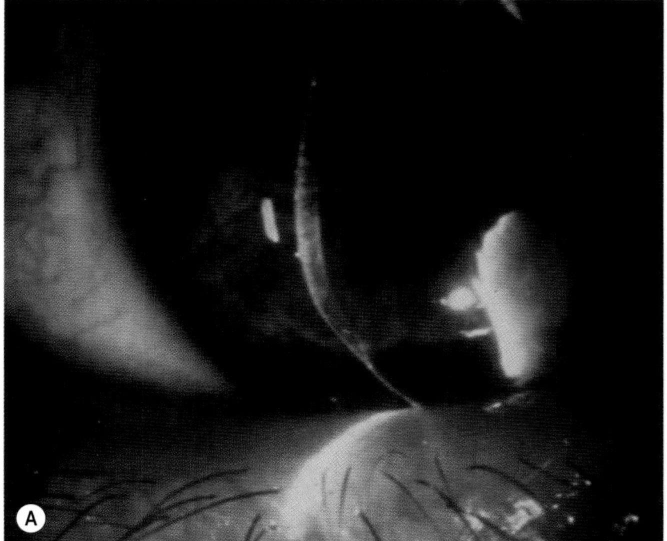

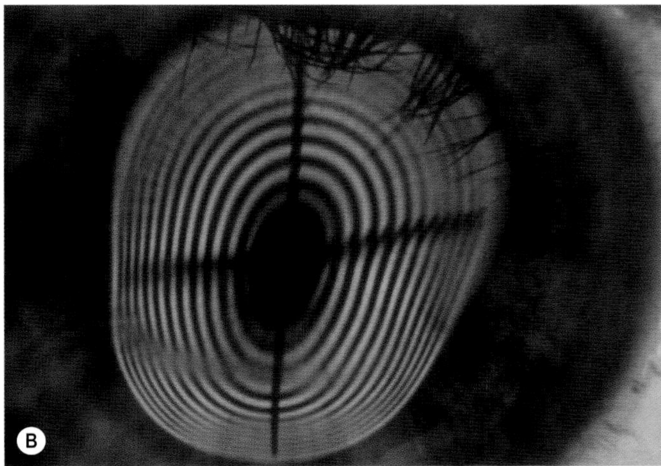

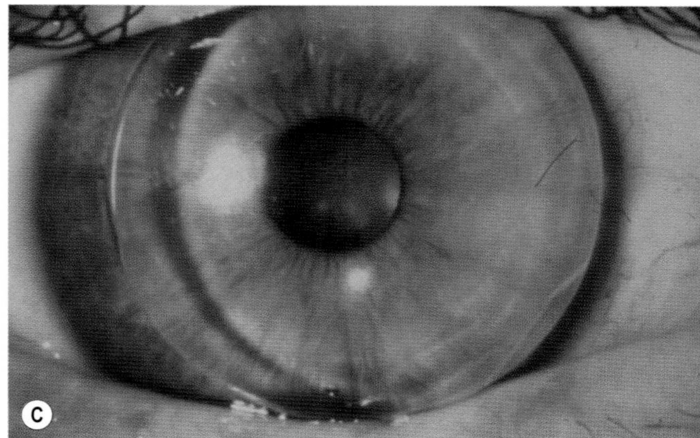

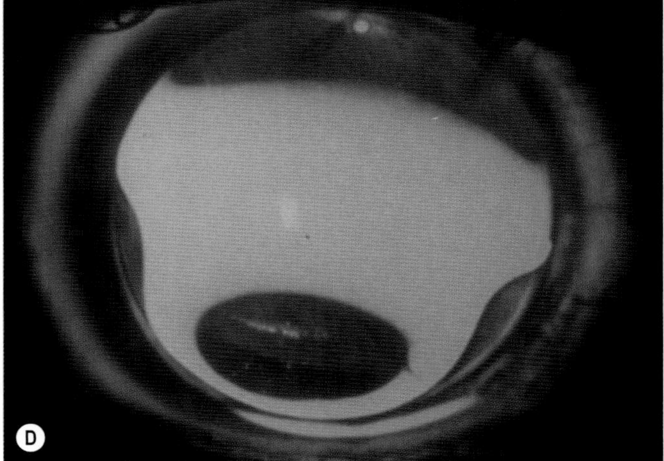

Figure 31.10 Bitoric rigid lens fitting in pellucid marginal degeneration. (A) Cornea viewed in optic section. (B) Placido image of cornea. (C) Bitoric rigid lens. (D) Fluorescein pattern indicates bearing of the inferior ectatic corneal zone against the lens (see text).

demonstrated that it can now be regarded as mandatory for hospital contact lens service departments to host, or have ready access to, a scleral lens facility (see Chapter 23).

Concurrent medication

Unpreserved unit dose eye drops are indicated for concurrent use with soft lenses. Preserved eye drops are rarely used in this situation, because of concerns that preservatives such as benzalkonium chloride can accumulate in the lens and be toxic to the corneal epithelium. This effect is usually of no clinical importance when disposable lenses are used for short periods. All topical drugs may be used with rigid lenses – both corneal and scleral. It is not known whether drugs achieve suitable concentrations in the ocular tissues when sealed scleral lenses are being worn. Ointment preparations and oily drops should not be used concurrently with contact lenses.

Drug delivery

Hydrogel lenses steeped in pilocarpine solutions (e.g. 4%, unpreserved) are sometimes used in the management of acute closed-angle glaucoma. This technique has also been used in the delivery of antibiotics, antiviral agents, epidermal growth factor and fibronectin (LeBourlais *et al.*, 1998).

Complications

The adverse effects of contact lenses used therapeutically are similar to those with lenses used generally (see Chapter 40), although the diseased or injured eye may be especially at risk. Complications of particular concern in therapeutic contact lens prescribing include hypoxia with or without neovascularization, sterile corneal infiltrates and suppurative keratitis. Careful follow-up is vital after the fitting of a lens for a therapeutic indication, and there is as yet no reason to vary the convention of examining the eye on the day after fitting and not more than 1 week after that. If unplanned-replacement lenses are used, spoilation may be observed to occur more quickly than with healthy eyes. Any change in the comfort or vision of the patient may be of great significance and instruction should be given to the patient to remove the lens in such circumstances, and to return to the clinic as an emergency if not rapidly relieved of the new symptoms.

Conclusions

One aim of this chapter was to dispel the misapprehension that the term 'therapeutic contact lens' is synonymous with a soft plano 'bandage' lens. All types of contact lenses have a potentially important therapeutic role to play in the relief of pain or discomfort and in facilitating the healing of injured or diseased ocular tissue.

References

Andrew, N. and Woodward, E. (1989) The bandage lens in bullous keratopathy. *Ophthal. Physiol. Opt.,* **9,** 66–68.

Bloomfield, S. E., Antonio, R. G., Forstot, S. L. *et al.* (1973) Treatment of filamentary keratitis with the soft contact lens. *Am. J. Ophthalmol.,* **76,** 978–982.

Bouchard, C. S. and Trimble, S. N. (1996) Indications and complications of therapeutic disposable Acuvue contact lenses. *Contact Lens Assoc. Ophthalmol. J.,* **22,** 2–6.

Brilakis, H. S. and Deutsch, T. A. (2000) Topical tetracaine with bandage soft contact lens pain control after photorefractive keratectomy. *J. Refract. Surg.,* **16,** 444–447.

Forooghian, F., Assaad, D. and Dixon, W. S. (2006) Successful conservative management of hydrops with perforation in pellucid marginal degeneration. *Can. J. Ophthalmol.,* **41,** 74–77.

Forstot, S. L. and Binder, P. S. (1979) Treatment of Thygeson's superficial punctate keratopathy with soft contact lenses. *Am. J. Ophthalmol.,* **88,** 186–192.

Gil-Cazorla, R., Teus, M. A. and Arranz-Márquez, E. (2008a) Comparison of silicone and non-silicone hydrogel soft contact lenses used as a bandage after LASEK. *J. Refract. Surg.,* **24,** 199–203.

Gil-Cazorla, R., Teus, M. A., Hernández-Verdejo, J. L. *et al.* (2008b) Comparative study of two silicone hydrogel contact lenses used as bandage contact lenses after LASEK. *Optom. Vis. Sci.,* **85,** 884–888.

LeBourlais, C., Acar, L., Zia, H. *et al.* (1998) Ophthalmic drug delivery systems – recent advances. *Prog. Ret. Eye Res.,* **17,** 1–18.

Lim, N. and Vogt, U. (2006) Comparison of conventional and silicone hydrogel contact lenses for bullous keratoplasty. *Eye Contact Lens,* **32,** 250–253.

Lim, L., Tan, D. T. and Chan, W. K. (2001) Therapeutic use of Bausch & Lomb PureVision contact lenses. *Contact Lens Assoc. Ophthalmol. J.,* **27,** 179–185.

Lin, P.-Y., Wu, C.-C. and Lee, S.-M. (2001) Combined phototherapeutic keratectomy and therapeutic contact lens for recurrent erosions in bullous keratopathy. *Brit. J. Ophthalmol.,* **85,** 908–911.

Liu, C. and Buckley, R. J. (1996) The Role of the Therapeutic contact lens in the management of recurrent corneal erosions: a review of treatment strategies. *Contact Lens Assoc. Ophthalmol. J.,* **22,** 79–82.

Pullum, K. and Buckley, R. J. (2007) Therapeutic and Ocular surface indications for scleral contact lenses. *The Ocular Surface* **5,** 40–49.

Romero-Rangel, T., Stavrou, P., Cotter, J. *et al.* (2000) Gas-permeable scleral contact lens therapy in ocular surface disease. *Am. J. Ophthalmol.,* **130,** 25–32.

Rubinstein, M. P. (1995) Disposable contact lenses as therapeutic devices. *J. Br. Contact Lens Assoc.,* **18,** 3–7.

Shoham, A., Tessler, Z., Finkelman, S. *et al.* (2000) Large soft contact lenses in the management of leaking blebs. *Contact Lens Assoc. Ophthalmol. J.,* **26,** 37–39.

Srur, M. and Dattas, D. (1997) The use of disposable contact lenses as therapeutic lenses. *Contact Lens Assoc. Ophthalmol. J.,* **23,** 1–5.

Tan, D., Pullum, K. and Buckley, R. J. (1995) Medical applications of scleral contact lenses: a retrospective analysis of 343 cases. *Cornea,* **14,** 121–129.

Williams, R. and Buckley, R. J. (1985) Pathogenesis and treatment of recurrent erosion. *Br. J. Ophthalmol.,* **69,** 435–440.

Yeh, S. and Smith, J. A. (2008) Management of acute hydrops with perforation in a patient with keratoconus and cone dystrophy: case report and literature review. *Cornea,* **9,** 1062–1065.

CHAPTER 32

Post-refractive surgery

Patrick J Caroline

Introduction

Fifty years of evolution in refractive surgery procedures has left in its wake a large group of patients with suboptimal visual results. Today, these patients are faced with three corrective options – glasses, contact lenses or further refractive surgery. For some of these individuals, where there is induced anisometropia, restoration of binocular vision may be achieved with contact lenses. Where there is induced irregular astigmatism, contact lenses, in particular rigid lenses, may provide the only option for visual rehabilitation (Alió *et al.*, 2002), as they are able to correct the residual refractive error and reduce the elevated total higher-order aberrations to more normal levels (Gemoules and Morris, 2007).

Types of refractive surgery

The number of different refractive surgical procedures continues to grow. Previous and current procedures are listed in Table 32.1. Each of these procedures modifies the corneal surface in a unique way, necessitating a rethinking of traditional lens designs and fitting techniques for optimal contact lens performance. Today laser-assisted *in situ* keratomileusis (LASIK) continues to be the dominant procedure for preoperative refractions from –8.00 to +3.00 D (Duffey and Leaming, 2005).

Contact lens fitting following radial keratotomy

Radial keratotomy (RK) is largely being phased out in favour of more sophisticated and predictable laser surgical procedures. Nevertheless, this technique is still indicated in certain circumstances and patients may therefore occasionally present for supplementary contact lens correction following RK.

Corneal topography

When radial incisions are placed into the mid peripheral cornea, the wounds gape open under the force of the intraocular pressure and stresses form within the corneal tissues (Figure 32.1). The gaping incisions are first filled with an epithelial plug, which is eventually replaced by a permanent wedge of fibroplastic scar tissue (Figure 32.2). This results in an overall increase in corneal surface area, although the corneal diameter remains unchanged.

There is a common misconception that the mid peripheral cornea steepens following RK. However, as the anterior cornea displaces to accommodate the gaping incisions, virtually the entire cornea, from limbus to limbus, flattens. The flattening effect is simply greater in the central cornea than in the periphery, resulting in the false impression of mid peripheral steepening.

The degree of wound gape and the resultant amount of corneal flattening are dictated by a number of surgical and biological factors, including the following:

- the number, depth and length of the incisions
- intraocular pressure forces
- stresses and biochemical properties within the corneal tissue
- patient age at the time of surgery
- individual wound-healing responses.

Rigid lenses

Following RK, the cornea may exhibit significant corneal flattening with only minimal mid peripheral flattening (approximately 0.1–0.2 mm flatter than its preoperative curvature). Therefore, in the fitting of a rigid lens, a back optic zone radius (BOZR) should be selected to align with the 'more normal' mid peripheral cornea, approximately 4.0 mm from the centre, along the horizontal meridian.

The radius of the post-operative mid peripheral cornea can be determined through corneal mapping or peripheral keratometry. Alternatively, a diagnostic lens can be selected with a BOZR that is 0.1–0.2 mm flatter than the preoperative flat K-reading can be evaluated. The appropriate BOZR should result in a fluorescein pattern that displays apical clearance over the flatter central cornea and a zone of mid peripheral bearing at the 3 and 9 o'clock locations (Figure 32.3). The lens should display unobstructed movement along the vertical meridian.

Lens decentration is a common problem following RK. It is often the result of uneven wound healing which creates geographic surface elevations on which the lens pivots

DOI: 10.1016/B978-0-7506-8869-7.00032-X

Table 32.1 Types of refractive surgery

Incisional	Laser	Other
Radial keratotomy (RK)	Photorefractive keratectomy (PRK)	Keratophakia
Astigmatic keratotomy (AK)	Laser-assisted *in situ* keratomileusis (LASIK)	Keratomileusis
Limbal relaxing incisions (LRI)	Laser-assisted subepithelial keratomileusis (LASEK) Laser thermokeratoplasty (LTK)	Epikeratophakia Thermokeratoplasty Conductive keratoplasty (CK) Automated lamellar keratoplasty Intracorneal ring segments (ICRS)

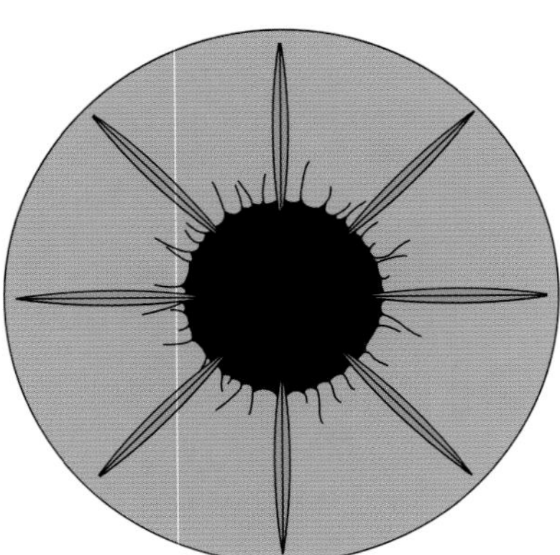

Figure 32.1 Wound gape created by symmetrically placed radial incisions.

(Figure 32.4). Lens decentration is best resolved by increasing the overall lens diameter to 10.5 mm or larger. Final lens power is best determined by performing a spherocylinder refraction over a well-centred diagnostic lens.

Astin (1991) warns that the cornea is malleable and prone to warpage during a period of up to 3 months following RK. She advised not to carry out lens fitting during this period unless it is medically necessary.

Soft lenses

Astin (1986) advises to wait for several months after RK surgery before fitting soft lenses, to allow the cornea to stabilize; she recommends fitting loose, high-water-content lenses. Vickery (1986) suggests that flat lens fits will tend to align more closely with the corneal contour and will avoid corneal compression following RK.

Incisional neovascularization is a common complication associated with the use of soft contact lenses following RK (Figure 32.5). This is especially true in the case of incisions that extend to or beyond the limbus. More modern surgical techniques, in which the incisions terminate short of the limbus, may be less prone to this complication. Today, incisional neovascularization can be minimized through the use of high-oxygen-permeability silicone hydrogel lenses used on a daily-wear basis.

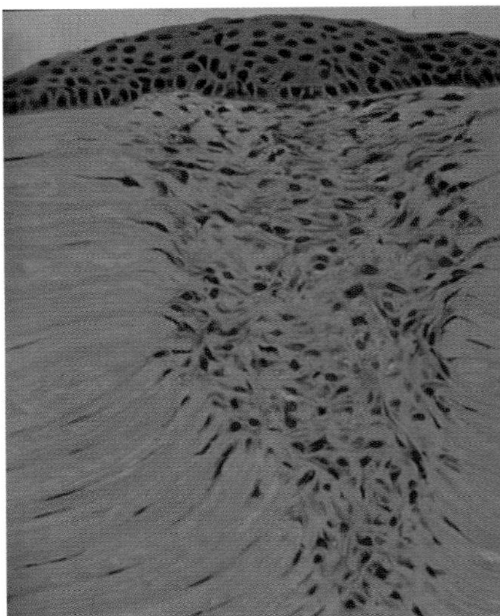

Figure 32.2 Wedge-shaped fibroplastic scar in a healed radial incision (cat eye).

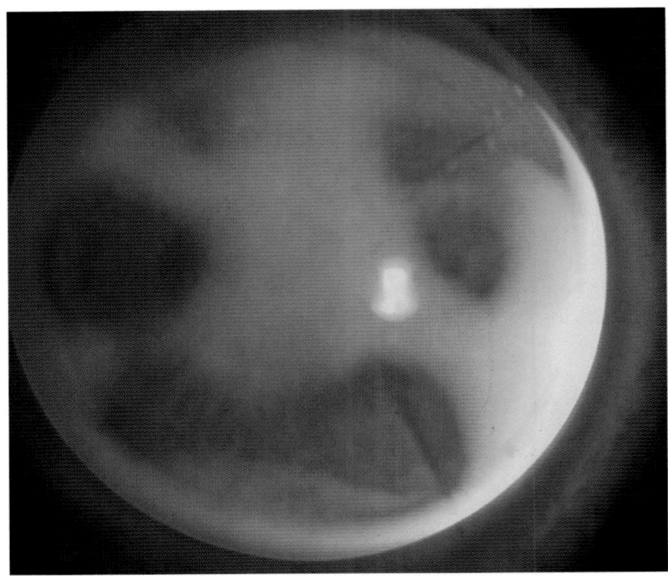

Figure 32.3 Fluorescein pattern post-radial keratotomy. The cornea has a central flat K of 8.76 mm and a mid peripheral curvature (4 mm temporal) of 7.94 mm. The lens has a back optic zone radius of 7.94 mm.

Contact lens fitting following photorefractive procedures

The contact lens management of the post-photorefractive keratectomy patient poses far fewer problems than those encountered after incisional keratotomy. Patients may present for contact lens fitting after having LASIK surgery performed on both eyes simultaneously. Bilateral LASIK is offered by 98% of surgeons in the USA (Waring *et al.*, 1999; Duffey and Leaming, 2005).

Contact lens fitting differs between incisional and laser procedures in the following respects:

- Following photorefractive keratectomy (PRK) or LASIK, the mid peripheral cornea remains relatively unchanged from its preoperative state.

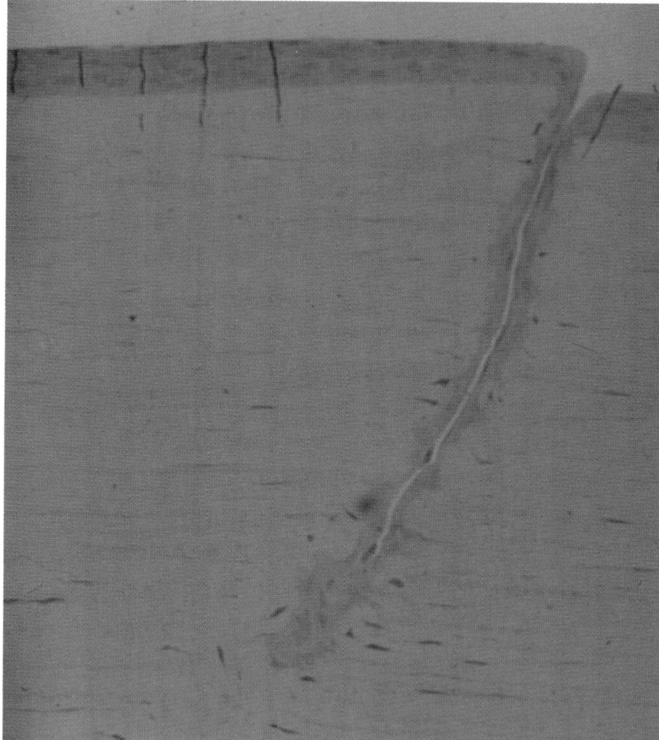

Figure 32.4 Pivot point created by uneven wound apposition, seen here at the top right corner of the tissue section (cat eye).

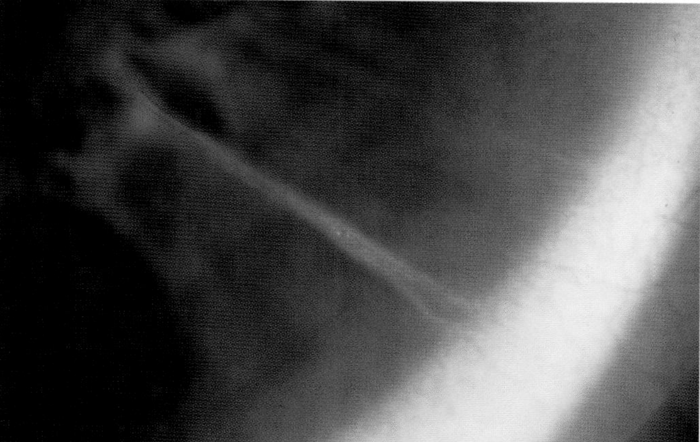

Figure 32.5 Incisional neovascularization secondary to the wearing of a low-water-content soft contact lens.

- A wider range of soft contact lens designs can be used following PRK or LASIK due to the absence of perilimbal incisions.
- The post-PRK and post-LASIK cornea does not have elevated mid peripheral pivot points secondary to incisional wound healing. These areas are the major cause of rigid lens decentration following RK.
- PRK and LASIK offer less diurnal fluctuation in visual acuity due to the stability of the peripheral cornea. This is especially important when soft contact lenses are used post-operatively.

In the experience of this author, the LASIK flap has presented few, if any, problems in the fitting or wearing of contact lenses. In fact, there has been no discernible difference with respect to contact lens fitting or physiological response between post-PRK and post-LASIK patients.

Gil-Cazorla *et al.* (2008) evaluated the clinical performance of two silicone hydrogel contact lens materials – PureVision and Acuvue Advance – as continuous-wear bandage lenses after laser-assisted subepithelial keratomileusis (LASEK). The purpose of the lenses is to protect the corneal epithelium during regrowth. There was no major clinical difference between the lenses, although patients report greater comfort with Acuvue Advance.

Tissue ablation and corneal topography

If RK is a tissue addition procedure, then PRK, LASIK and LASEK are tissue subtraction procedures. The amount of corneal tissue removed in a myopic laser procedure will play an important role in the post-surgical management of the patient with contact lenses. Tissue removal is determined by the Munnerlyn formula:

$$\text{Depth of ablation} = (\text{optic zone diameter})^2 \times (\text{refractive error})/3$$

Example:

Ablation diameter (optical zone diameter) = 6.0 mm
Optical zone squared (6.0 × 6.0) = 36
Multiplied by the desired correction (–6.00) = 216
Divided by 3 = 72
Thus, depth of the ablation =72 μm

The possibility that laser refractive surgery, particularly LASIK, results in irregular corneal astigmatism has been a concern ever since the excimer laser was introduced. However, the reality is that irregular astigmatism is a rare finding in both PRK and LASIK. The presence of irregular astigmatism can be diagnosed by improving poor spectacle-corrected visual acuity with a rigid contact lens. It may be induced by the creation of a suboptimal lamellar flap – too thin, irregular, bisected, buttonholed or a free flap. Flap striae are an important and often under-recognized cause of irregular astigmatism (Polack and Polack, 2003).

Rigid lens designs

Many patients who have undergone PRK or LASIK can be successfully fitted with traditional spherical or aspheric rigid lenses. With myopic ablations, the mid peripheral cornea (beyond the central 6.0–7.0 mm) remains unchanged. Therefore, the major concern in fitting rigid or soft contact lenses is the relative difference between the flatter central cornea and the steeper (normal) mid peripheral cornea. This difference creates few problems for patients who were low to moderate myopes prior to surgery. In such cases, the small amount of tissue ablated does not noticeably affect the contact lens fit or the on-eye lens dynamics. For example, a patient with a preoperative refractive error of –4.00 D might end up post-operatively –1.00 D undercorrected. The 3.00 D myopic reduction was produced by an ablation of approximately 36 μm of tissue (less than the thickness of the human epithelium). The minimal difference between the central and mid peripheral cornea creates few fitting and/or optical problems for a traditional rigid lens design.

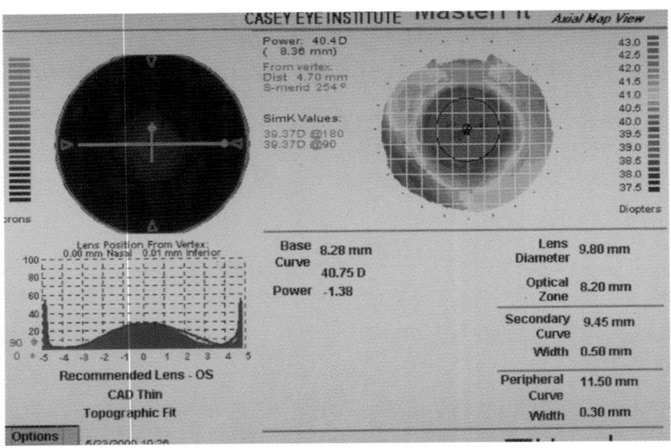

Figure 32.6 Simulated fluorescein pattern of a post-laser-assisted *in situ* keratomileusis (LASIK) eye with a –3.00 D correction.

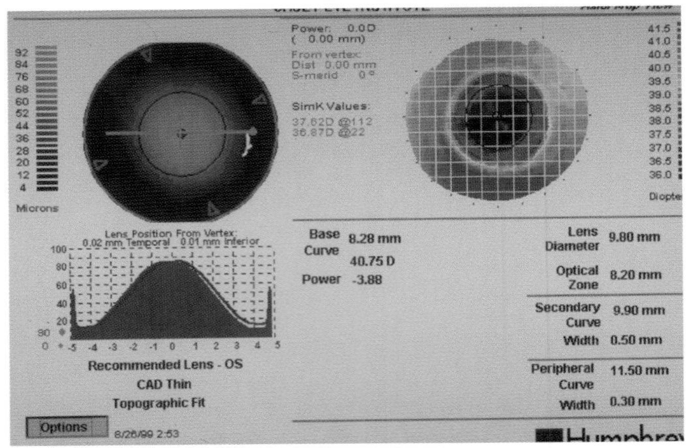

Figure 32.7 Simulated fluorescein pattern of a post-laser-assisted *in situ* keratomileusis (LASIK) eye with a –9.00 D correction.

These individuals are often best fitted with a BOZR designed to align the mid peripheral corneal topography 4.0 mm from the centre of the cornea (Figure 32.6).

Corneal shape following hyperopic laser correction is steeper, with a positive value for eccentricity often exceeding 0.5–0.7 (Gruenauer-Kloevekorn *et al.*, 2006). It may be necessary to consider a lens design usually reserved for keratoconus.

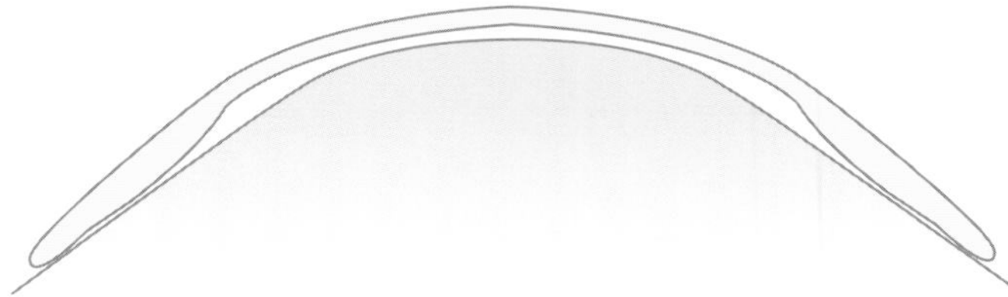

Figure 32.8 Reverse-geometry lens design.

Reverse-geometry rigid lens designs

A patient with a high preoperative refractive error, e.g. –10.00 D, might end up post-operatively –1.00 D. The –9.00 D myopic reduction required the removal of approximately 110 µm of corneal tissue. In this case, the difference between the central and mid peripheral cornea is such that a traditional rigid lens (designed to align with the mid peripheral cornea), may exhibit excessive apical clearance (Figure 32.7). The subsequent large volume of tears centrally can result in unstable optics and trapped bubbles can form beneath the centre of the lens.

In such situations, patients may be best managed with reverse-geometry lens designs (Lim *et al.*, 2000; Martin and Rodriguez, 2005) (Figure 32.8). A standard rigid design mimics the prolate shape of the normal, unoperated cornea, which is steeper in the centre than the periphery. The reverse-geometry design more closely parallels the post-refractive surgery topography (of a previously myopic eye) by incorporating a flat central radius of curvature with a steeper mid peripheral design (Figure 32.8). This creates a plateau configuration on the posterior lens surface, which dramatically decreases the volume of tear fluid present beneath the central portion of the lens (Szczotka, 1998).

With both PRK and LASIK, rigid lens fitting is best delayed until approximately 8–12 weeks after surgery. At this point, the refraction and topography have stabilized. At 3 months post-surgery, the integrity of the flap interface is usually sufficient to withstand the minor trauma associated with lens insertion and removal, as well as the normal on-eye movement that occurs with blinking.

Practitioners need to be aware of the level of corneal sensitivity following laser refractive surgery if contact lenses are to be fitted. The recovery of corneal sensitivity following PRK and LASIK was measured by Pérez-Santonja *et al.* (1999). Following PRK, a decrease in central corneal sensitivity was noted at 1 week, and had nearly recovered at 1 month after surgery. Following LASIK, there was a deep decrease in central corneal sensitivity at 1 week and 1 month after surgery. Corneal sensitivity values were found to be similar after 6 months – a finding in agreement with Benitez-del-Castillo *et al.* (2001). Darwish *et al.* (2007) examined subbasal nerve regeneration after LASEK using confocal microscopy and found corneal sensitivity had returned to normal levels after 3 months; however, subbasal nerves that were injured by LASEK had not returned to preoperative levels 6 months after surgery.

Patients frequently experience dry-eye symptoms after LASIK; however, the mechanisms that lead to these changes are not well understood. Tear film dysfunction has obvious implications if contact lenses are required after surgery. Yu *et al.* (2000) followed post-LASIK patients for 1 month and observed increased dry-eye symptoms, and reduced Schirmer test results, basal tear secretion and tear break-up time during this period. Benitez-del-Castillo *et al.* (2001) reported that tear secretion was reduced for a period of 9 months following LASIK surgery. After LASEK, Darwish *et al.* (2007) found tear break-up time had decreased significantly and had not returned to the preoperative level by 6 months after surgery. They found no significant differences in the phenol red thread test results before and after LASEK.

Soft lenses

Most of the currently available daily disposable or frequent-replacement soft lenses are viable options for the post-laser correction, either in high-water-content hydrogel or silicone hydrogel materials. However, after surgery a complex relationship exists between visual acuity, defocus (refractive error), diffraction and optical aberrations. The loss of post-operative central corneal asphericity can result in a form of spherical aberration (Hong and Thibos, 2000) which can be symptomatic - especially in patients with large pupils. Improved optical correction can be achieved with soft lens designs which incorporate aberration-correcting anterior aspheric optics.

Comparative performance of rigid versus soft lenses

Lim *et al.* (1999) evaluated the fitting of rigid and soft lenses following PRK. Patients with residual refractive errors greater than 2.00 D or visual acuity worse than 6/12 were enrolled; this amounted to 16 rigid lens wearers and 11 soft lens wearers. Twelve rigid lens wearers (75%) reported excellent visual quality and one reported fair visual quality. Eight soft lens patients (73%) reported excellent visual quality and three reported fair visual quality. The authors concluded that both lens types are viable options for the treatment of uncorrected refractive error following PRK.

Decentred ablations

Almost all patients with decentred ablations are left with varying degrees of uncorrected myopia. This is due to the eccentric position of the treatment zone away from the visual axis. Viewing through the edge of the ablation frequently results in a loss of best-corrected acuity, monocular diplopia and ghosting of distance images, especially under scotopic conditions.

The severity of symptoms often correlates with the size of the pupil. A decentred ablation with a large 6–7 mm pupil will produce more serious visual complaints than a similarly displaced ablation over a small 3–4 mm pupil.

Soft contact lenses rarely provide adequate optical correction in this small subset of patients. Optimal visual performance usually requires the use of a rigid lens design.

Conclusions

With time, new refractive surgery techniques will emerge, and old techniques will be abandoned or modified through modern technology. These procedures will come and go, yet the altered topographies left in their wake will remain for decades to come. Therefore, contact lenses will continue to play an important role in the lives of individuals whose corneas have been permanently compromised by refractive surgery. Whether contact lenses are used in lieu of, or in conjunction with, refractive surgery, the outcome can be a positive experience for the patient. With ongoing refinements in lens materials and designs, contact lens technology will continue to meet the challenges posed by future refractive surgery procedures.

References

Alió, J. L., Belda, J. I., Artola, A. *et al.* (2002) Contact lens fitting to correct irregular astigmatism after corneal refractive surgery. *J. Cataract Refract. Surg.*, **28,** 1750–1757.

Astin, C. L. K. (1986) Considerations in fitting contact lenses to patients who have undergone radial keratotomy. *Trans. Br. Contact Lens Assoc.*, **1,** 2–7.

Astin, C. L. K. (1991) Keratoreformation by contact lenses after radial keratotomy. *Ophthal. Physiol. Opt.*, **11,** 156–162.

Benitez-del-Castillo, J. M., del Rio, T., Iradier, T. *et al.* (2001) Decrease in tear secretion and corneal sensitivity after laser in situ keratomileusis. *Cornea,* **20,** 30–32.

Darwish, T., Brahma, A., Efron, N. *et al.* (2007) Sub-basal nerve regeneration after LASEK measured by confocal microscopy. *J. Refract. Surg.*, **23,** 709–715.

Duffey, R. J. and Leaming, D. (2005) US trends in refractive surgery: 2003 ISRS/AAO survey. *J. Refract. Surg.*, **21,** 87–91.

Gemoules, G. and Morris, K. M. (2007) Rigid gas-permeable contact lenses and severe higher-order aberrations in postsurgical corneas. *Eye Contact Lens,* **33,** 304–307.

Gil-Cazorla, R., Teus, M. A., Hernández-Verdejo, J. L. *et al.* (2008) Comparative study of two silicone hydrogel contact lenses used as bandage contact lenses after LASEK. *Optom. Vis. Sci.*, **85,** 884–888.

Gruenauer-Kloevekorn, C., Fischer, U., Kloevekorn-Norgall, K. *et al.* (2006) Varieties of contact lens fittings after complicated hyperopic and myopic laser in situ keratomileusis. *Eye Contact Lens,* **32,** 233–239.

Hong, X. and Thibos, L. N. (2000) Longitudinal evaluation of optical aberrations following laser in situ keratomileusis surgery. *J. Ref. Surg.*, **16,** S647–S650.

Lim, L., Siow, K., Chong, J. S. C. *et al.* (1999) Contact lens wear after photorefractive keratectomy: comparison between rigid gas permeable and soft contact lenses. *Contact Lens Assoc. Ophthalmol. J.*, **25,** 222–227.

Lim, L., Siow, K. L., Sakamoto, R. *et al.* (2000) Reverse geometry contact lens wear after photorefractive keratectomy, radial keratotomy, or penetrating keratoplasty. *Cornea,* **19,** 320–324.

Martin, R. and Rodriguez, G. (2005) Reverse geometry contact lens fitting after corneal refractive surgery. *J. Refract. Surg.*, **21,** 753–756.

Pérez-Santonja, J. J., Salka, H. F., Cardona, C. *et al.* (1999) Corneal sensitivity after photorefractive keratectomy and laser in situ keratomileusis for low myopia. *Am. J. Ophthalmol.*, **127,** 497–504.

Polack, P. J. and Polack, F. M. (2003) Management of irregular astigmatism induced by laser in situ keratomileusis. *Int. Ophthalmol. Clin.*, **43,** 129–140.

Szczotka, L. B. (1998) RGP RGLs for post-surgical corneas. *Contact Lens Spectrum,* **13,** 20.

Vickery, J. (1986) Post RK and the soft lens. *Contact Lens Forum,* **11**(10), 34–35.

Waring III, G. O., Carr, J. D. and Stulting, R. D. (1999) Prospective randomized comparison of simultaneous and sequential bilateral laser in situ keratomileusis for the correction of myopia. *Ophthalmology,* **106,** 732–738.

Yu, E. Y. W., Leung, A., Rao, S. *et al.* (2000) Effect of laser in situ keratomileusis on tear stability. *Ophthalmology,* **107,** 2131–2135.

33 CHAPTER

Post-keratoplasty

Barry A Weissman

Introduction

Corneal transplantation (keratoplasty or KP) is a surgical procedure by which diseased corneal tissue is removed and replaced by donor material (a corneal graft) (Figure 33.1).

Corneal transplantation resulting in relatively clear grafts was first reported in the ophthalmic literature with Reisinger's rabbit experiments (1824). Such homografts (or allografts) are transplants within the same species, that is, from one rabbit to another or from one human to another, and are the most common form of KP. Von Hippel (1888) made several unsuccessful attempts to graft a glass prosthesis but his work forms the basis of modern KP. Von Hippel and others also used animal corneas as donors for humans: these are heterografts, transplants from one species to another, and are commonly rejected. Zirm (1906) is credited with the first human corneal transplant (treating a leukoma due to a quicklime burn) to retain a moderate degree of transparency. The introduction of McCarey–Kaufman (MK) medium (McCarey and Kaufman, 1974; McCarey *et al.*, 1977) enabled donor human cornea to be stored for 3–4 days. Further advances based on tissue culture techniques extended the preservation of donor tissue for up to 30–40 days (Doughman *et al.*, 1976; Sperling, 1979, Doughman, 1980; Sperling *et al.*, 1981). Autografts, wherein one eye provides the donor cornea for the other, although rare for obvious reasons (the author has seen two human corneal autografts in his career; Figure 33.2), have limited, if any, risk of rejection. Artificial corneal grafts have progressed slowly from the time of von Hippel but have had some recent success (Figure 33.3).

Corneal grafts are performed for the following reasons:

- Optical – to restore visual function by removing scarred or irregular tissues (e.g. in keratoconus, post trauma and infection, corneal dystrophy).
- Therapeutic – to treat disease (e.g. to treat an infection by debulking).
- Tectonic – to restore, or preclude the loss of, globe integrity.
- Cosmetic – to improve appearance (e.g. eliminate an unsightly scar in a non-seeing eye).

The indications outlined above are not necessarily mutually exclusive.

Approximately 45 000 KP procedures are performed annually in the USA (Eye Bank Association of America, 2006) with another 2 500 in the UK (Rahman *et al.*, 2009).

Indications

The indications for corneal grafts include the following:

- Corneal oedema that is severe enough to affect visual function, and painful bullous keratopathy, usually a consequence of Fuchs' endothelial dystrophy or aphakic/pseudophakic endothelial failure.
- Keratoconus and other forms of corneal ectasia such as pellucid marginal degeneration and Terrien's degeneration. The criteria for performing KP may be when the condition is severe enough to limit vision with contact lens correction to 6/12 or worse, or when contact lens wear can no longer be tolerated for physical or physiological reasons. Approximately 20% of keratoconic patients will eventually come to benefit from corneal transplantation (Lass *et al.*, 1990).
- Corneal scars and interstitial keratitis, secondary to trauma and/or infection (e.g. herpetic keratitis).
- Visually debilitating forms of corneal dystrophy, such as granular, macular, lattice or Reis–Bücklers dystrophy.
- Congenital opacities, such as Peters' anomaly or buphthalmos secondary to congenital glaucoma.
- Previous graft rejection or failure.

Types of corneal graft

Full-thickness penetrating keratoplasty (PKP), utilizing a circular mechanical trephine, has been the standard of care in corneal transplantation for at least 50 years.

Superficial corneal diseases have been alternatively treated with anterior lamellar keratoplasty (LK) wherein, following initial partial-thickness trephination, a blunt blade is used mechanically to separate a deep plane in the

DOI: 10.1016/B978-0-7506-8869-7.00033-1

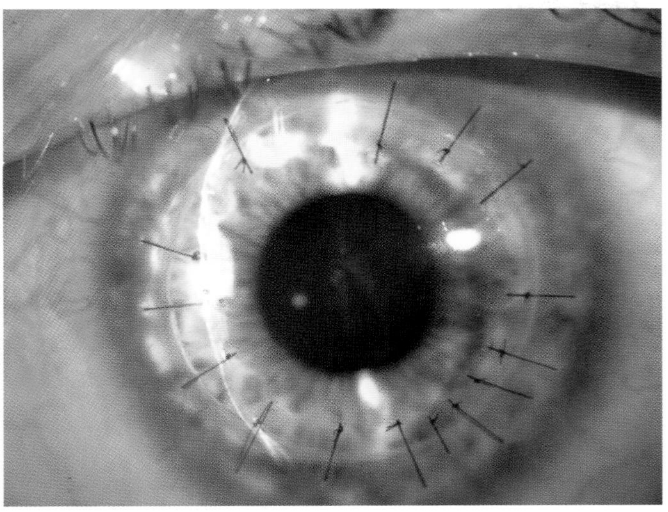

Figure 33.1 A penetrating keratoplasty with interrupted sutures.

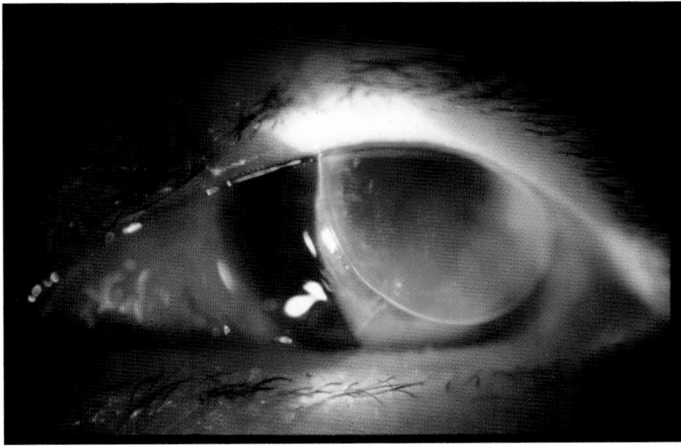

Figure 33.2 Corneal autograft. This patient had congenital lues and when the cornea of her good eye failed, it was grafted with a donor button taken from her contralateral, severely amblyopic eye (to enhance her chances of avoiding rejection) and that donor replaced with a traditional allograft.

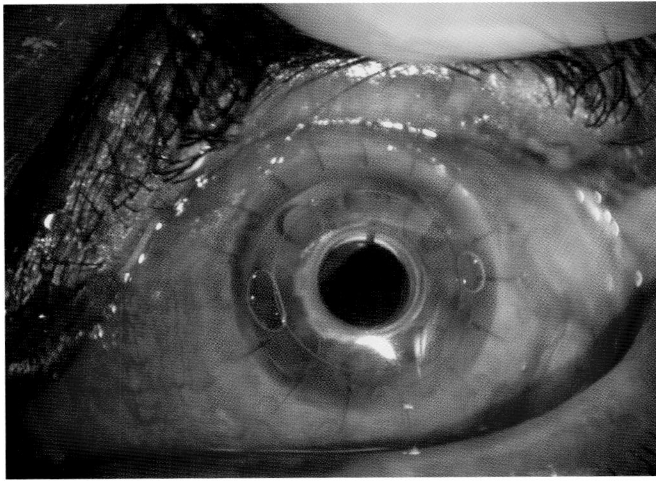

Figure 33.3 Dohlman keratoprosthesis. Note the bandage soft lens in place (by the bubbles seen in the 3/9 zones).

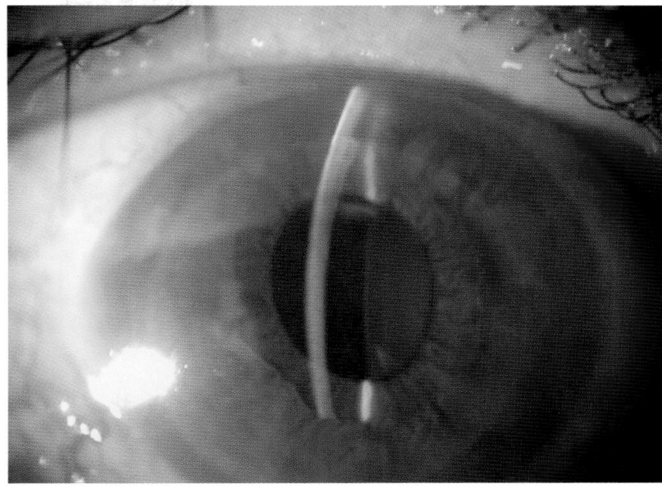

Figure 33.4 A cornea post Descemet's stripping endothelial keratoplasty (for treatment of the combination of iris naevus or Cogan–Reese syndrome; Chandler's syndrome; and essential iris atrophy, called ICE syndrome). Note increased corneal thickness extending into the anterior chamber seen in the optical section superiorly.

tissue to allow replacement of only the diseased superficial cornea. Deep lamellar keratoplasty (DLK) utilizes air, water or a microkeratome to separate the deep stromal fibres from Descemet's membrane (Archila, 1985; Price, 1989; Sugita and Kondo, 1997; Busin *et al.*, 2005). Both LK and DLK retain the host endothelium and thereby reduce rejection concerns. PKP, however, is both surgically less demanding and to date optically more successful, and hence has been the more common technique. Epikeratoplasty – wherein a donor cornea is applied to the anterior surface of the intact host stroma (epithelium removed) in an effort to address aphakia, keratoconus or high myopia – results in poor vision (secondary to interface problems) and has almost been abandoned. Patch grafts are used to seal corneal leaks.

Deep lamellar endothelial keratoplasty (DLEK) (Terry and Ousley, 2003; Watson *et al.*, 2004), whereby only the posterior cornea is removed (by femtosecond laser or mechanically), and more recently Descemet's stripping endothelial keratoplasty (DSEK) (Price and Price, 2006), have both been developed as LK procedures to replace only damaged posterior corneal tissues (as in Fuchs' dystrophy) (Figure 33.4), leaving the host anterior corneal surface smooth and intact; thus these patients may not require contact lens correction. Both DLEK and DSEK theoretically offer more rapid healing, more predictable refractive outcomes and better retention of corneal strength compared to PKP, but donor adherence may be challenging.

The IntraLase femtosecond laser also allows corneal surgeons to create complex, shaped PKP incisions (e.g. 'top hat,' 'mushroom,' 'zigzag') identical in both host and graft tissue. Called IntraLase-enabled keratoplasty or IEK, this procedure creates PKPs with customized edge designs and may minimize induced astigmatism and enhance wound strength. Fewer sutures may be required, healing is faster, and hopefully decreased regular and irregular astigmatism will enhance vision and reduce the need for contact lens correction, discussed below. The risk for displacement of the graft may also be reduced. Data collected from 23 initial IEK cases demonstrate improvement in vision compared to traditional trephine PKP: 3 months postoperatively, 45% of

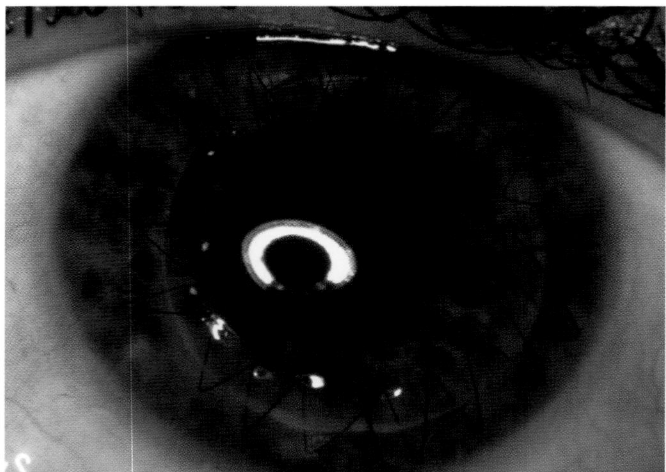

Figure 33.5 Irregular surface astigmatism in a graft, as indicated by the distorted reflex of a perfectly circular flash gun.

IEK patients were reported to have vision of 20/40 or better (IntraLase Corp., 2006), as opposed to 30% of almost 2 800 patients from a large study of traditional trephine PKP (Vail *et al.*, 1997).

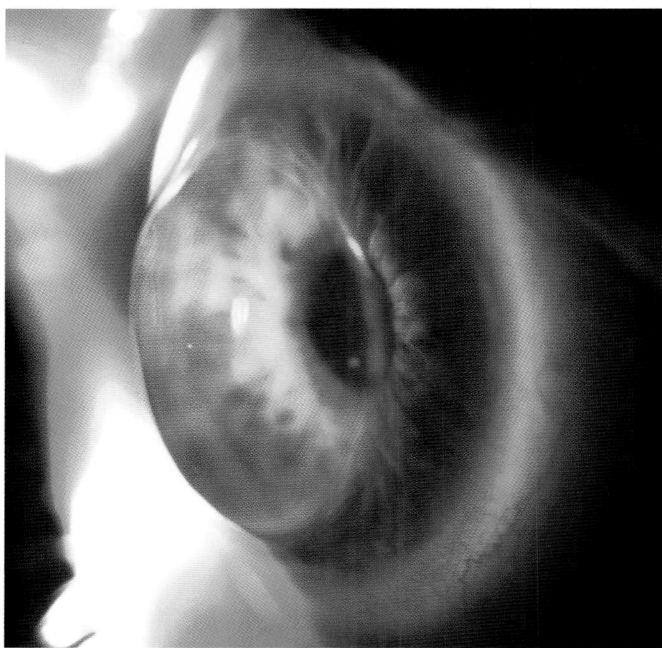

Figure 33.6 Proud graft totally elevated above the host corneal surface in a keratoconic eye.

Corneal topography following PKP

The main optical challenge following traditional PKP (and anterior corneal LK as well) has been irregular surface astigmatism (Figure 33.5). If IEK proves successful, this situation may change in the next decade, but for now, as the majority of PKPs worldwide continue to receive the traditional trephine procedure, we will discuss the current situation.

Waring *et al.* (1992) documented the prevalence of the various forms of corneal topography following trephine PKP as: 'prolate' (30%), 'oblate' (30%), 'mixed' (20%), asymmetric (10%) and 'steep to flat' (10%). Phillips (1997) discussed these corneal topographic outcomes in more clinically descriptive terminology, as follows: 'nipple' or steep; 'proud', whereby the graft is totally or partially elevated above the host corneal surface (Figure 33.6); 'sunken', whereby the graft is depressed below the host surface; 'tilted' or 'eccentric'. These outcomes are illustrated in Figure 33.7.

Hoppenreijs *et al.* (1993) suggest that causes of these topographic outcomes include:

- Suboptimal cutting of the donor, the host, or both.
- Eccentric placement of the graft.
- Elevation of the graft edge during healing, with poor wound approximation.
- Loosening of sutures.
- Localized abnormal healing.
- Initial corneal irregularity (e.g. keratoconus).

A second common optical problem following corneal grafts is anisometropia.

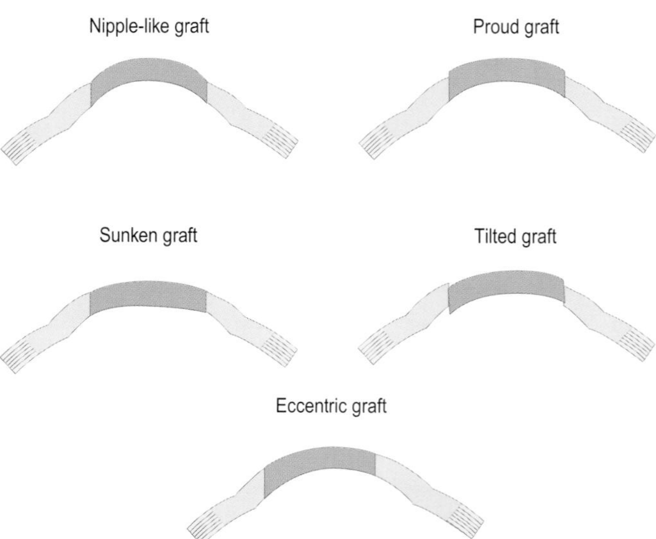

Figure 33.7 Graft profiles. (Adapted from Phillips, A. J. (1997) Postkeratoplasty contact lens fitting. In Contact Lenses for Pre- and Post-Surgery. (M. J. Harris ed.), pp. 97–132, Mosby.)

Suture techniques for PKP

Contact lens clinicians need a general appreciation of suture techniques used for KP because patients commonly present for fitting or aftercare visits with some or all sutures still in place. Sutures may be of the following forms:

- Running (or continuous) – a continuous suture forms a zigzag pattern across the host–graft interface, around the full circumference of the graft (Figure 33.8).
- Double running – two continuous sutures form a zigzag pattern across the host–graft interface that extends twice around the full circumference of the graft.
- Interrupted – a number of single sutures, commonly 16, equally spaced around the graft circumference (see Figure 33.1).

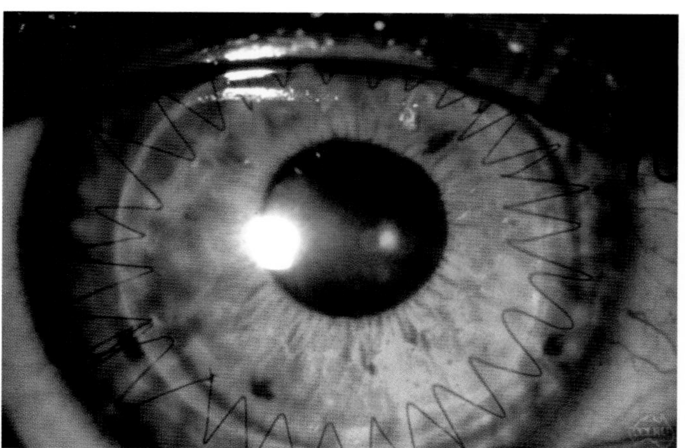

Figure 33.8 A penetrating keratoplasty with a single running suture.

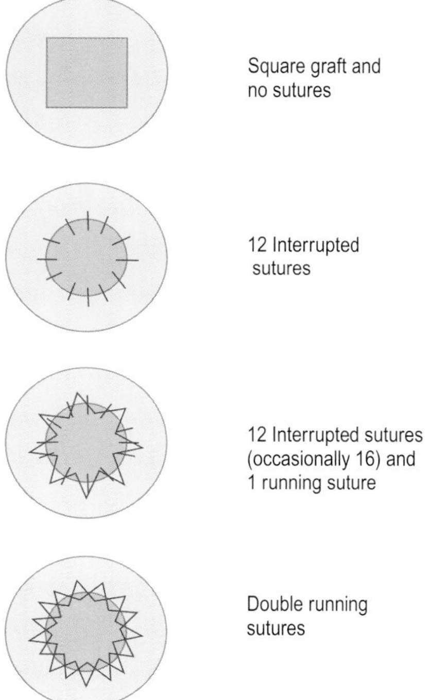

Figure 33.9 Grafts and sutures.

- Combination – both running and interrupted sutures are used.

These various forms of suturing are illustrated in Figure 33.9.

It appears that most surgeons use either double running or one running and several interrupted sutures as the technique of choice. Square grafts are rarely if ever performed now, but may be occasionally seen and followed. In a prospective study, astigmatism was found to be the least following double running sutures compared to interrupted or single running sutures 18 months after PKP (Kim *et al.*, 2008). At some point – commonly some 3–6 months after surgery – either one running suture, or the interrupted sutures, is/are removed, often selectively in an effort to moderate astigmatism. One running suture, or several interrupted sutures, is/are commonly left in place indefinitely, only to be removed if problems or breaks develop. Interrupted sutures alone are favoured when PKP must be attempted in the face of active anterior-segment inflammation or corneal neovascularization to permit later individual removal when appropriate. Adjunctive surgery, relaxing incisions, additional sutures, or even wedge resection procedures have been used with variable success to address postoperative astigmatism (Budak *et al.*, 1998).

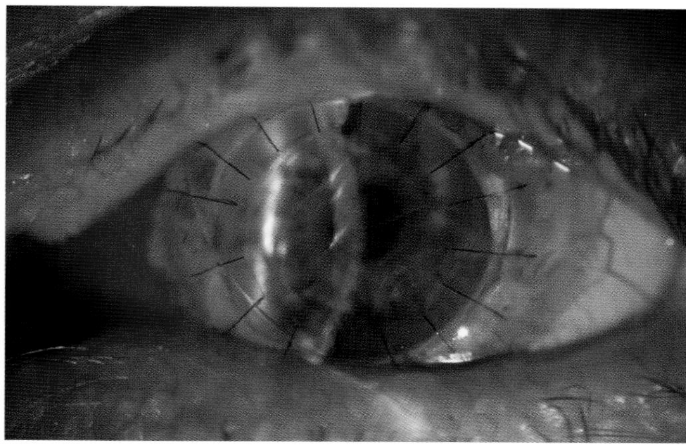

Figure 33.10 A bandage hydrogel lens used 1 day after surgery to cover a graft that has been secured with interrupted sutures.

Indications and contraindications for contact lens wear post corneal grafts

The indications for contact lens use following corneal grafts are primarily postoperative irregular or high astigmatism, and secondarily anisometropia (e.g. as will occur in aphakia). Between 20% and 60% of trephine-cut post-PKP patients benefit optically from contact lens wear (Ruben and Colbrook, 1979; Lass *et al.*, 1990; Smiddy *et al.*, 1992; Silbiger *et al.*, 1996; Wietharn and Driebe, 2004). Bandage hydrogel contact lenses are also sometimes used as drug delivery devices or to treat non-healing epithelial defects in the immediate postoperative period and for wound dehiscence at any time (Mannis and Zadnik, 1988) (Figure 33.10).

Contact lens contraindications are as follows:

- A good (or even just adequate) visual result with spectacle correction alone.
- Anticipated poor compliance with contact lens care.

The clinician should also be concerned about several other relative contraindications, including:

- Decreased corneal sensitivity – expected during the first year postoperatively (Ruben and Colbrook, 1979; Darwish *et al.*, 2007).
- Dry eyes – tear break-up time was found to be significantly shorter 3 and 12 months after keratoplasty (Darwish *et al.*, 2007).
- Blepharitis.
- Dacryocystitis.

Patients with collateral systemic diseases, such as acne rosacea and rheumatoid arthritis, which can both lead to dry eyes and increased risk of corneal ulcer/melts and neovascularization, need to be monitored carefully. Patients with diabetes or other immune system depressions, which can increase the risk of corneal infection, should also be approached with extra caution, and monitored frequently.

General concerns

Careful consideration needs to be given to the time period that should be allowed to elapse following surgery before contact lenses are fitted, if so indicated. Previous authors suggested 'a year post-surgery, when all sutures have been removed' (Soper *et al.*, 1964); however, this advice is not appropriate today because some sutures now are not removed unless they break or otherwise become problematic. The current approach, therefore, is that contact lenses can be fitted when the graft is considered to have healed sufficiently to tolerate lens wear (Wilson *et al.*, 1992). Contact lens application therefore may begin as early as 3–6 months postsurgery, and often with one or more sutures remaining. When sutures do come out during the postoperative course, after patients are already using contact lenses, the clinician should re-evaluate the patient before lens wear is resumed. A new fitting is occasionally indicated to address changes in corneal topography, optics, or both (more so with the removal of running sutures than with individual interrupted sutures, although surprises can occur) (Mathers *et al.*, 1991; Mader *et al.*, 1993; Langenbucher *et al.*, 2005).

Topical steroid treatment is known to potentiate secondary glaucoma, cataract and corneal infection, but many post corneal graft patients will continue to use topical steroids consistently or intermittently for the rest of their lives to suppress rejection. Hence, the clinician and patient must tolerate such risks and the patient should be reasonably monitored by both the corneal surgeon and the contact lens practitioner.

It is now accepted that extended wear of contact lenses may enhance the prevalence and severity of all the physiological complications of lens wear. These may be even more serious in the post-KP patient than the cosmetic contact lens patient, as many such complications potentiate graft rejection. The clinician must consider whether to advise extended or daily wear for each patient, accepting that some patients will be elderly or in other ways infirm and therefore unable to care for contact lenses. Under certain conditions, therefore, extended wear and its attendant risks may also need to be accepted by both clinician and patient.

Lens fitting techniques

Rigid lenses remain the overwhelming device of choice for the majority of post-KP patients because they efficiently and effectively optically mask most regular and irregular astigmatism. Soper *et al.* (1964) suggested that rigid lenses (then referring to non-oxygen-permeable polymethyl methacrylate) should be fitted so as to ride within the PKP, meaning that the overall diameter (OD) of the lens would probably be less than 7.5–8.0 mm. The subsequent introduction of rigid gas-permeable materials encouraged the use of lenses with larger ODs (9.0 mm to as much as 11.0 mm) that override the entire graft without causing hypoxic difficulties (Woodward, 1997). As rigid contact lenses tend to 'ride' towards and over the highest corneal point, larger-OD lenses allow enhanced stability and centration – which is still often difficult to achieve, especially on sunken or tilted PKPs. Excessively flat cornea topographies post-PKP, often associated with donor/hosts of equal diameter, may be especially difficult to fit with rigid lenses (Lagnado *et al.*, 2004). Ozbek and Cohen (2006) reported good results with the use of very-large-OD (11.2 mm) rigid lenses on a series of 27 irregular corneas (primary indication flat central and steep inferior corneal topography), including 6 post-PKP. They selected the initial base curve equal to the topographically determined central flat value and then modified their lenses as appropriate with the clinical goal of minimal lens decentration.

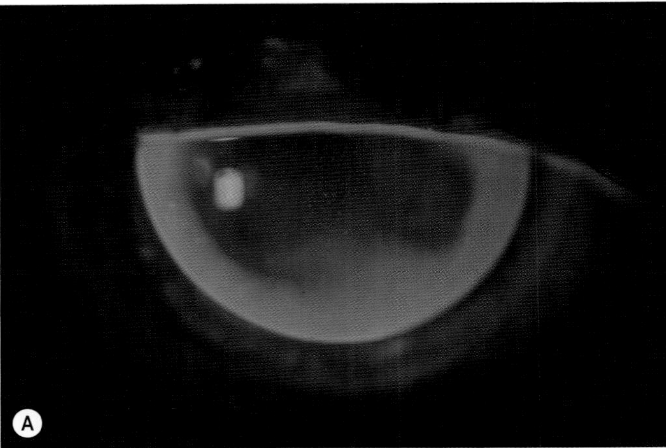

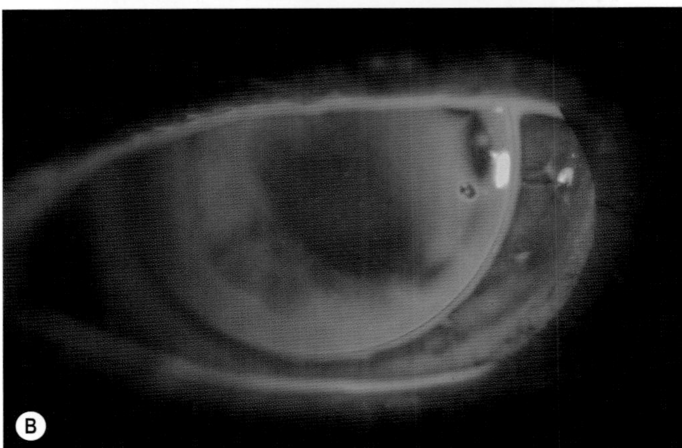

Figure 33.11 Examples of fluorescein patterns observed on fitting rigid lenses to corneas with imperfect grafts. (A) Plateau fit on proud graft. (B) Tilted sunken graft with small nipple; note that the contact lens partially rests on graft–host interface with running suture.

The back optic zone radius of a rigid lens should be selected, with initial assistance of keratometry or videokeratography measurements, so as to achieve some form of irregular corneal surface alignment, with neither excessive touch nor pooling of tears. Examples of fluorescein patterns obtained with rigid lenses fitted to imperfect corneal grafts are shown in Figure 33.11.

Toric and bitoric rigid designs are occasionally helpful in fitting PKP corneas exhibiting relatively regular astigmatism, and occasionally tilted and eccentric grafts. Weissman and Chun (1987) found that 7 of a series of 23 eyes fitted with bitoric design rigid lenses for irregular astigmatism were post-PKP and the majority of these (6 of 7 or 85%) were 'successful'.

Consideration needs to be given to edge design in fitting rigid lenses to graft corneas. Some corneal surfaces can be

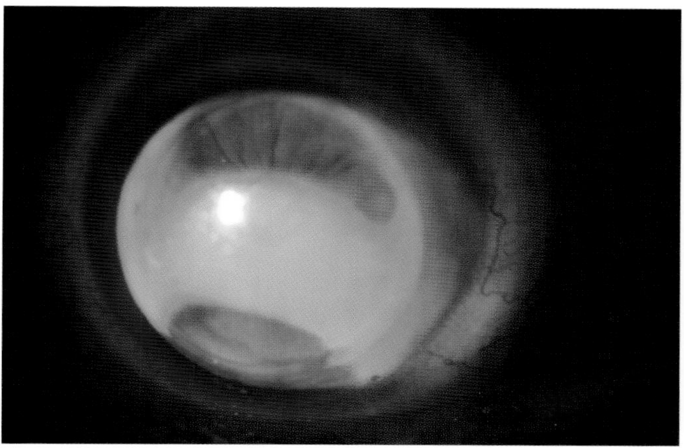

Figure 33.12 A hybrid lens (in this case a Synergeyes) is shown on a penetrating keratoplasty eye. Note arcuate areas of touch at the graft–host interface at both 12 and 6 o'clock as well as central corneal clearance of the tear film, or 'pooling', shown with high-molecular-weight Fluoresoft desirable in this kind of hybrid contact lens.

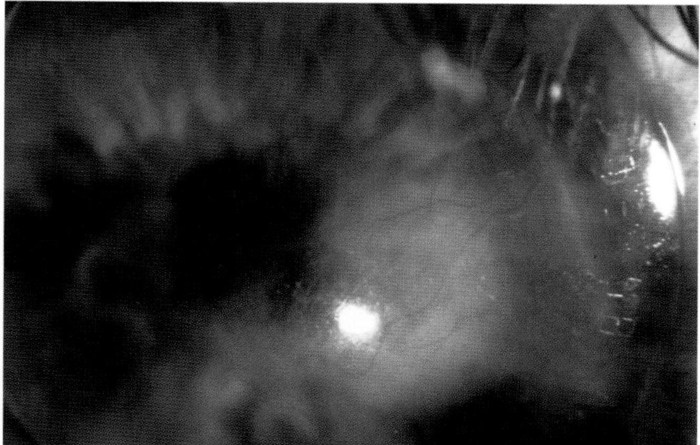

Figure 33.13 Vascularized graft fitted with high-oxygen-transmissibility rigid lens.

fitted with standard edge parameters. Many abnormal corneal shapes require flatter than standard, or steeper than standard, or even reverse-geometry edge designs (Lin *et al.*, 2003) to achieve mechanically acceptable corneal surface alignment, tear exchange and appropriate lens positioning.

Both Genvert *et al.* (1985) and Mannis *et al.* (1986) suggest that the overall success rate of rigid contact lens wear post-PKP approaches 80%.

Hydrogel contact lenses, both standard and in custom parameters, may be occasionally helpful, especially for patients who exhibit the following:

- High refractive errors with lesser degrees of astigmatism.
- Rigid lens intolerance.
- Acceptance of a less than optimal visual result.

Hybrid lens designs can be beneficial in post-PKP fitting; these include the following:

- 'piggyback' – where a top rigid lens is fitted upon a bottom hydrogel lens (Baldone, 1973); silicone hydrogels are often employed now as the bottom hydrogel lens to enhance oxygen supply (Weissman and Ye, 2006) and thereby decrease the stimulus to neovascularization
- Sofperm (formerly Saturn II) – a lens with a rigid centre and hydrophilic periphery ('skirt'), and the similar but newer Synergeyes design (Figure 33.12)
- scleral rigid lenses (Daniel, 1976; Schein *et al.*, 1990; see Chapter 23).

The above hybrid designs often allow optimal vision, similar to rigid lenses, but such lenses are expensive, complex in mechanical fitting, often lead to occlusive lens problems, and may induce hypoxia or binding, which in turn can increase the prevalence and severity of many complications, particularly neovascularization (Figure 33.13).

Continuing care and complications

Intraoperative and immediate postsurgery complications are not part of contact lens management and therefore are beyond the scope of this chapter. It is important to mention, however, that non-healing epithelial defects in the immediate postoperative period are sometimes managed with bandage hydrogel lenses used for extended wear, but only for overall time periods of a few days to a few weeks (see Figure 33.10).

The clinician who follows post-KP patients wearing contact lenses must be constantly vigilant for non-lens-related complications as well as pathology directly related to lens wear. Any complication can increase the risk of graft rejection and/or failure. Increased intraocular pressure, leading to glaucomatous damage to the corneal endothelium as well as the optic nerve – whether surgically induced or as a steroid response – is a good example (Foulks, 1987). Similarly, phakic PKP patients, especially those who are older, may suffer cataract within 5 years of surgery (Martin *et al.*, 1994).

Usual complications encountered in the care of post-PKP patients include:

- Microbial infection – sometimes associated with contact lens wear (in particular extended wear), corneal exposure, steroid use or loose/exposed sutures (Tseng and Ling, 1995).
- Corneal neovascularization – related to sutures, previous eye disease (e.g. blepharitis), large grafts, inflammation or contact lens wear (especially low-oxygen-transmissible and/or tight lenses and/or used on extended wear), probably potentiated by hypoxia or mechanical issues (Lemp, 1980; Dana *et al.*, 1995) (see Figure 33.13).
- Loose/exposed sutures – which can lead to localized abscesses and/or neovascularization, possibly induced by trauma during lens insertion/removals.
- Wound dehiscence – which can occur even years after successful PKP, and may occur spontaneously, following suture removal or even accidentally from trauma (e.g. associated with the use of mechanical contact lens removal devices: Ingraham *et al.*, 1998).
- Epithelial staining, abrasions or defects – which may or may not be related to contact lens wear.
- Papillary conjunctivitis – a common contact lens complication, but also associated with exposed sutures and corneal scars.

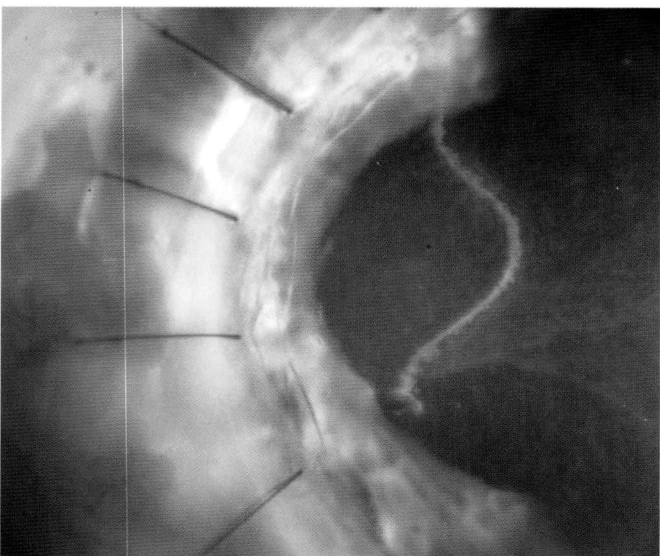

Figure 33.14 Vertical epithelial rejection line in a graft cornea stained with fluorescein.

- Retinal detachment – Aiello *et al.* (1993) found an almost 2% risk of detachment 2 years post-PKP in a cohort of 40 000 medical insurance recipients in the USA between 1984 and 1987.
- Uncontrolled glaucoma – typically surgically induced or a response to the use of steroids.

Graft rejection and failure

The clinician following post corneal graft patients for contact lens care must always be specifically alert for graft rejection and/or failure as well as other problems in both asymptomatic as well as symptomatic individuals. Symptoms of graft immunological rejection include any ocular inflammation, 'red eyes', pain and photophobia, but early rejection may be symptom-free (Kamp *et al.*, 1995).

Graft rejection can be epithelial, stromal or endothelial (Alldredge and Krachmer, 1981).

Epithelial rejection

Epithelial rejection appears as an elevated, undulating line that stains with fluorescein (Figure 33.14). The line represents a zone of donor epithelial destruction by leukocytes, and if left untreated, will march across the surface of the graft over several days or weeks. Although dramatic in appearance, epithelial rejection is not usually a major problem; the end result is the replacement of the donor epithelium by that of the host. Nevertheless, epithelial rejection should be managed with aggressive steroid treatment to decrease ocular inflammation, which may precipitate a secondary full-thickness rejection.

Stromal rejection

Stromal rejection is seen as patchy subepithelial infiltrates, similar to those seen in epidemic keratoconjunctivitis (Krachmer and Alldredge, 1978), and/or full-thickness corneal swelling and haze, usually associated with circumlimbal hyperaemia.

Endothelial rejection

A Khodadoust line and/or keratic precipitates are signs of endothelial rejection and will undoubtedly lead to an opaque cornea unless treated aggressively.

Anterior-chamber inflammation, indicated by the appearance of flare and cells, is another clinical sign of graft rejection.

The risk of rejection is believed to increase with the following:

- Any corneal neovascularization, but particularly deep stromal neovascularization, especially through the graft–host interface.
- Any ocular inflammation.
- Glaucoma.
- Certain diseases, such as active herpetic keratitis.
- Each subsequent corneal graft (when the patient undergoes multiple operations).

While Smiddy *et al.* (1992) suggested that rigid wear by itself does not increase the risk of rejection, Gomes *et al.* (1996) observed many complications in a series of 18 post-PKP patients fitted with rigid lenses. Problems observed over a 3-year period following surgery included corneal staining (8 cases), neovascularization (6 cases), graft rejection episodes (5 cases), papillary conjunctivitis (3 cases) and suture-related infiltrates (2 cases).

Graft failure

Graft failure (as distinct from immunological graft rejection), believed to represent the result of primary or secondary (e.g. glaucoma) endothelial decompensation, must also be considered. Failure can occur early or late, and may be the diagnosis when graft stromal oedema is seen without inflammation. Suspected graft failure should initially be treated with anti-inflammatory drugs (e.g. steroids) in case the diagnosis is really rejection, which may enable the KP to be saved.

Thompson *et al.* (2003) report an overall PKP survival rate of about 88% at 5 and 80% at 10 years postoperatively in a very large series (3992 consecutive eyes), with the highest risk of failure or rejection (about 4%) within the first 2 years but continuing at about 2% per year up through the 10-year point. PKPs for keratoconus had the best survival rates but endothelial failure was common for corneas grafted for pseudophakic bullous keratopathy and regrafts also had lower survival rates.

Other management issues

Several studies suggested that PKP topography changes with rigid wear, with the graft becoming both flatter and smoother (less astigmatic) (Manabe *et al.*, 1986; Wilson *et al.*, 1992; Sperber *et al.*, 1995). De Toledo *et al.* (2003), Szczotka-Flynn *et al.* (2004) and Lim *et al.* (2004), however, found increasing astigmatism with long-term follow-up of PKP for keratoconus, possibly due to keratoconus progression in the remaining host corneal (rim) tissue. Recurrent ectasia has been found in corneal grafts and is diagnosed on average two decades after the initial PK (Patel *et al.*, 2009). Hayashi and Hayashi (2006), on the other hand, found relative stability in corneal surface videotopography of 130 consecutive PKPs for a variety of diseases (31% keratoconus) studied with Fourier series analysis.

Corneal endothelial changes over time are not believed to be different from those expected of any PKP cornea without lens wear (Speaker *et al.*, 1991; Bourne and Shearer, 1995). Graft epithelial barrier function is maintained with post-PKP rigid lens wear (Boot *et al.*, 1991).

Collateral problems commonly encountered include blepharitis, meibomian gland dysfunction and dry eyes associated with acne rosacea or poor lid apposition. These conditions need to be managed aggressively with lid hygiene, artificial tears (preferably unpreserved and unit dose) or appropriate pulsed antibiotic treatment (both local and systemic). Additional surgery may be required, such as punctal occlusion or blepharoplasty. In general, strenuous efforts must be made to protect the graft from drying and to suppress inflammation, in order to avoid rejection episodes.

Dilated and fixed pupils are occasionally a sequela of intraocular surgery (Urrets-Zavalia syndrome: Tuft and Buckley, 1997), but usually do not pose any problems with respect to contact lens wear. Such patients rarely may benefit from an artificial pupil contact lens, but often this is more for cosmetic rather than visual reasons.

Contact lens results

Most trephine-cut post-PKP patients benefit optically from rigid contact lens wear (Ruben and Colbrook, 1979; Lass *et al.*, 1990; Smiddy *et al.*, 1992; Silbiger *et al.*, 1996; Wietharn and Driebe, 2004; Geerards *et al.*, 2006).

Ho *et al.* (1999) studied 40 post-PKP eyes (compared to 40 control eyes) and found that post-PKP eyes were more complex and time-consuming to fit successfully with rigid lenses than were 'normal' eyes, requiring more diagnostic contact lenses, more ordered contact lenses and more office visits than did control eyes. Contact lens wear success rate and complication rates (both lens and graft-related), however, were not significantly different in the two groups of eyes.

Conclusions

Over the past century, both PKP and LK have become accepted and frequently used surgical treatments for many corneal diseases. Although techniques had remained relatively stable during the second half of the 20th century, the last few years have seen the introduction of a set of new techniques, many of which hold promise for major improvements in outcomes and increased utilization. Sutton *et al.* (2008) found only 5.3% of patients required a rigid contact lens following KP for keratoconus. All others were able to attain at least 6/12 best corrected acuity 6 months postoperatively.

Nonetheless, for the near term, the anterior corneal surface commonly remains distorted following corneal grafts and therefore patients often benefit significantly from the optical enhancement afforded by the use of contact lenses – rigid lenses in particular. There are many potential post corneal graft complications, including corneal neovascularization, loose/exposed sutures, glaucoma, cataract, wound dehiscence, microbial infection, graft failure and rejection, and retinal detachment. The use of contact lenses can provoke additional complications, including enhanced risk of corneal neovascularization, loose/exposed sutures, wound dehiscence, epithelial defects, giant papillary conjunctivitis and other inflammatory conditions, and microbial infection. Many of these problems may potentiate graft rejection and/or failure. The risk/benefit ratio must therefore be considered carefully in each individual case, and professional supervision should occur at reasonable intervals, perhaps every 3–4 months, even in asymptomatic individuals.

In conclusion, Williams *et al.* (1991), reporting on 60 patients wearing contact lenses for more than 2 years following PKP, found that the majority (75%) were 'satisfied' with their outcomes, but those who were dissatisfied complained of both contact lens and graft problems.

Acknowledgement

I thank my colleague, Anthony J Aldave, MD, for his invaluable assistance in the preparation of this chapter.

References

Aiello, L. P., Javitt J. C. and Canner J. K. (1993) National outcomes of penetrating keratoplasty: risks of endophthalmitis and retinal detachment. *Arch. Ophthalmology,* **111,** 509–513.

Alldredge, O. C. and Krachmer, J. H. (1981) Clinical types of corneal transplant rejection; their manifestations, frequency, preoperative correlates and treatment. *Arch. Ophthalmology,* **99,** 599–604.

Archila, E. A. (1985) Deep lamellar keratoplasty dissection of host tissue with intrastromal air injection. *Cornea,* **3,** 217–218.

Baldone, J. A. (1973) The fitting of hard contact lenses onto soft contact lenses in certain diseased conditions. *Contact Lens Med. Bull.,* **6,** 15–17.

Boot, J. P., van Best, J., Stolwijk, T. R. *et al.* (1991) Epithelial permeability in corneal grafts by fluorophotometry. *Graefes Arch. Clin. Exp. Ophthalmol.,* **229,** 533–535.

Bourne, W. M. and Shearer D. R. (1995) Effects of long-term rigid contact lens wear on the endothelium of corneal transplants for keratoconus 10 years after penetrating keratoplasty. *Contact Lens Assoc. Ophthalmol. J.,* **21,** 265–267.

Budak, K., Friedman, N. J., Rhodes, L. *et al.* (1998) Peripheral radial incisions to treat inferior contact lens edge lift after penetrating keratoplasty for keratoconus. *J. Cataract Ref. Surg.,* **24,** 1529–1534.

Busin, M., Zambianchi, L. and Arffa, R. C. (2005) Microkeratome-assisted lamellar keratoplasty for the surgical treatment of keratoconus. *Ophthalmology,* **112,** 987–997.

Dana, M. R., Schaumberg, D. A., Kowal, V. O. *et al.* (1995) Corneal neovascularization after penetrating keratoplasty. *Cornea,* **14,** 604–609.

Daniel, R. (1976) Fitting contact lenses after keratoplasty. *Br. J. Ophthalmol.,* **60,** 263–265.

Darwish, T., Brahma, A., Efron, N. *et al.* (2007) Subbasal nerve regeneration after penetrating keratoplasty. *Cornea,* **26,** 935–940.

de Toledo, J. A., de la Paz, M., Barraquer, R. I. *et al.* (2003) Longterm progression of astigmatism after penetrating keratoplasty for keratoconus: evidence of late recurrence. *Cornea,* **22,** 317–323.

Doughman, D. J. (1980) Prolonged donor preservation in organ-culture: long-term clinical evaluation. *Trans. Am. Ophthalmol. Soc.,* **78:** 567–628.

Doughman, D. J., Harris, J. E. and Schmitt, K. M. (1976) Penetrating keratoplasty using 37°C organ-cultured cornea. *Trans. Am. Academy Ophthalmol. Otolaryngology,* **81,** 778–793.

Eye Bank Association of America. Available online at: http://www.restoresight.org/general/faqs.htm; accessed 14 November 2006.

Foulks, G. N. (1987) Glaucoma associated with penetrating keratoplasty. *Ophthalmology,* **94,** 871–874.

Geerards, A. J., Vreugdenhi, W. and Khazen, A. (2006) Incidence of rigid gas permeable contact lens wear after keratoplaty for keratoconus. *Eye and Contact Lens,* **32,** 207–210.

Genvert, G. I., Cohen, E. J., Arentsen, J. J. *et al.* (1985) Fitting gas permeable contact lenses after penetrating keratoplasty. *Am. J. Ophthalmol.,* **99,** 511–514.

Gomes, J. A., Rapuano, C. J. and Cohen, E. J. (1996) Topographic stability and safety of contact lens use after penetrating keratoplasty. *Contact Lens Assoc. Ophthalmol. J.,* **22,** 64–69.

Hayashi, K. and Hayashi, H. (2006) Longterm changes in corneal surface configuration after penetrating keratoplasty. *Am. J. Ophthalmol.,* **141,** 241–247.

Ho, S. K., Andaya, L. and Weissman, B. A. (1999) Complexity of contact lens fitting following penetrating keratoplasty. *Int. Contact Lens Clin.,* **26,** 163–167.

Hoppenreijs, V. P., Van Rij, G., Beekhuis, W. H. *et al.* (1993) Causes of high astigmatism after penetrating keratoplasty. *Doc. Ophthalmol.,* **85,** 21–34.

Ingraham, H. J., Perry, H. D., Epstein, A. B. *et al.* (1998) Suction cup/contact lens complications following penetrating keratoplasty. *Contact Lens Assoc. Ophthalmol. J.,* **24,** 59–62.

IntraLase Corp. Available online at: http://www.prnewswire.com; accessed 26 October 2006.

Kamp, M. T., Fink, N. E., Enger, C. *et al.* (1995) Patient reported symptoms associated with graft rejections in high risk patients in the Collaborative Corneal Transplantation Studies. *Cornea,* **14,** 43–48.

Kim, S. J., Wee, W. R., Lee, J. H. *et al.* (2008) The effect of different suturing techniques on astigmatism after penetrating keratoplasty. *J. Korean Med. Sci.,* **23,** 1015–1019.

Krachmer, J. H. and Alldredge, O. C. (1978) Subepithelial infiltrates as a probable sign of corneal transplant rejection. *Arch. Ophthalmol.,* **96,** 2234–2237.

Lagnado, R., Rubinstein, M. P., Maharajan, S. *et al.* (2004) Management options for the flat corneal graft. *Contact Lens and Anterior Eye,* **27,** 27–31.

Langenbucher, A., Naumann, G. O. H. and Seitz B. (2005) Spontaneous long-term changes of corneal power and astigmatism after suture removal after penetrating keratoplasty using a regression model. *Am. J. Ophthalmol,* **140,** 29–35.

Lass, J. H., Lemback, R. G., Park, S. B. *et al.* (1990) Clinical management of keratoconus. *Ophthalmology,* **97,** 433–445.

Lemp, M. A. (1980) The effect of extended wear aphakic hydrophilic contact lenses after penetrating keratoplasty. *Am. J. Ophthalmol.,* **90,** 331–335.

Lim, L., Pesudovs, K., Goggin, M. *et al.* (2004) Late onset post-keratoplasty astigmatism in patients with keratoconus. *Br. J. Ophthalmol.,* **88,** 371–376.

Lin, J. C., Cohen, E. J., Rapuano, C. J. *et al.* (2003) RK4 (reverse-geometry) contact lens fitting after penetrating keratoplasty. *Eye and Contact Lens,* **29,** 44–47.

Mader, T. H., Yuan, R., Lynn, M. J. *et al.* (1993) Changes in keratometric astigmatism after suture removal more than one year after penetrating keratoplasty. *Ophthalmology,* **100,** 119–127.

Manabe, R., Matsuda, M. and Suda, T. (1986) Photokeratoscopy in fitting contact lenses after penetrating keratoplasty. *Br. J. Ophthalmol.,* **70,** 55–59.

Mannis, M. J. and Zadnik, K. (1988) Hydrophilic contact lenses for wound stabilization in keratoplasty. *Contact Lens Assoc. Ophthalmol. J.,* **14,** 199–202.

Mannis, M. J., Zadnik, K. and Deutch, D. (1986) Rigid contact lens wear in the corneal transplant patient. *Contact Lens Assoc. Ophthalmol. J.,* **12,** 39–42.

Martin, T. P., Reed, J. W., Legault, C. *et al.* (1994) Cataract formation and cataract extraction after penetrating keratoplasty. *Ophthalmology,* **101,** 113–119.

Mathers, W. D., Gold, J. B., Kattan, H., *et al.* (1991) Corneal steepening with final suture removal after penetrating keratoplasty. *Cornea,* **10,** 221–223.

McCarey, B. E. and Kaufman, H. E. (1974) Improved corneal storage. *Invest. Ophthalmol. Vis. Sci.,* **13,**165–173.

McCarey, B. E., Meyer, R. F. and Kaufman, H. E. (1976) Improved corneal storage for penetrating keratoplasties in humans. *Annals Ophthalmol.,* **9,** 1488–1492.

Ozbek, Z. and Cohen, E. J. (2006) Use of intralimbal rigid gas permeable lenses for pellucid marginal degeneration, keratoconus, and after penetrating keratoplasty. *Eye and Contact Lens,* **32,** 33–36.

Patel, S. V., Malta, J. B., Banitt, M. R. *et al.* (2009) Recurrent ectasia in corneal grafts and outcomes of repeat keratoplasty for keratoconus. *Br. J. Ophthalmol.,* **93,** 191–197.

Phillips, A. J. (1997) Postkeratoplasty contact lens fitting. In *Contact Lenses for Pre- and Post-Surgery.* (M.J. Harris ed.), pp. 97–132, St Louis, MO: Mosby.

Price, F. W. (1989) Air lamellar keratoplasty. *Refractive and Corneal Surgery,* **5,** 240–243.

Price, F. W. and Price, M. O. (2006) Descemet's stripping with endothelial keratoplasty in 200 eyes; early challenges and techniques to enhance donor adherence. *J.Cataract Refract. Surg.,* **32,** 411–418.

Rahman, I., Carley, F., Hillarby, C. *et al.* (2009) Penetrating keratoplasty: indications, outcomes, and complications. *Eye,* **23,** 1288–1294.

Reisinger, F. (1824) Die Keratoplastik ein Versuch sur Erweiterung der Augenheil Kunst. Chapter XV in: *Baiersche Annalen Fuer abhan dlunger, Erfindungen und Beobachtungen Aus dem Gebiet der Chirurgie, Augenheil Kunst und Geburtshuelfe VI,* pp. 207–215, Sulzbach.

Ruben, M. and Colbrook, E. (1979) Keratoconus, keratoplasty curvatures and lens wear. *Br. J.Ophthalmol.,* **63,** 268–273.

Schein, O. D., Rosenthal, P. and Ducharme, C. (1990) A gas permeable scleral contact lens for visual rehabilitation. *Am. J. Ophthalmol.,* **109,** 318–322.

Silbiger, J. S., Cohen, E. J. and Laibson, P. R. (1996) The rate of visual recovery after penetrating keratoplasty for keratoconus. *Contact Lens Assoc. Ophthalmol. J.,* **22,** 266–269.

Smiddy, W. E., Hamburg, T. R., Kracher, G. P. *et al.* (1992) Visual correction following penetrating keratoplasty. *Ophthalmic Surg.,* **23,** 90–93.

Soper, J. W., Girard, L. J. and Sampson, W. G. (1964) Special designs and fitting techniques. In *Corneal Contact Lenses* (L.J. Girard ed.), pp. 317–318, St Louis, MO: Mosby.

Speaker, M. G., Cohen, E. J., Edelhouser, H. *et al.* (1991) Effect of gas-permeable contact lenses on the endothelium of corneal transplants. *Arch. Ophthalmol.,* **109,** 1703–1706.

Sperber, L. T., Lopatynsky, M. O. and Cohen, E. J. (1995) Corneal topography in contact lens wearers following penetrating keratoplasty. *Contact Lens Assoc. Ophthalmol. J.,* **21,** 183–190.

Sperling, S. (1979) Human corneal endothelium in organ culture. The influence of temperature and medium of incubation. *Acta Ophthalmologica,* **57,** 269–276.

Sperling, S., Oslen, T. and Ehlers, N. (1981) Fresh and cultured corneal grafts compared by post-operative thickness and endothelial cell density. *Acta Ophthalmologica,* **59,** 566–575.

Sugita, J. and Kondo, J. (1997) Deep lamellar keratoplasty with complete removal of pathological stroma for vision improvement. *Br. J. Ophthalmol.* **81,** 184–188.

Sutton, G., Hodge, C. and McGhee, C. N. (2008) Rapid visual recovery after penetrating keratoplasty for keratoconus. *Clin. Experiment. Ophthalmol.,* **36,** 725–730.

Szczotka-Flynn, L., McMahon, T. T., Lass, J. H., *et al.* (2004) Late stage progressive corneal astigmatism after penetrating keratoplasty for keratoconus. *Eye and Contact Lens,* **30,** 105–110.

Terry, M. A. and Ousley, P. J. (2003) In pursuit of emmetropia: spherical equivalent refraction results with deep lamellar endothelial keratoplasty (DLEK). *Cornea,* **22,** 619–626.

Thompson, R. W., Price, M. O., Bowers, P. J. *et al.* (2003) Long-term graft survival after penetrating keratoplasty. *Ophthalmology,* **110,** 1396–1402.

Tseng, S. H. and Ling, K. C. (1995) Late microbial keratitis after corneal transplantation. *Cornea* **14,** 591–594.

Tuft, S. J. and Buckley, R. J. (1997) Iris ischaemia following penetrating keratoplasty for keratoconus (Urrets-Zavalia syndrome). *Cornea,* **14,** 618–622.

Vail, A., Gore, S. M., Bradley, B. A. *et al.* (1997) Conclusions of the Corneal Transplant Follow Up Study. *Br. J. Ophthalmol.,* **81,** 631–636.

Von Hippel, A. (1888) Eine neue Methode der Hornhauttransplantation. *Von Graefe's Arch. Ophthalmol.,* **34,** 108–130.

Waring, G., Hannush, S., Bogan, S. *et al.* (1992) Classification of corneal topography with videokeratography. In *Corneal Topography Measuring and Modifying the Cornea* (D. Schanzlin, J. Robin eds), pp. 70–71, New York: Springer-Verlag.

Watson, S. L., Ramsay, A., Dart, J. K. *et al.* (2004) Comparison of deep lamellar keratoplasty and penetrating keratoplasty in patients with keratoconus. *Ophthalmology,* **111,** 1676–1682.

Weissman, B. A. and Chun, M. W. (1987) The use of spherical power effect bitoric rigid contact lenses in hospital practice. *J. Am. Optom. Assoc.,* **58,** 626–630.

Weissman, B. A. and Ye, P. (2006) Calculated tear layer oxygen tension under contact lenses offering resistance in series: piggyback and scleral lenses. *Contact Lens and Anterior Eye,* **29,** 231–237.

Wietharn, B. E. and Driebe, W. T. (2004) Fitting contact lenses for visual rehabilitation after penetrating keratoplasty. *Eye and Contact Lens,* **30,** 31–33.

Williams, K. A., Ash, J. K., Pararajasegaram, P. *et al.* (1991) Long-term outcome after corneal transplantation. Visual result and patient perception of success. *Ophthalmology,* **98,** 651–657.

Wilson, S. E., Friedman, R. S. and Klyce, S. D. (1992) Contact lens manipulation of corneal topography after penetrating keratoplasty: a preliminary study. *Contact Lens Assoc. Ophthalmol. J.,* **18,** 177–182.

Woodward, E. G. (1997) Postkeratoplasty. In *Contact Lenses,* 4th edn (A.J. Phillips and L. Speedwell eds), pp. 713–720, Oxford: Butterworth-Heinemann.

Zirm, E. (1906) Eine erfolgreiche totale Keratoplastik. *Arch. Ophthalmol.,* **64,** 580–591.

34 CHAPTER

Orthokeratology

Leo G Carney

Introduction

For whatever reason, many patients want to be able to see well and to function without the need for a refractive correction by glasses or contact lenses. The popularity of refractive surgery procedures with some patients is a clear indicator of that desire. Orthokeratology is one other manifestation of the ongoing attempts to meet this need. The fact that the cornea is the major optical contributor to the power of the eye, and is also the most accessible of the refractive elements of the eye, has made orthokeratology an obvious candidate for initiating refractive control.

It has long been known that the cornea can be deformed by the application of an external pressure, whether an acute pressure as in applanation tonometry or the more sustained pressure from wearing rigid contact lenses. Early studies on the wearing of polymethyl methacrylate (PMMA) lenses demonstrated that they can induce changes in corneal curvature, refractive error and visual acuity. The corneal changes were typically a central flattening, which often took weeks to return to normal. Corneal shape changes have also been demonstrated with the wearing of rigid gas-permeable contact lenses. In general, these changes include a reduction in corneal toricity and a tendency for the cornea to change from its aspheric shape to a more spherical one.

These corneal shape changes, when occurring in routine contact lens fittings, are normally considered an undesirable side-effect of a non-optimal lens fit. However, Jessen (1962) proposed the exploitation of this effect so as to induce useful corneal shape changes, which would eliminate or at least reduce myopic refractive errors.

While early orthokeratology procedures garnered some support, the lack of verifiable evidence on its clinical efficacy precluded general acceptance. More recently, the use of new innovative lens designs has given renewed impetus and interest in this technique.

Outcomes of earlier techniques

Throughout the 1960s and 1970s, an extensive literature on orthokeratology and its outcomes was produced. For the most part, these were anecdotal reports of success, and lacked any appropriate scientific analysis (Carney, 1994).

Some of the features of these early studies are:

- There was no single accepted approach to lens design and wearing protocol, but rather a multiplicity of techniques were advocated and accepted. There was no consensus on the most appropriate lens design, or on the number and timing of lens refittings.
- While some case reports suggested that myopia reductions of 4.00 D or more were feasible, the average reported in most studies was considerably less than that.
- The use of incomplete and inconsistent data was common, and control subjects were rarely included.
- The regression of any induced changes after ceasing lens wear was a major impediment to acceptance of the technique, and led to the concept of 'retainer' lens wear.

The lack of theoretical basis to the technique, the uncertainty of outcomes and the absence of controlled studies all acted to restrict enthusiasm for the technique and prevent its broad acceptance.

Independent studies

The lack of independent analysis of the early orthokeratology procedures was eventually addressed by some controlled clinical studies.

The first comprehensive study was by Kerns (1976, 1978). Further studies were reported by Binder *et al.* (1980) and Polse *et al.* (1983). While the experimental design and breadth of these studies varied, they nevertheless were reasonably consistent in their overall findings. As a result of those controlled clinical studies, the following findings emerged:

- The average myopia reduction was less than that generally reported from case studies, and indeed was of the order of 1.00 D or less.

DOI: 10.1016/B978-0-7506-8869-7.00034-3

- Inducing the refractive effect was slow, yet regression was rapid, and patients would require ongoing lens wear to retain any effect.
- The results were variable, and it was not possible to predict the response of individual patients.
- The quality of vision resulting from the refractive error shifts was variable and subjectively reported as being somewhat diminished.
- The tendency to induce significant corneal astigmatism, reported in the study of Kerns (1976, 1978), was an important complication when lenses decentred.

These reports helped to define better the outcomes of orthokeratology as practised to that time. The magnitude of refractive error change was usually quite limited, and would require ongoing use of contact lenses for part of most days for the effect to be retained. While orthokeratology continued to be utilized, it had a limited acceptance in general contact lens practice.

Modern orthokeratology

The advent and acceptance of keratorefractive surgery for the correction of refractive errors has ensured that interest in other non-surgical approaches, such as orthokeratology, has remained relevant. The resurgence of orthokeratology as a viable alternative to refractive surgery, or indeed traditional contact lens or spectacle corrections, is a consequence of three developments:

1. The availability of new lens designs, particularly reverse-geometry lenses, and the ability to design and manufacture lenses to produce a specific tear layer thickness profile.
2. The availability of videokeratographs to assist with contact lens design and to evaluate corneal shape changes.
3. The availability of new highly oxygen-permeable materials, allowing overnight lens wear.

Reverse-geometry lenses, which were originally developed by Wlodyga and Stoyen (cited by Mountford, 1997), have a secondary curve radius that is steeper than the base curve radius. These lenses offered the prospect of improved centration, and hence less corneal distortion. Importantly, the effectiveness of these lenses in inducing corneal shape changes was superior to earlier designs. They led to rapid, and more predictable, reductions in myopia.

Reverse-geometry lenses

Conventional orthokeratology fitting procedures used lenses designed with a base curve slightly flatter than the central corneal curvature. Myopia reduction took many months to achieve, and required frequent lens replacements. Lens centration was often unsatisfactory, and resulted in corneal distortion or increased astigmatism.

Reverse-geometry lenses have secondary curves that are steeper than the back optic zone radius (BOZR) (Figure 34.1). These lenses are manufactured in a range of optic zone diameters and with secondary curves of variable width and steepness compared to the BOZR (Mountford, 2004). This design allows for the lenses to be fitted with a much flatter central cornea relationship than usual, while maintaining good lens centration. The original design by Contex had a secondary curve which was steeper than the BOZR, and a peripheral curve to give the appropriate edge clearance. Newer designs can have a number of curves to give the reverse curve effect followed by one or more alignment curves (or a tangent curve) and peripheral curves. While there are numerous lens designs in use for orthokeratology, they are all based on the above principles with relatively minor variations in design.

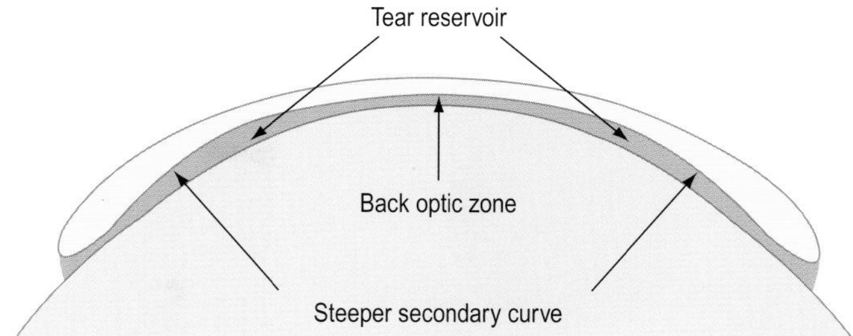

Figure 34.1 Reverse-geometry lens design, showing the steeper secondary curve and related tear reservoir.

Mountford (2004) advocated the fitting of these lenses based on corneal sagittal height measurement so that an improved balance between central touch and tear layer thickness could be established. He maintains that this approach removes the variability in assessment of fluorescein patterns and improves the efficacy of reverse-geometry lens designs.

The availability of materials with high gas permeability has also enhanced the general applicability of orthokeratology, permitting the wearing of orthokeratology lenses on an overnight basis. Current lenses are manufactured in a range of materials, including Equalens II (oxygen permeability of 85 Barrer), Boston XO (oxygen permeability of 100 Barrer) and Menicon Z (oxygen permeability of 165 Barrer). Lenses fabricated from these materials will minimize the hypoxic stress of closed-eye lens wear, but they will not necessarily overcome the other possible complications from overnight wear of any contact lens.

Indications and contraindications

Patient selection is just as important as for other contact lens fittings. However, in addition to the usual considerations, it is essential that realistic expectations about the magnitude of the expected improvement in unaided acuity, and the limitations on its stability, be established with prospective patients.

The usually accepted refractive error limitations are between 3.00 and 4.00 D of myopia, and 1.50 D of astigmatism. For the higher levels of ametropia, patients will need to accept that their unaided vision may be improved but will nevertheless be poorer than with a normal correction. Figure 34.2 shows the corneal topography results to be expected from the overnight wear of a well-centred orthokeratology lens.

Because the induced changes in central corneal shape can be achieved only over a limited optical zone, patients with large pupils in standard illumination may not be suitable candidates.

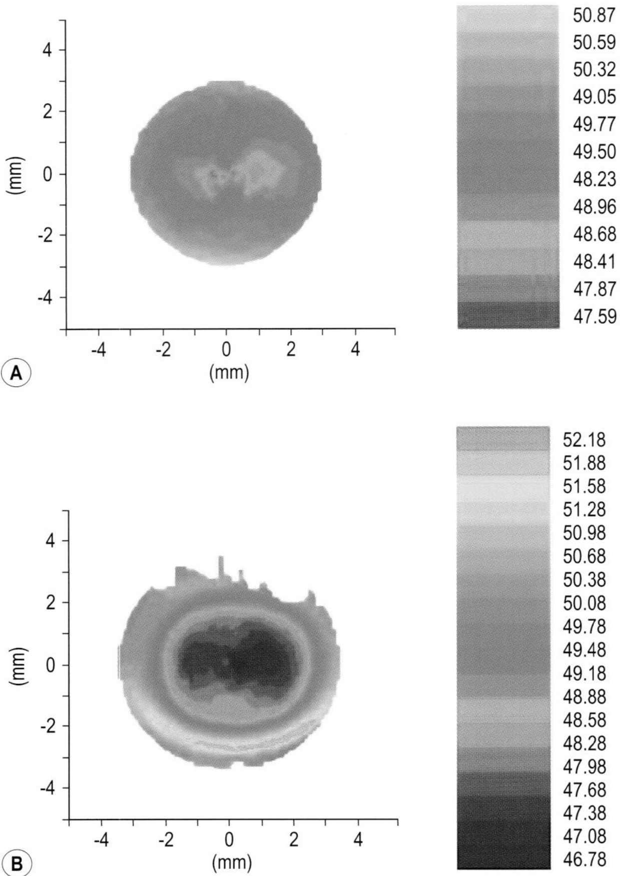

Figure 34.2 Corneal topography changes resulting from overnight wear of a well-fitting reverse-geometry lens design. (A) Pre-lens wear topography. (B) Topography 3 h post-lens removal after 1 night of lens wear.

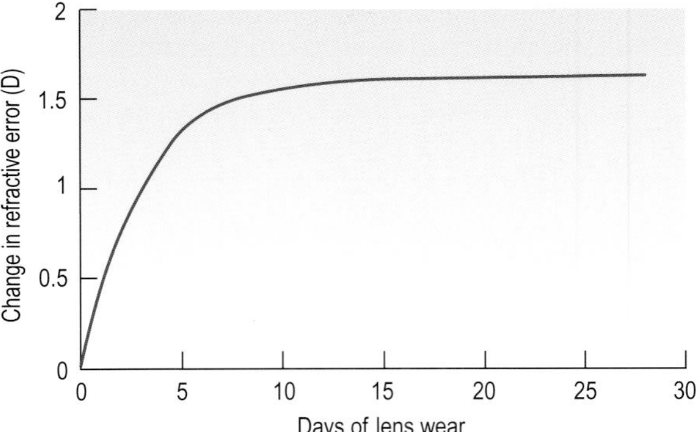

Figure 34.3 Model of the expected refractive change and its time course during wear of reverse-geometry lenses.

As with other lens fittings, good ocular health and the ability to handle and maintain the lenses are expected. Perhaps most important for prospective orthokeratology candidates is the motivation of the patient to see clearly without refractive correction, albeit with significant limitations on the extent and performance of the effect.

Outcomes of accelerated orthokeratology

The outcomes of accelerated orthokeratology can be measured with respect to the efficacy of the technique, the extent and time course of regression after lens removal and safety.

Efficacy

The efficacy of the use of reverse-geometry lenses, worn in both daily wear and overnight wear protocols, has been evaluated in a number of recent studies, examples of which are given here.

Swarbrick *et al.* (1998) fitted reverse-geometry lenses (OK74; Contex) manufactured in Airperm material to 6 young myopic subjects. The lenses were worn on a daily-wear basis for 28 days, and resulted in a myopia reduction of 1.71 ± 0.59 D. Lui and Edwards (2000) conducted a 100-day daily-wear trial on 14 subjects, again using the OK74 design in Airperm material. They reported a myopic reduction of 1.50 ± 0.45 D. Nichols *et al.* (2000) conducted a 60-day trial on overnight wear of the same Contex OK lenses, with 8 subjects completing the study. The reduction in subjective refraction 4 h after awakening was 1.83 ± 1.23 D. Using Paragon CRT lenses, Bernsten *et al.* (2005) found a reduction in myopia of 3.33 ± 0.96 D after 1 month of overnight lens wear.

These studies are therefore reasonably consistent in their estimation of the magnitude of refractive change, and in the variability of the response. While correction of greater amounts of myopia is sometimes reported, they are not what is to be expected in the usual application of current lenses.

Changes in corneal curvature and shape have also been evaluated in many studies, although differing techniques have been employed. Swarbrick *et al.* (1998) used the EyeSys corneal topographic mapping system, and found that the apical corneal power diminished by 1.19 ± 0.38 D. Over the central 5–6 mm zone of the cornea, there was significant central corneal flattening, which diminished towards the mid-periphery. Lui and Edwards (2000) used keratometry and the TMS-1 videokeratographer, and reported central corneal flattening of 0.14 ± 0.06 mm vertically and 0.12 ± 0.07 mm horizontally. Nichols *et al.* (2000) used both a Humphrey Atlas topographer and an Orbscan slit scan topographer, and reported a significant flattening of the apical radius of 0.20 ± 0.90 mm, together with a reduction in peripheral corneal flattening.

In general then, it is well established that changes in corneal shape and refractive error can be induced by the reverse-geometry lenses, and that the changes occur more rapidly than with earlier lens designs, with significant structural and optical change in as little as 15 min (Lu *et al.*, 2008). It is estimated that 75% of the required refractive change can on average be achieved with 1 night of lens wear with an end-point achieved within 7–10 nights of lens wear (Swarbrick, 2006). However, the average magnitude of the refractive change is still only about 2.00 D, and even this is subject to significant individual variability. The issue of predictability of these changes is still an important and unresolved one. A model of the average induced refractive change, and its time course, is shown in Figure 34.3.

Although corneal irregularities, such as a decentred treatment zone, are sometimes encountered, in general the corneal changes do not lead to losses of high-contrast visual acuity, low-contrast visual acuity or contrast sensitivity (Johnson *et al.*, 2007).

Regression

A major criticism of orthokeratology has been the lack of permanence and stability of any induced refractive changes. Modern orthokeratology techniques may be able to induce more rapid changes, but are they any more permanent? The brief answer appears to be that they are not.

For both daily wear and overnight wear of contact lenses, the refractive and vision changes show rapid regression when lenses are removed. Mountford (1998), in a retrospective study of 48 patients, found that after 90 days of overnight wear the regression of apical corneal power over approximately an 8 h period stabilized between 0.50 and 0.75 D per day, but with significant individual variation. Nichols *et al.* (2000) concluded from their study that the refractive outcomes after 60 days of overnight wear were sustained over an 8 h day. However, analysis of their findings shows that most changes were measured over only a 4 h period, and some changes - as indicated by autorefraction data - did show regression up to 0.50 D (Efron, 2000). On average, a regression of approximately 0.25–0.75 D is expected throughout the day after overnight lens wear, but this regression is greater in the early stages of orthokeratology lens use. Up to 90% of recovery towards the baseline refraction can be expected within 72 h of lens discontinuation (Barr *et al.*, 2004).

It is clear that, as was found in earlier evaluations, the corneal changes are not only quite limited in extent but are rarely lasting. Ongoing use of contact lenses, whether for overnight or daily wear, is still needed to sustain the refractive changes. The expected pattern of regression is illustrated in Figure 34.4.

Safety

Until recently, orthokeratology was considered to be a safe procedure with relatively few complications: the most frequently reported complication was corneal distortion or unwanted astigmatism. While this was a common outcome with earlier lens designs, and was a regular cause of discontinuation of lens wear, it is less prevalent with modern lens designs (Nichols *et al.*, 2000).

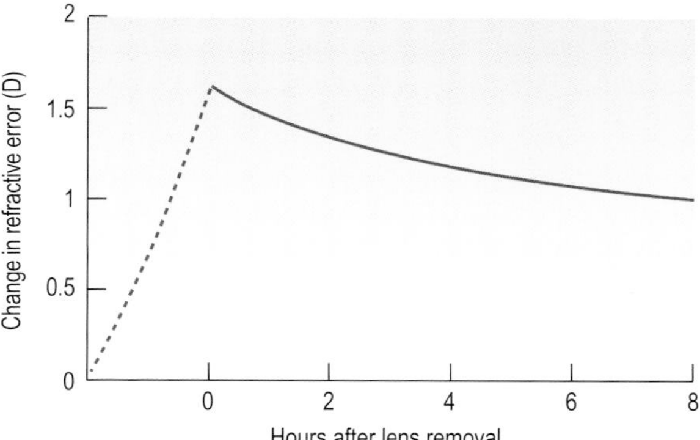

Figure 34.4 Model of the expected regression of refractive change during waking hours after overnight wear of reverse-geometry lenses.

Lum and Swarbrick (2007) reported the appearance of fibrillary lines in the anterior stroma of a 39-year-old Asian woman wearing overnight orthokeratology lenses. The fibrillary lines were fine, slightly curved and subepithelial, arranged in a band-like annulus in the corneal midperiphery. The lines were not associated with epithelial staining, although a marked Fischer–Schweitzer corneal mosaic was noted after blinking. Fibrillary lines are a relatively common finding in normal and keratoconic corneas and have been reported previously accompanying orthokeratology lens wear. Their origin is unknown and epithelial neural remodelling, corneal biomechanical stress and abrupt corneal curvature changes have been suggested as contributing factors. The appearance of fibrillary lines in the orthokeratology patient reported by Lum and Swarbrick (2007) had no adverse consequences on vision or ocular health, at least in the medium term.

Corneal complications can occur in orthokeratology, as in any form of contact lens wear. For example, corneal staining can be present, particularly after overnight lens wear. Occasional serious complications were reported (Swarbrick *et al.*, 1998), but these were mostly a general consequence of contact lens wear, and not the orthokeratology lens or procedures.

The potential for complications is undoubtedly greater when overnight use of contact lens is included, and indeed evidence of serious complications attributable to the overnight-wear modality has now been seen. While current studies suggest that oedema, neovascularizaton and other complications are unlikely, there is evidence that corneal integrity is compromised by the wearing regime. El Hage *et al.* (1999), for example, found that 71% of orthokeratology patients had an adverse response, although these were mostly of a minor nature.

In recent years, a number of cases of keratitis following overnight use of orthokeratology lenses have been reported (Watt and Swarbrick, 2007). The significance of epithelial thinning, as reported after wear of reverse-geometry lenses, in the occurrence of serious complications remains to be established (Swarbrick *et al.*, 1998). Overnight wear of any contact lens has previously been shown to be a major risk factor for keratitis (Holden and Lazon de la Jara, 2007), so the finding of complications in orthokeratology is perhaps not unexpected. Swarbrick (2006) has analysed the circumstances surrounding many of the reported cases, and points out that many are from one region of the globe and that there are indications of suboptimal practice in terms of lens design, lens material and lens care regimen. For example, *Acanthamoeba* keratitis in orthokeratology has been shown to be related to use of tap water for rinsing (Lee *et al.*, 2007).

Orthokeratology lenses have been shown to retain more bacteria than alignment-fit rigid lenses after bacteria-loaded overnight lens wear. This may increase the risk for an infection in orthokeratology patients if suitable conditions are present. Specific education on the cleaning of orthokeratology lenses is essential (Choo *et al.*, 2009). Cho *et al.* (2008) provided a comprehensive guideline for practitioners to improve their orthokeratology practice and minimize unnecessary or preventable complications as they believe that the key to safe orthokeratology lens wear is to update knowledge in the field continually, and to practise to the highest professional standards.

Accurate information on the prevalence of serious complications in orthokeratology is still not available, and the potential for their occurrence must be recognized and protected against (Van Meter *et al.*, 2008).

How orthokeratology works

Over the years, various empirical fitting techniques for orthokeratology have been developed. The lack of any strong theoretical basis for understanding the procedure, or the variables affecting its outcomes and its predictability, has been a significant drawback to its more general acceptance. Despite the development of new lens designs with their more rapidly induced changes, there is still no accepted understanding of the underlying corneal tissue changes or the mechanism of change.

The original concept of orthokeratology was based on the belief that a flat-fitting lens would induce central corneal flattening and hence a reduced level of myopia. As already mentioned, a common outcome of this approach was corneal distortion.

There is now good evidence that the corneal changes with reverse-geometry lenses are more complex than a mechanical bending of the cornea. Swarbrick *et al.* (1998) reported results of measurements of corneal shape and thickness changes after orthokeratology lens wear. They demonstrated that the myopia reduction was accompanied by a flattening of the central cornea, thinning of the central cornea and thickening of the mid peripheral cornea. The central thinning was mostly accounted for by epithelial changes, while the mid peripheral thickening was mostly a stromal effect. There were also differences in the time course of the various corneal changes, with corneal curvature and total thickness showing rapid changes and epithelial changes occurring more slowly. Stromal, but not epithelial, thickness changes during overnight wear of orthokeratology lenses has been shown to be related to oxygen transmissibility of the lenses (Haque *et al.*, 2007).

Cell compression, rather than cell movement or loss, may be the primary mechanism of central epithelial changes (Choo *et al.*, 2004). Swarbrick *et al.* (1998) suggest that the corneal curvature changes in orthokeratology result not from short-term corneal bending but from a longer-term redistribution of anterior corneal tissue. Posterior corneal curvature changes were found by Owens *et al.* (2004), which would suggest that corneal bending does have some role in the mechanism of change. However, using a Pentacam analysis system, Tsukiyama *et al.* (2008) have shown that overnight orthokeratology lens wear alters the anterior corneal shape rather than the posterior radius of the corneal curvature or the anterior-chamber depth.

Mountford (1997) hypothesized that it is the tear reservoir generated by the steeper secondary curves that primarily leads to the pressure changes responsible for the corneal tissue redistribution.

These corneal changes, whatever the mechanism, are clearly of a different nature to those resulting from the early flat-fitting lens designs. A schematic depiction of these contributions to the induced refractive changes is shown in Figure 34.5.

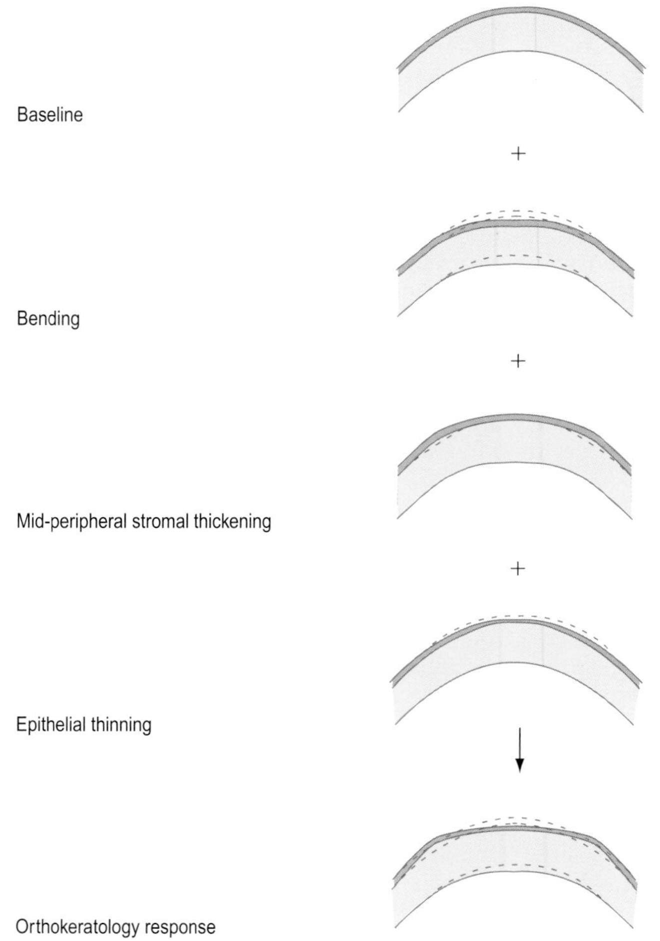

Figure 34.5 The change from baseline corneal shape and thickness can be modelled as a result of the composite effects of bending, mid peripheral stromal thickening and central epithelial thinning.

Determinants of success

A major drawback to the more general acceptance of orthokeratology has been the variability of responses and its general lack of predictability. While a number of ocular and contact lens characteristics have been proposed as candidates for influencing the refractive outcome, there have been no conclusive findings.

Carkeet *et al.* (1995) carried out an analysis of a range of ocular characteristics, including subjective refraction, corneal thickness profile, intraocular pressure, ocular rigidity and epithelial rigidity. The only significant finding was that orthokeratology success was related to the prefitting refractive error, with higher levels of myopia leading to reduced refractive change. Studies on corneal hysteresis and corneal resistance to deformation have failed to identify reliable and consistent effects of corneal biomechanics on orthokeratology outcomes (Chen *et al.*, 2009; Gonzalez-Meijome *et al.*, 2009).

The ocular characteristic most accepted as being of significance to the induced refractive change is the prefitting corneal shape. Mountford (1997) and others maintain that the practical limit of orthokeratology is defined by the corneal asphericity, since further corneal change is unlikely when the cornea achieves a spherical shape. A regression analysis of change in apical corneal power and initial corneal eccentricity directly related the induced corneal (and hence) refractive change to corneal shape. Near-spherical corneal shapes led to very little corneal power change (Mountford, 1997).

Correction of hyperopia

Orthokeratology techniques have been proposed as a means of correcting hyperopia as well as myopia. The principle here is to induce controlled amounts of central corneal steepening. The primary corneal change in hyperopic orthokeratology may be mid peripheral corneal thinning rather than central corneal thickening (Gifford and Swarbrick, 2008). Gifford *et al.* (2009) suggest that the mechanism of this thinning is corneal compression by the lens in the paracentral region as opposed to central postlens tear film suction.

These corneal steepening effects seem to be more difficult to induce and control compared to central corneal flattening. While such corneal changes can be produced, clinical results so far have not been compelling (Swarbrick *et al.*, 2004; Lu *et al.*, 2007).

Control of myopia progression in children

Since the early use of rigid contact lenses, there have been attempts not only to correct myopia optically but also to inhibit the progression of myopia in children. Evidence for this effect has been controversial. More recently, the efficacy of overnight orthokeratology lens wear in inhibiting myopia progression in children has been postulated. Cho *et al.* (2005) were the first to present evidence that overnight use of orthokeratology lenses in children not only temporarily corrects myopia but also restricts the axial length elongation, which leads to myopia progression. They acknowledged that their study suffered from similar drawbacks to early orthokeratology studies such as absence of appropriate control patients, but the finding has nevertheless prompted the uptake of orthokeratology approaches in populations with high levels of myopia and high myopia progression rates. Van Meter *et al.* (2008) reviewed the available literature and concluded that overnight orthokeratology for slowing the progression of myopia in children still needs well-designed and properly conducted controlled trials to investigate efficacy.

Correlations

The relationship between refractive changes and corneal curvature changes has been a matter of some conjecture. Numerous studies using early orthokeratology lens designs reported that the refractive change was greater than that expected from corneal power changes measured using keratometry. The reported ratio of these changes was often 2 : 1 or more.

This anomaly is most likely a consequence of the irregular nature of the induced corneal topographic changes. It is now apparent that the corneal shape changes are more marked in the central cornea, and diminish towards the mid-periphery (Swarbrick *et al.*, 1998), and hence keratometry results are somewhat unreliable. Similarly, the reported vision improvements were often much better than would be predicted from corneal curvature changes. As well as the above explanation, these vision reports were influenced by a lack of standardization of testing procedures, practice effects from repeated vision testing (McMonnies, 2001) and bias from the unmasked protocols often used (Carney, 1994).

These difficulties with correlating corneal curvature, refraction and vision were confirmed by Nichols *et al.* (2000) using overnight wear of reverse-geometry lenses. In that study, refraction was measured both subjectively and by autorefractor. A larger reduction in myopia was reported for subjective refraction than for autorefraction. The authors hypothesize that this finding is a consequence of the greater weight given to peripheral optical effects with autorefraction.

While the anomalies in correlations of corneal curvature, refraction and vision may all have the single basis of an irregular induced corneal shape, the findings still await a definitive optical analysis. In the meantime, the inability to derive significant correlations remains another contributor to the lack of predictability of orthokeratology.

Conclusions

A number of questions about current orthokeratology techniques can now be answered.

Is orthokeratology effective in modifying refractive errors?

The answer in terms of reducing myopia is a qualified yes. There is much evidence that correctly fitting reverse-geometry lenses will lead to a reduction in myopia. However, the level of the induced change is moderate, and averages less than 2.00 D; the procedure suffers from a lack of predictability in the magnitude of the change likely to be produced in any individual. The effect is transient.

Is orthokeratology safe?

The answer here is that, in general, the use of orthokeratology lenses brings with it the same risks as wearing any other form of contact lens. The corneal warpage often seen with earlier orthokeratology lens designs should not occur with modern designs. However, overnight wear of lenses brings with it the increased risk of keratitis (Morgan *et al.*, 2005; Watt and Swarbrick, 2007). It is possible that the use of orthokeratology lenses further increases the risks of complications from overnight lens wear because of diminished corneal integrity and epithelial thinning, but this is not yet proven.

Is orthokeratology clinically efficacious?

Limited reductions in myopia can certainly be achieved by orthokeratology. The refractive changes are transient, and with an overnight-wear regimen a significant proportion of the refractive effect is usually lost by the end of the following day. As well, the practitioner must invest in both new instrumentation and in developing appropriate expertise.

One view, then, is that given the limitations of the technique and its outcomes, particularly their transient nature, a better direction is to encourage appropriate use of conventional contact lens modalities. On the other hand, there are patients who strongly desire to function well without any refractive correction, and orthokeratology could then be seen as an alternative to the various forms of invasive and permanent refractive surgery. In this case, the patient must be made fully aware not only of the option of orthokeratology, but also its limitations, including the possibility, even if remote, of serious complications.

Acknowledgement

The assistance of Ms Julia Mainstone in developing the figures in this chapter is gratefully acknowledged.

References

Barr, J. T., Rah, M. J., Meyers, W. *et al.* (2004) Recovery of refractive error after corneal refractive therapy. *Eye Contact Lens,* **30,** 247–251.

Bernsten, D. A., Barr, J. T. and Mitchell, G. L. (2005) The effect of overnight corneal reshaping on higher-order aberrations and best-corrected visual acuity. *Optom. Vis. Sci.,* **82,** 490–497.

Binder, P. S., May, C. H. and Grant, S. C. (1980) An evaluation of orthokeratology. *Ophthalmology,* **87,** 729–744.

Carkeet, N. L., Mountford, J. A. and Carney, L. G. (1995) Predicting success with orthokeratology lens wear: a retrospective analysis of ocular characteristics. *Optom. Vis. Sci.,* **72,** 892–898.

Carney, L. G. (1994) Orthokeratology. In *Contact Lens Practice* (M. Ruben and M. Guillon, eds), pp. 877–888, London: Chapman & Hall.

Chen, D., Lam, A. K. C. and Cho, P. (2009) A pilot study on the corneal biomechanical changes in short-term orthokeratology. *Ophthal. Physiol. Opt.,* 29, 464–471.

Cho, P., Cheung, S. W. and Edwards, M. (2005) The longitudinal orthokeratology research in children (LORIC) in Hong Kong: a pilot study on refractive changes and myopia control. *Curr. Eye Res.,* **30,** 71–80.

Cho, P., Cheung, S. W., Mountford, J. *et al.* (2008) Good clinical practice in orthokeratology. *Cont. Lens Anterior Eye,* **31,** 17–28.

Choo, J., Caroline, P. and Harlin, D. (2004) How does the cornea change under corneal reshaping contact lenses? *Eye Contact Lens,* **30,** 211–213.

Choo, J. D., Holden, B. A., Papas, E. B. *et al.* (2009) Adhesion of *Pseudomonas aeruginosa* to orthokeratology and alignment lenses. *Optom. Vis. Sci,* **86,** 93–97.

Efron, N. (2000) Overnight orthokeratology (Correspondence). *Optom. Vis. Sci.,* **77,** 627–629.

El Hage, S., Leach, N. E. and Shahin, R. (1999) Controlled kerato-reformation (CRK): an alternative to refractive surgery. *Practical Optometry,* **10,** 230–236.

Gifford, P. and Swarbrick, H. A. (2008) Time course of corneal topographic changes in the first week of overnight hyperopic orthokeratology. *Optom. Vis. Sci.,* **85,** 1165–1171.

Gifford, P., Au, V., Hon, B. *et al.* (2009) Mechanism for corneal reshaping in hyperopic orthokeratology. *Optom. Vis. Sci.,* **86,** 306–311.

Gonzalez-Meijome, J. M., Villa-Collar, C., Querios, A. *et al.* (2008) Pilot study on the influence of corneal biomechanical properties over the short term in response to corneal refractive therapy for myopia. *Cornea,* 27, 421–426.

Haque, S., Fonn, D., Simpson, T. *et al.* (2007) Corneal refractive therapy with different lens materials, Part 1: corneal, stromal and epithelial thickness changes. *Optom. Vis. Sci.,* **84,** 343–348.

Holden, B. A. and Lazon de la Jara, P. (2007) Contact lenses: optimal vision – sub-optimal carrier? *Optom. Vis. Sci.,* **84,** 365–367.

Jessen, G. N. (1962) Orthofocus techniques. *Contacto,* **6,** 200–204.

Johnson, K. L., Carney, L. G., Mountford, J. A. *et al.* (2007) Visual performance after overnight orthokeratology. *Contact Lens Ant. Eye,* **30,** 29–36.

Kerns, R. (1976, 1978) Research in orthokeratology, Parts 1 to 8. *J. Am. Optom. Assoc.,* **47,** 1047–1051; **47,** 1275–1285; **47,** 1505–1515; **48,** 227–238; **48,** 345–359; **48,** 1134–1147; **48,** 1541–1553; **49,** 308–314.

Lee, J. E., Hahn, T. W., Oum, B. S. *et al.* (2007) *Acanthamoeba* keratitis related to orthokeratology. *Int. Ophthalmol.,* **27,** 45–49.

Lu, F., Sorbara, L., Simpson,T. *et al.* (2007) Corneal shape and optical performance after one night of corneal refractive therapy for hyperopia. *Optom. Vis. Sci.,* **84,** 357–364.

Lu, F., Simpson, T., Sorbara, L. *et al.* (2008) Malleability of the ocular surface in response to mechanical stress induced by orthokeratology contact lenses. *Cornea,* **27,** 133–141.

Lui, W-O. and Edwards, M. H. (2000) Orthokeratology in low myopia. Part 1: Efficacy and predictability. *Contact Lens Ant Eye,* **23,** 77–89.

Lum, E. and Swarbrick, H. (2007) Fibrillary lines in overnight orthokeratology. *Clin. Exp. Optom.,* **90,** 299–302.

McMonnies, C. W. (2001) Chart memory and visual acuity measurement. *Clin. Exp. Optom.* **84,** 26–34.

Morgan, P. B., Efron, N., Brennan, N. A. *et al.* (2005) Risk factors for the development of corneal infiltrative events associated with contact lens wear. *Invest. Ophthalmol. Vis. Sci.,* **46,** 3136–3143.

Mountford, J. A. (1997) Orthokeratology. In *Contact Lenses,* 4th edn (A. J. Phillips and L. Speedwell, eds), pp. 653–692, Oxford: Butterworth-Heinemann.

Mountford, J. A. (1998) Retention and regression of orthokeratology with time. *Int. Contact Lens Clin.,* **25,** 59–64.

Mountford, J. A. (2004) Design variables and fitting philosophies of reverse geometry lenses. In *Orthokeratology Principles and Practice* (J. Mountford, D. Ruston and T. Dave, eds), pp. 69–107, London: Butterworth Heinemann.

Nichols, J. J., Marsich, M. M., Nguyen, M. *et al.* (2000) Overnight orthokeratology. *Optom. Vis. Sci.,* **77,** 252–259.

Owens, H. A., Garner, L. F., Craig, J. P. *et al.* (2004) Posterior corneal changes with orthokeratology. *Optom. Vis. Sci.,* **81,** 421–426.

Polse, K. A., Brand, R. J., Vastine, D. W. *et al.* (1983) Corneal change accompanying orthokeratology. *Arch. Ophthalmol.,* **101,** 1873–1878.

Swarbrick, H. A. (2006) Orthokeratology review and update. *Clin. Exp. Optom.,* **89,** 124–143.

Swarbrick, H. A., Wong, G. and O'Leary, D. J. (1998) Corneal response to orthokeratology. *Optom. Vis. Sci.,* **75,** 791–799.

Swarbrick, H. A., Hiew, R., Kee, A. V. *et al.* (2004) Apical clearance rigid contact lenses induce corneal steepening. *Optom. Vis. Sci.,* **81,** 427–435.

Tsukiyama, J., Miyamoto, Y., Higaki, S. *et al.* (2008) Changes in the anterior and posterior radii of the corneal curvature and anterior chamber depth by orthokeratology. *Eye Contact Lens,* **34,** 17–20.

Van Meter, W. S., Musch, D. C., Jacobs, D. S. *et al.* (2008) Safety of overnight orthokeratology for myopia: a report by the American Academy of Ophthalmology. *Ophthalmology,* **115,** 2301–2313.

Watt, K. G. and Swarbrick, H. A. (2007) Trends in microbial keratitis associated with orthokeratology. *Eye Contact Lens,* **33,** 373–377; Discussion 382.

CHAPTER 35

Diabetes

Clare O'Donnell

Introduction

Diabetes mellitus may be defined as a chronic metabolic disorder that is characterized by elevation of blood glucose concentration. It is classified into two main types: type 1 (insulin-dependent) diabetes and type 2 (non-insulin-dependent) diabetes.

Diabetes affects around 3% of the world population. The incidence of diabetes is increasing, although the exact number of new cases diagnosed each year is difficult to ascertain. Type 1 diabetes accounts for approximately 20% of primary diabetes whereas type 2 diabetes accounts for 80%. The peak age of onset of type 1 diabetes is in the 10–14-year-old age group, whereas the incidence of type 2 diabetes increases with age.

The anterior eye

Retinopathy is the ocular complication that most commonly causes loss of vision in diabetic patients (Figure 35.1); however, structural abnormalities affecting the anterior eye have also been described.

In order to understand the possible effects of diabetes on the eye during contact lens wear, it is necessary to consider how the anterior eye of diabetic patients differs from that of non-diabetic patients.

Orbit

Patients with poorly controlled diabetes are more susceptible to bacterial and fungal infections of the orbit than non-diabetic patients. Those affected may present with ophthalmoplegia and proptosis.

Eyelids

Xanthelasma is a condition in which yellow deposits occur in the eyelid, and is thought to be due to abnormalities in lipid metabolism. Xanthelasmata occur at an earlier age and more frequently in patients with diabetes (Figure 35.2).

Ptosis can be an early sign of undiagnosed diabetes, the underlying cause being chronic tissue hypoxia. Ulcerative blepharitis, styes and meibomian cysts are also more commonly found in the diabetic population.

Tear film

Reduced tear secretion is often found in association with diabetes, and is perhaps related to dysfunction of the autonomic nervous system serving the lacrimal gland. Increased levels of secretory immunoglobulin A, lysozyme and glucose have been observed in the tear film of patients with diabetes. It has been suggested that increased tear glucose concentration could promote lens spoilation and the growth of microorganisms in diabetic contact lens wearers.

Since tear glucose concentration has been shown to mirror blood glucose concentration, it has been suggested that the measurement of tear glucose concentration could be used to monitor metabolic control non-invasively in diabetic patients. This could perhaps be carried out using contact lenses with a glucose-sensing agent (March *et al.*, 2004b; Domschke *et al.*, 2006). Using 'off-the-shelf' contact lenses embedded with new water-soluble, highly fluorescent and glucose-sensitive boronic acid containing fluorophores, Geddes (2004) found these lenses were able to track tear glucose levels, and so blood glucose levels.

Conjunctiva

Microaneurysms, capillary proliferation and vessel dilations have been noted in the conjunctivae of diabetic patients. These features are not unique to diabetes; they can occur in association with other systemic diseases such as hypertension and arteriosclerosis (L'Esperance and James, 1983). Conjunctival oxygen tension may be reduced in patients with advanced diabetic eye disease compared to those with milder retinal changes.

Iris

Iris changes associated with diabetes include the deposition of glycogen vacuoles in the iris pigment epithelium,

DOI: 10.1016/B978-0-7506-8869-7.00035-5

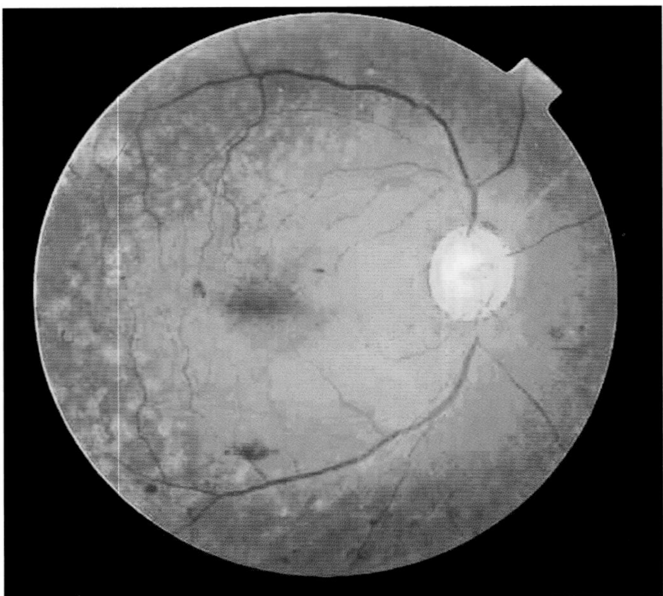

Figure 35.1 Diabetic retinopathy.

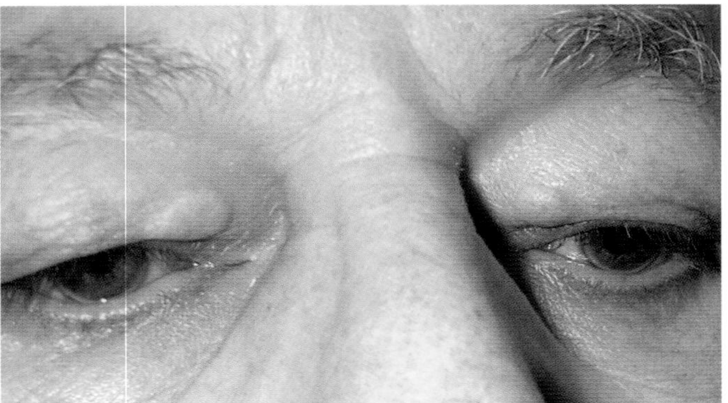

Figure 35.2 Diabetic patient with bilateral xanthelasmata.

pigment dispersion, iris atrophy and iris neovascularization.

Pupil

Pupil size and pupil reactions may be altered in diabetic patients with poor metabolic control. The pupil may be more difficult to dilate in diabetic patients with neuropathy.

Cornea

The ultrastructural and biochemical status of the cornea is altered in patients with diabetes (McNamara, 1997; O'Donnell and Efron, 1998; Wiemer *et al.*, 2007); some of the changes that have been described are summarized in Table 35.1.

Below is an account of alterations to the structure and function of the cornea that are of more immediate clinical relevance.

Table 35.1 Biochemical and structural changes associated with diabetes

Structure	Changes
Tears	Increased lysozyme Increased secretory immunoglobulin A Increased glucose concentration
Epithelium	Pleomorphism Increased cell size Thickened basement membrane Decreased adhesion of cells to basement membrane Decreased penetration of anchoring fibrils into stroma
Stroma	Increased thickness Glycosylation of collagen Increase in intermolecular spacing of collagen fibrils Increased autofluorescence
Descemet's layer	Folds Increased thickness
Endothelium	Polymegethism Pleomorphism Reduced Na-K-ATPase activity

Epithelium

The corneal epithelium is known to be particularly susceptible to mechanical trauma in diabetic patients (O'Leary and Millodot, 1981). Recurrent corneal epithelial defects, superficial punctate keratitis and prolonged epithelial healing rates have also been reported, particularly after ophthalmic surgery. Inadequate adhesion of cells to an abnormal underlying basement membrane, reduced corneal oxygen consumption and reduced corneal sensitivity have been implicated in many of the corneal epithelial complications observed.

Corneal nerves

Diabetes can cause a significant reduction in corneal sensitivity (O'Leary and Millodot, 1981). This sensory deficit is thought to occur due to a diffuse polyneuropathy. The extent of the reduction appears to relate to the duration of the diabetes, the age of the patient and the degree of diabetic metabolic control. Reduced corneal sensitivity has been linked with the development of corneal ulcers in diabetic patients (Lockwood *et al.*, 2006), and it is generally accepted that contact lens wear should be approached with caution in any patient with corneal hypoaesthesia. Such patients should be advised to remove lenses and to seek advice if they experience any discomfort.

Corneal confocal microscopy has been used to evaluate the alterations that occur in patients with diabetes. Researchers have reported structural changes to corneal nerves (Malik *et al.*, 2003; Kallinikos *et al.*, 2004) and others have related these changes to the reductions observed in corneal sensitivity (Rosenberg *et al.*, 2000). The alterations in nerve structure appear to be more pronounced in patients with diabetic polyneuropathy (Malik *et al.*, 2003) and patients with diabetic retinopathy (Mocan *et al.*, 2006). Quattrini *et al.* (2007) have shown that corneal confocal microscopy can quantify small fibre damage rapidly and non-invasively and it can detect earlier stages of nerve damage compared with currently used techniques. This may make it an ideal

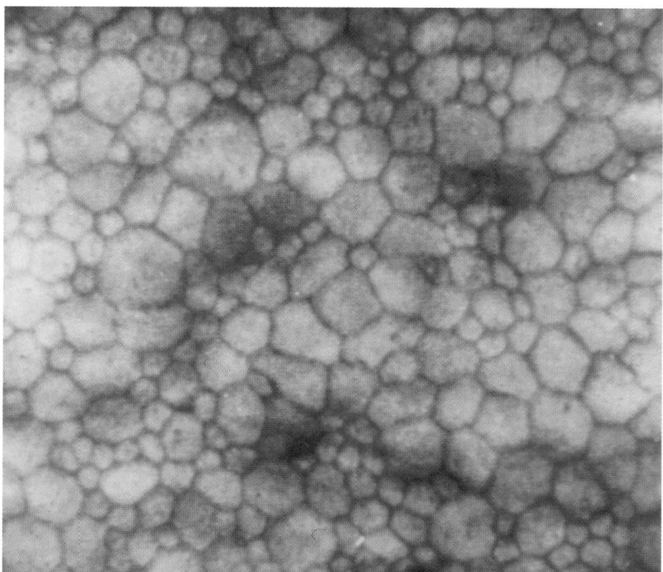

Figure 35.3 Endothelial polymegethism.

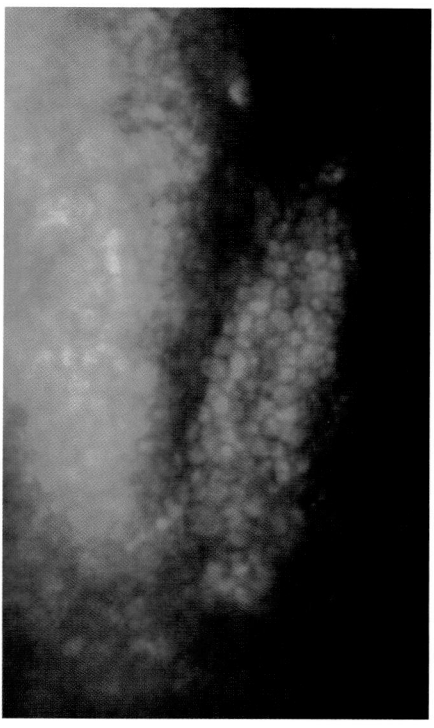

Figure 35.4 A single diagonally oriented endothelial fold.

technique to diagnose accurately and assess progression of human diabetic neuropathy.

Endothelium

Studies of corneal endothelial morphology in diabetic humans and animals have revealed increased levels of polymegethism and pleomorphism (Figure 35.3).

Most researchers have failed to demonstrate significant reductions in endothelial cell density among diabetic patients (O'Donnell and Efron, 2004a), which contrasts with the findings of Lee *et al.* (2006).

The appearance of folds in Descemet's membrane has been reported in diabetic patients (Figure 35.4). When associated with diabetes, vertical folds often appear in the central corneal endothelium of both eyes. Folds due to diabetes appear to be enduring, unlike folds due to contact lens-induced corneal oedema, which disappear after lens removal (O'Donnell *et al.*, 2001).

Corneal hydration control

Corneal thickness is often increased in diabetic patients (Skaff *et al.*, 1995; McNamara *et al.*, 1998; Lee *et al.*, 2006). Abnormal function of the corneal endothelium has been postulated as the cause, perhaps as a direct result of the accumulation of glucose and sorbitol (McNamara, 1997).

Increased corneal epithelial and endothelial permeability to fluorescein has been reported in patients with diabetes compared to non-diabetic control subjects. It has been suggested that the limiting layers of the diabetic cornea function normally during everyday conditions, but may have a reduced ability to cope with the stress induced by ophthalmic surgery or long-term contact lens wear (McNamara, 1997).

Investigators have used pachymetry to monitor the recovery response to oedema induced by contact lenses of low oxygen transmissibility. This approach has demonstrated reduced absolute corneal swelling (O'Donnell and Efron, 2006) and prolonged recovery times from oedema in diabetic patients compared with normal controls. Since the rate of recovery from corneal oedema is reduced in diabetic patients, it has been suggested that care should be taken when prescribing contact lenses for such patients. However, it could be argued that these studies do not identify any obvious problems arising in diabetic patients wearing contact lenses with high oxygen transmissibility on a daily-wear basis.

Microbial keratitis

Schein *et al.* (1989) found that diabetic patients using contact lenses have an increased risk of developing microbial keratitis, although the magnitude of the increased risk was not stated. In view of this, diabetic contact lens wearers should be advised to seek immediate advice if they develop a painful red eye or other symptoms suggestive of corneal ulceration.

Panretinal photocoagulation

Corneal complications such as reduced corneal sensitivity, corneal erosions and keratitis have been reported following panretinal photocoagulation (PRP). (This procedure has also been associated with other complications such as visual field loss, persistent mydriasis, iritis, iris atrophy, lens opacities, shallowing of the anterior chamber and accommodative palsy.) Corneal endothelial cell loss after PRP has also been documented.

Ocular response to contact lenses

Given the alterations to the anterior segment that accompany diabetes, an important issue to be addressed is whether or not cosmetic contact lenses should be prescribed for diabetic patients.

The results of a prospective, controlled study have demonstrated that daily-wear soft contact lenses can be a viable mode of vision correction for patients with diabetes. O'Donnell *et al.* (2001) and March *et al.* (2004a) suggest that practitioners should not expect to see adverse clinical signs in diabetic contact lens wearers that are any different from those seen in non-diabetic lens wearers. If adverse signs are detected in a diabetic lens wearer, they should not be attributed solely to the fact the patient has diabetes; however, the predisposition of the diabetic patient to corneal infection should always be borne in mind.

Special considerations

Roughening of the fingertips caused by home blood glucose monitoring could lead to damage to the lens surface during cleaning, and patients should therefore be reminded to inspect contact lenses for damage prior to lens insertion. Fingernails should be kept short and smooth to reduce the risk of corneal erosion (O'Donnell and Efron, 1998).

Prescribing contact lenses

Although there are established trends in contact lens prescribing for the general population, clinical opinion is divided as to which type of contact lens is most appropriate for diabetic patients. In view of the fragility of the corneal epithelium, rigid contact lenses were previously not recommended for diabetic patients since corneal abrasion occurs more frequently with rigid contact lenses. However, rigid lenses have certain advantages over soft lenses. The likelihood of toxins and potential pathogens becoming trapped beneath the lens is reduced with a rigid lens compared to a soft lens. Rigid lenses are also more durable and less prone to tearing or splitting compared to soft contact lenses.

The results of a survey conducted in the UK indicated that practitioners believed that rigid lenses are the safest form of contact lens for diabetic patients (Veys *et al.*, 1997). This survey was conducted prior to the availability of silicone hydrogel contact lenses. The reason for rigid lenses being favoured for diabetic patients was a perceived reduced risk of infection with these lenses compared to soft lenses. Practitioners stated that important factors to be considered when fitting contact lenses to diabetic patients include the degree of metabolic control and the contact lens wear time.

Compliance

O'Donnell and Efron (2004b) investigated the notion that diabetic contact lens wearers may represent a special group displaying higher levels of compliance with their lens care regimens as a result of learned behaviour relating to maintenance of their diabetic condition. To test this hypothesis, a prospective, single-centre, controlled, masked study was performed whereby 29 diabetic contact lens patients and 29 non-diabetic control subjects were issued with disposable hydrogel contact lenses and a multipurpose lens care regimen. All participants were given identical instruction on lens care and maintenance. Compliance levels were assessed at a 12-month aftercare appointment by demonstration and questionnaire. Twenty-four different aspects of compliance were scored, 12 by observation and 12 by questionnaire report, of which only two showed a significant difference between the diabetic and control groups. Although the combined population of contact lens wearers was generally compliant, there were examples of non-compliance in both groups. Neither the duration of diabetes nor the degree of metabolic control appeared to have a significant effect on compliance. The results suggest that eye care practitioners cannot assume that diabetic patients will be more compliant with contact lens care and maintenance than non-diabetic patients.

Contact lens wear in patients with other systemic disease

Patients with any systemic disease known to affect the anterior eye adversely potentially face problems during contact lens wear. Conditions such as thyroid deficiency, hyperthyroidism, rheumatoid arthritis, atopic eczema, psoriasis and acne rosacea may affect suitability for contact lenses. In general, these conditions, when managed, do not contraindicate contact lens wear but may influence the lens type or the wear schedule selected. Patients with allergies can achieve success with contact lenses but may require more frequent lens replacement or more frequent aftercare examinations, since these patients are more susceptible to lens-induced discomfort and lid problems. There is no contraindication to fitting contact lenses to patients who are human immunodeficiency virus (HIV)-positive providing the anterior eye is healthy. Practitioners should wear protective gloves if they have open skin lesions. If the patient has progressed to acquired immunodeficiency syndrome (AIDS), the increased risk of opportunistic infection should be considered and contact lens fitting approached with extreme caution.

Corneal scarring or thinning

Where a patient suffers from any condition resulting in an irregular corneal surface, contact lenses may prove to be the only practical method of vision correction. In such cases, rigid lenses are usually the lens of choice (O'Callaghan and Phillips, 1994). Careful slit-lamp examination together with a detailed history will alert the practitioner to those patients susceptible to corneal perforation.

Keratoconjunctivitis sicca

Patients with systemic conditions resulting in dry eye may require ocular lubricants, tear supplements, dietary and environmental modifications and ultimately punctal occlusion. Since the successful wearing of any form of contact lens requires a well-lubricated surface, contact lens materials offering good wettability should be selected.

Handling problems

Restrictions of mobility as in rheumatoid arthritis or 'diabetic hand syndrome' may make the handling of contact lenses difficult (Figure 35.5).

Patients should be encouraged to handle their own lenses whenever possible. When handling becomes impossible, a

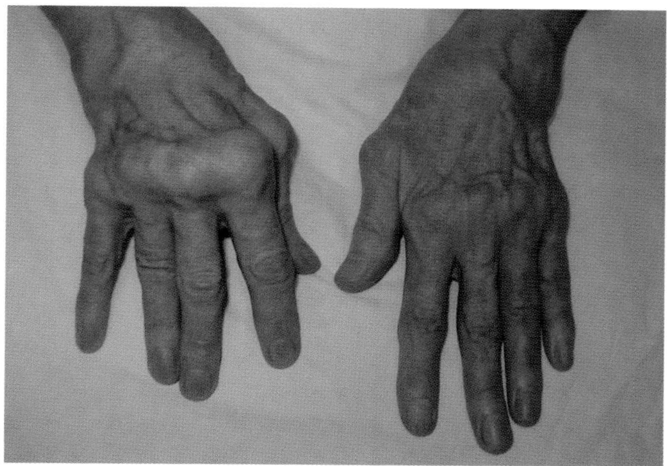

Figure 35.5 Deformation of the knuckles and finger joints in a patient with rheumatoid arthritis.

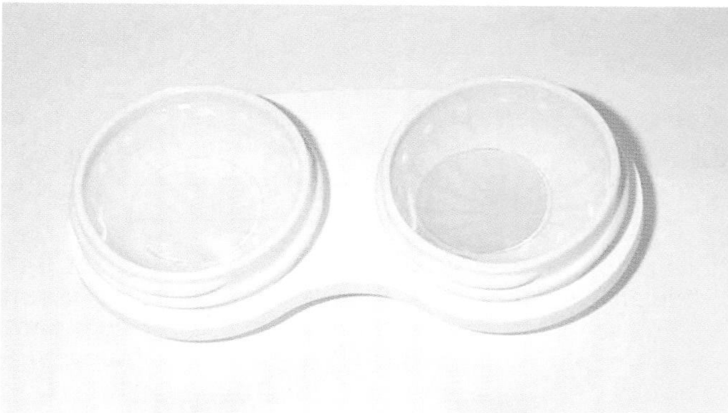

Figure 35.6 Pink discoloration of hydrogel contact lenses (in the right side of the lens case) can be observed with medications such as rifampicin. The left side of the lens case contains an unaffected lens.

relative or neighbour may provide assistance, and periods of extended or continuous wear may be appropriate.

Ocular side-effects of therapy

The ocular complications of both prescription and over-the-counter medications - such as decongestants, antihistamines and oral contraceptives - should be taken into consideration. Possible side-effects of medications include dry eye, photosensitivity, corneal and contact lens deposition, punctate keratopathy, subconjunctival haemorrhage and discoloration of contact lenses (Figure 35.6).

Conclusion

When considering whether to proceed with contact lens fitting in patients with systemic disease affecting the anterior eye, the practitioner needs to conduct a risk-benefit analysis. Where an increased risk of ocular complications has been ascertained, the patient should be informed of the risks and the benefits of contact lens wear. The importance of complying with recommendations for lens care and maintenance, wearing schedules and attending follow-up visits should also be emphasized. A thorough understanding of the ocular and systemic history, careful examination during fitting and follow-up to exclude the possibility of external eye disease, and the use of superior contact lens products will increase the likelihood of success for all prospective contact lens wearers.

References

Domschke, A., March, W., Kabilan, S. *et al.* (2006) Initial clinical testing of a holographic non-invasive contact lens glucose sensor. *Diab. Technol. Thera.,* **6,** 49–52.

Geddes, C. (2004) Ophthalmic glucose monitoring using disposable contact lenses. *Conf. Proc. IEEE Eng. Med. Biol. Soc.,* **7,** 5122.

Kallinikos, P., Berhanu, M., O'Donnell, C. *et al.* (2004) Corneal nerve tortuosity in diabetic patients with neuropathy. *Invest. Ophthalmol. Vis. Sci.,* **24,** 418–422.

L'Esperance, F. A. and James, W. A. (1983) The eye and diabetes mellitus. In *Diabetes Mellitus* (M. Ellenberg and H. Rifkin, eds), pp. 725–757, New York: Medical Examination Publishing Co.

Lee, J. S., Oum, B. S., Choi, H. Y. *et al.* (2006) Differences in corneal thickness and corneal endothelium related to duration in diabetes. *Eye,* **20,** 315–318.

Lockwood, A., Hope-Ross, M. and Chell, P. (2006) Neurotrophic keratopathy and diabetes mellitus. *Eye,* **20,** 837–839.

Malik, R. A., Kallinikos, P., Abbott, C. A. *et al.* (2003) Corneal confocal microscopy: a non-invasive surrogate of nerve fibre damage and repair in diabetic patients. *Diabetologia,* **46,** 683–688.

March, W., Long, B., Hofmann, W. *et al.* (2004a) Safety of contact lenses in patients with diabetes. *Diab. Technol. Thera.,* **6,** 49–52.

March, W., Mueller, A. and Herbrechtsmeier, P. (2004b) Clinical trial of a non-invasive contact lens glucose sensor. *Diab. Technol. Thera.,* **6,** 782–789.

McNamara, N. A. (1997) Effects of diabetes on anterior ocular structure and function. *Int. Contact Lens Clin.,* **24,** 81–90.

McNamara, N. A., Brand, R. J., Polse, K. A. *et al.* (1998) Corneal function during normal and high serum glucose levels in diabetes. *Invest. Ophthalmol. Vis. Sci.,* **39,** 3–17.

Mocan, M. C, Durukan, I., Irkec, M. *et al.* (2006) Morphologic alterations of both the stromal and subbasal nerves in the corneas of patients with diabetes. *Cornea,* **25,** 769–773.

O'Callaghan, G. J. and Phillips, A. (1994) Rheumatoid arthritis and the contact lens wearer. *Clin. Exp. Optom.,* **77,** 137–143.

O'Donnell, C. and Efron, N. (1998) Contact lens wear and diabetes mellitus. *Contact Lens Ant. Eye,* **21,** 19–26.

O'Donnell, C. and Efron, N. (2004a) Corneal endothelial cell morphometry and corneal thickness in diabetic contact lens wearers. *Optom. Vis. Sci.,* **81,** 858–862.

O'Donnell, C. and Efron, N. (2004b) Non-compliance with lens care and maintenance in diabetic contact lens wearers. *Ophthal. Physiol. Opt.,* **24,** 504–510.

O'Donnell, C. and Efron, N. (2006) Corneal hydration control in contact lens wearers with diabetes mellitus. *Optom. Vis. Sci.,* **83,** 22–26.

O'Donnell, C., Efron, N. and Boulton, A. J. (2001) A prospective study of contact lens wear in diabetes mellitus. *Ophthal. Physiol. Opt.,* **21,** 127–138.

O'Leary, D. J. and Millodot, M. (1981) Abnormal epithelial fragility in diabetes and in contact lens wear. *Acta Ophthalmol.,* **59,** 827–833.

Quattrini, C., Tavakoli, M., Jeziorska, M. *et al.* (2007) Surrogate markers of small fiber damage in human diabetic neuropathy. *Diabetes,* **56,** 2148–2154.

Rosenberg, M. E., Tervo, T. M., Immonen, I. J. *et al.* (2000) Corneal structure and sensitivity in type 1 diabetes mellitus. *Invest. Ophthalmol. Vis. Sci.,* **41,** 2915–2921.

Schein, O. D., Glynn, R. J., Poggio, E. C. *et al.* (1989) The relative risk of ulcerative keratitis among users of daily-wear and extended-wear soft contact lenses: a case-control study. *New Engl. J. Med.,* **321,** 773–778.

Skaff, A., Cullen, A. P., Doughty, M. J. *et al.* (1995) Corneal swelling and recovery following wear of thick hydrogel contact lenses in insulin-dependent diabetics. *Ophthal. Physiol. Opt.,* **15,** 287–297.

Veys, J., Efron, N. and Boulton, A. (1997) A survey of contact lens wear among diabetic patients in the United Kingdom. *Contact Lens Ant. Eye,* **20,** S27–S33.

Wiemer, N. G., Dubbelman, M., Kostense, P. J. *et al.* (2007) The influence of chronic diabetes mellitus on the thickness and the shape of the anterior and posterior surface of the cornea. *Cornea,* **26,** 1165–1170.

PART: VI

Patient examination and management

CHAPTER 36

History taking

Keith H Edwards

Introduction

The initial assessment of a prospective contact lens wearer has a number of objectives, which can be summarized as follows:

- To determine suitability for contact lens wear based on:
  - An analysis of patient-specific indications and contraindications.
  - A risk/benefit analysis for the individual patient.
- To provide patient education on lens types and likely suitability.
- To record baseline information:
  - That is relevant for future management.
  - For subsequent justification of clinical decision-making.

When considered in conjunction with the outcomes of the preliminary examination and refraction, the results of this assessment will indicate the suitability of the patient for contact lens wear and will guide the selection of the most appropriate lens type and wearing modality.

The *College of Optometrists Members' Handbook* (Anonymous, 2007) advises members of their responsibilities when fitting contact lenses, which include:

- In addition to the responsibilities related to the eye examination, the optometrist examining a patient wishing to wear contact lenses has a duty to assess the patient's suitability for contact lenses and to advise and inform the patient about contact lens wear.
- Following the preliminary assessment the optometrist has a duty to ensure that each individual contact lens wearer is fitted with the most appropriate lens type to meet his or her needs (including occupational, lifestyle and cosmetic requirements) and to give optimum vision for the required use.
- The optometrist has a duty to provide the patient with an appropriate lens care regimen, instruction on the use and wear of lenses, and instructions and information on the care, wearing, treatment, cleaning and maintenance of the lens or lenses.
- An optometrist has a duty to ensure that he or she always works within his or her limit of clinical competency, especially when engaging in specialist areas of contact lens practice.

Some aspects of these responsibilities may relate to the lens fitting process, dispensing or follow-up but many need to be considered during the initial history taking.

Indications and contraindications for contact lens wear

As part of the assessment, any specific indications or contraindications for contact lens wear must be established. These are best considered in the following categories.

Anatomical

In elective fitting (i.e. non-therapeutic use) there are few anatomical features that influence the suitability for contact lenses. However extremely steep or flat corneas or extremes of corneal astigmatism may present particular fitting difficulties that could increase the time spent on fitting. With bifocal fitting, lower-lid tension and position may be critical to the visual outcome and pupil size may also influence fitting success. In such cases, the implications for likely success and the increased fitting time and expense should be explained carefully.

In specific anatomical conditions, lenses may be used as a therapeutic device to prevent corneal desiccation or damage or to alleviate ocular conditions such as ptosis (see Chapter 31). In other less marked anomalies, particularly to the lids, a decision must be taken on whether elective contact lens wear will be adversely affected by the anomalies present.

Ocular health

Since a contact lens will come into intimate contact with the ocular surfaces, it is essential that there are no presenting ocular conditions that might be aggravated or exacerbated

DOI: 10.1016/B978-0-7506-8869-7.00036-7

by lens wear. Ocular surface disorders such as recurrent infection, irregular corneal surface or recurrent erosions may be relative contraindications for elective contact lens wear depending on severity. However in severe cases of ocular surface disorders, the protection afforded by a therapeutic lens may become a significant indication.

Perhaps the most widely noted symptom of contact lens wearers is a sensation of dryness. Contact lenses will disrupt the normal tear film (Korb, 1994; Korb *et al.*, 1996) and it is important to pay particular attention to both the quantity and quality of the tears before offering advice on suitability for contact lens wear. McMonnies (1986) constructed a dry-eye questionnaire to identify patients who had a tendency to ocular sicca. This questionnaire approach was designed to identify both those with current problems and those who might develop symptoms associated with provocative factors such as contact lens wear. Robboy and Orsborn (1989) validated the questionnaire as a good predictor of those patients likely to complain of dry-eye symptoms. The format of a typical dry-eye questionnaire is given in Appendix J.

Meibomian gland dysfunction is a significant factor in contact lens intolerance (Korb and Henriquez, 1980). Hom *et al.* (1990), in a study of 398 patients, found that meibomian gland dysfunction had a positive correlation with age. They found an overall prevalence of 39% but with a variation from less than 19% in under-20-year-olds and over 67% in those over 65 years. Careful examination of the lid margins is therefore critical, particularly when fitting older patients.

General health

There are numerous health problems that may influence the suitability for contact lenses, including those that have direct effect on the ocular tissues and those that may cause secondary problems. In addition, several systemic medications may influence the tear film and thus the ability to wear lenses comfortably.

Allergies

Those who are susceptible to allergies may experience problems from two sources. Kari and Haahtela (1992) found that those with atopy may be more intolerant to contact lens wear by a factor of five times compared to non-atopic wearers. It is also suggested that wearing time should be limited during the allergy season. Those with other more specific allergies are most at risk from reactions to the chemicals within preservative-based lens care systems. These chemicals can interact with deposits on the lens surface, creating an allergic-type response. In such cases preservative-free systems or daily disposable lenses might be indicated. A review article by Lemp (2008) provides further insights into the management of contact lens wear in the allergic patient.

Chronic infection

Those with chronic sinusitis or catarrh may be more at risk of developing infection secondary to corneal abrasion (Lowther and Snyder, 1992) and the associated mucus in the tears may cause visual problems from lens surface wetting anomalies as well as blocking the nasolacrimal ducts and causing epiphora.

Metabolic disorders

Disorders of metabolism may have varying effects on the eye and its physiology. Hyperthyroidism with its associated exophthalmos may create problems in tear film distribution while diabetes may influence the stability of refractive error, corneal deturgescence and epithelial wound healing. An informed decision on fitting diabetics is not necessarily very easy (see Chapter 35).

Pregnancy

Due to hormonal changes during pregnancy and lactation, patients may be prone to corneal oedema and mucus build-up. Comfort and overall tolerance can be reduced, although the response of a previously adapted lens wearer during pregnancy may often be good. It is less desirable to commence fitting lenses during pregnancy and lactation. It is widely believed that disruption to the tear film can also occur during puberty, menopause and while taking oral contraceptives or hormone replacement therapy. This can give rise to chronic or transient problems with tolerance. Brennan and Efron (1989) found that those on oral contraceptives reported dryness more frequently while a study by Tomlinson *et al.* (2001) could find no difference in tear physiology or subjective comfort during their respective menstrual cycles in groups of young females who were using oral contraceptives or age-matched groups not using oral contraceptives.

Systemic medication

As well as the systemic conditions that can affect tolerance to lenses, medication used in the treatment or control of those conditions can also have undesirable side-effects. These generally affect the tear film, either causing symptoms of dryness or in some cases colouring the tears and causing soft lens discoloration (e.g. rifampicin). Table 36.1 shows the most common drugs associated with tear film anomalies. Recently new drugs designed to treat acne vulgaris and rosacea have added to the problems of contact lens wearers. These drugs can create a significant dry-eye effect through their targeting of sebaceous secretions (Suss *et al.*, 1992; Anonymous, 2005a); contact lenses are specifically mentioned as being susceptible to discomfort during the period of medication. The use of lubricants and discontinuation of lens wear are recommended in such cases (Anonymous, 2005b).

Where systemic medication has caused ocular side-effects, specific lens material choices can prevent further sequelae from developing. Astin (2001) reported a case of amiodarone keratopathy where an ultraviolet-absorbing material was used to protect against the possibility of medically induced photosensitivity.

Psychological factors including motivation

In addition to the main anatomical and health-related issues, it is important to judge the motivation to wear contact lenses and the personality type of the potential wearer. Contact lenses are considered to give a more normal cosmetic appearance and may contribute significantly to overall appearance, particularly when the refractive error is high. In addition, there are cases where lenses can be used specifically to conceal significant cosmetic defects

Table 36.1 Medications that can affect tear film, causing symptoms of dry eye

Drug category	Example
Antibiotics	Tetracycline
Antihistamines	Allergy medications Sinus medications Sleep medications Diet medications
Antihypertensives	Methyldopate hydrochloride Reserpine
Antiperspirants (long-term)	
Belladonna alkaloids	Bellergal Donnatal Pro-Banthine
Beta-blockers (topical)	
Oral contraceptives	
Botulinum toxin	
Dermatological medication	Isotretinoin
Diuretics	Chlorothiazides Furosemide Hydrochlorthiazide
Psychotomimetics	Diazepam Amitriptyline Thioridazine Chlordiazepoxide

(After Lowther, G. E. and Snyder, C., 1992. In Contact Lens Procedures and Techniques. Butterworth-Heinemann)

such as iris anomalies, corneal opacities, inoperable squint or microphthalmos.

Since patient compliance with practitioner instruction will be a major concern in patient management, it is important to judge the prospective patient's ability to understand the full implications of lens wear. It is also important that the patient's expectations that drive motivation are realistic and achievable. These may relate to visual outcomes, management of the refractive error (through potential myopia control from conventional rigid lenses or orthokeratology) or cosmetic appearance. A thorough understanding of the patient's expected outcomes will help in the appropriate management of those expectations and the delivery of an acceptable result.

A particularly exacting personality type may find the adaptation period and the initial learning of handling techniques too intrusive to outweigh the overall benefits of lens wear.

Lifestyle/occupational issues

In addition to motivational and psychological factors, consideration must be given to lifestyle and occupational issues. Often contact lenses are believed to be inappropriate for certain occupations and, while this may be true for particularly contaminated atmospheres, contact lenses may provide some protection against both foreign bodies and chemicals (Nilsson and Andersson, 1982; Nilsson, 1989) or may offer no obvious disadvantages (e.g. in the Fire Service; Owen *et al.*, 1997a, b).

However hygiene is important and this must be of the highest order. Additionally, lens handling requires some degree of dexterity, while particularly rough or callused hands may damage lenses during the handling and cleaning process.

Financial considerations

Finally it is important that the patient understands the financial implications not only of the fitting but the continuing clinical care and the ongoing costs of lens care solutions and lens replacements. Fitting lenses to a patient without the financial means to care for them will inevitably lead to non-compliance and increase the potential for adverse events to occur.

The case history

With both a patient new to contact lenses and a contact lens patient new to the practice, a detailed case history is the basis for all future clinical decisions. It is therefore important that it is both thorough and well documented. In order to determine suitability for lenses, information must be gained to judge the balance of presenting indications and contraindications and offer advice on lens type and wearing modality. For the existing wearer, additional information must be attained that will help an understanding of previous lens-wearing history and any future potential complications. The exact nature of the history taking differs with lens wearers and neophytes.

Non-lens wearers

A full ocular history, including age of first correction and spectacle-wearing habits, will help to gauge general suitability for lenses. For example, a prospective wearer who only wears spectacles intermittently may not be an obvious choice for contact lens wear. However, if that intermittent wear is driven by a dislike of the cosmetic effect of spectacles, then contact lenses become a more obvious choice. Existing use of spectacles for distance and near use may give some indications of whether the patient will have to adapt to significant changes in accommodation and convergence once contact lens wear is initiated. This may be particularly relevant to early presbyopic myopes who may either take their spectacles off to read or have insufficient reserves of accommodation to cope with the additional accommodative demands in contact lenses compared to spectacles.

Previous ophthalmological, orthoptic or general practitioner treatment will give clues about past ocular status that might influence the clinical decision-making process. General health and use of medication are also significant. A positive family ocular or general health history also adds additional information about future potential risks that may relate to contact lens wear or more general patient management. It may be appropriate to ask whether the patient is a smoker since this seems to be associated with a higher risk of microbial keratitis (Schein *et al.*, 1989). Questioning about specific allergies will help to guide choice of lens modality, frequency of replacement and care system.

Symptoms with the present spectacles will also give information that may help to differentiate specific contact lens symptoms in the future from pre-existing problems.

Contact lens-specific questions will include why the patient wants contact lenses and what is expected from lens wear. Questions on leisure activities and occupation will help determine the type of lens most suitable and also provide an opportunity to offer advice on eye protection if appropriate. In more complex fittings such as bifocals or torics it may also help to determine whether an acceptable visual outcome is likely to result from a particular lens type.

This information, when taken in conjunction with refractive and binocular vision results, will lead to informed advice being offered to the patient on suitability for lenses and the most appropriate lens type, wearing modality and care system.

Previous lens wearer

When the patient is an existing contact lens wearer, the questioning used for the non-wearer is still appropriate. However, there is additional lens-specific information that is also required. The type of lens worn, the time since fitting, changes in lens type (e.g. from rigid to soft or from spherical to toric) all start to build a picture of the lens-wearing history. When such changes have been made it is useful to determine the patient's understanding of why they were necessary. It is important to determine what modality of wear, frequency of replacement and choice of care system were recommended by the previous practitioner(s) and whether the patient actually complied with those recommendations. Average daily wearing time, number of nights of overnight wear and the number of hours of wear at the time of consultation all help determine the significance of any clinical signs seen during subsequent ocular examination. In particular it is important to understand the patient's primary complaint (if any) and any other symptoms that are present at the first consultation as well as the reasons why care is no longer being provided by the original practitioner. Knowing the length of time since the last contact lens assessment will help in the judgement of the severity of any ocular changes as well as indicating likely future patient compliance. The routine questioning is summarized in Table 36.2.

As with all history taking, it is important to use follow-up questions to get as much information as possible relevant to understanding the patient history and making informed clinical decisions. This is particularly true where there are presenting patient problems and follows the same pattern as for general aftercare (see Chapter 39).

Table 36.2 Initial history taking for the contact lens wearer and non-wearer

Patient new to lenses	Existing contact lens wearer
Age at first correction	As new patients plus:
Use of spectacles	Date of first contact lens correction
Full-time/part-time	Type of lens worn
Recency of current prescription	At initial fitting
Ocular history	Currently
Medical treatment	Modality recommended
Hospital treatment	Daily or overnight wear
Orthoptic treatment	Replacement frequency recommended
General health history	Care system recommended
Medication	Compliance with recommendations
Prescribed or over-the-counter	Average/maximum wearing time
Family ocular history	Number of nights worn without removal
Family general health history	Hours of continuous wear at time of visit
Smoker – yes/no	Patient's primary complaint
Allergies	Other symptoms/signs
Motivation for lens wear	Reason for discontinuation of previous care
Expectations of lens wear	Date of last appointment
Occupational/recreational activities	

Patient education, risk/benefit analysis and informed consent

When fitting patients new to lenses as well as those being refitted, it is important to get informed consent. Essentially this requires that the patient has a reasonable understanding of the main benefits of contact lens wear as well as the potential risks that accompany lens wear.

Part of this process involves educating the patient on the various lens types and any that might be particularly suited (or unsuited) to the patient's particular needs. Information on wearing schedules and use of lenses in overnight wear, appropriate lens care systems and replacement intervals are all relevant factors in the patient's decision to proceed with lens fitting. While there are many positive features to contact lenses, including visual, cosmetic and potentially psychological benefits, the patient must be warned of possible adverse events. Risks of suffering microbial keratitis have been well documented but the incidence rates may mean little to the lay public. Equally risks from cross-contamination, such as variant Creutzfeldt–Jakob disease, are almost impossible to quantify because of insufficient data but should be drawn to the attention of patients for whom diagnostic lenses are necessary, as much to protect the practitioner as the patient.

Since there are so many factors that might be relevant to the decision on contact lens wear, it is difficult to know how much information to provide. In general, it is not necessary to disclose every possible risk, only those that a reasonable person or a member of the profession would expect to be told (Rosenwasser, 1991). Patients may need specific advice on aspects such as driving with monovision or where a particular undesirable outcome is not unexpected. Equally, it should be remembered that a minor can neither give informed consent nor contract to pay for services.

In some countries, it is common practice to ask the patient to sign a consent form, but the legal protection that this affords is questionable.

Patients experience anxiety during contact lens consultations. This is typically associated with poor attention. Therefore, optometrists should not assume that patients remember what they are told during the consultation (Court *et al.*, 2008) and practitioners should provide written instructions to their patients (see Chapter 38).

Record keeping

During the whole process of the initial assessment and history taking, information is being gathered on which clinical decisions on patient suitability will be made. As with all clinical processes, suitable records are essential. These records not only offer insight into the ocular status of the patient presenting for fitting but also give credence to the clinical decisions being made. In the event of a dispute with the patient, they can be invaluable in showing the maintenance of good clinical standards and the provision of the standard of care expected. Detailed consideration is beyond the scope of this chapter but is given elsewhere (Lewis and Edwards, 1995; Edwards, 1998).

In essence record keeping should include all relevant patient information relating to the primary and significant secondary complaints as well as all the tests conducted in response to that information. The records should clearly indicate the clinical decision being made and the basis of that decision (i.e. diagnosis). A written record of all the advice offered to the patient should be included. As a general rule, it should not be forgotten that potential and existing contact lens wearers are just as prone to general ophthalmic problems as the rest of the population and non-contact lens causes of patient visual and ocular problems should not be overlooked.

Practitioners should conduct all the appropriate testing necessary to test their working clinical hypothesis about the cause of the presenting problems. Where testing suggests that the hypothesis is flawed, the data should be re-examined and other possibilities assessed through further testing. At a minimum, the records should reflect this process and include all test results that rule a probable or possible diagnosis in or out of consideration. If this procedure is followed, there can be no doubts about whether the standard of care has been delivered.

Conclusions

The initial assessment and history taking form the cornerstone on which all subsequent clinical decisions will be built. It is important that this aspect of patient care is conducted thoroughly and to the highest standards. Time spent on this initial stage of the patient assessment may prevent much wasted time later in the management of the patient, when clinical decisions have been made inadvisedly.

Sound and thorough record keeping will ensure both good continuity of care and a good defence in the unlikely event of patient complaint.

References

Anonymous (2005a) Accutane: Patient Information Sheet. Rockville: Food & Drug Administration.

Anonymous (2005b) Roaccutane: Consumer Medicine Information. Sydney: F Hoffman La Roche.

Anonymous (2007) The College of Optometrists Members' Handbook. The College of Optometrists. London.

Astin, C. L. (2001) Amiodarone keratopathy and rigid contact lens wear. *Cont. Lens Anterior Eye,* **24,** 80–82.

Brennan, N. A. and Efron, N. (1989) Symptomatology of HEMA contact lens wear. *Optom. Vis. Sci.,* **66,** 834–838.

Court, H., Greenland, K. and Margrain, T. H. (2008) Evaluating patient anxiety levels during contact lens fitting. *Optom. Vis. Sci.,* **85,** 574–580.

Edwards, K. (1998). Lessons in litigation. *Optician,* **216**(5672), 24–27.

Hom, M. M., Martinson, J. R., Knapp, L. L. *et al.* (1990) Prevalence of Meibomian gland dysfunction. *Optom. Vis. Sci.,* **67,** 710–712.

Kari, O. and Haahtela, T. (1992) Is atopy a risk factor for the use of contact lenses? *Allergy,* **47,** 295–298.

Korb, D. R. (1994) Tear film-contact lens interactions. *Adv. Exp. Med. Biol.,* **350,** 403–410.

Korb, D. R. and Henriquez, A. S. (1980) Meibomian gland dysfunction and contact lens intolerance. *J. Am. Optom. Assoc.,* **51,** 243–251.

Korb, D. R., Greiner, J. V. and Glonek, T. (1996) Tear film lipid layer formation: implications for contact lens wear. *Optom. Vis. Sci.,* **73,** 189–192.

Lemp, M. A. (2008) Contact lenses and allergy. *Curr. Opin. Allergy Clin. Immunol.,* **8,** 457–460.

Lewis, B. and Edwards, K. (1995) Record keeping - best practice or best defence? *Optometry Today,* **35**(22), 18–23.

Lowther, G. E. (1997) *Dryness, Tears and Contact Lens Wear. Contact Lens Update Series,* Boston: Butterworth-Heinemann.

Lowther, G. E. and Snyder, C. (1992) *Contact Lens Procedures and Techniques.* Stoneham, MA: Butterworth-Heinemann.

McMonnies, C. (1986) Key questions in a dry eye history. *J. Am. Optom. Assoc.,* **57,** 512–517.

Nilsson, S. E. (1989) Review of contact lenses in relation to the work environment. *J. Brit. Contact Lens Assoc.,* **12,** 15–19.

Nilsson, S. and Andersson, L. (1982) The use of contact lenses in environments with organic solvents, acids or alkalies. *Acta Ophthalmol.,* **60,** 599–608.

Owen, C. G., Margrain, T. H., and Woodward, E. G. (1997a) Use of contact lenses by firefighters. Part 1: Questionnaire data. *Ophthalmic Physiol. Opt.,* **17,** 102–111.

Owen, C. G., Margrain, T. H., and Woodward, E. G. (1997b) Use of contact lenses by firefighters: Part 2. Clinical evaluation. *Ophthalmic Physiol. Opt.,* **17,** 205–215.

Robboy, M. and Orsborn, G. (1989) The response of marginal dry eye lens wearers to a dry eye survey. *Contact Lens J.,* **17,** 8–9.

Rosenwasser, H. M. (1991) *Malpractice and Contact Lenses.* Boston, MA: Butterworth-Heinemann

Schein, O. D., Glynn, R. J., Poggio, E. C. *et al.* (1989) The relative risk of ulcerative keratitis among users of daily-wear and extended-wear soft contact lenses. A case-control study. Microbial Keratitis Study Group. *N. Engl. J. Med.,* **321,** 773–778.

Suss, R., Ruzicka, T., and Scheiffarth, O. F. (1992) [Why is 13-*cis*-retinoic acid (Roaccutane) contraindicated in contact lens patients?] *Hautarzt,* **43,** 521.

Tomlinson, A., Pearce, E. I., Simmons, P. A., *et al.* (2001) Effect of oral contraceptives on tear physiology. *Ophthalmic Physiol. Opt.,* **21,** 9–16.

37 CHAPTER

Preliminary examination

Adrian S Bruce

Introduction

The preliminary examination includes the taking of a full history and initial patient assessment (see Chapter 36), ocular measurements, refraction and supplementary tests. The examination enables the practitioner to advise patients on their suitability for contact lens wear and, if it is decided to go ahead with lens fitting, of appropriate lens choices. While it is rare that a patient cannot be fitted with contact lenses, the information obtained from the preliminary examination is vital in the selection of the most suitable lens material, replacement frequency, wear modality (daily or extended wear), care system and wearing time.

This chapter provides an overview of the typical full routine of the preliminary contact lens examination, following case history, and comments on the interpretation of the information obtained. Details of the instrumentation referred to in this chapter can be found in Chapter 4.

Measurement of vision

After the case history, vision should always be the first measurement in the preliminary examination. In this way, the vision measurement will be most indicative of the habitual vision of the patient and will be unaffected by the lights and ocular manipulations associated with later test procedures. An additional, but equally important, reason to establish a baseline measure of vision is for medicolegal reasons.

The computer-presented visual acuity chart has advantages above other types of vision chart for contact lens practice (Figure 37.1).

Computer-generated optotypes can be randomized to prevent the contact lens patient from learning the letter sequences at successive visits. In addition, computerized vision charts can usually present letters down to 6/3 – a level of vision that can be achieved by many younger contact lens wearers.

Vision should be measured with and without the habitual distance spectacles of the patient at both distance and near. The level of vision will be useful information to relate to the history, refraction and the binocular vision examination. The unaided vision is of interest because patients who are commonly or intermittently uncorrected will compare that to the level of acuity they achieve with contact lenses.

Retinoscopy and subjective refraction

The first phase of the refraction may be retinoscopy. While not necessarily performed routinely, retinoscopy can give valuable information since it is an objective technique. This procedure also allows a qualitative assessment of the optics of the eye. Possible indications for retinoscopy include:

- vision with spectacles of less than 6/6
- astigmatism of higher levels, or changing magnitude or direction of astigmatism, where keratoconus may be suspected
- looking for clues of corneal irregularity, such as a scissors reflex
- pseudomyopia, whereby less minus may be revealed.

The subjective refraction may be best performed in a trial frame, since many contact lens patients are young and the trial frame may be less likely to induce accommodation than the phoropter. Even if 6/6 vision is achieved, it is useful to check the subjective refraction in each eye with the previous spectacles or contact lenses that the patient presents with, as they may reveal excess minus power that could account for symptoms unrelated to visual acuity (such as asthenopia or binocular vision problems).

It is necessary with non-presbyopic patients to adopt a technique with the refraction so as to relax their accommodation. Measuring a blur function is one such method, whereby the addition of +0.50 D or +0.75 D lenses is expected to blur the 6/6 line significantly.

Anatomical measurements

Measurements of the dimensions of anatomical structures of the anterior eye should be routinely made for contact lens fitting. Because of the differences in fitting characteristics between soft and rigid lenses, different sets of

DOI: 10.1016/B978-0-7506-8869-7.00037-9

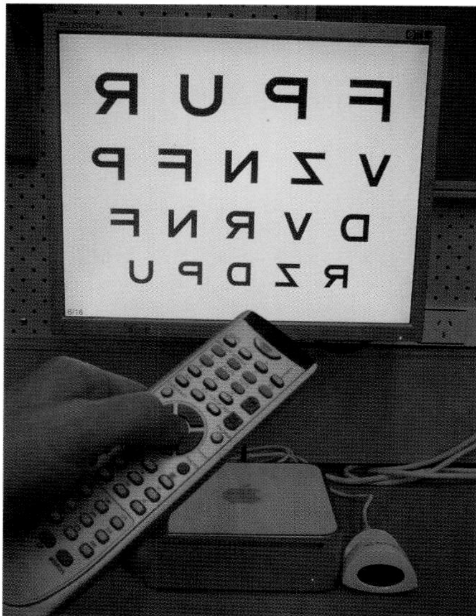

Figure 37.1 2020 Vision (www.canelasoftware.com) computerized visual acuity chart. The letters on the screen are reversed for mirror display.

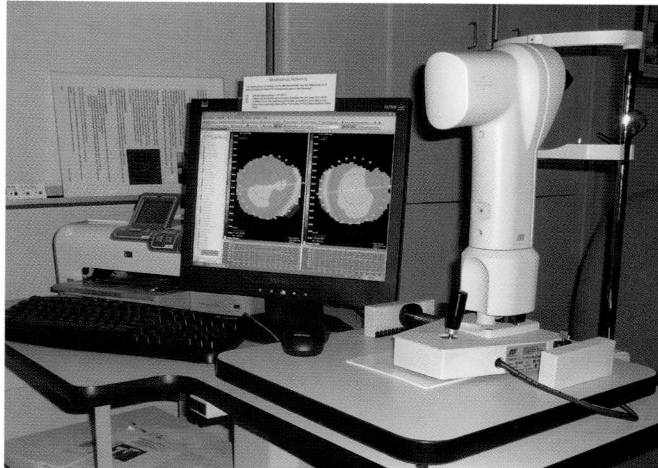

Figure 37.2 Medmont E300 corneal topography instrument (www.medmont.com.au).

measurements are often required. For rigid lens fitting in particular, it is useful to make a diagram of the upper and lower eyelid positions in relation to the cornea. Typically, the lower eyelid sits at the inferior limbus and the upper eyelid partly covers the superior limbus. Assessment of lid geometry assists in the selection of lens diameter for the optimization of lens comfort. Possible lid geometries include:

- Most often, the upper eyelid covers the superior limbus by 1–2 mm, and the lower eyelid is very near the inferior limbus (Bruce, 2006).
- Low inferior lid position.
- Narrow palpebral aperture – low superior lid.
- Wide palpebral aperture – high superior lid.

Protocols for anatomical measurement when fitting soft and rigid lenses are given in Chapters 9 and 16, respectively.

Keratometry

Keratometry is a standard part of the contact lens preliminary examination (Figure 37.2). It allows measurement of the curvature of the central 3 mm of the cornea.

For soft lens fitting, particularly disposable lenses which might, for example, be available in only two back optic zone radii (BOZR), the assessment is often used simply to identify steeper corneas, which require the lens with the steeper (smaller) BOZR.

In rigid lens fitting the keratometry readings are used directly to select the BOZR of the initial trial lens. The amount of keratometric astigmatism should be compared with the ocular astigmatism. This identifies lenticular or irregular astigmatism, which may be the cause of residual astigmatism in rigid lens wear.

Keratometry is a simple, rapid and non-invasive test, but it does have some limitations. It only measures at one corneal radius, it assumes a spherical cornea with regular astigmatism (i.e. that the principal axes are orthogonal) and it has a limited range of powers (36.00–53.00 D).

Extreme corneal powers can be measured by interposing a −1.00 D lens (for low corneal powers, i.e. very flat corneas) or a +1.25 D lens (for high corneal powers, i.e. very steep corneas) in front of the entrance aperture of the keratometer (on the patient side of the instrument). The doubled mires are aligned in the usual way, and the keratometer reading is converted to the actual corneal power using tables such as those given in Appendix E.

Corneal topography

Corneal topography projects a set of illuminated concentric rings (Placido disc) on to the cornea, enabling most of the corneal surface to be measured. Especially in the assessment of conditions such as keratoconus, it is preferable to use corneal topography in order to gain a comprehensive appreciation of the shape of the cornea (see Chapter 4).

With corneal topography, keratoconus is indicated if one or more of the following observations are found:

- A difference in corneal power of ≥1.50 D at locations 3 mm above and below the visual axis.
- An apical corneal power ≥47.00 D.
- Interocular asymmetry in apical corneal power ≥1.00 D (Bruce and Bohl, 1992).

Corneal topography maps may be displayed in a number of ways. The most common format is known as the axial map, where all curvatures are calculated in reference to the visual axis of the patient. Axial maps are useful in the diagnosis of a range of corneal conditions (Figure 37.3).

A tangential map is considered to be more accurate, although not as easy to interpret for diagnostic purposes. Tangential maps are based on local curvature at each corneal point and more sensitive for detecting localized changes (e.g. keratoconus, post surgical). In addition, tangential maps show the true position of the corneal apex.

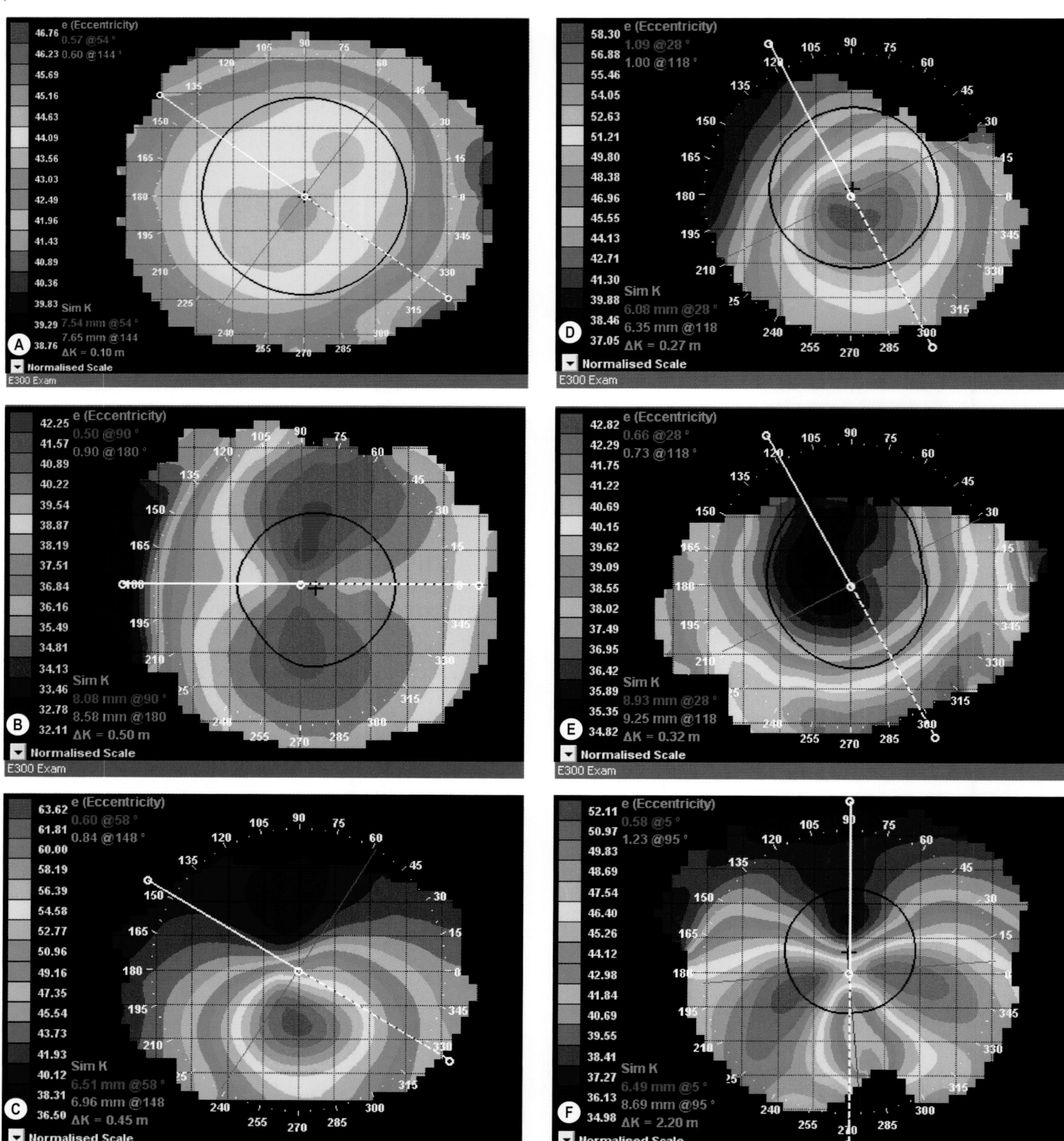

Figure 37.3 Corneal topography maps. (A) Normal eye; (B) with-the-rule 'hourglass' astigmatism; (C) keratoconus with inferior located cone; (D) keratoconus with central 'nipple' cone; (E) postoperative refractive surgery for myopia (laser *in situ* keratomileusis: LASIK); (F) pellucid marginal degeneration, 'walrus moustache' pattern.

Slit-lamp biomicroscopy

In the preliminary examination, biomicroscopy is used to assess the health of the anterior eye, and more specifically to screen for conditions or features that may be relevant to contact lens wear. It is also important to record baseline appearance of the eyes prior to inserting any lenses for medicolegal reasons.

Six areas of the anterior eye should be assessed in the preliminary examination, and any signs should be recon-

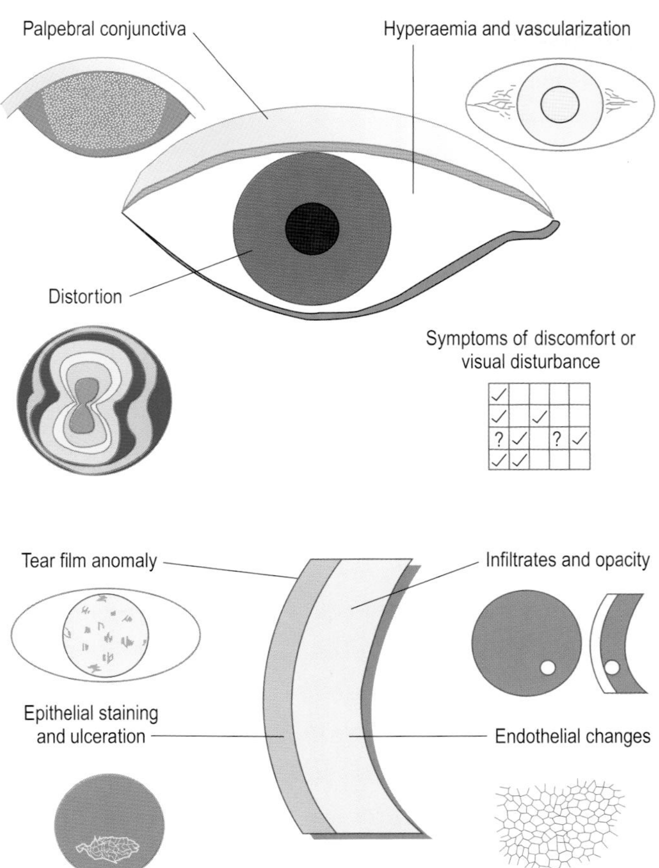

Figure 37.4 Considerations in the assessment of the anterior eye. There are six primary areas to examine with the slit lamp, as well as considering corneal shape and symptoms. (Adapted from Bruce, A. S. and Brennan, N. A. (2000) A Guide to Clinical Contact Lens Management, 3rd edn. CIBA Vision.)

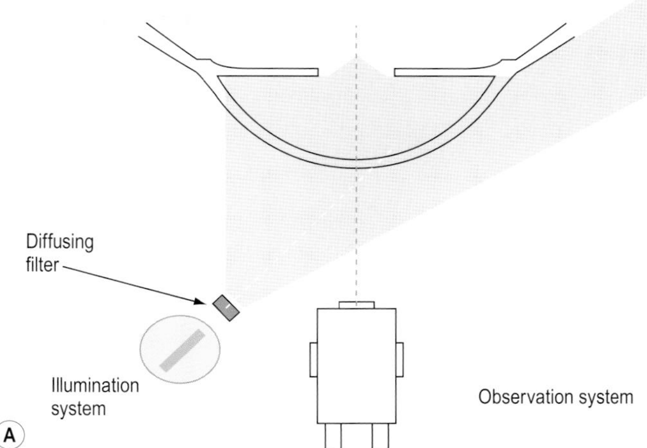

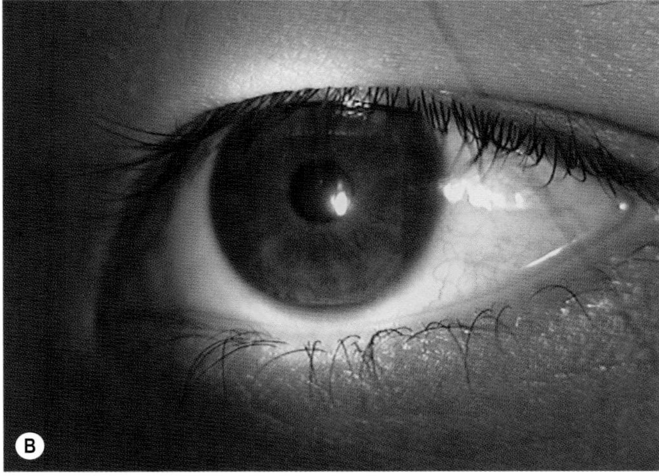

Figure 37.5 (A) Diffuse illumination slit-lamp technique. (Adapted from Jones, L. W. and Jones, D. A. (2001) Slit lamp biomicroscopy. In The Cornea: its Examination in Contact Lens Practice (N. Efron, ed.), pp. 1–49, Butterworth-Heinemann.) (B) Diffuse illumination view of the cornea.

ciled with symptoms and assessment of the corneal curvature (Figure 37.4).

Characteristics of the normal anterior eye, and the severity of any abnormalities that are detected, can be recorded with the assistance of grading scales (see Chapter 39). Efron and McCubbin (2007) have demonstrated that effective grading can be undertaken in a few seconds, which means that this important clinical practice will not consume undue amounts of valuable chair time.

A normal technique is to use a variety of illumination methods - such as those described below (Jones and Jones, 2001) - and cobalt blue light for fluorescein staining.

Diffuse wide beam

A ground-glass filter is placed in the focused light beam of the slit lamp. This will defocus and diffuse the light to give a broad, even illumination over the entire field of view and is generally used to provide low-magnification views of the opaque tissues of the anterior segment, including the bulbar conjunctiva, sclera, iris, eyelid margins and the tarsal conjunctiva of the everted lids (Figure 37.5).

Unusual signs in these tissues could include dilated blood vessels in the bulbar conjunctiva, pigmented areas in the conjunctiva or eyelids, roughness or opacity of the conjunctiva and abnormal eyelash position or orientation. Such signs could be indicative of conditions such as trichiasis, bulbar injection, pterygium or papillary conjunctivitis.

In assessing the eyelid margins, consider the apposition of the lids and puncta against the globe. Also look for clear glands near the base of the lashes, and flaking or scaling of the eyelid skin. These may indicate the presence of ectropion, blepharitis or epiphora.

Direct focal illumination

This describes any illumination technique where the slit beam and viewing system are focused coincidentally. The illumination beam is turned up as brightly as possible (ensuring that the patient remains comfortable) and placed at a separation of 40–60° on the side of the microscope corresponding to the section of the cornea to be viewed. The beam is swept smoothly across the ocular surface. Typically a beam width of 2–3 mm is chosen initially and this may be reduced so as to bring more contrast (due to less light scatter) to an area of interest. Whilst scanning the external

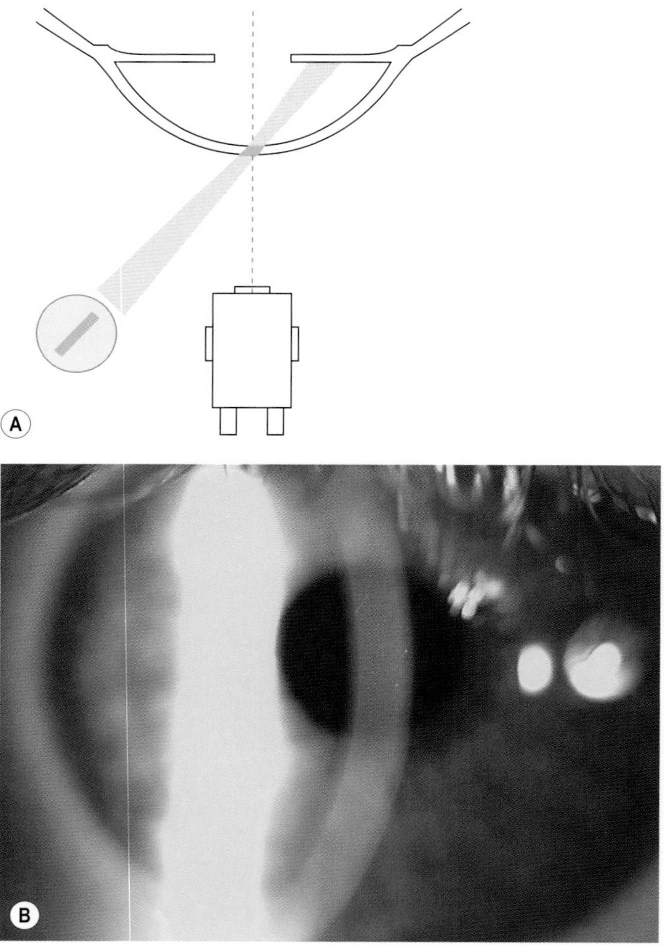

Figure 37.6 (A) Parallelepiped slit-lamp technique. (Adapted from Jones, L. W. and Jones, D. A. (2001) Slit lamp biomicroscopy. In The Cornea: its Examination in Contact Lens Practice (N. Efron, ed.), pp. 1–49, Butterworth-Heinemann.) (B) Parallelepiped illumination view of the cornea.

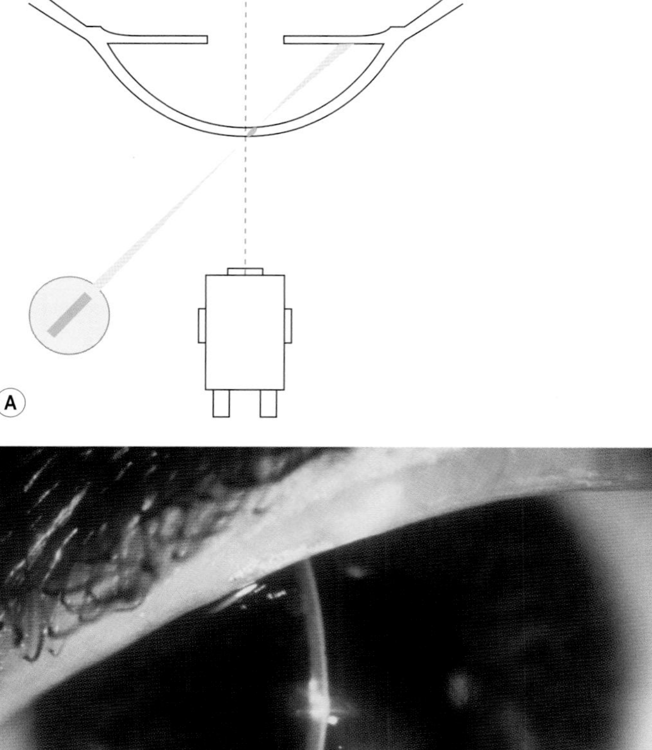

Figure 37.7 (A) Optic section slit-lamp technique. (Adapted from Jones, L. W. and Jones, D. A. (2001) Slit lamp biomicroscopy. In The Cornea: its Examination in Contact Lens Practice (N. Efron, ed.), pp. 1–49, Butterworth-Heinemann.) (B) Optic section view of a corneal foreign-body injury.

ocular surface, a low-to-medium magnification is initially chosen and the magnification is increased if any area of interest needs to be examined more closely.

Parallelepiped

Using the set-up described above, a 0.1–1.0 mm wide illuminating beam is scanned over the ocular surface (Figure 37.6).

This permits assessment of the location, width and height of any object within the cornea or adjacent structures. The parallelepiped is the most commonly used direct illumination technique and is employed, for example, to assess corneal scarring, infiltrates and corneal staining.

Optic section

Once an area or object of interest is located the beam width is narrowed to approximately 0.02–0.1 mm to cross-section the corneal tissue. This provides the ability to assess accurately the depth of an object within the corneal layers (Figure 37.7).

Typical uses include assessment of the depth of a foreign body, location of a corneal scar and determining whether tissue within an area of staining is excavated, flat or raised.

Oblique illumination

This is infrequently used in contact lens practice, but is nonetheless a useful technique. Oblique illumination is achieved by setting up a parallelepiped and then moving the illumination system away from the observation system until the angle between them is close to 90°. The illumination arm is adjusted until the light beam is almost tangential to the object of interest. Any raised areas cast a shadow, and this technique is particularly useful for viewing subtle defects within the iris architecture and subtle changes to the epithelial surface.

Specular reflection

This is a specific case of a parallelepiped set-up, where the angle of the incident slit beam is equal to the angle of the observation axis through one of the oculars. At this angle

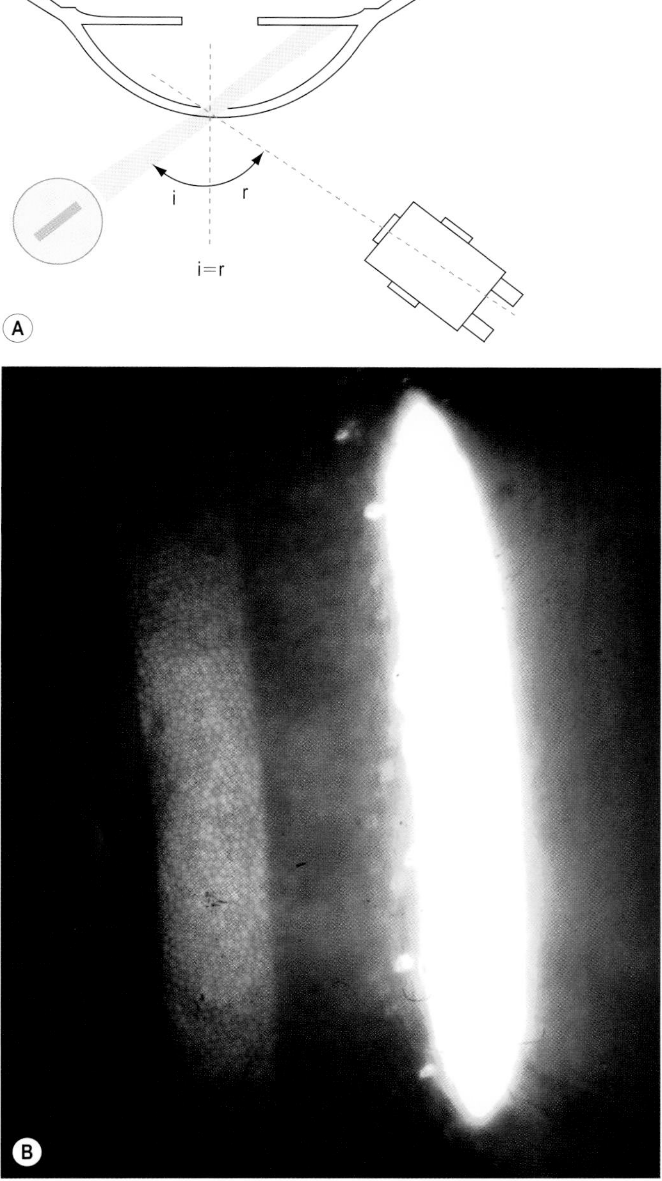

Figure 37.8 (A) Specular reflection slit-lamp technique. (Adapted from Jones, L. W. and Jones, D. A. (2001) Slit lamp biomicroscopy. In The Cornea: its Examination in Contact Lens Practice (N. Efron, ed.), pp. 1–49, Butterworth-Heinemann.) (B) Specular reflection view of the corneal endothelium. *i* = angle of incidence; *r* = angle of reflection.

(typically 40–50°) the illumination beam is reflected from the smooth surfaces of the anterior segment and provides a mirror-like reflection (Figure 37.8).

Such specular images occur at every interface between structures of different refractive indices. The technique of specular reflection is used in the preliminary examination to view the corneal endothelium, and may reveal changes such as endothelial blebs, guttae and polymegethism. However, even at 40× magnification only a gross clinical judgement of the endothelium can be made, as individual cells can barely be seen. The tear film lipid layer and the inferior tear meniscus can also be readily examined, as well as the anterior surface of the crystalline lens. If a contact lens is being worn, front surface wetting break-up time can be assessed and the postlens tear film may be observed using specular reflection (Little and Bruce, 1994).

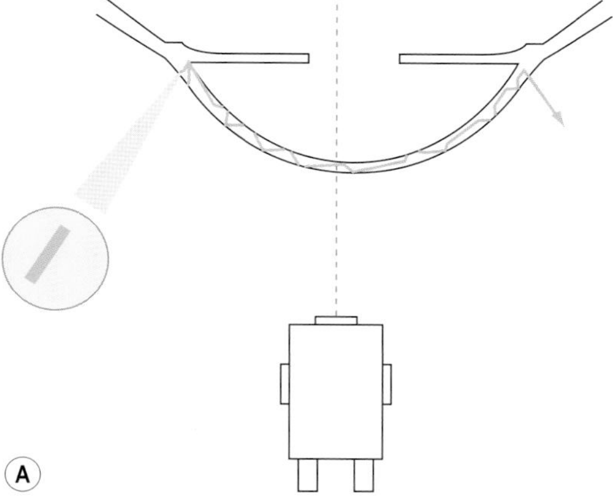

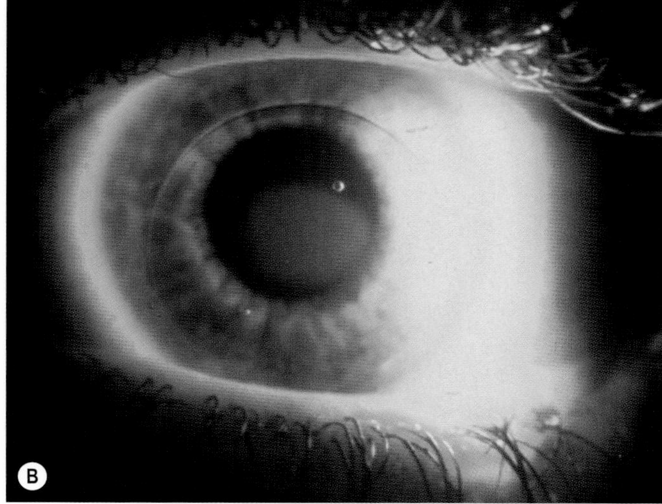

Figure 37.9 (A) Sclerotic scatter slit-lamp technique. (Adapted from Jones, L. W. and Jones, D. A. (2001) Slit lamp biomicroscopy. In The Cornea: its Examination in Contact Lens Practice (N. Efron, ed.), pp. 1–49, Butterworth-Heinemann.) (B) Central corneal oedema viewed using sclerotic scatter.

Indirect illumination

This refers to any technique where the focus of the illuminating beam does not coincide with the focal point of the observation system. Indirect illumination can be achieved by 'uncoupling' the instrument and manually displacing the slit beam to the side. However, it is possible to effect indirect illumination without uncoupling the instrument; this is achieved by directing a slit beam on to a section of the cornea adjacent to that of interest, and to direct gaze to the side of the directly illuminated section.

Two specific types of indirect illumination are possible: sclerotic scatter and retroillumination.

Sclerotic scatter

This technique is used to investigate any subtle changes in corneal clarity occurring over a large area, such as central

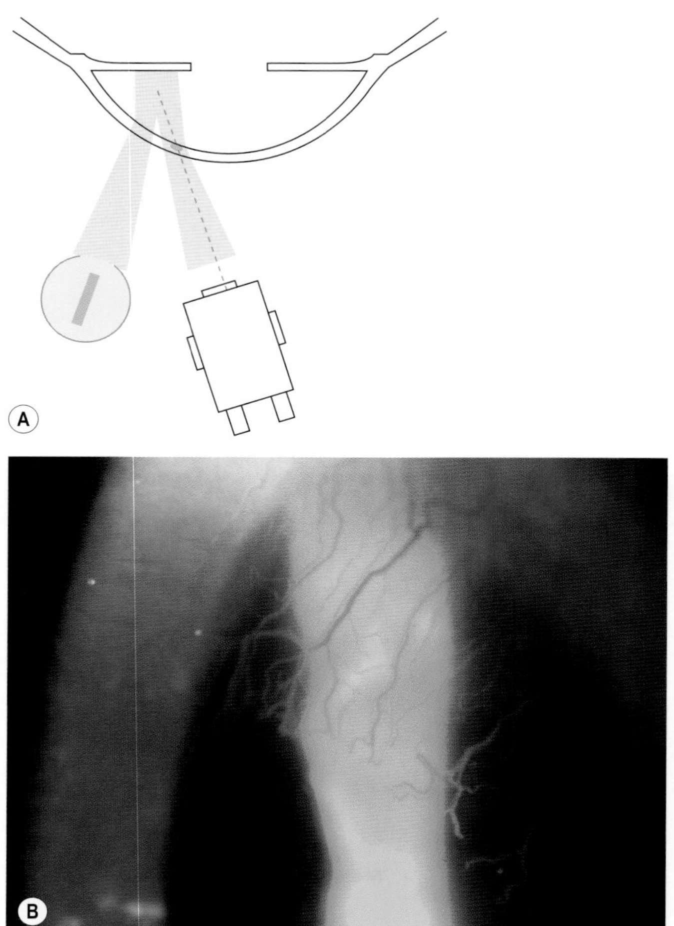

Figure 37.10 (A) Direct retroillumination slit-lamp technique. (Adapted from Jones, L. W. and Jones, D. A. (2001) Slit lamp biomicroscopy. In The Cornea: its Examination in Contact Lens Practice (N. Efron, ed.), pp. 1–49, Butterworth-Heinemann.) (B) Vessels viewed by direct retroillumination against the bright iris in the background.

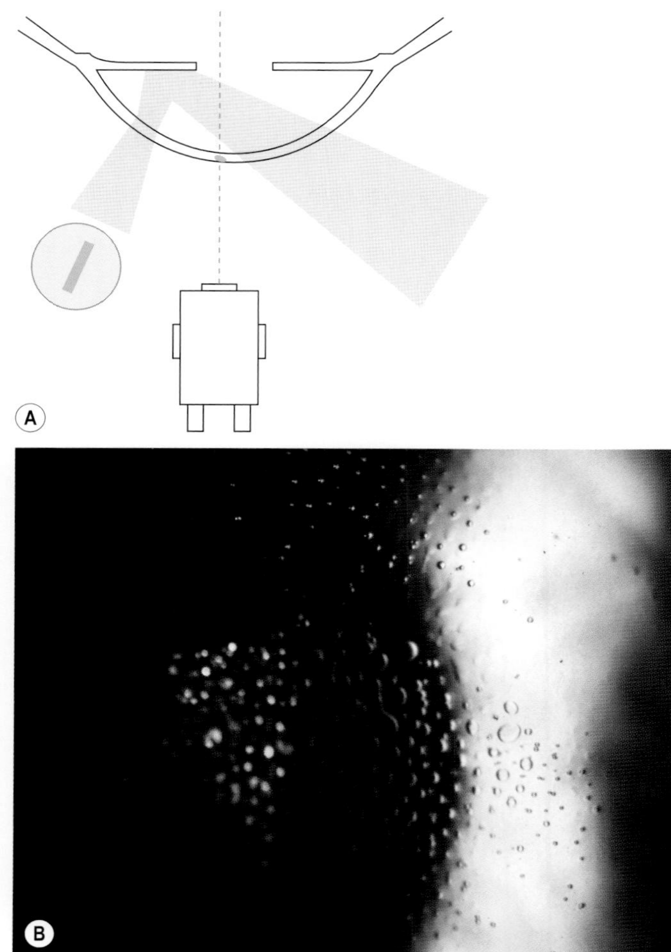

Figure 37.11 (A) Indirect retroillumination slit-lamp technique. (Adapted from Jones, L. W. and Jones, D. A. (2001) Slit lamp biomicroscopy. In The Cornea: its Examination in Contact Lens Practice (N. Efron, ed.), pp. 1–49, Butterworth-Heinemann.) (B) Dimple veiling viewed by indirect retroillumination against the dark pupil in the background.

corneal oedema. The slit lamp is set up for a wide-angle parallelepiped (45–60°) and the viewing system is focused centrally. The beam is manually offset ('uncoupled') and focused on the limbus. The slit beam is totally internally reflected across the cornea and a bright limbal glow is seen around the entire cornea (Figure 37.9).

Any specific area of abnormality, such as a corneal scar, will interrupt the beam in its passage and produce a light reflection in the otherwise dark cornea.

Retroillumination

This refers to any technique in which light is reflected from the iris, anterior lens surface or retina, and is used to back-illuminate an area more anteriorly positioned. The area may be seen against a light background (direct retroillumination; Figure 37.10) or a dark background (indirect retroillumination; Figure 37.11), depending on whether or not the illumination and viewing systems are coincident.

Direct retroillumination is used most often, whereby corneal opacities will appear black against a bright field. This technique is particularly useful for examining epithelial microcysts, neovascularization, scars, degenerations and dystrophies.

Fluorescein staining

Slit-lamp examination using the vital stain fluorescein, observed in cobalt blue light and a yellow Wratten or Boston observation filter, allows the assessment of ocular surface defects and irregularities. The cornea, bulbar conjunctiva and tarsal conjunctiva may be assessed. Tarsal papillae and roughness, as well as a wide variety of corneal changes, such as desiccation, may be detected.

Tear film evaluation

There are six clinical categories of technique for diagnosis of tear film impairment (the six Ss) (Mainstone *et al.*, 1996):

1. *Symptoms* and history – quantify with the dry-eye survey, such as that shown in Appendix J.
2. *Slit-lamp* biomicroscopy – including tear meniscus height assessment and lipid layer interferometry in

specular reflection. The Keeler Tearscope offers additional useful qualitative information.

3. Tear *stability* tests – most notably fluorescein or non-invasive break-up time. If contact lenses are being worn, tear stability may be assessed using the specular reflection of the slit-lamp beam, or using the mires of the keratometer or topographer (Bruce *et al.*, 2001).
4. Ocular *surface* evaluation – in particular staining with fluorescein and lissamine green.
5. Lid *surfacing* assessment – including blink rate and completeness.
6. Tests of tear *secretion* or quantity – such as the Schirmer and more recently the cotton thread tests (Zone Quick, Menicon).

A thorough analysis of any symptoms and related history is perhaps the most important of the above tests. The two most common causes of dry eye are aqueous deficiency (with reduced tear secretion) and meibomian gland dysfunction (with coloured lipid layer patterns in specular reflection).

Ophthalmoscopy

An ocular fundus exam is a routine part of an initial patient examination for screening ocular disease. Examination of the ocular media in retroillumination with a +10.00 D lens addition to the ophthalmoscope also shows cataract or corneal abnormalities.

A mydriatic fundus examination is often beneficial, enabling assessment of the optic disc with stereopsis and visualization of the retinal periphery. Mydriasis may also be used if there is a reduction in visual acuity, or symptoms of flashes or floaters, among other indications.

Binocular vision assessment

Contact lens wear may exacerbate the effect of a pre-existing accommodation or convergence insufficiency; the optical basis for this is explained in Chapter 3. In essence, there may be differences in vergence and accommodation demand between contact lenses and spectacles. In higher degrees of myopia, the contact lenses can require greater accommodation and convergence by the wearer for near activities. Depending upon age, the patient may also need to be advised that a near correction is required at an earlier age.

If the patient has pre-existing symptoms of difficulty with near vision, then accommodation and vergence performance should be assessed. Measures should be compared with age norms for accommodative amplitude, near point of convergence, distance and near heterophoria, relative near accommodation and vergence reserves at near.

Supplementary tests

There are a number of tests that will not be routinely conducted on all contact lens patients but may be performed on indication.

Corneal sensitivity

If there is reason to suspect that the patient may have anaesthetic corneas, then corneal sensitivity should be assessed. Possible indications could be a history of ocular surgery or corneal infection. Sensitivity may be simply checked clinically, using a wisp of sterile cotton wool touched to the cornea. Approach from the side, so that the patient does not see it coming, and avoid touching the lashes. A normal blink reflex should result from touching the cotton wool to either the corneal apex or limbus. A more sophisticated technique – the Cochet–Bonnet aesthesiometer – can be used to quantify the extent of the deficit of corneal sensitivity.

Visual fields

Testing of visual fields should be conducted if the patient has peripheral vision symptoms, if there are questionable fundus signs or if there is an unexplained reduction in acuity. Contact lenses can improve or restrict the visual field, depending upon the type. For example, contact lenses can remove the mid peripheral scotoma associated with spectacles in hyperopia, while opaque, coloured soft lenses can cause a slight depression in the visual field (Bruce and Vingrys, 1990).

Tonometry

Whether the measurement of intraocular pressure is carried out routinely on patients under 40 years of age, or on indication, will vary between different clinical situations. Although the onset of glaucoma typically occurs in patients over 40 years of age, the clinical examination of a younger patient that reveals extensive optic disc cupping (0.5), or asymmetry of cupping (difference 0.2), may be an indication for performing tonometry.

Stereopsis

Measurement of stereopsis is indicated when binocularity is particularly important to contact lens wear. A good example is contact lens monovision correction for presbyopia, where the monocular near-vision correction can disrupt binocularity. A test of stereopsis can quantify the extent of this disruption (Collins and Bruce, 1994).

Colour vision testing

Red–green colour deficiencies occur in an estimated 8% of male and 0.5% of female patients. It is therefore worthwhile assessing colour vision at least once on all contact lens patients.

Conclusions

The preliminary examination of a prospective contact lens patient is in many respects similar to that which would be conducted on any healthy patient seeking a general eye examination. Perhaps the key distinction is that, in the case of a contact lens patient, consideration is being given to prescribing an appliance that will come into direct contact with the ocular tissues. In this regard, a thorough examination with the slit-lamp biomicroscope is perhaps the cornerstone of the preliminary examination. Certainly, the information obtained at this initial visit is of paramount importance because it will provide the baseline findings against which all future observations of the effects of lens wear will be assessed.

References

Bruce, A. S. (2006) Rigid gas-permeable lens fitting and eyelid geometry (CD-ROM). In *Manual of Contact Lens Fitting and Prescribing with CD-ROM,* 3rd edn. (M. Hom and A.S. Bruce eds), Boston, MA: Butterworth-Heinemann Elsevier.

Bruce, A. S. and Bohl, G. N. (1992) Topographic modelling system in assessment of keratoconus. *Clin. Exp. Optom.,* **75,** 149–152.

Bruce, A. S. and Brennan, N. A. (2000) *A Guide to Clinical Contact Lens Management,* 3rd edn. Duluth, GA: CIBA Vision.

Bruce, A. S. and Vingrys, A. J. (1990) Does a coloured contact lens change the visual sensitivity of patients? *Clin. Exp. Optom.,* **73,** 200–204.

Bruce A. S., Golding T. R. and Mainstone, J. C. (2001) Analysis of tear film breakup on etafilcon A hydrogel lenses. *Biomaterials,* **22,** 3249–3256.

Collins, M. J. and Bruce, A. S. (1994) Factors influencing performance in monovision. *J. Br. Contact Lens Assoc.,* **17,** 83–89.

Efron, N. and McCubbin, S. (2007) Grading contact lens complications under time constraints. *Optom. Vis. Sci.,* **84,** 1082–1086.

Jones, L. W. and Jones, D.A. (2001) Slit lamp biomicroscopy. In *The Cornea: its Examination in Contact Lens Practice* (N. Efron, ed.), pp. 1–49, Oxford: Butterworth-Heinemann.

Little, S. A. and Bruce, A. S. (1994) Hydrogel (Acuvue) lens movement is influenced by the postlens tear film. *Optom. Vis. Sci.,* **71,** 364–370.

Mainstone, J. C., Golding, T. R. and Bruce, A. S. (1996) Tear meniscus measurement in the diagnosis of dry eye. *Curr. Eye Res.,* **15,** 653–661.

CHAPTER 38

Patient education

Sarah L Morgan

Introduction

The quality of instruction and advice given to a patient contributes to the success or failure of the new wearer (Ettinger, 1993). Therefore, the importance of the dispensing visit should not be underestimated, and this chapter will cover some of the key aspects of this activity.

Objectives

Proper and careful tuition of a patient at a dispensing visit will facilitate confident lens handling by the patient and will help nurture a sound appreciation of how lenses should perform and how to manage various situations that can arise in contact lens wear. Certainly, poor patient education can result in premature discontinuation from lens wear and increase the likelihood of unscheduled visits to the practice.

The dispensing visit seeks to:

- Teach the patient the correct methods of lens application and removal.
- Explain the methods that optimize lens comfort, such as understanding when a lens is inside out or the removal of postlens debris.
- Inform the patient about the likely adaptation issues that may be encountered.
- Outline the correct use of the prescribed care regimen.

Timing

The availability of diagnostic lens banks has negated the need for individual lens ordering (with the exception of more specialized lenses such as soft toric lenses and the majority of rigid lenses) and has made both the fitting and dispensing appointment possible on the same day. Some patients are so motivated following their first experience of contact lens wear that the dispensing can take place immediately after the initial trial fitting. On the other hand, rescheduling the dispensing visit for another day has the benefits of giving the patient a break after the fitting visit, and allows the patient to read through some preliminary literature about the contact lenses.

Creating the optimum teaching environment

A trained member of support staff as opposed to the practitioner commonly adopts the teaching role; this person is sometimes referred to as the contact lens hygienist. Having a trained member of the support staff undertaking this task can have several advantages. Some patients feel pressured to have to 'perform' in front of the practitioner whereas they may feel more relaxed with a member of the support staff. The delegation of this role requires careful selection of personnel who can be relied upon to provide accurate information to the patient and refer back to the practitioner when necessary (Morgan, 2008).

The teaching area

Patients who have elected to wear contact lenses are often apprehensive about the process of lens application and removal. For this reason, the teaching room should be of a comfortable temperature and well ventilated, as many patients become quite anxious in their frustrations if they do not apply the lens on the first attempt. The area should be reasonably private – perhaps screened off from the rest of the practice – and it is essential that the instructor and the patient are free from incidental interruptions. Patients require careful attention when they first handle lenses, and the instructor must not be taken away or distracted from this supervisory task.

Good lighting is important, along with suitable seating for both the patient and the instructor, as flexibility to be able to sit on each side of the patient is needed (Figure 38.1).

The chair of the patient should be set at a desk such that the knees of the patient can fit comfortably under the desk. This is helpful if the patient accidentally drops the lens during handling.

DOI: 10.1016/B978-0-7506-8869-7.00038-0

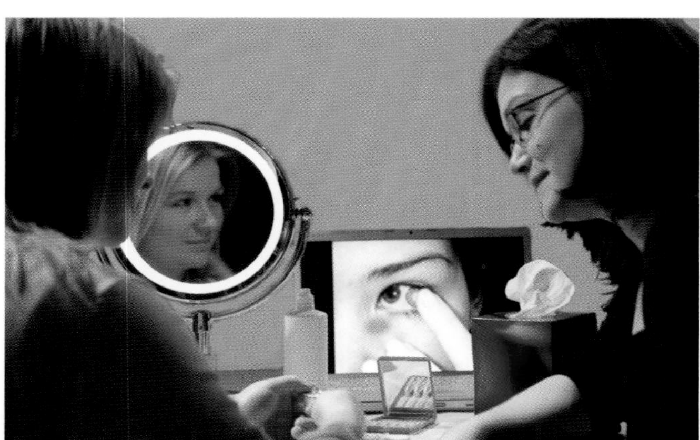

Figure 38.1 The teaching area should be well illuminated, with seating for both patient and instructor and with all necessary accoutrements immediately to hand.

Accoutrements

An illuminated, double-sided (with one side that magnifies), height-adjustable and tilting mirror is ideal. The teaching area must be prepared in advance of the lesson, so that all necessary items are to hand:

- Contact lenses – cross-checked with the record card and spectacle prescription.
- Lens case – which may be supplied with the solutions.
- Trial pack of solutions – sufficient for the needs of the patient until the first scheduled aftercare visit.
- Additional solution – for rinsing during the lesson.
- Comfort drops – to help alleviate any ocular discomfort.
- Box of tissues – with a spare box available.
- Hand-washing facilities – soap (in pump dispenser) and lint-free paper towels.
- Mirror as described above – cleaned and free from fingerprints.
- Appropriately sized plastic bag – for the patient to carry away lenses, solutions and accompanying literature.

Patient instruction

Contact lens handling can be a very frustrating experience for the novice patient. Accordingly, patience and communication skills are the most critical personality traits of the member of staff chosen to instruct contact lens patients. The instruction session should not be rushed, and the patient should feel comfortable asking questions.

Hand grooming and hygiene

The nails of all fingers that are likely to be involved in lens manipulation should be cut short and filed smooth to avoid both lens damage and the potential for corneal insult. It is imperative that the importance of hand washing prior to lens handling is reinforced throughout the instruction phase. The best way of achieving this without appearing to be patronizing to the patient is for the instructor to wash his/her hands prior to lens handling, in full view of the patient. A very brief explanation as to why this is so important – the prevention of lens contamination and reducing the risks of infection – can be given to the patient. The patient can then be invited to wash his/her hands. At all future instruction or aftercare visits, patients should be prompted to wash their hands if they forget to do this before proceeding to handle lenses.

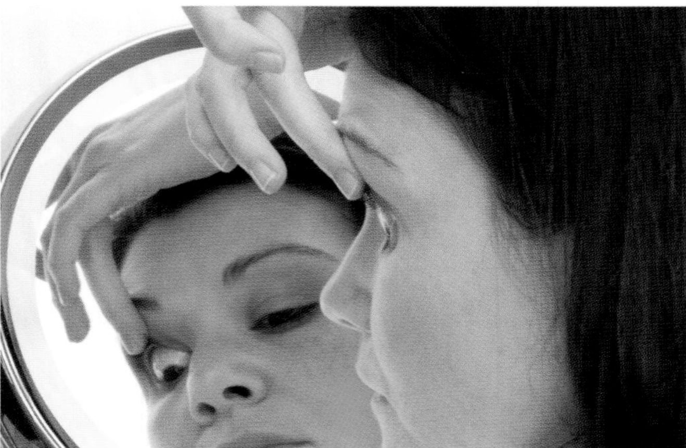

Figure 38.2 Taking control of the upper lid.

Lid manipulation

Touching the eye area can be awkward for many patients. The patient must first practise how to overcome the natural blink reflex, and this can be achieved by way of a 'dry run', in that the patient is not handling the lens at first. It is usual for the instructor to perform each part of the handling process before the patient tries. Effective upper-lid control is crucial to lens application.

Most patients will prefer to apply lenses on to each eye using the same hand, whereas some will use the right hand to apply the right lens and the left hand to apply the left lens. Consider, by way of example, a 'dry run' for lens application on to the right eye with the right hand. The patient is given the following instructions:

> *In order to take control of your right upper lid, look downwards so that the whole of the upper lid is exposed. Next, bringing your left hand vertically over your forehead, place the finger tip of your middle finger on your lid margin closest to the eyelashes and gently draw the lid upwards and hold it against your brow bone (Figure 38.2).*
>
> *Now look straight into the mirror, and place the middle finger of your right hand on the middle of your lower lid and gently retract the lower lid (Figure 38.3). (This further increases the palpebral aperture and helps to stabilize the hand applying the lens.) The forefinger of your right hand is then free to apply the lens directly on to your eye.*

Once the patient has mastered lid manipulation, lens handling can be taught.

Lens inspection

Practitioners routinely inspect lenses prior to application for evidence of lens damage, debris and whether a soft lens

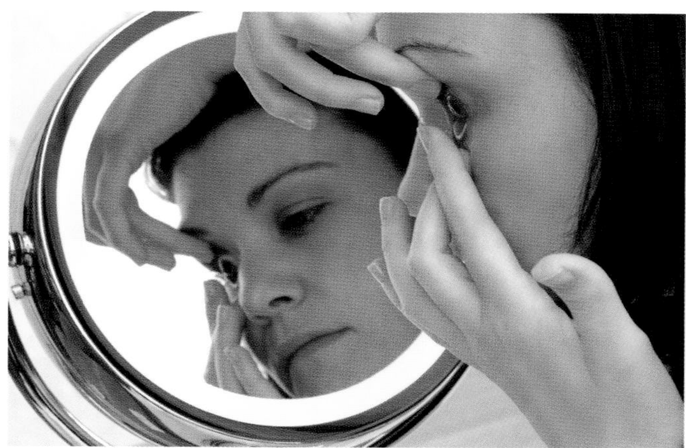

Figure 38.3 With both lids retracted the patient is ready to apply the lens.

is inside out or not. Patients need this basic level of instruction, even to the level of detail of explaining how to remove the lens from the lens packaging (in the case of disposable soft lenses) and also how to replace and remove a lens carefully from the lens case to avoid lens damage; this is particularly relevant to basket-style cases for soft lenses, which clip shut, and barrel cases with lens supports for rigid lenses. Patients need reassurance that a soft contact lens applied inside-out is not harmful, but such a lens may be slightly uncomfortable and may be prone to move excessively, which in turn can affect vision performance and in some cases cause the lens to be blinked out.

For the experienced contact lens practitioner, careful passive inspection of the lens on the tip of the finger will reveal whether the lens is inside out or not. However, for the novice, assessing soft lens inversion can be difficult. An active approach can be more enlightening; the lens is allowed to dehydrate for a few seconds, and then, with the lens placed in the crease of the palm of the hand, the lens edges are moved together by cupping the hand as if intending to fold it in half – the 'taco test', as a lens which is the right way round curls up rather like a taco shell. If the lens edges appear to curl towards each other, the lens is the right way around (Figure 38.4A), and if the edges appear to curl outwards, the lens is probably inside out (Figure 38.4B). Typically, a practitioner would utilize this technique by placing the lens on the tip of the finger; however, by definition, a new wearer finds lens manipulation a challenge so the hand technique is both easier to teach and more practical for the patient.

It may be necessary to invert the lens repeatedly in order to confirm this; the drier the lens becomes, the more apparent the inversion status of the lens will be.

Some manufacturers mark their lenses with an inversion indicator. When viewed from a designated aspect, a small pattern or number sequence can be observed in the correct orientation. If the lens is inverted, the pattern or number sequence will be reversed (incorrect) when viewed from the same aspect. Patients should be advised of any other markings on the lenses, and their purpose if known (such as toric lens scribe marks) so that they are aware that these features are meant to be present on the lens and are not a hair or defect.

When handling lenses, the forefinger applying the lens needs to be as dry as possible. On removing the lens from the case or packaging, it should be placed in the palm of the opposite hand to help drain off excess solution. The lens can then be 'scooped up' from the palm by the side of the fingertip of the forefinger with some aid from the forefinger and thumb of the opposite hand. Tissues on the desk – preferably lint-free – can be used to dab the forefinger dry during this process. In the case of soft lenses, the lens may need to be lifted off the forefinger to dry the fingertip to prevent the lens from sagging back over a wet fingertip due to surface tension. The complete circumference of the lens should be sitting proud of the finger.

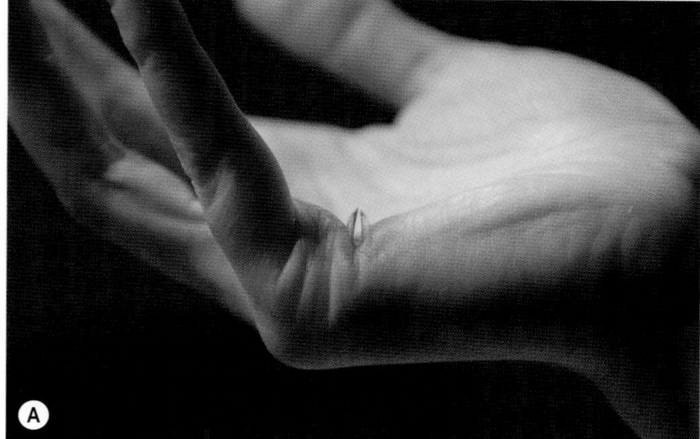

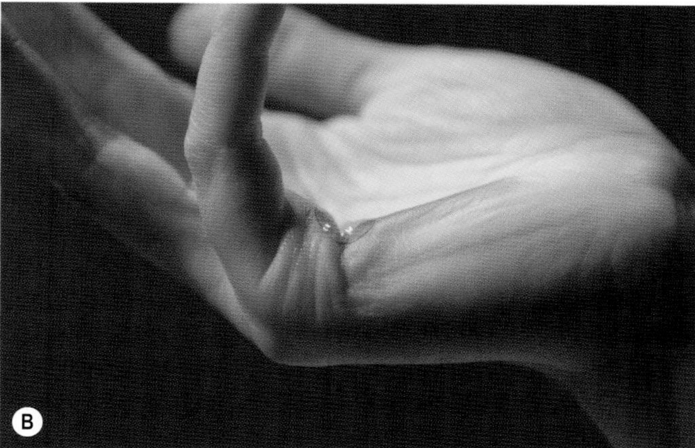

Figure 38.4 A simple technique for checking if a soft lens is inverted. (A) Right way; (B) wrong way.

Lens application

Soft lens application requires a slow-motion approach. The patient must not release the upper lid too soon, as this can lead to the lens being ejected due to air trapped behind the lens. The instructor should sit beside the patient rather than across the desk because, firstly, this is less confrontational, and secondly, a better view of the actions of the patient is possible. When the right lens is applied and removed, the instructor should sit on the right side of the patient and vice versa. The patient should be directed to apply the lower edge of a soft contact lens to the area 1–2 mm below the limbus at an angle of 45° having vaulted the lower lid (Figure 38.5).

Once contact with the tear film has been made, the contact lens is attracted to the cornea. If there are any air bubbles underneath the lens, these can be overcome by the patient

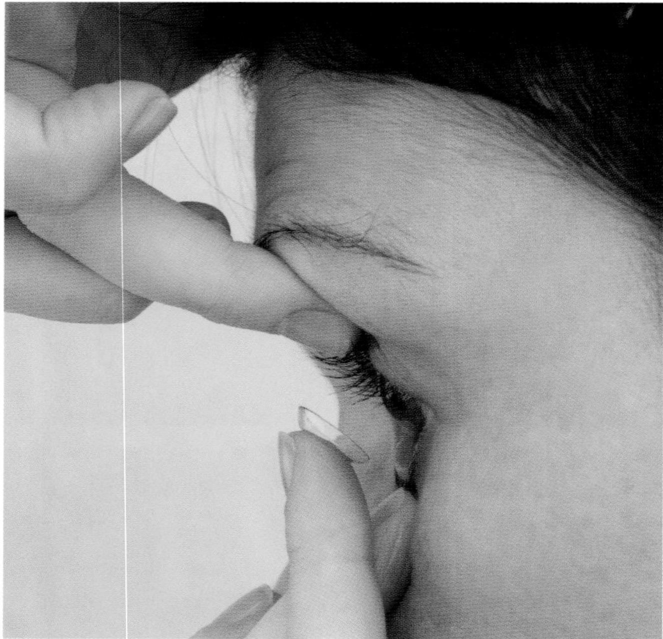

Figure 38.5 The lens is best applied at an angle of 45° to the cornea.

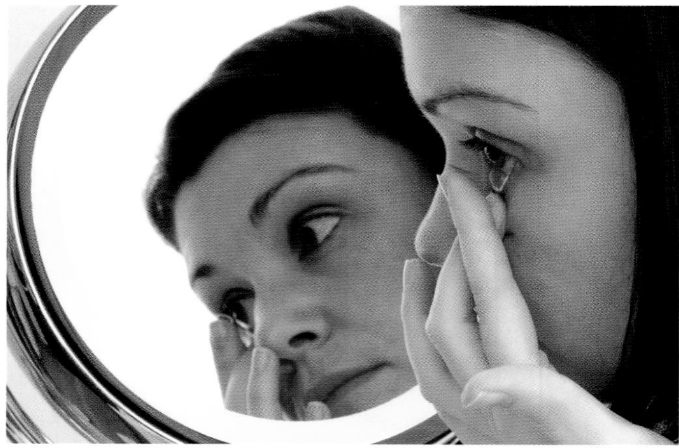

Figure 38.6 One-handed lens application.

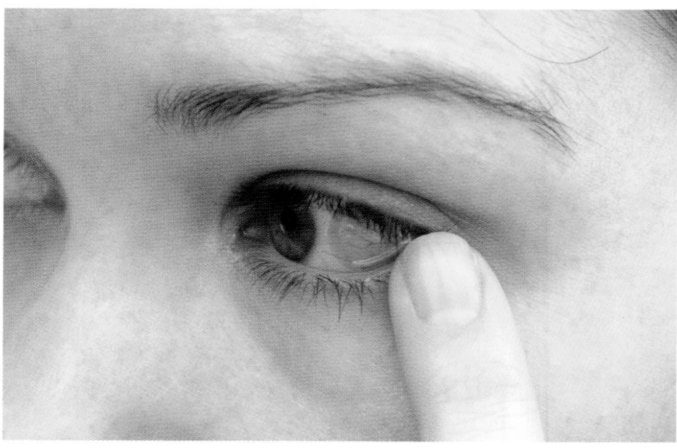

Figure 38.7 Displacing a soft contact lens laterally is a useful technique for removing debris from behind the lens.

looking downwards and slowly releasing the upper lid whilst still looking down and then closing the eye tight so as to squeeze out the remaining air.

A rigid lens, being of smaller diameter, is easier to apply, and its shape remains consistent throughout handling. Rigid lenses should be placed directly on to the central cornea as failure to do so can lead to the lens being displaced on to the conjunctiva.

Some patients have flexibility problems with their arms and/or hands, so common-sense adaptations to the usual recommended approach will need to be made. For example, one-handed application can be achieved with the patient dipping the chin towards the chest and looking upwards into the mirror. This serves to provide a larger area inferior to the limbus on which to apply a soft lens, and the lens, once applied, can be manipulated into place. A rigid lens can be applied directly on to the cornea using this method (Figure 38.6).

Having applied the lens, the patient can check that it is in position by covering the other eye and checking that vision is as clear as expected. For patients wearing monovision correction, the near lens should be applied first so that application of the distance lens is easier. In other cases, developing a habit of handling the right lens first for both application and removal helps to avoid mixing up the two lenses.

Tips on comfort and lens recentring

Contact lenses can attract debris during lens preparation prior to application and wearers can experience some mild lens awareness. In the case of soft lenses, sliding the lens temporally on to the conjunctiva can relieve this (Figure 38.7).

For the right eye, the patient looks directly into the mirror and turns the head to the right whilst maintaining a straight-ahead gaze. This helps to expose a large area of temporal conjunctiva on to which the lens can be displaced. Using the right hand, the patient displaces the inferior lid slightly with the middle finger and slides the lens completely off the cornea on to the temporal conjunctiva using the forefinger. The patient will usually experience instant relief from any previous foreign-body sensation. At this point, the patient blinks three to five times, which washes the tear film over the cornea, thereby displacing any unwanted debris. The lens can be manually repositioned on to the cornea, or alternatively the patient can look temporally with a couple of blinks, which will achieve the same result. If this type of discomfort is experienced on application of a rigid lens, the lens should be removed, rinsed and reapplied. With soft lenses, if a foreign-body sensation persists after this technique has been tried, the lens should be removed, rinsed and inspected for any signs of damage; the lens can then be reapplied if all looks well (or replaced if damaged).

If a rigid lens is decentred from the cornea on to the conjunctiva, the patient must attempt to manoeuvre the lens on to the cornea by holding the upper and lower edges of the lens through the lids and gently lifting the lens edges to allow tears to flow underneath the lens which in turn helps to release the lens and allows manipulation back on to the cornea. Locating the lens in the first instance may require careful observation using the mirror as well as

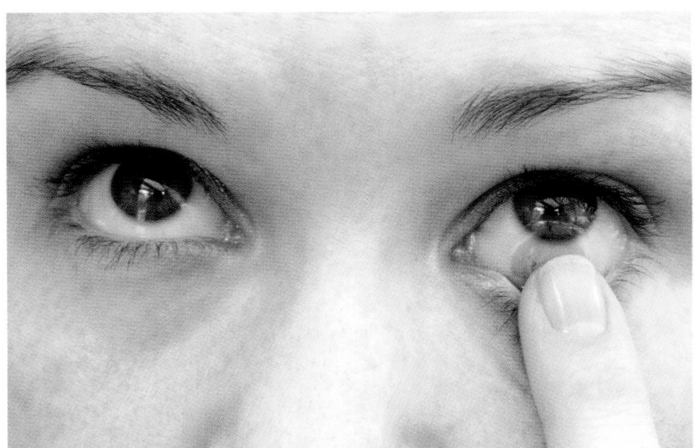

Figure 38.8 A soft lens should be displaced downwards prior to removal.

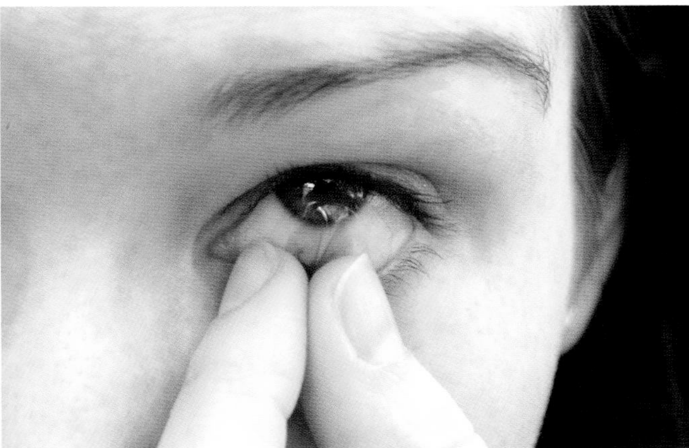

Figure 38.9 Soft lens removal.

lifting the upper lid to investigate if the lens has been displaced vertically. Patients must be informed that contact lenses can never 'disappear behind their eyes' and 'float into their brain', which is a commonly held misconception. Most rigid lenses can be felt through the lid because of their rigidity, whereas soft lenses can be more difficult to locate, especially if they have folded in half before being swept up under the upper lid. The instillation of comfort drops may suffice or saline solution (via an eye bath) can be helpful in releasing lenses in this situation.

Lens removal

Whilst soft lenses are more difficult to apply than rigid lenses, they can be easier to remove. Soft lens removal must be achievable in any situation, so it is recommended that patients learn how to remove lenses without the aid of a mirror. The chance of causing a corneal abrasion on lens removal must be given consideration; thus, removal of soft lenses from the more resilient conjunctiva is preferable. The back surface of a soft lens is designed to align closely with the cornea, so displacing the lens on to the conjunctiva helps to loosen the attachment of the lens, thereby aiding removal.

To remove a soft lens from the right eye, the patient rests the middle finger of his/her preferred hand on the lower-lid margin, displacing it away from the globe slightly, looks upwards and then slides the lens downwards on to the inferior conjunctiva using the forefinger (Figure 38.8).

Whilst still touching the lens with the forefinger, the thumb of the same hand can be brought in to pinch the lens off the conjunctiva, thereby completing lens removal (Figure 38.9).

Sometimes a few attempts are necessary with instructor guidance until the patient becomes aware of the sensation of lens displacement and of gripping the lens between the thumb and forefinger.

The technique for rigid lens removal is patient-dependent. Some patients can more easily spring the lens out using their lids; others, however, need to employ a different method.

The blink technique

This technique utilizes the natural narrowing of the palpebral aperture and lid margin tension to get behind the lens to 'flip' it out (Figure 38.10).

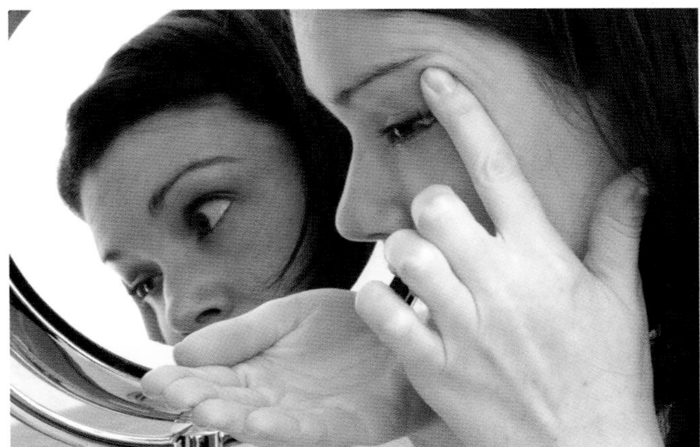

Figure 38.10 The blink technique for rigid lens removal.

With this technique, the patient first stares very wide to ensure the lid margins are beyond and not over the lens edge. The eye of the patient needs to be as central as possible in the palpebral aperture to achieve this. The patient then places the forefinger only on the outer canthus whilst pulling temporally to make the lids taut. Once the patient feels the edge of the lens, a forceful blink may flip the lens out. Sometimes it is necessary for the patient to look slightly nasally in order to position the cornea and lens in an area of narrower aperture.

The two-handed technique

This method involves manually tensioning the lids against the lens edge (Figure 38.11).

For the right eye, the patient positions the forefinger of the left hand on the middle edge of the upper lid and the forefinger of the right hand on the middle edge of the lower lid. The lids are first moved apart to ensure that the lens is free to move, and they are then moved into the globe to tighten against the lens edge. Slightly more pressure is applied to the upper lid in order to flip the lens out over the lower lid with the top of the lens being released first. Care must be taken such that the lens edge is not forced into the cornea itself.

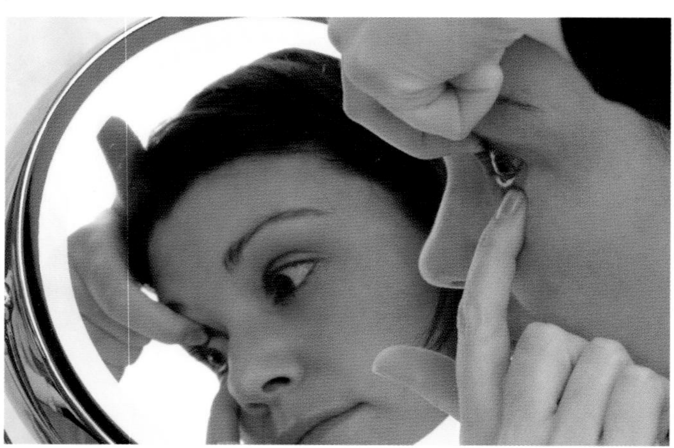

Figure 38.11 The two-handed technique for rigid lens removal.

Suction holders

Special rigid lens suction holders are available, although these have three key disadvantages:

1. If patients are only able to remove the lens with the aid of this device, they will be unable to remove the lens in an emergency without it
2. An inexperienced wearer may fail to attach the suction holder to the lens and bring the holder in contact with either the cornea or conjunctiva
3. Proper hygiene of the suction cup is required: it may be an additional source of contamination of the contact lenses (Boost and Cho, 2005).

In these respects, the use of suction holders is not advocated.

Patients must be able to remove their contact lenses safely before taking them away. For new wearers, performing this routine three times is recommended. For existing wearers new to the practice or having been fitted with a new lens with subtly different handling characteristics, demonstrating their established technique once usually suffices. Some practitioners, when refitting patients who are new to the practice, assume that they follow a good routine with respect to lens wear and care. It may be prudent in an age of litigation that all patients undergo some degree of in-practice training as well as signing an informed consent form so that there is a written record that the patient understands the correct protocols for lens wear and care. Periodically, all established lens wearers may be updated in this way to ensure they are aware of current advice and the recommended practice protocols.

Care products

The full care regimen should be demonstrated from start to finish, explaining why each step is necessary as well as what could happen if the routine is not strictly adhered to. The patient should be handed written information about the care products being dispensed; this may be information that is supplied by the manufacturer and/or material prepared by the practitioner.

Having applied and removed lenses a couple of times, the patient may appreciate a comfort drop in each eye. This serves to demonstrate the benefit of ocular lubricants as well as teaching the patient how to instil comfort drops when wearing lenses. Instances in which comfort drops provide symptomatic relief – such as during prolonged near work when blink rates are reduced, and in smoky atmospheres – can be discussed. The dangers of using tap water and saliva as rewetting agents can be outlined (Shovlin, 1990), as well as the appropriateness or otherwise of using prescribed and over-the-counter eye drops when wearing lenses. Patients should be aware that persistent lens discomfort should not be ignored, and that lens removal in this instance is indicated.

Cosmetics

For contact lens wearers using cosmetics, advice from the practitioner about their safe use should be given. Contact lenses can readily become soiled or damaged as a result of contamination from various cosmetic products (Tlachac, 1994).

Some tips for cosmetic use by lens wearers (Association of Contact Lens Manufacturers, 2009):

- Always wash your hands before handling your lenses; avoid perfumed or medicated soaps.
- Insert your contact lenses before applying make-up. This will help you to see what you are doing while applying your cosmetics.
- Close your eyes when applying loose powder, to keep it from getting in your eyes.
- Stay away from make-up and cleansers that can leave a greasy film on lenses. The same goes for hand creams and lotions; put these on after handling your lenses.
- Avoid using 'lash extender' mascaras, as they contain fibres that can flake off and get into your eyes, causing possible irritation.
- Cream or liquid blushers, eyeshadows and eyeliners are preferable since they do not contain gritty substances that can irritate your eyes. If you use powdered eyeshadow, make sure to apply it with a wet applicator. Do not use frosted shadows, as they contain tinsel, an ingredient that will stain your lenses.
- Never apply your eyeliner on the inside part of your lid. It could get on your contact lenses, blurring vision and irritating your eyes.
- Look out for cosmetics designed especially for contact lens wearers.
- It is best not to use hairsprays and other aerosol products after inserting your lenses. If you find it necessary to apply hairspray when you are wearing lenses, close your eyes.
- Store your make-up properly, making sure lids are tightly sealed. Replace mascara and applicators at least every 3 months to avoid bacteria build-up.

Wearing schedules

In the past, all patients were advised to adopt a wearing schedule, which means progressively increasing lens wearing time when wearing lenses for the first time, or after not having worn lenses for a prolonged period. The said purpose of advising adherence to a wearing schedule was to allow patients to adapt to lenses. Failure to adapt to early-generation, low-oxygen-performance polymethyl methacrylate (PMMA) and thick soft lenses – by exceeding the adaptation wearing schedule – resulted in worsening discomfort and red and watery eyes towards the end of the wearing period. The physiological basis of this adaptation process remains unclear, but appears to be related to the effects of lens-induced hypoxia.

Soft lenses

The introduction of 1-day disposable soft lenses in the mid-1990s has meant that a number of patients wear their lenses on a part-time basis. Soft contact lens wearers used to be advised to wear their lenses for no more than 4 h on the first day and increase the next consecutive wearing days by no more than 2 h each day up to a maximum of 12 h wear per day. New modalities and improvements in soft lens materials and designs have now largely rendered this approach redundant.

Some gradual adaptation may be advised if the patient is working towards full-time wear or when a patient is particularly sensitive to lens wear. Inevitably, the more frequently lenses are worn, the greater the level of adaptation. Patients should be warned not to overwear daily-wear non-silicone hydrogel soft contact lenses in spite of how comfortable they may feel.

For new lens wearers embarking on continuous wear of lenses, a week of daily wear is advised prior to sleeping in them (Maldonado-Codina *et al.*, 2005). This serves two purposes: (1) ensuring the patient is adapted to lens wear; and (2) ensuring the patient is proficient in lens handling.

Rigid lenses

Rigid lenses require a longer adaptation period. Topical anaesthetics have been advocated by some practitioners to alleviate discomfort during the fitting appointment and the dispensing visit (Bennett *et al.*, 1998). Nominally, patients are instructed to wear lenses on the first day for about 2 h, building up by an extra 2 h per day. Some practitioners accelerate this process by advising patients to wear lenses in the morning, followed by a break during the afternoon, and then to recommence wear in the evening. The adaptation process is patient-dependent, and the patient's own level of comfort can act as a guide.

It sometimes takes a few days for the surface of rigid lenses to attain an optimal level of wettability and comfort for a variety of reasons. First, some hydrophobic polishing compounds may not have been completely removed from the lens surface prior to delivery (thorough lens cleaning prior to dispensing the lens to the patient can alleviate such problems). Second, until becoming coated with natural constituents of the tears, rigid lenses may remain slightly hydrophobic on the first day of wear, especially if they have been delivered in a dry state (storing rigid lenses in solution for about 24 h prior to dispensing will minimize this effect) (Bourassa and Benjamin, 1992).

Recognizing an emergency

Patients need to know how to identify an emergency situation when wearing lenses. At the same time, new wearers need to be aware of normal adaptation symptoms such as mild foreign-body sensation and intermittent blurring of vision. If a contact lens wearer is concerned that there is a problem, he/she can be advised to check that the eyes 'look good, feel good and see good (well)'. This easy-to-remember adage refers to the following:

- 'Look good' – there is no more ocular redness than normal.
- 'Feel good' – their eyes feel comfortable prior to and after lens application.
- 'See good (well)' – their vision is what they would usually expect (each eye checked monocularly).

Any significant redness when accompanied by pain needs urgent practitioner attention which may also require medical treatment, especially if the redness and pain do not ease following lens removal. Visual losses should not automatically be put down to contact lens wear, as there may be some form of ocular pathology present that is unrelated to lens wear.

Patient discharge

A useful strategy to instil confidence in patients who have never worn lenses previously is to have the patient apply his/her lenses at the conclusion of the training session, and to leave the practice wearing the lenses. The patient will then be forced to confront the challenge of lens handling (at least lens removal in the first instance), rather than, as might occur, putting the lenses aside until enough courage can be mustered to wear lenses at a later date.

An aftercare appointment should be made before the patient leaves the practice with the new contact lenses. The patient must appreciate that ongoing success with contact lenses is dependent upon several factors, such as adaptation to the lenses, compliance with the instructions given and attendance for regular aftercare visits. It should be impressed upon the patient that, whilst good vision and comfort are indicators of success, this does not automatically prove optimum product choice and individual compatibility. All wearers must be made aware of the importance of regular biomicroscopic examination. The standard strategy for encouraging compliance with the requirement to return for regular aftercare visits is to restrict the supply of lenses issued to the patient to correspond with the desired time period between aftercare appointments. Patients should also be made aware of the regularity of contact lens types and ancillary products becoming available, so attendance for aftercare visits ensures that they are advised about the most up-to-date product choices for their individual needs.

Informed consent

Informed consent means that a patient embarking on contact lens wear should be made aware of both the risks and benefits of contact lens wear as well as having the opportunity to ask questions (Rosenwasser, 1991; Roberts *et al.*, 2005). The information provided verbally should be reinforced with written material. As well as providing the patient with information about the recommended lenses and/or solution system of choice, the practitioner must also have discussed the possible alternatives.

A comprehensive list of every possible contact lens complication does not need to be discussed, but a practitioner is required to discuss those that a reasonable person or members of the profession would expect to be told. A practitioner would be expected to mention the more common non-serious aspects of lens wear, such as the normal adaptation symptoms, in addition to the less common risks that could lead to a serious complication such as visual loss from corneal infection.

Prospective wearers should also be made aware of the consequences of not following the recommended instructions. This may be perceived by some practitioners as a negative approach, as it does not present contact lenses in a positive light. However, discussing such possible scenarios will preclude patients from claiming lack of informed consent if they are non-compliant with advice. There is no legal stipulation regarding the provision of information when prescribing a contact lens; however, providing information and obtaining informed consent form part of good clinical practice. Whilst written consent is not evidence that informed discussion has taken place, written agreements can be used to provide a basis for the process.

A standard form can be used, which the patient signs to acknowledge that he/she has been given the necessary advice and instructions (Rosenwasser, 1991). The patient should be given a copy of this with the other copy retained in the records. In the case of minors, the form should be signed by both the child (where possible) and the parent or guardian.

Conclusion

The success of the dispensing visit is fundamental to the future welfare of the contact lens patient. Careful preparation and skilful instruction are involved in setting the patient on the road to success. Whilst this function is commonly and appropriately delegated to support staff, the practitioner must feel confident in the training and instruction routine so that all aspects of contact lens wear and care are covered. Written information in addition to booklets provided by manufacturers are essential accompaniments for this visit as well as a requirement of signing the statement of informed consent.

References

Association of Contact Lens Manufacturers (ACLM). (2009) Lens and Makeup Care. Available online at: www.aclm.org.uk.

Bennett, E. S., Smythe, J., Henry, V. A. *et al.* (1998) Effect of topical anesthetic use on initial patient satisfaction and overall success with rigid gas permeable contact lenses. *Optom. Vis. Sci.*, **75,** 800–805.

Boost, M. V. and Cho, P. (2005) Microbial flora of tears of orthokeratology patients, and microbial contamination of contact lenses and contact lens accessories. *Optom. Vis. Sci.*, **82,** 451–458.

Bourassa, S. and Benjamin, W. J. (1992) RGP wettability: the first day could be the worst day. *Int. Contact Lens Clin.*, **19,** 25–34.

Ettinger, E. R. (1993) *Professional Communications in Eye Care*, Boston, MA: Butterworth-Heinemann.

Maldonado-Codina, C., Morgan, P. B., Efron, N. *et al.* (2005) Comparative clinical performance of rigid versus soft hyper *Dk* contact lenses used for continuous wear. *Optom. Vis. Sci.*, **82,** 536–548.

Morgan, S. (2008) *The Complete Optometric Assistant.* Edinburgh: Butterworth-Heinemann.

Roberts, A., Kaye, A. E., Kaye, R. A. *et al.* (2005) Informed consent and medical devices: the case of the contact lens. *Br. J. Ophthalmol.*, **89,** 782–783.

Rosenwasser, H. M. (1991) *Malpractice and Contact Lenses*, Boston, MA: Butterworth-Heinemann.

Shovlin, J. P. (1990) *Acanthamoeba* keratitis in rigid lens wearers: the issue of tap water rinses. *Int. Contact Lens Clin.*, **17,** 47–49.

Tlachac, C. A. (1994) Cosmetics and contact lenses. *Optom Clin.*, **4,** 35–45.

CHAPTER 39

Aftercare

Loretta B Szczotka-Flynn and Nathan Efron

Introduction

Contact lenses are generally very well tolerated by the majority of patients; however, appropriate aftercare of the contact lens patient is essential to ensure that long-term success is maintained. Aftercare procedures are equally as important as the original lens fitting because the lenses that were fitted initially may develop unanticipated complications, which require correction at any time during postfitting patient care. In fact, it is commonly held that contact lens aftercare represents a continuum and as such can never be considered to be complete.

Postfitting care can be considered as 'early' or 'late' aftercare. Early aftercare usually encompasses the first 3 months after lens dispensing and is generally considered part of the initial lens fitting, during which parameters are often modified, early toxic or allergic reactions are identified and patients are adapting to lens wear. Late aftercare includes 6-month and annual progress evaluations, which assess contact lens effects on corneal shape and physiology. Lenses are reordered or replaced as needed. The late aftercare visits are critical to evaluate the patient for signs of lens-induced pathology, such as papillary conjunctivitis, blepharoptosis, neovascularization, polymegethism, corneal warpage and refractive error change. All aftercare visits should assess the patient for compliance as well. Routine ophthalmic examinations also should be performed as necessary during the aftercare visit for conditions unrelated to lens wear.

This chapter will offer a measure of the standard of care required of an aftercare visit by highlighting the procedures and strategies that can be employed at every aftercare visit in order to investigate efficiently and accurately the contact lens-wearing eye and arrive at the precise diagnosis if there are any problems. Occasionally, patients will present with complaints of poor vision, discomfort or red eyes. Ocular changes associated with such symptoms may or may not be detected by examining the eye and vision with standard clinical instruments such as the phoropter, slit-lamp biomicroscope and keratometer. If subclinical ocular changes are responsible for such lens-related complaints, they may only be detected using specific problem-solving strategies, and often with the use of advanced equipment. Therefore, strategies and advanced procedures used in the investigation of symptomatic as well as preclinical ocular changes associated with contact lens wear are also highlighted. Some instruments are only found in research and teaching institutions, but others are affordable enough to become part of the key devices that contact lens practitioners can add to their practices for routine pre- and postfitting care.

DOI: 10.1016/B978-0-7506-8869-7.00039-2

Recommended visit schedules

Aftercare schedules will vary based on lens type, mode of wear and underlying corneal physiology. For example, patients wearing rigid lenses should be examined more frequently during the first few months of lens wear. Patients using lenses for extended wear must be monitored more frequently, with the initial visits in the early morning to assess lens adherence (Figure 39.1), excessive overnight corneal swelling or infiltrative responses.

Additionally, patients with corneal pathology such as keratoconus, corneal dystrophy, postkeratoplasty, post

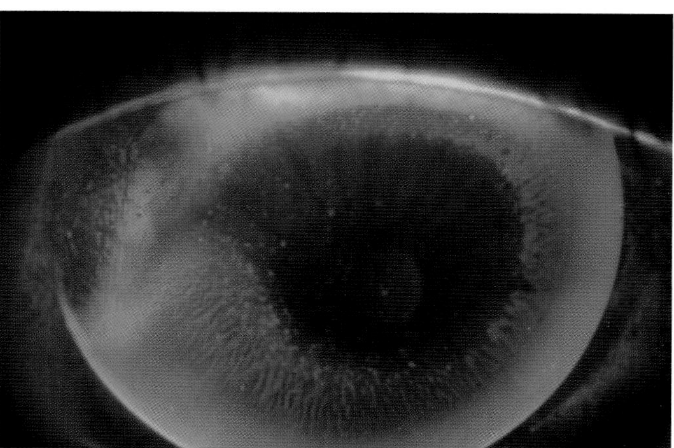

Figure 39.1 Fluorescein reveals binding of a rigid lens to the cornea. This was observed in the morning following overnight lens wear.

Table 39.1 Suggested aftercare schedules

Soft lens: daily wear	Soft lens: extended wear	Rigid lens: daily wear	Rigid lens: extended wear	Therapeutic use
1–2 weeks	1 day (a.m. visit)	1–2 weeks	1 day (a.m. visit)	1 week
1 month	1 week	1 month	1 week	3–4 weeks
3 months	1 month	2 months	2 weeks	2 months
6 months	3 months	3 months	1 month	3 months
Every 6–12 months thereafter	Every 3 months thereafter	6 months Every 6–12 months thereafter	3 months Every 3 months thereafter	6 months Every 6 months thereafter

refractive surgery or patients using contact lenses for other therapeutic applications such as aphakia, high ametropia or paediatric contact lens fitting, generally require more frequent aftercare as part of their management compared with uncomplicated cosmetic lens wearers.

Table 39.1 lists the recommended schedule of visits based on lens type, modality or therapeutic requirement for contact lens wear.

These recommendations are based on a survey of the literature and common clinical practice, and are listed in reference to the suggested mode of lens wear.

Preparing for the aftercare visit

Certain preparations need to be made before the aftercare appointment. The previous record cards of the patient should be reviewed beforehand so that the practitioner can become familiar with the case history, anticipate any potential problems and devise an appropriate history-taking strategy. It is common practice that record cards for contact lens aftercare examinations are separate from the comprehensive examination encounter form. Initial contact lens fitting forms can be combined with progress evaluation forms if space allows. The aftercare evaluation form should be designed to facilitate the recording of the recommended postfitting procedures, and an undesignated space should be provided for general notes.

Before acquiring any patient-abstracted information, it is critical to include some patient demographics and appointment information. Along with patient names and identification numbers, age is an important variable to document, as this will assist in identifying presbyopic symptoms. The appointment date as well as time should be recorded. This allows more accurate postexamination reviews if adverse reactions are noted at a certain time of day. For example, extended-wear patients typically are required to have initial extended-wear progress checks within 2 h of awakening because stromal oedema and lens adherence, especially with low-*Dk* lenses, will only be apparent at this time. Silicone hydrogel wearers should have initial progess checks within the first 2–4 h of lens insertion to document any asymptomatic corneal staining induced from unanticipated lens–solution interactions (Andrasko and Ryen, 2008). Rigid lens patients are usually examined later in the day because lens-induced pathology is likely to become more evident the longer the lens is worn.

Expected parameters of contact lenses worn to the aftercare visit should be at hand; these are typically carried over from the previous visit. This strategy is not always accurate because patients can present wearing a previous pair of lenses, or lenses that have become switched between the eyes; however, it affords an important point of reference during case history and compliance review.

Aftercare procedures while lenses are worn

The general strategy adopted for aftercare visits is to consider the procedures in two phases: those conducted with the patient wearing lenses (assuming that the patient presents wearing lenses) and those conducted following lens removal. Certainly, patients should present to all aftercare visits while wearing lenses, unless a complication warrants lens discontinuation. It is rarely necessary to conduct all possible aftercare procedures at every follow-up visit. Essential procedures (such as those outlined below) generally should be performed; these can be supplemented with ancillary testing to solve specific problems. The aftercare visit may on occasions be very brief; for example, if a patient presents with a minor problem soon after having been given a full aftercare examination and the solution is straightforward, it may only be necessary to see the patient for a few minutes. The only caveat here is that, for medicolegal reasons, vision should always be measured if the patient enters the consulting room, no matter how brief the visit.

History taking

The case history is crucial to assess patient compliance and to begin to formulate an opinion about the cause of any possible contact lens-related complications that have developed. The information obtained should include, at minimum, a subjective assessment of vision (including extent and duration of any morning or postlens removal blur), comfort, wearing time and care regimen. Additionally, it is important to elicit symptoms such as redness, tearing, photophobia or discharge if they are present. In the early aftercare phase, these series of questions are imperative to establish if there is an incompatibility with solutions or lenses.

During the late aftercare phases – in addition to all of the above case history – it is good practice to review medications used by the patient and to ascertain if any general allergic responses have been encountered, to ensure that these circumstances have not changed since the last visit. Additionally, patients can be invited to describe their chief complaint (if any) and review the overall lens-wearing history. A more detailed account of contact lens history taking can be found in Chapter 36.

Visual acuity

Presenting distance and near visual acuity with contact lenses should be recorded monocularly and binocularly with the consulting room lights on. This should be undertaken at each visit and the results compared to those expected from the dispensing visit or previous progress check. Visual acuity should be recorded prior to the utilization of any bright lights or disclosure dyes, which can induce lacrimation or lens misalignment.

Overrefraction

As with any subjective refraction, initial objective retinoscopy provides the starting point for the subjective overrefraction. Retinoscopy can also provide invaluable information when qualitatively viewing the red reflex over the lenses. Features such as optical zone edges or bifocal segments within the entrance pupil can be observed and correlated with patient complaints. Distortions or small visual obstructions induced from lens deposits, scratches, warped lenses or lens lift-off from the corneal surface may also be detected during overretinoscopy. Lastly, ocular pathology of new onset since the last visit, such as a posterior subcapsular cataract, can be easily detected by viewing the red reflex.

A subjective spherocylindrical refraction over the contact lenses is an important measure which should be recorded at every visit. At any aftercare visit, overrefraction can reveal required power changes due to unanticipated lacrimal lens formations, lens rotation, changes in refractive error, patient-induced lens power changes, lens warpage or lens flexure. The duochrome test is especially useful in determining the refractive end-point of an eye wearing a contact lens.

A useful clinical technique during subjective refraction is to obtain both spherical and spherocylindrical end-points independently (rather than merely calculating the best-sphere refraction from the spherocylindrical end-point). In cases of spherical lens fitting, spherical power modifications can be demonstrated and the resultant visual acuity measured. If vision is inadequate following a spherical overrefraction, a spherocylindrical overrefraction should be performed and a toric lens fit initiated if warranted. In soft toric or rigid front surface toric lens fitting, a spherocylindrical overrefraction can assist in determining the magnitude and direction of any cylinder mislocation (Lindsay *et al.*, 1997).

A repeatable cylindrical overrefraction obtained over a spherical rigid lens suggests lens flexure. Thin rigid lenses can flex approximately one-third of the corneal toricity. The probability of flexure increases with steeper and larger lenses. Flexure has been thought to increase with materials of higher oxygen permeability (*Dk*), but a study of current rigid materials across a range of *Dk* values (from 15 to 151 Barrer) failed to find a difference in flexure when measured by overrefraction (Lin and Snyder, 1999). Flexure can be confirmed by manual or automated keratometry over the lenses. A cylindrical overrefraction over a back toric rigid lens results from a crossed-cylinder effect and careful review of the measured cylindrical power and axis suggests either over- or undercorrected cylindrical correction, misaligned cylinder axes or residual lenticular cylinder.

Overkeratometry

Overkeratometry while the lenses are worn will provide an index of lens flexure over a spherical rigid lens. Since the anterior lens surface is being measured, the absolute keratometer readings will not correlate with the baseline corneal measurements. The degree and location of detected cylinder should correlate with the overrefraction if lens flexure is the suspected cause of residual astigmatism over a spherical lens on a toric cornea.

Overkeratometry is believed by some practitioners to be a useful aid in determining the lens–cornea relationship in soft lens fitting. Certainly, the clarity, consistency and shape of the mires that are reflected off the anterior soft lens surface can be useful for problem solving. For example, overkeratometry can help detect a steep or flat-fitting soft lens even though the lens fit may be judged to be clinically acceptable upon biomicroscopic examination. In a steep-fitting relationship, sustained overkeratometry observation can reveal distorted mires that become more irregular as the eye is left open between blinks. Additionally, the mire quality improves immediately after the blink when the lens has temporarily improved drapage over the cornea. In a flat fit, the opposite occurs; the mires blur immediately after blinking due to excessive lens movement and the mire quality improves as the eye remains open and the lens stabilizes (Figure 39.2).

External examination

General inspection of the eye under an Anglepoise lamp will reveal the presence of any general ocular pathology, such as red eye, conjunctival oedema or indeed almost any form of pathology if severe enough. Also, evaluating the head posture, blink habits and palpebral aperture of the patient can provide important information on lens adaptation and lid effects. New rigid lens wearers often present with partial blinks or a narrowing of their palpebral aperture in an attempt to decrease lid sensations. Rigid contact lens wear has also been shown to induce true acquired non-senile blepharoptosis from mechanical manipulation of the eyelids, or mild contact lens-induced lid inflammation (see Chapter 40).

Slit-lamp biomicroscopy

During the biomicroscopy evaluation while contact lenses are worn, the lens surface is first examined, followed by an evaluation of the lens fitting characteristics, and finally an assessment is made of possible interactions between the lens and eye.

Lens surface assessment

Both rigid and soft lenses should be inspected for surface quality, deposit formation, tear film interactions, and gross surface or edge defects. Clinically, it is very useful to

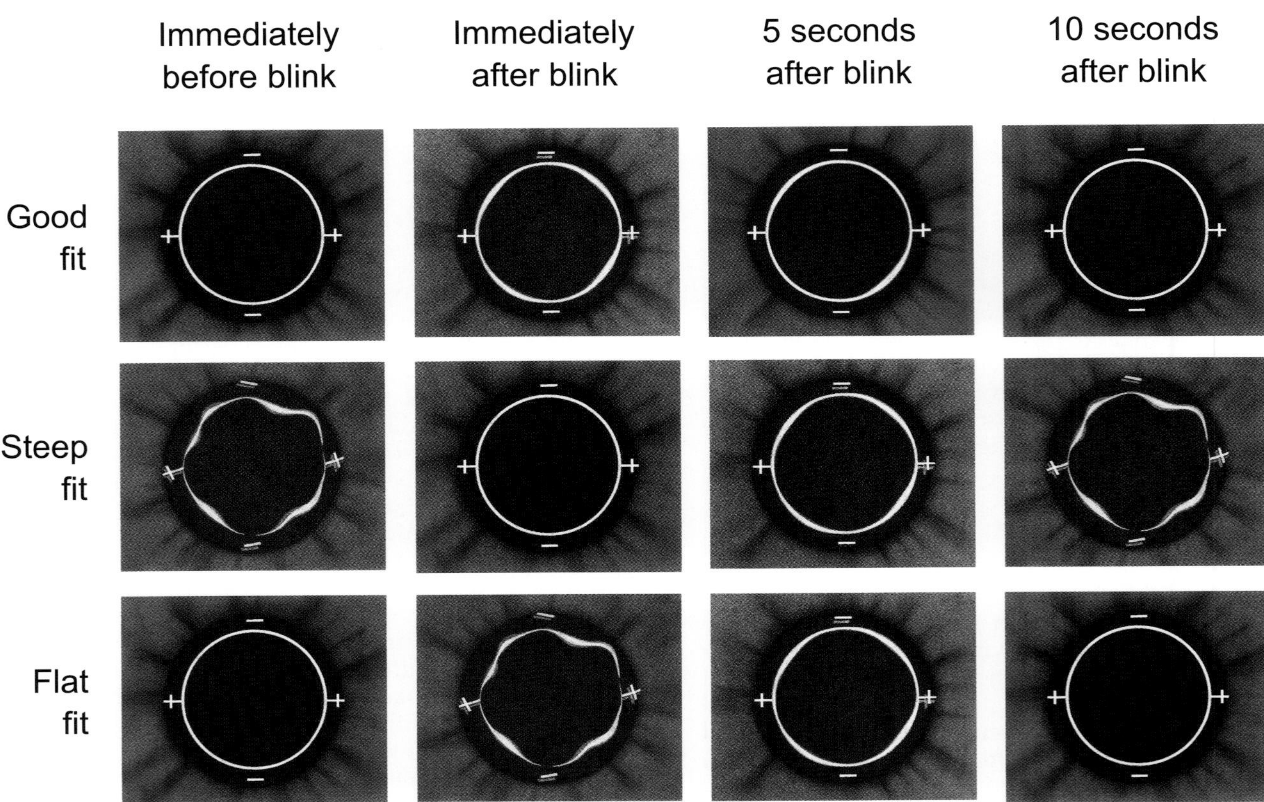

Figure 39.2 Appearance of keratometer mires reflecting off the surface of good, steep- and flat-fitting lenses, observed immediately before a blink, and immediately, 5 s and 10 s after a blink.

observe the characteristics of the tear film and anterior lens surface between blinks. All hydrogel lenses form mucoprotein deposits, which begin to form as soon as the lens is inserted. Tear film constituent deposition and coating is also expected; however, the analysis at this stage is aimed at determining whether the specific lens–cornea interaction in the patient being examined has resulted in the formation of a biocompatible coating, and if it has, whether there has been any adverse reaction as a result. A decision can then be made as to whether the lens replacement frequency needs to be increased.

Although the majority of deposits on hydroxyethyl methacrylate (HEMA)-based materials are mucoprotein, silicone hydrogel lenses may suffer from incompatible lipid deposition. It is estimated that there are more than 45 individual lipids within the tear film and the chemistry of the relatively hydrophobic silicone hydrogel materials has resulted in clinicians needing to understand the deposition of lipids on to contact lenses and how they may best manage these interactions (Lorentz and Jones, 2007). Thus, silicone hydrogel lenses should be closely observed for deposition even in the early refitting phase. Although these lenses deposit minimal amounts of protein (Suwala *et al.*, 2007), about 13% of patients wearing silicone hydrogel lenses exhibit clinically significant lipid deposition on new lenses, even though they may not have had this problem with previous HEMA-based materials (Nichols, 2006).

Although it is clinically difficult to assess lens and tear film interactions, a biomicroscopy method for assessing tear break-up time using white light has been suggested. It is assumed that an intact and smooth tear film coating on the anterior surface of a lens (indicated by longer tear break-up times) enhances the biocompatibility of the lens and thus promotes comfort and tolerance. The patient is instructed to refrain from blinking and the examiner records the time to observe disruption of the tear film as evidenced by a disruption of the white-light specular reflex from the anterior lens surface. Generally, break-up times of greater than 5 s should be observed on clean or mildly coated lenses. Break-up times of 4 s or less are usually associated with visible deposits and may indicate that the lens should be replaced more regularly or that the lens material is incompatible with the ocular surface of the patient (Hart, 1987).

Obvious non-wetting of rigid lenses is easily detectable during the biomicroscopy evaluation and should correlate with patient symptoms of discomfort, hazy vision and the frequent need for lens removal and cleaning (Figure 39.3).

Rigid lens non-wetting is occasionally noticed during lens dispensing; this may be related to improper preparation of the lens by the manufacturing laboratory that supplied the lens. Causes of manufacturing-related non-wetting include residual pitch and improper polishing. Non-wetting detected in late aftercare visits may be secondary to organic causes such as cosmetics, moisturizers, inappropriate lens care or adverse chemical interactions between incompatible solutions.

Other lens surface changes that should be assessed include deposit formations and surface hazing. Deposit formations have been discussed in Chapter 19, and usually indicate that more frequent lens replacement, or a change of lens material, is necessary. Symptoms caused by rigid

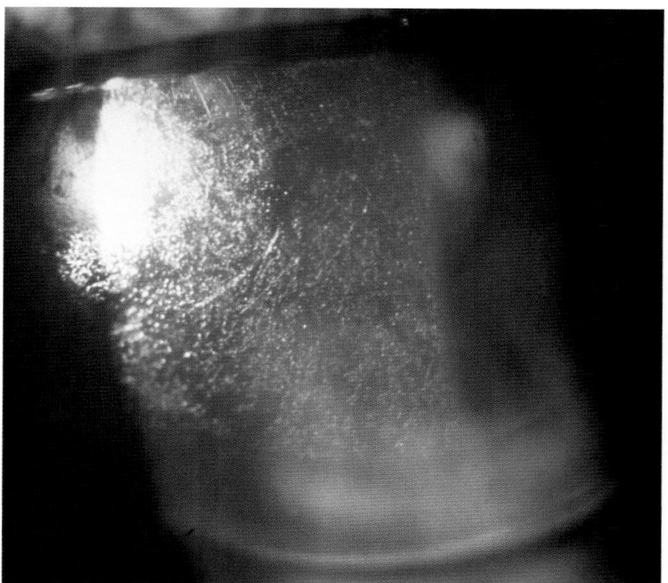

Figure 39.3 Deposition on the surface of a rigid lens, presumed to be denatured protein.

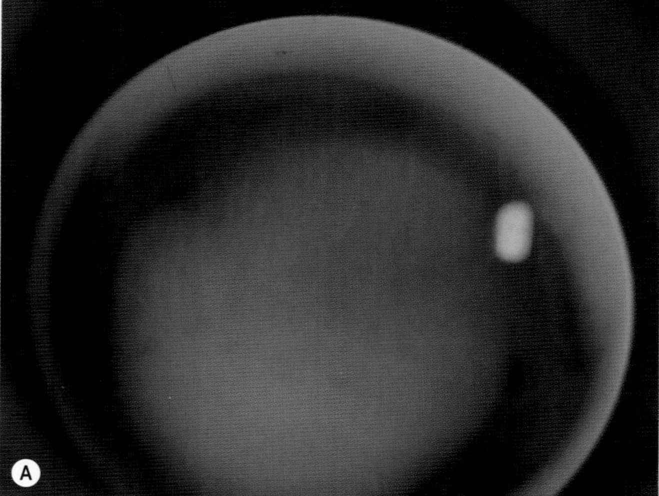

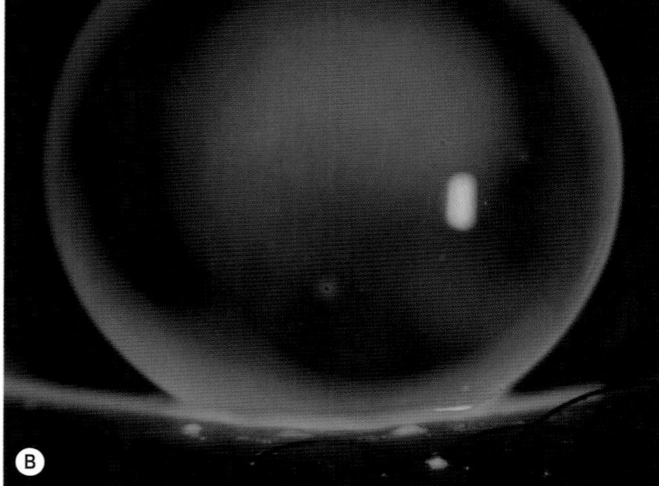

Figure 39.4 (A) Rigid lens fluorescein pattern at initial lens dispensing, showing apical clearance. (B) Same patient and lens as in (A), seen at an aftercare visit 2 weeks later, after adapting somewhat to lens wear. Note that mild corneal touch is now evident; this may have been masked by excessive tearing during lens fitting.

lens surface hazing include lens dryness and variable vision; this problem is thought to be due to excess tear film evaporation from the anterior lens surface, resulting in surface drying. Surface hazing on rigid lenses in the early aftercare phases may be an indication to change the lens material. In general, silicone acrylate and fluorosilicone acrylate materials behave differently, with the latter exhibiting greater tear film retention.

Lens fitting characteristics

Lens movement and centration should be evaluated as described in Chapters 9 and 16 for soft and rigid lenses, respectively. Deviations from the initially desired fitting approach should be assessed and changes made to lens parameters as needed. However, practitioners should anticipate the possibility of a slight alteration of in-eye soft lens (HEMA-based) performance towards the end of each day, as the lens dehydrates (Efron *et al.*, 1987). Lens fitting may also alter towards the end of the wearing cycle of disposable soft lenses. This is due to an 'ageing effect', whereby there is a gradual loss of water over the life of the lens (Morgan and Efron, 2000). This water loss can possibly alter the lens dimensions and have an impact on lens movement and comfort.

For rigid lenses, a fluorescein pattern evaluation should always be performed, with either the Burton lamp, the slit-lamp biomicroscope, or both. It should be noted that with the Burton lamp it is not possible to observe the fluorescein patterns of rigid lenses made from materials that deliberately or inadvertently absorb ultraviolet light. When the slit-lamp biomicroscope is used, the appearance of the fluorescein pattern can be enhanced by introducing a cobalt blue filter into the illumination system and a yellow barrier filter (Wratten number 12 yellow) into the observation system.

The fluorescein pattern should be assessed at every routine rigid lens aftercare visit to establish if the lens fit has changed. In the early aftercare phase, fluorescein pattern interpretations can vary as patients adapt to their lenses and reflex tearing subsides. It is not uncommon for a lens to be judged fit with apical clearance at a dispensing visit, yet observed to be fit with apical touch at a progress evaluation (Figure 39.4).

Because corneal shape and posterior lens tear film thickness may change as the patient adapts to new lenses (which will influence the interpretation of the lens fit), it is wise not to alter lens parameters until the fitting relationships have stabilized, typically at least 2–4 weeks after lens fitting.

Lens–eye interactions

With the lens in the eye, there is an opportunity to look for any adverse interactions between the lens and ocular surface. In the case of 3 and 9 o'clock corneal staining, the tissue compromise would be expected to be aligned with the position of the lateral edges of a rigid lens. In the context of lens fitting, the peripheral system of a rigid lens may appear steeper at a follow-up visit than initially

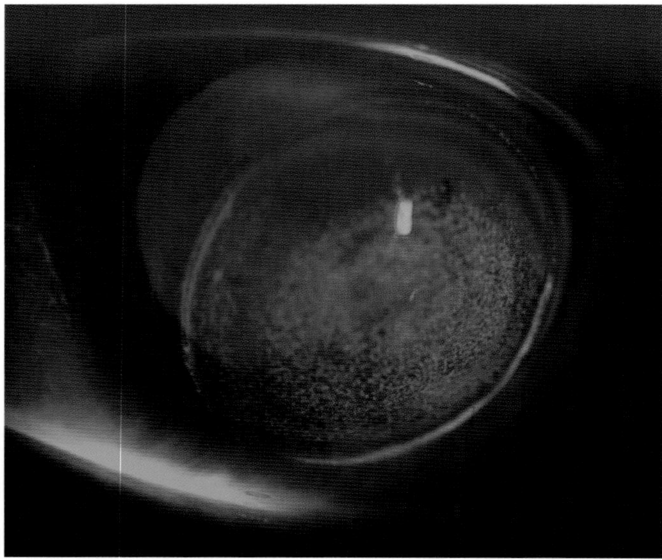

Figure 39.5 Epithelial indentation ring immediately following lens removal, revealed with the aid of fluorescein, indicating an extremely steep-fitting lens and/or a strongly adherent lens.

documented once reflex tearing has subsided; this can be detected by insufficient edge clearance, peripheral seal-off or even an epithelial indentation ring (Figure 39.5).

A conjunctival indentation ring induced by a tight-fitting soft lens would be expected to coincide with the position of the lens circumference. Higher-modulus silicone hydrogel lenses may also create asymptomatic conjunctival imprints or conjunctival flaps at the edge of the lens. Corneal staining induced by a lens defect is likely to be observed in the proximity of that defect. It would be difficult to reconcile many of the adverse reactions described above with lens performance and location if these reactions were first detected after the lens had been removed.

Aftercare procedures following lens removal

At this juncture, the lenses need to be removed from the eyes of the patient. Patients should be invited to remove their lenses and demonstrate what they would do generally in their habitual lens maintenance environment. This provides an opportunity to observe and evaluate the general level of hygiene, lens-handling skills, appropriate solution usage and general compliance. Any improper or irregular procedures should be either raised at this point or noted for later discussion with the patient. A series of tests that parallel those performed with the patient wearing lenses can now be undertaken with the lenses removed.

Uncorrected vision

An initial measure of uncorrected vision can be reconciled against the presenting visual acuity, the magnitude and nature of the refractive error and the subsequent subjective refraction. It should be noted that vision may be significantly degraded – beyond that attributable to uncorrected refractive error – during the first 15 min following lens removal. This is due to the fact that the tear layer is disrupted following lens removal, and it takes about 15 min to recover (Faber *et al.*, 1991).

Refraction

Contact lens-induced alterations in corneal curvature can significantly alter the refractive error with associated changes in visual acuity. Retinoscopy should be initially performed to serve as the starting point of the subjective refraction, to observe the optical quality of the eye and to detect aberrations or distortions on the corneal surface induced by the contact lens. The refractive error should be expected to remain constant or to progress slowly over time, and should be unaffected by lens wear. Also, visual acuity should remain correctable to prefitting levels. Reduced visual acuity may signal the presence of ocular pathology or lens-induced warpage if correlated with corneal curvature changes, as described later in this chapter. An average of a one-line decrease in best corrected visual acuity attributable to contact lens-induced topographic abnormalities has been reported (Ruiz-Montenegro *et al.*, 1993).

Specific refractive error changes have been documented with certain lens types and wearing schedules. Myopic progression associated with daily wear of hydrogel lenses with low oxygen permeability was reported in early clinical trials (Barnett and Rengstorff, 1977). An average of 0.30 D increase in myopia has been reported after 9 months of extended wear of low-*Dk* soft lenses, presumably due to hypoxic-driven corneal oedema (Binder, 1983; Dumbleton *et al.*, 1999). Conversely, extended wear with silicone hydrogel materials has no impact on refractive error, and may even be associated with a hyperopic shift from central corneal flattening in some patients (Dumbleton *et al.*, 1999). In fact, orthokeratology-like induced topographic changes have been documented with silicone hydrogel lenses that are typically of high powers and/or worn inside-out (Szczotka-Flynn, 2004; Caroline and Andre, 2005).

Refractive error changes have been reported in adult patients who have monocular blur intentionally induced with monovision contact lens correction. Specifically, studies show that approximately one-third of patients can expect changes in anisometropia between 0.50 and 1.25 D after wearing monovision contact lenses (Wick and Westin, 1999).

Keratometry and corneal topography

Corneal shape changes and/or warpage may appear with any type of contact lens secondary to mechanical stress or lens interference with corneal metabolism (Holden *et al.*, 1985a; Wilson *et al.*, 1990; Ruiz-Montenegro *et al.*, 1993; Smolek *et al.*, 1994; Sarzynski *et al.*, 1997). It is important to be able to identify these corneal changes correctly before they create severe visual consequences. Also, careful corneal curvature assessment is a good predictor of lens fit and physiology. Manual or automated keratometry may simply reveal numerical changes from the prefitting values, or an increase or decrease in corneal astigmatism. A general consensus is that changes greater than ±1.00 D from baseline are clinically significant, and in such cases the fit should be investigated for potential alteration to prevent potentially long-term corneal moulding. Additionally, manual keratometry can detect surface irregularity by assessment

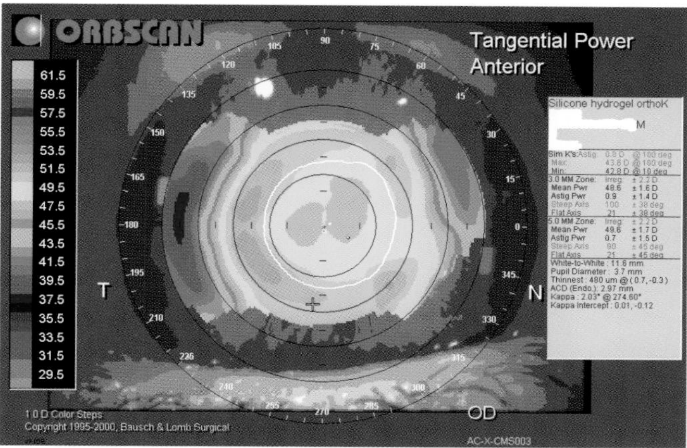

Figure 39.6 Oblate corneal shape induced unintentionally in a lotrafilcon A extended-wear contact lens user.

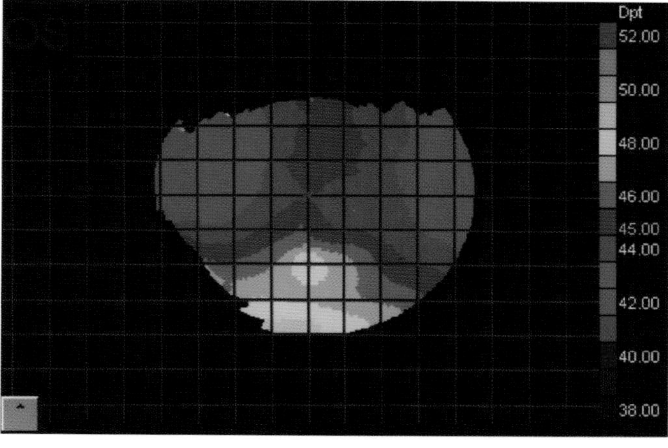

Figure 39.7 Inferior corneal steepening secondary to corneal warpage from long-term rigid lens wear.

of mire distortion. In fact, the quality of the mires should be graded at every progress check (see Appendix K).

A better technique to assess changes in corneal curvature is corneal topography. One of the most valuable applications of this technology is to monitor the stability of the cornea after both short- and long-term lens wear. Subtle corneal steepening or sphericalization that is undetectable with keratometry may characterize early corneal changes due to contact lens wear. Serial topography and topographic difference maps may reveal such subtle changes over time.

Occasionally, contact lenses can distort the corneal surface, resulting in transient or permanent corneal warpage. Most forms of distortion can be traced back to the fit and/or material of the lens. Different forms of corneal distortion can be detected, and often can be classified into one of three categories: (1) a shift from a prolate to an oblate shape; (2) inferior corneal steepening; and (3) 'smile' impression arcs.

Oblate shape

The normal cornea is a prolate shape; it is steeper in the centre and flattens aspherically in the periphery. Long-term flat-fitting lenses can permanently shift the cornea to an oblate shape by flattening the central cornea and secondarily steepening the periphery. This type of warpage may not be detected with keratometry or manifest refraction if the astigmatism is regular and the patient remains correctable to 6/6. Only corneal topography can reveal the oblate shape, which can create difficulty in rigid lens fitting and problem solving. As mentioned previously, silicone hydrogel lenses can induce a transient oblate corneal shape and a related decrease of myopia. Figure 39.6 shows an example of this phenomenon where a high myope wore a high-modulus silicone hydrogel lens for 30-day continuous wear, and 3 months after entering this mode of wear central corneal flattening and 1 D of decreased myopia were detected.

Inferior steepening

Long-term wear of polymethyl methacrylate (PMMA), low-*Dk* rigid lenses or superiorly decentred rigid lenses can cause inferior corneal steeping and give the appearance of keratoconus (Figure 39.7).

Lebow and Grohe (1999) compared the topography findings of 100 eyes with either keratoconus or contact lens-induced warpage. They concluded that keratoconic eyes have high shape factors, extremely high corneal irregularity measures and steep toric mean reference curvatures, whereas contact lens-induced warpage is characterized by almost spherical shape factors, elevated corneal irregularity measures and normal toric mean reference curvatures.

Even hydrogel lenses can cause severe shape changes, often due to corneal hypoxia with secondary tissue swelling, which can also give the appearance of inferior corneal steepening and pseudokeratoconus. Figure 39.8A shows the topography of a patient after sleeping in group 4 hydrogel lenses on a weekly basis for 6 months. Note the inferior steepening, which mimics keratoconus. After discontinuing all lens wear, her topography returned to normal in 3 weeks (Figure 39.8B).

This example illustrates how topography can reveal inferior corneal steepening. Some topography systems have introduced keratoconus detection software that attempts to detect and possibly differentiate keratoconus suspects from contact lens-induced corneal warpage, using paradigms such as those identified by Lebow and Grohe (1999), as described above.

Impression arcs

Rigid lens-induced arcuate corneal shape changes are most often located in the inferior third of the cornea and are commonly encountered if topography is routinely performed. These changes are referred to as 'smile' patterns because the resultant topographic plot gives the impression of a smiling face. In traditional rigid lens fitting, a flattened arcuate compression ring usually signifies unintended corneal moulding from the inferior edge of a superiorly decentred rigid lens. Just outside the lens edge, an arcuate zone of steepening appears (Figure 39.9).

If the patient reports spectacle blur, this may suggest intermittent lens adhesion, and an attempt should be made to flatten the posterior curves for improved corneal stability. Difference maps are helpful in quantifying the amount of such lens-induced corneal changes (Figure 39.10).

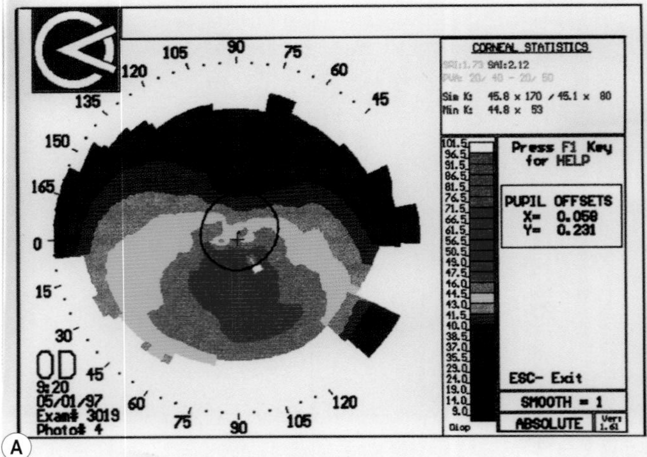

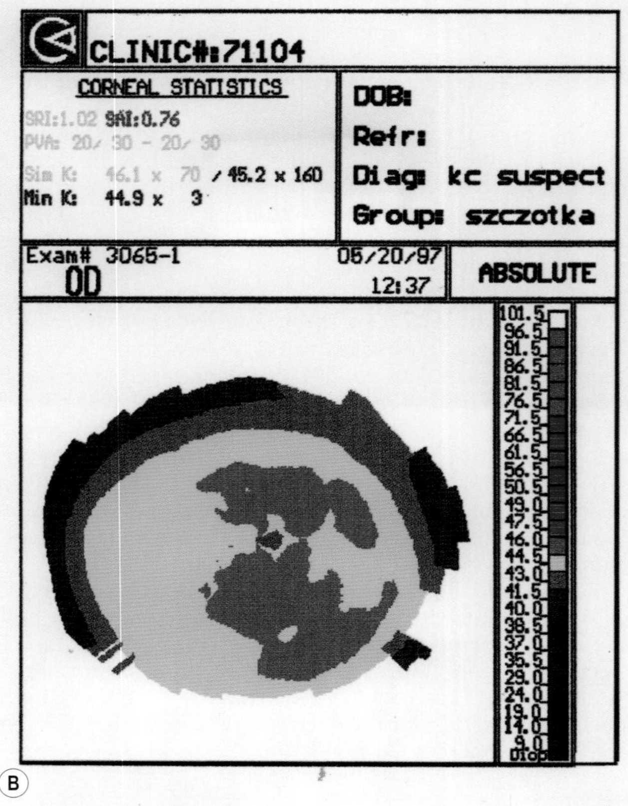

Figure 39.8 (A) Pseudokeratoconus pattern due to soft lens-induced hypoxia. (B) Same eye as represented in (A) after 3 weeks without lens wear; note the resolution of corneal distortion.

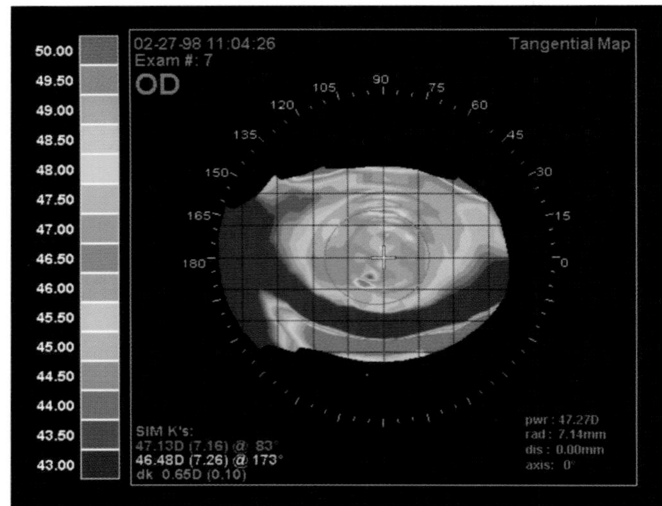

Figure 39.9 Inferior arcuate 'smile' corneal distortion caused by a decentred rigid lens.

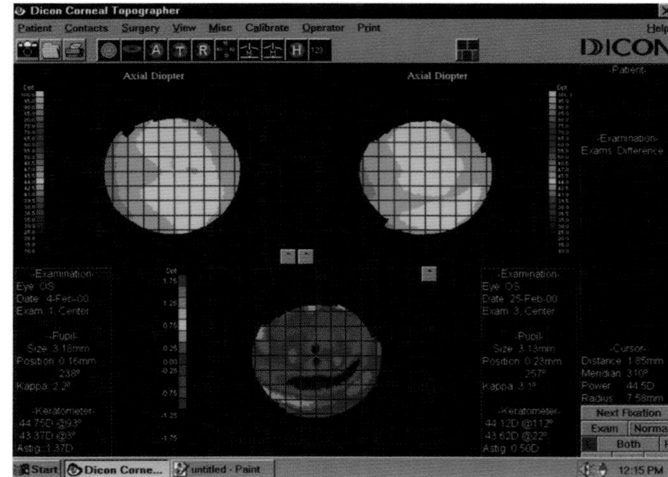

Figure 39.10 Topography difference map denoting the amount of corneal curvature change at an aftercare visit, which took place 3 weeks after dispensing a new rigid lens.

Once corneal warpage or clinically significant shape changes have been detected, the aftercare strategy should focus on adjusting the lens fit and monitoring the cornea for resolution. Soft lens-induced corneal curvature changes have been shown to stabilize between 6 and 18 weeks after discontinuing lens use (Sarzynski *et al.*, 1997). In rigid lens-induced corneal warpage, up to 6 months may be required for a return to stable corneal topography (Wilson *et al.*, 1996). If refitting a long-term PMMA contact lens wearer into rigid lenses, improved corneal health is be expected and spectacle-corrected acuity may improve, but the general topographic patterns of corneal warpage may not improve significantly (Novo *et al.*, 1995).

Posterior corneal elevation

Corneal topography has really evolved as a gold-standard method of measuring and following the cornea during contact lens fitting, and most devices used in practice are Placido-based systems. However, state-of-the-art elevation-based systems that can image the posterior corneal surface have evolved and are now increasingly found in more centres. The advantage to the contact lens patient is the ability to screen for abnormally high posterior surface elevation which would not have been detected with anterior-surface topography. Contact lenses can rarely alter the posterior corneal surface elevation; however, having access to such a measurement can help differentiate early keratoconus, posterior keratoconus (Figure 39.11) and postsurgical ectasia from other conditions causing decreased acuity

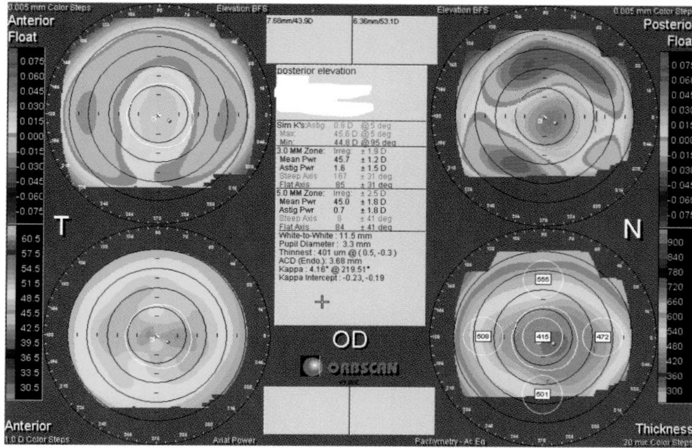

Figure 39.11 Abnormal posterior corneal elevation in an otherwise asymptomatic myopic contact lens wearer. The high posterior elevation results in central corneal thinning.

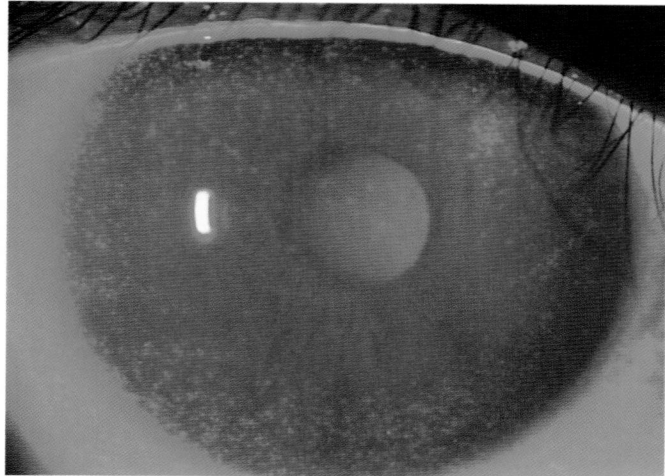

Figure 39.12 Corneal staining in a silicone hydrogel lens wearer using a multipurpose cleaning and storage solution.

which could not be detected with anterior-surface topography. Thus, in aftercare procedures, the best patients to utilize this instrumentation on are refractive surgery patients who resumed contact lens wear and have a decrease in visual acuity (to screen for posterior corneal ectasia), and other patients who have decreased visual acuity which cannot be accounted for by any other pathology after a complete dilated exam has been performed.

Using the Orbscan instrument, the average amount of maximum posterior elevation is about 21–28 µm in non-diseased eyes. In a series of 140 normal eyes examined by Wei *et al.* (2006), the maximum posterior elevation was never greater than 46 µm. Therefore, if using the Orbscan instrument, a posterior elevation greater than 50 µm is clearly out of the range of normal. Some feel that a posterior elevation greater than 40 µm, when coupled with positive findings on other topographic screening programmes, is a cause for concern (Rao *et al.*, 2002). The Pentacam instrument differs from Orbscan and generally provides much lower values for posterior corneal elevation. If using this instrument, suggested cutpoints to delineate forme fruste KC range from 15.5–32 µm.

Slit-lamp biomicroscopy

Biomicroscopy with fluorescein instillation and upper-lid eversion is essential at each aftercare visit. The clinical technique of slit-lamp biomicroscopy as it specifically applies to contact lens wear has been described in Chapter 37. The various ocular complications associated with contact lens wear are described in Chapter 40.

During each aftercare visit, a general anterior-segment examination should be performed and any significant findings carefully noted on the record card. The general anterior-segment examination includes an assessment of the lids and adnexa, conjunctiva, cornea, tear film, anterior chamber, iris and lens. Additionally, the progress evaluation form should contain a clinical grade of the severity of any observed tissue change under evaluation (see section on grading scales, below).

With silicone hydrogel lenses encompassing more of the contact lens market, it is important at this stage to screen for lens–solution incompatibility. This can be detected by the presence of corneal staining, as seen in Figure 39.12. It is most evident 2 h after lens insertion in silicone hydrogel wearers who utilize a multipurpose solution (Jones *et al.*, 2002; Garofalo *et al.*, 2005; Andrasko and Ryen, 2008).

Lens inspection and verification

Lens inspection and verification is an important final step of the aftercare visit. Lenses can be inspected using a 10× hand loupe or a binocular microscope. Alternatively, the lens can be retained using rubber-tipped tweezers and held in position adjacent to the brow rest of a slit-lamp biomicroscope. A broad beam is used to illuminate the lens, which is best viewed against a dark background.

The techniques of soft and rigid lens verification are described in Chapters 8 and 15. Rigid lens verification is important because these lenses can steepen or flatten with time and may be susceptible to warpage. An assessment made on a patient who – unknown to the practitioner – is wearing a distorted lens, may result in that practitioner reordering a lens of inappropriate parameters. Additionally, rigid lens power changes have been shown to be induced as a result of overzealous lens cleaning by patients. For example, increased minus power in rigid lenses can result from aggressive digital cleaning with abrasive cleaners on silicone acrylate lenses (O'Donnell, 1994; Woods and Efron, 1999). Soft lenses can also be verified in cases of suspected lens mix-up or to characterize the key features of the lens of a patient who may be new to the practice.

Additional procedures

Additional procedures, which may not be readily available to all contact lens clinicians, include corneal thickness measurements (pachymetry) and endothelial specular microscopy. If available, these techniques afford valuable information that can have an impact on the management of contact lens patients at early and late aftercare visits. Digital slit-lamp imaging is a valuable method of recording clinical information; this technique is described in Chapter 41.

Pachymetry

Ultrasonic pachymetry has largely replaced optical pachymetry for measuring corneal thickness in clinical practice. Ultrasonic pachymetry has the advantage of ease of use, allowing ancillary staff to operate the apparatus proficiently with only modest training. The small size of an ultrasonic pachymeter makes it portable and convenient. During contact lens aftercare, the primary application of an ultrasound pachymeter is to assess corneal swelling in extended-wear patients.

It is a well-established finding that, with no lens wear, the cornea swells by an average of 2–4% overnight during sleep (eye closure). In extended wear with traditional hydrogel lenses, an average of about 10% corneal swelling has been documented. This level of oedema is difficult or impossible to detect with the slit-lamp biomicroscope. However, it is important to be able to measure low levels of oedema when prescribing and following patients in extended wear. Indeed, some practitioners use the corneal swelling response as an indicator of successful extended-wear candidates. Solomon (1996) has advocated the use of ultrasonic pachymetry to measure corneal thickness changes after one night of lens wear as the basis of a 'stress test' for extended-wear lenses. This is essentially a 'provocative test' to identify patients who are at risk for developing significant oxygen deprivation, as indicated by the oedema response. If more than 5% swelling occurs, the patient should be discouraged from continuing in extended wear (Solomon, 1996).

Corneal thickness may also be determined from some of the elevation-based topographic systems such as Orbscan II or Pentacam or even optical coherence tomography. However, clinicians should be aware that corneal thickness measurements are influenced by the method of measurement and that, although highly correlated, instruments such as ultrasound pachymetry, anterior-segment optical coherence tomography and Orbscan II should not be used interchangeably for the assessment of corneal thickness (Li *et al.*, 2007).

Corneal endothelial analysis

Specular microscopy is an *in vivo* technique of viewing the corneal endothelium. It is a standard method for determining cell loss or changes in cell size (polymegethism) or cell shape (pleomorphism) with ageing (Laing *et al.*, 1976) and following contact lens wear (Carlson *et al.*, 1988). In the contact lens practice, the major function of this device is to evaluate the short-term endothelial response ('blebs') (Holden *et al.*, 1985b), and, more importantly, the long-term endothelial response to contact lens wear (polymegethism and pleomorphism, referenced to age-matched normals) (Carlson *et al.*, 1988) during the aftercare visits. These endothelial responses to contact lens wear are described in Chapter 40.

Other tests as required

Although the patient may be presenting for an eye examination relating to contact lens wear, practitioners have an obligation to be cognizant of all possible causes of reported signs and symptoms, which on occasion may be unrelated to lens wear. If time is available, and/or the signs and symptoms are marked, it may be necessary to undertake a procedure that normally relates to a primary eye care examination, such as visual fields, ophthalmoscopy, tonometry, gonioscopy, binocular vision assessment, corneal sensitivity, Tearscope evaluation and colour vision assessment. If, for whatever reason, these techniques cannot be undertaken at the time of the aftercare visit, another appointment should be made, or the patient should be referred for specialist attention, as appropriate.

Discussion with patient

A critical aspect of the aftercare visit is the final discussion with the patient concerning the outcome of the consultation. The patient should be given reassurances as appropriate – for example, that the cause of the signs/symptoms has been identified (assuming this to be the case) and that the remedial action recommended should solve the problem. An explanation should be given to the patient as to why changes are being made – for example, that lenses are being changed because the patient has become more myopic through natural progression. The patient should be invited to ask any questions. Potential or actual aspects of non-compliance detected during the examination can be raised with the patient, and good practice reinforced. The essence of this discussion should be noted on the record card (Veys *et al.*, 2001). Finally, patients should be instructed of the date and time of their next aftercare appointment, and they should be instructed to wear their lenses to the next aftercare visit and to bring their lens case, solutions and any other paraphernalia associated with lens wear.

Grading scales

As an aid to accurate record keeping, health care practitioners of all disciplines often resort to the use of standardized grading scales of various conditions. Presented in Appendix K are the Efron grading scales for contact lens complications (Efron, 2000); these provide a simple, convenient and accurate means by which clinicians can record and communicate the severity of complications of contact lens wear. The Efron grading scales were painted by an ophthalmic artist; the advantage of using painted (versus photographic) grading scales is that greater clarity can be achieved because the precise level of severity can be depicted, all other factors can be kept constant, potentially confounding artefacts can be avoided and artistic licence can be adopted. The grading assigned to a particular condition can serve as a reference against which any future tissue change may be assessed, and can therefore influence clinical decision making. These grading scales may act as a standard clinical reference for describing the severity of contact lens complications.

Grading scale design

The primary design criteria upon which the Efron grading scales are based are simplicity, convenience and ease of use by clinicians. Sixteen sets of grading images are depicted in two panels, each comprising eight complications. These 16 grading scales cover the key anterior ocular complications of contact lens wear. Those shown on the panel beginning with 'conjunctival redness' are frequently encountered;

Table 39.2 Magnification of complications (relative to a whole cornea being × 1) depicted in the Efron grading scales

Complication	Magnification	Image depicted in Figure 39.13
Corneal staining	1×	A
Corneal ulcer	1×	B
Corneal infiltrates	1×	C
Corneal neovascularization	1×	D
Papillary conjunctivitis	1×	E
Meibomian gland dysfunction	1×	F
Blepharitis	1×	G
Superior limbic keratoconjunctivitis	2×	H
Limbal redness	2×	I
Conjunctival staining	2×	J
Conjunctival redness	2×	K
Corneal distortion	2×	L
Corneal oedema	40×	M
Epithelial microcysts	100×	N
Endothelial blebs	200×	O
Endothelial polymegethism	600×	P

those in the other panel are less common and thus less likely to be graded routinely. On each panel, complications are depicted in the approximate order that they would be encountered in the course of a typical slit-lamp examination of the eye. Each complication is illustrated in five stages of increasing severity, from 0 to 4, with 'traffic light' colour banding from green (normal) to red (severe). The severity of the complications is based on an appraisal of accumulated evidence in the literature and clinical experience.

Image size

Each complication has been painted to an equivalent level of magnification that addresses the compromise between being high enough to depict the key features of the tissue changes, and being low enough to relate to what practitioners can observe with available clinical techniques. The approximate magnification of each complication (relative to a whole cornea depicted as 1×) is given in Table 39.2.

Figure 39.13 shows the 16 complications at grade 4 severity (each of which is identified by a letter code in Table 39.2) and indicates the approximate magnification of the images with a series of size boxes.

A consequence of these magnification levels is that, although epithelial microcysts and endothelial blebs can be detected and graded at 40× magnification on a slit-lamp biomicroscope, they will not be viewed at the resolution depicted. Furthermore, endothelial polymegethism can only be assessed with the aid of an endothelial microscope. All other complications can be viewed at the resolution depicted and are capable of being graded by direct observation and/or using a slit-lamp biomicroscope up to 40× magnification.

How to grade

Grading is a simple procedure that can be undertaken with little additional chair time (Efron and McCubbin, 2007). The tissue change of interest should be observed directly or with the aid of a slit-lamp biomicroscope, under low and/or high magnification as required, and the grade of severity should be estimated to the nearest 0.1 scale unit. For example, a tissue change that is judged to be considerably more severe than grade 2, but not quite as severe as grade 3, may be assigned a grade of 2.8 or 2.9. Although this procedure can sometimes be difficult (Efron and Chaudry, 2007), grading to the nearest 0.1 scale unit (rather than simply assigning a whole-digit grade of 0, 1, 2, 3 or 4) affords much greater precision and increases the sensitivity of the grading scale for detecting real changes or differences in severity. Objective, automated grading is also possible using digital image capture and analysis (Peterson and Wolffsohn, 2009).

How to record grading

Various grading scales are available, so it is important to designate clearly the grading system used and the specific tissue change being graded. A more expedient approach would be to print or stamp the 16 tissue changes on to a record card, each with an accompanying box, for entering the assigned grade. It may be necessary to make additional annotations to describe the condition more fully – for example, to indicate the location of the pathology. Increasingly, practitioners are using computers for clinical record keeping. Specially designed software for this purpose could include either the picture-based grading scales or computer morphs of the images. The latter have been shown to offer considerable utility in terms of recording gradings (Efron *et al.*, 2002).

Interpretation of grading

The five-stage 0–4 grading scale is based on a universally accepted concept whereby a higher numeric grade denotes greater clinical severity. This schema can be applied to any tissue change. The designation and general interpretation of each grading step are shown in Table 39.3; it must be recognized that these are only very general guidelines, and are not intended to replace sound professional judgement.

There are two exceptions with respect to the above interpretation. Corneal ulceration may require urgent action when detected or even suspected at any level of severity. Endothelial blebs require no clinical action, even at grade 4.

When using grading scales for the first time, a confidence range of about 1.2 is to be expected (Efron *et al.*, 2001); however, with experience, this confidence range may reduce to 0.7 grading scale units. In general, a change or difference of more than about 1.0 grading scale unit, or a level of severity of more than grade 2, is considered to be clinically significant. Practitioners can determine their own grading precision using a grading tutor (Efron and Morgan, 2001).

Determinants of grading performance

Reliable and accurate grading of contact lens complications is thought to be a function of three attributes, which

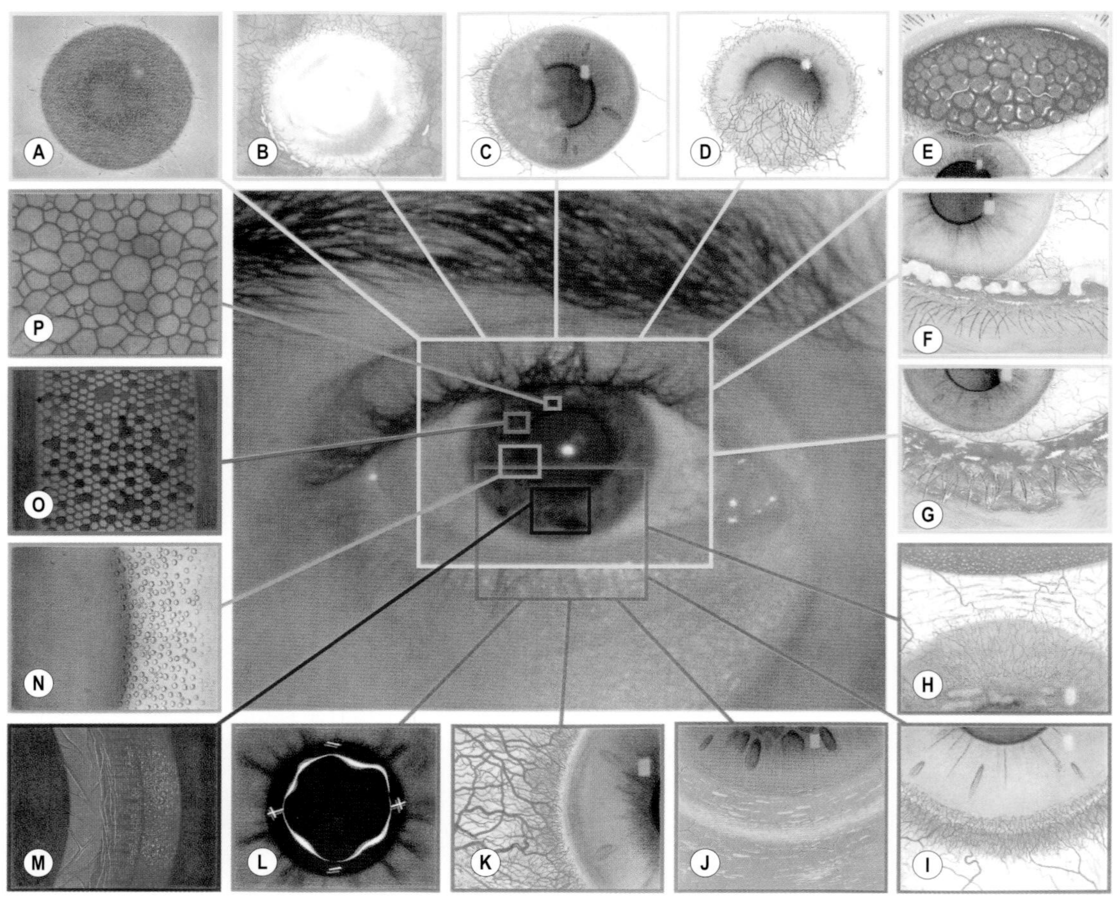

Figure 39.13 The 16 complications represented in the Efron grading scales (presented in full in Appendix K), depicted here at grade 4 severity. The approximate magnification of each complication (relative to the whole cornea being 1× magnification) is indicated by coloured boxes interposed over the image of the eye. The 16 complications are labelled with a letter code and are identified in Table 39.2.

Table 39.3 Designation and interpretation of the various levels of severity depicted in the Efron grading scales

Grade	Severity	Colour band	Clinical interpretation
0	Normal	Green	Clinical action not required
1	Trace	Lime	Clinical action rarely required
2	Mild	Yellow	Clinical action possibly required
3	Moderate	Orange	Clinical action usually required
4	Severe	Red	Clinical action certainly required

collectively constitute the 'clinical skills set' (Efron *et al.*, 2003a):

1. knowledge – the broad knowledge base that underpins the clinical task, e.g. that attribute gained after optometric training
2. training – the pedagogic experience of teaching and guided learning, e.g. lectures, tutorials, workshops, directed learning
3. experience – the repeated use of a grading scale over time, e.g. that attribute gained with unguided learning by 'trial and error'.

Efron *et al.* (2003a) found that those without ophthalmic training (engineering students) were able to grade as accurately as optometrists, although less reliably and with less confidence. They concluded that the possession of a relevant clinical skills set ensures that one is more reliable and confident when grading contact lens complications. Further studies revealed that grading reliability is not enhanced by training but does improve with experience (Efron *et al.*, 2003b).

General approaches to solving problems

Patient-reported symptoms generally fall into three broad categories, relating to the following:

1. Appearance of the eyes – for example, 'my eyes have been quite red lately'.
2. Ocular discomfort – for example, 'the lenses are irritating my eyes'.
3. Poor visual quality – for example, 'everything seems a little hazy'.

Indeed, it was probably the realization that this is the classical pattern of symptomatology in contact lens practice that led to the adoption of the catchphrase advice that is often related to patients – to check periodically that one's eyes 'look good, feel good and see good (well)' (see Chapter 38). It is pertinent, therefore, to consider strategies for solving problems relating to these categories of symptoms.

Eye redness

Conjunctival redness is so obvious and easily recognizable that it is perhaps the only sign of contact lens wear that is also reported as a symptom by patients. Indeed, excessive eye redness is cosmetically unsightly and is generally perceived as a potential disadvantage of wearing contact lenses. It is recognized in eye care generally that the clinical presentation of a 'red eye' can be one of the most difficult cases to solve due to the numerous possible causes that are known. This problem may be even more complex in a contact lens wearer because there are many additional contact lens-related causes of red eye.

Characterizing eye redness

Throughout the literature, the terms hyperaemia, injection, vascularity and redness are used as synonyms. These terms are defined as follows:

- Hyperaemia – increased blood in a part, resulting in distension of the blood vessels (Osol, 1973).
- Injection – a state of hyperaemia (Osol, 1973).
- Vascularity – the quality of vessels (Osol, 1973).
- Redness – of or approaching the colour seen at the least-refracted end of the spectrum, of shades varying from crimson to bright brown and orange (Sykes, 1976).

In strict terms, 'hyperaemia' or 'injection' is the cause and 'redness' is the effect. That is, an increased volume of blood in the conjunctival vessels (hyperaemia or injection) causes an increased appearance of redness. The term 'vascularity' is somewhat ambiguous and could represent both the cause and effect.

Strategies for diagnosing and solving eye redness

When a contact lens-wearing patient presents with a red eye as a primary complaint, the initial diagnostic step is to determine whether or not the problem is related to lens wear. This can often be simply solved by removing the lens; eye redness should dissipate rapidly if the problem is purely lens-related. However, the possibility that the lens was somehow exacerbating a complication unrelated to lens wear itself should not be discounted.

Another differential diagnosis that may be necessary when presented with an extremely red eye is to determine to what extent the redness is due to conjunctival injection or ciliary flush. Two simple tests can be applied. A sterile cotton bud can be held lightly against the bulbar conjunctiva in the region of redness and gently moved from side to side. The conjunctival vessels will move but the ciliary vessels will remain in a fixed position. It can then be determined whether the redness relates primarily to the 'moving' vessels (indicating conjunctival involvement) or the 'static' vessels (indicating ciliary involvement).

An alternative test is to instil a decongestant into the eye (Jose *et al.*, 1984). The effect of a decongestant is limited to the superficial conjunctival vessels; these drugs have no effect on the deeper ciliary vessels. Thus, if the instillation of a decongestant alleviates eye redness, the condition is primarily conjunctival. If the decongestant has no impact on the appearance of the eye, then the redness can be attributed to excessive ciliary flush.

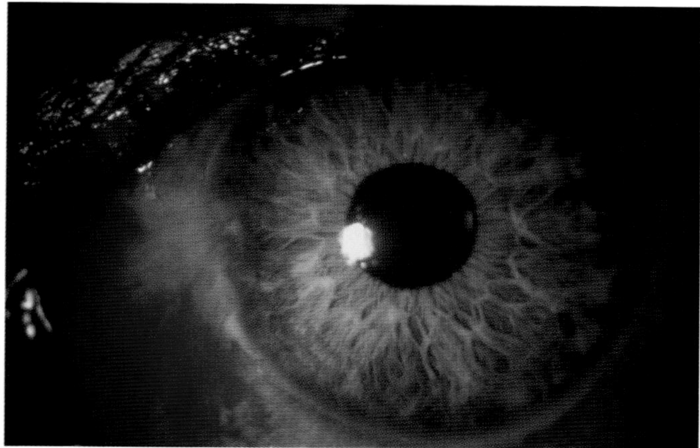

Figure 39.14 Conjunctival haemorrhage in the eye of a soft lens wearer who was struck in the eye by a squash ball. Note the clear avascular zone around the limbus.

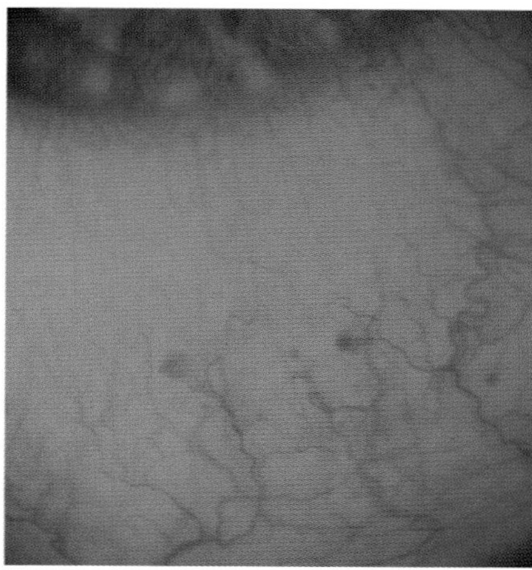

Figure 39.15 Small conjunctival haemorrhages observed in a patient wearing soft lenses.

A subconjunctival haemorrhage can be easily differentiated from conjunctival and/or ciliary hyperaemia because of the stark appearance of an intensely 'blood-red' eye and the lack of hyperaemia around the limbus (Figure 39.14).

Small haemorrhages of individual conjunctival vessels can also increase conjunctival redness (Figure 39.15), but again these are self-evident and differential diagnosis from vascular engorgement is clear.

Assuming that a given case of eye redness is lens-related, it is necessary to determine whether the source of the problem is the cornea or conjunctiva. Conjunctival redness associated with a quiet limbus and absence of pain indicates a primary conjunctival problem. Conjunctival redness associated with an injected limbus and severe pain

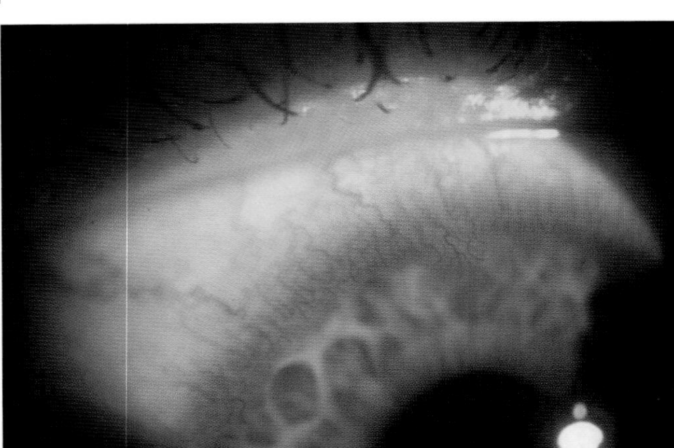

Figure 39.16 Limbal redness suggestive of corneal pathology.

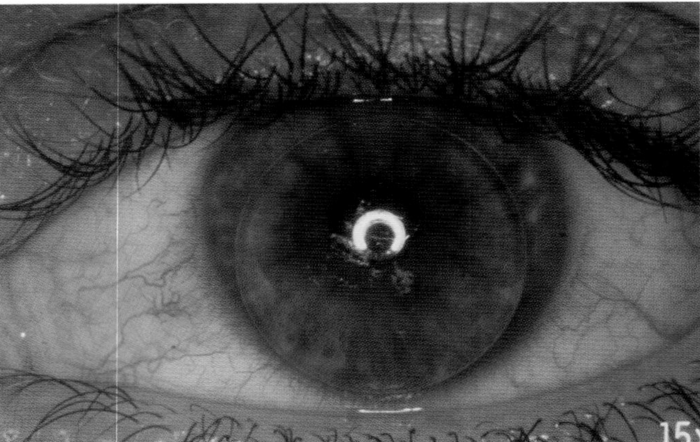

Figure 39.17 Combination of limbal and bulbar conjunctival redness in a rigid lens wearer, possibly due to 3 and 9 o'clock staining (i.e. corneal involvement) and conjunctival desiccation (i.e. conjunctival involvement).

indicates corneal involvement, or indeed a problem that is related exclusively to the cornea (Figure 39.16).

Redness of both the limbus and bulbar conjunctiva may indicate a coexistence of corneal and conjunctival pathology (Figure 39.17).

Careful examination of the anterior ocular structures with a slit-lamp biomicroscope, and inspection of the lens at high magnification, will generally reveal the cause of the problem. It may also be necessary to prescribe different care systems and differentially diagnose the effects of various solutions over time.

If the red eye is deemed to be unrelated to lens wear, then other possible causes must be investigated. This may involve a full ocular examination involving the use of direct and indirect ophthalmoscopy and tonometry.

Discomfort

The most common patient symptom that will confront a contact lens practitioner is that of discomfort, and in particular, 'dryness' (Brennan and Efron, 1989; Begley *et al.*, 2000). Reconciliation of patient symptoms with clinical signs is a constant challenge to all health care practitioners. There is always the potential to devote undue attention to a complaint that bears little significance to the well-being of the patient, or conversely to give token consideration to a symptom arising from a potentially serious condition. Furthermore, there are many signs that the clinician detects that also have a major influence upon patient management but for which the patient shows no or minimal symptoms. Conditions that may be asymptomatic, such as corneal neovascularization, microcystic oedema and endothelial polymegethism, are important pathophysiological signs that require some form of treatment – however, the most rewarding management plans, from the perspective of the patient, are those that alleviate discomfort.

During adaptation to contact lens wear, soft lenses offer a greater level of comfort than rigid lenses. Indeed, a study that assessed comfort of hydrogel lenses over short wearing periods found that more than half of lens wearers were unaware of the presence of the lens in their eyes at any given moment (Efron *et al.*, 1986). Both soft and rigid lenses are very comfortable once the patient has adapted to the lenses. Nonetheless, occasions will arise when lenses become less comfortable. Because of the subjective nature of discomfort symptoms, most reports in the literature concerning this topic have been anecdotal. Here, a systematic approach for quantification of discomfort is outlined, and management strategies for solving this problem are advanced.

The neural mechanisms by which the conjunctiva and cornea produce ocular sensibilities during contact lens wear have yet to be elucidated. Certainly, these mechanisms are somewhat imprecise. For example, ocular sensibilities are often poorly differentiated such that the description and localization of an abnormal event in the eye by a patient are often inaccurate. It is therefore not surprising that patient reports of ocular sensations can be confusing to the practitioner. In the absence of major anomalies of the lens or eye, the comfort of the lens appears to depend upon the interaction between the lid and lens.

The exact nature of the stimulus that gives rise to the sensation of dryness is also unclear and the reasons for the high frequency of this symptom in contact lens wearers are a matter for speculation, given that it is the least frequently reported symptom of non-lens wearers (McMonnies and Ho, 1986). Since there are no specific 'dryness receptors' in human tissue, the ocular sensation of 'dryness' must be a response to specific coding of afferent neural inputs. One may hypothesize that 'dryness' results from an interference with tear physiology and structure by the contact lens – the specific mechanism being an increased tear evaporation and faster break-up of the tear film. The sensation may also arise from the neural misinterpretation of stimuli seemingly unrelated to dryness, such as direct mechanical interaction of the lens with the ocular tissues, lens dehydration or vasodilation and the subsequent rise in local temperature (Efron and Brennan, 1996).

Characterizing symptoms of discomfort

Patients can employ one or more of a myriad of descriptions to describe symptoms of discomfort during contact lens wear. Terms that may be used include:

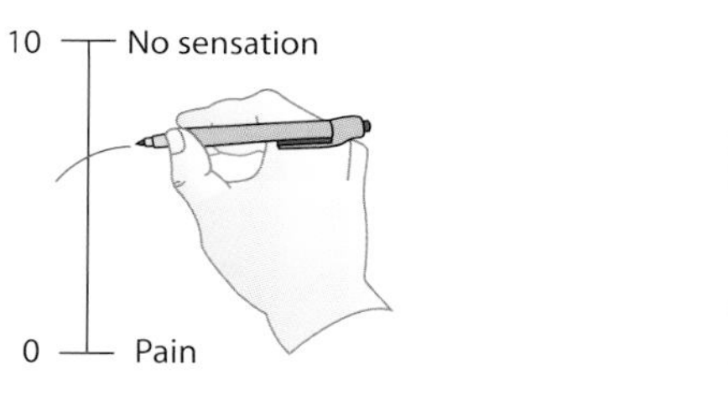

Figure 39.18 Vertical analogue scale used to quantify subjective comfort, whereby a higher number indicates greater comfort.

- scratchy
- dry
- watery
- itchy
- gritty
- hot
- cold
- burning
- tired
- irritated
- uncomfortable
- sore
- hurting
- aching
- painful.

A systematic approach can be applied for quantifying the level of subjective discomfort experienced during lens wear. Specifically, the severity of discomfort can be described in three ways:

1. Nominal – purely descriptive terms are used, such as mild or severe.
2. Ordinal – the level of severity is ranked on a scale of discrete steps; e.g. grades 0, 1, 2, 3 or 4. Descriptors may be employed for the extreme grades as a guide; e.g. grade 0 means 'no sensation' and grade 4 means 'extreme pain'.
3. Analogue – where the level of comfort is indicated on a continuous scale. A popular technique employed in contact lens research is the vertical analogue comfort scale (Figure 39.18). The patient is invited to mark the position on a vertical scale corresponding to the level of comfort. (The reason why the scale is oriented vertically is to avoid potential bias that may invalidate the use of a horizontal scale, as a result of 'handedness'.) The distance along the scale from the zero position is measured and taken as an index of the degree of comfort (so the higher the score, the more comfortable the lens).

Strategies for solving symptoms relating to discomfort

The following strategies can be employed to determine whether the discomfort is eye- or lens-related:

- Always be on the lookout for concurrent ocular pathology that may be unrelated to lens wear (e.g. glaucoma).
- Consider the laterality of the discomfort – for example, discomfort due to a toxic reaction to a contact lens solution would be expected to be bilateral, whereas discomfort due to a damaged contact lens would be expected to be unilateral.
- Remove the lenses – persistent discomfort following lens removal suggests an ocular problem, whereas relief of discomfort following lens removal suggests a lens problem.
- Swap the lenses between the eyes – an ocular problem is indicated if unilateral discomfort remains in the same eye after the lenses have been swapped; a lens-related problem is indicated if unilateral discomfort swaps to the other eye after the lenses have been swapped.
- Prescribe ocular lubricants – relief after an ocular lubricant has been instilled into the sore eye suggests a mechanical or abrasive source of the discomfort.

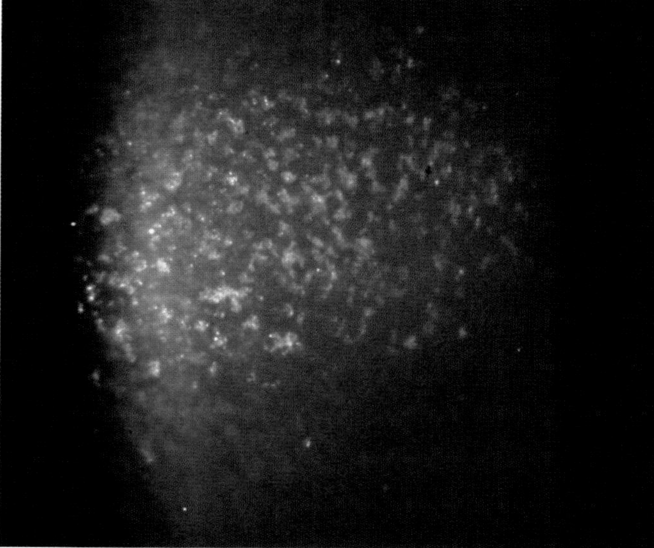

Figure 39.19 Epithelial desiccation caused by a hyperthin experimental soft lens.

There are many possible causes of lens-related discomfort. These causes, and strategies for alleviating the problem, include:

- Poor-fitting lenses – change to a better-fitting lens; specifically, a lens of larger diameter and/or steeper base curve may move less and therefore be more comfortable.
- Physical defects in lenses – replace the lens and/or change to a superior product.
- Particulate matter partially embedded in lenses – replace the lens.
- Foreign bodies beneath lenses – rinse the lens.
- End-of-day dryness in hydrogel lens wear – use a silicone hydrogel lens to enable longer weaaring times (Dumbleton *et al.*, 2008).
- A toric soft lens might be slightly less comfortable than its spherical equivalent because of thick stabilization zones – employ a toric design with a thinner profile.
- Dehydration of hyperthin soft lenses can lead to epithelial drying and discomfort (Figure 39.19) – refit the patient with a thicker lens.
- Older lenses tend to feel more dry – replace lenses more frequently.
- Lenses with surface deposits can be uncomfortable – replace the lens and increase the replacement frequency.

If a patient complains of lens discomfort, and there is no apparent cause after having carefully examined the lens and eye, the lens should be thoroughly cleaned with a surfactant cleaner, rinsed in saline and reinserted into the eye. If the discomfort persists, the lens may contain a subclinical defect or it may have a microscopic foreign body embedded in the back surface. In either case, the lens should be discarded.

Various forms of contact lens-related ocular pathology can cause discomfort; it should be noted that the apparent severity of the tissue pathology does not necessarily correlate with the degree of discomfort suffered by the patient. Such conditions include the following:

- Corneal epithelial microcysts – may cause slight discomfort.
- Corneal stromal oedema – moderate oedema (5% swelling) can cause mild discomfort but severe oedema (20% swelling) can be very painful, although the pain may be attributed to associated pathology such as an anterior uveal reaction. Oedema associated with the corneal exhaustion syndrome may be very uncomfortable.
- Acute red eye – occurs in extended-wear patients, and can be very painful; lens removal often gives immediate relief.
- Superior limbic keratoconjunctivitis – causes increased lens awareness and itching; symptoms are alleviated by ceasing lens wear.
- Infectious keratitis – can be very painful, especially *Acanthamoeba* keratitis, where patients can be suicidal.
- Tear film dysfunction – discomfort is due to lens surface drying (Versura *et al.*, 2000); ocular lubricants can provide short-term relief.

Ocular discomfort during contact lens wear may be due to the use of associated lens care products. Specifically, the discomfort may be related to:

- solution pH and tonicity
- solution toxicity (Figure 39.20)
- solution allergy
- lens denaturation due to thermal disinfection (rarely used today)
- residual unneutralized hydrogen peroxide
- hydrogen peroxide burn.

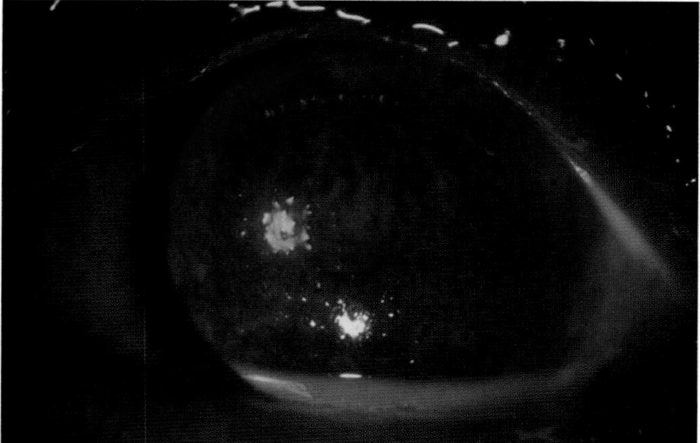

Figure 39.20 Severe toxicity reaction due to the patient inadvertently introducing a soft lens cleaning solution directly into the eye (having mistaken this for a wetting solution). Severe corneal staining is revealed with fluorescein.

Poor vision

Contact lenses are fitted to correct defects of vision. It is therefore paradoxical that, of all the topics discussed in the contact lens literature, the issue of vision correction receives relatively little attention. The causes of vision loss during contact lens wear are not always obvious, and a definitive diagnosis may be difficult due to the transient or inconsistent nature of the problem (Brennan and Efron, 1996). A wide variety of factors may lead to vision problems during contact lens wear; in this section, consideration will be given to ways in which vision loss can be denoted, and suggestions will be offered for strategies to determine the cause of suboptimal vision during contact lens wear.

Characterizing symptoms of poor vision

In addition to measuring vision with and without contact lenses, additional descriptive information relating to symptoms of poor vision should be obtained from the patient, such as:

- Severity – mild or severe.
- Consistency – constant or fluctuating.
- Onset – immediate or delayed.
- Proximity – difficulty at distance or near.
- Persistence – whether the problem persists throughout the period of lens wear and/or following lens removal.
- Description – whether the problem is best described as blur, haze, glare or some other descriptor.

Other techniques for assessing vision may help characterize the problem. These include:

- Contrast sensitivity function – may be suppressed during adaptation, but otherwise should be no different from that obtained with the best corrected spectacle prescription.
- High- and low-contrast acuity charts (Figure 39.21) – reduced acuity with a high-contrast chart suggests a refractive problem, whereas reduced acuity with a low-contrast chart indicates a 'non-refractive' problem, such as poor lens fit, ocular pathology or excess lens deposition.
- Glare sensitivity test – a bright light is positioned next to a low-contrast eye chart facing the patient; reduced vision under this condition indicates glare sensitivity, which can be due to conditions that scatter light, such

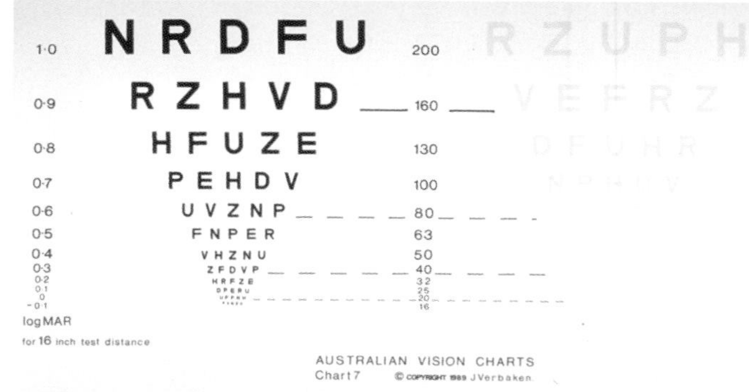

Figure 39.21 High-contrast (letters on the left) and low-contrast (letters on the right) logMAR visual acuity chart.

as epithelial oedema, epithelial microcysts and anterior-chamber flare.

Strategies for solving symptoms relating to poor vision

After the symptoms of poor vision with contact lenses have been fully characterized, the following general strategies can be employed to help resolve the problem:

- Restoration of vision immediately after lens removal (with a corrective trial lens before the eye) suggests a lens-related problem.
- Sustained vision loss after lens removal (with a corrective trial lens before the eye) suggests an ocular problem (which may or may not be related to lens wear) (Figure 39.22).

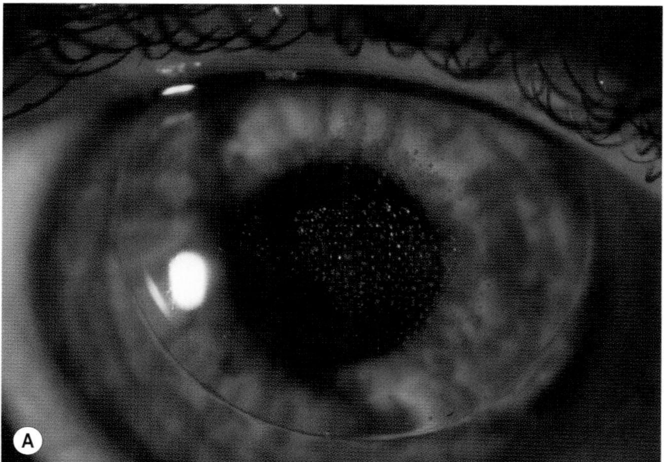

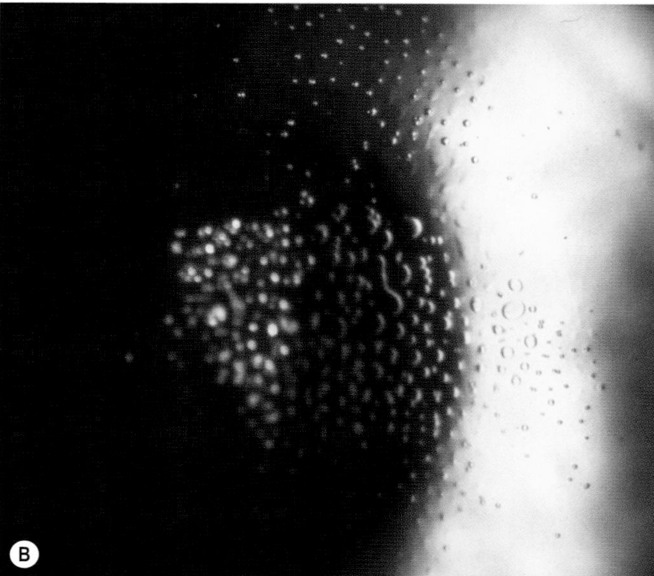

Figure 39.22 An unusual case of vision loss with rigid lenses. (A) A fine stippled appearance is evident using the slit lamp with general diffuse illumination. (B) A high-magnification photograph taken through the slit-lamp eyepiece confirms a case of extensive dimple veiling, due to bubble formations beneath the lens. On questioning, it was discovered that the lens was sprayed with 'fizzy' aerosol saline prior to lens insertion. Vision recovered after a few hours.

- Unilateral vision loss may be due to the lens or uniocular pathology.
- Bilateral vision loss may be due to a refractive cause or to general ocular pathology (e.g. toxic or allergic solution reaction) or systemic disease (e.g. diabetes).
- Worse vision immediately after a blink may signal excessive lens movement and either a flat fit (corrected by fitting the lens more steeply) or inappropriate lens rotation in the case of a soft toric lens (corrected by employing better lens stabilization techniques). This indicator is correlated with the appearance of keratometer mires before and after the blink (discussed above; see Figure 39.2).
- Improved vision immediately after a blink may signal a tight fit (corrected by fitting the lens more loosely).

The following causes of vision loss with contact lenses relate to spherical refractive error:

- Patients may be unaware that the lens has become displaced from the cornea on to the sclera, or even lost from the eye, leaving vision uncorrected – inspect the eye.
- Shifts in refractive error can reduce vision – check the refraction.
- Lens power may have been ordered, and therefore supplied, incorrectly – check the record card against the power specified on the lens box.
- Lens power may have been ordered correctly but supplied incorrectly – check the record card against the power specified on the lens box.
- Lens power may be incorrect (manufacturing/packaging error) – measure the power of the lens and check this against the power specified on the lens box.
- The tear layer beneath a rigid lens can have significant optical power – reconcile ocular refraction, overrefraction, keratometry readings, lens parameters and observed fluorescein pattern.
- Flexure of thick soft lenses can induce power shifts – fit lenses that are thinner and/or made of a material of lower modulus.

An uncorrected astigmatic component of a refraction with contact lenses can be due to:

- An astigmatic shift in refraction.
- Residual uncorrected astigmatism.
- Mislocation of toric lens cylinder axis.
- Lens power may have been ordered, and therefore supplied, incorrectly – check the record card against the power specified on the lens box.
- Lens power may have been ordered correctly but supplied incorrectly – check the record card against the power specified on the lens box.
- Lens power may be incorrect (manufacturing/packaging error) – measure the power of the lens and check this against the power specified on the lens box.
- Corneal warpage.

Contact lens correction of presbyopia entails a variety of visual compromises, such as:

- Monovision correction – degrades stereopsis at near.
- Alternating-vision bifocal lenses – incomplete or improper lens translation will compromise vision.

- Simultaneous-vision bifocal lenses – the visual system may have difficulty in processing clear and blurred images on the same region of retina; non-optimal pupil size will degrade vision.

Most non-optical causes of vision loss relate to problems of poor lens fitting, such as the following:

- Flat-fitting lenses will decentre away from the pupil.
- Excessive postlens movement can degrade vision.
- Steep-fitting lenses may buckle in the centre and degrade vision.
- Hyperthin soft lenses can dehydrate the epithelium, leading to vision loss.
- Lenses of low oxygen transmissibility can induce gross oedema, leading to vision loss.
- Poor lens surface quality – due to manufacturing problems, lens deposits or excessive surface drying – can degrade vision (Tutt *et al.*, 2000).

A variety of pathological and non-pathological ocular problems relating to lens wear can cause vision loss, including:

- corneal infection
- tear film dysfunction
- corneal epithelial desiccation
- corneal epithelial oedema
- corneal stromal oedema
- corneal stromal infiltrates
- corneal neovascularization
- corneal warpage
- binocular vision problems.

Conclusions

Aftercare examinations should be undertaken routinely on all contact lens wearers, on the basis that 'prevention is better than cure'. A thoughtful approach to these visits should, in most cases, result in the early detection of subclinical problems. Remedial action can often be undertaken without the patient being aware that a problem exists.

Patients can present for unscheduled visits complaining of one or more of a large number of possible problems – for reasons that are not necessarily the fault of the patient or practitioner. A strategic approach can be adopted, whereby patient-reported problems are considered in the context of three broad categories – eye appearance (redness), discomfort and poor vision. This approach should facilitate an efficient determination of a likely cause and appropriate remedial action can be put into effect. The outcome – whether any action taken is related to prevention or cure – should be a happy patient who is motivated to continue to derive the undoubted benefits of contact lenses.

References

Andrasko, G. and Ryen, K. (2008) Corneal staining and comfort observed with traditional and silicone hydrogel lenses and multipurpose solution combinations. *Optometry*, **79**, 444–454. Comment in: *Optometry*, **80**, 116–117; author reply 117–118.

Barnett, W. A. and Rengstorff, R. H. (1977) Adaptation to hydrogel contact lenses: variations in myopia and corneal curvature measurements. *J. Am. Optom. Assoc.*, **48**, 363–366.

Begley, C. G., Caffery, B., Nichols, K. K. *et al.* (2000) Responses of contact lens wearers to a dry eye survey. *Optom. Vis. Sci.*, **77**, 40–46.

Binder, P. S. (1983) Myopic extended wear with the Hydrocurve II soft contact lens. *Ophthalmology*, **90**, 623–626.

Brennan, N. A. and Efron, N. (1989) Symptomatology of HEMA contact lens wear. *Optom. Vis. Sci.*, **66**, 834–838.

Brennan, N. A. and Efron, N. (1996) Visual problems with contact lenses. In *Contact Lenses: Treatment Options for Ocular Disease* (M. G. Harris, ed.). In *Mosby's Optometry Problem Solving Series* (R. London, series ed.), pp. 123–138, London: Mosby.

Carlson, K. H., Bourne, W. M., Brubaker, R. F. (1988) Effect of long-term contact lens wear on corneal endothelial cell morphology and function. *Invest. Ophthalmol. Vis. Sci.*, **29**, 185–193.

Caroline, P. and Andre, M. (2005) Topographical changes after everted silicone hydrogel wear. *Contact Lens Spectrum*, **20**(6).

de Sanctis, U., Loiacono, C., Richiardi, L., *et al.* (2008) Sensitivity and Specificity of Posterior Corneal Elevation Measured by Pentacam in Discriminating Keratoconus/Subclinical Keratoconus. Ophthalmology, 115, 1534–1539 and Mihaltz, K., Kovacs, I., takacs, A., Nagy, Z. Evaluation of Keratometric, Pachymetirc, and Elevation Parameters of Keratoconus Corneas with Pentacam. Cornea. 2009 Aug 29. Epub ahead of print.

Dumbleton, K., Chalmers, R., Richter, D. *et al.* (1999) Changes in myopic refractive error with nine months extended wear of hydrogel lenses with high and low oxygen permeability. *Optom. Vis. Sci.*, **76**, 845–849.

Dumbleton, K. A., Woods, C. A., Jones, L. W. *et al.* (2008) Comfort and adaptation to silicone hydrogel lenses for daily wear. *Eye Contact Lens.*, **34**, 215–223.

Efron, N. (2000*) Efron Grading Scales for Contact Lens Complications. Millennium Edition, January 1, 2000.* Hamble, Southampton: Biocompatibles-Hydron.

Efron, N. and Brennan, N. A. (1996) Comfort problems with contact lenses. In *Contact Lenses: Treatment Options for Ocular Disease* (M. G. Harris, ed.). In *Mosby's Optometry Problem Solving Series* (R. London, series ed.), pp. 139–157, London: Mosby.

Efron, N. and Chaudry, A. (2007) Grading static versus dynamic images of contact lens complications. *Clin. Exp. Optom.*, **90**, 361–366.

Efron, N. and McCubbin, S. (2007) Grading contact lens complications under time constraints. *Optom. Vis. Sci.* **84**, 1082–1086.

Efron, N. and Morgan, P. B. (2001) The Efron Grading Tutor. In *Contact Lens Complications CD – an Interactive Multi-media Tool* (by N. Efron and P. B. Morgan). Oxford: Butterworth-Heinemann.

Efron, N., Brennan, N. A., Currie, J. M., *et al.* (1986) Determinants of the initial comfort of hydrogel contact lenses. *Am. J. Optom. Physiol. Opt.* **63**, 819–823.

Efron, N., Brennan, N. A., Bruce, A. S. *et al.* (1987) Dehydration of hydrogel lenses under normal wearing conditions. *Contact Lens Assoc. Ophthalmol. J.*, **13**, 152–156.

Efron, N., Morgan, P. B. and Katsara, S. S. (2001) Validation of grading scales for contact lens complications. *Ophthal. Physiol. Opt.*, **21**, 17–29.

Efron, N., Morgan, P. B. and Jagpal, R. (2002) Validation of computer morphs for grading contact lens complications. *Ophthal. Physiol. Opt.*, **22**, 341–349.

Efron, N., Morgan, P. B. and Jagpal, R. (2003a) The combined influence of knowledge, training and experience when grading contact lens complications. *Ophthal. Physiol. Opt.* **23,** 79–85.

Efron, N., Morgan, P. B., Farmer, C. *et al.* (2003b) Experience and training as determinants of grading reliability when assessing the severity of contact lens complications. *Ophthal. Physiol. Opt.,* **23,** 119–124.

Faber, E., Golding, T. R., Lowe, R. *et al.* (1991) Effect of hydrogel lens wear on tear film stability. *Optom. Vis. Sci.,* **68,** 380–384.

Garofalo, R. J., Dassanayake, N., Carey, C., *et al.* (2005) Corneal staining and subjective symptoms with multipurpose solutions as a function of time. *Eye Contact Lens,* **31,** 166–174.

Hart, D. E. (1987) Surface interactions on hydrogel contact lenses. Scanning electron microscopy. *J. Am. Optom. Assoc.,* **55,** 962–974.

Holden, B. A., Sweeney, D. F., Vannas, A. *et al.* (1985a) Effects of long term extended wear contact lens wear on the human cornea. *Invest. Ophthalmol. Vis. Sci.,* **26,** 1489–1501.

Holden, B. A., Williams, L. and Zantos, S. G. (1985b) The etiology of transient endothelial changes in the human cornea. *Invest. Ophthalmol. Vis. Sci.,* **26,** 1354–1360.

Jones, L., MacDougall, N. and Sorbara, L. G. (2002) Asymptomatic corneal staining associated with the use of balafilcon silicone-hydrogel contact lenses disinfected with a polyaminopropyl biguanide-preserved care regimen. *Optom. Vis. Sci.,* **79,** 753–761.

Jose, J. G., Polse, K. A. and Holden, E. K. (1984) *Optometric Pharmacology,* Orlando, FL: Grune & Stratton.

Laing, R. A., Sandstrom, M. M., Berrospi, A. R. *et al.* (1976) Changes in the corneal endothelium as a function of age. *Exp. Eye Res.,* **22,** 587–594.

Lebow, K. A. and Grohe, R. M. (1999) Differentiating contact lens induced warpage from keratoconus using corneal topography. *Contact Lens Assoc. Ophthalmol. J.,* **25,** 114–122.

Li, E. Y., Mohamed, S., Leung, C. K. *et al.* (2007) Agreement among 3 Methods to Measure Corneal Thickness: Ultrasound Pachymetry, Orbscan II, and Visante Anterior Segment Optical Coherence Tomography. *Ophthalmology,* **114,** 1842–1847.

Lin, M. C. and Snyder, C. (1999) Flexure and residual astigmatism with RGP lenses of low, medium, and high oxygen permeability. *Int. Contact Lens Clin.,* **26,** 5–9.

Lindsay, R. G., Bruce, A. S., Brennan, N. A. *et al.* (1997) Determining axis misalignment and power errors of toric soft lenses. *Int. Contact Lens Clin.,* **24,** 101–107.

Lorentz, H. and Jones, L. (2007) Lipid deposition on hydrogel contact lenses: how history can help us today. *Optom. Vis. Sci.,* **84,** 286–295.

McMonnies, C. W. and Ho, A. (1986) Marginal dry eye diagnosis: history versus biomicroscopy. In *The Preocular Tear Film in Health, Disease, and Contact Lens Wear* (F. Holly, ed.), pp. 32–40. Lubbock, TX: The Dry Eye Institute.

Morgan, P. B. and Efron, N. (2000) Hydrogel contact lens ageing. *Contact Lens Assoc. Ophthalmol. J.,* **26,** 85–90.

Nichols, J. J. (2006) Deposition rates and lens care influence on galyfilcon A silicone hydrogel lenses. *Optom. Vis. Sci.,* **83,** 751–757.

Novo, A., Pavlopoulos, G. and Feldman, S. (1995) Corneal topographic changes after refitting polymethylmethacrylate contact lens wearers into rigid gas permeable materials. *Contact Lens Assoc. Ophthalmol. J.,* **21,** 47–51.

O'Donnell, J. J. (1994) Patient-induced power changes in rigid gas permeable contact lenses: a case report and literature review. *J. Am. Optom. Assoc.,* **65,** 772–773.

Osol, A. (ed.) (1973) Blakiston's Pocket Medical Dictionary, 3rd edn, New York: McGraw-Hill.

Peterson, R. C. and Wolffsohn, J. S. (2009) Objective grading of the anterior eye. *Optom. Vis. Sci.,* **86,** 273–278.

Rao, S., Raviv, T., Majmudar, P. *et al.* (2002) Role of Orbscan II in screening keratoconus suspects before refractive surgery. *Ophthalmology,* **109,** 1642–1646.

Ruiz-Montenegro, J., Mafra, C. H., Wilson, S. E. *et al.* (1993) Corneal topographic alterations in normal contact lens wear. *Ophthalmology,* **100,** 128–134.

Sarzynski, A., Gorski, K. and Gierek-Ciaciura, S. (1997) Changes in corneal curvature in soft contact lens users. *Klin. Oczna.,* **99,** 323–326.

Smolek, M. K., Klyce, S. D. and Maeda, N. (1994) Keratoconus and contact lens induced corneal warpage analysis using the keratomorphic diagram. *Invest. Ophthalmol. Vis. Sci.,* **35,** 4192–4204.

Solomon, O. D. (1996) Corneal stress test for extended wear. *Contact Lens Assoc. Ophthalmol. J.,* **22,** 75–78.

Suwala, M., Glasier, M. A., Subbaraman, L. N. *et al.* (2007) Quantity and conformation of lysozyme deposited on conventional and silicone hydrogel contact lens materials using an in vitro model. *Eye Contact Lens,* **33,** 138–143.

Szczotka-Flynn, L. (2004) Unintended Ortho-K effect from silicone hydrogel lenses. *Contact Lens Spectrum,* **19**(8).

Sykes, J. B. (ed.) (1976) *The Concise Oxford Dictionary of Current English,* 6th edn, Oxford: Clarendon Press.

Tutt, R., Bradley, A., Begley, C. *et al.* (2000) Optical and visual impact of tear break-up in human eyes. *Invest. Ophthalmol. Vis. Sci.,* **41,** 4117–4123.

Versura, P., Bernabini, B., Torreggiani, A. *et al.* (2000) Frequent replacement and conventional daily wear soft contact lens symptomatic patients: tear film and ocular surface changes. *Int. J. Artif. Organs,* **23,** 629–636.

Veys, J., Meyler, J. and Davies, I. (2001) Contact lens aftercare. *Optician,* **220**(5779), 28–34.

Wei, R., Lim, L., Chan, W. *et al.* (2006) Evaluation of Orbscan II corneal topography in individuals with myopia. *Ophthalmology,* **113,** 117–183.

Wick, B. and Westin, E. (1999) Change in refractive anisometropia in presbyopic adults wearing monovision contact lens correction. *Optom. Vis. Sci.,* **76,** 33–39.

Wilson, S. E., Lin, D. T., Kleiss, S. D. *et al.* (1990) Topographic changes in contact lens induced corneal warpage. *Ophthalmology,* **97,** 734–744.

Wilson, S., Calossi, A., Verzella, F. *et al.* (1996) Corneal warpage resolution after refitting an RGP contact lens wearer into hydrophilic high water content material. *Contact Lens Assoc. Ophthalmol. J.,* **22,** 242–244.

Woods, C. and Efron, N. (1999) The parameter stability of a high Dk rigid lens material. *Contact Lens Ant. Eye,* **22,** 14–18.

40 CHAPTER

Complications

Nathan Efron

Introduction

Just as contact lenses have become easier to fit over the past century, our knowledge base of the ocular response to lens wear has expanded exponentially over the same period. Thus, there has been a commensurate shift in emphasis in contact lens practice away from the technical skills of lens fitting (although these are certainly still required) and more towards the theoretical knowledge and clinical diagnostic skills required for aftercare management and problem-solving.

Contact lenses can adversely affect most of the anterior ocular structures, and the conditions described in this chapter are categorized in terms of these anatomical structures. This schema reflects the natural approach to clinical decision-making, whereby the initial observation and consideration of a problem begin with an examination of the affected ocular tissue.

This chapter will review the key ocular responses to contact lens wear, some of which can have serious ocular consequences (e.g. microbial keratitis), and some of which are benign (e.g. endothelial blebs). Each of these conditions can present in various levels of severity, so to assist the reader in gaining an appreciation of this, attention is drawn to the Efron grading scales for contact lens complications in Appendix K. Throughout this chapter, references will be made to various grades of severity referenced against a five-point scale that extends from 0 (normal) to 4 (severe). More details on the application of the use of grading scales in practice are given in Chapter 39.

Eyelids

The eyelids can impact upon, and be affected by, a contact lens-wearing eye by way of their pattern of movement (e.g. blinking), their physical state (e.g. ptosis), their general state of health and the condition of the eyelashes. Each of these factors will be considered in turn.

Blinking

Contact lenses elicit reflex blinking during lens insertion, removal and other instances of manual manipulation. Also, as a result of a reflex blink, contact lenses may mislocate or become dislodged from the eye. Both soft and rigid lens wear cause the spontaneous blink rate to increase (Carney and Hill, 1984; Hill and Carney, 1984). In rigid lens wear, this change may be more related to reflex blinking rather than spontaneous blinking; that is, the increased blink rate may be a result of continual irritation caused by the lens edge buffeting against the lid margin. Such alterations to blink rate are not thought to be permanent.

Contact lenses can affect the pattern of blinking. A decrease in the frequency of occurrence of long-duration interblink periods occurs in association with rigid lens wear, but not soft lens wear. Neither rigid nor soft lens wear alters the proportion of complete, incomplete, twitch and forced blinks. Infrequent or incomplete blinking with contact lenses (Figure 40.1) can cause a number of problems, including lens surface drying and deposition, epithelial desiccation, post-lens tear stagnation, hypoxia and hypercapnia, and 3 and 9 o'clock staining. Faults in lens design and fitting can interfere with proper blink-mediated lid–lens interaction. Fewer complete eyeblinks, more incomplete eyeblinks and more eyeblink attempts were observed in rigid lens wearers with 3- and 9-o'clock staining compared with those with minimal staining and non-wearers (van der Worp *et al.*, 2008).

There are essentially two options when faced with a clinical problem relating to non-pathological disorders of spontaneous blinking activity associated with contact lens wear, such as infrequent and/or infrequent blinking. These options are to train patients to modify their blinking activity (Collins *et al.*, 1987), and/or to alter the lens type or lens fit.

Practitioners should always be alert to the possibility that apparent anomalies in the type or pattern of blinking activity in a contact lens wearer may be attributable to unrelated disease states. Interruptions to the neural input and/or muscular systems of the eyelids can adversely affect normal spontaneous blinking activity. For example, patients with Parkinson's disease exhibit a low blink rate. Increased mechanical resistance to eyelid movement as in Graves' disease can also reduce blink frequency. Local pathology of the eyelids, such as ptosis, chalazia and carcinomas, can alter eyelid function and movement, and hence interfere with normal blinking activity. It is therefore essential to rule out the possibility of unrelated pathology before ascribing blinking dysfunction to contact lens wear.

DOI: 10.1016/B978-0-7506-8869-7.00040-9

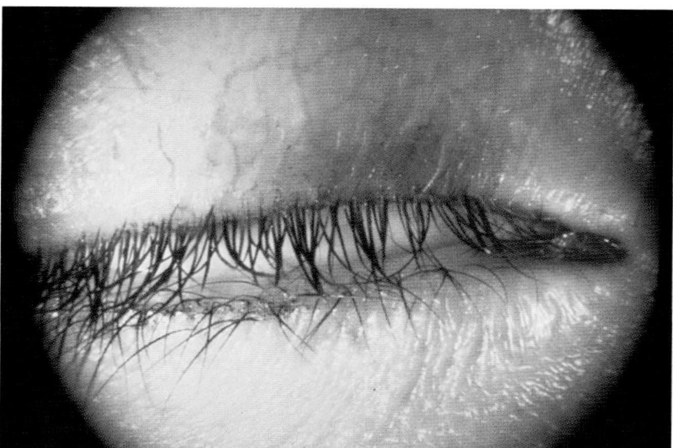

Figure 40.1 Incomplete blink in a soft lens wearer.

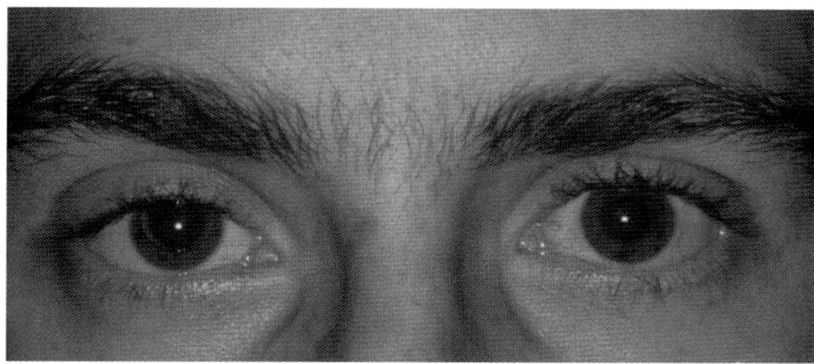

Figure 40.2 Unilateral right-eye ptosis induced by the wearing of a rigid lens in the right eye for 4 weeks on an extended-wear basis; the left eye wore a soft lens. Note that the gap between the skin fold (just beneath the eyebrows) and the upper-lid margin is greater in the right eye than the left.

Ptosis

The classical appearance of ptosis is of a narrowing of the palpebral fissure and a relatively large gap between the upper-lid margin and the skin fold at the top of the eyelid (Figure 40.2). Fonn *et al.* (1996) measured the palpebral aperture size to be 10.10 ± 1.11 mm in non-wearers and 9.76 ± 0.99 mm in rigid lens wearers; it was unaltered in soft lens wearers. According to van den Bosch and Lemij (1992), clinically significant ptosis occurs when the distance between the centre of the pupil and the lower margin of the upper lid is less than 2.8 mm. Using this criterion, contact lens-induced ptosis (CLIP) occurs in about 10% of rigid lens wearers (van den Bosch and Lemij, 1992). The ptosis takes 4–6 weeks to develop fully, and is generally noticed by patients in advanced cases. There are no associated signs or symptoms.

A number of mechanisms have been advanced as possible causes of CLIP. Those involving some form of dysfunction of the aponeurosis include forced-lid repeated squeezing and lateral eyelid stretching during lens removal, rigid lens displacement of the tarsus and blink-induced eye rubbing (Fujiwara *et al.*, 2001). Non-aponeurogenic causes of CLIP include lens-induced lid oedema, blepharospasm and papillary conjunctivitis. Watanabe *et al.* (2006) suggest that CLIP is often attributable to fibrosis in Müller muscle.

To differentiate between these possible causes, patients demonstrating CLIP should be required to cease lens wear

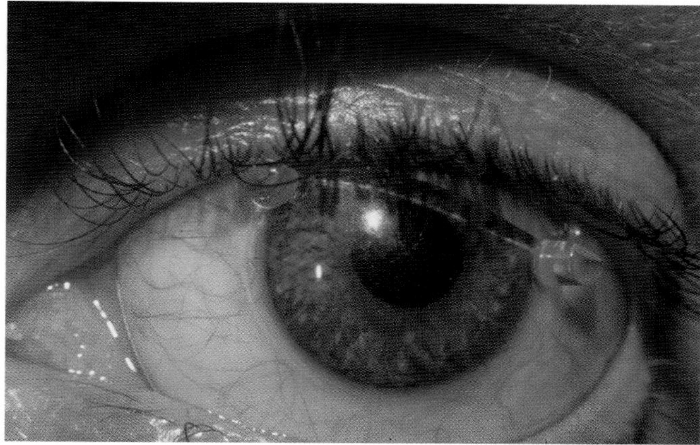

Figure 40.3 Scleral lens with 'ptosis crutch' in the form of two lugs and a shelf.

for at least 1 month (to detect any trends towards recovery) and perhaps as long as 3 months (to demonstrate complete resolution). If the CLIP partially or completely resolves after ceasing lens wear for 1 month, then the cause is lid oedema and/or involuntary blepharospasm, and the patient may need to be refitted with soft lenses (which do not induce ptosis). The eyelids should also be inverted to determine if papillary conjunctivitis is involved, and if so, appropriate action should be taken to alleviate the condition. If the ptosis persists after resolution of the papillary conjunctivitis, or after ceasing lens wear for 1 month, then the cause is most likely damage to the aponeurosis or Müller muscle, whereby surgical correction is the preferred option. Management strategies available to patients with severe CLIP who do not wish to undergo lid surgery include being fitted with a 'ptosis crutch' (Figure 40.3).

The prognosis for recovery from aponeurogenic CLIP is poor; the condition can only be reversed by surgical correction or other management options as described above. The prognosis for recovery from non-aponeurogenic CLIP is good. If the cause of ptosis is papillary conjunctivitis, the time course of resolution of the ptosis will parallel the time course of recovery of the papillary conjunctivitis.

If a contact lens wearer presents with ptosis, the numerous other possible causes of this condition must be considered so that the appropriate course of management can be adopted.

Meibomian gland dysfunction

The oily secretion from the normal meibomian gland is generally clear. The key diagnostic feature of contact lens-associated meibomian gland dysfunction (CL-MGD) is a change in the appearance of the clear oil expressed from healthy meibomian glands to a cloudy creamy yellow appearance (Figure 40.4). Frothing or foaming of the lower tear meniscus is sometimes observed in CL-MGD, especially towards the outer canthus (Figure 40.5). This appearance is accompanied by symptoms of smeary vision, greasy lenses, dry eyes and reduced tolerance to lens wear (Ong, 1996). In severe cases where the meibomian orifices are blocked, there may be an absence of gland secretion. Long-standing cases of CL-MGD may be associated with additional signs such as irregularity, distortion and thickening of eyelid margins, slight distension of glands, mild to

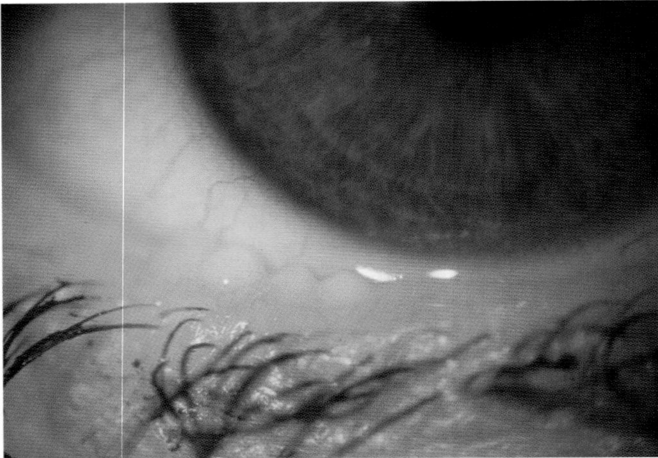

Figure 40.4 Inspissated meibomian gland secretion in the lower lid of a female patient wearing rigid lenses.

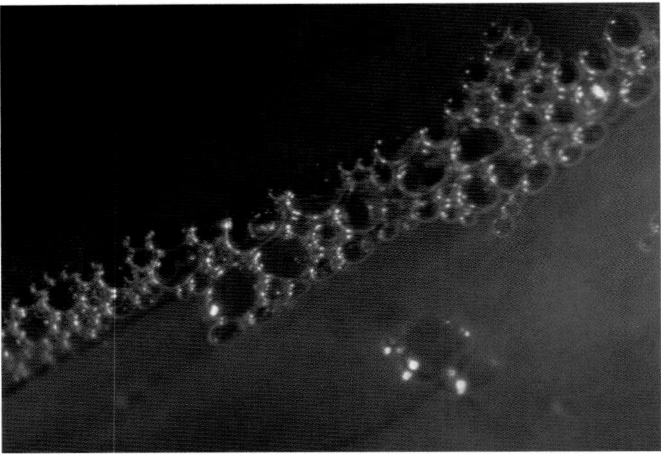

Figure 40.5 Frothing in the tear film due to meibomian gland dysfunction.

moderate papillary hypertrophy, vascular changes and chronic chalazia. The prevalence of CL-MGD is unrelated to gender but increases with age.

Associated signs of CL-MGD include all those which arise from clinical diagnostic procedures that are designed to indicate the integrity or otherwise of the lipid layer. Specifically, patients suffering from CL-MGD may display a reduced tear break-up time (measured either with fluorescein or non-invasively). Examination of the tear layer in specular reflection using a Tearscope may reveal a contaminated lipid pattern, which is exacerbated by the use of cosmetic eye make-up. Symptoms of blurred or greasy vision can probably be attributed to adhesion of waxy dysfunctional meibomian oils to the surface of the contact lens; this can lead to lens surface drying, lens dehydration and sensations of dryness.

Theories for the aetiology of CL-MGD include, firstly, that it is due to excess eye rubbing causing chronic damage to meibomian glands, and, secondly, that it occurs secondary to papillary conjunctivitis. From a tissue pathology standpoint, MGD is characterized by increased keratinization of the epithelial walls of meibomian gland ducts. As might be expected, therefore, this condition is often observed in combination with seborrhoeic dermatitis and acne rosacea. This leads to the formation of keratinized epithelial plugs that create a physical blockage in meibomian ducts, which in turn restricts or prevents the outflow of meibomian oils. Arita *et al.* (2009) have shown that contact lens wear is associated with a decrease in the number of functional meibomian glands, and that this decrease is proportional to the duration of lens wear.

Although the underlying cause of meibomian gland dysfunction cannot be treated, it is possible to provide symptomatic relief by adopting one or more of the following procedures, all of which should be undertaken with contact lenses removed:

- Application of warm compresses.
- Lid scrubs.
- Mechanical expression.
- Prescription of antibiotics.
- Use of artificial tears.
- Omega-3 dietary supplements.
- Use of surfactant lens cleaners.

By adopting these procedures, CL-MGD can be kept under good control and adverse symptoms minimized (Paugh *et al.*, 1990; Macsai, 2008).

Eyelash disorders

Disorders of the eyelashes (cilia), and of associated structures at the base of the eyelashes such as the eyelash follicles, glands of Zeis and Moll, and skin of the lid margin, have implications with respect to contact lens wear. An external hordeolum (stye) presents as a discrete, tender swelling of the anterior lid margin; specifically, it is an inflammation of the tissue lining the lash follicle and/or an associated gland of Zeis or Moll. Contact lenses may add to the discomfort due to the mechanical effect of the lens, and patients may prefer to cease lens wear during the acute phase of the formation of a stye.

Blepharitis is classified as being either anterior or posterior. Posterior blepharitis is a disorder of the meibomian glands; this was considered earlier. Anterior blepharitis is directly related to infections of the base of the eyelashes and manifests in two forms – staphylococcal and seborrhoeic. Staphylococcal anterior blepharitis is caused by a chronic staphylococcal infection of the eyelash follicles. The lid margins are covered in shiny brittle scales (Figure 40.6), and patients may complain of burning, dryness, itching, foreign-body sensations and mild photophobia. Management strategies include antibiotic ointment, promoting lid hygiene (Keys, 1996), application of weak topical steroids and artificial tears. Seborrhoeic anterior blepharitis is due to a disorder of the glands of Zeis and Moll. The signs and symptoms are similar but less severe than for staphylococcal anterior blepharitis. Contact lens wear is generally contraindicated during an acute phase of anterior blepharitis, especially if the cornea is compromised. Attention to lens cleaning is critical to prevent continued recontamination of the eye. Daily disposable contact lenses will eliminate the problem of recontamination by contact lenses.

Infestation of the eyelashes by mites or lice can lead to signs and symptoms that closely resemble marginal blepharitis. Typical symptoms include pruritus, burning, crusting, itching, swelling of the lid margins and loss and

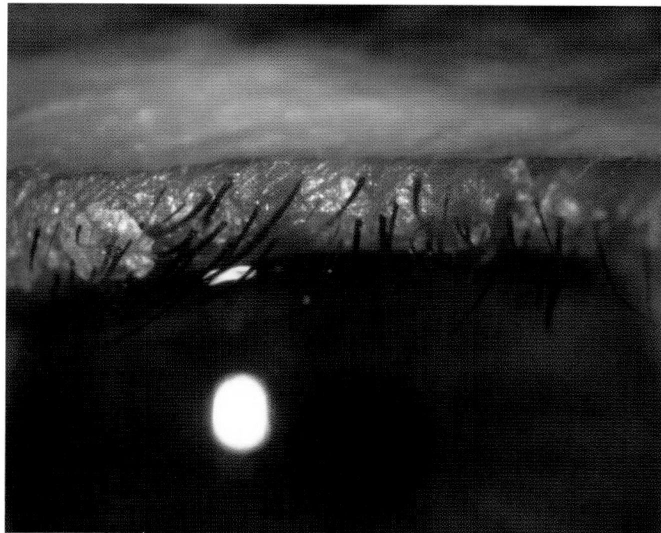

Figure 40.6 Staphylococcal anterior blepharitis.

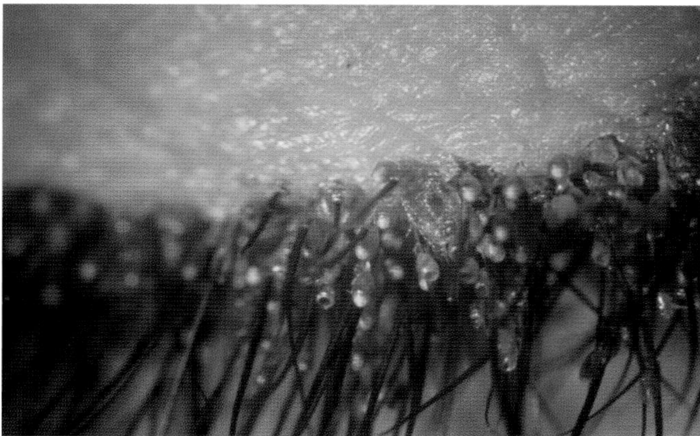

Figure 40.7 A nearly transparent crab louse can be seen at the root of the lashes, surrounded by nits encapsulated in shells, and some empty shells.

easy removal of lashes. The itching often parallels the 10-day mite reproductive cycle.

The pubic or 'crab' louse (*Phthirus pubis*) has two pairs of strong grasping claws on the central and hind legs, allowing it to hold on to eyelashes with considerable tenacity. Crab louse infestation (phthiriasis) is considered to be a venereal disease because it is passed on by sexual contact, although infestation from contaminated bedding and towels is another possible mode of transfer.

Signs of phthiriasis include pruritus of the lid margins, blepharitis, marked conjunctival injection, madarosis and the presence of lice as well as oval, greyish-white nit shells attached to the base of lashes (Figure 40.7). Additional signs include preauricular lymphadenopathy and secondary infection along the lid margins at the site of lice bites. The most predominant symptom is intense itching. The initial course of action is to attempt to remove as many mites and mite eggs as possible. Patients should be advised to engage in vigorous lid scrubbing twice daily using commercially available preparations. In general, contact lens wearers presenting with parasitic infestation of the eyelids should be treated in the same way as similarly infested non-lens-wearers (Caroline *et al.*, 1991).

Tear film

The functions of the tear film during contact lens wear can be categorized as follows:

- Optical – the tear film maintains an optically uniform interface between the air and the anterior surface of the lens.
- Mechanical – the tear film acts as a vehicle for the continual blink-mediated removal of intrinsic and extrinsic debris and particulate matter from the front of the lens and from beneath the lens.
- Lubricant – the tear film ensures a smooth movement of the eyelids over the front surface of the lens, and of the lens over the globe, during blinking.
- Bactericidal – the tear film contains defence mechanisms in the form of proteins, antibodies, phagocytotic cells and other immunodefence mechanisms that prevent contact lens-induced infection.
- Nutritional – the tear film supplies the corneal epithelium with necessary supplies of oxygen, glucose, amino acids and vitamins beneath contact lenses via the lid–lens tear pump.
- Waste removal – the tear film acts as an intermediate reservoir for the removal of corneal metabolic byproducts, such as carbon dioxide and lactate, from beneath the lens via the lid–lens tear pump.

This section will outline how these functions can be compromised during lens wear leading to the primary problem of dryness and the secondary problem of mucus ball formation. Techniques for detecting and resolving these problems are also considered.

Dry eye

Of all the symptoms experienced by contact lens wearers, that of 'dryness' is reported most frequently (Brennan and Efron, 1989); about half of all wearers have symptoms of dryness and discomfort (Fonn, 2007). A major difficulty in assessing the symptom of 'dryness' is that there may be many stimuli that elicit this sensation; that is, it can not be assumed that the cause of a patient symptom of 'dryness' is necessarily due to the eye being dry. Because there are no specific 'dryness receptors' in human tissue, ocular dryness must be a response to specific coding of afferent neural inputs. Aside from an actual dry eye, reports of 'dryness' may arise from the neural misinterpretation of stimuli that are unrelated to dry eye, such as vasodilation induced by mechanical irritation of ocular tissues by deposits on the lens surface. Thus, the condition of 'dry eye' may be related to a broad spectrum of tear film abnormalities in addition to a reduced tear volume.

A prudent initial approach in dealing with a tentative diagnosis of contact lens-induced dry eye is to apply a comprehensive questionnaire that draws in other systemic correlates of dryness, such as dryness of other mucous membranes of the body, use of medications, effect of different challenging environments and times when dryness

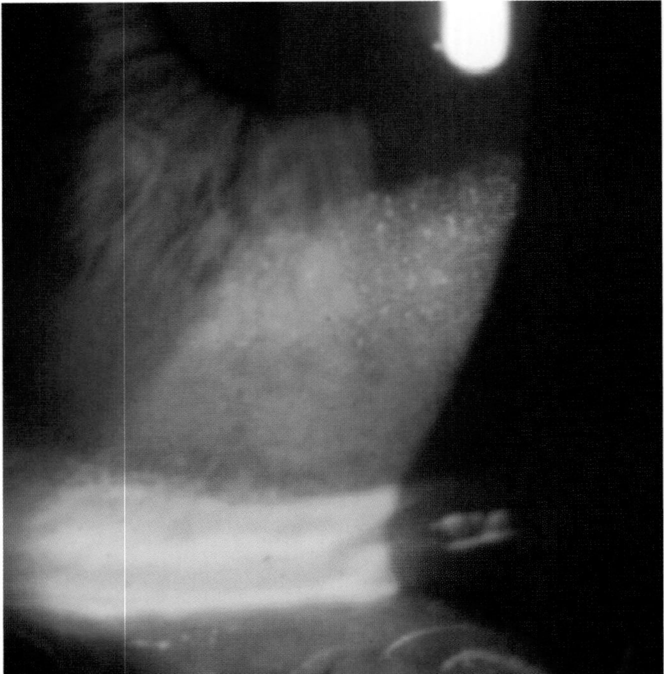

Figure 40.8 Inferior desiccation staining in a patient wearing soft lenses and suffering from dry-eye symptoms.

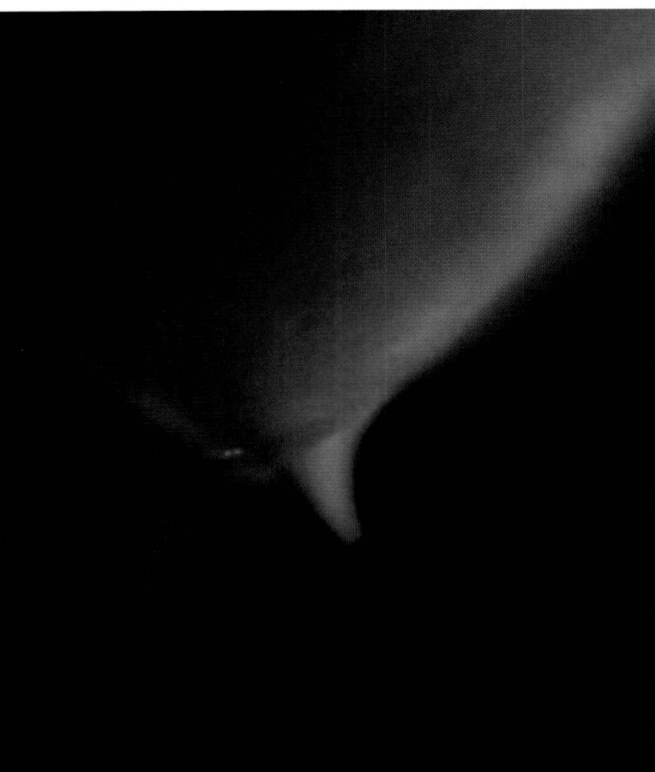

Figure 40.9 Healthy lower lacrimal tear prism, stained with fluorescein.

is noted. Such questionnaires can help identify a true dry-eye situation in prospective or current contact lens wearers and thus form a clinical rationale for more detailed assessment.

The most fundamental test that a clinician can apply when investigating contact lens-related dry eye is to observe the tear film using the slit-lamp biomicroscope. The overall integrity of the tears during lens wear can be assessed by observing the general flow of tears over the lens surface following a blink, as indicated by the movement of tear debris. A sluggish movement may indicate an aqueous-deficient, mucus-rich and/or lipid-rich tear film, and the amount of debris provides an indication of the level of contamination of the tears – for example, from overuse of cosmetics. A sluggish and/or contaminated tear film is potentially problematic, and could result in increased deposit formation, intermittent blurred vision and symptoms of dryness. Incomplete blinking in soft lens wearers can lead to lens dehydration and consequent epithelial staining of the inferior cornea, corresponding to the position of the palpebral aperture (Figure 40.8).

The volume of tears in prospective and current contact lens wearers can be assessed by observing the height of the lower lacrimal tear prism. Mainstone *et al.* (1996) found that measurements of tear meniscus radius of curvature and height (Figure 40.9) correlated well with results of the cotton thread test, non-invasive tear break-up time and ocular surface staining scores, demonstrating the value of such an assessment in diagnosing contact lens-associated dry eye. Tear volumes in dry-eye symptomatic wearers are lower than asymptomatic wearers, resulting in the sensation of dryness (Chen *et al.*, 2009). A wide-field, cold cathode light source, which is available as a hand-held instrument known as a Tearscope, can be used to assess tear quality during lens wear.

Most of the strategies that are applied to alleviating signs and symptoms of dry eye of the non-lens-wearing eye can also be applied to the eye during contact lens wear. The characteristics of a contact lens that is most suited for a patient experiencing dry-eye problems are as follows:

- A soft lens – for full corneal coverage (although some patients report relief from dry-eye symptoms after changing from a soft lens to a rigid lens).
- A lens that displays minimal in-eye dehydration – to prevent ocular surface desiccation.
- A lens that is replaced frequently – for optimal, deposit-free surface characteristics.

Numerous other strategies have been advocated for alleviating contact lens-related dry eye, including avoidance of preservatives in care solutions, avoidance of solutions altogether via the use of one-day disposable lenses, use of rewetting drops, periodic lens rehydration, use of nutritional supplements, control of evaporation, prevention of excess tear drainage (with punctal plugs), use of tear stimulants, reducing wearing time and ceasing lens wear.

Mucin balls

Approximately 50% of patients who wear silicone hydrogel lenses on an extended-wear basis display a peculiar phenomenon known as mucin balls. These formations can be observed in the post-lens tear film as small discrete particles, or 'plugs', and are similar in appearance to tear film debris. In some patients, as many as 200 mucin balls can be observed. At high magnification (×40), mucin balls can be seen to be of variable size and to take on a characteristic

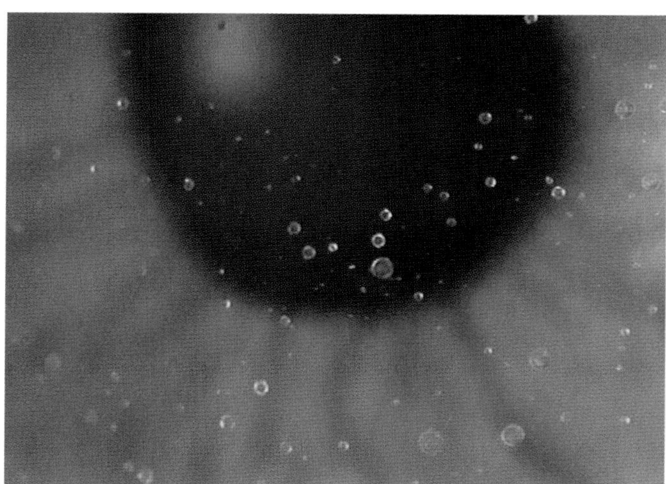

Figure 40.10 Mucin balls displaying characteristic 'doughnut' appearance.

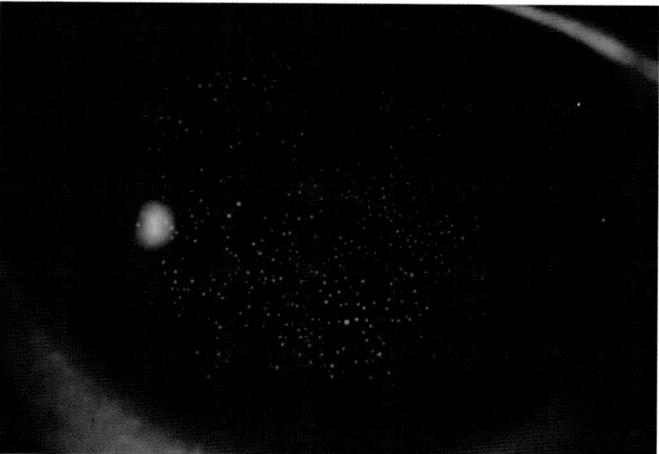

Figure 40.11 Mucin balls and fluid-filled pits staining with fluorescein.

'flattened doughnut' shape, with a thin circular annulus and broad central depression (Figure 40.10). They are observed in greater numbers in patients who sleep in silicone hydrogel lenses. Mucin balls are immovable beneath the lens and appear to be stuck to the epithelium. A higher number of mucin balls is associated with a looser lens fit (Dumbleton, 2003). Mucin balls generally increase in number over the first months of lens wear and remain constant thereafter.

Mucin balls cause no discomfort or loss of vision, and appear to be of no immediate consequence with respect to ocular health (Pritchard *et al.*, 2000). However, there may be cause for concern in the long term. Confocal microscopy, with magnification of up to 650×, has shown mucin balls can penetrate the full thickness of the epithelium, leading to activation of keratocytes in the underlying anterior stroma (Efron, 2007). The precorneal mucin layer is also known to be an important defence mechanism against infection, by way of preventing attachment of microorganisms to the corneal surface and facilitating the entrapment and removal of microorganisms in the course of the natural turnover of mucus, whereby the mucus is constantly being aggregated, rolled up and flushed from the eye (Fleiszig *et al.*, 1994). Lens-induced mucin ball production may therefore represent a compromise to this important protective mechanism.

Mucin balls are composed primarily of collapsed mucin, as well as some lipid and tear proteins (Millar *et al.*, 2003). The mechanism by which mucin balls form beneath the lens may in part be related to a physicochemical phenomenon caused by the plasma-treated surface of silicone hydrogel lenses. Specifically, the lipophilic surface of these lenses establishes a complex interfacial relationship with the tear film which creates a shearing force that has the effect of rolling up tear mucus into small spheres. The mechanical vehicles facilitating such events may be rapid eye movements during sleep and blink-induced lens movement upon awakening. The relatively high modulus of silicone hydrogel lenses may also contribute to the above mechanism (Tan *et al.*, 2003). In addition, the more viscous, mucus-rich nature of the closed-eye post-lens tear film is probably of aetiological significance in the formation of mucin balls.

Following lens removal, some mucin balls remain 'stuck' to the epithelium and some are washed away with blinking

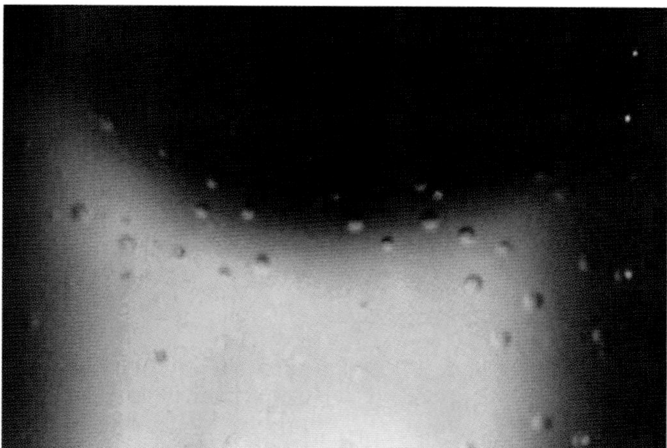

Figure 40.12 Fluid-filled epithelial pits caused by mucin balls displaying unreversed illumination.

but leave behind pits in the epithelial surface which fill with tear aqueous. Both the remaining mucin balls and surface fluid-filled pits stain with fluorescein (Figure 40.11). When viewed at ×40 magnification, the fluid-filled pits give rise to the optical phenomenon of unreversed illumination, which is due to the fact that they are composed of a material (tear aqueous) of lower refractive index than the surrounding epithelial tissue (Figure 40.12). This appearance is almost identical to dimple veiling caused by air bubbles trapped beneath rigid lenses. Mucin ball-induced fluid-filled pits can therefore can be differentiated from epithelial microcysts, which display reversed illumination. Mucin ball-induced fluid-filled pits will stain heavily with fluorescein and give the appearance of an extensive punctate keratitis, whereas epithelial microcysts do not stain except for a few small spots caused by some microcysts breaking through the epithelial surface.

Conjunctiva

As a tissue that is in direct apposition with a contact lens, the conjunctiva has an important role to play in the

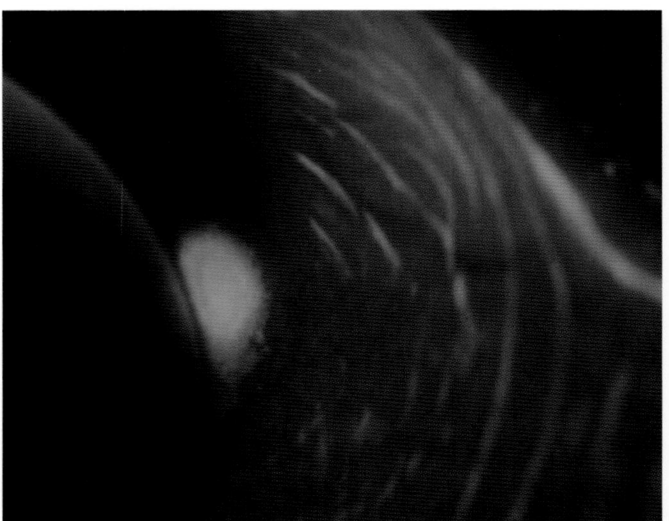

Figure 40.13 Fluorescein fills natural folds in the conjunctiva.

maintenance of successful lens wear. Unlike the cornea, it is a vascularized tissue and is thus capable of mobilizing rapid and often dramatic defence mechanisms, which will in turn serve to resolve the problem and at the same time send a strong signal (e.g. red eye) to the lens wearer and clinician of the existence of a physiological disturbance that requires attention.

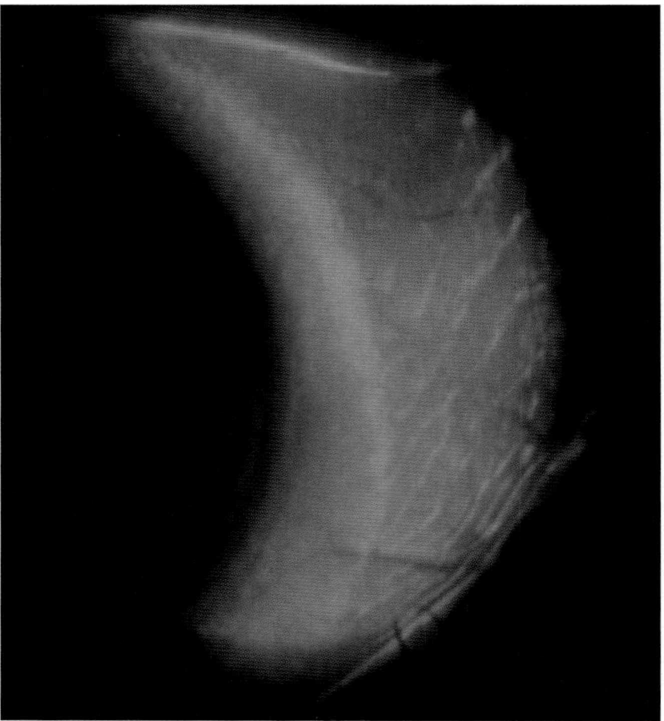

Figure 40.14 Conjunctival staining caused by compression from the edge of a tight-fitting soft lens.

Conjunctival staining

Lakkis and Brennan (1996) evaluated 50 hydrogel lens wearers and 50 non-lens-wearing control subjects for conjunctival staining and symptoms. These disregarded parallel line patterns, which are attributed to pooling of fluorescein in natural conjunctival folds (Figure 40.13). They found that 98% of all subjects displayed some degree of clinically significant conjunctival staining, but only 12% of the non-wearers versus 62% of the lens wearers exhibited staining greater than grade 1. The symptom of dryness was associated with increased conjunctival staining. Brautaset *et al.* (2008) reported observing conjunctival staining in 33% of 338 adapted hydrogel contact lens wearers.

An imprint can be created on the conjunctiva as a result of chafing or physical compression by the edge of a soft lens. Chafing may be due to a lens edge design that causes the edge to 'dig in' to the conjunctiva. Defects in the lens edge have also been demonstrated to cause increased conjunctival staining (Efron and Veys, 1992). Fitting a lens with a different edge design and a 'defect-free' edge will alleviate this problem.

Compression staining will usually be accompanied by a tight-fitting and/or a decentred lens. This manifests as a broad ring of heavy conjunctival staining corresponding to the lens edge, which is clearly evident following lens removal (Figure 40.14). Conjunctival vessels distal to the lens edge may be engorged. The patient is usually asymptomatic. This condition can be solved by refitting the patient with a lens of greater back optic zone radius.

Instillation of fluorescein in a dry-eye patient may reveal the presence of a desiccation staining on the conjunctiva, which manifests as a series of diffuse punctate lesions within the interpalpebral zone. The condition will return to normal soon after removing the lens, but long-term resolution may require a combination of treating the underlying cause of the dry eye and refitting the patient with lenses that will facilitate complete conjunctival wetting.

A conjunctival epithelial flap may be seen in patients wearing silicone hydrogel contact lenses. These arcuate formations on the conjunctiva are composed of sheets of cells detached from the underlying conjunctiva, which probably form as a result of physical irritation by the edge of lenses of higher modulus (Graham *et al.*, 2009). They are seen more in patients wearing lenses on an extended-wear basis (Santodomingo-Rubido *et al.*, 2008). These flaps are asymptomatic, and their clinical significance is unclear.

Compromise to the conjunctiva as revealed by fluorescein staining is of concern because of recent demonstrations of morphological changes to the conjunctival epithelium associated with lens wear. These changes include alterations to conjunctival cell shape, nuclear morphology and chromatin condensation (Knop and Bremitt, 1992), and are reported to be more prevalent in symptomatic lens wearers (Aragona *et al.*, 1998). Soft lens wear is also associated with a reduction in goblet cell density (Knop and Bremitt, 1992; Conner *et al.*, 1997); this could lead to a reduction in mucin production, which in turn could explain and perhaps further exacerbate pre-existing symptoms of dryness.

Conjunctival redness

The clinical presentation of a 'red eye' can be one of the most difficult cases to solve due to the numerous possible causes that are known. This problem may be even more complex in a contact lens wearer because of the wide variety of

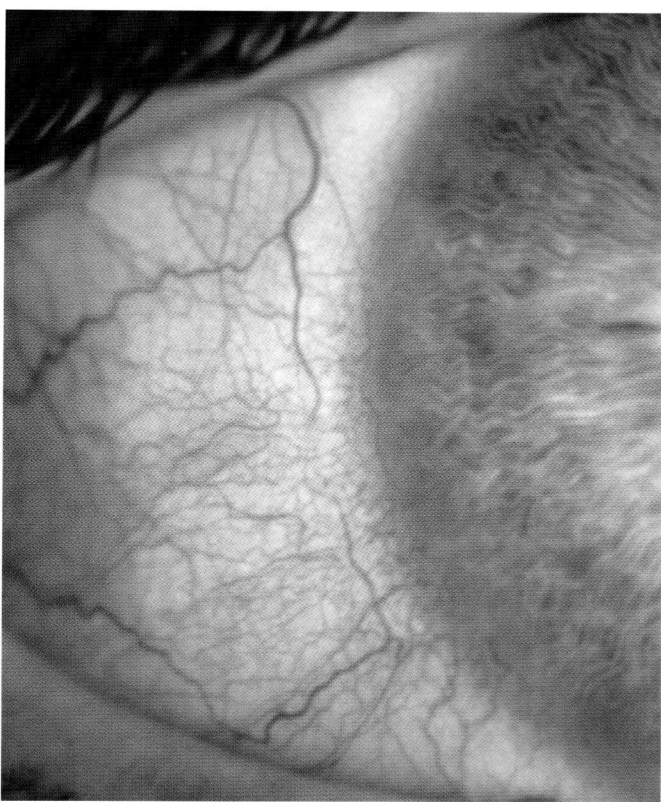

Figure 40.15 Bulbar conjunctival hyperaemia.

causes of contact lens-related red eye. Conjunctival redness in lens wearers is generally asymptomatic, but patients may complain of itchiness, congestion, non-specific mild irritation or a warm or cold feeling (Figure 40.15). The existence of pain usually indicates corneal involvement or other tissue pathology (e.g. uveitis or scleritis).

The amount of conjunctival redness induced by contact lenses is less with silicone hydrogel lenses versus conventional hydrogel lenses. In a 4-week study of patients who had not worn lenses previously, Maldonado-Codina *et al.* (2004) observed that conventional hydrogel lenses caused an increase in conjunctival redness of about 0.3 grading scale units (Efron scale) whereas silicone hydrogel lenses induced no change in redness.

The conjunctiva has a rich plexus of arterioles which contain a thick layer of smooth muscle that is richly enervated with sympathetic nerve fibres. The smooth muscle, as well as being under central autonomic control, can be influenced by numerous local changes. Vasodilation refers to enlargement in the circumference of a vessel due to relaxation of its smooth-muscle layer, which leads to decreased resistance and increased blood flow through the vessel (active hyperaemia). Since blood vessels can be observed directly through the transparent conjunctiva, this leads to an appearance of increased redness (less white sclera is visible).

A contact lens can have a local mechanical effect on the conjunctiva, resulting in increased redness. As a device that can interfere with normal metabolic processes of the cornea and conjunctiva, and is used in association with various solutions, a contact lens can affect the level of conjunctival redness via a local chemical or toxic effect (Figure 40.16).

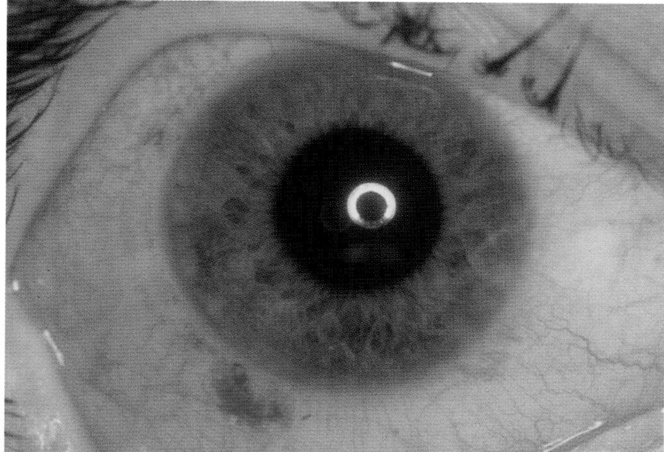

Figure 40.16 General bulbar conjunctival redness, limbal redness and inferior limbal haemorrhages. Adverse reaction to an experimental disinfecting solution in a 22-year-old female soft lens wearer.

Local infection and inflammation can cause eye redness. Accordingly, treatment options fall into four broad categories:

1. Alterations to the type, design and modality of lens wear.
2. Alterations to care systems.
3. Improving ocular hygiene.
4. Prescription of pharmaceutical agents.

The prognosis for recovery from chronic contact lens-induced redness after removal of lenses and cessation of wear is good. Holden *et al.* (1986) found that, following approximately 5 years of extended hydrogel lens wear, general conjunctival redness resolved within 2 days. In general, removal of any noxious stimulus, including a contact lens, will lead to a very rapid recovery of eye redness to normal levels.

Papillary conjunctivitis

This condition refers to the appearance of localized swellings, or papillae, on the tarsal conjunctiva. Papillae are primarily observed in the upper eyelid, and can only be viewed by everting the lid. Rarely, papillae can be observed on the lower tarsus by pulling the lower lid firmly down. In soft lens wearers, papillae are more numerous; they are located more towards the upper tarsal plate (that is, closer to the fold of the everted lid), and the apex of the papillae takes on a more rounded form (Figure 40.17). In rigid lens wearers, papillae are flatter and are located more towards the lash margin, with few papillae being present on the upper tarsal plate. Papillae often appear as round light reflexes, giving an irregular specular reflection (Allansmith *et al.*, 1977).

In the early stages (less than grade 2) of contact lens-induced papillary conjunctivitis (CLPC), the tarsal conjunctiva may be indistinguishable from the normal tarsal conjunctiva apart from increased redness. In advanced cases (greater than grade 2), papillae can exceed 1 mm in diameter and often take on a bright red/orange hue. The distribution of papillae can be more readily appreciated with the aid of fluorescein (Figure 40.18). The hexagonal/

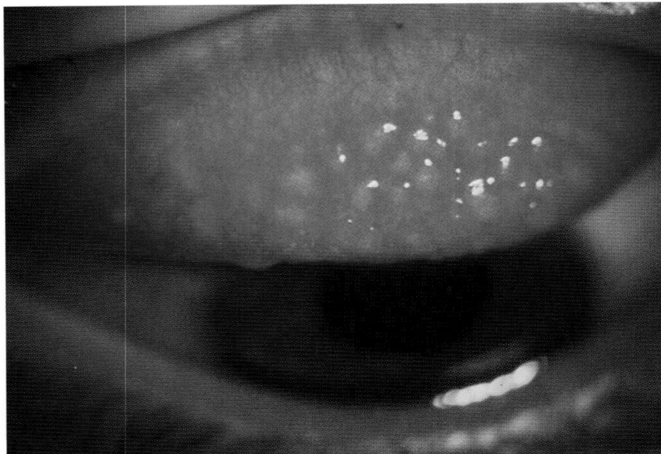

Figure 40.17 Everted eyelid revealing the presence of contact lens-induced papillary conjunctivitis.

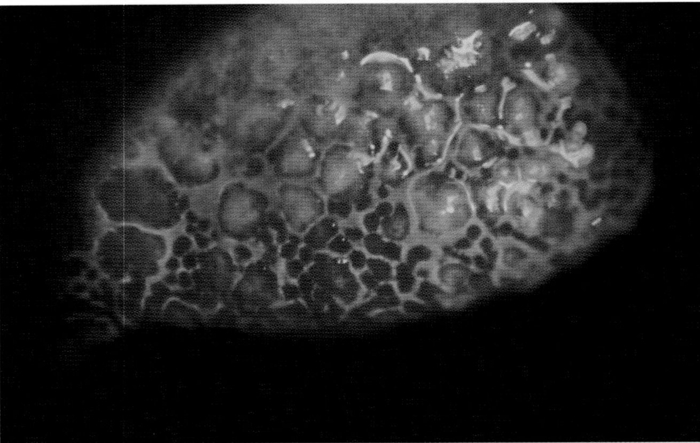

Figure 40.18 Distribution of papillae as revealed by fluorescein. Same eye as in Figure 40.17.

pentagonal shape is lost in favour of a more rounded appearance, with a flattened or even slightly depressed apex or tip. A tuft of convoluted capillary vessels is often observed at the apex of papillae; this vascular tuft will typically stain with fluorescein. Other signs in severe CLPC (greater than grade 3) include conjunctival oedema, excessive mucus and mild ptosis. The cornea may display punctate staining and superior infiltrates. Injection of the superior limbus may also be apparent.

Skotnitsky *et al.* (2006) have proposed that two distinct clinical presentations of CLPC are observed in hydrogel lens wearers – local and general. This classification is based on location and extent of papillae, whereby CLPC is classified as local if papillae are present in one to two areas of the tarsal conjunctiva and general if papillae occur in three or more areas. CLPC is less commonly associated with silicone hydrogel lens wear (Sorbara *et al.*, 2009).

There is general concordance between the severity of signs and symptoms. In the early stages of CLPC, patients may complain of discomfort towards the end of the wearing period, slight itching, excess mucus upon awakening, intermittent blurring and a slight but non-variable vision loss while wearing lenses. As the condition progresses, patients report itching, discomfort and excessive lens movement.

Key factors implicated in the aetiology of CLPC include lens-induced mechanical irritation, and immediate and delayed hypersensitivity. There is often a link with meibomian gland dysfunction, and atopic patients may be more susceptible to developing the condition.

Treatment options include:

- Altering the lens material.
- Replacing lenses more frequently (Porazinski *et al.*, 1999).
- Altering or eliminating the care system.
- Improving ocular hygiene.
- Treating any associated meibomian gland dysfunction.
- Prescribing pharmaceutical agents such as soft steroids (e.g. loteprednol etabonate), mast cell stabilizers (e.g. 4% cromolyn sodium), combined antihistamine/mast cell stabilizers (e.g. olopatadine hydrochloride 0.1% or ketotifen fumarate 0.025%).
- Dispensing ocular lubricants for symptomatic relief.
- Reducing wearing time.
- Suspending or ceasing lens wear.

Compared with planned-replacement hydrogel lenses, daily disposable hydrogel lenses reduce the risk of papillary conjunctivitis by 50% (Radford *et al.*, 2009).

The prognosis for recovery from CLPC after removal of lenses and cessation of wear is good, with symptoms disappearing within 5 days to 2 weeks of lens removal, and redness and excess mucus resolving over a similar time course. Resolution of papillae takes place over a much longer time course – typically many weeks and as long as 6 months. The more severe the condition, the longer the recovery period. In the longer term, however, the prognosis is less good. The condition can recur, especially in atopic patients who appear to have a propensity for developing CLPC.

Limbus

The limbus is of particular significance in contact lens wear because it is a complex anatomical entity by way of it being a transition zone between the cornea and conjunctiva, and it is the region of the anterior eye that is often in close proximity to the edge of both rigid and soft lenses.

Limbal redness

Assuming that a given case of eye redness is lens-related, it is necessary to determine whether the source of the problem is the cornea or conjunctiva. Conjunctival redness associated with a quiet limbus and absence of pain indicates a primary conjunctival problem. Conjunctival redness associated with an injected limbus and corneal pain indicates more corneal involvement, or indeed a problem that is related exclusively to the cornea. Careful slit-lamp examination of the anterior ocular structures, and inspection of the contact lens at high magnification, will generally reveal the cause of the problem. It may also be necessary to prescribe different care systems and differentially diagnose the effects of various solutions over time.

In the absence of any clinically observable ocular pathology, corneal hypoxia is the likely cause of excessive limbal redness (Figure 40.19). Hypoxia stimulates the release of inflammatory mediators from the limbal vessel walls

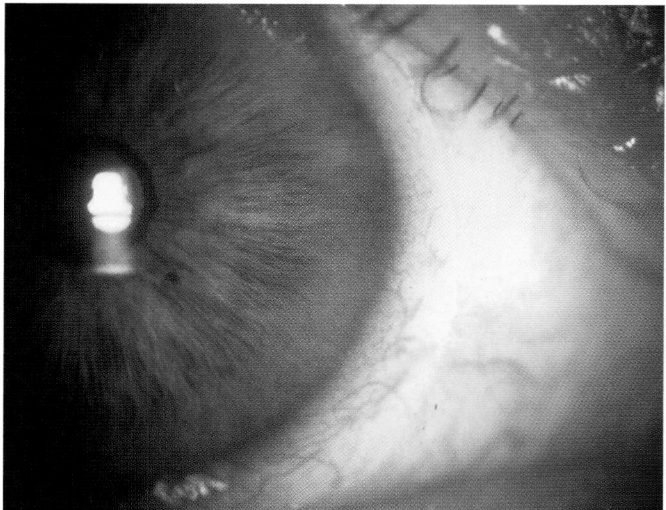

Figure 40.19 Circumlimbal redness due to hypoxia induced by a soft lens of low oxygen transmissibility.

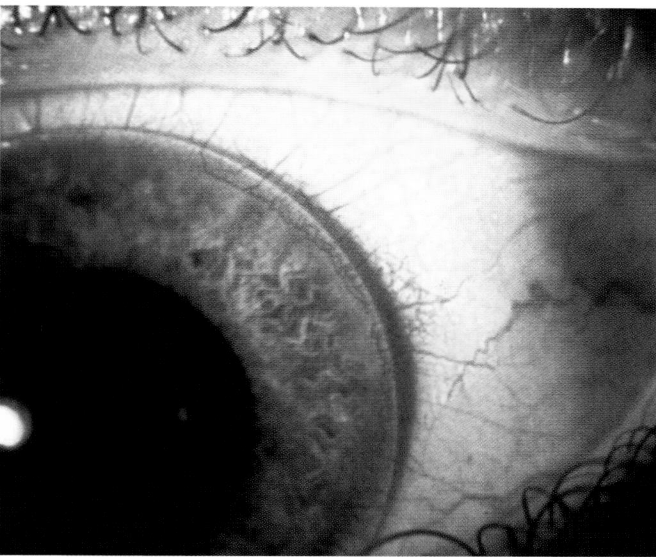

Figure 40.20 Limbal redness due to direct physical irritation from the thick edge of a soft lens that is of insuffcent diameter for this patient.

leading to vasodilatation; this is an automatic reaction designed to facilitate a greater flow of oxygenated blood to the distressed tissue. This mechanism fails in the case of the limbus because limbal blood flow contributes little to corneal oxygenation; the cornea derives virtually all of its oxygen supply from the atmosphere. The result, therefore, is contact lens-induced hypoxia maintaining chronic limbal vessel engorgement in a vain attempt to reoxygenate the cornea.

Papas (1998) has demonstrated a significant relationship between the oxygen transmissibility of the peripheral region of the lens and limbal redness. Indeed, one of the key benefits of high-permeability silicone hydrogel lenses is that they induce very low levels of limbal redness (Maldonado-Codina *et al.*, 2004).

Although hypoxia is presumed to be the key determinant of limbal redness, practitioners should be alert to the possibility of other causes, such as poor lens edge design (Figure 40.20) or pathology of the anterior ocular structures, especially the cornea.

The prognosis for recovery from chronic contact lens-induced limbal redness after removal of lenses and cessation of wear is good. Holden *et al.* (1986) found that, following approximately 5 years of extended lens wear, general conjunctival redness resolved within 2 days, whereas recovery from limbal redness had a longer time course, taking about 7 days to resolve.

Vascularized limbal keratitis

This condition is observed in patients wearing rigid contact lenses on an extended-wear basis. It manifests as a limbal inflammation – typically at either the 3 or 9 o'clock positions – and an encroachment of limbal vessels (Figure 40.21). The adjacent conjunctiva may be oedematous and hyperaemic, and the lesion may be surrounded by fine superficial punctate epithelial staining and mild corneal infiltration (Figure 40.22) (Grohe and Lebow, 1989). The patient may be only mildly symptomatic, complaining of ocular dryness. The problem may be exacerbated if the lens surface is crazed or deposited (Miller, 1995).

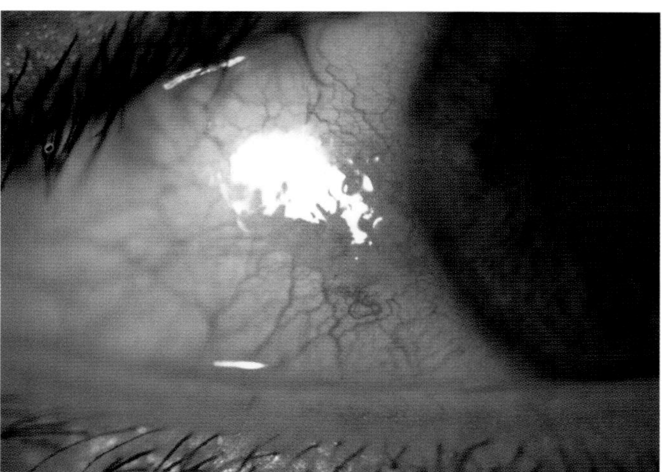

Figure 40.21 Vascularized limbal keratitis in a rigid lens wearer.

This condition often occurs in regions of the limbus that have become desiccated due to poor wetting of the ocular surface. This problem is caused by bridging of the lids away from the globe, thus preventing the lids from distributing tears over the affected area. In this regard, vascularized limbal keratitis may be an advanced form of 3 and 9 o'clock staining. In late stages of this condition, the lesion can become slightly raised, in the form of a thickened mass of epithelial tissue through which blood vessels traverse at various depths (Figure 40.23) (Grohe and Lebow, 1989). This epithelial hypertrophy may be related to the fact that the limbus contains a high concentration of stem cells, creating a greater capacity for epithelial cell mitosis and movement. Also, the limbus hosts a vast array of immunological mechanisms mediated via the reticuloendothelial system in limbal vessels.

Vascularized limbal keratitis is reversible, and cessation of lens wear for a few weeks will allow most of the pathology to resolve. Converting the patient from extended wear

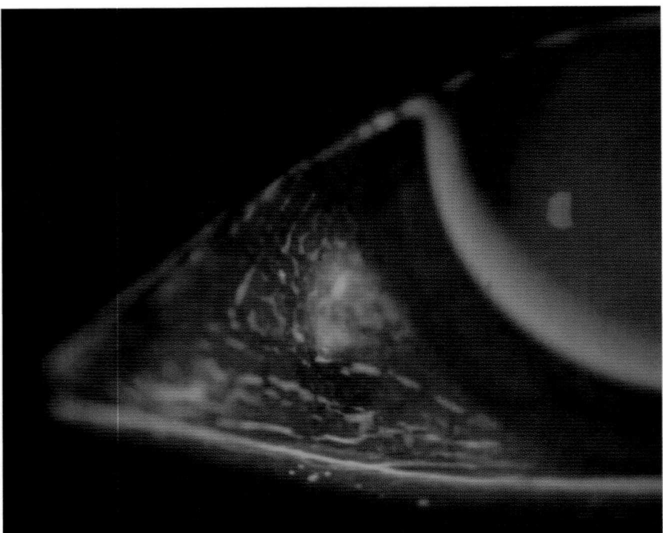

Figure 40.22 Epithelial mass in vascularized limbal keratitis staining with fluorescein (same patient as in Figure 40.21).

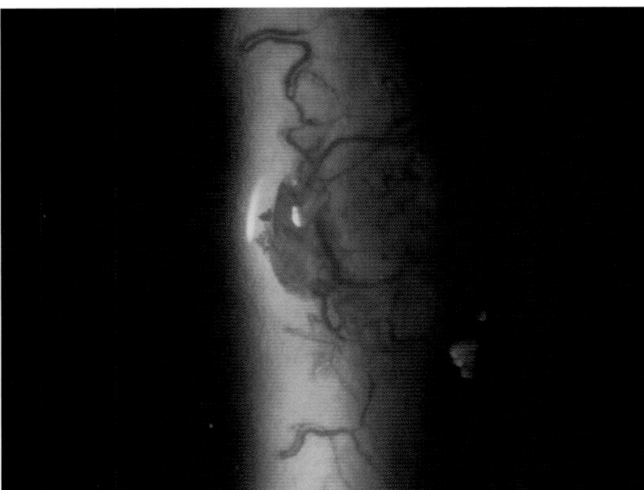

Figure 40.23 High-magnification view (×40) of epithelial mass in vascularized limbal keratitis.

to daily wear, and refitting with a smaller-diameter lens, may prevent the problem from recurring. Changing from rigid to soft lenses will certainly eliminate the problem.

Superior limbic keratoconjunctivitis

In its mild form, contact lens-induced superior limbic keratoconjunctivitis (CLSLK) is easy to overlook. The condition is confined to the superior limbal area and as such is hidden by the upper lid in primary gaze. The proper procedure for observing this condition is to lift the upper lid while the patient gazes down.

A myriad of signs are observed in the region of the superior limbus in patients with CLSLK; these include:

- punctate epithelial fluorescein staining
- epithelial rose bengal staining
- intraepithelial opacities

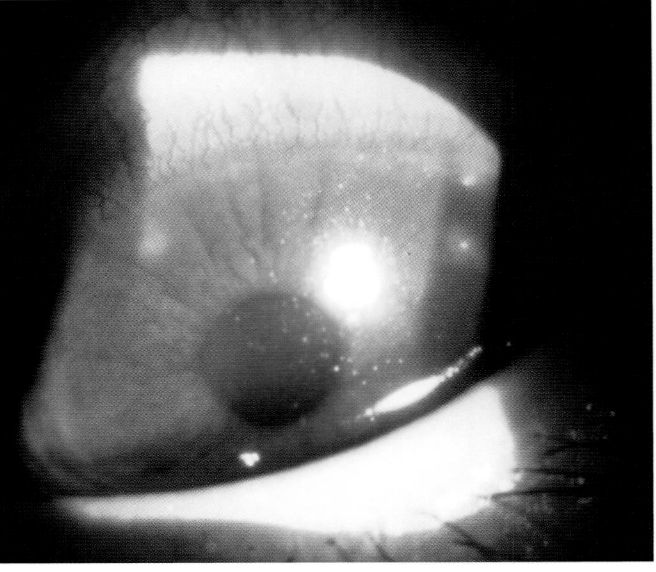

Figure 40.24 Early stage of superior limbic keratoconjunctivitis (grade 1.0) showing superior limbal hyperaemia, focal infiltrates, increased lacrimation (indicated by full lacrimal river) and epithelial decompensation (indicated by hazy slit-lamp reflex).

- subepithelial haze
- epithelial dulling
- microcysts
- infiltrates and irregularities
- stromal fibrovascular micropannus
- fine subepithelial linear opacities
- limbal oedema
- hypertrophy
- fluorescein staining
- vascular injection
- poor wetting
- punctate staining
- hyperaemia
- chemosis and irregular thickening of the superior bulbar conjunctiva
- papillary and follicular hypertrophy
- hyperaemia and petechiae of the upper tarsal conjunctiva
- corneal filaments
- corneal warpage and astigmatism
- corneal pseudodendrites (Figure 40.24) (Stenson, 1983).

The tissue compromise progresses from the limbus to the centre of the cornea in a V-shaped pattern with the apex directed towards the pupil centre (Figure 40.25).

Symptoms of CLSLK include increased lens awareness, lens intolerance, foreign-body sensation, burning, itching, photophobia, redness, increased lacrimation, slight mucus secretion and slight loss of vision. This condition is uncommon, and occurs mostly in soft lens wearers. It is almost always bilateral, and the specific signs often display symmetry between the eyes. There is considerable variability in the time course of onset of the condition; signs usually becomes manifest between 2 months and 2 years after commencement of lens wear.

The primary aetiological factor in the development of CLSLK is thimerosal hypersensitivity (Wilson *et al.*, 1981)

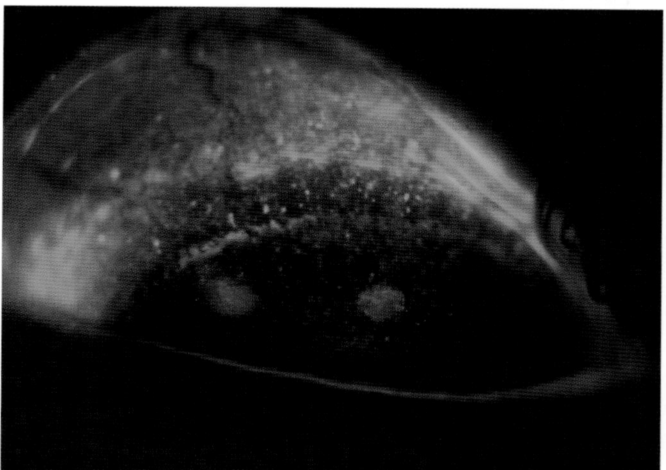

Figure 40.25 Fluorescein reveals tissue compromise in superior limbic keratoconjunctivitis (grade 2.3).

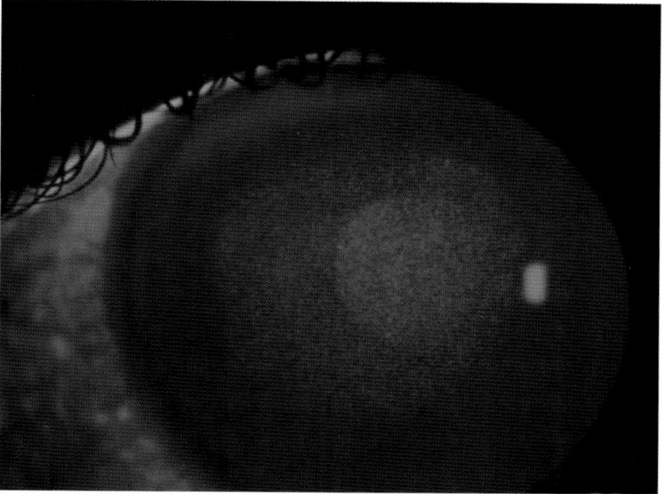

Figure 40.26 Extensive superficial punctate epithelial staining.

– a preservative that is no longer used in contact lens care solutions. Provocative tests in thimerosal-sensitized patients result in general circumlimbal redness (not just confined to the superior limbus), meaning that contact lens wear must be having an impact on the clinical presentation of CLSLK, which is confined to the superior limbus. Although other factors perhaps play a minor role by initiating, modulating or exacerbating the condition, it is unlikely that CLSLK will develop in the absence of ocular contact with thimerosal. Other factors implicated in the aetiology of CLSLK include thimerosal toxicity, mechanical effects, lens deposits and hypoxia beneath the upper lid.

Patients suffering from CLSLK may be advised to cease lens wear for 2–4 weeks if less than grade 2 and up to 3 months in severe cases (greater than grade 2). All previously worn lenses should be discarded. Refitting can be undertaken when the corneal haze has largely resolved and the corneal surface is smooth (less than grade 1); however, a vascular pannus may be permanent. Lens wear can be resumed in the presence of a vascular pannus as long as the patient is monitored closely to check for the absence of further vascular encroachment. Thimerosal and any other potentially allergenic preservatives should be excluded from the care system. Single-use daily disposable lenses are the best option. Ocular lubricants in the form of drops or ointments may provide symptomatic relief during the recovery phase, further to a positive placebo effect in a naturally anxious patient. Clinical signs and visual acuity will resolve within about 4 months of cessation of lens wear, although this can vary between 3 weeks and 9 months.

Corneal epithelium

The corneal epithelium is in direct contact with a contact lens, and is thus susceptible to physical trauma. Being highly metabolically active, the epithelium is also sensitive to metabolic insult. In the case of contact lens wear, the primary metabolic insult is an interference with normal tissue respiration. Many of the complications that are observed throughout the full depth of the cornea are mediated by the epithelium.

Epithelial staining

Epithelial staining is not strictly a condition in itself – rather, it is a general term that refers to the appearance of tissue disruption and other pathophysiological changes in the anterior eye, as revealed with the aid of one or more of a number of dyes, such as fluorescein, rose bengal, lissamine green, fluorexon or alcian blue. Fluorescein has by far the greatest utility in contact lens practice, so the terms 'epithelial staining' and 'corneal staining' are taken to mean staining with fluorescein, unless stated otherwise.

Epithelial staining following instillation of fluorescein is observed under cobalt blue light as a bright green fluorescence, which can be described as 'punctate' (spot-like) (Figure 40.26), 'diffuse' (spots merging together) and 'coalescent' (large regions of confluence). The staining pattern may be described according to the following groups of type descriptors: arcuate, linear or dimpled; superior, inferior, temporal, nasal or central; and deep or superficial (Korb and Korb, 1970). Staining 'syndromes' include inferior epithelial arcuate lesion ('smile stain'), superior epithelial arcuate lesion (otherwise known as 'epithelial splitting') and exposure keratitis. An 'epithelial plug' refers to a large coalescent field of full-thickness epithelial loss. Observed areas of fluorescence are believed to indicate one of three phenomena: (1) fluorescein entering damaged cells; (2) fluorescein entering intercellular spaces; or (3) fluorescein filling gaps in the epithelial surface that are created when epithelial cells are displaced (Wilson *et al.*, 1995); however, Morgan and Maldonado-Codina (2009) point out that our clinical understanding and interpretation of corneal surface fluorescence are based upon assumption, extrapolation and clinical intuition rather than solid evidence-based science underpinning the basic causative mechanisms of this phenomenon.

Severe staining (grades 3 and 4) may be accompanied by bulbar conjunctival redness and chemosis, limbal redness, excessive lacrimation and, in some cases stromal infiltrates, depending on the cause of the problem. Visual acuity is generally unaffected by epithelial staining, although a slight loss might be expected in extreme cases (grade 4). There is no clear relationship between the severity of staining and the degree of ocular discomfort.

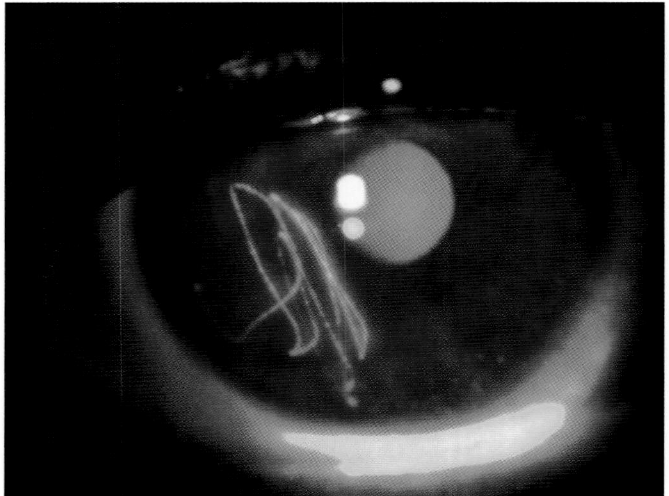

Figure 40.27 Foreign-body track stain in a rigid lens wearer revealed with the aid of fluorescein.

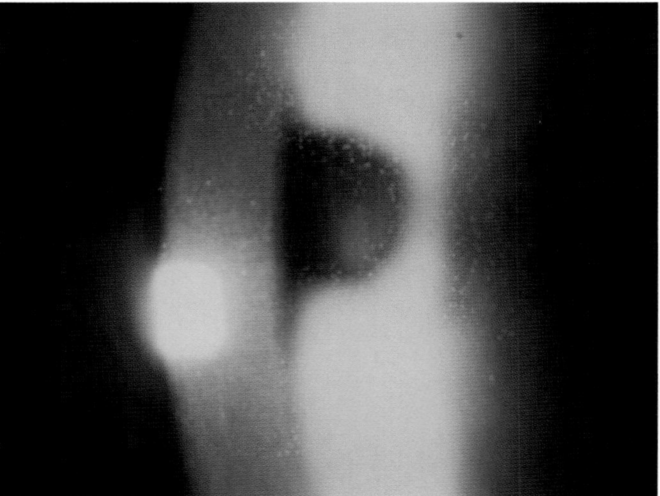

Figure 40.28 Extensive formation of epithelial microcysts in a soft lens wearer.

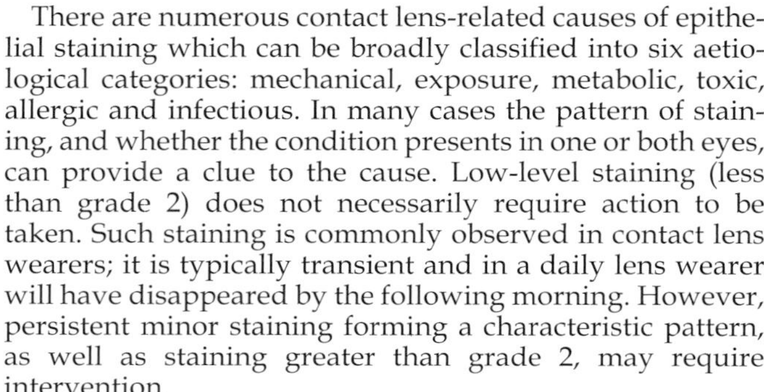

There are numerous contact lens-related causes of epithelial staining which can be broadly classified into six aetiological categories: mechanical, exposure, metabolic, toxic, allergic and infectious. In many cases the pattern of staining, and whether the condition presents in one or both eyes, can provide a clue to the cause. Low-level staining (less than grade 2) does not necessarily require action to be taken. Such staining is commonly observed in contact lens wearers; it is typically transient and in a daily lens wearer will have disappeared by the following morning. However, persistent minor staining forming a characteristic pattern, as well as staining greater than grade 2, may require intervention.

Management strategies are generally self-evident if the cause can be discerned. For example, mechanical trauma due to a foreign body trapped beneath a rigid lens (Figure 40.27) can be resolved by removing and rinsing the lens and rinsing the eye; exposure keratitis causing 3 and 9 o'clock staining in a rigid lens wearer can be resolved by fitting soft lenses; epitheliopathy due to metabolic disturbance can be solved by fitting a lens of higher oxygen transmissibility; staining due to toxicity or allergy can be resolved by eliminating the toxic or allergic agent; and staining associated with an infection is treated by applying the appropriate antimicrobial therapy. Recovery from epithelial staining generally occurs within hours or days of removal of the offending source, but will be more prolonged if lenses are worn during the recovery period.

Microcysts

Microcysts appear as minute scattered grey opaque dots when viewed with the slit-lamp biomicroscope using low magnification and focal illumination (Figure 40.28), and as transparent refractile inclusions with indirect retroillumination. They are generally of a uniform spherical or ovoid shape and are in the order of 20 μm in diameter. At high magnification (×40) using the observation technique of marginal retroillumination, microcysts can be observed to display a characteristic optical phenomenon known as 'reversed illumination'; that is, the distribution of light within the microcyst is opposite to the light distribution of the background (Figure 40.29). This indicates that the microcyst is acting as a converging refractor; therefore, it must consist of material that is of a higher refractive index than the surrounding epithelium. Microcysts probably represent apoptotic (dead) cells which either become phagocytosed (ingested) by living neighbouring cells, or remain involuted in the intercellular spaces. In a process similar to that which occurs in Cogan's microcystic dystrophy, the epithelial basement membrane reduplicates and folds, forming intraepithelial sheets that eventually detach from the basement membrane and encapsulate the cellular debris (Holden and Sweeney, 1991).

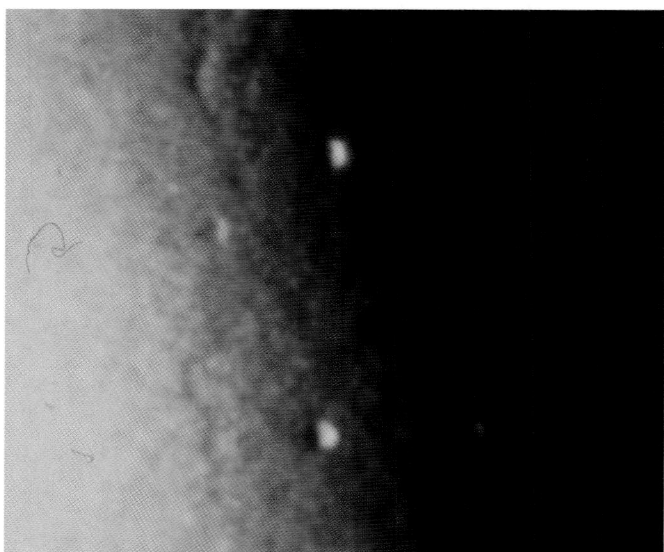

Figure 40.29 High-magnification image (×200) of two epithelial microcysts, displaying reversed illumination.

Microcysts primarily represent visible evidence of chronic tissue metabolic stress and altered cellular growth patterns. These changes are presumed to be caused by a combination of the direct effects of hypoxia, and tissue acidosis created by the indirect effects of hypoxia (producing lactic acid) and hypercapnia (producing carbonic acid). They may also have a mechanical aetiology; Efron and Veys (1992) provided evidence that lens-induced mechanical trauma can induce microcysts.

Whilst the presence of microcysts is not thought to be dangerous, their existence in large numbers is worrying as this is representative of epithelial metabolic distress. Based on the working hypothesis that the severity of the microcyst response is related to the level of hypoxia/hypercapnia induced by lens wear, a variety of strategies can be employed in an attempt to minimize the number of microcysts. Strategies that are likely to be successful include refitting with high-oxygen-transmissibility silicone hydrogel lenses (Covey *et al.*, 2001; Keay *et al.*, 2001; Brennan *et al.*, 2007), decreasing the frequency of overnight wear, changing from extended wear to daily wear, changing from soft to rigid lenses and avoiding defective lenses.

The prognosis for eliminating microcysts is good, but the time course is peculiar. Following cessation of lens wear, there is an initial increase over a 7-day period in the number of microcysts, followed by a subsequent decrease. The initial increase in microcysts is thought to be due to an initial resurgence in epithelial metabolism and growth, resulting in an accelerated removal of cellular debris (formation of microcysts) and a rapid movement of microcysts towards the surface. This is followed by a gradual decrease as the existing microcysts are completely eliminated from the cornea over a period of 3–5 months (Holden *et al.*, 1985a).

Vacuoles

When the cornea is severely compromised, such as in the case of severe stromal oedema or an extensive microcyst response, the epithelium can also become oedematous; this manifests as the appearance of small fluid vacuoles in the epithelium. By observing the cornea using indirect retroillumination on the slit-lamp biomicroscope, fluid vacuoles can be observed to display 'unreversed illumination'; that is, the distribution of light within the microcyst is the same as the light distribution of the background (Figure 40.30). This indicates that the microcyst is acting as a diverging refractor; therefore, it must consist of material that is of a lower refractive index (fluid) than the surrounding epithelial tissue (Zantos, 1983).

The aetiology of epithelial fluid vacuoles is twofold. Epithelial oedema follows traumatic loss of surface epithelial cells. The fluid barrier (zonula occludens) that is normally found between surface epithelial cells is breached, resulting in the movement of fluid into the deeper layers of the epithelium. Since the cells are tightly fitted and attach snugly together, the oedema may not occur instantly nor be widespread. Epithelial oedema can also form as a result of hypotonic ocular exposure, which can compromise the integrity of the fluid barrier. Animal studies have demonstrated the coexistence of epithelial oedema and thinning following periods of rigid lens wear.

The flare observed with fluorescein in and around corneal abrasions is epithelial oedema. Histopathological evaluation of corneas following hypotonic exposure demonstrates that the oedema is extracellular and is present throughout the full thickness of the epithelium (Krutsinger and Bergmanson, 1985). Reflex tears are of low tonicity and may also provoke epithelial oedema, such as during adaptation to rigid lenses.

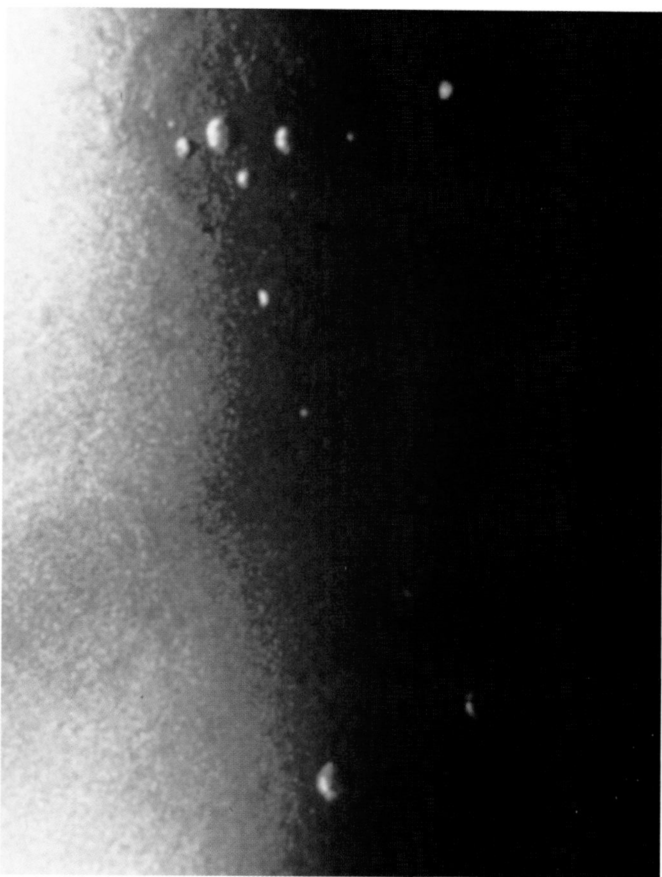

Figure 40.30 Epithelial vacuoles, displaying unreversed illumination.

Breakdown of the corneal fluid barrier, as indicated by the presence of fluid vacuoles, can lead to secondary problems. For example, contaminated low-tonicity water – such as that which may be found in a hot tub – has an association with contracting an *Acanthamoeba* keratitis. The amoeba may use the spaces created between cells by the oedematous state to gain entry to the cornea. This scenario is possible in both contact lens wearers and non-lens wearers. Fluid vacuoles can break through the anterior epithelial surface, leading to a very painful condition (Figure 40.31). Practitioners should therefore take action to eliminate fluid vacuoles from the epithelium by treating the underlying cause, which generally equates to the prescription of highly gas-permeable contact lenses that afford optimal corneal oxygenation.

Wrinkling

Corneal wrinkling is a rare but severe ocular complication of contact lens wear, characterized by the appearance of a series of deep parallel grooves, giving the impression of a 'wrinkled' cornea. In white light, the ridges of the wrinkles can be seen as bright reflexes (Figure 40.32). The case described by Lowe and Brennan (1987) took the form of two linear wave patterns of fluorescein pooling across the cornea and intersecting at an angle of 70°. Several discrete spots of fluorescence were observed at the points of intersection of the two wave patterns.

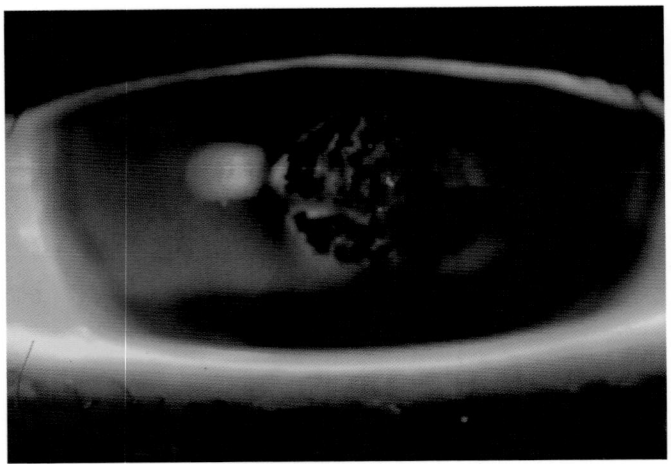

Figure 40.31 Vacuole eruption through anterior layers. The patient had been wearing high-oxygen-transmissibility rigid lenses on an extended-wear basis for 3 years, and awoke one day with stinging and blurred vision.

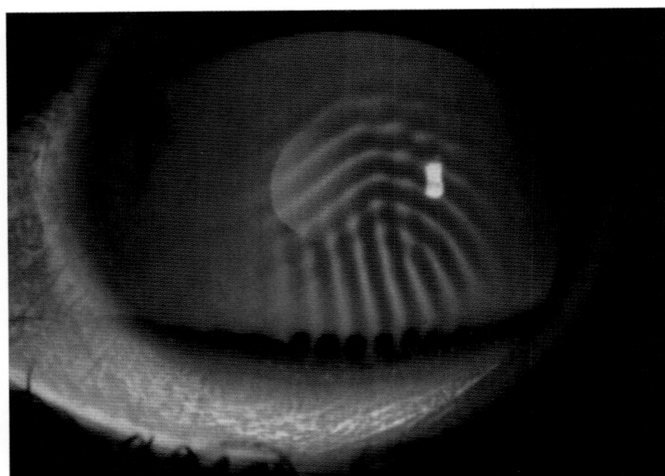

Figure 40.33 Corneal wrinkling pattern revealed by fluorescein.

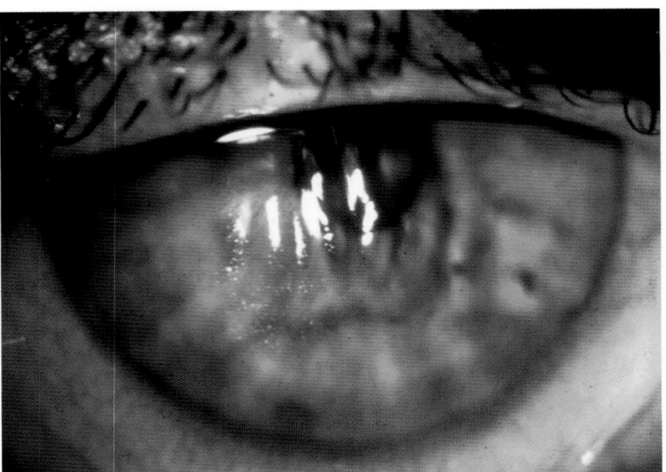

Figure 40.32 Severe corneal wrinkling.

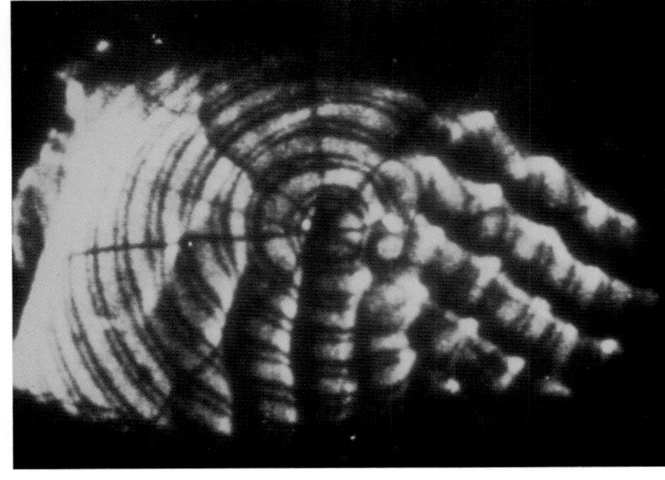

Figure 40.34 Photokeratogram of cornea showing extreme wrinkling.

This condition is observed in patients wearing steeply fitted, highly elastic, ultrathin, mid-water-content lenses. In the two cases described in the literature (Quinn, 1982; Lowe and Brennan, 1987), the lenses that induced corneal wrinkling were custom-made and were not standard commercial products. Excessive elastic forces are thought to draw corneal tissue inwards from the limbus, causing the cornea essentially to 'collapse' in a concertina-like fashion, creating a wrinkled appearance. These forces could be derived from intrinsic elastic energy created when a relatively steep lens is compressed against the eye and then attempts to return to its original shape, and it is noteworthy in this regard that the lens used by Lowe and Brennan (1987) had a fairly steep base curve of 8.20 mm. Corneal wrinkling may also have an osmotic aetiology in view of the observation that complete evaporation of the tear film in normal humans can cause an almost identical corneal wrinkling and vision loss to lens-induced wrinkling.

As one would expect with such a dramatic distortion of the corneal surface, vision loss is dramatic. Indeed, vision drops to less than 6/60 within 5 min of lens insertion. The condition is also extremely painful. Clinical evaluation of corneal wrinkling is best achieved by slit-lamp examination under white light and with fluorescein under cobalt blue light. Computerized videokeratoscopy can provide useful supplementary information by viewing both the unprocessed image of the reflected mires and the processed, colour-coded surface map.

Lowe and Brennan (1987) argue that corneal wrinkling involves the epithelium and anterior stroma. This view is based upon their observations of the extreme variance in intensity of fluorescence across the ridges of a wrinkled cornea (Figure 40.33), implying deep furrows, and the extreme distortion of photokeratometric mires (Figure 40.34). The intensity of the wrinkling pattern increased with time following a blink, indicating fluorescein pooling within deep troughs.

The treatment protocol for a patient experiencing corneal wrinkling is to cease lens wear immediately. Although the appearance of wrinkling will indeed have disappeared within 24 hours, the patient should not wear lenses for 1 week as a precaution so as to allow possible subclinical compromise to resolve. The patient should then be refitted with a soft lens that is devoid of inherently high elastic forces. Alternatively, rigid lenses can be fitted because corneal wrinkling does not occur with such lenses.

The time course of recovery of corneal wrinkling has been demonstrated to be directly related to the period of lens wear that induced the changes. Lowe and Brennan (1987) noted that corneal wrinkling took 3, 90 and 240 min to recover following 5, 90 and 300 min of lens wear, respectively.

Corneal stroma

The stroma constitutes 90% of corneal thickness and is a key component of the structural integrity of the globe. As it is normally clear and transparent, the stroma can be directly observed in exquisite detail with the slit-lamp biomicroscope and confocal microscope, providing a privileged insight into adverse tissue reactions (and a decided clinical decision-making advantage) that is not available during the examination of other tissues in the human body.

Oedema

Oedema refers to an increase in the fluid content of tissue. Since the cornea is only able to swell in the anterior–posterior direction – as a result of the collagen fibre network in the stroma – the physical dimensions of the cornea can only increase in that dimension – that is, in thickness. The human cornea experiences about 3.5% oedema during sleep. With hydrogel lenses, daytime corneal oedema typically varies between 1 and 6%, and the level of overnight oedema measured upon awakening generally falls in the range 5–13% (Holden *et al.*, 1983). Silicone hydrogel lenses induce less than 4% overnight oedema, which is only slightly more than occurs when sleeping without lenses (Sweeney *et al.*, 2004; Martin *et al.*, 2008).

Clinicians can estimate the magnitude of corneal oedema by careful observation with the slit-lamp biomicroscope, as a number of structural changes can be identified that correlate with various levels of oedema. Using direct focal illumination, striae appear as fine, wispy, white, vertically oriented lines in the posterior stroma when the level of oedema reaches about 5% (grade 2). Striae are thought to represent fluid separation of the predominantly vertically arranged collagen fibrils in the posterior stroma. Folds can be observed – using specular reflection technique – in the endothelial mosaic as a combination of depressed grooves or raised ridges, or as a general area of apparent buckling, when the level of oedema reaches about 8% (grade 3) (Figure 40.35). It is thought that folds indicate a physical buckling of the posterior stromal layers in response to high levels of oedema. Folds can also be observed with the confocal microscope as a series of parallel lines crossing the stroma orthogonally (Figure 40.36). The stroma takes on a hazy, milky or granular appearance when the level of oedema reaches about 15% (grade 4); such high levels of oedema are often associated with other signs and symptoms of ocular distress.

Contact lenses potentially restrict corneal oxygen availability, creating a hypoxic environment at the anterior corneal surface. To conserve energy, the corneal epithelium begins to respire anaerobically. Lactate, a byproduct of anaerobic metabolism, increases in concentration and moves posteriorly into the corneal stroma. This creates an osmotic load that is balanced by an increased movement of water into the stroma. The sudden influx of water cannot be matched by the removal of water from the stroma by the endothelial pump, resulting in corneal oedema (Klyce, 1981).

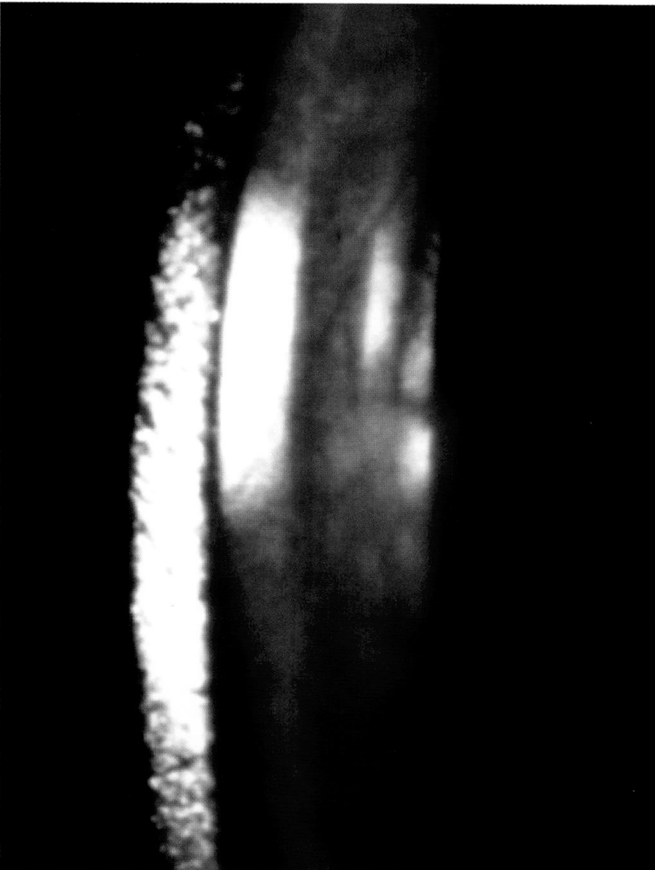

Figure 40.35 Stromal folds observed using a slit-lamp biomicroscope (×30).

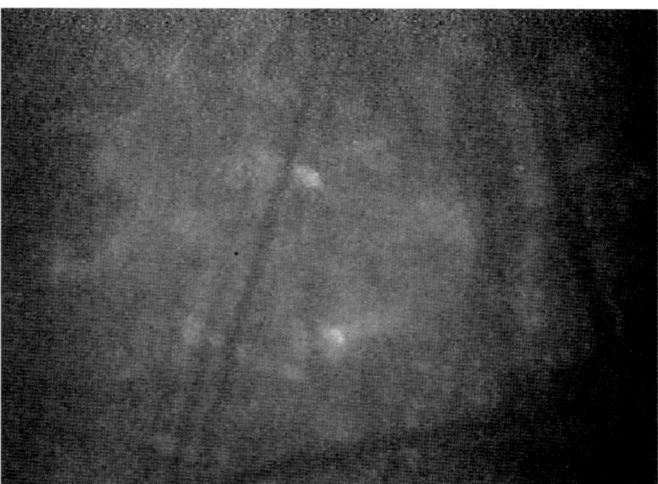

Figure 40.36 Stromal folds observed using a confocal microscope (×680).

The key strategy for reducing the oedema response is to increase corneal oxygen availability during lens wear. Rigid lens oedema can be alleviated by increasing lens oxygen transmissibility; or fitting a lens of flatter base curve, greater edge lift or smaller diameter so as to increase lens-mediated tear exchange. Hydrogel soft lens oedema can be alleviated by hydrogel lenses of higher oxygen transmissibility, flattening the base curve or reducing lens diameter. General strategies for reducing oedema include changing from extended to daily wear; changing from soft to rigid lenses; fitting silicone hydrogel lenses, or reducing wearing time.

In general, the prognosis for recovery of the cornea from lens-induced oedema is excellent. The oedema induced when a patient wears a contact lens for the first time will resolve within 4 hours of the lens being removed. Chronic lens-induced oedema can take up to 7 days to resolve (Holden *et al.*, 1985a).

Thinning

Although low levels of oedema during the day may appear to be harmless, there is a growing body of evidence indicating that chronic oedema may compromise the physiological integrity of the cornea in the long term. It is now clear that long-term wear of conventional hydrogel lenses can induce thinning of the stroma. Whereas the extent of stromal oedema varies with the prevailing level of corneal oxygenation and dissipates upon removal of hypoxic stress, stromal thinning is a chronic and irreversible tissue change observed in patients who have worn lenses for many years.

Stromal thinning was formally defined for the first time by Holden *et al.* (1985a), although it had been reported anecdotally by earlier workers. Holden *et al.* (1985a) detected stromal thinning by measuring the presenting corneal thickness of patients who had been wearing a lens in one eye only on an extended-wear basis for an average of 5 years, due to unilateral myopia or amblyopia. Upon ceasing lens wear, it was noted that corneal thickness in the lens-wearing eye decreased to a steady-state level that was thinner than the fellow non-wearing eye. Assuming that the corneas of both eyes were the same prior to lens wear (this was validated in a non-lens-wearing control group of unilateral myopes and amblyopes), the only assumption that can be drawn is that contact lenses induce stromal thinning. The revelation of stromal thinning has facilitated interpretation of data from earlier longitudinal lens-wearing studies which incorrectly ascribed a progressive decrease in corneal thickness over time as representing some form of adaptation. Iskeleli *et al.* (2006) found that central corneal thickness was significantly thinner in patients wearing long-term low-oxygen-transmissibility rigid lenses compared to no contact lens wear and soft contact lenses with a water content of 55%. Central corneal thickness was also decreased significantly in long-term soft contact lens wear with a water content of 38% compared to 55%.

Contact lens-induced stromal thinning can be of clinical significance. For example, patients who have worn contact lenses for many years may be precluded from undergoing laser ablative refractive surgery if too much thinning has occurred.

The phenomenon of contact lens-induced stromal thinning does not confound or invalidate interpretation of the clinical signs of oedema discussed above. Striae, folds and haze represent a given level of oedema irrespective of whether or not the stroma has thinned.

It is presumed that stromal thinning is due to the effects of chronic oedema, and two mechanisms may be postulated to explain how this might occur. Firstly, stromal keratocytes may lose their ability to synthesize new stromal tissue due to the direct effects of tissue hypoxia, and/or the indirect effects of chronic lens-induced tissue acidosis due to an accumulation of lactic acid and carbonic acid. Secondly, constantly elevated levels of lactic acid associated with chronic oedema may lead to some dissolution of the mucopolysaccharide ground substance of the stroma. Recent evidence obtained using confocal microscopy, demonstrating loss of stromal keratocytes following hydrogel lens wear (Jalbert and Stapleton, 1999; Efron *et al.*, 2001; Kallinikos and Efron, 2004; Kallinikos *et al.*, 2006), lends support to the former theory (Figure 40.37).

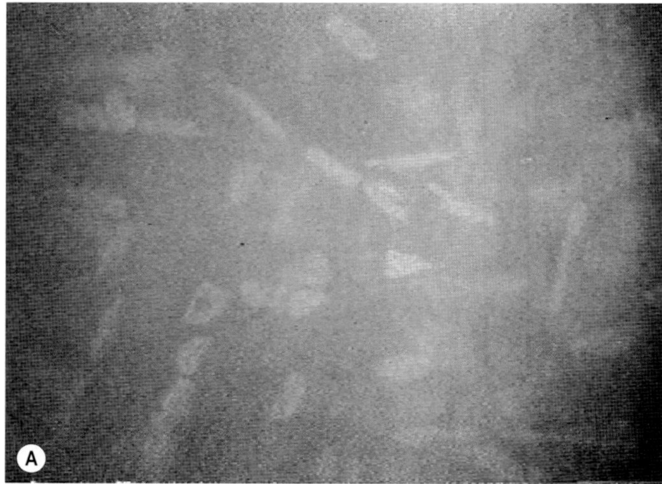

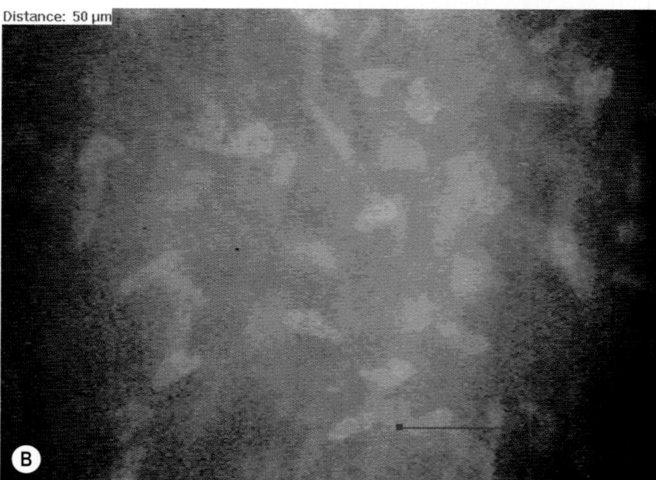

Figure 40.37 (A) Confocal microscopic images of the posterior stroma in a contact lens wearer. (B) An age- and sex-matched non-lens-wearing control subject. (×300.)

Deep stromal opacities

A number of authors have noted apparently benign, deep stromal opacities (DSOs) in the corneas of contact lens wearers (Brooks *et al.*, 1986; Gobbels *et al.*, 1989; Remeijer *et al.*, 1990; Loveridge and Larke, 1992; Holland *et al.*, 1995; Pimenides *et al.*, 1996). The opacities have been variously described as being white, grey, brown, blue and cyan in colour, and cloudy, scar-like, lattice-like and stellate-like in

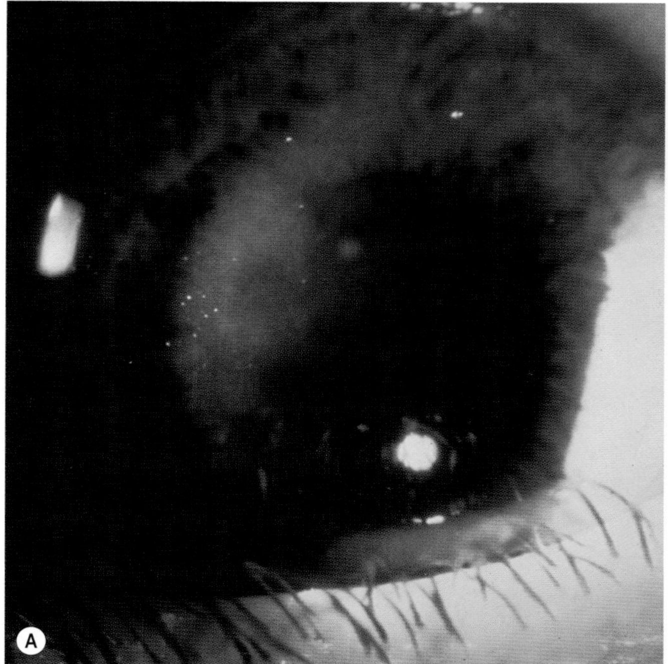

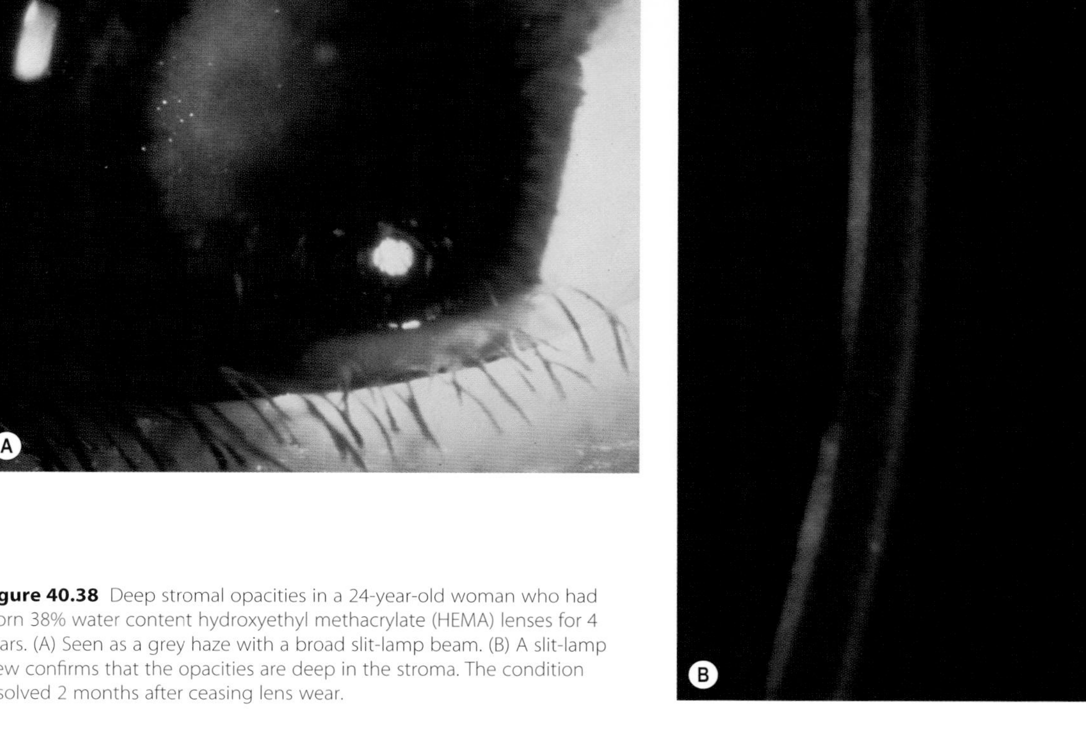

Figure 40.38 Deep stromal opacities in a 24-year-old woman who had worn 38% water content hydroxyethyl methacrylate (HEMA) lenses for 4 years. (A) Seen as a grey haze with a broad slit-lamp beam. (B) A slit-lamp view confirms that the opacities are deep in the stroma. The condition resolved 2 months after ceasing lens wear.

form. They are sometimes associated with folds and striae in Descemet's layer, and with deep stromal vascularization (Loveridge and Larke, 1992). It is possible to distinguish DSOs from infiltrates (which typically reside in the anterior half of the stroma) because DSOs are invariably located deep in the stroma (Figure 40.38). However, DSOs can take on a similar appearance to certain forms of posterior stromal dystrophy, and some of the reported cases of DSO may have been confused with dystrophies. The aetiology of this condition is unknown but probably varied (Loveridge and Larke, 1992).

Examination of the living human cornea at very high magnification (680×) using a confocal microscope has revealed the presence of highly reflective 'microdot deposits' throughout the corneal stroma (Böhnke and Masters, 1997; Trittibach *et al.*, 2005) (Figure 40.39); these microdots may be a subclinical correlate of DSOs. According to Böhnke and Masters (1997), microdots are small, discrete, brightly reflective spots or dots scattered throughout the stroma; they are generally round or oval in shape, and vary in diameter from about 1 to 4 μm. In patients who had worn soft contact lens for an average of 26 years, panstromal microdot deposits were observed with a mean grade of 3.1 (range, 1–4). In the control group, none of 29 patients had stromal microdot deposits. The authors concluded that stromal microdot degeneration may be the early stage of a significant corneal disease, which eventually may affect large numbers of patients after decades of contact lens wear.

Mutalib (2000) conducted an experiment in an attempt to replicate the findings of Böhnke and Masters (1997). The corneas of one eye of 13 patients (age 32 ± 7 years) who had worn contact lenses for an average of 8.2 years were imaged using the confocal microscope, as were the corneas of one eye of 13 age- and sex-matched control subjects who had never worn contact lenses. Microdot deposits were observed in the stroma of all 13 lens wearers, with a mean severity of grade 2.0 ± 1.1. In the control group, microdots were observed in 10 of the 13 subjects, with a mean severity in the 10 eyes displaying microdots of 1.5 ± 0.7. The difference in the severity of microdots was statistically significant. The microdots had an identical appearance in lens-wearing and control subjects, apart from the difference in grading. They were all fairly similar in size (1–2 μm diameter).

The fact that microdot deposits are observed in all subjects, whether contact lenses have been worn or not, suggests that this phenomenon cannot be properly characterized as a disease (Efron, 2005). However, the higher grading assigned to microdots in lens wearers indicates that contact lens wear is exacerbating otherwise normal corneal morphological features. Deep corneal opacities seen with the slit-lamp biomicroscope may be a gross manifestation

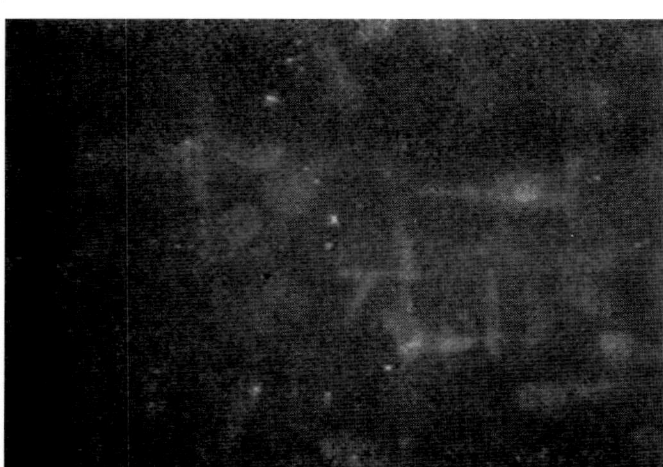

Figure 40.39 Microdot deposits (bright white spots) observed in the posterior stroma of a contact lens wearer.

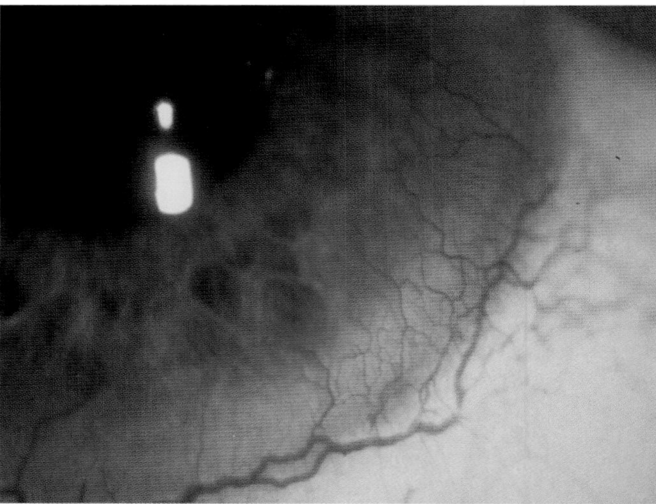

Figure 40.40 Superficial stromal neovascularization.

of microdot formation – for example, by way of a massive aggregation of microdots in the deep stroma.

It should also be recognized that it is not possible at present to determine whether the appearance of DSOs and of microdots is related to the contact lenses or to solutions used in conjunction with lens wear.

Neovascularization

Corneal neovascularization can be defined as the formation and extension of vascular capillaries within and into previously avascular regions of the cornea. Superficial neovascularization is the most common of the various forms of contact lens-induced vascular response (Figure 40.40). Vision loss is rare and will only occur if vessels encroach the pupillary axis or if there has been an extensive leakage of lipid into the stroma (grade 4). Deep stromal neovascularization develops insidiously, usually in an already-compromised cornea (e.g. keratoconus), and may also progress in the absence of acute symptoms (Shah *et al.*, 1998) (Figure 40.41).

A pannus is a thick plexus of vessels typically observed at the superior limbus. Two forms of pannus may be observed in contact lens wearers – active (inflammatory) and fibrovascular (degenerative). An active pannus is avascular and is composed of subepithelial inflammatory cells. In the later stages it may be associated with secondary scarring of the stroma.

In contact lens-induced corneal neovascularization, vessel lumina are approximately 15–80 μm in diameter and contain erythrocytes and sometimes leukocytes. Numerous extravascular leukocytes are observed around blood vessels, and the surrounding stromal lamellae are disorganized and separated with lines of keratocytes lying between them. The overlying corneal epithelium is often affected, with general oedema, cell loss and the presence of large fluid-filled vesicles. The underlying Descemet's layer and endothelium are apparently unaffected (Madigan *et al.*, 1990).

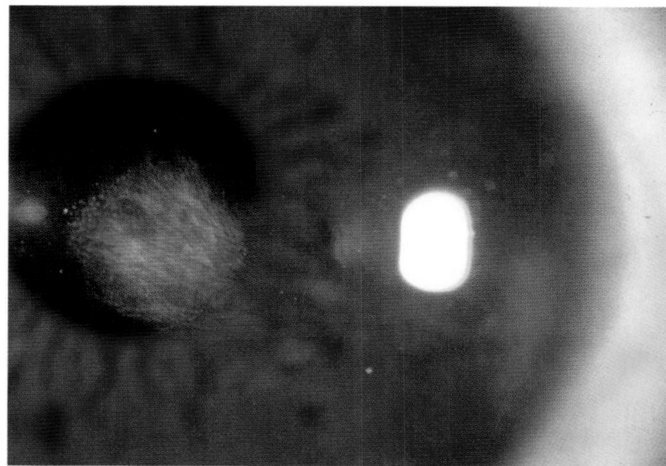

Figure 40.41 Deep stromal neovascularization, progressing to the site of a corneal ulcer.

Contact lens-induced corneal neovascularization can be explained in terms of a dual aetiology model. Chronic hypoxia induces stromal oedema, which 'softens' the stroma and renders this tissue more susceptible to vascular penetration. Some secondary factor must act to stimulate vessel growth – for example, this could be mechanical injury to the epithelium, resulting in a release of enzymes. Inflammatory cells migrate to this site and release vasostimulating agents that cause vessels to grow in that direction.

Efron (1987) reviewed the early literature and calculated that the limits of 'normal' or 'expected' vascular ingrowth (i.e. less than grade 1), measured from the limit of visible iris, were 0.2, 0.4, 0.6 and 1.4 mm for no wear, daily-wear rigid, daily-wear hydrogel and extended-wear hydrogel regimes, respectively. There have been no reports of neovascularization being induced by silicone hydrogel lenses in the first decade after their introduction to the market (Bergenske *et al.*, 2007).

If corneal neovascularization is a primary concern, the prescription of lenses with design features known to provide minimal interference with corneal physiology is indicated, namely: high oxygen transmissibility (to minimize oedema and metabolic acidosis), minimal mechanical effect (as judged by patient comfort) and good movement (to avoid venous stasis resulting from limbal compression in soft lenses). Care systems likely to induce toxic or allergic responses should be avoided, and regular aftercare visits are essential. Other options to be considered include changing from extended wear to daily wear, changing from hydrogel to rigid or silicone hydrogel lenses, replacing lenses more frequently, reducing wearing time or even ceasing lens wear.

Cessation of lens wear will halt the progression of vessel infiltration into the cornea, but empty 'ghost' vessels may remain in place for months or years. Resumption of lens wear in a previously vascularized cornea will result in immediate refilling of the vessels. Thus, in advanced cases of neovascularization, long-term cessation of lens wear is indicated until ghost vessels can no longer be detected.

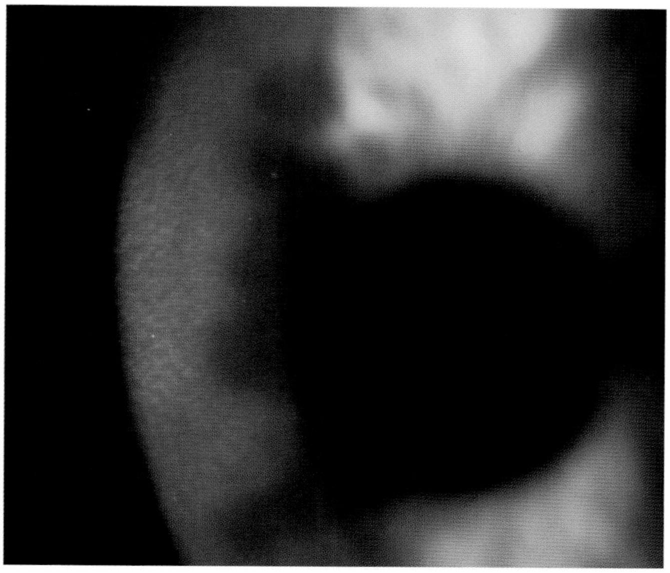

Figure 40.42 Broad band of sterile infiltrative keratitis in a soft lens wearer attributed to hypoxia.

Keratitis

Keratitis refers to inflammation of the cornea. From the perspective of the aetiology and pathology of contact lens-associated keratitis, it is possible to characterize a condition as being either sterile (non-infectious) or microbial (infectious). However, the difficulty with this approach is that, from a clinical perspective, it is virtually impossible to distinguish between the two in the early stages of the disease. To complicate matters further, some researchers have sought to classify sterile keratitis into four subgroups – the so-called contact lens peripheral ulcer, contact lens-associated red eye, infiltrative keratitis and asymptomatic infiltrative keratitis (Sweeney *et al.*, 2003). Subsequent research has shown that it is virtually impossible to differentiate these conditions clinically (Efron and Morgan, 2006a). These approaches have now been abandoned in favour of considering all corneal infiltrative events – from the mildest symptomatic infiltrate to severe microbial keratitis – as a potential disease continuum, and to treat less severe events with caution, as possible cases of microbial keratitis (Efron and Morgan, 2006b).

From an aetiological perspective, contact lens-associated sterile keratitis can result from a variety of mechanisms, such as solution toxicity, bacterial endotoxicity (as distinct from infectivity), immunological reaction, trauma, hypoxia and metabolic disturbance (Figure 40.42). Other aetiological factors include breakdown of trapped post-lens tear film debris, lens deposits and poor patient hygiene. The condition may be ulcerative (Figure 40.43) or non-ulcerative.

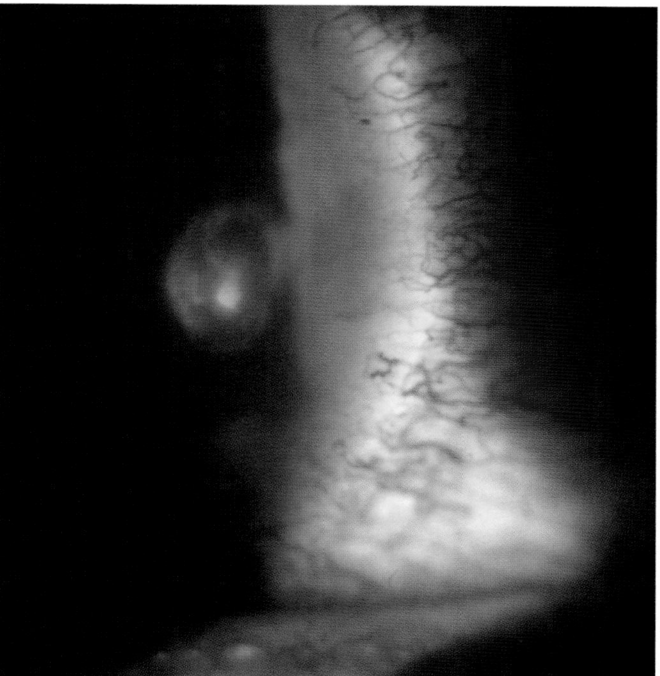

Figure 40.43 Contact lens-associated sterile ulcerative keratitis.

Histopathological analysis of human tissue from patients suffering from sterile keratitis reveals focal areas of epithelial loss, attenuated epithelium and stromal infiltration with polymorphonuclear leukocytes; Bowman's layer is unaffected (Holden *et al.*, 1999).

Contact lens associated microbial (infectious) keratitis can be ulcerative (e.g. *Pseudomonas aeruginosa* keratitis) or non-ulcerative (e.g. epidemic keratoconjunctivitis); the latter form is not *caused* by contact lens wear and will not be considered further here. A positive culture result for bacteria, virus, fungus or amoeba will provide strong evidence that the keratitis is infectious (microbial), but a negative culture result simply means that microbial agents could not be detected in the tissue. In the latter case, a keratitis may still be classified clinically as 'infectious' based upon associated signs and symptoms (Aasuri *et al.*, 2003).

An early symptom of keratitis is a foreign-body sensation in the eyes associated with an increasing desire to remove

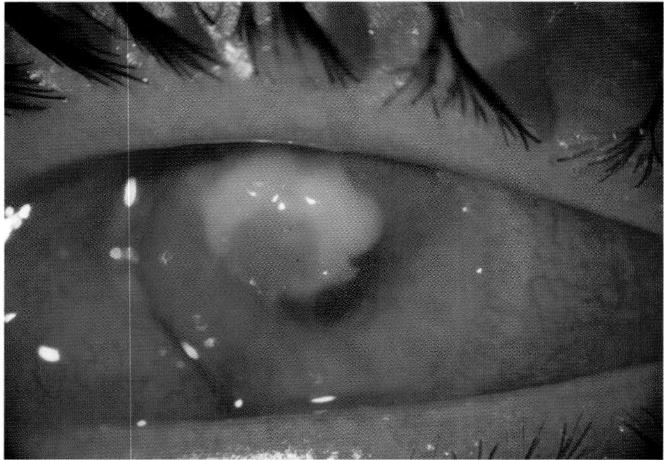

Figure 40.44 Advanced microbial keratitis in a soft lens wearer. The corneal ulcer displays a 'soupy' appearance typical of Gram-negative bacterial keratitis; the lesion was culture-positive for *Pseudomonas aeruginosa*.

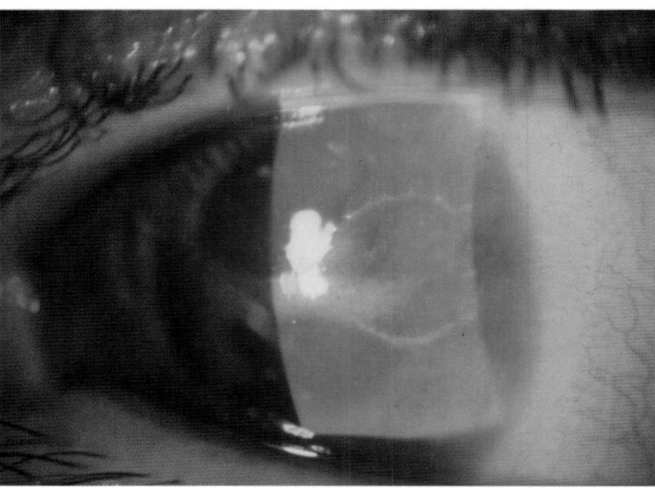

Figure 40.45 Characteristic pattern of radial keratoneuritis in a soft lens wearer with *Acanthamoeba* keratitis.

the lenses. Continuing or worsening discomfort following lens removal should lead a clinician to suspect microbial keratitis, with associated symptoms including pain, eye redness, swollen lids, increased lacrimation, photophobia, discharge and loss of vision. Conversely, if the condition is self-limiting and signs and symptoms eventually resolve without any clinical or therapeutic intervention, the condition can retrospectively be deemed to have been a case of sterile keratitis. However, a mild keratitis, in the early stages of development, should never be diagnosed as a sterile keratitis (or one of the so-called subcategories referred to above). Sterile keratitis is a condition that can only be diagnosed retrospectively. So, if a patient presents with ocular discomfort and infiltrates are evident in the cornea, no matter how apparently mild or innocuous, the case should be considered as a potential microbial keratitis and managed accordingly (Efron and Morgan, 2006b).

Bacterial keratitis (e.g. *Pseudomonas*) can have a rapid and devastating time course. Epithelial and stromal haze, lacrimation and limbal redness adjacent to the lesion will be noticed initially, followed by anterior chamber flare, iritis, hypopyon and a serous or mucopurulent discharge. If not properly treated, the stroma can melt away, leading to corneal perforation in a matter of days (Figure 40.44). The time course of *Acanthamoeba* keratitis is not as rapid; typical signs include corneal staining, pseudodendrites, epithelial and anterior stromal infiltrates which may be focal or diffuse and a classic radial keratoneuritis – this being a circular formation of opacification that becomes apparent relatively early in the disease process (Figure 40.45). A fully developed corneal ulcer may take weeks to form (Moore *et al.*, 1985).

The factors leading to the development of microbial keratitis, and strategies for minimizing the risk of developing this condition, are essentially the same as those discussed above in relation to the aetiology of sterile keratitis, with the obvious additional factor of microbial invasion of corneal tissue. Other risk factors for microbial keratitis include male gender, diabetes, tobacco use and travel to warm climates (Morgan *et al.*, 2005).

A corneal scraping is usually performed to determine if the condition is infectious and possibly to identify the offending microorganism. Medical therapies may include the use of antibiotics, mydriatics, collagenase inhibitors, non-steroidal anti-inflammatory agents, analgesics, tissue adhesives, debridement, bandage lenses and collagen shields. Steroids may be prescribed with extreme caution in the late healing phase to dampen the host response. Surgical interventions include penetrating graft, which may need to be performed in the case of large perforations or non-healing deep central ulceration, or possibly lamellar graft. The prognosis for recovery from microbial keratitis is variable, ranging from a few weeks in the case of *Pseudomonas* keratitis, to many months of regression and recurrence in the case of *Acanthamoeba* keratitis.

Warpage

Videokeratographic corneal mapping techniques reveal that all forms of contact lens wear are capable of inducing small changes in corneal topography. These shape changes, which are generally referred to as 'warpage', are primarily mediated by the stroma, which is the main structural entity of the cornea (the epithelium and endothelium offer little mechanical resistance to deforming forces).

The degree of irregularity of corneal surface shape can be expressed by various mathematical indices. For example, the surface asymmetry index (SAI) provides a quantitative measure of the radial symmetry of the four central videokeratoscope mires surrounding the vertex of the cornea. The higher the degree of central corneal symmetry, the lower the SAI. Ruiz-Montenegro *et al.* (1993) reported SAI mean values (± standard error of mean) associated with the following forms of lens wear: polymethyl methacrylate (PMMA) 0.86 ± 0.22; daily-wear rigid 0.48 ± 0.09; daily-wear hydrogel 0.48 ± 0.11; extended-wear hydrogel 0.46 ± 0.08; and non-lens-wearing controls 0.35 ± 0.03. The SAI was significantly greater than the control group for all forms of lens wear except for daily-wear hydrogel.

The surface regularity index (SRI) is a measure of central and paracentral corneal irregularity derived from the summation of fluctuations in corneal power that occur along semimeridians of the 10 central photokeratoscope mires. The more regular the anterior surface of the central cornea, the lower the SRI. The SRI is highly correlated with best spectacle-corrected visual acuity. Ruiz-Montenegro *et al.* (1993) reported SRI mean values (± standard error of mean) associated with the following forms of lens wear: PMMA 1.17 ± 0.34; daily-wear rigid 0.93 ± 0.18; daily-wear hydrogel 0.52 ± 0.08; extended-wear hydrogel 0.51 ± 0.06; and non-lens-wearing controls 0.41 ± 0.04. The SRI was significantly greater than the control group for PMMA and daily rigid lens wear but not for daily or extended hydrogel lens wear.

All known forms of contact lens-induced warpage can be explained in terms of three underlying pathological mechanisms that primarily act on the stroma. These mechanisms are: (1) physical pressure on the cornea exerted either by the lens and/or eyelids; (2) contact lens-induced stromal oedema; and (3) mucus binding beneath rigid lenses. The relative contributions of these factors will govern the type and extent of topographical alteration (Carney, 1975).

Rigid lenses can induce clinically significant warpage, which may be especially evident in patients with higher prescriptions requiring thicker lenses or unusual lens designs (Figure 40.46). Such lenses will impart greater physical and hypoxic stress on the cornea compared with thinner lenses made of the same material. Altering the parameters of a rigid lens can reduce the physical impact of the lens on the cornea and thus minimize corneal shape changes. Of course, in any case of rigid lens-induced warpage, refitting into soft lenses will usually provide a cure because soft lenses are known to have little or no effect on corneal topography.

The prognosis for recovery of normal corneal topography is highly variable and dependent upon the cause, magnitude and duration of the lens-induced deformation. The time course of recovery from physical forces on the cornea is difficult to predict. Recovery from chronic lens-induced oedema is known to occur within 7 days of cessation of lens wear; thus, recovery from oedema-mediated warpage would be expected to follow a similar time course. Hashemi *et al.* (2008) suggest that a 2-week contact lens-free period is adequate for the cornea to stabilize; however, they suggest that it is difficult to predict the minimum time needed for each individual patient.

Corneal endothelium

As the tissue layer responsible for corneal hydration control, the endothelium must be kept healthy so as to avoid chronic oedema-related problems and the added risk of compromise during ocular surgery. It is only in the past 30 years that it has been recognized that the endothelium can be affected by contact lens wear.

Bedewing

Contact lens-associated endothelial bedewing (CLEB) is characterized by the appearance of small particles in or on the endothelium in the region of the inferior central cornea, immediately below the lower pupil margin (Figure 40.47). The area of bedewing can vary in shape. For example, CLEB may appear as an oval cluster of particles or a less discrete dispersed formation. The condition is usually bilateral. The cells invariably display reversed illumination (see discussion on microcysts, above, for an explanation of this phenomenon), suggesting that bedewing represents inflammatory cells rather than intracellular endothelial oedema (which would display unreversed illumination). When viewed in direct illumination, CLEB can appear as fine white precipitates or as an orange/brown dusting of cells. The colour of the particles can give a clue to the length of time they have been present; newly deposited cells

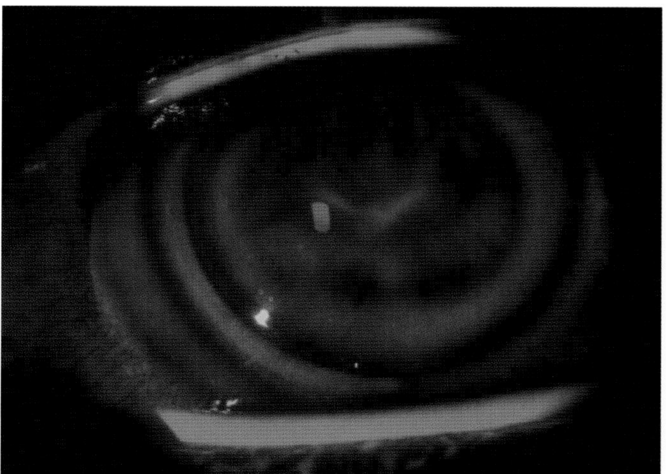

Figure 40.46 Fluorescein pattern showing severe corneal warpage in the form of several concentric bands of deep corneal indentation. This deformation was evident immediately after removal of an immobile hybrid lens (rigid centre and hydrophilic surround annulus). The patient was keratoconic and required a prescription of –34.00 D. The lens caused extreme pain.

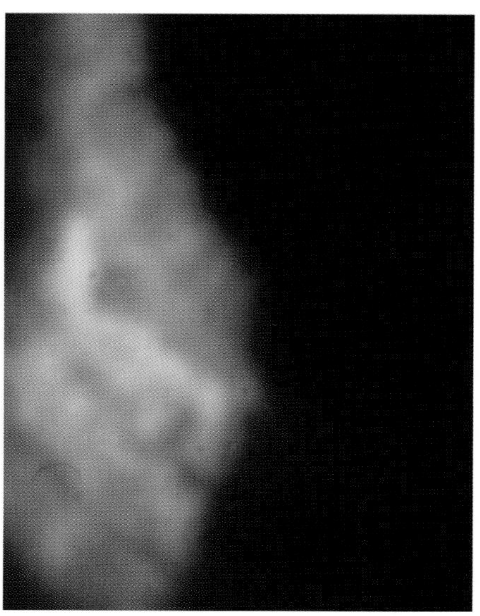

Figure 40.47 Endothelial bedewing.

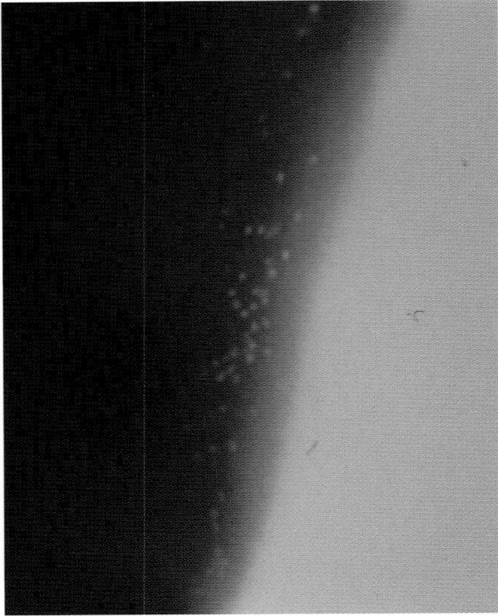

Figure 40.48 Endothelial bedewing observed at high magnification (×40).

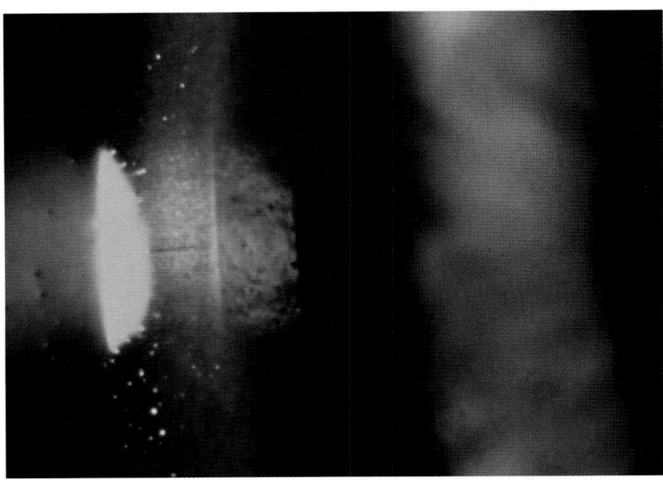

Figure 40.49 Endothelial blebs can be seen in specular reflection (×40) immediately to the left of the dark band running down the centre of the picture.

are often whitish in colour (Figure 40.48), but these become pigmented over time. The cells can become engulfed within the endothelium over time (Bergmanson and Weissman, 1992).

The following signs may coexist with CLEB: conjunctival injection, epithelial erosion, epithelial oedema and reduced corneal transparency. The main associated feature of endothelial bedewing is either total or partial intolerance to lens wear. Some patients may present after having recently abandoned lens wear. Patients may also complain of 'fogging' of vision or stinging.

On the assumption that CLEB represents a mild inflammatory uveal response, the origin of the inflammatory cells is likely to be the iris and/or ciliary body. During inflammation, vascular permeability is increased and inflammatory cells leave vessels in the iris and ciliary body and float around in the aqueous until they come to rest on the endothelial surface. One would therefore expect to observe mild aqueous flare occasionally in patients with CLEB, but this does not appear to have been reported. This mild inflammatory status probably causes lens intolerance.

Patient management is guided by symptomatology rather than clinical signs. Wearing time should be reduced to a level that represents the balance between the needs of the patient to wear lenses for a desired length of time each day versus the level of discomfort that can be tolerated (McMonnies and Zantos, 1979). The presence of inflammatory cells on the endothelial surface should be viewed with great caution by clinicians, because the condition may not necessarily be related to lens wear. Certainly, all forms of uveitis should be considered and tests should be conducted to exclude such possibilities. In all cases of CLEB, intraocular pressures should be measured because some inflammatory cells may have migrated into the anterior angle, creating a blockage of aqueous outflow. Gonioscopy is also indicated, especially if intraocular pressure is elevated.

The pattern of recovery from CLEB is variable. In some cases bedewing will completely disappear within 4 months, and in other cases it may change little over a much longer time period. Lens intolerance may persist for many months in some patients, even after the bedewing has disappeared (McMonnies and Zantos, 1979).

Blebs

The endothelial mosaic undergoes a dramatic alteration in appearance in all lens wearers within minutes of inserting a contact lens. These changes can only just be resolved when observed under the highest magnification possible (×40) using the slit-lamp biomicroscope (Figure 40.49). When viewed at much greater magnification (×200), a number of black, non-reflecting areas can be seen in the endothelial mosaic corresponding to the position of individual cells or groups of cells (Figure 40.50). These are called blebs. There is also an apparent increase in the separation between cells (Zantos and Holden, 1977). There is a large variation in the intensity of the response between patients.

Blebs can be seen within 10 min of lens insertion. The number of blebs peaks in 20–30 min (grade 3), then decreases to a lower level after about 45–60 min. A low-level bleb response (grade 1–2) can be observed throughout the remainder of the wearing period. Hydrogel lenses cause a greater bleb response than rigid lenses, and hydrogel lenses of greater average thickness also induce a greater response than thinner lenses. Brennan *et al.* (2008) demonstrated the percentage area of blebs in response to overnight wear of a 38% water-content hydrogel lens to be 8%, whereas the percentage area of blebs in response to overnight wear of three silicone hydrogel lenses ranged from 1.6 to 2.0%. The percentage area of blebs in response to open-eye wear of silicone hydrogel lenses was 0.4%.

The appearance of blebs can be explained as follows. When the endothelium is viewed using specular reflection, light rays reflect from the tissue plane corresponding to the interface between the posterior surface of the endothelium

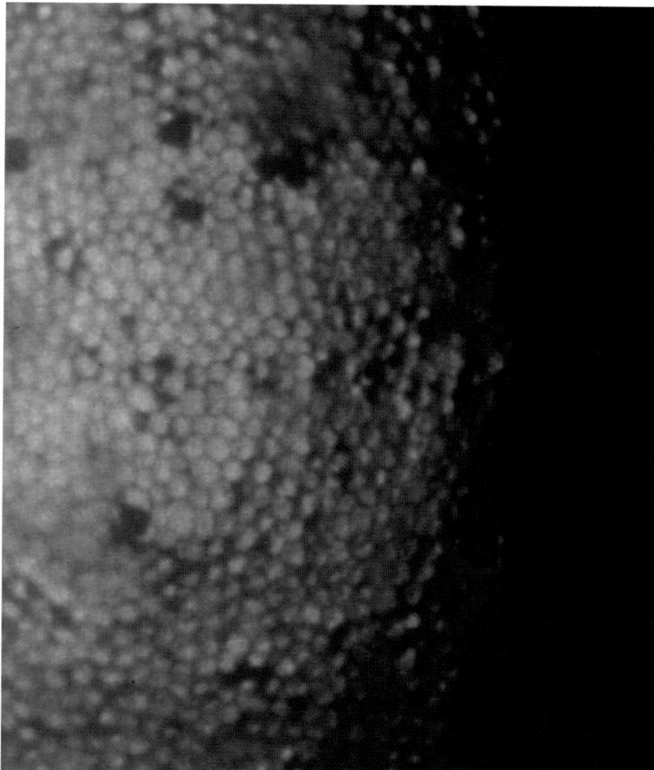

Figure 40.50 Endothelial blebs viewed at ×200 magnification.

and the aqueous humour. This interface acts as the reflective surface because it represents a significant change in tissue refractive index. The light rays that are reflected from this interface give rise to an observed image of an essentially flat (or slightly undulating) and featureless endothelial cell mosaic. Light rays which strike 'blebbed' endothelial cells will be deflected away from the observation path, leaving a corresponding area of darkness. Thus, an endothelial bleb is simply an individual endothelial cell (or group of adjacent cells) that has become swollen and bulged in the direction of the aqueous humour, giving rise to the compelling optical illusion that the cell (or cells) has disappeared.

Endothelial blebs are caused by a local acidic pH change at the endothelium. Two separate factors induce an acidic shift in the cornea during contact lens wear: (1) an increase in carbonic acid due to retardation of carbon dioxide efflux (hypercapnia) by a contact lens; and (2) increased levels of lactic acid as a result of lens-induced oxygen deprivation (hypoxia) and the consequent increase in anaerobic metabolism (Holden *et al.*, 1985c). All cells in the human body function optimally when surrounded by extracellular fluid that is maintained within an acceptable range of pH, temperature, tonicity and ion balance. The carbonic acid and lactic acid alter the physiological status of the environment surrounding the endothelial cells by shifting pH in the acidic direction. This induces changes in membrane permeability and/or membrane pump activity, resulting in a net movement of water into certain endothelial cells when the threshold for a change in membrane permeability is exceeded for those cells. The resultant cellular oedema in such cells is observed as 'blebbing'.

Despite their stunning clinical appearance, blebs are asymptomatic and thought to be of little clinical significance. After removal of a contact lens, blebs disappear within minutes.

Polymegethism

The human corneal endothelium is a single-cell layer that appears as an ordered mosaic of primarily hexagonal-shaped cells (Figure 40.51A). A significant variation in apparent size of cells is referred to as endothelial polymegethism (Figure 40.51B). ('Polymegethism' is derived from the Greek word *megethos* meaning 'size'; *poly* means 'many'). The extent of polymegethism increases throughout life; consequently, the degree of lens-induced polymegethism should be taken to mean the degree of change in excess of that expected for a given age.

It is difficult to assess the integrity of the endothelium using a slit-lamp biomicroscope, because individual endothelial cells are just beyond the limit of resolution. Thus, a normal endothelial mosaic can only be seen as a speckled or textured field. Endothelial polymegethism of a severity greater than grade 2 can sometimes be detected because some of the larger cells can be seen (Figure 40.52). Inspection of the endothelium is best undertaken using instruments designed specifically for high-magnification imaging, such as the specular endothelial microscope or confocal microscope.

Sweeney (1992) has drawn an anecdotal association between endothelial polymegethism and a condition which she termed 'corneal exhaustion syndrome'. This is a condition in which patients who have worn hydrogel contact lenses for many years suddenly develop a severe intolerance to lens wear characterized by ocular discomfort, reduced vision, photophobia and an excessive oedema response. These patients also displayed a distorted endothelial mosaic and moderate to severe polymegethism. Bergmanson (1992), however, has observed that the endothelium of contact lens wearers showed some inter- and intracellular oedema; the cells were otherwise of a healthy appearance containing normal, undamaged organelles. He argues that endothelial polymegethism is a non-problematic adaptation to chronic metabolic stress.

The suggestion that endothelial polymegethism is a benign tissue change has been challenged by researchers who have demonstrated a link between endothelial polymegethism and corneal hydration control (Nieuwendaal *et al.*, 1994). Recovery from oedema is significantly slower in the corneas of contact lens wearers than in matched controls who have corneas with lower levels of polymegethism.

It is likely that the aetiology of endothelial polymegethism – contact lens-induced endothelial acidosis – is precisely the same as the aetiology of endothelial blebs, whereby the former represents a chronic response and the latter represents an acute response to the same stimuli. Endothelial acidosis may induce changes in membrane permeability and/or membrane pump activity, resulting in water movement that acts to elongate endothelial cell walls. A reconfiguration of cell shape then occurs in order to preserve cell volume, resulting in the appearance of

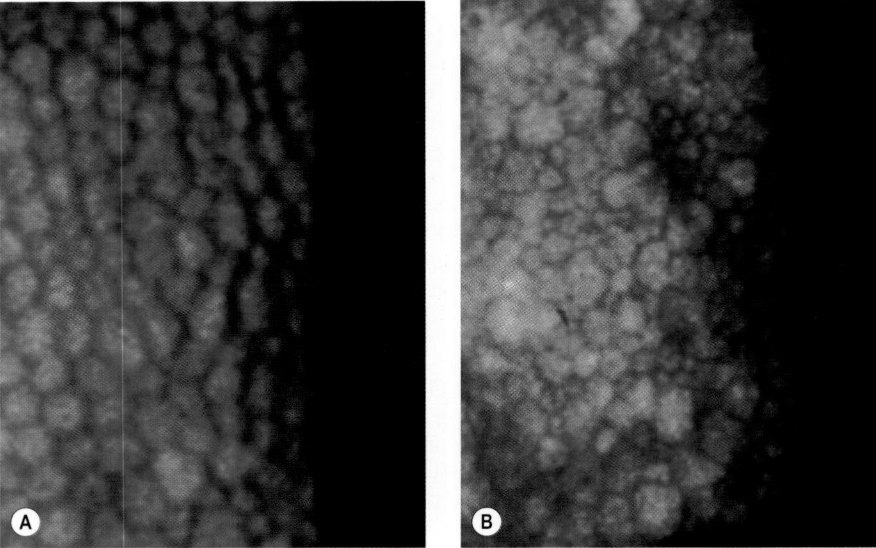

Figure 40.51 (A) Normal endothelial mosaic. (B) Endothelium displaying severe (grade 3.5) polymegethism.

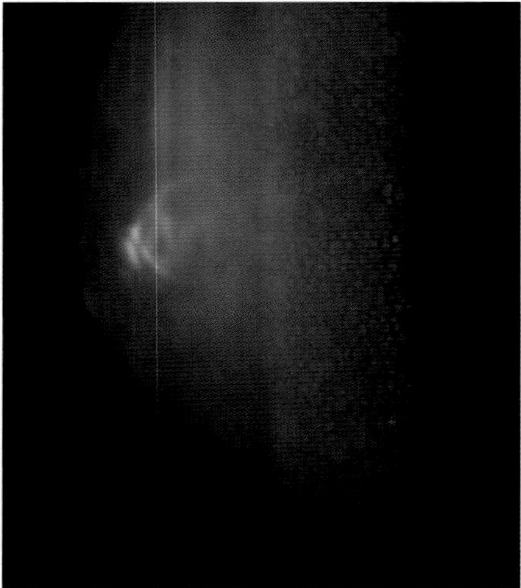

Figure 40.52 Enlarged view of the endothelium as seen with a slit-lamp biomicroscope, showing polymegethism induced by 10 years of soft contact lens wear.

polymegethism at the apical surface of the endothelium (Bergmanson, 1992).

Lenses of higher oxygen performance will induce lower levels of polymegethism (Holden *et al.*, 1985a). Doughty *et al.* (2005) found no significant change in endothelial polymegethism after 6 months of silicone hydrogel lens wear. From a clinical perspective, it is essential to take note of the presence of significant endothelial polymegethism and to take action to minimize the metabolic stress to the cornea known to be associated with this change.

Strategies for alleviating contact lens-induced hypoxia and hypercapnia include the following:

- Fitting lenses of higher oxygen transmissibility, such as silicone hydrogel lenses.
- Sleeping in extended-wear lenses less frequently.
- Changing from extended lens wear to daily lens wear.
- Reducing lens wearing time.
- Fitting rigid lenses with more movement and edge lift (to enhance oxygen-enriching tear exchange).

The prognosis for recovery from endothelial polymegethism is poor. Holden *et al.* (1985b) were unable to detect a recovery from endothelial polymegethism 6 months after removal and cessation of wear of high-water-content hydrogel contact lenses that had previously been worn on an extended-wear basis for an average of 5 years.

Conclusions

This chapter has provided key clinical insights into some of the more common contact lens complications. Many other rare conditions and interesting variations of the complications discussed above have not been considered. The reader is therefore directed to textbooks devoted exclusively to this subject for more detailed information, and encouraged to monitor the ophthalmic literature constantly. As more sophisticated tools continue to be developed that can be used to study the ocular response of the living eye to contact lens wear – such as confocal microscopy and optical coherence tomography (see Chapter 4) – it is certain that further tissue reactions and complications will be discovered.

References

Aasuri, M. K., Venkata, N. and Kumar, V. M. (2003) Differential diagnosis of microbial keratitis and contact lens-induced peripheral ulcer. *Eye Contact Lens,* **29**(1 Suppl), S60–62.

Allansmith, M. R., Korb, D. R., Greiner, J. V. *et al.* (1977) Giant papillary conjunctivitis in contact lens wearers. *Am. J. Ophthalmol.,* **83,** 697–708.

Aragona, P., Ferreri, G., Micali, A. *et al.* (1998) Morphological changes of the conjunctival epithelium in contact lens wearers evaluated by impression cytology. *Eye,* **12,** 461–466.

Arita, R., Itoh, K., Inoue, K. *et al.* (2009) Contact lens wear is associated with decrease of meibomian glands. *Ophthalmology,* **116,** 379–384.

Bergenske, P., Long, B., Dillehay, S. *et al.* (2007) Long-term clinical results: 3 years of up to 30-night continuous wear of lotrafilcon A silicone hydrogel and daily wear of low-*Dk/t* hydrogel lenses. *Eye Contact Lens,* **33,** 74–80.

Bergmanson, J. P. G. (1992) Histopathological analysis of corneal endothelial polymegethism. *Cornea,* **11,** 133–142.

Bergmanson, J. P. G. and Weissman, B. A. (1992) Hypoxic changes in corneal endothelium. Ch. 3. In *Complications of Contact Lens Wear* (A. Tomlinson, ed.) p. 52. St Louis, MO: Mosby Year Book.

Böhnke, M. and Masters, B. R. (1997) Long term contact lens wear induces a corneal degeneration with microdot deposits in the corneal stroma. *Ophthalmology,* **104,** 1887–1896.

Brautaset, R. L., Nilsson, M., Leach, N. *et al.* (2008) Corneal and conjunctival epithelial staining in hydrogel contact lens wearers. *Eye Contact Lens,* **34,** 312–316.

Brennan, N. A. and Efron, N. (1989) Symptomatology of HEMA contact lens wear. *Optom. Vis. Sci.,* **66,** 834–838.

Brennan, N. A., Coles, M. L., Connor, H. R. *et al.* (2007) 12-month prospective clinical trial of comfilcon A silicone-hydrogel contact lenses worn on a 30-day continuous wear basis. *Cont. Lens Anterior Eye,* **30,** 108–118.

Brennan, N. A., Coles, M. L., Connor, H. R. *et al.* (2008) Short-term corneal endothelial response to wear of silicone-hydrogel contact lenses in East Asian eyes. *Eye Contact Lens,* **34,** 317–321.

Brooks, A. M. V., Westmore, R., Grant, G. *et al.* (1986) Deep corneal stromal opacities with contact lenses. *Aust. New Zeal. J. Ophthalmol.,* **14,** 243–249.

Carney, L. G. (1975) The basis of corneal shape change during contact lens wear. *Am. J. Optom.,* **52,** 445–454.

Carney, L. G. and Hill, R. M. (1984) Variation in blinking behaviour during soft lens wear. *Int. Contact Lens Clin.,* **11,** 250–253.

Caroline, P. J., Kame, R. T. and Hatashida, J. K. (1991) Pediculosis parasitic infestation in a contact lens wearer. *Clin. Eye Vis. Care,* **3,** 82–86.

Chen, Q., Wang, J., Shen, M. *et al.* (2009) Lower volumes of tear menisci are associated with dry eye symptoms in contact lens wearers. *Invest. Ophthalmol. Vis. Sci.,* **50,** 3159–3163.

Collins, M., Heron, H. and Larson, R. (1987) Blinking patterns in soft contact lens wearers can be altered with training. *Am. J. Optom. Physiol. Opt.,* **64,** 100–103.

Conner, C., Campbell, J. and Steel, S. (1997) The effects of disposable daily wear contact lenses on goblet cell count. *Contact Lens Assoc. Ophthalmol. J.,* **23,** 37–39.

Covey, M., Sweeney, D. F., Terry, R. *et al.* (2001) Hypoxic effects on the anterior eye of high-*Dk* soft contact lens wearers are negligible. *Optom. Vis. Sci.,* **78,** 95–99.

Doughty, M. J., Aakre, B. M., Ystenaes, A. E. *et al.* (2005) Short-term adaptation of the human corneal endothelium to continuous wear of silicone hydrogel (lotrafilcon A) contact lenses after daily hydrogel lens wear. *Optom. Vis. Sci.,* **82,** 473–480.

Dumbleton, K. (2003) Noninflammatory silicone hydrogel contact lens complications. *Eye Contact Lens,* **29,** S186–189.

Efron, N. (1987) Vascular response of the cornea to contact lens wear. *J. Am. Optom. Assoc.,* **58,** 836–846.

Efron, N. (2005) Microdot stromal degenerations. *Eye Contact Lens,* **31,** 46.

Efron, N. (2007) Contact lens-induced changes in the anterior eye as observed in vivo with the confocal microscope. *Prog. Retin. Eye Res.,* **26,** 398–436.

Efron, N. and Morgan, P. B. (2006a) Can subtypes of contact lens-associated corneal infiltrative events be clinically differentiated? *Cornea,* **25,** 540–544.

Efron, N. and Morgan, P. B. (2006b) Rethinking contact lens associated keratitis. *Clin. Exp. Optom.,* **89,** 280–298.

Efron, N. and Veys, J. (1992) Defects in disposable contact lenses can compromise ocular integrity. *Int. Contact Lens Clin.,* **19,** 8–18.

Efron, N., Hollingsworth, J., Koh, H. H. *et al.* (2001) Confocal microscopy. Ch. 3. In *The Cornea: its Examination in Contact Lens Practice.* (N. Efron, ed.) Oxford: Butterworth-Heinemann.

Fleiszig, S. M. J., Zaidi, T. S. and Ramphal, R. (1994) Modulation of *P. aeruginosa* adherence to the corneal surface by mucus. *Infect. Immun.,* **62,** 1799–1804.

Fonn, D. (2007) Targeting contact lens induced dryness and discomfort: what properties will make lenses more comfortable. *Optom. Vis. Sci.,* **84,** 279–285.

Fonn, D., Pritchard, N. and Garnett, B. (1996) Palpebral aperture sizes of rigid and soft contact lens wearers compared with nonwearers. *Optom. Vis. Sci.,* **73,** 211–214.

Fujiwara, T. I., Matsuo, K., Kondoh, S. *et al.* (2001) Etiology and pathogenesis of aponeurotic blepharoptosis. *Ann. Plastic Surg.,* **46,** 29–35.

Gobbels, M., Wahning, A. and Spitznas, M. (1989) Endothelial function in contact lens-induced deep corneal opacities. *Fortschr. Ophthalmol.,* **86,** 448–450.

Graham, A. D., Truong, T. N. and Lin, M. C. (2009) Conjunctival epithelial flap in continuous contact lens wear. *Optom. Vis. Sci.,* **86,** 324–331.

Grohe, R. M. and Lebow, K. A. (1989) Vascularized limbal keratitis. *Int. Contact Lens Clin.,* **16,** 197–203.

Hashemi, H., Firoozabadi, M. R., Mehravaran, S. *et al.* (2008) Corneal stability after discontinued soft contact lens wear. *Cont. Lens Anterior Eye,* **31,** 122–125.

Hill, R. M. and Carney, L. G. (1984) The effects of hard lens wear on blinking behaviour. *Int. Contact Lens Clin.,* **11,** 242–248.

Holden, B. A. and Sweeney, D. F. (1991) The significance of the epithelial microcyst response: a review. *Optom. Vis. Sci.,* **68,** 703–707.

Holden, B. A., Mertz, G. W. and McNally, J. J. (1983) Corneal swelling response to contact lenses worn under extended wear conditions. *Invest. Ophthalmol. Vis. Sci.,* **24,** 218–226.

Holden, B. A., Sweeney, D. F., Vannas, A. *et al.* (1985a) Effects of long-term extended contact lens wear on the human cornea. *Invest. Ophthalmol. Vis. Sci.,* **26,** 1489–1501.

Holden, B. A., Vannas, A., Nilsson, K. T. *et al.* (1985b) Epithelial and endothelial effects from the extended wear of contact lenses. *Curr. Eye Res.,* **4,** 739–742.

Holden, B. A., Williams, L. and Zantos, S. G. (1985c) The etiology of transient endothelial changes in the human cornea. *Invest. Ophthalmol. Vis. Sci.,* **26,** 1354–1359.

Holden, B. A., Sweeney, D. F., Swarbrick, H. A. *et al.* (1986) The vascular response to long-term extended contact lens wear. *Clin. Exp. Optom.,* **69,** 112–119.

Holden, B. A., Reddy, M. K., Sankaridurg, P. R. *et al.* (1999) Contact lens-induced peripheral ulcers with extended wear of disposable hydrogel lenses: histopathologic observations on the nature and type of corneal infiltrate. *Cornea,* **18,** 538–543.

Holland, E. J., Lee, R. M., Bucci, F. A. *et al.* (1995) Mottled cyan opacification of the posterior cornea in contact lens wearers. *Am. J. Ophthalmol.,* **119,** 620–626.

Iskeleli, G., Onur, U., Ustundag, C. *et al.* (2006) Comparison of corneal thickness of long-term contact lens wearers for different types of contact lenses. *Eye Contact Lens,* **32,** 219–222.

Jalbert, I. and Stapleton, F. (1999) Effect of lens wear on corneal stroma: preliminary findings. *Aust. New Zeal. J. Ophthalmol.,* **27,** 211–213.

Kallinikos, P. and Efron, N. (2004) On the etiology of keratocyte loss during contact lens wear. *Invest. Ophthalmol. Vis. Sci.,* **45,** 3011–3020.

Kallinikos, P., Morgan, P. and Efron, N. (2006) Assessment of stromal keratocytes and tear film inflammatory mediators during extended wear of contact lenses. *Cornea,* **25,** 1–10.

Keay, L., Jalbert, I., Sweeney, D. F. *et al.* (2001) Microcysts: clinical significance and differential diagnosis. *Optometry,* **72,** 452–460.

Keys, J. E. (1996) A comparative study of eyelid cleaning regimens in chronic blepharitis. *Contact Lens Assoc. Ophthalmol. J.,* **22,** 209–213.

Klyce, S. D. (1981) Stromal lactate accumulation can account for corneal oedema osmotically following epithelial hypoxia in the rabbit. *J. Physiol.,* **332,** 49–64.

Knop, E. and Bremitt, H. (1992) Conjunctival cytology in asymptomatic wearers of soft contact lenses. *Graefe's Arch. Clin. Exp. Ophthalmol.,* **230,** 340–347.

Korb, D. R. and Korb, J. M. E. (1970) Corneal staining prior to contact lens wearing. *J. Am. Optom. Assoc.,* **41,** 228–234.

Krutsinger, B. D. and Bergmanson, J. P. G. (1985) Corneal epithelial response to hypotonic exposure. *Int. Eye Care,* **1,** 440–443.

Lakkis, C. and Brennan, N.A. (1996) Bulbar conjunctival fluorescein staining in hydrogel contact lens wearers. *Contact Lens Assoc. Ophthalmol. J.,* 22, 189–194.

Loveridge, R. and Larke, J. (1992) Deep stromal opacification: a review. *J. Br. Contact Lens Assoc.,* **15,** 109–139.

Lowe, R. and Brennan, N. A. (1987) Corneal wrinkling caused by a thin medium water content lens. *Int. Contact Lens Clin.,* **10,** 403–408.

Macsai, M. S. (2008) The role of omega-3 dietary supplementation in blepharitis and meibomian gland dysfunction (an AOS thesis). *Trans. Am. Ophthalmol. Soc.,* **106,** 336–356.

Madigan, M. C., Penfold, P. L., Holden, B. A. *et al.* (1990) Ultrastructural features of contact lens-induced deep corneal neovascularisation and associated stromal leucocytes. *Cornea,* **9,** 144–151.

Mainstone, J. C., Bruce, A. S. and Golding, T. R. (1996) Tear meniscus measurements in the diagnosis of dry eye. *Curr. Eye Res.,* **15,** 653–661.

Maldonado-Codina, C., Morgan, P. B., Schnider, C. M., *et al.* (2004) Short-term physiologic response in neophyte subjects fitted with hydrogel and silicone hydrogel contact lenses. *Optom. Vis. Sci.,* **81,** 911–921.

Martin, R., de Juan, V., Rodriguez, G. *et al.* (2008) Contact lens-induced corneal peripheral swelling differences with extended wear. *Cornea,* **27,** 976–979.

McMonnies, C. W. and Zantos, S. G. (1979) Endothelial bedewing of the cornea in association with contact lens wear. *Br. J. Ophthalmol.,* **63,** 478–482.

Millar, T. J., Papas, E. B., Ozkan, J. *et al.* (2003) Clinical appearance and microscopic analysis of mucin balls associated with contact lens wear. *Cornea,* **22,** 740–745.

Miller, W. L. (1995) Rigid gas permeable defects associated with an isolated case of vascularized limbal keratitis. *Int. Contact Lens Clin.,* **22,** 209–212.

Moore, M. B., McCulley, J. P., Luckenbach, M. (1985) *Acanthamoeba* keratitis associated with soft contact lenses. *Am. J. Ophthalmol.,* **100,** 396–403.

Morgan, P. B. and Maldonado-Codina, C. (2009) Corneal staining: do we really understand what we are seeing? *Cont. Lens Anterior Eye,* **32,** 48–54.

Morgan, P. B., Efron, N., Brennan, N. A. (2005) Risk factors for the development of corneal infiltrative events associated with contact lens wear. *Invest. Ophthalmol. Vis. Sci.,* **46,** 3136–3143.

Mutalib, H. A. (2000) Confocal microscopy of the cornea during contact lens wear. PhD Thesis, University of Manchester Institute of Science and Technology, Manchester, United Kingdom.

Nieuwendaal, C. P., Odenthal, M. T. P., Kok, J. H. C. *et al.* (1994) Morphology and function of the corneal endothelium after long-term contact lens wear. *Invest. Ophthalmol. Vis. Sci.,* **35,** 3071–3077.

Ong, B. L. (1996) Relation between contact lens wear and meibomian gland dysfunction. *Optom. Vis. Sci.,* **73,** 208–210.

Papas, E. (1998) On the relationship between soft contact lens oxygen transmissibility and induced limbal hyperaemia. *Exp. Eye. Res.,* **67,** 125–231.

Paugh, J. R., Knapp, L. L and Martinson, J. R. (1990) Meibomian therapy in problematic contact lens wear. *Optom. Vis. Sci.,* **67,** 803–806.

Pimenides, P., Steele, C. F., McGhee, C. N. J. *et al.* (1996) Deep corneal stromal opacities associated with long term contact lens wear. *Br. J. Ophthalmol.,* **80,** 21–24.

Porazinski, A. D. and Donshik, P. C. (1999) Giant papillary conjunctivitis in frequent replacement contact lens wearers: a retrospective study. *Contact Lens Assoc. Ophthalmol. J.,* **25,** 142–147.

Pritchard, N., Jones, L., Dumbleton, K. *et al.* (2000) Epithelial inclusions in association with mucin ball development in high-oxygen permeability hydrogel lenses. *Optom. Vis. Sci.,* **77,** 68–72.

Quinn, T. G. (1982) Epithelial folds. *Int. Contact Lens Clin.,* **9,** 365–366.

Radford, C. F., Minassian, D., Dart, J. K. *et al.* (2009) Risk factors for nonulcerative contact lens complications in an ophthalmic accident and emergency department: a case-control study. *Ophthalmology,* **116,** 385–392.

Remeijer, L., Van Rij, G., Beekhuis, W. H. *et al.* (1990) Deep corneal stromal opacities in long-term contact lens wear. *Ophthalmology,* **97,** 281–285.

Ruiz-Montenegro, J., Mafr, C. H. and Wilson, S. E. (1993) Corneal topographic alterations in normal contact lens wearers. *Ophthalmology,* **100,** 128–134.

Santodomingo-Rubido, J., Wolffsohn, J. and Gilmartin, B. (2008) Conjunctival epithelial flaps with 18 months of silicone hydrogel contact lens wear. *Eye Contact Lens,* **34,** 35–38.

Shah, S. S., Yeung, K. K. and Weissman, B. A. (1998) Contact lens-related deep stromal vascularization. *Int. Contact Lens Clin.,* **25,** 128–136.

Skotnitsky, C. C., Naduvilath, T. J., Sweeney, D. F. *et al.* (2006) Two presentations of contact lens-induced papillary conjunctivitis (CLPC) in hydrogel lens wear: local and general. *Optom. Vis. Sci.,* **83,** 27–36.

Sorbara, L., Jones, L., Williams-Lyn, D. (2009) Contact lens induced papillary conjunctivitis with silicone hydrogel lenses. *Cont. Lens Anterior Eye,* **32,** 93–96.

Stenson, S. (1983) Superior limbic keratoconjunctivitis associated with soft contact lens wear. *Arch. Ophthalmol.,* **101,** 402–404.

Sweeney, D. F. (1992) Corneal exhaustion syndrome with long-term wear of contact lenses. *Optom. Vis. Sci.,* **69,** 601–608.

Sweeney, D. F., Du Toit, R., Keay, L. *et al.* (2004) Clinical performance of silicone hydrogel lenses. Ch. 5. In *Silicone Hydrogels: Continuous-Wear Contact Lenses* (D. F. Sweeney, ed.), 2nd edn, pp. 90–149. Edinburgh: Butterworth-Heinemann.

Sweeney, D. F., Jalbert, I., Covey, M. *et al.* (2003) Clinical characterization of corneal infiltrative events observed with soft contact lens wear. *Cornea,* **22,** 435–442.

Tan, J., Keay, L., Jalbert, I. *et al.* (2003) Mucin balls with wear of conventional and silicone hydrogel contact lenses. *Optom. Vis. Sci.,* **80,** 291–297.

Trittibach, P., Cadez, R., Eschmann, R. *et al* (2005) Determination of microdot stromal degenerations within corneas of long-term contact lens wearers by confocal microscopy. *Eye Contact Lens,* **30,** 127–131.

van den Bosch, W. A. and Lemij, H. G. (1992) Blepharoptosis induced by prolonged hard contact lens wear. *Ophthalmology,* **99,** 1759–1765.

van Der Worp, E., De Brabander, J., Swarbrick, H. *et al.* (2008) Eyeblink frequency and type in relation to 3- and 9-o'clock staining and gas permeable contact lens variables. *Optom. Vis. Sci.,* **85,** 857–866.

Watanabe, A., Araki, B., Noso, K. *et al.* (2006) Histopathology of blepharoptosis induced by prolonged hard contact lens wear. *Am. J. Ophthalmol.,* **141,** 1092–1096.

Wilson, L. A., McNatt, J. and Reitschel, R. (1981) Delayed hypersensitivity to thiomersal in soft contact lens wearers. *Ophthalmology,* **81,** 804–809.

Wilson, G., Ren, H. and Laurent, J. (1995) Corneal epithelial fluorescein staining. *J. Am. Optom. Assoc.,* **66,** 435–439.

Zantos, S. G. (1983) Cystic formations in the corneal epithelium during extended wear of contact lenses. *Int. Contact Lens Clin.,* **10,** 128–137.

Zantos, S. G. and Holden, B. A. (1977) Transient endothelial changes soon after wearing soft contact lenses. *Am. J. Optom. Physiol. Opt.,* **54,** 856–858.

Digital imaging

Adrian S Bruce and Milton M Hom

Introduction

Digital imaging has quickly become a ubiquitous part of modern life, particularly due to the growing popularity of camera phones and consumer digital cameras. Inside the consulting room, digital imaging has also been demonstrating phenomenal growth and diversity.

'Digital imaging' refers to the electronic form of capturing and displaying pictures, by using a combination of computer and camera. In contact lens practice, digital imaging is most often used to document contact lens fittings and ocular pathology. As with all forms of technology, cameras and computer systems become better in quality, cheaper to set up and easier to operate as time goes on. This chapter shows how to set up a digital imaging system, illustrates the results that can be obtained and outlines the benefits for contact lens practice.

Photodocumentation has traditionally been used by contact lens practitioners primarily for the purposes of publications, presentations and for teaching purposes; however, with the advent of digital imaging, photodocumentation has become easier and it is being used increasingly for routine electronic medical records, and to assist in real-time patient education. In addition, photodocumentation is valuable in referrals and in documentation in cases of potential legal action (Schwartz, 1998).

In summary, photodocumentation enhances communication with other practitioners and with patients, as well as enhancing the accuracy of clinical records. The merits of photodocumentation are numerous. Digital imaging has taken photodocumentation to another level.

Previous imaging methods

Traditionally, the imaging system of choice for contact lens practice was a photographic 35 mm film slit-lamp biomicroscope. A photographic slit lamp differs from a conventional slit lamp in that a flash tube is built into the illumination system. The flash is necessary to provide sufficient illumination for correct exposure of photographic film. The camera is mounted on the slit lamp with a beam splitter attached to the observation system. Photographic slit lamps were not widely used in clinical practice because they were difficult to use and substantially more expensive than conventional models. One of the most difficult aspects in photographic slit-lamp technique was obtaining proper lighting. The learning curve was steep because of the guesswork involved in setting up the illumination.

Video recording may also be used for imaging (Hammack, 1995). A video camera is mounted on a slit lamp and the image is saved with videotape or a video printer. A built-in slit-flash system is not required; thus, video recording systems can be retrofitted to many slit lamps. Video-based systems allow instant imaging, which assists patient education. A disadvantage of a videotape type of system was cumbersome editing. Finding the exact location on the tape to make edits could be very time-consuming. Editing done on the computer has greatly simplified everything.

Despite this array of high-technology and high-quality alternatives, the most common method for recording contact lens fittings or ocular changes remains the use of handwritten notes and diagrams. In recent years these have been improved somewhat with the advent of formal grading scales (Efron *et al.*, 2001; Pritchard *et al.*, 2003) (see Chapter 39 and Appendix K). One problem with notes and diagrams is variability between observers. Even amongst the same observer, over a long interval between visits, some interpretation of the notes may be required.

Principles of digital imaging

The basic principle of digital imaging is that a light-sensitive silicon computer chip is used instead of film in a camera. The silicon chip is known as a charge-coupled device (CCD), and forms the light-sensitive element in video and digital cameras. The image can be instantly

DOI: 10.1016/B978-0-7506-8869-7.00041-0

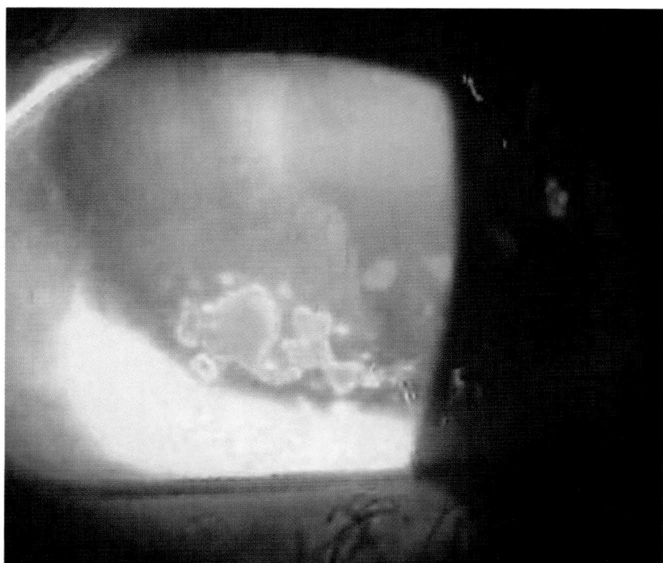

Figure 41.1 Image of corneal staining taken through the eyepiece of a slit lamp with a Palm Treo mobile telephone. Such digital imaging is highly convenient, although the quality is limited.

displayed on a computer screen, viewed by the practitioner and patient, then stored or printed.

Digital imaging is so common now that most mobile telephones include a digital camera. Although the quality of such cameras may not be ideal, the convenience and utility are indications of the progress in digital imaging in recent years. Figure 41.1 shows an image of corneal staining taken through a slit lamp with a mobile telephone digital camera.

Previous reviews of digital imaging have discussed the issues of image resolution and colour depth (Cox, 1995; Meyler and Burnett-Hodd, 1998) and these are therefore not covered in great depth here. A digital image may be characterized in three main ways:

1. The image resolution refers to the image dimensions (width × height) in units of the number of dots (pixels). Common resolutions are 640 × 480 or 1280 × 960, although larger images from digital still cameras are common.
2. The colour depth is the number of colours that may be specified for each pixel. For true colour this should be in the thousands or millions.
3. The file format for an image describes the way it is saved on disk and affects its compatibility with different programs for viewing and e-mailing. The internet standard image file format is jpeg, and carries the benefit of small file size, high definition and broad compatibility with internet e-mail and browser software.

Benefits of digital imaging for contact lens practice

There are numerous features and benefits with digital imaging (Table 41.1). These include the following:

Table 41.1 Summary of features of digital imaging

Instant result
Zero cost per image
Educate patients
Make prints for referral
Store many images on computer
Make movies as well as stills
Transfer over the internet
Image copies have no loss of quality

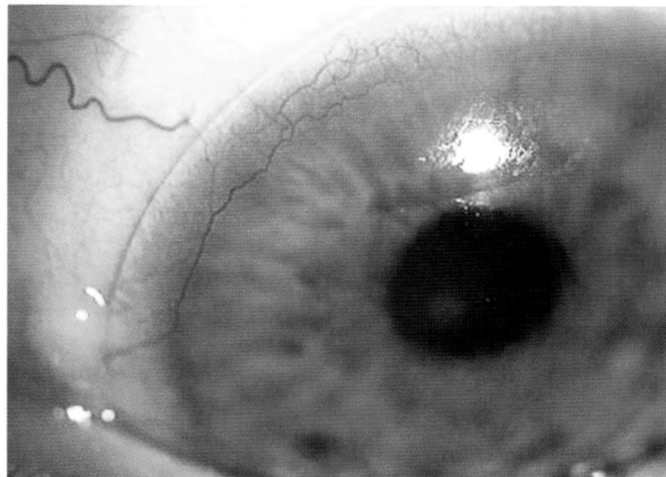

Figure 41.2 Corneal neovascularization.

- Instant imaging – digital imaging avoids the delay required for film processing in conventional photography. Thus any error in image focus or exposure can be corrected immediately. The main drawback to good photodocumentation (proper illumination) is easier to rectify when the feedback is instant.
- Patient education – there is a benefit in the patient immediately seeing his or her own condition. An example is the demonstration of limbal neovascularization (Figure 41.2). The patient 'wow' factor is beneficial to practice growth.
- Image manipulation and quantification – after an image is captured, the brightness, contrast or colour may be enhanced (see below). Furthermore, image parameters can be quantified by the computer, e.g. blood vessel length, scar dimensions and cup/disc ratio. However, care must be taken not to alter an image that may be legal evidence. Image-editing software is available off-the-shelf and can correct brightness and contrast with a click of a button.
- Video movies – dynamic conditions such as contact lens fittings or certain dynamic forms of pathology evaluation can be captured as a short movie on the computer. For example, a movie enables recording of the intricacies of lid interactions and the effects of lens centration on fluorescein patterns. Lens performance is

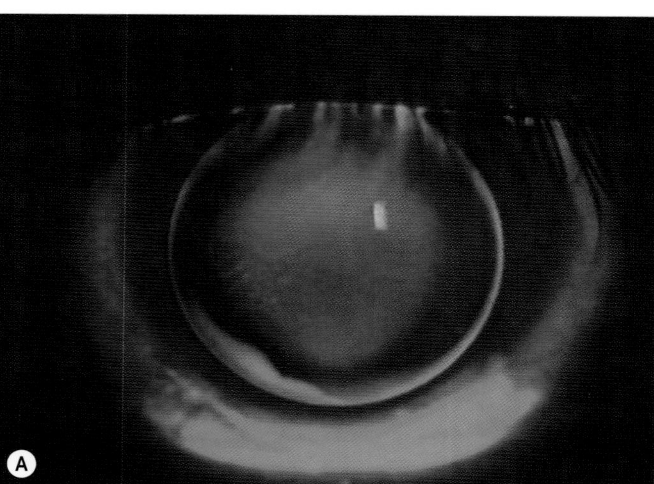

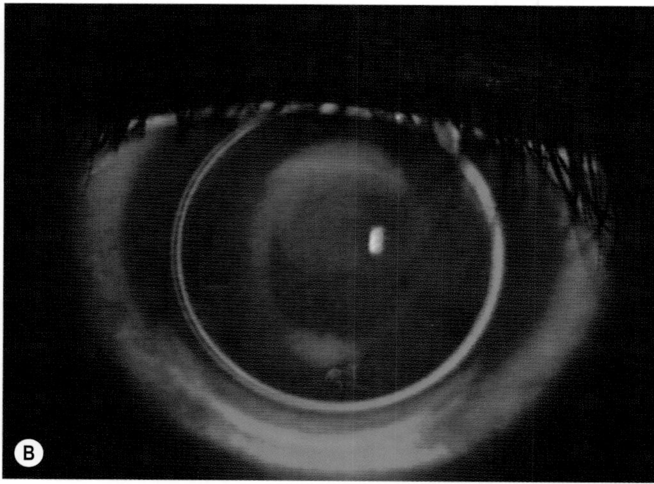

Figure 41.3 Keratoconic fitting. (A) Rigid spherical lens fitting on keratoconic cornea (Quadcurve design; back optic zone radius 6.70 mm; total diameter 9.00 mm; back optic zone diameter 6.80 mm). (B) Rigid spherical lens with toric periphery fitting on keratoconic cornea (Quadcurve design; back optic zone radius 6.70 mm; total diameter 8.80 mm; back optic zone diameter 6.60 mm; periphery +0.6/1.2(0.5), +1.9/2.4(0.3), +4.0/4.5(0.3)).

much easier to understand and interpret when a moving (versus static) image is presented.

Once the digital image has been captured in an electronic format; this opens up the following possibilities:

- Paperless office – many contact lens practices are using electronic medical records for patient visits. Digital imaging is a logical adjunct to electronic records. With the internet, patient records can be accessed at more than one office location.
- Minimal image costs – once a digital imaging system is set up, an image can be captured instantly and at no additional cost. With modern computers having multigigabyte hard-disk capacity, many thousands of images may be easily stored and retrieved.
- Image transfer – increasingly, clinicians are communicating by e-mail. A digital image is already on the computer and this makes attachment to an e-mail easy. E-mail has made consultations with colleagues from all over the world accessible.
- Presentations – images can be transferred to computer presentation programs, which are used for training and delivering lectures. Digital images can easily be dropped into Powerpoint and Keynote presentation programs (see Table 41.1).

Examples of digital imaging in contact lens practice

Limbal neovascularization

The eye featured in Figure 41.3 showed significant superior superficial corneal neovascularization related to wear of a low-water-content high-minus-prescription lens. In this instance digital imaging served two main purposes. The image was shown to the patient at the time of the consultation, to explain the condition and to reinforce management. The image was also used as a reference against which any subsequent changes in the vessels were assessed.

Rigid lens fitting

Quadcurve lenses with toric peripheral curves were used to fit the keratoconic eye featured in Figure 41.3. A number of lenses were ordered and digital images were recorded of each fit; this enabled an accurate record of each lens fitting.

More complex rigid lens fluorescein patterns such as these would have been difficult to characterize via a hand-drawn diagram.

Refractive surgery on disposable contact lens wearer

A highly myopic patient (–10.00 D) had been wearing disposable hydrogel lenses for several years. The patient then underwent unilateral excimer photorefractive keratectomy, which unfortunately resulted in regression and some scarring (Figure 41.4A).

Two years later, the patient successfully had a further photorefractive keratectomy procedure performed on the same eye in order to reduce the scarring (Figure 41.4B). The patient now has a prescription of –2.00 D in that eye and is relatively happy with the outcome.

Illumination methods for slit-lamp digital imaging

There are four commonly used illumination techniques for photodocumentation:

1. Diffuser – this is best for opaque tissues, such as the conjunctiva, sclera and eyelids. It is used in conjunction with a full-width slit, and the brightness of the beam is varied for optimum exposure.

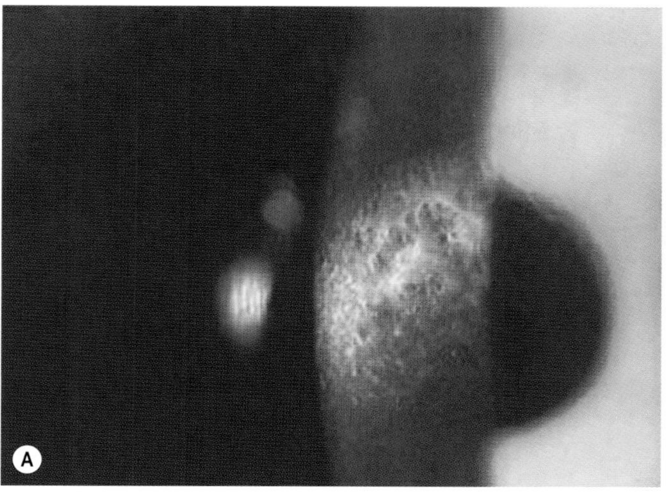

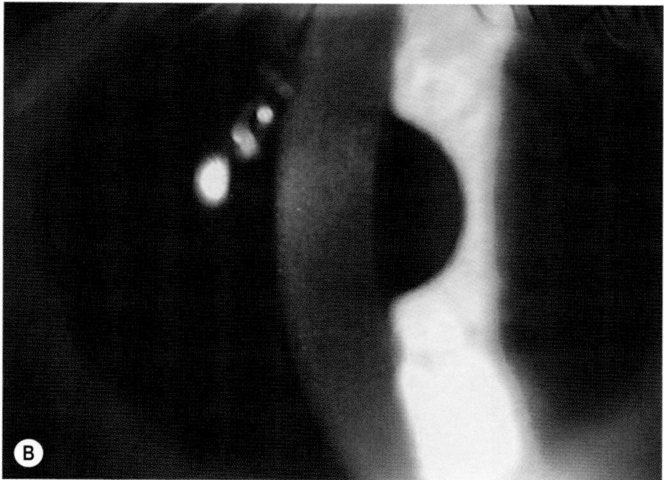

Figure 41.4 Excimer photorefractive keratectomy. (A) Corneal scarring after first refractive surgery procedure. (B) Reduction in corneal scarring after second surgical procedure.

2. Slit section – this is most useful for transparent tissues. An angled slit beam gives a dark-field background to highlight features. A slit section can also be used with retroillumination to highlight opaque tissue changes.
3. Fluorescein staining – surface defects are best shown with the combination of a cobalt blue illumination filter and a yellow barrier filter with a wide slit beam.
4. Tear film assessment – specular illumination with the slit lamp or other instrument will show lipid layer patterns, tear film thickness and break-up (Nichols *et al.*, 2002).

Examples of digital images for each of the illumination types are shown in Figure 41.5.

Commercial digital imaging systems

Contact lens practitioners wishing to enter the world of digital imaging have the choice of purchasing a commercially produced system or building their own system.

A commercially produced digital imaging system can be defined as a ready-to-use integrated system, sold by an ophthalmic equipment supplier. It will typically consist of a slit-lamp biomicroscope with video camera, or digital still camera, beam splitter and a personal computer with database and image manipulation software. Commercial systems are also available that may adapt to the practitioner's existing slit lamp (Table 41.2).

A commercial digital imaging system is probably the best alternative for practitioners who are not so familiar with computers. These systems have the benefit of a relatively simple interface and an easy-to-use database for managing records. The company supplying the equipment will have taken care of the technical issues related to setting up image acquisition by the computer from the video camera.

Table 41.2 Some commercial digital imaging slit-lamp systems

Slit-lamp system	Type	Link
SL 990 Digital Vision System	Video Firewire	www.csophthalmic.com www.dfv.com.au
Haag-Streit Imaging Module IM-900	Video Firewire	www.haag-streit.com www.haag-streit-usa.com
Topcon SL-D7/D8Z Imaging System	Still USB	www.topconmedical.com
Mayo Multimedia Turnkey System	Video Firewire	www.mayoimaging.com
Veatch Ophthalmic Instruments ReSeeVit System	Video Firewire	http://www.veatchinstruments.com/
Marco iDoc	Video Firewire	www.marco.com
Marco Snapshot	Still USB	www.marco.com

Some of these links were located from the Review of Optometry Product Source website: http://www.revoptom.com/productguide.asp.

'Build-your-own' digital imaging system

Many of the components required for a build-your-own system are available from consumer outlets; therefore, it is a realistic proposition for practitioners with a technical interest to build their own system. In most cases the components are modular and easily connected. Perhaps the best reason to consider building your own digital imaging system is the lower overall cost – around half the price, as a result of not having to pay for a customized database program or for the assembly of the system.

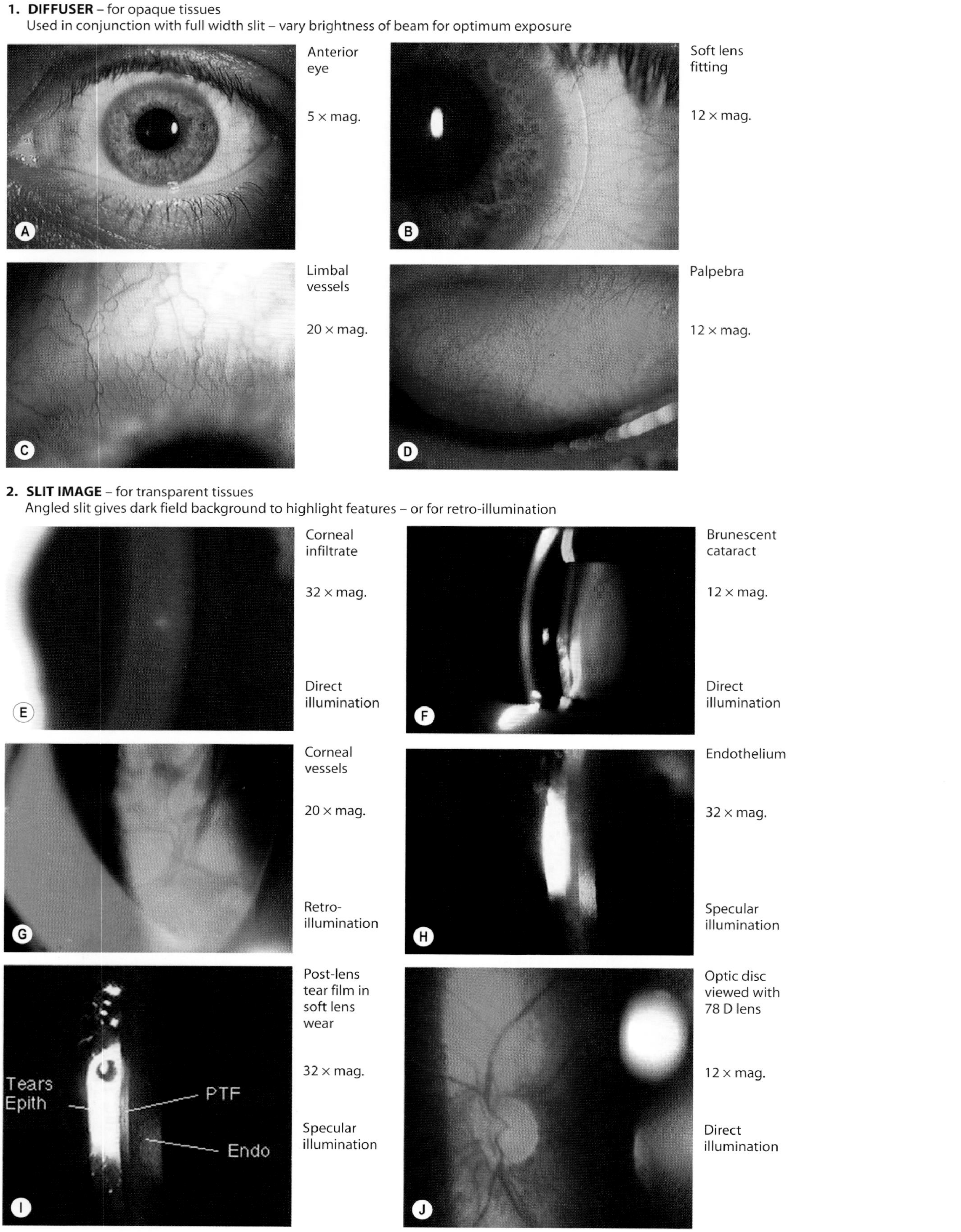

1. **DIFFUSER** – for opaque tissues
Used in conjunction with full width slit – vary brightness of beam for optimum exposure

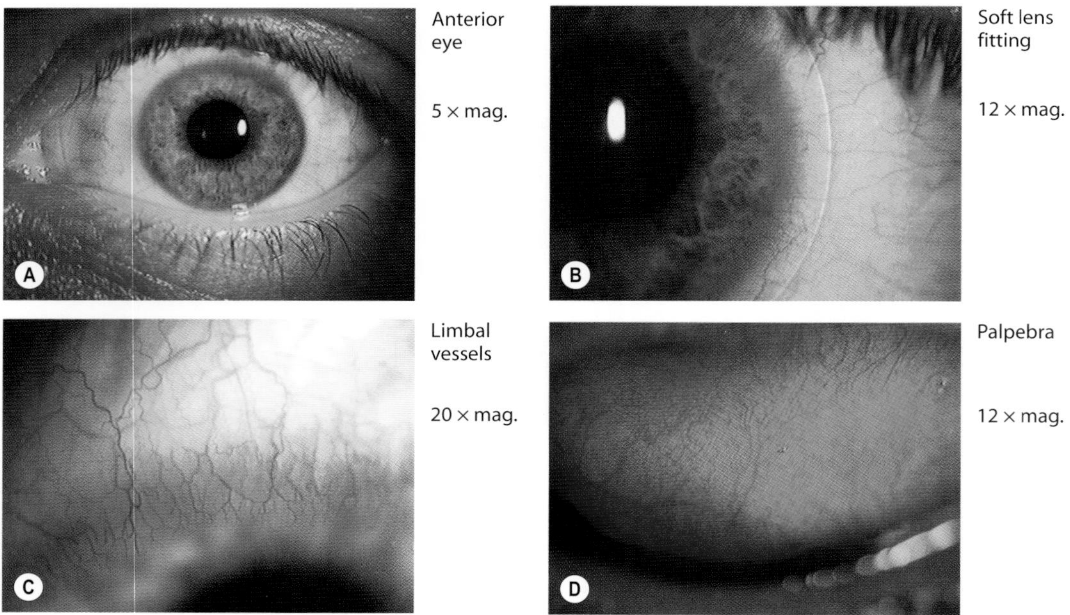

A: Anterior eye — 5 × mag.

B: Soft lens fitting — 12 × mag.

C: Limbal vessels — 20 × mag.

D: Palpebra — 12 × mag.

2. **SLIT IMAGE** – for transparent tissues
Angled slit gives dark field background to highlight features – or for retro-illumination

E: Corneal infiltrate — 32 × mag. — Direct illumination

F: Brunescent cataract — 12 × mag. — Direct illumination

G: Corneal vessels — 20 × mag. — Retro-illumination

H: Endothelium — 32 × mag. — Specular illumination

I: Post-lens tear film in soft lens wear — 32 × mag. — Specular illumination

Tears
Epith
PTF
Endo

J: Optic disc viewed with 78 D lens — 12 × mag. — Direct illumination

Figure 41.5 Slit-lamp photography: illumination and magnification guide.

3. FLUORESCEIN STAINING
Cobalt blue illumination filter, yellow barrier filter, high slit brightness; wide slit width

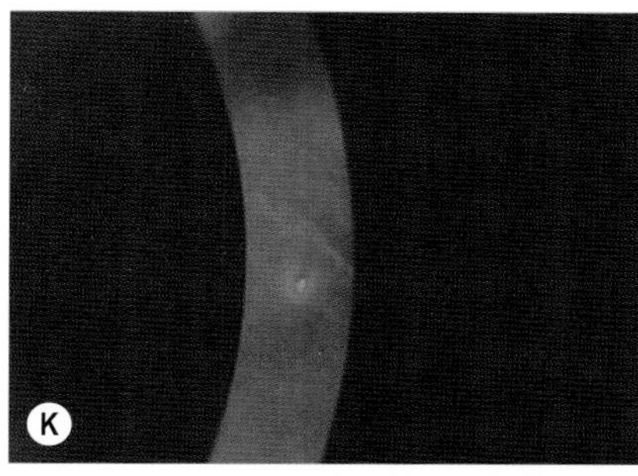

Corneal punctate staining

20 × mag.

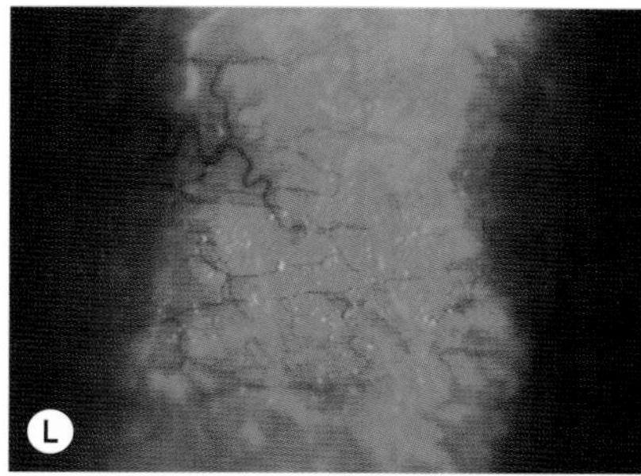

Bulbar conjunctival staining

20 × mag.

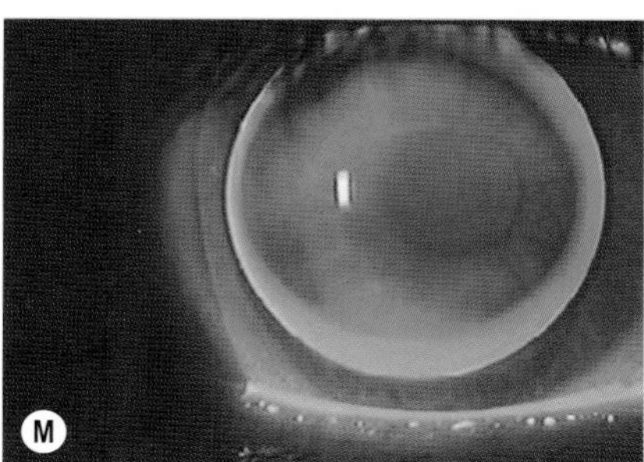

Rigid lens fitting

8 × mag.

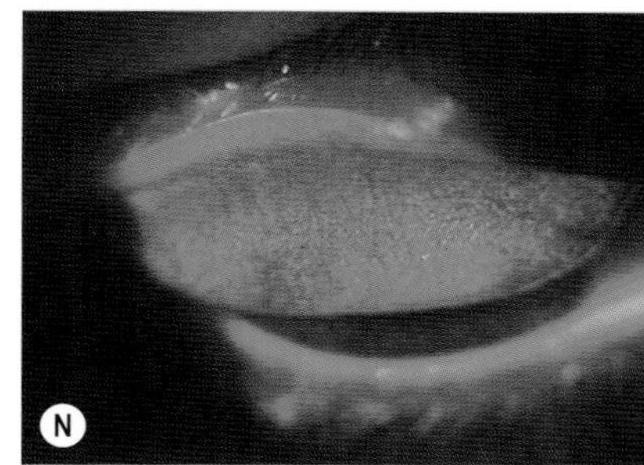

Palpebral conjunctiva – early papillary conjunctivitis

5 × mag.

4. TEAR-FILM OBSERVATION WITH THE KEELER TEARSCOPE

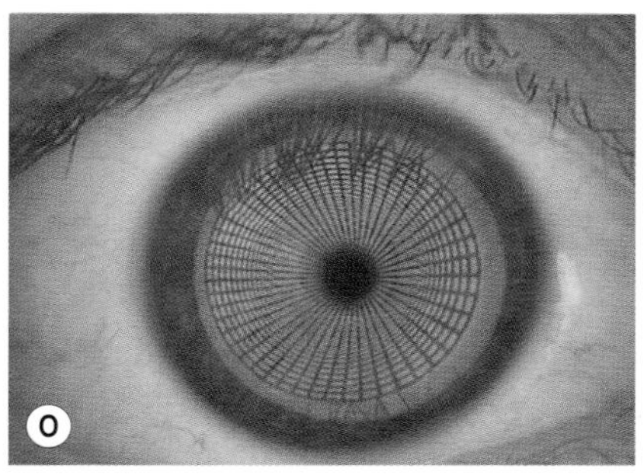

Tearscope mires for break-up time

5 × mag.

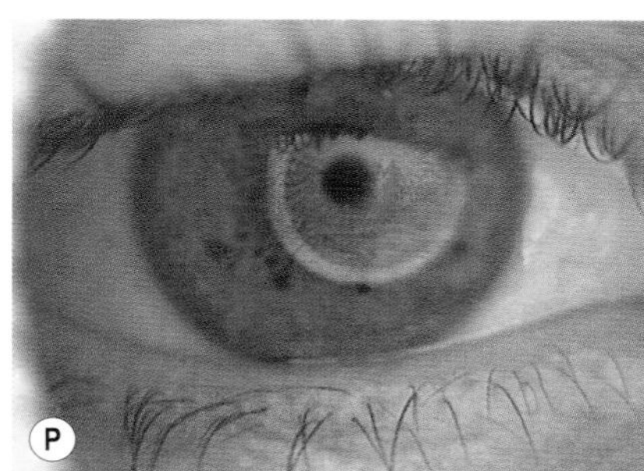

Lipid layer of tear film, located in a different focal plane to the Tearscope mires

5 × mag.

Figure 41.5 *Continued*

A do-it-yourself system is easier to upgrade. Most of the turn-key systems have imaging optics that are at lower resolution than those you can find on your own. For instance, an off-the-shelf digital camera will usually offer higher resolutions and lower costs than the turn-key system. Many times, changing the camera is all that is required to upgrade.

In essence, digital imaging in contact lens practice can take three forms – employing a video slit lamp, a digital still camera slit lamp or an anterior eye camera.

Video slit-lamp imaging system

The most common approach for contact lens work is to use a video slit lamp to capture the image, then a personal computer with a video capture facility to digitize the image. The image can then be displayed on the computer, saved or printed. This option has the benefits of good low-light performance, live image preview and the facility for digital movie capture (Meyler and Burnett-Hodd, 1998).

The two key steps are to connect a video camera to the slit lamp and to input the video signal into the computer. If a beam splitter is available for the slit lamp, then the remainder of the system is relatively inexpensive.

Digital video camera and beam splitter

The permanent connection of a video camera to a slit lamp requires a beam splitter in the slit-lamp observation system. If it is intended to use an existing slit lamp, it will be necessary to check with a slit-lamp supplier whether a suitable beam splitter is available.

Some slit lamps come with a built-in beam splitter as standard, like the Haag-Streit BD900 slit lamp (Figure 41.6). This is a neat design, since it is in line with the observation system and makes it easy to connect a video (CCD) camera. Other slit lamps have a modular design, like the Zeiss SL120 or CSO SL990, and the beam splitter and camera can be readily added together. Contact information for these manufacturers is in Table 41.2.

For these types of beam splitter a video camera must be selected. A good solution is a single- or three-CCD

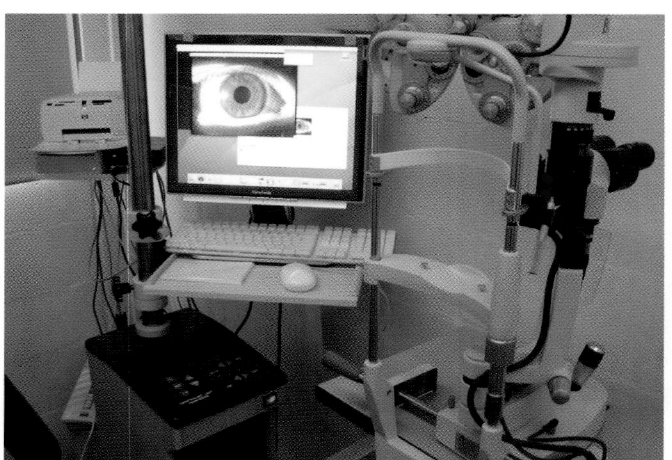

Figure 41.6 Haag-Streit BD900 video slit lamp, with compact off-the-shelf imaging system. There is an Apple Mac Mini running BTVPro software, interfaced to a Canopus ADVC-90 for video conversion, HP compact photo printer and flat-panel LCD display.

microcamera with separate power supply. These are known as 'lipstick' cameras, due to their compact size, making them suited for an ophthalmic instrument. The low-light performance, resolution and colour rendering are acceptable for most slit-lamp applications. If a video camera with a digital (Firewire or USB) output is selected, then it will directly connect to your computer.

Computer and video digitizer

Almost any current or recent model computer can be used for digital imaging, running either Windows XP/Vista, or Mac OS X 10.3–10.5. The Apple Mac Mini (www.apple.com) is ideal for the consulting room, since it is both small and quiet, being about the size of five compact disc cases stacked on top of each other. If you prefer a Windows computer or need the compatibility, consider a laptop computer, as they are also relatively compact and quiet. Desktop Windows machines have the advantage of low cost, but they take up much space.

There are also numerous choices in video digitizers:

- Firewire (IEEE 1394) – the Firewire plug is installed on some computers. If available, this interface is ideal, since the Firewire plug was specifically designed for high-speed (400 Mb/s) connection to a digital video camcorder or video converter. Digital video cameras have the Firewire plug, rather than the traditional analogue video composite or s-video plugs. If your slit lamp has an analogue video camera, then use a Firewire video converter, for example the Canopus ADVC-55 (www.canopus.us).
- USB video digitizer – this is an inexpensive external converter that simply plugs into the USB plug on all computers. The video slit-lamp plug (s-VHS or composite video) plugs into the USB video converter.
- PCI video digitizer card – which is installed internally into the computer. This method offers higher quality, but at a slightly higher cost. An example is a MiroMotion PCI video input card.

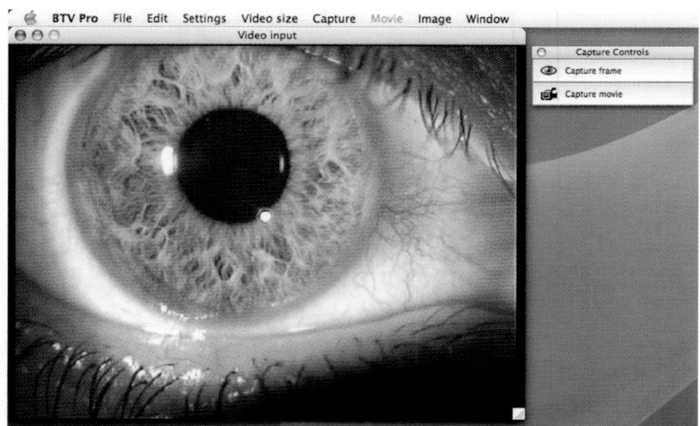

Figure 41.7 BTVPro software interface for both still image and video capture.

Software for still images

Many of the video digitizer devices will come with bundled software for image acquisition. Furthermore, your practice electronic medical records software may support image acquisition and there are third-party digital imaging packages for ophthalmic use, for example Medmont Studio (www.medmont.com). In essence, the key features the software needs to support are video display, capture, saving and printing. Desirable features for the software include database functions for linking the image to patient details and image modification functions for contrast, brightness and so on. A simple low-cost program for the Mac Mini mentioned above is BTVPro (www.bensoftware.com) (Figure 41.7).

Image files are saved in jpeg format with a naming convention of 'condition/eye/patient number', to enable files to be readily found later. Other software may be used to adjust the image brightness, contrast or colour rendition to be optimized prior to saving (see section on image editing, below).

Recording digital movies

Contact lens practice is photogenic not only for still images, but also for dynamic movies. Two important uses for movies include recording the dynamic procedures involved in lens fittings, and showing corneal complications as the light source is moved or scanned. Other interesting non-contact-lens-related pathology where motion is useful includes anomalies of the pupils, eye movements and vitreous.

The program Adobe Premiere is suitable for capturing movies and manipulating them, and the software is bundled with many of the video digitizer PCI boards. Video can be captured to QuickTime, AVI or other movie file formats. Quicktime Player Pro (www.apple.com), or BTVPro, referred to above, may also be used. With the large hard disks common in modern computers, the larger file sizes associated with video capture are no longer an issue. Available on Mac OS X is the program iMovie HD (www.apple.com). This simple program has enough features to handle most editing tasks.

File back-up

Whatever system is used, it is vital to have a means of backing up the data stored on the slit-lamp-interfaced computer, for example by using a recordable CD-RW or DVD-RW or a removable USB hard disk or flash memory drive. Recently, the costs of external hard drive systems have become very reasonable. Attaching an external several-hundred-gig drive is convenient and easy to do. It is appropriate to store anterior eye images at between 1280 × 811 and 767 × 569 pixel resolution and at up to 1 : 70 jpeg compression without significant loss of resolution (Peterson and Wolffsohn, 2005).

Printer

There is a wide range of printers available, each with unique benefits. For contact lens private practice work, an inkjet printer is appealing because of its compact size, low capital cost and high-quality prints. If quarter-page (postcard) size images are made for attachment to record cards or referral letters, then both the speed and cost per print are moderate.

Digital still camera slit-lamp imaging system

The alternative approach to a video camera for slit-lamp imaging is via a digital still camera. The advantage of a digital still camera is that a higher-resolution image can be created. Consumer digital still cameras afford high-resolution (3 million pixels or more), good low-light performance and options for attaching to instruments. For example, the Nikon Coolpix camera (www.nikon.com) has traditionally been popular in ophthalmic applications, in part because of the thread mount on the front of the lens to assist attachment to the slit lamp and the video-out plug for image preview on an external monitor. Alternative model digital still cameras can be used by holding them to the slit-lamp eyepiece (Figure 41.8A) or for capturing images of lenses via the camera macro lens (Figure 41.8B).

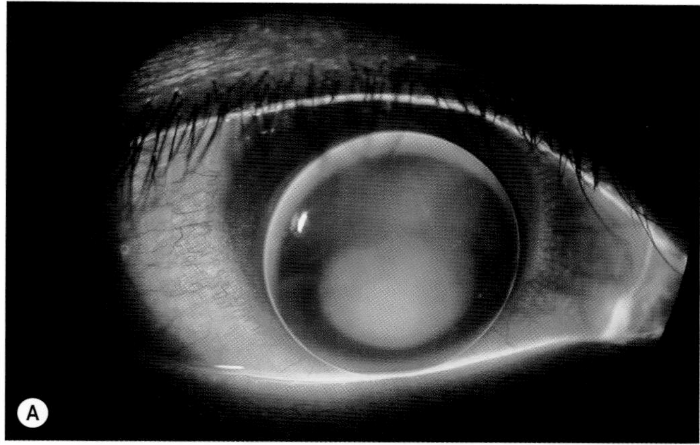

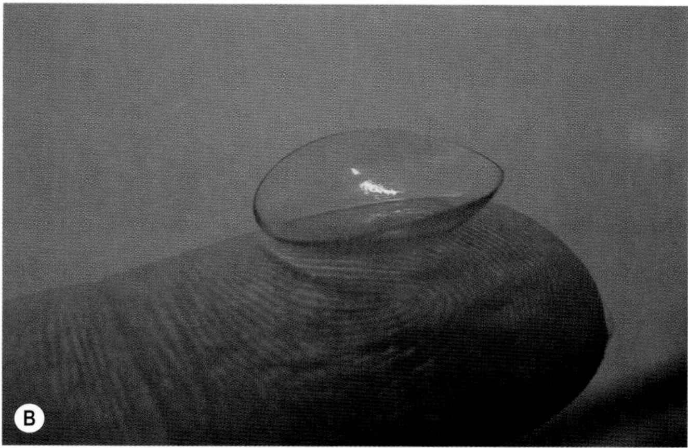

Figure 41.8 (A) Image of a rigid lens fit captured through the slit-lamp eyepiece using a Ricoh RDC-5300 digital still camera. (B) Image of contact lens taken using the close-up macro lens of a Ricoh RDC-5300 digital still camera.

Fundus camera

Digital fundus (retinal) cameras are becoming more common in clinical practice, as the ease of use and image quality have improved, and costs have come down. It is useful to remember that digital fundus cameras will give high-quality images of the anterior eye as well, by simply inserting the high-plus (often +10.00 D) dioptre compensation lens. The plus lens enables focus on the anterior eye, and excellent images may be obtained of opaque tissues such as the sclera, everted palpebra, pigmented lesions, corneal opacities and eyelid skin (Figure 41.9). To date fundus cameras do not usually include a cobalt blue filter, making fluorescein images difficult.

OCT anterior segment

The newest imaging technology for contact lens practice is optical coherence tomography (OCT), which gives a three-dimensional scan and image of the anterior eye. OCT is a significant advance because accurate measurements of the anterior eye may be made, although the initial instruments are expensive.

Zeiss Visante (www.zeiss.com) anterior-segment imaging uses a 1310 nm infrared laser to image the anterior segment. The laser is able to penetrate contact lenses, cornea and sclera, but not pigmented tissues. Axial resolution is 18 μm and transverse resolution is 50 μm. It can image a volume up to 16 × 16 × 6 mm depth. Image examples are shown in Figures 41.10 and 41.11.

The SL-OCT from Heidelberg Engineering (www.heidelbergengineering.com) also provides high-precision assessments of the anterior segment, and is cleverly integrated into a conventional slit-lamp instrument.

Other instruments

Confocal microscopy is a specialized contact microscopy technique for corneal imaging. It gives magnification up to 400× with a small field of view. The technique shows the detail of individual cells in each layer of the cornea, allowing *in vivo* assessment of the effects of contact lenses, corneal infections, inflammations and dystrophies. Available instruments include the Nidek Confoscan4 (www.nidek.com) and Heidelberg Laser Scanning Confocal Microscope (www.heidelbergengineering.com).

Other instruments that are perhaps more targeted at measurement, and less at imaging, include the Pentacam, which uses a rotating Scheimpflug camera (www.oculususa.com) and the Orbscan II, which uses a scanning slit beam for corneal and anterior-chamber assessment (www.zyoptix.com).

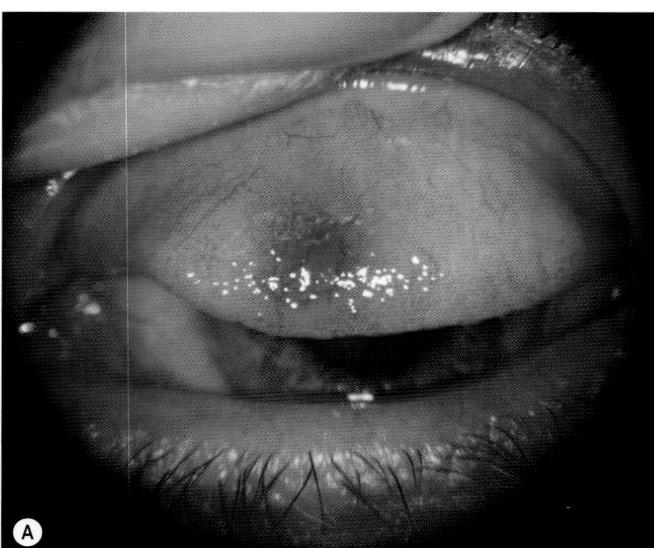

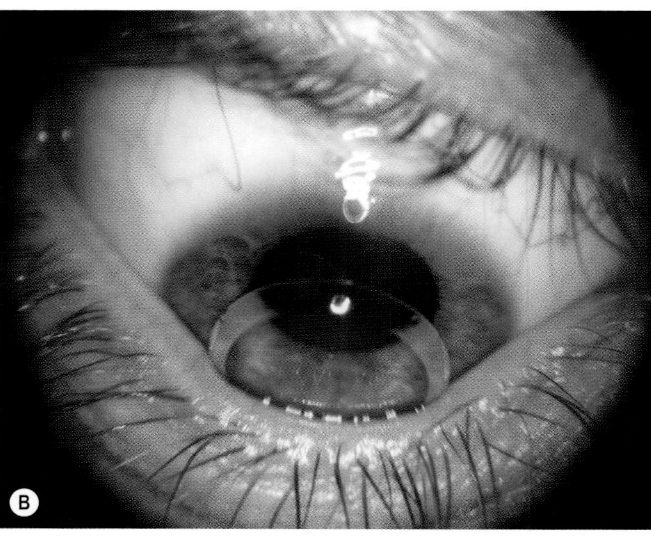

Figure 41.9 (A) Palpebral conjunctiva with papillae, imaged using a Canon DGi fundus camera with the +10.00 auxiliary lens inserted. The flash highlights the peaks of the papillae when the everted eyelid is angled appropriately. (B) Rigid lens in keratoconus, imaged with the same method as in (A). In downgaze, Munson's sign is apparent.

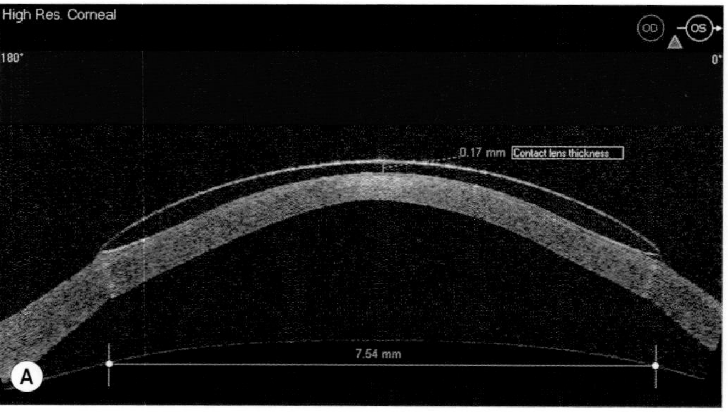

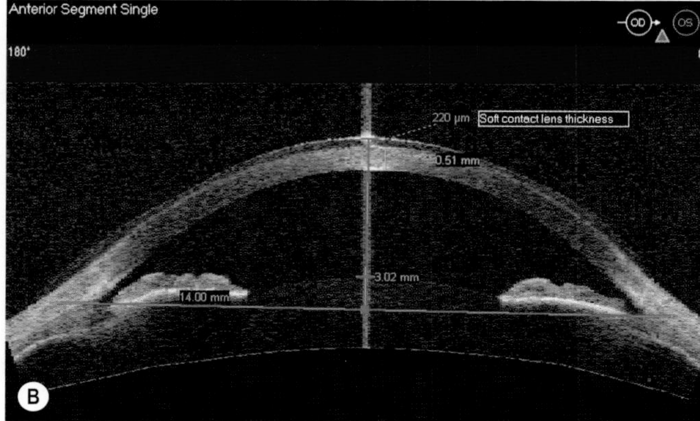

Figure 41.10 Optical coherence tomography (OCT) images of contact lenses. (A) Horizontal line scan (10 × 3 mm) of a rigid contact lens in moderate keratoconus. The central corneal thickness is 0.38 mm. (B) Horizontal line scan (16 × 6 mm) of a disposable soft contact lens for moderate hyperopia.

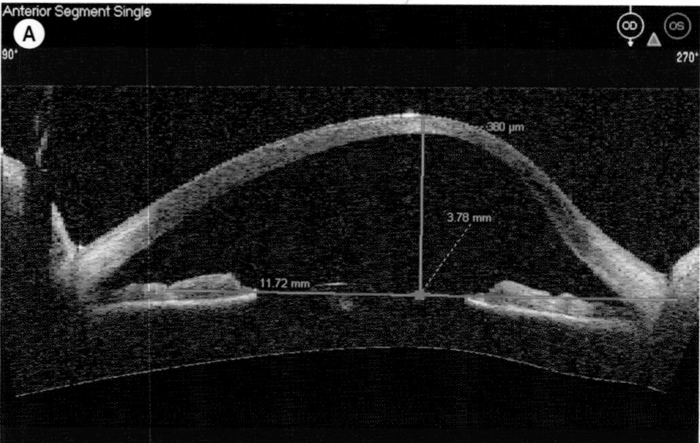

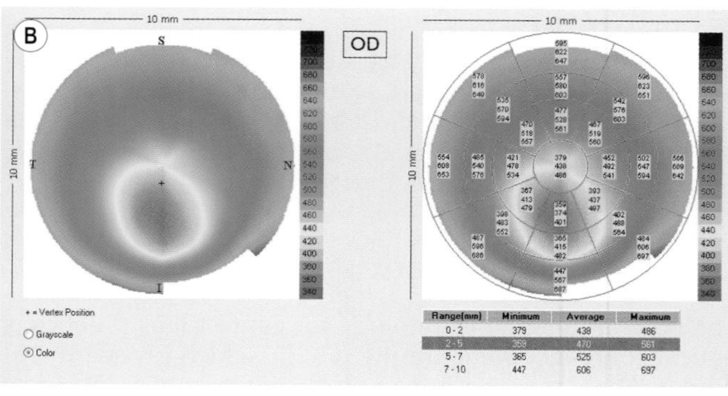

Figure 41.11 Optical coherence tomography (OCT) images in keratoconus. (A) Vertical line scan showing the cone profile, corneal thinning and increased anterior-chamber depth. (B) Map of corneal thickness in the same patient showing inferior corneal thinning.

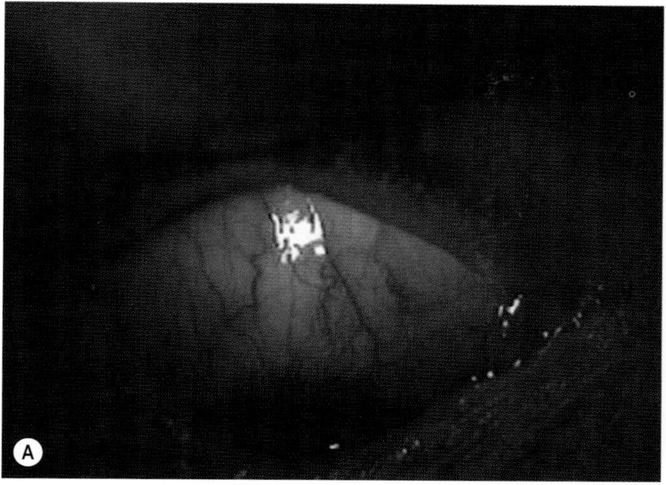

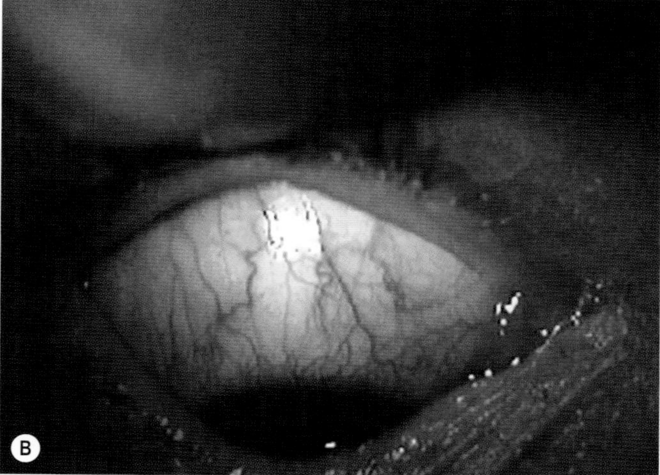

Figure 41.12 Image enhancement. (A) The original dull image. (B) The same image after brightness and contrast enhancement.

Image editing

Digital images have the advantage of image manipulation. There are many image-editing programs available on the market today. Basic image-editing capabilities are offered as a software feature in some commercial slit-lamp packages. Key editing applications with respect to contact lens imaging include the following:

- Brightness and contrast correction – images that are underexposed can be corrected easily with image editing (Figure 41.12).
- The lightest pixel and darkest pixel in the picture specify each end of the spectrum. The remaining pixels are rescaled to fill out the rest of the spectrum (Hom and Bruce, 1998).
- Fluorescein pattern analysis – fluorescein pattern images can be analysed by colour (Costa and Franco, 1998). Objective methods can be used to determine the fit of a lens (flat, steep, aligned). The fluorescein pattern is analysed by RGB colour channels. The histograms of the blue and green channels can be used to differentiate between a flat, steep and aligned (on-*K*) fit (Hom and Bruce, 1998).
- Tear layer thickness analysis – tear layer thickness under the lens can be determined by the intensity of the fluorescence. The thinner tear layers are dark. Thicker tear layers are brighter. Reducing the colour depth of a fluorescein pattern separates the colour differences between the thick and thin tear layers (Figure 41.13). The different thickness areas are made even more distinct by applying new colours. The corneal topography underneath a rigid lens can be interpolated with this technique (Hom and Bruce, 1998).

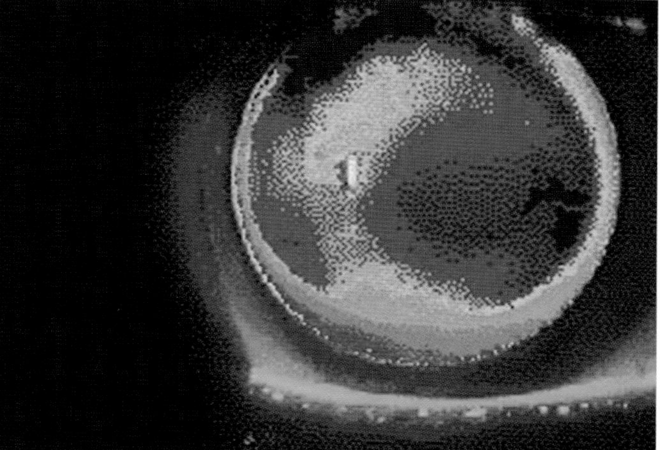

Figure 41.13 Tear layer thickness pattern (see text).

Conclusion

Digital photography is a hugely advantageous technique for contact lens practice. Both commercial and do-it-yourself digital imaging systems may be used. These systems have become simpler and less expensive over time.

This chapter has demonstrated the great potential and versatility of digital image capture systems for the accurate recording and sharing of clinical information relating to contact lens practice. The future is bright for digital imaging and the advantages are invaluable. Some day, we hope all contact lens practices will enjoy the enhancements it offers.

References

Costa, M. F. M. and Franco, S. (1998) Improving the contact lens fitting evaluation by the application of image-processing techniques. *Int. Contact Lens Clin.*, **25,** 22–27.

Cox, I. (1995) Digital imaging in contact lens practice. *Int. Contact Lens Clin.*, **22,** 62–66.

Efron, N., Morgan, P. B. and Katsara, S. S. (2001) Validation of grading scales for contact lens complications. *Ophthal. Physiol. Opt.*, **21,** 17–29.

Hammack, G. G. (1995) Updated video equipment recommendations for slit lamp videography. *Int. Contact Lens Clin.*, **22,** 54–61.

Hom, M. M. and Bruce, A. S. (1998) Image-editing techniques for anterior segment and contact lenses. *Int. Contact Lens Clin.*, **25,** 46–49.

Meyler, J. and Burnett-Hodd, N. (1998) The use of digital image capture in contact lens practice. *Contact Lens Ant. Eye,* **21,** S3–S11.

Nichols J. J., Nichols K. K., Puent B. *et al.* (2002) Evaluation of tear film interference patterns and measures of tear break-up time. *Optom. Vis. Sci.,* **79,** 363–369.

Peterson, R. C. and Wolffsohn, J. S. (2005) The effect of digital image resolution and compression on anterior eye imaging. *Br. J. Ophthalmol.*, **89,** 828–830.

Pritchard, N., Young, G., Coleman, S. *et al.* (2003) Subjective and objective measures of corneal staining related to multipurpose systems. *Cont. Lens Anterior Eye,* **26,** 3–9.

Schwartz, C. A. (1998) Photodocumentation: Optimizing today's contact lens practice. *Contact Lens Spectrum,* **13,** 24–29.

CHAPTER 42

Compliance

Nathan Efron

Introduction

Patients are often lying when they say they have regularly taken the prescribed medicine.

Hippocrates, 400 BC

The issue that Hippocrates was highlighting was that of compliance – an important field of medicine that has been the subject of medical research since the beginning of the 20th century. In the contact lens field, studies of compliance commenced only in the mid-1980s, with the first peer-reviewed journal article on this topic being published in 1986 by Collins and Carney.

Although patients sometimes unwittingly, carelessly or even recklessly contribute to their own misfortune (Figure 42.1), the model offered by Hippocrates is perhaps a little too simplistic. Sackett and Hayes (1976) defined compliance as 'the extent to which a patient's behaviour coincides with the clinical prescription'. This is a more instructive definition in that it highlights the critical importance of the practitioner–patient relationship in avoiding adverse events. This chapter will review the field of compliance as it relates to contact lens wear and will conclude with the presentation of a contact lens-specific compliance model.

Consequences of non-compliance

Although full compliance with practitioner instructions does not guarantee trouble-free lens wear (Najjar *et al.*, 2004), it is worth considering the possible consequences of non-compliance because the conclusions from such an analysis provide the rationale for studying this topic. In general, non-compliance will result in the following adverse effects: reduction of treatment efficacy; secondary problems; incorrect prescribing; wasting of practitioner chair time; and wasting of patient time. Clearly, health care delivery will be enhanced if the above adverse consequences of non-compliance can be minimized or eliminated.

Extent and pattern of non-compliance

It is not possible simply to characterize the behaviour of a patient as compliant or non-compliant, because there will be variations in the pattern of non-compliance over time, and extent of non-compliance at a given instance in time. Such cases are difficult to deal with, because the non-compliant behaviour may continue undetected for some time. There is a greater likelihood of detecting consistent and/or total non-compliant behaviours at an aftercare visit.

Duration of the prescription

In the general health care field, the extent of non-compliance has been found to be related to the duration of the prescription. For short-term medication (e.g. a 9-day course of antibiotics) about 20–30% of patients will be non-compliant. Higher rates of non-compliance are found for long-term regimens: 30–40% of patients are non-compliant with preventive or prophylactic measures (e.g. using sun protection creams outdoors in patients susceptible to skin cancer) and greater than 50% of patients do not adhere to advice relating to long-term therapy (e.g. ongoing medication for chronic hypertension) (DiMatteo and DiNicola, 1982; Claydon and Efron, 1994b).

The prescription of contact lenses and contact lens care systems is akin to a long-term preventive measure; it is therefore not surprising that numerous studies have concluded that about 40–90% of contact lens wearers are non-compliant in at least some aspects of their contact lens care regimens (Claydon and Efron, 1994a). That is, the contact lens literature is in broad agreement with estimates of patient non-compliance documented in the general medical literature.

Erroneous contact lens procedures

A complete documentation of the ways in which contact lens patients have been shown to be non-compliant with their wear and care protocols is beyond the scope of this chapter. However, it is of interest to peruse a summary list, compiled from data reviewed by Claydon and Efron (1994a), of the types of transgressions that can occur:

- 62% keep solutions too long.
- 40% never clean the lens case.
- 36% irregularly clean lenses.
- 30% do not disinfect lenses daily.

DOI: 10.1016/B978-0-7506-8869-7.00042-2

- 30% do not wash hands before handling lenses.
- 27% wear lenses too long.
- 10% never rinse the lens after cleaning.
- 8% never clean lenses.
- 3% clean lenses in tap water.

Ky *et al.* (1988) attribute such transgressions to a lack of understanding of proper care procedures.

Compliance with the incorrect prescription

The vast majority of practitioners endeavour to dispense the correct and proper prescription; it would be unethical to do otherwise. However, in the past there have been well-documented contact lens-related cases of practitioners dispensing the incorrect prescription based on misinformation or a misinterpretation (Efron *et al.*, 1991; Matthews *et al.*, 1992). An example of this was a recommendation to soak disposable lenses overnight in unpreserved saline solution (instead of a multipurpose disinfecting solution) based upon the mistaken belief that frequent lens replacement obviates the need for daily lens disinfection. In developing regions where practitioner knowledge is minimal, such as China, rates of non-compliance and consequent ocular complications of contact lens wear are high (Fan *et al.*, 1995).

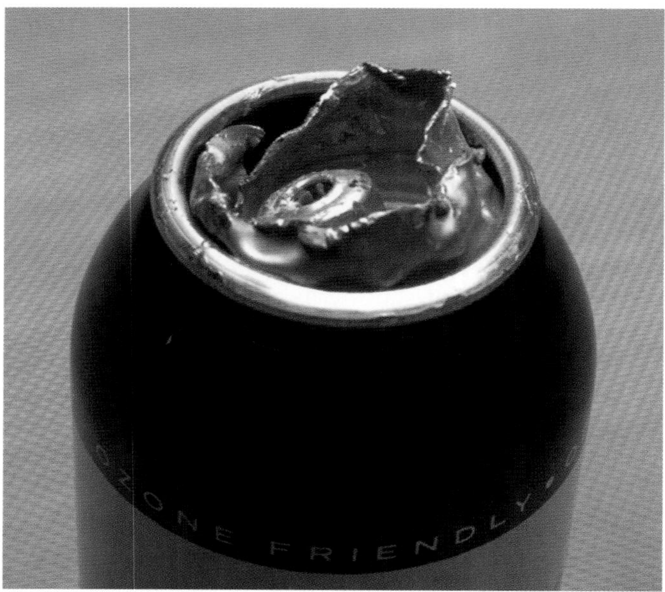

Figure 42.1 Reckless attempt by a patient to obtain residual solution from a can of aerosol saline (because the nozzle had ceased to function) by sawing the top off.

Whether inadvertent or deliberate, incorrect prescribing is a reality that must be considered in order to provide a comprehensive analysis of non-compliance. Figure 42.2 is a flow diagram that reveals five possible outcomes based upon the assumption that an incorrect prescription (or incorrect advice) has been dispensed to the patient. A tick indicates the likelihood of a positive outcome, and a cross indicates the likelihood of a negative outcome.

If the patient is compliant with the incorrect prescription, a negative outcome, such as ocular irritation, is more likely. A patient may also be non-compliant with the incorrect prescription. Non-compliance can be deliberate or unintentional, and a patient can be deliberately non-compliant in a rational or irrational manner. Unintentional non-compliance can be due to forgetfulness or a misunderstanding of the instructions. It is unlikely that unintentional non-compliance will result in correct procedures being readopted because of the plethora of random and most likely erroneous procedures that are theoretically available.

Compliance with the correct prescription

A patient being non-compliant with the correct prescription probably constitutes the classical view taken by practitioners. Figure 42.3 is a flow diagram that reveals five possible outcomes based upon the assumption that a correct prescription (or correct advice) has been issued. If the patient is compliant with the correct prescription, a positive outcome is more likely. Conversely, a negative outcome is likely if a patient is non-compliant with the correct prescription.

Investigation of strategies for compliance enhancement

Vincent (1971) conducted a study on a large cohort of glaucoma patients who were specifically told that if they did

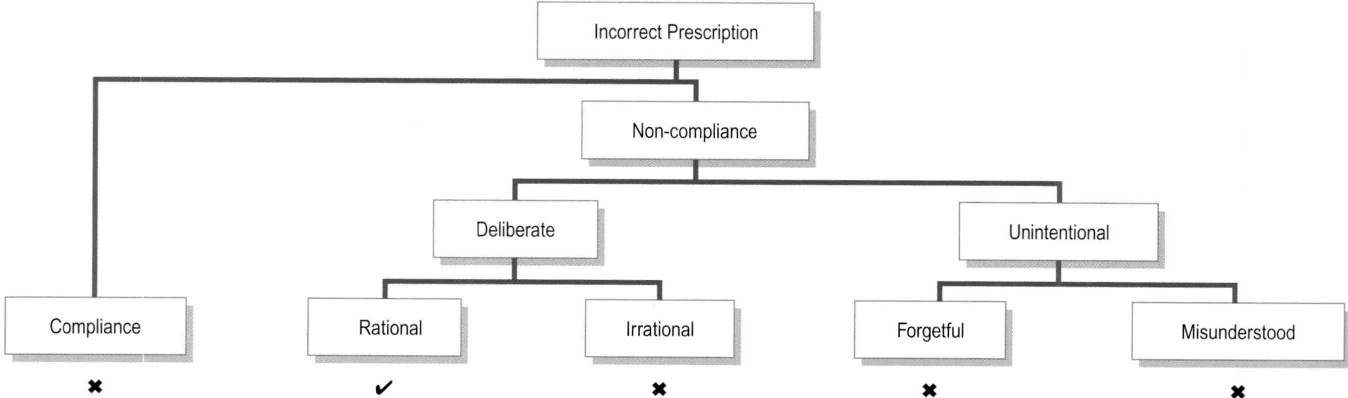

Figure 42.2 Consequences of compliance with the incorrect prescription (a tick indicates the likelihood of a positive outcome and a cross indicates the likelihood of a negative outcome).

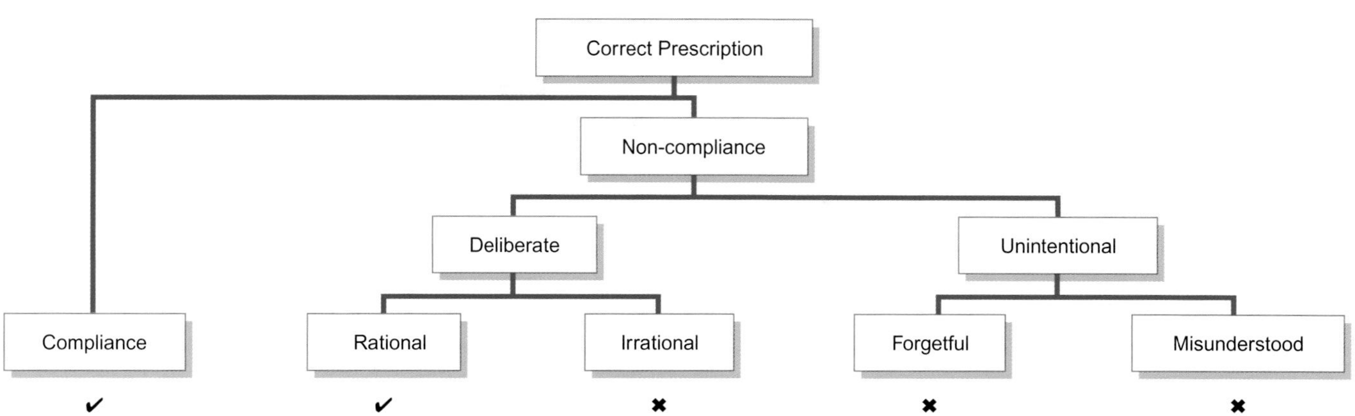

Figure 42.3 Consequences of compliance with the correct prescription (a tick indicates the likelihood of a positive outcome and a cross indicates the likelihood of a negative outcome).

not comply with the instruction to instil three drops of topical medication into their eyes daily they could go blind. The outcome of the study was that 50% of patients did not comply often enough, and that there was no improvement in compliance in those who lost sight in one eye.

In the light of such results, one may wonder whether anything can be done to improve compliance among contact lens wearers, especially in view of the fact that the consequences of non-compliance, such as the development of a corneal ulcer, carry a very low absolute risk. A more logical approach might be to assume that there will always be a certain level of non-compliance, and that contact lenses and lens care systems should be designed to have a sufficient level of redundancy, or safety margin, to account for this.

Notwithstanding the above reservations, the search for viable compliance enhancement strategies needs to continue in view of the known adverse consequences of non-compliance.

Because contact lens wearers typically overestimate their level of compliance (Donshik *et al.*, 2007), strategies in addition to the use of questionnaires must be adopted to derive an accurate picture of the level of adherence to instruction. Such strategies include observation and scoring of patient actions and procedures in a clinical situation and direct determination of the number of lenses used or care solution volumes remaining over fixed time frames.

Improving initial patient education

Claydon *et al.* (1997) conducted a 12-month study on 80 patients who were randomly divided into two groups. One group was given standard verbal instructions, and the other group was subjected to a compliance enhancement strategy. Handwashing was the only procedure that improved to an extent that was statistically verifiable. The intensity of initial education had no bearing on the integrity of the anterior ocular structures. Thus, the compliance enhancement strategy failed, indicating that a level of instruction in excess of that typically being offered at the present time is likely to be redundant in terms of enhancing compliance.

There may be other benefits of a thorough initial education, such as: (1) raising awareness of lens types and lens care products; (2) reinforcing brand loyalty (if this is of interest); and (3) enhancing the patient–practitioner relationship. Although an enhanced initial instruction will not improve compliance, benefits of reinstruction are clear. Compliance can be enhanced by constantly reminding patients of correct procedures at aftercare visits (Capellani and Boyce, 1999). Radford *et al.* (1993) demonstrated that such an approach improved the rate of compliance in one study group from 44% to 90%.

Periodic self-review

Yung *et al.* (2007) administered a regular self-review exercise on proper lens handling to a group of 60 lens wearers once every 3 months for 12 months. The levels of compliance and contamination of contact lenses and lens care accessories between test and control groups were compared at the end of the 12-month period to evaluate the effect of the intervention. All showed some degree of non-compliance in the care of their contact lenses and lens accessories. Most (about 60%) were non-compliant with at least six of a total of 15 lens care procedures. The most common non-compliant behaviour among contact lens wearers was associated with the care of the lens case. By the end of the study period, the compliance enhancement strategy did not appear to have had a significant effect on the behaviour of the subjects, except for improvement in the care of lens cases.

Reducing cost

Sheard *et al.* (1995) conducted a 4-month study on 59 patients who were randomly divided into two groups. The 'full-pay' group paid the full retail price of lens care products, whereas the 'nominal-pay' group paid a nominal fee for their lens care products. They found that reducing cost did not affect compliance as measured by solution usage or procedure demonstration. Had this experiment been conducted the other way around – by determining the level of compliance as the cost of care products is increased – it would have been possible to determine a threshold cost above which patients become dangerously non-compliant. Of course, such an experimental approach is not possible.

The ability of patients to pay for health care was studied by de Andrade Sobrinho and Carvalho (2003), and related to the extent of compliance with contact lens care and wear regimens. The authors found no correlation, and concluded that socioeconomic factors do not seem to have an impact on compliance with contact lens care routines.

Predicting non-compliance

Many of the problems relating to non-compliant patient behaviour could be overcome if it were possible to predict which patients were less likely to be compliant. Unfortunately, most attempts at identifying such predictors have been unsuccessful. For example, Davidson and Akingbehin (1980) failed to find an association in general ophthalmological practice between non-compliance and the following personal and sociological characteristics: age, sex, race, occupation or socioeconomic status.

Interestingly, Chun and Weissman (1987) were able to identify one potentially useful predictor of non-compliance relating to contact lens wear – patient age. They found that patients under the age of 30 years and over the age of 50 years were more likely to display non-compliant behaviour. Thus, practitioners ought to be alert to compliance-related issues when dealing with contact lens patients in these age ranges.

Claydon (1995) investigated the possibility that measurement of certain personality traits can be used to predict a likelihood or otherwise of compliance. She conducted a study in which the level of compliance with a simple contact lens regimen was measured on 48 contact lens wearers using demonstration and questionnaire techniques. The subjects also completed a psychological test known as the 16PF inventory (Cattell *et al.*, 1988) and the data were examined for possible associations. No overall correlations linking personality with compliance were revealed, although some interesting individual correlations were found. The personality trait adherence was found to be associated with the thoroughness of case cleaning and surfactant cleaning. The personality trait extroversion was found to be associated with the thoroughness of disinfecting and handwashing. Further work in this area may eventually lead to the formulation of a useful predictive test that can be applied clinically, such as a simple 10-question test that can predict the likelihood of compliance.

Cardona and Llovet (2004) used an oral and written comprehension test to establish the comprehension skills typology of contact lens wearers, thus allowing for the appropriate type of instructions (oral or written) to be given to each patient in accordance with their particular abilities. These authors suggested that this approach could enhance compliance among contact lens wearers.

The notion that contact lens wearers who are under strict life-preserving medical regimes and understand the value of general medical compliance will be more compliant with their contact lens wear behaviours was tested by O'Donnell and Efron (2004). Specifically, they hypothesized that diabetic contact lens wearers may represent a special group displaying higher levels of compliance with their lens care regimens as a result of learned behaviour relating to maintenance of their diabetic condition. Although the combined population of 29 diabetic and 29 non-diabetic contact lens wearers was generally found to be compliant, there were examples of non-compliance in both groups. Neither the duration of diabetes nor the degree of metabolic control appeared to have a significant effect on compliance. The results suggest that associated health compliance behaviours are poor predictors of compliance with instructions relating to contact lens wear and care.

A compliance enhancement model

Notwithstanding the difficulties discussed above in devising strategies to enhance or predict compliance, it is possible to construct a specific model for compliance enhancement in a contact lens setting based upon a wealth of evidence published in the contact lens field, and drawing upon the extensive literature defining the determinants of compliance in general health care. This model comprises four components: (1) the clinic and the practitioner; (2) the patient; (3) the advice that is given; and (4) the contact lens industry. In essence, the model amounts to a set of general principles and guidelines for enhancing compliance. Each component of the model will be considered in turn.

The clinic and practitioner

The clinic must have the following qualities:

- Staff should be informed and aware of key issues.
- Advice given should be consistent over time and between personnel.
- Appointment times should be individualized (as opposed to block booking).
- Waiting times should be minimal.
- There should be continuity of care wherever possible.
- The clinical environment should be warm and friendly.

Important qualities of the practitioner are as follows:

- Project a devotion to eye care (virtually all eye care practitioners are devoted to eye care, but this is not always outwardly projected).
- Listen effectively to what the patient has to say.
- Use minimum jargon.
- Emphasize key points, especially following delivery of a long and perhaps complex set of instructions.
- Set specific and realistic goals for patients to aim at.
- Adopt strategies to motivate patients.

Strategies for optimizing the effectiveness of the aftercare visit include:

- Sending appointment reminders.
- Advising patients of the importance of regular check-ups.
- Providing feedback and reward to patients.
- Repetition of key information.
- Stimulating the patient's interest in vision.
- Providing in-practice information via leaflets, posters and videos.

The patient

A valuable approach to learning patient attitudes is to explore their health beliefs (Sokol *et al.*, 1990) using a compliance decision tree. Figure 42.4 is a diagram of such a decision tree. The answers to the sequence of questions posed in the decision tree will indicate whether or not the patient is likely to be compliant with a contact lens system.

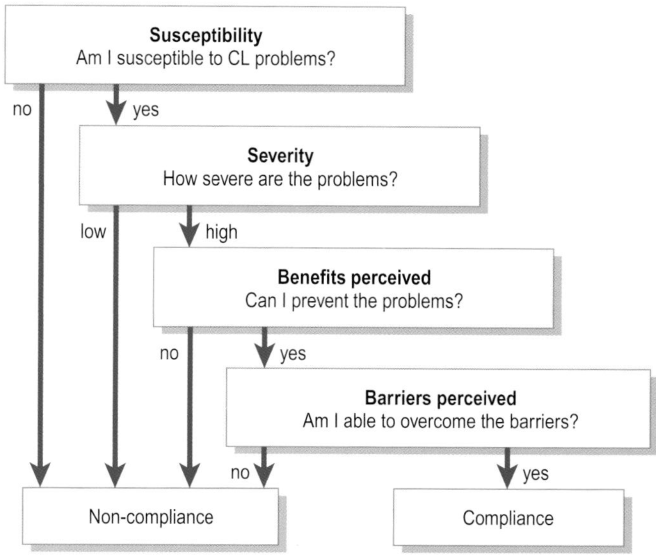

Figure 42.4 The decision tree which can be used to explore how the health beliefs of a contact lens (CL) patient may influence his/her level of compliance.

For example, Fan *et al.* (2002) found that, among contact lens wearers, those who had previously suffered from lens-related microbial keratitis believed more strongly than controls who had never suffered from keratitis in the perceived benefit of checking initially with the optometrist for the correct method of lens cleaning.

If it is determined that the health beliefs of the patient are likely to lead to non-compliance, steps should be taken to modify the specific beliefs that are erroneous. This can be achieved via a variety of strategies, such as talking persuasively, supplying pertinent information or utilizing a health care contract that emphasizes the responsibilities of the patient for achieving safe and comfortable ocular health during lens wear.

The advice

Care systems should be simple and easy to understand, tailored for the individual, ritualized and not too expensive. Advice given to patients should be verbal and written. Printed material should be readable and well illustrated. Clearly illustrated sequential steps with minimum wording will aid understanding and interpretation. Written material should also contain warnings; obviously, a balance must be found whereby patients are alerted to possible dangers but are not frightened away from wearing lenses.

The contact lens industry

An important role is played by the contact lens industry in compliance enhancement – a role that falls into three broad categories:

1. Pricing policy – it is self-evident that prohibitive pricing will produce a general disincentive to purchase all of the required products and to use them as required. The contact lens care industry thus has an obligation to contain prices as far as economically possible.
2. Product support – clear and unambiguous packaging and simple and clear instructions are thought to be important contributing factors to compliance enhancement; such issues are the sole responsibility of the contact lens industry. Many companies provide attractive starter packs which motivate patients.
3. Research and development – contact lens care systems should be designed to be effective, as distinct from the usual practice of designing systems that are merely efficacious. An efficacious system is one which can be demonstrated to work under ideal situations, that is, assuming full patient compliance. An efficient system is one which will work in a 'real-world' scenario, allowing for a certain level of non-compliance. This chapter has established that full compliance does not exist. All patients will be at least partially non-compliant in some aspect of their care regimen. If one accepts this argument then it behoves the contact lens industry to develop effective contact lens care systems.

Conclusion

Patient compliance with contact lens wear and care is a complex issue; it is difficult to enhance and it is impossible to predict. As a result, we must continue to rely on the outcome of models constructed from the general medical literature and what little has been determined from contact lens research. Practitioners are invited to contemplate all of the issues highlighted in this chapter when faced with adverse ocular reactions to contact lens wear; although the patient may well be at fault, it is important to avoid taking the easy option of 'blaming the victim'!

References

Capellani, J. P. and Boyce, P. (1999) Are you missing these telltale signs of non-compliance? *Rev. Optom.*, **138,** 51–54.

Cardona, G. and Llovet, I. (2004) Compliance amongst contact lens wearers: comprehension skills and reinforcement with written instructions. *Cont. Lens Anterior Eye,* **27,** 75–81.

Cattell, R. B., Eber, H. W. and Tatsuoka, M. M. (1988) *Handbook for the 16PF,* Champaign, IL: Institute for Personality and Ability Testing.

Chun, M. W. and Weissman, B. A. (1987) Compliance in contact lens care. *Am. J. Optom. Physiol. Opt.*, **64,** 274–276.

Claydon, B. E. (1995) *A Prospective Study of Non-Compliance in Contact Lens Wear,* PhD Thesis, University of Manchester Institute of Science and Technology, United Kingdom.

Claydon, B. E. and Efron, N. (1994a) Non-compliance in contact lens wear. *Ophthal. Physiol. Opt.*, **14,** 356–364.

Claydon, B. E. and Efron, N. (1994b) Non-compliance in general health care. *Ophthal. Physiol. Opt.*, **14,** 257–264.

Claydon, B. E., Efron, N. and Woods, C. A. (1997) A prospective study of the effect of education on non-compliant behaviour in contact lens wear. *Ophthal. Physiol. Opt.*, **17,** 137–146.

Collins, M. J. and Carney, L. G. (1986) Compliance with care and maintenance procedures among contact lens wearers. *Clin. Exp. Optom.*, **69,** 174–177.

Davidson, S. and Akingbehin, T. (1980) Compliance in ophthalmology. *Trans. Ophthalmol. Soc. U.K.*, **100,** 286–290.

de Andrade Sobrinho, M. V. and Carvalho, R. A. (2003) Do the economic and social factors play an important role in relation to the compliance of contact lenses care routines? *Eye Contact Lens,* **29,** 210–212.

DiMatteo, M. R. and DiNicola, D. D. (1982) *Achieving Patient Compliance.* New York: Pergamon Press.

Donshik, P. C., Ehlers, W. H., Anderson, L. D. *et al.* (2007) Strategies to better engage, educate, and empower patient compliance and safe lens wear: compliance: what we know, what we do not know, and what we need to know. *Eye Contact Lens,* **33,** 430–433.

Efron, N., Wohl, A., Toma, N. *et al.* (1991) *Pseudomonas* corneal ulcers associated with daily wear of disposable hydrogel contact lenses. *Int. Contact Lens Clin.*, **18,** 46–52.

Fan, L., Jia, Q., Jie, C. *et al.* (1995) The compliance of Chinese contact lens wearers. *Int. Contact Lens. Clin.*, **22,** 188–192.

Fan, D. S., Houang, E. S., Lam, D. S. *et al.* (2002) Health belief and health practice in contact lens wear – a dichotomy? *Contact Lens Assoc. Ophthalmol. J.*, **28,** 36–39. Erratum in: *Contact Lens Assoc. Ophthalmol. J.*, **28**(3) (following table of contents).

Ky, W., Scherick, K. and Stenson, S. (1988) Clinical survey of lens care in contact lens patients. *Contact Lens Assoc. Ophthalmol. J.*, **24,** 216–219.

Matthews, T. D., Frazer, D. G., Minassian, D. C. *et al.* (1992) Risks of keratitis and patterns of use with disposable contact lenses. *Arch. Ophthalmol.*, **110,** 1559–1562.

Najjar, D. M., Aktan, S. G., Rapuano, C. J. *et al.* (2004) Contact lens-related corneal ulcers in compliant patients. *Am. J. Ophthalmol.*, **137,** 170–172.

O'Donnell, C. and Efron, N. (2004) Non-compliance with lens care and maintenance in diabetic contact lens wearers. *Ophthalmic Physiol. Opt.*, **24,** 504–510.

Radford, C. F., Woodward, E. G. and Stapleton, F. (1993) Contact lens hygiene compliance in a university population. *J. Br. Contact Lens Assoc.*, **16,** 105–111.

Sackett, D. L. and Heyes, R. B. (1976) *Compliance with Therapeutic Regimens.* Baltimore, MD: John Hopkins University Press.

Sheard, G., Efron, N. and Claydon, B. E. (1995) Does solution cost affect compliance among contact lens wearers? *J. Br. Contact Lens Assoc.*, **18,** 59–64.

Sokol, J., Meir, M. G. and Bloom, S. (1990) A study of patient compliance in a contact lens wearing population. *Contact Lens Assoc. Ophthalmol. J.*, **16,** 209–213.

Vincent, P. (1971) Factors influencing patient non-compliance: a theoretical approach. *Nursing Res.*, **20,** 509–516.

Yung, M. S., Boost, M., Cho, P. *et al.* (2007) The effect of a compliance enhancement strategy (self-review) on the level of lens care compliance and contamination of contact lenses and lens care accessories. *Clin. Exp. Optom.*, **90,** 190–202.

CHAPTER 43

Practice management

Nizar K Hirji

Introduction

Contact lens practice by definition resides within an optometric practice embracing, amongst other products and services, the prescribing, fitting and dispensing of contact lenses and associated products and services. Thus, practice management issues that have an impact on contact lens practice are firstly all those that have an impact on an optometric practice, and additionally, if it is possible to separate them, those issues that are regarded as more the domain of contact lens practice.

Practice management may be defined as that activity concerned with planning, organizing and controlling the non-clinical activities of an optometric enterprise to ensure predefined outcomes and goals, through the effective use of the available physical, financial and human resources. The supply of optometric goods and services ranges from very tangible goods (e.g. supply of a contact lens case) to entirely intangible services such as a contact lens consultation (e.g. aftercare).

In managing the contact lens 'service product', for want of a better descriptor, it is important to appreciate that what is involved is primarily the provision of professional services. A detailed description of the characteristics that separate a professional service-oriented business like contact lens practice from a product-oriented business is beyond the scope of this chapter and detailed elsewhere (Hirji, 1999). These characteristics place special management demands on optometric and contact lens practices.

The key elements that determine the management issues in a primarily service-oriented enterprise such as a contact lens practice can be categorized according to the following six Ps:

1. Practice location and accommodation.
2. Personnel at the practice.
3. Products and services provided.
4. Pricing – fees and charges.
5. Promotional issues.
6. Processes.

These issues have to be considered within the framework of the wider legal, political, economic and institutional environment within which optometry has to operate. This chapter will thus confine itself to a limited overview of these issues. The model adopted here will be that of a contact lens service being provided within optometric practice. It is recognized, of course, that contact lens practice can be effected in a variety of settings, such as medical practices, hospitals and dispensing outlets. Nevertheless, the principles of efficient management highlighted here can be applied to all of these situations.

Practice location and accommodation

In contact lens practice, the patient participates, in person, in the buying process. It is therefore important to be located as conveniently to the patient as possible. The decision regarding the location of the practice is crucial, not only in terms of the ease of access for potential patients and customers, but also because a wrong or a poor decision cannot easily be reversed – unlike decisions on pricing or product choice. The costs of a mistake include financial losses involved in acquiring and running a practice (e.g. fixtures and fittings, launch costs), and – just as important to many businesses – the indirect cost of not keeping a competitor out of a better location. The suitability of a particular practice location is based on the estimated potential for attracting patients and customers in a given catchment area and the location of competitors.

Sophisticated models using a variety of information, including census data, family expenditure surveys and geodemographic characteristics, have been developed to help quantify catchment areas and the desirability of differing sites. Checklists with key considerations listed may also be used to help the decision-making process with or without computer modelling. Other good sources of information about an area include local authorities (e.g. planning department, electoral office, rating office, clerks office), estate agents and the local and national press. Having decided on the location, it is important to ensure that the physical site will be able to accommodate a contact lens practice, including a waiting area, consulting and data collection rooms, spectacle and contact lens dispensaries, staff room, storage/stock room and washrooms.

DOI: 10.1016/B978-0-7506-8869-7.00043-4

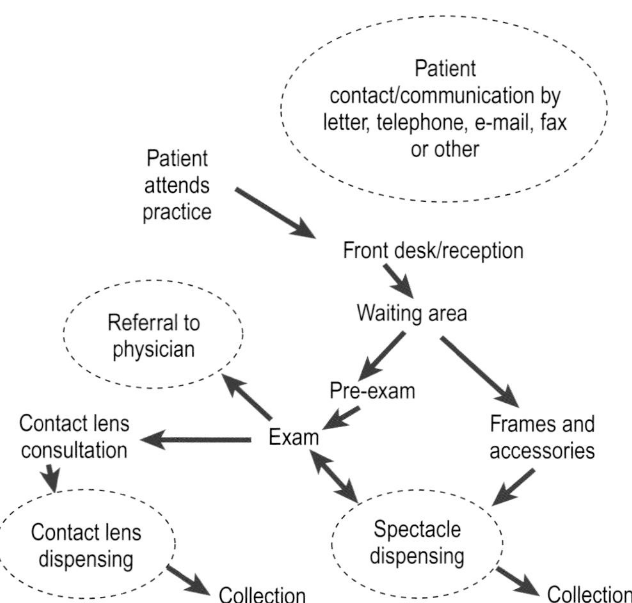

Figure 43.1 Activity and information flow in contact lens practice.

Layout

The layout of the practice will be governed by the physical limitations of the site and the sequence and order of activities that the patient undergoes during a visit to the practice. Figure 43.1 illustrates the principal integrated activities of an optometric practice with contact lenses as part of the product/service range.

Reception area and front desk

This is the first person contact position for the visiting patient, and should be a welcoming point as well as a help desk. The reception area will also often be the last point of contact before the patient leaves the practice.

Waiting area

The waiting area needs to be comfortable, with sufficient seating to accommodate potential patients and customers. A rule of thumb worth considering is that this area should be furnished and decorated to be just marginally 'better' than the front room of the patients and customers attending the practice.

Consulting room

Depending on the patient workload of the practice, more than one room may be dedicated to the consultation and examination activity. Increasingly, delegation of data collection tasks (e.g. non-contact tonometry, visual field analysis, autorefraction) to support staff means that an area or room will be utilized for this pre-exam screening or adjunct data collection.

The consulting room will have all the equipment found in a modern optometric practice with an emphasis on anterior-eye evaluation/recording. In addition to this, it will be necessary to have some contact lens verification equipment, and if a speciality practice, possibly a corneal topographer. The need for specialist diagnostic fitting sets and materials (e.g. preformed rigid scleral lenses, bifocal lenses, eye impression materials) will be dictated by the profile of patients attending the practice.

Spectacle dispensary

Every contact lens-wearing patient is an optometric patient who happens to be using contact lenses. All contact lens wearers require spectacles. The spectacle dispensary should thus be able to provide for the functional and aesthetic needs of the patient, just as any optometric practice would.

Contact lens dispensary

The contact lens dispensing area is where patients will attend for instructions and practice of placement and removal of contact lenses on to and from their eyes (see Chapter 38). It is also here that patients will receive their (starter) contact lens care systems, advice on wear, care and hygiene with respect to their contact lenses, and complete the paperwork. It should therefore have the furniture, facilities, materials and equipment to allow this to happen effectively. Employing videos and CD-ROMs in this area to support the education process along with written materials is now a common practice.

Personnel at the practice

Contact lens practices rely on individuals to deliver their professional services and products to patients and customers. Thus, at a minimum level of practice activity, it will be necessary to employ someone to provide reception and general administrative support with respect to the day-to-day activities of the practice. At the other end of the spectrum, a busy large practice in a shopping centre location may employ additional optometrists, dispensing staff, contact lens hygienists, technicians, optical receptionists/advisors, secretaries and cleaners. It is important to remember that many more individuals will need to be employed to cover the practice requirements in terms of hours per day, particularly as part-time employment increases. The issues of managing the practice staff take increasingly more prominence as the size and the activity of the practice increase (ACAS, 1994).

Recruitment and selection

Once a vacancy has been identified, and additional hours of staff time are justified, it is essential to establish the duties of the new member of staff. Having decided the qualifications, training needs and skills that are required to do the job, it is useful to prepare a job description and then to decide on the type of person who would ideally be recruited to fill this vacancy – that is, a person specification. Two good methods of producing the specification include Roger's seven-point plan (Roger, 1951), taking account of:

1. physical make-up
2. attainments
3. general intelligence
4. special aptitudes
5. interests
6. disposition
7. circumstances.

Table 43.1 Example of a person specification – Fraser's fivefold grading

Essential qualities	Desirable qualities
1. Impact on other people	
(appearance, speech and manner)	Smart presentation
Clean and tidy presentation	Gets on well with young adults
Good writing and speech	
2. Qualifications and experience	
(education, training and work experience)	Experience in medical reception or pharmacy
GCSE English and mathematics	Experience of data input and output
Able to work on a computer	
3. Innate abilities	
(aptitude for learning)	Able to prioritize and decide on action
Quick to grasp ideas and views	
4. Motivation	
(consistency, determination and success in achieving goals)	Interested in a potential career in optics
Interested in health care and general cosmesis	
5. Adjustment	
(emotional stability, ability to handle stress and ability to get on with people)	Comfortable with the pressures of day-to-day practice activities and the demands of patients and practitioners
Friendly and able to work as part of a team	

(Adapted from Hirji, N. K., 1999 Business Awareness for Optometrists – a Primer, Butterworth-Heinemann)

and Fraser's five-point grading (Fraser, 1958), which covers:

1. impact on others
2. qualifications or acquired knowledge
3. innate abilities
4. motivation
5. adjustment or emotional balance.

Table 43.1 describes an example of a person specification for a receptionist in a practice that wants to develop a contact lens interest.

Selection then involves choosing the right person by interviewing short-listed candidates with a view to selecting the applicant who has the skills, abilities, aptitude and personal qualities to do the job. The job description and the person specification will decide the major selection criteria normally considered during the interview process.

Contract of employment

A contract of employment is simply the legal agreement between the employer and the employee, clarifying their mutual obligations. The law provides the employee with a number of employment rights and imposes some statutory obligations on the employer. Contracts do not have to be in writing. However, employment law in the UK has gone slightly further, and even where a verbal contract may exist, there is a requirement for employers to give any employee taken on for 1 month or more a written statement setting out the main employment particulars within 2 months of the starting date of employment. Covered by common and contract law, contracts of employment are governed by the Employment Rights Act (1996).

Discipline and dismissal

A practice handbook that sets out basic information about the policies and facilities of the practice can act as a clear guide for all staff to providing optometric and contact lens services. It should be an easily accessible set of ground rules that promote a good working environment in the practice. If a case of misconduct (breach of rules that merits disciplinary action) arises, the rules in the handbook will be invaluable as to the expected conduct. Table 43.2 gives an outline disciplinary procedure.

Training staff

Training embraces the identification and development of employee potential for job satisfaction, improvement, practice value creation and ultimately improved patient care. It can often be the driver of improvements and has the potential to bring about reduced costs, increased value and practice profitability. Ultimately, training is about getting people to do different things or to do things differently.

For training to be effective for a contact lens practice, however, it must be:

- Valid – relevant to contact lens-related jobs in the practice.
- Capable of solving problems – identified as needing resolution in practice.
- Focused on objectives – either at the individual or at the job/practice level.
- Measurable – its results can be gauged directly or indirectly.

Improvements that training and development bring should hopefully result in reduced costs and increased value and profits through (for example):

- Improved efficiency – doing the job correctly, accurately and with care at the outset reduces replacements, unplanned rescheduling and revisits to the practice by patients. This improves utilization of resources and practice output overall.
- Improved quality – enhances the reputation of the practice, and reduces complaints, costs of returns, refunds and credits.
- Less wastage and reworking – not only is the material not wasted but the greater cost saving is in the staff costs, time the equipment is occupied and ancillary costs in reworking the job by the laboratory (e.g. a complete pair of spectacles, alternative set of contact lenses).
- Improved consulting room and equipment utilization – consulting room occupancy and equipment use dictate the capacity of the practice to conduct eye exams and contact lens consultations. An unnecessarily occupied or indeed unoccupied consulting room is costly.
- Reduced time taken to do jobs – less time taken to produce same or better-quality products will translate to reduced staff costs relative to sales revenues.

Table 43.2 Outline disciplinary procedures

Offence	Action	Details
Minor misconduct	Verbal discussion (informal)	Counsel and help employee improve. Keep a note
Minor misconduct	Stage 1 Verbal warning (formal)	Advise of reason for the warning Advise that this is a first stage of the disciplinary procedure and the right of appeal Keep a note of the warning for say 6 months and then repeal subject to satisfactory conduct and performance
Repeated minor misconduct or serious misconduct	Stage 2 Written warning	Advise of reason for warning Give details of the improvement required and the timescale Advise that this is the second stage of the disciplinary procedure and the right of appeal Keep a note of the warning for say 6 months and then repeal subject to satisfactory conduct and performance
Repeated minor/serious misconduct or gross misconduct – in which case suspension with pay may be invoked until investigation is completed	Stage 3 Final written warning Stage 4 Dismissal	Advise of reason for warning Explain that dismissal will occur if there is no satisfactory improvement Advise of the right of appeal Keep a note of the warning for say 12 months and then repeal subject to satisfactory conduct and performance Give the reason for dismissal Give the date of termination of employment Advise of the right of appeal

(Adapted from Torrington, D. and Hall, L., 1987 Personnel Management – a New Approach, Prentice-Hall & ACAS (1994) Employing People – The ACAS Handbook for Small Firms, ACAS Publications)

- Improved time management – translates to improved patient scheduling and staff usage, which will lead to reduced staff costs relative to sales revenues.
- Reduced staff turnover – costs of recruitment, selection, training and reduced efficiency not unnecessarily incurred.
- Reduced accidents and equipment down time – reduces costs to practice in terms of costs in sick pay, down time of equipment, compensation claims, insurance premiums, unscheduled service costs and replacements.
- Reduced sickness and absenteeism – greater job satisfaction means better staff morale and efficient teamwork.

Training alone is not the driver of these benefits. Other factors that affect these issues include economic, political and employment situations locally and nationally.

An important decision for the practice owner–manager is to decide what training can be done by the practice itself and what external support will be required.

Products and services provided

Income generated in an optometric practice is derived from provision and sales of:

- Eye examinations – the vast majority of patients attend for eye examinations, which is the key value driver in optometric practice. Only after a complete eye exam is conducted are contact lenses prescribed and dispensed.
- Spectacle dispensing – regardless of how much contact lens activity a practice has, the supply of complete spectacles will always be a necessary part of contact lens practice.
- Contact lenses – apart from a stock of 'off-the-shelf' designs, the practice may need to have to hand specialist contact designs and products.
- Accessories – a range of appropriate contact lens care systems and other accessories need to be available, such as sunglasses, spectacle chains, contact lens and spectacle cases.
- Subscription schemes – both contact lens wearers and spectacle-wearing patients benefit from service agreement schemes, which enable them to obtain replacement products and specific professional services at preferential terms. Such schemes are now common and maintain a degree of continuity to the practice.

Pricing – fees and charges

The very personal and individual nature of both services and products involved in contact lens practice means that mass production approaches cannot be applied without risking negative effects to the practice. When making pricing decisions, three elements normally need to be taken into account: the practice cost base, the patients and customers to the practice, and the competition. The fees and charges of the practice will generally be a compromise between what the business needs to cover costs, what the patients and customers expect to pay for the services and the products, and what the competition charges. Pricing issues are further confounded by the fact that not every owner–optometrist will seek to maximize profits, nor is detailed information about costs, competition and the potential patient/customer easily available to the practice.

Speciality–commodity continuum

The concept of the speciality–commodity continuum applies to both contact lens products and services. At one extreme is the service product consisting of a speciality service which is highly differentiated from the rest of the competition, whilst at the other extreme is a commodity.

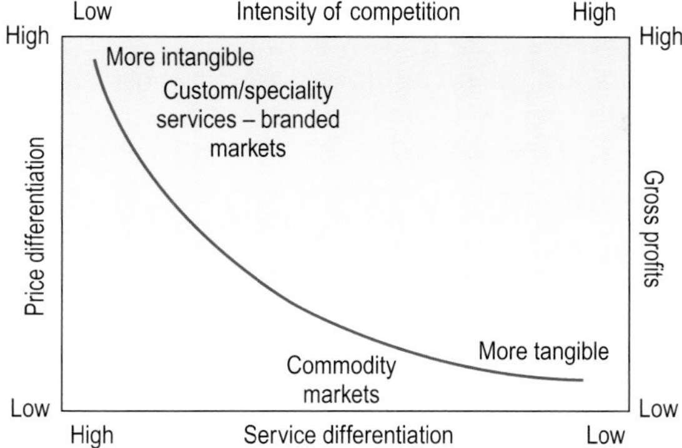

Figure 43.2 The speciality–commodity continuum.

Figure 43.2 illustrates this speciality–commodity continuum as a conceptual map, describing some of the characteristics of the competition, gross profits, price differentiation and image differentiation associated with the two extremes.

Optometric practices would be best served by ensuring that contact lens products and services do not slide to the extreme commodity end. It is worth noting the features of a commodity, which include self-determination of need, self-management of use, non-invasive with little (perceived) potential for harm, non-regulated and price determined by market forces.

Professional model

Developing a fees and charges schedule is never an easy task. Once one subscribes to the need to move away from the commodity end of the market where competition relies primarily on purchase decisions based only on price, to the speciality end, then the need for a professional model for fees and charges becomes paramount. One way to do this is to establish the expenses overhead per hour for the practice (chair time). Knowing the actual chair time required for differing types of contact lens services (e.g. spherical rigid lenses, soft lenses, daily/monthly disposable soft lenses, toric and bifocal lenses), allowing for potential unscheduled visits, adding the contact lens material and care system costs (duly marked up, say 20–35%), and any other handling charges, this figure can then be used to calculate the fees and charges for any service product provided by the practice. With the advent of mail-order contact lenses, internet trading and an increasing trend for contact lenses to be considered as a commodity, it is important to adopt a transparent fees and charges schedule that is competitive on a like-for-like basis without eroding the professional fees dimension.

Promotional issues

Communicating the availability of products and services that have been identified as 'needs and wants' by patients and customers, at a price that creates sustained value for the practice, is what promotions are about. A variety of options are open to the optometrist–owner to communicate with existing and potential contact lens patients and customers. The mix of these will often be determined by which stage the practice is at in its life cycle. For example, a new practice with mostly new patients will rely more on external promotions, whilst an existing mature practice will rely more on internal communications and promotions.

Internal

Internal promotions embrace all aspects of communication to existing contact lens patients and include the spectrum from personal contact at the practice – which embraces the practice ambience and point-of-sale literature – through to special mailings. Personal communication is by far the most significant mode of internal contact with the patient, and can adopt the following guises:

- The recall letter – with careful database management, it is possible not only to send out recall letters for routine contact lens aftercare visits, but also to tailor promotions of specific products and services to patients by criteria other than clinical need.
- Special mailings – some practitioners will send patients thank you cards for referrals and cards on the arrival of a new family member.
- Practice newsletters – both via conventional mail and e-mail – are increasingly used and are indeed a good way of educating and maintaining contact with patients, and keeping them aware about the practice, its personnel and its activities.

The use of a website as an internal communication tool merits some mention. Practice websites, and electronic mail, will increasingly play a role in allowing patient education, e-mail recall letters, e-promotions and opportunities for patients to contact the practice to order sun wear, contact lens accessories and replacement products, to book an appointment and even to submit medical history. Similarly, it makes sense to consider a contact lens aftercare appointment reminder communication via e-mail or SMS.

External

These promotions include all activities where potential contact lens patients might be exposed to the activities, personnel or products at the practice. These include national and regional newspapers, trade and professional magazines, radio and television broadcasts, telephone directories, exhibitions and health fairs, direct mail, public relations, speaking engagements and the worldwide web. This last method enables practices to broaden their catchment area, offer sun wear, contact lens accessories, frames and spectacles along with practice information and opportunities to book appointments online.

Processes

These are the procedures, mechanisms and routines that the practice adopts to provide the services and products to patients and customers. Although in contact lens practice the people element is critical, no amount of attention and effort from staff will overcome unsatisfactory process configuration. For example, no matter how well members of staff do their job – or what equipment one uses for the data collection – if the process of, say, booking appointments is too cumbersome or inaccurate, then patient dissatisfaction is inevitable, as is ineffective clinical care. Generally, the greater the complexity and divergence (variability of the steps/sequences) of the task, the more it is usually necessary to empower the staff to exercise their judgement in the best interest of the patient and the practice.

A variety of processes are employed in managing patients, products, money and personnel. They are too numerous to include in full, so a selection of key contact lens activity-oriented processes is mentioned here.

Managing patients

Patients who attend for contact lens services have requirements in addition to their needs as routine optometric patients, and will thus place special demands on the processes of the practice. These range from appointment scheduling through to the transfer of records and clinical details.

Contracts, service agreements and informed consent

A contract is an agreement between parties (two or more) that is enforceable by law. Four essential elements need to be present for a contract to be legally enforceable; specifically, there must be:

1. the existence of both an offer and an acceptance
2. an intention by both parties to create a legally enforceable relationship
3. clear and certain terms and conditions, for the courts to be able to enforce them
4. consideration – that is to say, each party has agreed to contribute to the deal – for example, the practitioner promises to provide agreed professional services to the patient, such as eye examination, contact lens fitting, supply and aftercare, and the patient in turn promises to pay the agreed fees.

In an attempt to clarify the terms and conditions, to educate the patient and to generate documentary evidence, practitioners have produced a variety of contact lens service/subscription agreements and policy documents. These generally range from describing what is included in the fees and charges, to what is included in prepaid contact lens service subscriptions (for regular optometric and contact lens reviews and replacement of contact lenses).

Contracts, such as those mentioned above, do not have to be in writing. They can be verbal, as long as the above elements are present and enforceable by the law (in theory). However, in practice it is a real challenge without written documentation.

The doctrine of informed consent is an aspect of health care generally that is constantly evolving, and arises from the fact that touching another person (during an optometric consultation) without consent may be regarded as offensive or harmful, for which damages could be claimed and awarded. In medicine this has often translated to mean consent to medical procedures. In reality, it is an approach to practising defensively, and if a claim of negligence arises, it could be shown that the patient knew and consented to what was done, as a potential means of defence. Although the USA has adopted an approach whereby the fullest possible information as to the treatment/procedure is given to the patient to make informed choices, the English courts tend to look at approved practice amongst professionals when deciding what the patient should be told of the risks/procedures. Nevertheless, it would be prudent to keep patients as well informed as is reasonably possible, to ensure long-term success in contact lens practice.

Patient scheduling

The eye examination is the key value driver in any optometric practice, whilst staff costs are the key costs. Effective practice resource management without compromising clinical care is often dependent on the use of appropriate appointment scheduling methods. There are three principal approaches commonly found in practice:

1. Traditional – patients here are booked in at regular intervals with equal times set aside for each consultation. For example, patients are booked in every 20 min, starting and ending at a given time. It is simple and that is why it is used so often. However, it does not allow for patients who require longer consultations or patients who require less time. It is thus possible to end up with unproductive portions of time when less time with a patient is needed, and long waiting queues if a patient requires a longer consultation.
2. Block system – this is not often used in optometry but is found in hospitals and general medical practice. This method involves scheduling multiple patients in the same time slot. For example, there would be three patients booked at 9.00 a.m. and then none until 10.00 a.m., when there would be three more patients booked, and so on. Individuals who have experienced this approach are often disgruntled to find that they have the same appointment slot as others.
3. Mixed – some practices find a mixture of traditional and block booking to be a workable combination, using the block system for scheduling shorter 15-min visits (e.g. groups of children, some contact lens follow-up visits) and 20-min scheduling for routine eye exam consultations.

The challenge is to schedule patients so that the down time and the time taken to 'settle in' in the consulting room do not curb the consultation time of the practitioner. In contact lens practice, appointments are normally scheduled for eye examinations, preliminary examination and initial fitting, evaluation after diagnostic lens wear (return), collection/hygiene, routine aftercare and unscheduled visits (urgent, emergency).

Patient education

Contact lens practice has a particular responsibility to instruct patients on the wear, care and hygiene with respect to contact lenses. Anyone who has been in contact lens practice will concur that good patient education is key to successful contact lens wear. It is thus not surprising that significant resources are often dedicated to this function in contact lens practice. This may include a dedicated area/room, and a dedicated and appropriately trained individual (contact lens hygienist) to instruct and educate one or more patients at a time on placement and removal of lenses, wearing schedules, caring for lenses and cases, general hygiene and lid hygiene. It is also in this area that any service agreements and details of emergency cover are discussed and issued. Increasingly, practices provide both verbal and written instructions, and some also lend videos and CD-ROMs for patients to view and review the procedures in their own home. It is logical for this information to be made available and downloadable from practice websites for patients.

Records on patient web pages

The internet has already significantly altered the way in which one can promote contact lens practice. Practice websites carrying information and offering access to the supply of contact lenses and other optical products online directly to patients are already here. This is an expected reaction to counter mail-order and online supply of optical products by non-optometrists and non-opticians. However, from a patient perspective, it is worth bearing in mind that the internet also offers the possibility to store personal medical and associated records in one easily accessible location. This would then enable any health care practitioner, anywhere in the world, to access these records with the consent of the patient and protected by using an appropriate password. It is thus not too far-fetched for patients to ask that their contact lens/optometric data be uploaded to their personal health web pages in the future.

Managing contact lens products

The tangible products that contact lens practices supply include all those products normally supplied in general optometric practice, plus contact lenses, contact lens care systems and associated products. In view of recent concerns about the transmission of new variant Creutzfeldt–Jakob disease (see Chapter 18), the use of empirically fitted rigid lenses is now the preferred option, and the use of stock disposable soft and silicone hydrogel lenses a practical alternative. It is thus necessary for contact lens practices to stock a variety of lens types for fitting and possibly initial supply. However, it must be borne in mind that this stock, if paid for by the practice, is only creating value if sold. Similarly, the stocking of a variety of contact lens care systems and accessories is essential in providing a complete service. Like contact lenses, stock that is held in the practice only creates value if it is sold or supplied to patients and customers. Bar-coding of contact lenses and care systems will help manage the inventory of both contact lenses and solutions; however, the value of this process in the absence of a standardized bar-coding scheme is somewhat limited.

Managing money

Income to the practice will accrue from patients, customers and third-party payments (national and private health insurance, driving licence authorities, employers). It is therefore important that records are kept of every transaction and that there is no hindrance for receiving these payments by any method (e.g. cash, credit cards, cheques, direct debit, standing order, electronic transfer of funds) (Holmes and Sugden, 1986). Of these methods, the use of direct debits in prepaid subscription schemes has proved to be a particularly useful option. Similarly, the practice will need to pay its suppliers (e.g. laboratories, prescription houses, various forms of sales tax, telephone, printing and stationery) and its staff.

The provision of contact lens services, like optometric services, is indeed a provision of professional time. The supply of products is secondary to this, and it is appropriate to adopt an accounting method that mirrors this approach. The Association of Optometrists in the UK has published guidance on such an approach and the reader is referred to this (Hayes *et al.*, 1999).

The use of computers in practice management and in particular practice finances is beyond the scope of this chapter. Suffice it to say that many 'off-the-shelf' software options are available and adaptable, whilst others dedicated to optometric practice management and incorporating the special needs for contact lens practice are also available. Figure 43.3 illustrates practice activity where computers may be utilized.

Lens ordering

A majority of lenses prescribed today are obtained initially from in-office inventories of disposable lenses. Once the patient is satisfied with the lenses fitted, an order must be placed with the manufacturer, or a third-party distributor, for an appropriate ongoing supply (typically for 3 or 6 months). There is clearly a wide assortment of technical means of placing an order, which parallels modes of modern communication – that is, a written order posted in the mail (rarely used these days), telephone, fax and the internet. The latter two modes of communication are preferred because there is less likelihood of confusion, and a clear audit trail for checking, if the order is issued in textual form. Patients are often looking to order replacement lenses online. If patients were able to do this from a practice website, patient retention is likely to be enhanced (McNelis, 2009).

Disposable soft lenses are typically specified by manufacturer, lens trade name and lens power. If the lens is available in a variety of parameters, then the parameter of choice obviously needs to be specified also. More detailed information is generally required for custom-made soft lenses and rigid lenses. As a general rule, the more details that are supplied when ordering a custom-designed lens, the greater the likelihood that the lens delivered will be as required.

Professional regulation

The manner in which a practitioner fits and supplies contact lenses may be controlled by various regulations. In the UK, the General Optical Council (GOC), by the powers vested in it by the Opticians Act 1985 section 31, has made rules regulating the prescription, supply and fitting of contact lenses by registered optometrists, opticians or companies and their employees.

The Rules on the Fitting of Contact Lenses 1985 cover the details with respect to the circumstances in which trainee optometrists or opticians may fit contact lenses. The Contact Lens (Qualifications etc.) Rules 1988 provide for a minimum level of education, training and qualification before a registered optometrist or optician can undertake the fitting of contact lenses in the UK. The Contact Lens (Specification) Rules 1989 require that an optometrist or optician who fits contact lenses shall on completion of the fitting give the patient a written specification of the lenses in sufficient detail to enable the lens to be replicated.

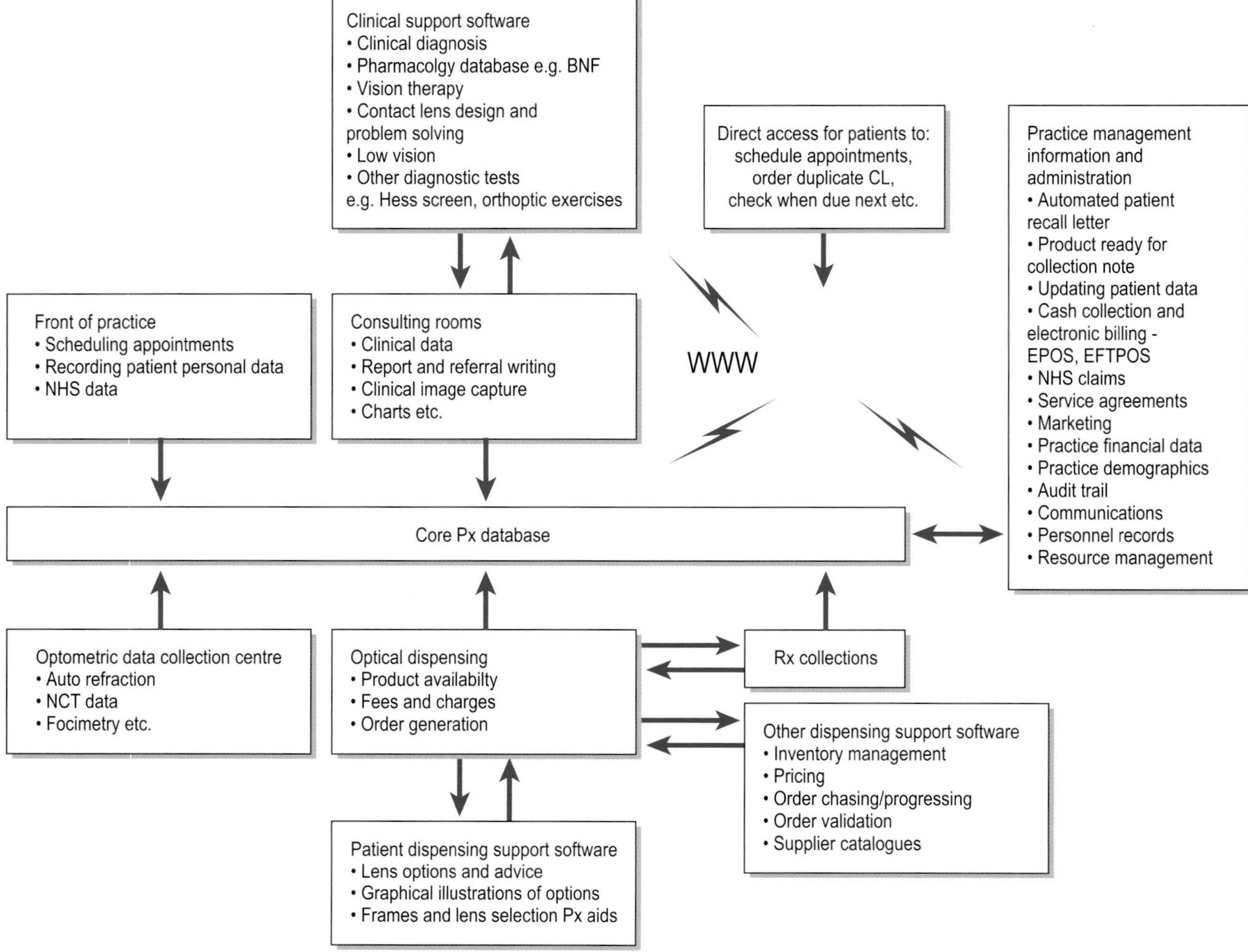

Figure 43.3 Practice activity where computers may be utilized. BNF = *British National Formulary*; CL = contact lens; EPOS = electronic point of sale; EFTPOS; electronic funds transfer at point of sale; NHS = National Health Service; Px = patient; Rx = prescription; NCT = non-contact tonometry; VFA = visual field analyser. (Adapted from Hirji, N. K. (1999) Business Awareness for Optometrists – a Primer, Butterworth-Heinemann.)

The Opticians Act 1989 (Amendment) Order 2005, made under section 60 of the Health Act, 1999, amends the Opticians Act 1989 and came into effect with its supporting Rules on 30 June/1 July 2005. This was the first of the series of orders that the government made to modernize the health care professions in the UK and significantly affects the provision of optometric and optical care and the framework within which the optical professions practise and optical businesses operate (Hirji and Clarkson, 2006). This order improves significantly the way in which the GOC can discharge its duty of protecting the public by bringing about the changes that affect registration, recognition of specialisms, professional indemnity insurance, continuing education and training, registrants' fitness to practise and supply contact lenses and allows the GOC to seek additional relevant information about the registrant, including character. It redefines the role of the GOC as the overseer of 'professional education, conduct and performance among registrants'.

All contact lens fitting and aftercare remain entirely the domain of registered practitioners, including the fitting of zero-powered contact lenses (plano cosmetic lenses), which when completed obliges the practitioner to provide a specification of the contact lenses prescribed (subject to the Data Protection Act 1988) which has to include the following information (SI 2005/1481):

- The name and address of the patient.
- If the patient has not attained the age of 16 on the day the specification is issued, his/her date of birth.
- The name of the practitioner and his/her registration number in the GOC register or General Medical Council register.
- The address from which the practitioner practises.
- The name of the practice on whose premises the fitting was done.
- The date the fitting was completed.
- Sufficient details of any lens fitted to enable a person who fits or supplies a contact lens to replicate the lens.
- The date the specification expires.

and such information of a clinical nature as that prescribing practitioner considers to be necessary in the particular case.

This closes the loophole that existed for non-registrants to fit and supply zero-powered cosmetic contact lenses prior to this order. However duplicate contact lenses can be purchased by the public from unregistered suppliers, in person, via mail order or through internet-enabled enterprises as a result of this order except for:

- Minors.
- Those registered severely visually impaired.
- Those who are visually impaired.

in which case supply can only be by a registrant.

There are, however, conditions imposed, which include the following: that the transaction is the result of:

- A valid verified original contact lens specification from a registered practitioner, submitted either in writing or electronically.
- For the use of the person named in the specification.
- Before the expiry date mentioned in the specification and that the supply is under the direction of a registered optometric/optical practitioner or a medical practitioner.

'General direction' in this context was described during the passage of the legislation through parliament as meaning that a registered practitioner is employed in the management chain of the supplier's business and accountable for what goes on between the supplier and the purchaser, ultimately answerable to the GOC and therefore providing a measure of protection to the public which was hitherto absent. The seller (whether registered or unregistered) must also make reasonable arrangements for the person who is purchasing the contact lenses from the seller to receive aftercare. The supply of zero-powered cosmetic contact lenses is also covered by bringing this area under the auspices of the GOC. The supply of contact lenses by suppliers and manufacturers to registrants and others, and not directly to patients would not, however, be subject to such requirements. It should also be noted that it remains a defence to any prosecution under the relevant section to demonstrate that the lenses were sold as an antique (except where the seller had reason to believe that the lenses would be used to correct, remedy or relieve a defect of sight) (Hirji and Clarkson, 2006).

On 30 October 2006, the GOC released a statement setting out the GOC's view that, whilst the sale of prescription (sight-correcting) contact lenses may be supplied under the 'general direction' of a GOC registrant or a medical practitioner, a 'supervised sale' is a requirement for the sale of plano (zero-powered) contact lenses. The statement also affirms the GOC position that a supervisor (a registered optometrist, dispensing optician or medical practitioner) must be able to exercise professional skill and judgement as a clinician. In the absence of any statutory definition of 'supervision', however, the GOC will consider the issue of whether a sale was made under 'supervision' on a case-by-case basis, involving expert clinical opinion as appropriate. Also, the GOC asked the professional optical bodies to provide a detailed guideline on their interpretation of the meaning of 'supervision' (February 2007). Finally, in the press release of the same date, the GOC states that only in the supply of corrective lenses will the purchaser be required to provide a valid 'specification' for the supply to be legal (Hirji and Clarkson, 2007). The College of Optometrists and the Association of British Dispensing Opticians now provide guidance on their interpretation of 'supervision' (essentially that the practitioner should be in a position to exercise clinical judgement and intervene, and ensure appropriate aftercare arrangements are made) and 'general direction' (essentially that the practitioner should ensure and be satisfied that procedures are in place to safeguard the patient, that the supplier (person) is appropriately trained, that the lenses supplied meet the specifications and that appropriate aftercare arrangements are made) (College of Optometrists, 2007). This guidance has been accepted by the GOC.

Conclusions

A key aim of this book has been to describe the great clinical and intellectual challenges involved in contact lens practice. This chapter has outlined the principles involved in managing an eye-care practice that engages in contact lens fitting. By providing an organized and efficient service to patients, and paying proper attention to staff management and support, contact lens practice can be enjoyable and profitable as well as being clinically challenging.

References

ACAS (1994) *Employing People – The ACAS Handbook for Small Firms*, ACAS Publications.

College of Optometrists (2007) Code of Ethics and Guidance for Professional Conduct Guidance (Revised Feb 2007) Section 28. Available online at: http://www.college-optometrists.org/index.aspx/pcms/site.publication.Ethics_Guidelines.recent/displayAmount/5/page/4/.

Fraser, J. M. (1958) *A Handbook of Employment Interviewing*. Cited by Torrington and Hall (1987).

Hayes, I., Cornwell-Kelly, M., Hunter, I. and Smith, J. (1999) Accounting for VAT. *Optometry Today,* **39,** 15 January, 1–12.

Hirji, N.K. (1999) *Business Awareness for Optometrists – a Primer,* Oxford: Butterworth-Heinemann.

Hirji, N.K. and Clarkson, R. (2006) ' The Opticians Act 1989 (Amendment) Order 2005 – So what's the story?' *Contact Lens Anterior Eye,* **29,** 217–222.

Hirji, N. K. and Clarkson R. (2007) 'Order of Change' *Optician* **233**(6094), 28–32.

Holmes, G. and Sugden, A. (1986) *Interpreting Company Reports and Accounts,* 3rd edn. Cambridge: Woodhead-Faulkner.

McNelis, K. (2009) Use technology to improve your contact lens practice. *Ophthalmology Times.* **34,** February 15.

Roger, A. (1951) The Seven-Point Plan. Cited by Torrington and Hall (1987).

Torrington, D. and Hall, L. (1987) *Personnel Management – a New Approach,* New Jersey: Prentice-Hall.

Appendices

Appendix A
Contact lens design and specifications

Figure A.1 Plan and cross-sectional view of a minus-powered contact lens with a single curve front surface and bicurve back surface.

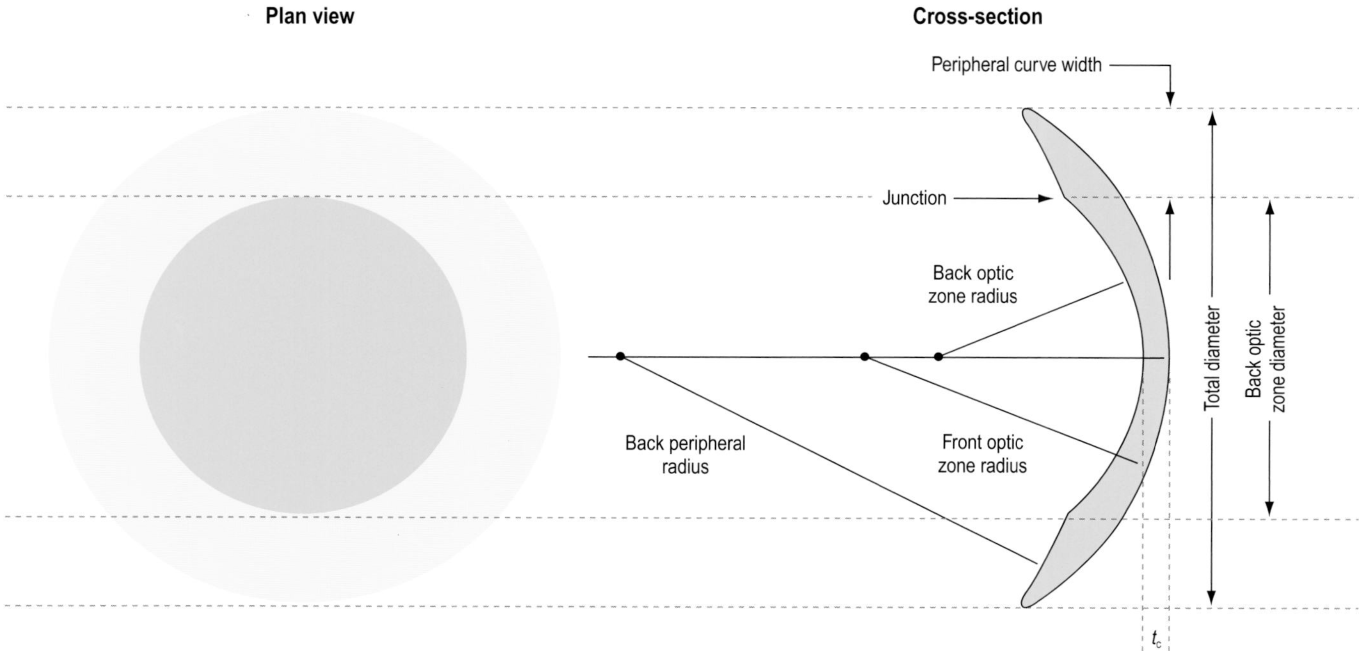

Terms, symbols and abbreviations used to describe contact lenses

Term	Symbol	Abbreviation
Back optic zone radius	r_0	BOZR
Back peripheral radius	$r_1, r_2, \ldots$	BPR1, BPR2, ...
Front optic zone radius	r_{a0}	FOZR
Front peripheral radius	$r_{a1}, r_{a2}, \ldots$	FPR1, FPR2, ...
Back optic zone diameter	$\O_0$	BOZD
Back peripheral zone diameters	$\O_1, \O_2, \ldots$	BPZD1, BPZD2, ...
Total diameter	$\O_T$	TD
Front optic zone diameter	$\O_{a0}$	FOZD
Front peripheral zone diameters	$\O_{a1}, \O_{a2}, \ldots$	FPZD1, FPZD2, ...
Geometric centre thickness	t_c	tc
Carrier junction thickness	t_{a0}	tj
Peripheral junction thickness	$t_{a1}, t_{a2}, \ldots$	ta1, ta2, ...
Radial edge thickness	t_e	RET
Axial edge thickness	t_{ak}	AET
Radial edge lift	l_r	REL
Axial edge lift	l_a	AEL
Front vertex power	F_v	FVP
Back vertex power	F'_v	BVP
Oxygen flux	j	j
Oxygen permeability	Dk	Dk
Oxygen transmissibility	Dk/t	Dk/t

- The terms and symbols outlined above were obtained from the following standard: ISO8320–1986 Optics and optical instruments – contact lenses – vocabulary and symbols.
- (The abbreviations given above were modified from those suggested by: Hough, T., 2000 A Guide to Contact Lens Standards. British Contact Lens Association)

Appendix B
Contact lens tolerances

Table A Dimensional tolerances for soft, polymethyl methacrylate (PMMA) and rigid lenses (all units in mm)

Dimension	Soft lenses	PMMA lenses	Rigid lenses
Back optic zone radius	±0.20	±0.025	±0.05
Back optic zone radii of toroidal surfaces where the difference in radii is:			
<0.20		±0.25	±0.05
0.2–0.4		±0.35	±0.06
0.4–0.6		±0.55	±0.07
>0.6		±0.75	±0.09
Sagitta at specified diameter	±0.05		
Back optic zone diameter	±0.20	±0.025	±0.05
Back peripheral radius		±0.10	±0.10
Front peripheral radius		±0.10	±0.10
Back peripheral diameter		±0.20	±0.20
Total diameter	±0.20	±0.10	±0.10
Front optic zone diameter	±0.20	±0.20	±0.20
Bifocal segment height		–0.10 to +0.20	–0.10 to +0.20
Centre thickness		±0.02	±0.02
Centre thickness, where the nominal value is:			
≤0.10	±0.010 + 10%		
>0.10	±0.015 + 5%		

Table B Optical tolerances for soft, polymethyl methacrylate (PMMA) and rigid lenses

Dimension	Soft lenses	PMMA lenses	Rigid lenses
Back vertex power			
≤5 D		±0.12 D	±0.12 D
≤10 D	±0.25 D	±0.18 D	±0.18 D
≤15 D		±0.25 D	±0.25 D
≤20 D	±0.50 D	±0.37 D	±0.37 D
>20 D	±1.00 D	±0.50 D	±0.50 D
Cylinder power			
≤0.2	±0.25 D	±0.25 D	±0.25 D
2–4	±0.37 D	±0.37 D	±0.37 D
>4	±0.50 D	±0.50 D	±0.50 D
Cylinder axis	±5°	±5°	±5°
Prismatic error (measured at the geometric centre of the optic zone)			
Back vertex power ≤6 D		±0.25 cm/m	±0.25 cm/m
Back vertex power >6 D		±0.50 cm/m	±0.50 cm/m
Prescribed prism		±0.25 cm/m	±0.25 cm/m

Table C Material property tolerances for soft lenses

Material property	Tolerance
Refractive index	±0.005
Water content	±2%
Oxygen permeability	±20%

- The tolerances outlined in this appendix were obtained from the following standards:
  ISO 8321-1: 1991 Optics and optical instruments – contact lenses – part 1: specification for rigid corneal and scleral contact lenses.
  BS EN ISO 8321-2: 2000 (BS 7208-24:2000) Ophthalmic optics – specifications for material, optical and dimensional properties of contact lenses – part 2: single-vision hydrogel contact lenses.
- PMMA tolerances are given here because trial lens fitting sets are often fabricated from this material due to its resilience.
- See also: Hough, T. (2000) *A Guide to Contact Lens Standards.* British Contact Lens Association.

Appendix C
Vertex distance correction

Effective power (D) of plus- and minus-prescription spectacle lenses at the corneal plane for various vertex distances (mm)*. Courtesy of Adrian S Bruce.

Spec Rx	Power (D) at corneal plane for different vertex distances (mm)									
	8 mm		10 mm		12 mm		14 mm		16 mm	
	plus	minus	plus	minus	plus	minus	plus	minus	plus	minus
4.00	4.13	3.88	4.17	3.85	4.20	3.82	4.24	3.79	4.27	3.76
4.25	4.40	4.11	4.44	4.08	4.48	4.04	4.52	4.01	4.56	3.98
4.50	4.67	4.34	4.71	4.31	4.76	4.27	4.80	4.23	4.85	4.20
4.75	4.94	4.58	4.99	4.53	5.04	4.49	5.09	4.45	5.14	4.41
5.00	5.21	4.81	5.26	4.76	5.32	4.72	5.38	4.67	5.43	4.63
5.25	5.48	5.04	5.54	4.99	5.60	4.94	5.67	4.89	5.73	4.84
5.50	5.75	5.27	5.82	5.21	5.89	5.16	5.96	5.11	6.03	5.06
5.75	6.03	5.50	6.10	5.44	6.18	5.38	6.25	5.32	6.33	5.27
6.00	6.30	5.73	6.38	5.66	6.47	5.60	6.55	5.54	6.64	5.47
6.25	6.58	5.95	6.67	5.88	6.76	5.81	6.85	5.75	6.94	5.68
6.50	6.86	6.18	6.95	6.10	7.05	6.03	7.15	5.96	7.25	5.89
6.75	7.14	6.40	7.24	6.32	7.34	6.24	7.45	6.17	7.57	6.09
7.00	7.42	6.63	7.53	6.54	7.64	6.46	7.76	6.38	7.88	6.29
7.25	7.70	6.85	7.82	6.76	7.94	6.67	8.07	6.58	8.20	6.50
7.50	7.98	7.08	8.11	6.98	8.24	6.88	8.38	6.79	8.52	6.70
7.75	8.26	7.30	8.40	7.19	8.54	7.09	8.69	6.99	8.85	6.90
8.00	8.55	7.52	8.70	7.41	8.85	7.30	9.01	7.19	9.17	7.09
8.25	8.83	7.74	8.99	7.62	9.16	7.51	9.33	7.40	9.50	7.29
8.50	9.12	7.96	9.29	7.83	9.47	7.71	9.65	7.60	9.84	7.48
8.75	9.41	8.18	9.59	8.05	9.78	7.92	9.97	7.80	10.17	7.68
9.00	9.70	8.40	9.89	8.26	10.09	8.12	10.30	7.99	10.51	7.87
9.25	9.99	8.61	10.19	8.47	10.40	8.33	10.63	8.19	10.86	8.06
9.50	10.28	8.83	10.50	8.68	10.72	8.53	10.96	8.38	11.20	8.25
9.75	10.57	9.04	10.80	8.88	11.04	8.73	11.29	8.58	11.55	8.43
10.00	10.87	9.26	11.11	9.09	11.36	8.93	11.63	8.77	11.90	8.62
10.25	11.17	9.47	11.42	9.30	11.69	9.13	11.97	8.96	12.26	8.81
10.50	11.46	9.69	11.73	9.50	12.01	9.33	12.31	9.15	12.62	8.99
10.75	11.76	9.90	12.04	9.71	12.34	9.52	12.65	9.34	12.98	9.17
11.00	12.06	10.11	12.36	9.91	12.67	9.72	13.00	9.53	13.35	9.35
11.25	12.36	10.32	12.68	10.11	13.01	9.91	13.35	9.72	13.72	9.53
11.50	12.67	10.53	12.99	10.31	13.34	10.11	13.71	9.91	14.09	9.71
11.75	12.97	10.74	13.31	10.51	13.68	10.30	14.06	10.09	14.47	9.89
12.00	13.27	10.95	13.64	10.71	14.02	10.49	14.42	10.27	14.85	10.07
12.25	13.58	11.16	13.96	10.91	14.36	10.68	14.79	10.46	15.24	10.24
12.50	13.89	11.36	14.29	11.11	14.71	10.87	15.15	10.64	15.63	10.42
12.75	14.20	11.57	14.61	11.31	15.05	11.06	15.52	10.82	16.02	10.59

Spec Rx	Power (D) at corneal plane for different vertex distances (mm)									
	8 mm		10 mm		12 mm		14 mm		16 mm	
	plus	minus	plus	minus	plus	minus	plus	minus	plus	minus
13.00	14.51	11.78	14.94	11.50	15.40	11.25	15.89	11.00	16.41	10.76
13.25	14.82	11.98	15.27	11.70	15.76	11.43	16.27	11.18	16.81	10.93
13.50	15.13	12.18	15.61	11.89	16.11	11.62	16.65	11.35	17.22	11.10
13.75	15.45	12.39	15.94	12.09	16.47	11.80	17.03	11.53	17.63	11.27
14.00	15.77	12.59	16.28	12.28	16.83	11.99	17.41	11.71	18.04	11.44
14.25	16.08	12.79	16.62	12.47	17.19	12.17	17.80	11.88	18.46	11.60
14.50	16.40	12.99	16.96	12.66	17.55	12.35	18.19	12.05	18.88	11.77
14.75	16.72	13.19	17.30	12.85	17.92	12.53	18.59	12.23	19.31	11.93
15.00	17.05	13.39	17.65	13.04	18.29	12.71	18.99	12.40	19.74	12.10
15.25	17.37	13.59	17.99	13.23	18.67	12.89	19.39	12.57	20.17	12.26
15.50	17.69	13.79	18.34	13.42	19.04	13.07	19.80	12.74	20.61	12.42
15.75	18.02	13.99	18.69	13.61	19.42	13.25	20.21	12.90	21.06	12.58
16.00	18.35	14.18	19.05	13.79	19.80	13.42	20.62	13.07	21.51	12.74
16.25	18.68	14.38	19.40	13.98	20.19	13.60	21.04	13.24	21.96	12.90
16.50	19.01	14.58	19.76	14.16	20.57	13.77	21.46	13.40	22.42	13.05
16.75	19.34	14.77	20.12	14.35	20.96	13.95	21.88	13.57	22.88	13.21
17.00	19.68	14.96	20.48	14.53	21.36	14.12	22.31	13.73	23.35	13.36
17.25	20.01	15.16	20.85	14.71	21.75	14.29	22.74	13.89	23.83	13.52
17.50	20.35	15.35	21.21	14.89	22.15	14.46	23.18	14.06	24.31	13.67
17.75	20.69	15.54	21.58	15.07	22.55	14.63	23.62	14.22	24.79	13.82
18.00	21.03	15.73	21.95	15.25	22.96	14.80	24.06	14.38	25.28	13.98
18.25	21.37	15.92	22.32	15.43	23.37	14.97	24.51	14.54	25.78	14.13
18.50	21.71	16.11	22.70	15.61	23.78	15.14	24.97	14.69	26.28	14.27
18.75	22.06	16.30	23.08	15.79	24.19	15.31	25.42	14.85	26.79	14.42
19.00	22.41	16.49	23.46	15.97	24.61	15.47	25.89	15.01	27.30	14.57
19.25	22.75	16.68	23.84	16.14	25.03	15.64	26.35	15.16	27.82	14.72
19.50	23.10	16.87	24.22	16.32	25.46	15.80	26.82	15.32	28.34	14.86
19.75	23.46	17.06	24.61	16.49	25.88	15.97	27.30	15.47	28.87	15.01
20.00	23.81	17.24	25.00	16.67	26.32	16.13	27.78	15.63	29.41	15.15

* Based on the equation: OR = SR/(1 − [d × SR]), where:
OR = ocular refraction
SR = spectacle refraction
d = vertex distance (m)
The lens powers enclosed within the heavy border relate to the standard vertex distance of 12 mm that will apply in most cases.

Appendix D
Corneal curvature – corneal power conversion

Conversion between corneal front surface radius of curvature (*r*; mm) and corneal power (*K*; D)*. Courtesy of Adrian S Bruce.

r (mm)	*K* (D)	*r* (mm)	*K* (D)	*r* (mm)	*K* (D)	*r* (mm)	*K* (D)	*r* (mm)	*K* (D)
6.30	53.57	6.99	48.28	7.63	44.23	8.27	40.81	8.91	37.88
6.36	53.07	7.00	48.21	7.64	44.18	8.28	40.76	8.92	37.84
6.37	52.98	7.01	48.15	7.65	44.12	8.29	40.71	8.93	37.79
6.38	52.90	7.02	48.08	7.66	44.06	8.30	40.66	8.94	37.75
6.39	52.82	7.03	48.01	7.67	44.00	8.31	40.61	8.95	37.71
6.40	52.73	7.04	47.94	7.68	43.95	8.32	40.56	8.96	37.67
6.41	52.65	7.05	47.87	7.69	43.89	8.33	40.52	8.97	37.63
6.42	52.57	7.06	47.80	7.70	43.83	8.34	40.47	8.98	37.58
6.43	52.49	7.07	47.74	7.71	43.77	8.35	40.42	8.99	37.54
6.44	52.41	7.08	47.67	7.72	43.72	8.36	40.37	9.00	37.50
6.45	52.33	7.09	47.60	7.73	43.66	8.37	40.32	9.01	37.46
6.46	52.24	7.10	47.54	7.74	43.60	8.38	40.27	9.02	37.42
6.47	52.16	7.11	47.47	7.75	43.55	8.39	40.23	9.03	37.38
6.48	52.08	7.12	47.40	7.76	43.49	8.40	40.18	9.04	37.33
6.49	52.00	7.13	47.34	7.77	43.44	8.41	40.13	9.05	37.29
6.50	51.92	7.14	47.27	7.78	43.38	8.42	40.08	9.06	37.25
6.51	51.84	7.15	47.20	7.79	43.32	8.43	40.04	9.07	37.21
6.52	51.76	7.16	47.14	7.80	43.27	8.44	39.99	9.08	37.17
6.53	51.68	7.17	47.07	7.81	43.21	8.45	39.94	9.09	37.13
6.54	51.61	7.18	47.01	7.82	43.16	8.46	39.89	9.10	37.09
6.55	51.53	7.19	46.94	7.83	43.10	8.47	39.85	9.11	37.05
6.56	51.45	7.20	46.88	7.84	43.05	8.48	39.80	9.12	37.01
6.57	51.37	7.21	46.81	7.85	42.99	8.49	39.75	9.13	36.97
6.58	51.29	7.22	46.75	7.86	42.94	8.50	39.71	9.14	36.93
6.59	51.21	7.23	46.68	7.87	42.88	8.51	39.66	9.15	36.89
6.60	51.14	7.24	46.62	7.88	42.83	8.52	39.61	9.16	36.84
6.61	51.06	7.25	46.55	7.89	42.78	8.53	39.57	9.17	36.80
6.62	50.98	7.26	46.49	7.90	42.72	8.54	39.52	9.18	36.76
6.63	50.90	7.27	46.42	7.91	42.67	8.55	39.47	9.19	36.72
6.64	50.83	7.28	46.36	7.92	42.61	8.56	39.43	9.20	36.68
6.65	50.75	7.29	46.30	7.93	42.56	8.57	39.38	9.21	36.64
6.66	50.68	7.30	46.23	7.94	42.51	8.58	39.34	9.22	36.61
6.67	50.60	7.31	46.17	7.95	42.45	8.59	39.29	9.23	36.57
6.68	50.52	7.32	46.11	7.96	42.40	8.60	39.24	9.24	36.53
6.69	50.45	7.33	46.04	7.97	42.35	8.61	39.20	9.25	36.49
6.70	50.37	7.34	45.98	7.98	42.29	8.62	39.15	9.26	36.45
6.71	50.30	7.35	45.92	7.99	42.24	8.63	39.11	9.27	36.41
6.72	50.22	7.36	45.86	8.00	42.19	8.64	39.06	9.28	36.37
6.73	50.15	7.37	45.79	8.01	42.13	8.65	39.02	9.29	36.33

r (mm)	*K* (D)	*r* (mm)	*K* (D)	*r* (mm)	*K* (D)	*r* (mm)	*K* (D)	*r* (mm)	*K* (D)
6.74	50.07	7.38	45.73	8.02	42.08	8.66	38.97	9.30	36.29
6.75	50.00	7.39	45.67	8.03	42.03	8.67	38.93	9.31	36.25
6.76	49.93	7.40	45.61	8.04	41.98	8.68	38.88	9.32	36.21
6.77	49.85	7.41	45.55	8.05	41.93	8.69	38.84	9.33	36.17
6.78	49.78	7.42	45.49	8.06	41.87	8.70	38.79	9.34	36.13
6.79	49.71	7.43	45.42	8.07	41.82	8.71	38.75	9.35	36.10
6.80	49.63	7.44	45.36	8.08	41.77	8.72	38.70	9.36	36.06
6.81	49.56	7.45	45.30	8.09	41.72	8.73	38.66	9.37	36.02
6.82	49.49	7.46	45.24	8.10	41.67	8.74	38.62	9.38	35.98
6.83	49.41	7.47	45.18	8.11	41.62	8.75	38.57	9.39	35.94
6.84	49.34	7.48	45.12	8.12	41.56	8.76	38.53	9.40	35.90
6.85	49.27	7.49	45.06	8.13	41.51	8.77	38.48	9.41	35.87
6.86	49.20	7.50	45.00	8.14	41.46	8.78	38.44	9.42	35.83
6.87	49.13	7.51	44.94	8.15	41.41	8.79	38.40	9.43	35.79
6.88	49.06	7.52	44.88	8.16	41.36	8.80	38.35	9.44	35.75
6.89	48.98	7.53	44.82	8.17	41.31	8.81	38.31	9.45	35.71
6.90	48.91	7.54	44.76	8.18	41.26	8.82	38.27	9.46	35.68
6.91	48.84	7.55	44.70	8.19	41.21	8.83	38.22	9.47	35.64
6.92	48.77	7.56	44.64	8.20	41.16	8.84	38.18	9.48	35.60
6.93	48.70	7.57	44.58	8.21	41.11	8.85	38.14	9.49	35.56
6.94	48.63	7.58	44.53	8.22	41.06	8.86	38.09	9.50	35.53
6.95	48.56	7.59	44.47	8.23	41.01	8.87	38.05	9.51	35.49
6.96	48.49	7.60	44.41	8.24	40.96	8.88	38.01	9.52	35.45
6.97	48.42	7.61	44.35	8.25	40.91	8.89	37.96	9.53	35.41
6.98	48.35	7.62	44.29	8.26	40.86	8.90	37.92	9.54	35.38

* Based on the equation: Surface power (D) = (1.3375 – 1.0)/radius (m)

Appendix E
Extended keratometer range conversion

Conversion of keratometer reading (D) to its extended value (D) when a +1.25 D lens (for steep corneas) or a −1.00 D lens (for flat corneas) is held in front of the keratometer*. Courtesy of Adrian S Bruce.

Steep corneas (using a +1.25 D lens)[†]					
Keratometer reading (D)	Extended value (D)	Keratometer reading (D)	Extended value (D)	Keratometer reading (D)	Extended value (D)
43.00	50.13	46.13	53.78	49.25	57.42
43.13	50.28	46.25	53.92	49.38	57.57
43.25	50.42	46.38	54.07	49.50	57.71
43.38	50.57	46.50	54.21	49.63	57.86
43.50	50.72	46.63	54.36	49.75	58.00
43.63	50.86	46.75	54.51	49.88	58.15
43.75	51.01	46.88	54.65	50.00	58.30
43.88	51.15	47.00	54.80	50.13	58.44
44.00	51.30	47.13	54.94	50.25	58.59
44.13	51.44	47.25	55.09	50.38	58.73
44.25	51.59	47.38	55.23	50.50	58.88
44.38	51.74	47.50	55.38	50.63	59.02
44.50	51.88	47.63	55.53	50.75	59.17
44.63	52.03	47.75	55.67	50.88	59.32
44.75	52.17	47.88	55.82	51.00	59.46
44.88	52.32	48.00	55.96	51.13	59.61
45.00	52.47	48.13	56.11	51.25	59.75
45.13	52.61	48.25	56.25	51.38	59.90
45.25	52.76	48.38	56.40	51.50	60.04
45.38	52.90	48.50	56.55	51.63	60.19
45.50	53.05	48.63	56.69	51.75	60.34
45.63	53.19	48.75	56.84	51.88	60.48
45.75	53.34	48.88	56.98	52.00	60.63
45.88	53.49	49.00	57.13		
46.00	53.63	49.13	57.27		

[†]Based on the equation: Extended = (1.166 × Keratometer) − 0.005

Flat corneas (using a − 1.00 D lens)[‡]					
Keratometer reading (D)	**Extended value (D)**	**Keratometer reading (D)**	**Extended value (D)**	**Keratometer reading (D)**	**Extended value (D)**
36.00	30.87	38.12	32.70	40.25	34.52
36.12	30.98	38.25	32.80	40.37	34.63
36.25	31.09	38.37	32.91	40.50	34.73
36.37	31.19	38.50	33.02	40.62	34.84
36.50	31.30	38.62	33.12	40.75	34.95
36.62	31.41	38.75	33.23	40.87	35.06
36.75	31.52	38.87	33.34	41.00	35.16
36.87	31.62	39.00	33.45	41.12	35.27
37.00	31.73	39.12	33.55	41.25	35.38
37.12	31.84	39.25	33.66	41.37	35.48
37.25	31.94	39.37	33.77	41.50	35.59
37.37	32.05	39.50	33.88	41.62	35.70
37.50	32.16	39.62	33.98	41.75	35.81
37.62	32.27	39.75	34.09	41.87	35.91
37.75	32.37	39.87	34.20	42.00	36.02
37.87	32.48	40.00	34.30		
38.00	32.59	40.12	34.41		

[‡]Based on the equation: Extended = (1.858 × keratometer) −0.014

* (Derived from data in: Mandell, R.B., 1988 Dioptral and mm curves for extended keratometer range. Appendix 7. In: *Contact Lens Practice*, 4th edn. pp. 998–999. Springfield, IL: Charles C. Thomas)

Appendix F
Soft lens average thickness

The body of the table contains the average thickness (mm) of soft lenses of given centre thickness (mm) and lens power (D), based on the assumptions given at the foot of the table. Courtesy of Adrian S Bruce.

Centre thickness (mm)	Average thickness (mm) for various lens powers (D)											
	+8.00	+6.00	+4.00	+2.00	−2.00	−4.00	−6.00	−8.00	−10.00	−12.00	−14.00	−16.00
0.03					0.047	0.062	0.075	0.088	0.099	0.110	0.121	0.131
0.04					0.057	0.073	0.087	0.100	0.113	0.124	0.136	0.147
0.05					0.067	0.084	0.098	0.112	0.125	0.137	0.149	0.160
0.06					0.077	0.094	0.109	0.124	0.137	0.150	0.162	0.174
0.07					0.087	0.104	0.120	0.135	0.148	0.162	0.174	0.186
0.08				0.052	0.097	0.114	0.130	0.145	0.160	0.173	0.186	0.199
0.09				0.062	0.107	0.124	0.141	0.156	0.171	0.184	0.198	0.210
0.10				0.072	0.116	0.134	0.151	0.167	0.181	0.195	0.209	0.222
0.11				0.082	0.126	0.144	0.161	0.177	0.192	0.206	0.220	0.233
0.12				0.091	0.136	0.154	0.171	0.187	0.203	0.217	0.231	0.245
0.13			0.071	0.101	0.145	0.164	0.181	0.198	0.213	0.228	0.242	0.256
0.14			0.082	0.111	0.155	0.174	0.191	0.208	0.223	0.238	0.253	0.267
0.15			0.093	0.121	0.165	0.184	0.201	0.218	0.234	0.249	0.263	0.278
0.16			0.103	0.131	0.174	0.193	0.211	0.228	0.244	0.259	0.274	0.288
0.17		0.078	0.113	0.140	0.184	0.203	0.221	0.238	0.254	0.269	0.284	0.299
0.18		0.090	0.123	0.150	0.194	0.213	0.231	0.248	0.264	0.280	0.295	0.309
0.19		0.101	0.134	0.160	0.203	0.223	0.241	0.258	0.274	0.290	0.305	0.320
0.20		0.112	0.144	0.169	0.213	0.232	0.250	0.268	0.284	0.300	0.315	0.330
0.21		0.123	0.153	0.179	0.223	0.242	0.260	0.278	0.294	0.310	0.326	0.341
0.22	0.094	0.134	0.163	0.189	0.232	0.252	0.270	0.287	0.304	0.320	0.336	0.351
0.23	0.107	0.144	0.173	0.198	0.242	0.261	0.280	0.297	0.314	0.330	0.346	0.361
0.24	0.119	0.155	0.183	0.208	0.251	0.271	0.290	0.307	0.324	0.340	0.356	0.372
0.25	0.131	0.165	0.193	0.218	0.261	0.281	0.299	0.317	0.334	0.350	0.366	0.382

Assumptions:
- Back optic zone radius = 8.7 mm
- Optic zone diameter = 8.00 mm
- Refractive index (n) = 1.48 – 0.0015 × water content
- Water content = 55%
  - (Note: variations to 38% and 74% only affect average thickness by ± 0.03 mm)
- Minimum thickness at edge of optic zone for plus lenses = 0.03 mm

(Based on the theory outlined in: Brennan, N.A., 1984 Average thickness of a hydrogel lens for gas transmissibility calculations. *Am. J. Optom. Physiol. Opt.*, **61**, 627–635)

Appendix G
Soft lens oxygen performance

Conversion between soft (hydrogel) lens water content (%), Barrer (Fatt units) and ISO oxygen permeability (*Dk*) values, and Fatt oxygen transmissibility (*Dk/t*) values for various lens thicknesses. Courtesy of Adrian S Bruce.

Water content (%)	*Dk* Barrer units* at 35°C	*Dk* ISO units[†] at 35°C	*Dk/t*[‡] at 35°C (based on Barrer units) for various lens thicknesses (*t*, mm)												
			0.03	0.04	0.05	0.06	0.07	0.08	0.09	0.10	0.12	0.15	0.20	0.25	0.30
35	6.7	5.0	22.3	16.8	13.4	11.2	9.6	8.4	7.4	6.7	5.6	4.5	3.4	2.7	2.2
36	7.0	5.2	23.2	17.4	13.9	11.6	10.0	8.7	7.7	7.0	5.8	4.6	3.5	2.8	2.3
37	7.3	5.4	24.2	18.1	14.5	12.1	10.4	9.1	8.1	7.3	6.0	4.8	3.6	2.9	2.4
38	7.5	5.7	25.2	18.9	15.1	12.6	10.8	9.4	8.4	7.5	6.3	5.0	3.8	3.0	2.5
39	7.9	5.9		19.6	15.7	13.1	11.2	9.8	8.7	7.9	6.5	5.2	3.9	3.1	2.6
40	8.2	6.1		20.4	16.3	13.6	11.7	10.2	9.1	8.2	6.8	5.4	4.1	3.3	2.7
41	8.5	6.4		21.3	17.0	14.2	12.1	10.6	9.4	8.5	7.1	5.7	4.3	3.4	2.8
42	8.8	6.6		22.1	17.7	14.7	12.6	11.1	9.8	8.8	7.4	5.9	4.4	3.5	2.9
43	9.2	6.9		23.0	18.4	15.3	13.2	11.5	10.2	9.2	7.7	6.1	4.6	3.7	3.1
44	9.6	7.2		23.9	19.2	16.0	13.7	12.0	10.6	9.6	8.0	6.4	4.8	3.8	3.2
45	10.0	7.5		24.9	19.9	16.6	14.2	12.5	11.1	10.0	8.3	6.6	5.0	4.0	3.3
46	10.4	7.8			20.7	17.3	14.8	13.0	11.5	10.4	8.6	6.9	5.2	4.1	3.5
47	10.8	8.1			21.6	18.0	15.4	13.5	12.0	10.8	9.0	7.2	5.4	4.3	3.6
48	11.2	8.4			22.5	18.7	16.0	14.0	12.5	11.2	9.4	7.5	5.6	4.5	3.7
49	11.7	8.8			23.4	19.5	16.7	14.6	13.0	11.7	9.7	7.8	5.8	4.7	3.9
50	12.2	9.1			24.3	20.3	17.4	15.2	13.5	12.2	10.1	8.1	6.1	4.9	4.1
51	12.6	9.5				21.1	18.1	15.8	14.1	12.6	10.5	8.4	6.3	5.1	4.2
52	13.2	9.9				21.9	18.8	16.5	14.6	13.2	11.0	8.8	6.6	5.3	4.4
53	13.7	10.3				22.8	19.6	17.1	15.2	13.7	11.4	9.1	6.8	5.5	4.6
54	14.2	10.7				23.7	20.4	17.8	15.8	14.2	11.9	9.5	7.1	5.7	4.7
55	14.8	11.1				24.7	21.2	18.5	16.5	14.8	12.4	9.9	7.4	5.9	4.9
56	15.4	11.6					22.0	19.3	17.1	15.4	12.9	10.3	7.7	6.2	5.1
57	16.1	12.0					22.9	20.1	17.8	16.1	13.4	10.7	8.0	6.4	5.4
58	16.7	12.5					23.9	20.9	18.6	16.7	13.9	11.1	8.4	6.7	5.6
59	17.4	13.0					24.8	21.7	19.3	17.4	14.5	11.6	8.7	7.0	5.8
60	18.1	13.6					25.8	22.6	20.1	18.1	15.1	12.1	9.0	7.2	6.0
61	18.8	14.1						23.5	20.9	18.8	15.7	12.5	9.4	7.5	6.3
62	19.6	14.7						24.5	21.7	19.6	16.3	13.0	9.8	7.8	6.5
63	20.4	15.3							22.6	20.4	17.0	13.6	10.2	8.1	6.8
64	21.2	15.9							23.5	21.2	17.7	14.1	10.6	8.5	7.1
65	22.1	16.5							24.5	22.1	18.4	14.7	11.0	8.8	7.4
66	22.9	17.2								22.9	19.1	15.3	11.5	9.2	7.6
67	23.9	17.9								23.9	19.9	15.9	11.9	9.5	8.0
68	24.8	18.6								24.8	20.7	16.6	12.4	9.9	8.3
69	25.8	19.4								25.8	21.5	17.2	12.9	10.3	8.6
70	26.9	20.2								26.9	22.4	17.9	13.4	10.8	9.0

Continued

Water content (%)	*Dk* Barrer units* at 35°C	*Dk* ISO units† at 35°C	*Dk/t*‡ at 35°C (based on Barrer units) for various lens thicknesses (*t*, mm)												
			0.03	0.04	0.05	0.06	0.07	0.08	0.09	0.10	0.12	0.15	0.20	0.25	0.30
71	28.0	21.0									23.3	18.7	14.0	11.2	9.3
72	29.1	21.8									24.3	19.4	14.6	11.6	9.7
73	30.3	22.7									25.2	20.2	15.1	12.1	10.1
74	31.5	23.6										21.0	15.8	12.6	10.5
75	32.8	24.6										21.9	16.4	13.1	10.9
76	34.1	25.6										22.7	17.1	13.6	11.4
77	35.5	26.6										23.7	17.8	14.2	11.8
78	36.9	27.7										24.6	18.5	14.8	12.3
79	38.4	28.8											19.2	15.4	12.8
80	40.0	30.0											20.0	16.0	13.3

* Traditional units of oxygen permeability are: $\times 10^{-11}$ ($cm^2 \times ml\ O_2$)/($s \times ml \times mmHg$), or Barrer.
† ISO units of oxygen permeability are: $\times 10^{-11}$ ($cm^2 \times ml\ O_2$)/($s \times ml \times hPa$).
‡ Traditional units of oxygen transmissibility are: $\times 10^{-9}$ ($cm \times ml\ O_2$)/($s \times ml \times mmHg$), or Barrer/cm.

- For lenses $\leq \pm$ 1.50 D: average thickness = centre thickness.
- *Dk/t* values for thicknesses below a minimum manufacturable thickness are not shown.
- Data in this table are based on the Morgan–Efron equation, which corrects for boundary and edge effect errors during polarographic measurement: $Dk = 1.67 \times 10^{-11} \exp^{0.0397WC}$ [Morgan, P.B. and Efron, N., 1998 The oxygen performance of contemporary hydrogel contact lenses. *Contact Lens Ant. Eye,* 21, 3–6]
- The shaded cells represent *Dk/t* values that are considered to be adequate for open-eye (daily) lens wear; that is, *Dk/t* <12 Barrer/cm [Benjamin W.J., 1996 Downsizing of *Dk* and *Dk/L*: The difficulty in using hPa instead of mmHg. *Int. Contact Lens Clin*., **23**, 188–189]
- The data in this table do not apply to silicone hydrogel lenses, which are described by a water content–*Dk* relationship that is essentially the inverse of that which is used here to describe hydrogel lenses.

Appendix H
Constant edge clearance rigid lens designs

The theoretical edge clearances shown at the head of each table are for a lens fitted with 10 μm central clearance on a cornea with a shape factor of 0.85. Courtesy of Graeme Young.*

8.40 mm diameter – 69 μm edge clearance

BOZR	7.00	7.10	7.20	7.30	7.40	7.50	7.60	7.70	7.80	7.90	8.00	8.10	8.20	8.30	8.40	8.50
BOZD	7.40	7.40	7.40	7.40	7.40	7.40	7.40	7.40	7.40	7.40	7.40	7.40	7.40	7.40	7.40	7.40
BPR1	7.80	7.90	8.05	8.20	8.30	8.45	8.60	8.75	8.90	9.00	9.15	9.25	9.40	9.50	9.65	9.80
BPZD1	8.00	8.00	8.00	8.00	8.00	8.00	8.00	8.00	8.00	8.00	8.00	8.00	8.00	8.00	8.00	8.00
BPR2	9.80	10.10	10.30	10.50	10.90	11.20	11.40	11.70	12.00	12.40	12.60	13.10	13.40	13.80	14.10	14.40
TD	8.40	8.40	8.40	8.40	8.40	8.40	8.40	8.40	8.40	8.40	8.40	8.40	8.40	8.40	8.40	8.40

8.80 mm diameter – 73 μm edge clearance

BOZR	7.00	7.10	7.20	7.30	7.40	7.50	7.60	7.70	7.80	7.90	8.00	8.10	8.20	8.30	8.40	8.50
BOZD	7.60	7.60	7.60	7.60	7.60	7.60	7.60	7.60	7.60	7.60	7.60	7.60	7.60	7.60	7.60	7.60
BPR1	7.70	7.85	7.95	8.10	8.20	8.35	8.45	8.60	8.75	8.90	9.00	9.15	9.25	9.40	8.55	9.65
BPZD1	8.30	8.30	8.30	8.30	8.30	8.30	8.30	8.30	8.30	8.30	8.30	8.30	8.30	8.30	8.30	8.30
BPR2	8.90	9.10	9.30	9.50	9.80	10.00	10.30	10.40	10.70	10.80	11.10	11.40	11.70	11.90	12.10	12.50
TD	8.80	8.80	8.80	8.80	8.80	8.80	8.80	8.80	8.80	8.80	8.80	8.80	8.80	8.80	8.80	8.80

9.20 mm diameter – 80 μm edge clearance

BOZR	7.00	7.10	7.20	7.30	7.40	7.50	7.60	7.70	7.80	7.90	8.00	8.10	8.20	8.30	8.40	8.50
BOZD	7.80	7.80	7.80	7.80	7.80	7.80	7.80	7.80	7.80	7.80	7.80	7.80	7.80	7.80	7.80	7.80
BPR1	7.60	7.70	7.85	7.95	8.10	8.20	8.35	8.45	8.60	8.70	8.85	8.95	9.10	9.20	9.35	9.47
BPZD1	8.60	8.60	8.60	8.60	8.60	8.60	8.60	8.60	8.60	8.60	8.60	8.60	8.60	8.60	8.60	8.60
BPR2	8.60	8.80	9.00	9.20	9.40	9.60	9.80	10.00	10.20	10.40	10.60	10.90	11.10	11.30	11.60	11.83
TD	9.20	9.20	9.20	9.20	9.20	9.20	9.20	9.20	9.20	9.20	9.20	9.20	9.20	9.20	9.20	9.20

9.60 mm diameter – 90 μm edge clearance

BOZR	7.00	7.10	7.20	7.30	7.40	7.50	7.60	7.70	7.80	7.90	8.00	8.10	8.20	8.30	8.40	8.50
BOZD	8.00	8.00	8.00	8.00	8.00	8.00	8.00	8.00	8.00	8.00	8.00	8.00	8.00	8.00	8.00	8.00
BPR1	7.60	7.70	7.80	7.95	8.10	8.20	8.30	8.45	8.55	8.70	8.85	8.95	9.10	9.20	9.35	9.50
BPZD1	8.90	8.90	8.90	8.90	8.90	8.90	8.90	8.90	8.90	8.90	8.90	8.90	8.90	8.90	8.90	8.90
BPR2	8.30	8.50	8.70	8.90	9.00	9.30	9.50	9.70	9.90	10.10	10.20	10.50	10.60	10.90	11.00	11.20
TD	9.60	9.60	9.60	9.60	9.60	9.60	9.60	9.60	9.60	9.60	9.60	9.60	9.60	9.60	9.60	9.60

10.00 mm diameter – 105 μm edge clearance

BOZR	7.00	7.10	7.20	7.30	7.40	7.50	7.60	7.70	7.80	7.90	8.00	8.10	8.20	8.30	8.40	8.50
BOZD	8.20	8.20	8.20	8.20	8.20	8.20	8.20	8.20	8.20	8.20	8.20	8.20	8.20	8.20	8.20	8.20
BPR1	7.65	7.70	7.80	7.95	8.10	8.20	8.35	8.45	8.65	8.70	8.85	9.00	9.15	9.25	9.40	9.50
BPZD1	8.90	8.90	8.90	8.90	8.90	8.90	8.90	8.90	8.90	8.90	8.90	8.90	8.90	8.90	8.90	8.90
BPR2	8.00	8.15	8.35	8.50	8.60	8.80	8.90	9.10	9.15	9.45	9.60	9.75	9.90	10.10	10.25	10.45
BPZD2	9.50	9.50	9.50	9.50	9.50	9.50	9.50	9.50	9.50	9.50	9.50	9.50	9.50	9.50	9.50	9.50
BPR3	8.10	8.30	8.40	8.60	8.80	9.00	9.20	9.30	9.50	9.70	9.80	10.00	10.20	10.40	10.50	10.70
TD	10.00	10.00	10.00	10.00	10.00	10.00	10.00	10.00	10.00	10.00	10.00	10.00	10.00	10.00	10.00	10.00

* (Based on the design concept of Guillon, M., Lydon, D. P. M. and Sammons, W. A., 1983 Designing rigid gas-permeable contact lenses using the edge clearance technique. *J. Br. Contact Lens Assoc.*, **6**, 19–25)

Appendix I
Soft toric lens misalignment demonstrator

This table demonstrates the residual refractive error induced by mislocation of toric lenses of given cylindrical powers, based upon an ocular refraction of plano/–cyl × 180. (Courtesy of Adrian Bruce)

Example
- Ocular refraction (required refractive correction) is: plano/–1.00 × 180
- A lens is placed on the eye of back vertex power: plano/–1.00 × 180
- An overrefracton yields a residual error of: +0.34/–0.68 × 35
- From the table, a mislocation is indicated of: –20°
- The lens back vertex power in situ is: plano/–1.00 × 160

Mislocation (–)(°)	–1.00 D cylinder	–2.00 D cylinder	–3.00 D cylinder
5	0.09/–0.17 × 42.5	0.17/–0.35 × 42.5	0.26/–0.52 × 42.5
10	0.17/–0.35 × 40.0	0.35/–0.69 × 40.0	0.52/–1.04 × 40.0
15	0.26/–0.52 × 37.5	0.52/–1.04 × 37.5	0.78/–1.55 × 37.5
20	0.34/–0.68 × 35.0	0.68/–1.37 × 35.0	1.03/–2.05 × 35.0
25	0.42/–0.85 × 32.5	0.85/–1.69 × 32.5	1.27/–2.54 × 32.5
30	0.50/–1.00 × 30.0	1.00/–2.00 × 30.0	1.50/–3.00 × 30.0
35	0.57/–1.15 × 27.5	1.15/–2.29 × 27.5	1.72/–3.44 × 27.5
40	0.64/–1.29 × 25.0	1.29/–2.57 × 25.0	1.93/–3.86 × 25.0
45	0.71/–1.41 × 22.5	1.41/–2.83 × 22.5	2.12/–4.24 × 22.5
50	0.77/–1.53 × 20.0	1.53/–3.06 × 20.0	2.30/–4.60 × 20.0
55	0.82/–1.64 × 17.5	1.64/–3.28 × 17.5	2.46/–4.91 × 17.5
60	0.87/–1.73 × 15.0	1.73/–3.46 × 15.0	2.60/–5.20 × 15.0
65	0.91/–1.81 × 12.5	1.81/–3.63 × 12.5	2.72/–5.44 × 12.5
70	0.94/–1.88 × 10.0	1.88/–3.76 × 10.0	2.82/–5.64 × 10.0
75	0.97/–1.93 × 7.5	1.93/–3.86 × 7.5	2.90/–5.80 × 7.5
80	0.98/–1.97 × 5.0	1.97/–3.94 × 5.0	2.95/–5.91 × 5.0
85	1.00/–1.99 × 2.5	1.99/–3.98 × 2.5	2.99/–5.98 × 2.5
90	1.00/–2.00 × 0.0	2.00/–4.00 × 0.0	3.00/–6.00 × 0.0

Generated using the formulae in:
(Lindsay, R.G., Bruce, A.S., Brennan, N.A. and Pianta, M.J., 1997 Determining axis misalignment and power errors of toric soft lenses. *Int. Contact Lens. Clin.*, **24**, 101–107)

Rules of thumb for soft toric mislocation:
1. The spherical equivalent is zero if the error is purely due to axis misalignment.
2. The direction of lens misalignment is always opposite to the axis of the overrefraction, relative to the prescribed cylinder axis.
3. LARS: 'left add, right subtract'. When allowing for nasal rotation in the right eye, the amount of rotation should be subtracted from the required cylinder axis and vice versa for the left eye.

Appendix J
Dry-eye questionnaire

A typical dry-eye questionnaire. Courtesy of Keith H Edwards. (Adapted with permission from: Lowther, G. E., 1997 Examination of patients and predicting tear-film related problems with hydrogel lens wear. In: *Dryness, Tears and Contact Lens Wear.* pp. 23–53. Oxford: Butterworth-Heinemann)

Symptom	Frequency			
	Never	Sometimes	Often	Constantly
Sandy or gritty feeling				
Burning				
Dryness				
Soreness				
Scratchiness				
Itching				
Eye discomfort on waking				
Tearing (watery eyes)				
Foreign-body sensation				
Eye pain				
Redness				
Mucus discharge				
Light sensitivity				
Blurred vision				
Infection of lids or eye				
Hayfever				
Other allergy				
Nasal congestion				
Cough				
Bronchitis				
Cold symptoms				
Sinus congestion				
Dryness of throat/mouth/vagina				
Trouble swallowing food				
Asthma symptoms				
Joint pain				
Muscle pain				

Do your eyes seem overly sensitive to:							
Cigarette smoke	☐	Swimming	☐	Smog	☐	Alcohol	☐
Air conditioning	☐	Sunshine	☐	Heater and air blowers	☐	Wind	☐
Dust	☐	Use of VDUs	☐	Pollen	☐	Eye drops	☐

General questions relating to dry eye	Yes	No
Do you wear contact lenses?		
Have you previously tried to wear contact lenses?		
Do you use artificial tears or drops?		
Have you ever been told you sleep with your eyes open?		
Have you ever been treated for dry eyes?		
Do you take antihistamines?		
Do you take birth control pills?		
Are you taking diuretics (water pills)?		
Are you taking any other medication (prescribed or over-the-counter)? If yes, give brand and reason for taking medication		

Condition	Have you or any blood relative had any of the following?		
	Yourself	Relative	Relationship
Arthritis			
Thyroid disease			
Lupus			
Sarcoidosis			
Asthma			
Sjögren's syndrome			
Skin disorders			
Heart disease			
Hypertension			
Gout			
Cataract			
Diabetes			
Glaucoma			

Appendix K
Efron grading scales for contact lens complications

The grading scales presented on the following two pages were devised by Professor Nathan Efron and painted by the ophthalmic artist, Terry R Tarrant.

These grading scales are designed to assist practitioners to quantify the level of severity of a variety of contact lens complications. The eight complications on the left-hand page are those that are more likely to be encountered in contact lens practice. Many of these complications are graded routinely by some practitioners. The complications on the right-hand page are less commonly encountered in contact lens practice, and represent pathology that is rare or unusual.

An explanation as to how to use these grading scales is given in Chapter 39.

The development of these grading scales was kindly sponsored by CooperVision.

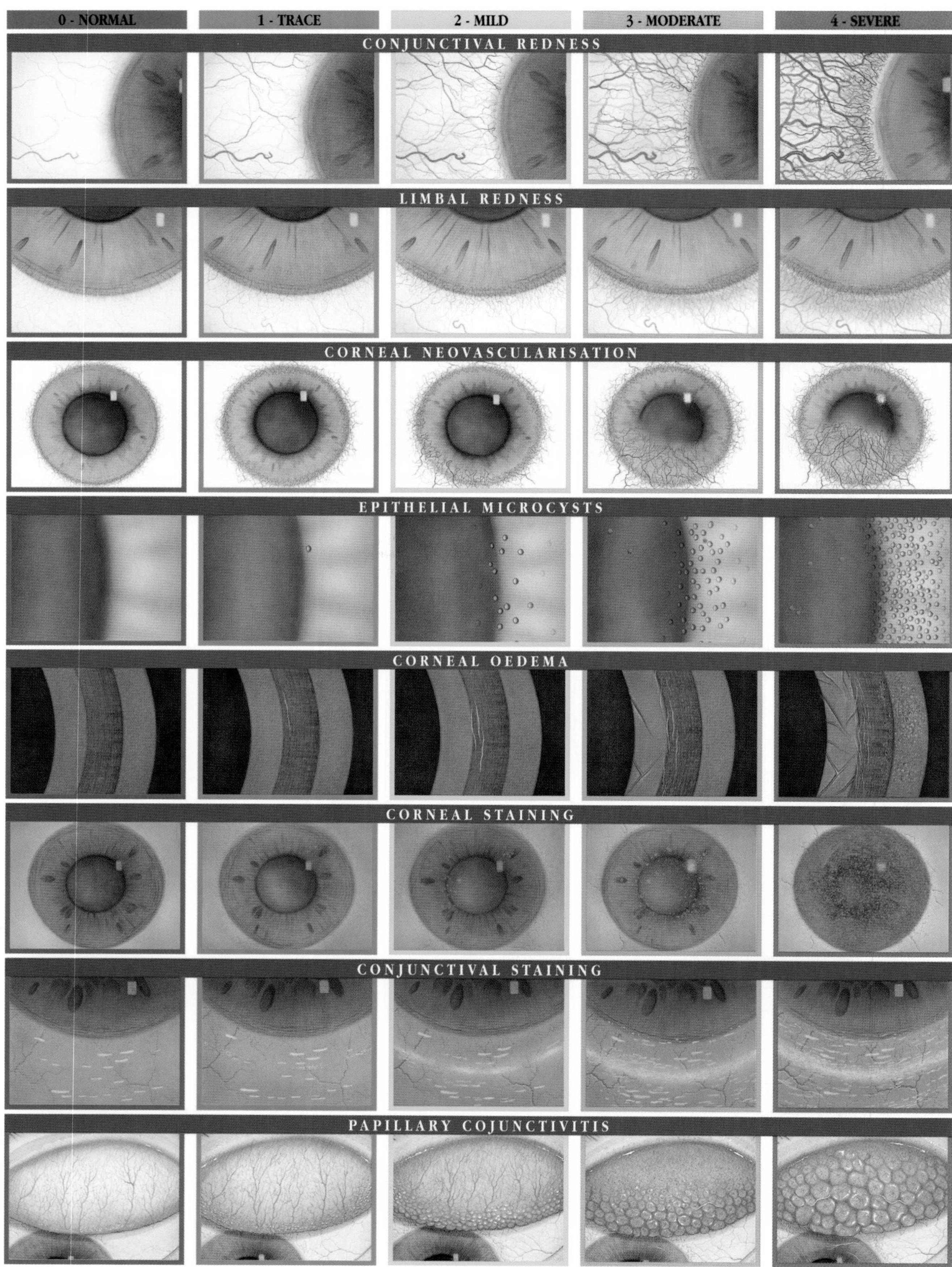
0 - NORMAL
1 - TRACE
2 - MILD
3 - MODERATE
4 - SEVERE
CONJUNCTIVAL REDNESS
LIMBAL REDNESS
CORNEAL NEOVASCULARISATION
EPITHELIAL MICROCYSTS
CORNEAL OEDEMA
CORNEAL STAINING
CONJUNCTIVAL STAINING
PAPILLARY COJUNCTIVITIS

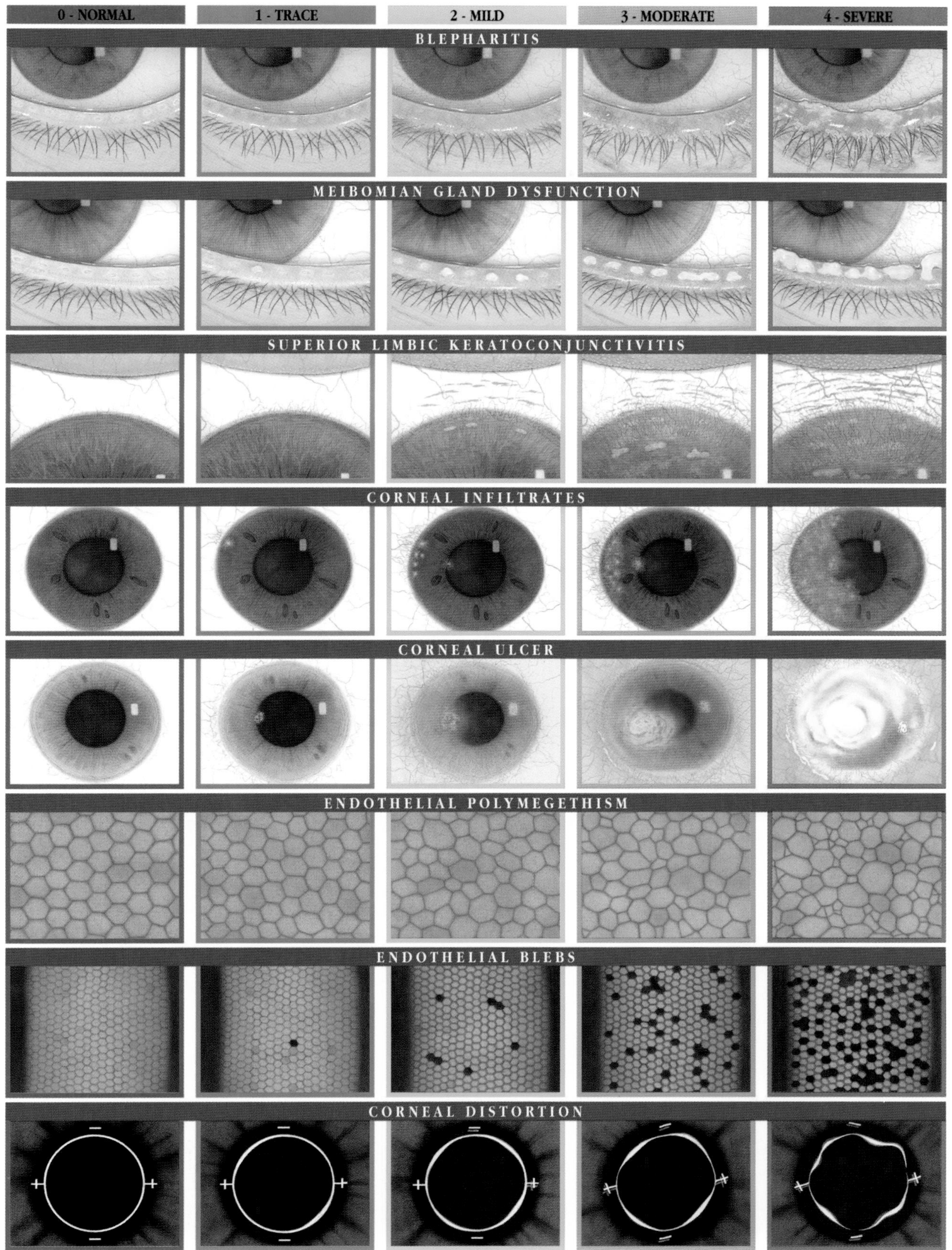
0 - NORMAL
1 - TRACE
2 - MILD
3 - MODERATE
4 - SEVERE
BLEPHARITIS
MEIBOMIAN GLAND DYSFUNCTION
SUPERIOR LIMBIC KERATOCONJUNCTIVITIS
CORNEAL INFILTRATES
CORNEAL ULCER
ENDOTHELIAL POLYMEGETHISM
ENDOTHELIAL BLEBS
CORNEAL DISTORTION

Index

Notes

1. All references are to eyes, except where otherwise indicated
2. **Bold** page numbers indicate **chapter** extents
3. *Italic* page numbers indicate *illustrations, diagrams and tables.* There are frequently textual references on the same pages.
4. Sub-entries are in alphabetical order, except where chronological order is occasionally more significant